369 0160716

LIBRARY
ACCESSION No.

This book is due for return on or before the last date shown below.

MONKLANDS HOSPITAL
AIRDRIE ML6 0JS

WID

D1422520

Diagnostic Pathology of Infectious Disease

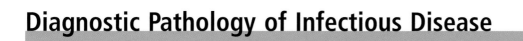

Diagnostic Pathology of Infectious Disease

Richard L. Kradin, MD

Associate Professor of Pathology and Medicine
Department of Pathology
Harvard Medical School

Associate Pathologist and Associate Physician
Pulmonary/Critical Care Unit
Massachusetts General Hospital
Boston, Massachusetts

SAUNDERS

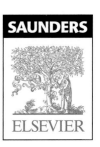

ELSEVIER

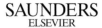

1600 John F. Kennedy Blvd.
Ste 1800
Philadelphia, PA 19103-2899

DIAGNOSTIC PATHOLOGY OF INFECTIOUS DISEASE ISBN: 978-1-4160-3429-2

Copyright © 2010 Elsevier Inc. All rights reserved.

No part of this publication may be reproduced or transmitted in any form or by any means, electronic or mechanical, including photocopying, recording, or any information storage and retrieval system, without permission in writing from the Publisher. Details on how to seek permission, further information about the Publisher's permissions policies, and our arrangements with organizations such as the Copyright Clearance Center and the Copyright Licensing Agency can be found at our website: www.elsevier.com/permissions.

This book and the individual contributions contained in it are protected under copyright by the Publisher (other than as may be noted herein).

Notices

Knowledge and best practice in this field are constantly changing. As new research and experience broaden our understanding, changes in research methods, professional practices, or medical treatment may become necessary.

Practitioners and researchers must always rely on their own experience and knowledge in evaluating and using any information, methods, compounds, or experiments described herein. In using such information or methods they should be mindful of their own safety and the safety of others, including parties for whom they have a professional responsibility.

With respect to any drug or pharmaceutical products identified, readers are advised to check the most current information provided (i) on procedures featured or (ii) by the manufacturer of each product to be administered, to verify the recommended dose or formula, the method and duration of administration, and contraindications. It is the responsibility of practitioners, relying on their own experience and knowledge of their patients, to make diagnoses, to determine dosages and the best treatment for each individual patient, and to take all appropriate safety precautions.

To the fullest extent of the law, neither the Publisher nor the authors, contributors, or editors assume any liability for any injury and/or damage to persons or property as a matter of product liability, negligence, or otherwise, or from any use or operation of any methods, products, instructions, or ideas contained in the material herein.

Library of Congress Cataloging-in-Publication Data
Diagnostic pathology of infectious disease / [edited by] Richard L. Kradin.—1st ed.
        p. ; cm.
    Includes bibliographical references.
    ISBN 978-1-4160-3429-2
1. Communicable diseases–Diagnosis.   2. Diagnosis, Laboratory.   I. Kradin, Richard L.
    [DNLM: 1. Communicable Diseases–diagnosis.   2. Clinical Laboratory Techniques.
3. Communicable Diseases–pathology.   WC 100 D536 2010]
    RC113.3.D53 2010
    616.9′0475—dc22

                                                      2009042846

Acquisitions Editor: William Schmitt
Developmental Editor: Kathryn DeFrancesco
Publishing Services Manager: Linda Van Pelt
Project Manager: Sharon Lee
Design Direction: Louis Forgione

Printed in China

Last digit is the print number: 9 8 7 6 5 4 3 2 1

Working together to grow
libraries in developing countries

www.elsevier.com | www.bookaid.org | www.sabre.org

ELSEVIER   BOOK AID International   Sabre Foundation

Dedication

I dedicate this textbook to
my wife, Karen, and our six children: Rachel, Sarah, Ben,
Michael (×2), and Daniel, who have all been consistently
supportive of the many gyrations that
my career has taken.

Contributors

H. Thomas Aretz, MD
Associate Professor of Pathology
Harvard Medical School
Affiliate Pathologist
Massachusetts General Hospital
Boston, Massachusetts
8. Cardiac Infections

Sandra Camelo-Piragua, MD
Clinical Fellow in Pathology
Harvard Medical School
Massachusetts General Hospital
Boston, Massachusetts
18. Infections of the Nervous System

Elizabeth G. Demicco, MD
Clinical Fellow in Pathology
Harvard Medical School
Massachusetts General Hospital
Boston, Massachusetts
14. Infections of Joints, Synovium-Lined Structures,
*   and Soft Tissue*

Alton B. Farris, MD
Clinical Fellow in Pathology
Harvard Medical School
Massachusetts General Hospital
Boston, Massachusetts
5. Ultrastructural Diagnosis of Infection
15. Genitourinary Infectious Disease Pathology

Judith A. Ferry, MD
Associate Professor of Pathology
Harvard Medical School
Associate Pathologist
Massachusetts General Hospital
Boston, Massachusetts
11. Infectious Lymphadenitis

Jay A. Fishman, MD
Associate Director, MGH Transplantation Center
Director, Transplant Infectious Disease & Compromised Host
   Program
Massachusetts General Hospital
Associate Professor of Medicine
Harvard Medical School
Boston, Massachusetts
3. The Biopsy in the Diagnosis of Infection: Clinical Approach

Robert P. Hasserjian, MD
Associate Professor of Pathology
Harvard Medical School
Associate Pathologist
Massachusetts General Hospital
Boston, Massachusetts
12. Infectious Diseases of the Bone Marrow and Spleen

E. Tessa Hedley-Whyte, MD
Professor of Pathology
Harvard Medical School
Neuropathologist
Departments of Pathology and Neurology
Massachusetts General Hospital
Boston, Massachusetts
18. Infections of the Nervous System

A. John Iafrate, MD
Assistant Professor of Pathology
Harvard Medical School
Massachusetts General Hospital
Boston, Massachusetts
2. General Principles in the Diagnosis of Infection

Matthew M. Johnson, MD
Clinical Fellow in Pathology
Harvard Medical School
Massachusetts General Hospital
Boston, Massachusetts
6. Ear, Nose, and Throat Infections

Susan V. Kattapuram
Department of Radiology
Harvard Medical School
Massachusetts General Hospital
Boston, Massachusetts
13. Bone Infections
14. Infections of Joints, Synovium-Lined Structures,
*   and Soft Tissue*

Richard L. Kradin, MD
Associate Professor of Pathology and Medicine
Department of Pathology
Harvard Medical School
Associate Pathologist and Associate Physician
Pulmonary/Critical Care Unit
Massachusetts General Hospital
Boston, Massachusetts
1. Introduction
2. General Principles in the Diagnosis of Infection
7. Pulmonary Infections
8. Cardiac Infections
9. Infections of the Gastrointestinal Tract
14. Infections of Joints, Synovium-Lined Structures,
*   and Soft Tissue*

Gregory Lauwers, MD
Associate Professor of Pathology
Harvard Medical School
Director of Gastrointestinal Pathology
Massachusetts General Hospital
Boston, Massachusetts
9. Infections of the Gastrointestinal Tract

Alice Z. C. Lobo, MD
Research Fellow
Dermatopathology Division
Department of Pathology
Massachusetts General Hospital
Boston, Massachusetts
19. Skin Infections

Eugene J. Mark, MD
Professor of Pathology
Harvard Medical School
Massachusetts General Hospital
Boston, Massachusetts
7. Pulmonary Infections

Martin C. Mihm, MD, FACP, FRCPI
Clinical Professor of Dermatology and Pathology
Harvard Medical School
Senior Dermatopathologist
Massachusetts General Hospital
Boston, Massachusetts
19. Skin Infections

Mari Mino-Kenudson, MD
Assistant Professor of Pathology
Harvard Medical School
Massachusetts General Hospital
Boston, Massachusetts
9. Infections of the Gastrointestinal Tract

Joseph Misdraji, MD
Assistant Professor of Pathology
Harvard Medical School
Massachusetts General Hospital
Boston, Massachusetts
10. Liver and Bile Duct

Gunnlaugur Petur Nielsen, MD
Associate Professor of Pathology
Harvard Medical School
Director of Electron Microscope Unit
Department of Pathology
Massachusetts General Hospital
Boston, Massachusetts
5. Ultrastructural Diagnosis of Infection
13. Bone Infections
15. Genitourinary Infectious Disease Pathology

Carlos Nicolas Prieto-Granada, MD
Research Fellow
Department of Pathology
Tufts Medical Center
Boston, Massachusetts
19. Skin Infections

Drucilla J. Roberts, MD
Associate Professor of Pathology
Harvard Medical School
Head of Obstetric and Perinatal Pathology
Massachusetts General Hospital
Boston, Massachusetts
17. Perinatal Infections

Andrew E. Rosenberg, MD
Associate Professor of Pathology
Harvard Medical School
Head of Bone & Soft Tissue
Department of Pathology
Massachusetts General Hospital
Boston, Massachusetts
13. Bone Infections
14. Infections of Joints, Synovium-Lined Structures,
*   and Soft Tissue*

Vicki J. Schnadig, MD
Professor, Department of Pathology
Director, Division of Cytopathology
University of Texas Medical Branch
Galveston, Texas
4. Cytopathology of Infectious and Inflammatory Diseases

Rosemary Tambouret, MD
Assistant Professor of Pathology
Harvard Medical School
Massachusetts General Hospital
Boston, Massachusetts
16. Gynecologic Infections

Preface

During my residency in internal medicine some 30 years ago, I was strongly drawn to the clinical practice of infectious disease. My teachers at the University of Pennsylvania were astute clinicians, formidably knowledgeable, and keen observers. During my subsequent training in anatomic pathology at the Massachusetts General Hospital, I considered a career in infectious disease pathology but was hard-pressed to identify it as a viable independent specialty. As a result, I compromised and devoted the next years of my training to specialty interests in both pulmonary medicine and lung pathology, in part because I was aware that many infections affect the lungs.

My subsequent training included research in cellular immunology, and I learned that the primary principles of host defense had largely evolved in response and in parallel to the challenges of infection. Relatively late in my career, I volunteered for the job of being a dedicated expert in infectious disease pathology, and as there was no competition, I got it. In many respects it has proved to be the most rewarding role of my career.

Most surgical pathology departments today are primarily focused on the field of neoplasia; infection has largely become the domain of the microbiology laboratory. Yet the amount of infectious disease pathology that is seen regularly in the practice of surgical pathology in most hospitals is substantial, varied, and diagnostically challenging. In a single week, I often see tens of cases of infection, some of them common, others extraordinary and exotic. It is my considered opinion that the challenges of expert infectious disease pathology diagnosis rival and frequently exceed those of diagnostic tumor pathology.

The nuances of the specialty are unique. They include a degree of clinical expertise, the knowledge of how diseases are geographically distributed, experience in identifying the varied morphological features of a host of pathogens, awareness of how in-host responses vary with levels of immunosuppression, and recognizing when one is not dealing with infection in responses that can mimic it. While most surgical pathologists manage to do a very reasonable job in diagnosing infection, most would admit that their level of sophistication in this area is too frequently limited.

Whereas most textbooks on the topic of infectious disease pathology emphasize details of microbial identification, it is evident that the practicing surgical pathologist primarily needs a firm grounding in recognizing the spectrum of histological responses by the host that can be seen in infection. In a hospital such as my own where pathologists are sub-specialized, surgical pathologists become well versed in how to diagnose the infections that frequently present in their organ of specialized interest. This is unfortunate for those of us who choose to practice infectious disease pathology as a primary subspecialty, as many interesting cases never reach my microscope. But this is easily remedied by maintaining a working relationship with the hospital clinical infectious disease specialists, who invariably make me aware of the cases of interest!

Frankly, few busy pathologists have the time or the inclination to specialize in infection, yet it is just this group that needs access to a single handy resource that will help them to establish an accurate diagnosis. That was the rationale for the present text. As I have noted elsewhere, this text may not invariably provide the level of detail that may be gleaned in the in-depth study of infectious disease morphology. For example, exhaustive detail has not been included with respect to the diagnosis of rare parasitic disorders, but there are already excellent textbooks available that can address these features. This is also not a source book on the molecular aspects of infection; this too can be found elsewhere. What the reader will find here, hopefully, is a practical, accessible, and well illustrated text of the surgical pathology of infection.

Acknowledgments

It is difficult to know where to begin with respect to acknowledgments. Perhaps the best place is with my fellow authors, with one exception, all colleagues in the Massachusetts General Hospital Surgical Pathology Unit of the Department of Pathology. If truth be told, some of them were initially reticent to sign up for the project. Their reasons varied: some were busy, few had a strong primary interest in infection, and so on. But what I knew after many years of working with them was that they are all expert diagnosticians and that once on board they would produce quality chapters, as they did. I hope that it was not too much of a hardship for them and that they have as a result become more comfortable with their own expertise in this area of surgical pathology.

The MGH Infectious Disease Unit is simply superb. I attend their weekly case conferences and am always impressed by the insight that they bring to the diagnosis and management of challenging cases. They have been consistently supportive of my activities, and I hope that I have added to their experience of the study and treatment of infectious disease. I must specifically thank Dr. Jay Fishman, a wise clinician with a good sense of humor who agreed, late in the process, to contribute an important chapter to this text.

My colleagues in the MGH Pulmonary/Critical Care Unit and most especially, Dr. Walter O'Donnell, who has shown a consistent interest in pulmonary infectious disease pathology and has been a source of erudition and support.

Dr. Eugene J. Mark, my colleague and co-author for many years in MGH Pulmonary and Autopsy Pathology, who encouraged me to develop this area of expertise.

The Infectious Disease Pathology Branch at the Armed Forces Institute of Pathology, which has made enormous contributions to the area of diagnostic surgical pathology of infection, and where I spent an enjoyable week some years back reviewing their extraordinary slide collection.

Drs. Sherif Zaki, Francis Chandler, and David Walker, whose lectures on infectious disease pathology at the MGH were both instructive and inspiring to those interested in this area.

To the late Dr. Walter Putschar, whose steadfast approach to discovering the truth was an inspiration, especially with respect to his knowledge of exotic parasitic infections.

To the staff of the London School of Hygiene and Tropical Medicine, who gave me the opportunity to study for a Diplomate in Tropical Infectious Diseases.

To the editorial staff at Elsevier, including Bill Schmitt, who recognized the merit in this project, and Katie DeFrancesco, who has patiently shepherded it along.

Contents

Introduction

Richard L. Kradin

Infectious diseases account for the majority of human diseases. Indeed, in much of the world, infection is the leading cause of debilitating chronic disease and death. In recent decades, medicine has witnessed great strides in the diagnosis and treatment of infection, but it has also seen the emergence of new and deadly pathogens, including the human immunodeficiency virus, that have profoundly influenced how modern medicine is practiced. New treatment modalities including potent immunosuppressive regimens that weaken host defenses have contributed to this emergence of new pathogens and to the recrudescence of others that would normally not be considered pathogens.

In response to the challenge of infection, surgical pathologists are increasingly called on to render diagnoses from both cytology specimens and biopsy specimens. In an effort to decrease patient morbidity with respect to the biopsy procedure, both noninvasive and minimally invasive approaches have been developed that challenge the practicing pathologist to opine on the basis of smaller samples. Furthermore, in addition to establishing the cause of infection, the pathologist must consider a range of disorders in the differential diagnosis with regard to underlying factors that might predispose the host to infection and can mimic the histology of infection. Finally, the histologic response to infection may be the best indication of immunocompetence and indicate prognosis.

Biopsy samples from immunosuppressed hosts can be difficult to assess with accuracy, and they constitute a challenge that some might wish to avoid. Whereas the microbiology laboratory and medical specialists have become increasingly skilled in the diagnosis of infectious diseases, the same has not been uniformly true of surgical pathologists, who may prefer to defer to their clinical colleagues in this area. This is compounded by a trend among surgical pathologists to focus primarily in their practice on the diagnosis of neoplasia, where surgical pathologists maintain preeminent expertise. Their choice is fostered by the frustration of trying to identify small numbers of small pathogens, the delay in diagnosis that results from ancillary histochemical staining and other testing, and difficulties in diagnosing organisms with accuracy due to the morphologic distortions that can ensue after antimicrobial therapies. Taken together, the time, effort, and expense of diagnosing infection can at times seem nongratifying for a busy surgical pathologist.

Nevertheless, the ubiquity of infectious diseases makes it highly unlikely that surgical pathologists can avoid being confronted with their diagnosis in practice, so it behooves them to be aware of the intricacies of how infection manifests in situ. The primary aim of this text is to rekindle the interest that most surgical pathologists once held for the pathologic diagnosis of infectious diseases. Although this may seem like a tall order, it is certainly a worthy one.

The text is organized unlike most other textbooks of infectious disease pathology. The editor has long recognized that most subspecialists in surgical pathology establish expertise in diagnosing the infections that primarily affect the organ system of their specialty, although they may confess to limited interest in the details of infectious diagnosis in other tissues. For this reason, this text has been primarily organized based on organ systems rather than a litany of specific infectious organisms. As a consequence, the reader will be exposed to these disorders as they are actually encountered in a subspecialty practice of pathology. The nuances of infectious diagnoses are presented together with their differential diagnosis, so that the reader can better glean from the text how to narrow the differential diagnosis in practice.

The text includes a preliminary discussion of the types of inflammatory responses that can be elicited by various microorganisms and how host defenses modify these responses. There is a detailed explanation of how to apply histochemical stains differentially in order to narrow the differential diagnosis with respect to microbial morphology. The roles of immunohistochemical staining, in situ hybridization, and the polymerase chain reaction are discussed before the discussion of each of the major organ systems.

Because many microorganisms can affect a variety of human tissues, there is necessarily some redundancy in their description. However, on balance, the superimposed constraints of tissue microanatomy lead to diversity with respect to the morphologic appearances of infection at different sites, so that repetitiveness in this regard has a didactic purpose. In addition, for the busy practitioner, this text may be used as a single resource concerning infection in an organ system of specific interest, in a case-dependent fashion, without having to consult a series of subspecialty texts.

This text is meant to be functionally complete but not encyclopedic. There is much information regarding the clinical, epidemiologic, and mechanistic bases of infection that will not be found here. In addition, some exotic parasitic disorders have not been included. Other texts that include these data are available, and a pathologist may wish to refer to them at times. However, for the most part, all that is required to diagnose the vast majority of infections can be found in the pages of this text.

One final point: The diagnosis of infection is in many respects comparable to that of neoplasia—it requires experience. The morphologic appearances of infection are at least as diverse as those of malignancy. The variations encountered are virtually inexhaustible, and no textbook can suffice to illustrate all that may be encountered in practice. At times textbooks tend to focus on one aspect of an infection, and the inexperienced pathologist in this area may be misled, expecting to encounter examples that are comparable to those within selected illustrations. Let the reader be forewarned that this text cannot replace experience. But, once the diverse appearances of infection are appreciated and accepted, the surgical pathologist may derive substantial pleasure from pondering its fine distinctions and take pride in the growing sense of competence that develops from experience in this area.

General Principles in the Diagnosis of Infection

Richard L. Kradin and A. John Iafrate

Introduction

The identification of infection in biopsied tissues is the primary responsibility of the surgical pathologist. In an age when both noninvasive and minimally invasive approaches and techniques have increased, it is important to revisit the role of the biopsy in the diagnosis of infection (Table 2-1). Isolating microorganisms in the microbiology laboratory is a sensitive and accurate approach to their identification, but it has several important limitations. First, it cannot distinguish infection from colonization, nor can it ascertain the significance of the isolated organism. Only the presence of an organism in situ, together with an expected inflammatory response by the host, constitutes acceptable evidence of its role in infection.

For example, consider how to interpret the clinical significance of a fungus isolated from the airways of a patient with bronchiectasis who also has a new pulmonary infiltrate in the setting of immunosuppression. Is the fungal isolate the likely cause of the opportunistic infection, or might it be a benign commensal? Studies have attempted to address this question[1] with guidelines formulated for practice, but these are indeed merely "guidelines," because only identification of a potential pathogen within a site of infection can provide substantive evidence that the fungus is an invasive pathogen. For this and other reasons to be addressed in this text, the pathologic diagnosis of infection is a critical element in formulating optimal therapy.

Sampling

Tissue sampling is fundamentally important in the diagnosis of infection. All excised tissues should be considered as potentially infective. This approach fosters due diligence with respect to the possibility of contagion, as well as thoughtful concern as to how the tissues will be handled to optimize the chances of establishing an accurate diagnosis (Table 2-2). Samples of excised tissues should be harvested by sterile technique and sent to the microbiology laboratory with information concerning the types of organism that are being considered diagnostically. Directions to consider anaerobic and fastidious species should be clearly stated.

The surgical pathologist must ascertain that all diagnostic possibilities have been considered. Consultation with an infectious disease specialist can be invaluable in ensuring that specimens are properly handled *ab initio*. What must be avoided is thoughtlessly placing a biopsy specimen directly into formalin fixative without first considering a diagnosis of infection.

Touch imprints should be routinely prepared and can be stained in the frozen-section suite or in the microbiology laboratory. In general, 5 to 10 touch imprints will suffice, with sampling from the most suspicious portions of the biopsy specimen (e.g., areas of necrosis or suppuration).

Harvesting a portion of the biopsy specimen for ultrastructural analysis can foster the accurate diagnosis of many organisms (e.g., viruses, *Tropheryma whippelii*, microsporidia).[2] Specimens may be harvested for polymerase chain reaction (PCR) testing to establish the diagnosis of others (e.g., *Coxiella*, mycobacteria, rickettsia).[3]

The rapid diagnosis of a frozen section can help to focus the diagnostic workup. All of the pertinent histochemical and ancillary studies can ideally be ordered before the permanent sections are processed, to avoid undue delay in diagnosis.

Diagnosing Infection In Situ

Because host immune mechanisms can greatly amplify the host response, the actual numbers of pathogens present in tissues is frequently surprisingly small. This means that many sections may need to be examined before a pathogen is identified. Although

Table 2-1 Role of the Surgical Pathologist in the Diagnosis of Infection

Establish morphologic diagnosis of infection

Assess immunocompetence of the host

Narrow the differential diagnosis of possible pathogens

Confirm results of microbiologic cultures

Refute the relevance of microbiologic cultures

Establish diagnosis unrelated to infection

Identify concomitant infection in a primary inflammatory or neoplastic disorder

Identify new pathogens

Table 2-2 Optimal Handling of Tissue Biopsies: Always Consider Infection!

Make touch imprints for histochemical staining

Handle samples for microbiologic culture with sterile technique

Harvest samples for ultrastructural examination in glutaraldehyde fixative

Harvest fresh samples for appropriate polymerase chain reaction assays

Freeze portion of biopsy specimen for research

After all of this is done, place biopsy specimen in formalin

Table 2-3 Tissue Responses to Infection

Type of Inflammation	Example
Exudative inflammation	Pyogenic bacteria
Necrotizing inflammation	Gram-negative bacteria, amebiasis
Granulomatous inflammation	Mycobacteria, fungi
Histiocytic inflammation	*Rhodococcus, Legionella,* Whipple's disease
Eosinophilic inflammation	Fungi, parasites
Cytopathic changes	Viruses
No response	Host anergy

few surgical pathologists would balk at the idea of ordering additional sections to exclude malignancy in a biopsy they deemed suspicious, it is not uncommon for a pathologist to examine only a single histochemically stained tissue section in the diagnostic process of infection.[4] More egregious is the fantasy that the causative infectious agent will eventually be diagnosed by the microbiology laboratory, so there is no need for the surgical pathologist to belabor the process.

This approach is wrong-minded for several reasons. First, the microbiology laboratory may fail to identify a causative organism.[5] Second, the organism isolated by the laboratory may not represent the actual infective agent in vivo. The analogy is the role for Gram staining of secretions in chronically intubated patients to determine whether there is a neutrophilic exudate consistent with infection and whether there is a predominating organism—steps that can promote the choice of appropriate antibiotic therapy.[6] In this setting, undue emphasis on culture results can lead to a seemingly endless process of adding or eliminating antibiotics in patients who are merely colonized by bacteria and not actually infected. Treatment decisions that do not take into account the host response and dominating organisms will tend to favor the production of increasingly antibiotic-resistant isolates and may potentially compromise public health. This is only one of several compelling reasons to consider diagnostic biopsies in patients with infections in situations that do not readily yield to noninvasive approaches.

Potential Limits of Biopsy Interpretation

Despite the merits of examining biopsy specimens in the diagnosis of infection, one must be aware of those situations in which the sensitivity and specificity of histochemically stained sections is limited. An example is tuberculosis, in which biopsies can fail to demonstrate mycobacteria in almost half of cases.[7] But even in this setting, the appearance of the inflammatory response in situ should foster a working diagnosis that is often sufficiently reliable to institute empirical treatment.

Classification of Patterns of Infection

There is currently no uniformly accepted classification schema for the histologic patterns of response yielded by microorganisms. The inflammatory response in infection is a function of the host response, which is in turn a function of (1) the anatomy of the affected organ, (2) the virulence factors produced by the infective agent, and (3) host immunocompetence. The surgical pathologist must be aware that a single species of microorganism may be capable of evoking a variety of different patterns of inflammation. An example is the broad spectrum of disorders produced in response to infection with *Aspergillus* spp., which ranges from benign colonization, to hypersensitivity responses, to malignant angioinvasive infection.[8]

The characteristic types of inflammation elicited by infection (Table 2-3) can be broadly categorized as follows.

1. **Pyogenic responses.** In these responses, neutrophils predominate, leading to pus formation. They are evoked primarily by bacteria, although viruses and fungi can also elicit them (Fig. 2-1).

2. **Necrotizing inflammation.** Tissue necrosis can occur in several forms. In certain infections, such as those caused by amebas or gram-negative bacteria, liquefactive necrosis is frequently seen (Fig. 2-2). Other forms, such as ischemic, mummefactive, and caseous necrosis, are often seen in mycobacterial and fungal infections.

3. **Granulomatous inflammation.** This response is characterized by the presence of epithelioid macrophages with multikaryon (giant cell) formation. It appears to reflect cell-mediated immunity to poorly catabolized antigens and is evoked by mycobacteria, fungi, and parasites (Fig. 2-3).

4. **Histiocytic inflammation.** These responses are characterized primarily by the presence of foamy macrophages and are a prominent component of infections caused by *Legionella*,

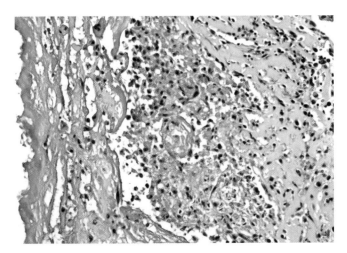

Figure 2-1. Pyogenic response in acute infective endocarditis due to *Streptococcus* spp. with neutrophilic exudate. (×400)

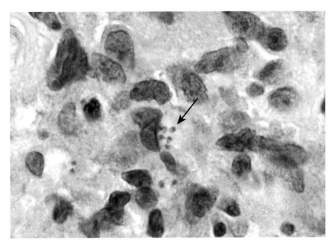

Figure 2-4. Histiocytic response shows "foamy" macrophages containing *Leishmania donovani* (*arrow*). (×600)

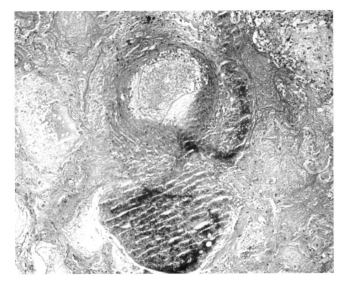

Figure 2-2. Necrotizing response to *Pseudomonas aeruginosa,* showing liquefactive destruction of lung tissue. (×250)

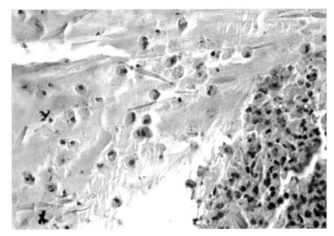

Figure 2-5. Eosinophilic response to *Aspergillus fumigatus.* (×400)

Rhodococcus, Calymmatobacterium, Leishmania, and *T. whippelii* (Fig. 2-4). In patients who are severely immunocompromised, organisms that normally elicit granulomatous inflammation may instead evoke histiocytic infiltrates.

5. **Eosinophilic inflammation.** This is seen in response to multicellular parasites and certain fungi (Fig. 2-5).

6. **Cytopathic changes.** Although this is not properly a type of inflammation, cytopathic changes do reflect a response to viral infection. Nuclear inclusions are part of the response to DNA viruses, whereas cytologic inclusions are seen with some RNA and DNA viral infections, such as cytomegalovirus (Fig. 2-6).

7. **Null responses.** In the setting of profound immunosuppression, one may not see inflammation; only the uninhibited growth of microorganisms is apparent (Fig. 2-7).

This classification schema is only a crude approximation, because overlap patterns of inflammation are common, as with necrotizing granulomatous inflammation, granulohistiocytic inflammation (Fig. 2-8), and granulomatous inflammation with tissue eosinophilia (Fig. 2-9). The primary didactic element is

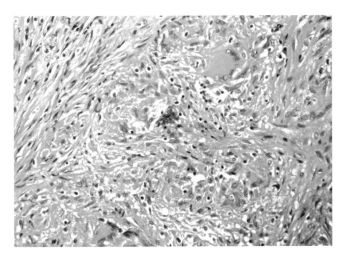

Figure 2-3. Granulomatous response to *Mycobacterium tuberculosis.* (×25)

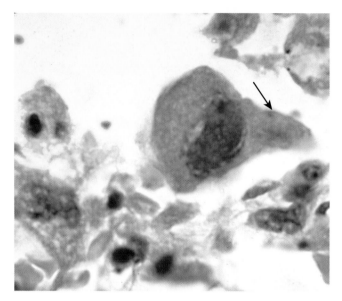

Figure 2-6. Cytopathic response to *Cytomegalovirus* with both nuclear and cytoplasmic (*arrow*) inclusions. (×600)

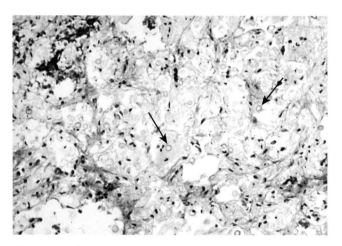

Figure 2-7. Null response to *Cryptococcus neoformans* (*arrows*). (×400)

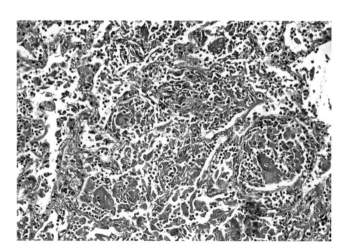

Figure 2-8. Granulohistiocytic response to *Blastomyces dermatitidis*. (×250)

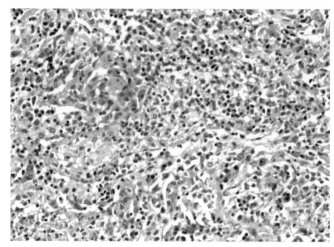

Figure 2-9. Granulomatous response with tissue eosinophilia due to *Coccidioides immitis*. (×250)

that careful consideration of the histological response in situ can help to narrow what would otherwise be a very broad differential diagnosis and can also provide invaluable information concerning host immunocompetence. For this reason, surgical pathologists must develop expertise concerning the inflammatory patterns that can accompany reduced immunocompetence resulting from genetic factors, age, toxins, and drugs, because they can skew the expected pattern of inflammation and at times confound the diagnosis.

Histochemical Stains

The identification of microorganisms in biopsy samples is enhanced by the selective application of widely available histochemical stains (Table 2-4). Pathologists should be aware of the spectrum of histochemical staining by microorganisms and knowledgeable with respect to how to formulate combinations of stains to enhance diagnostic specificity.[9]

Hematoxylin and Eosin

The majority of pathogens can be identified with the standard hematoxylin and eosin (H&E) stain. These include cytopathic viruses, some bacteria, most fungi, and virtually all parasites (Table 2-5).

Gram Stain

The tissue Gram stain is a congener of the Gram stain used routinely to identify organisms in body secretions and fluids. The Brown-Hopps stain is currently the preparation of choice, because it enhances gram-negative bacteria and rickettsia to a greater degree than the Brown-Brenn. In addition, the latter can be hazardous to technical personnel and has largely fallen into disfavor. The tissue Gram stain colors the cell walls of gram-positive bacteria a deep violaceous blue (Fig. 2-10A) and gram-

Table 2-4 Histochemical Staining Characteristics of Microbes

Organism	Staining Characteristics
Viruses	
Influenza	No cytopathic change
Coronavirus (SARS)	No cytopathic change
Adenovirus	H&E (smudge cells); IHC
Cytomegalovirus	H&E (intranuclear and cytoplasmic inclusions); IHC; PAS and GMS (intracytoplasmic inclusions)
Herpesvirus	H&E (intranuclear inclusions); IHC
Measles	H&E (intranuclear inclusions, polykaryons)
Respiratory syncytial virus	H&E (polykaryons); IHC
Parainfluenza	H&E (intracytoplasmic inclusions)
Bacteria	
Gram-positive	Tissue Gram, GMS (all)
Gram-negative	Tissue Gram, GMS (some)
Legionella	Silver impregnation
Nocardia	Tissue Gram, GMS, modified ZN
Actinomyces	Tissue Gram, GMS
Mycobacteria tuberculosis	ZN and modified ZN; PCR
Atypical mycobacteria	Modified ZN, ± ZN, PCR
Fungi	
Histoplasma	GMS, PAS
Cryptococcus	H&E, GMS, PAS, mucicarmine; Fontana, IHC
Blastomyces	H&E, GMS, PAS, mucicarmine (weak)
Coccidiomyces	H&E, GMS, PAS
Candida	H&E, GMS, PAS, Gram stain; IHC
Aspergillus	H&E, GMS, PAS, IHC
Zygomyces	H&E, GMS, PAS
Pseudeallescheria	H&E, GMS, PAS
Alternaria and dematiaceous fungi	H&E, GMS, PAS, Fontana
Parasites	
Protozoa	H&E, PAS, Gram stain (microsporidia); IHC (*Toxoplasma*),
Metazoans	H&E, trichrome stain
Echinococcus	GMS in chitinous wall, modified ZN (hooklets)
Paragonimiasis	Ova birefringent
Schistosomiasis	Lateral and terminal spines stain with modified ZN

GMS, Gomori methenamine silver stain; H&E, hematoxylin and eosin stain; IHC, immunohistochemical methods; PAS, periodic acid–Schiff stain. PCR, polymerase chain reaction; SARS, severe acute respiratory syndrome; ZN, Ziehl-Neelsen stain.

Table 2-5 Microbes That Can Be Identified with Hematoxylin and Eosin Stain

Cytopathic viruses
Bacteria in colonies or in "granules"
Most fungi
Parasites

negative bacteria a pale salmon pink (see Fig. 2-10B). Consequently, it is far easier to detect gram-positive species, and one must be careful not to overlook the presence of faintly stained gram-negative species. Gram variability is a potential pitfall in interpretation, because it can raise the specter of polymicrobial infection. Attention to the uniform morphologic characteristics of stained organisms is the best way to avoid being misled by this phenomenon.

Nonbacterial pathogens can also be identified with the Gram stain. The blastoconidia (yeast) of *Candida* spp. (Fig. 2-11A) and the microconidia of *Aspergillus* spp. (see Fig. 2-11B) are gram-positive, and this feature can help in distinguishing these species from other fungi. Microsporidia can be well demonstrated as gram-positive intracellular inclusions within cells (Fig. 2-12).

Silver Impregnation

The impregnation of tissue sections with silver constitutes the basis of the Warthin-Starry, Dieterle, and Steiner stains. There is some controversy among experts as to whether these stains are equally efficacious in the identification of certain organisms, such as *Bartonella* spp., but in general they yield comparable results. In theory, all eubacteria, including mycobacteria, will stain positively with silver impregnation. However, in our experience, they do not do so reliably, and this approach cannot be recommended as a screening tool. In general, bacteria are enhanced both colorimetrically and in size by the deposition of silver salts on their cell walls, making them easier to identify but at times causing confusion in interpretation. Background staining presents a problem in interpretation, but the morphologic regularity of eubacteria usually allows for accurate identification, once experience has been established with the technique.

Certain weakly gram-reactive or non–gram-reactive bacteria cannot be demonstrated reliably by any other histochemical method. These include *Treponema* spp. (Fig. 2-13), *Borrelia* spp., *Bartonella* spp., *Leptospira* spp., and *Calymmatobacterium*. Weakly staining gram-negative bacteria, including *Legionella* spp., *Burkholderia* spp., *Francisella* spp., and *Helicobacter*, are also best demonstrated by silver impregnation.

Fungal Stains

The Gomori methenamine silver (GMS) and Gridley stains are the preferred methods for demonstrating fungi (Table 2-6). Because certain fungi demonstrated by GMS do not consistently stain well with periodic acid–Schiff (PAS), the latter should be

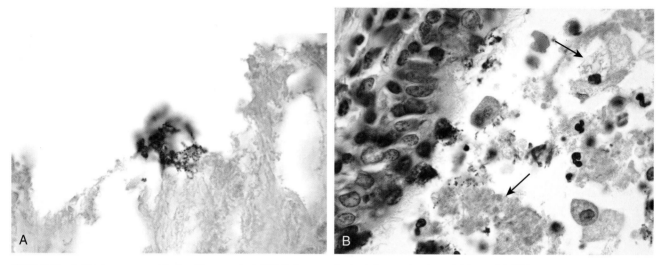

Figure 2-10. A, *Streptococcus* spp. stain deep blue-magenta. (×600) **B,** Gram-negative bacteria are pale salmon-pink (*arrows*). (×600)

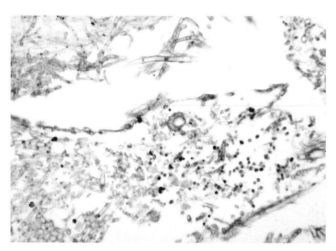

Figure 2-11. The microconidia of *Aspergillus fumigatus* stain intensely gram-positive. (×250)

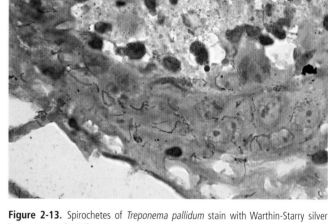

Figure 2-13. Spirochetes of *Treponema pallidum* stain with Warthin-Starry silver impregnation. (×400)

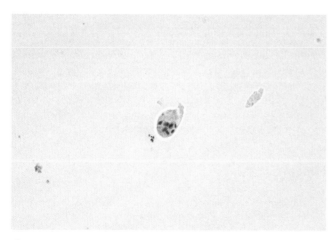

Figure 2-12. Gram-positive intracytoplasmic microsporidia. (×400)

reserved as a secondary approach, but it can at times enhance morphologic detail. Although the GMS is often counterstained with methyl green for contrast, other counterstains can be applied. It is possible, for example, to counterstain with H&E; this allows for a detailed assessment of the cellular immune response and promotes accurate identification of intravascular and perineural invasion by organisms.

All gram-positive bacteria, including the actinomycetes, stain with GMS (Fig. 2-14), as do some encapsulated gram-negative bacteria, such as *Klebsiella* spp. Bacteria that have been treated before tissue sampling (e.g., infective endocarditis), may not be well decorated by the Gram stain, but they often retain their GMS positivity. For this reason, both stains should be examined before excluding a gram-positive bacterial infection. The actinomycetes, including mycobacteria, are gram-positive eubacteria and consequently also stain with GMS. The GMS is the stain of choice for demonstrating *Pneumocystis jiroveci* (Fig. 2-15), and it highlights the trophozoites of *Entamoeba*

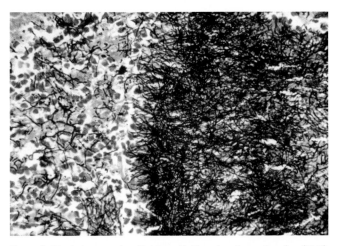

Figure 2-14. *Actinomyces israelii* stains with Gomori methenamine silver (GMS). (×250)

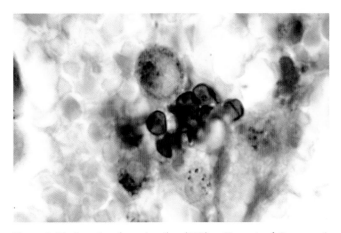

Figure 2-15. Gomori methenamine silver (GMS)-positive cysts of *Pneumocystis jiroveci.* (×600)

Table 2-6 Fungal Identification in Tissue

Organism	Size (Width in μm)	Defining Morphology
Histoplasma capsulatum	2-5	Narrow-neck bud
Cryptococcus neoformans	5-20	Narrow-neck bud
Blastomyces dermatitidis	15-30	Broad-based bud
Candida glabrata	3-5	Budding, no pseudohyphae
Candida spp.	2-3	Yeast, pseudohyphae, hyphae
Aspergillus spp.	3-5	Acute-angle branching, septate, conidial head
Zygomyces spp.	5-8	Right-angle branching, ribbons, pauciseptate
Pseudallescheria spp.	3-4	Acute-angle branch, septate, terminal chlamydospore, pigmented conidia
Fusarium spp.	4-5	Acute and right-angle branch, septate, narrowed branch points
Coccidioides immitis	20-200	Endosporulation

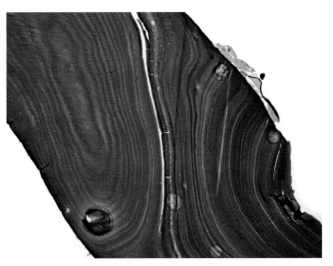

Figure 2-16. Gomori methenamine silver (GMS)-positive wall of cyst produced by *Echinococcus granulosus.* (×200)

histolytica, encysted amebas, the intracytoplasmic inclusions of cytomegalovirus-infected cells, the polar bodies of microsporidia, and the cyst wall of *Echinococcus* spp. (Fig. 2-16).

Acid-Fast Bacteria Stains

The Ziehl-Neelsen (ZN) stain and its modifications historically have been essential tools in the identification of mycobacteria.[3] *Mycobacterium* spp. (Fig. 2-17A) are also GMS-positive (see Fig. 2-17B), and some atypical mycobacteria, such as *Mycobacterium avium-intracellulare* complex (MAC), also stain with PAS. The

modified stain for acid-fast bacteria (Fite-Faraco or Putt's) detects mycobacterial antigens that are sensitive to strong acid, a step in the decolorization of the ZN stain. For this reason, it can be used to screen for all mycobacteria and may be required to detect certain atypical mycobacteria, such as *Mycobacterium leprae*, as well as *Nocardia*, *Rhodococcus*, and *Legionella micdadei*. The cortical spines of *Schistosoma* spp. (Fig. 2-18), the hooklets of *Echinococcus*, and the spores of *Cryptosporidium* also stain well, but variably, with modified acid-fast bacillus stains.

Connective Tissue Stains

Masson's trichrome, Movat's pentachrome, and Wilder reticulin stains can be useful ancillary methods for classifying helminthic infections (Fig. 2-19). The inclusions of cytomegalovirus are demonstrated well by trichrome stains. The reticulin stain demonstrates the details of most helminths, the amasti-

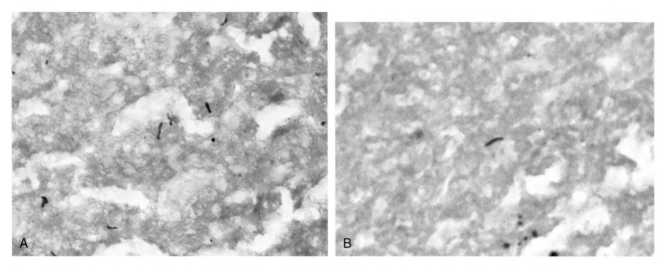

Figure 2-17. *Mycobacterium tuberculosis* stains with Ziehl-Neelsen stain (×600) **(A)** and Gomori methenamine silver (GMS) stain (×600) **(B)**.

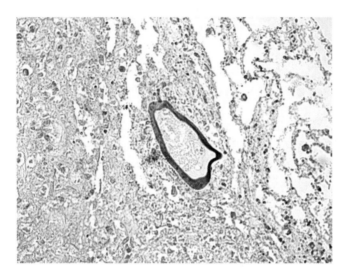

Figure 2-18. Cortical spine of ovum of *Schistosoma mansoni* stains positive with Fite-Faraco stain. (×600)

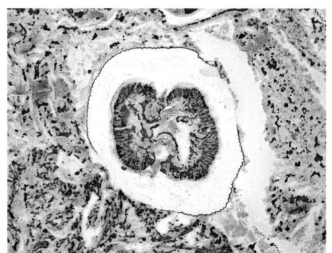

Figure 2-19. Wilder reticulin stain highlights *Dirofilaria immitis.* (×150)

gotes of trypanosomes, and the rod-shaped kinetoplast of *Leishmania* spp.

Giemsa Stains

Giemsa stains and their variants can help in identifying a wide spectrum of pathogens, including protozoa, bacteria, chlamydia, and rickettsia. However, the small size of some of these organisms (e.g., rickettsiae) limits the degree of confidence in establishing an accurate diagnosis, and prior experience in diagnosing these infections is essential.[10]

Mucicarmine

Several fungi, most notably *Cryptococcus, Blastomyces,* and *Rhinosporidium,* exhibit mucicarminophilia, either in their secreted capsules (*Cryptococcus*) or in their cell walls. Mucicarminophilia

is an essential feature in the diagnosis of *Cryptococcus;* however, this staining, although invariably present, may be difficult to detect in capsule-deficient variants (Fig. 2-20).[11]

Melanin Stains

The Fontana-Masson stain demonstrates pre-melanin precursors within the cell wall of *Cryptococcus neoformans* and is an essential confirmatory approach to the in situ identification of capsular-deficient forms (Fig. 2-21).[12] All dematiaceous fungi are positive with Fontana-Masson, and this stain can help to confirm the impression of pigmentation seen in H&E sections.

Viral Inclusion Body Stains

A number of stains (e.g., Feulgen) can detect viral inclusions with cells. However, none adds considerably to the H&E stain

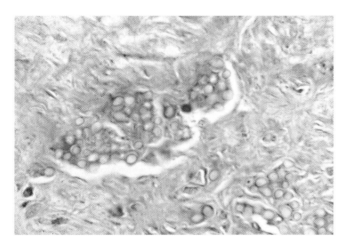

Figure 2-20. Mucicarmine stain decorates the capsule of *Cryptococcus neoformans.* (×400)

Table 2-7 Immunohistochemical Stains Commercially Available for Microbe Identification in Paraffin-Embedded Tissues

Fungi	Viruses and Bacteria
Aspergillus (genus only)	Herpesvirus 1 (cross-reacts herpesvirus 2)
Cryptococcus	Varicella-zoster
Histoplasma	Cytomegalovirus
Candida spp.	Respiratory syncytial virus
Coccidioides immitis	Adenovirus
Pneumocystis jiroveci	Epstein-Barr (Epstein-Barr encoded RNA)
Pseudallescheria boydii	Actinomycetes
Zygomycoses (genus only)	*Actinomyces israelii*
Sporothrix schenckii	*Actinomyces naeslundii*
Trichosporon	*Arachnia propionica*

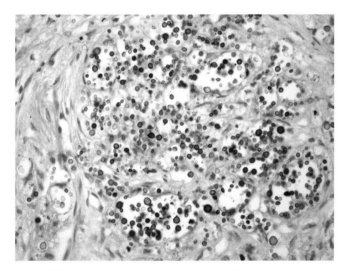

Figure 2-21. Fontana-Masson stain assists in the identification of an "acapsular" variant of *Cryptococcus neoformans.* (×400)

in this regard, and they are rarely adopted in practice, especially since confirmatory immunostains have become more widely available.

Immunohistochemical Methods

A large number of immunostains are available that can be helpful in the identification of microorganisms (Table 2-7).[13] Many of these are commercially available and currently enjoy wide popularity in diagnostic pathology laboratories. Others are available reliably only at highly specialized centers such as the Centers for Disease Control and Prevention. Development of new immunohistochemical techniques can be a worthwhile but labor-intensive task. Because there is wide cross-reactivity among fungal species and among bacteria, it is critical to establish the potential cross-reactivity of any new antibody and its relative specificity.[14] Nevertheless, it may at times be possible to limit the use of a reagent to a narrow range of differential diagnostic possibilities

(e.g., to distinguish *Aspergillus* spp. from *Pseudallescheria boydii* infection).

Molecular Diagnostics

Molecular techniques continue to dramatically reshape clinical microbiology practice. Currently, molecular techniques involving the identification of microbial nucleic acids are critical to the management of a growing number of infectious agents, most importantly the chronic viral infections, including human immunodeficiency virus (HIV), hepatitis B virus, and hepatitis C virus. HIV management is a prototype for the implementation of molecular medicine, because the diagnosis can be made using reverse transcriptase–polymerase chain reaction (RT-PCR) amplification of viral RNA, antiviral therapy regimens can be adjusted based on serial RT-PCR viral load measurements, and resistance mutations can be detected by sequencing of the viral genes targeted by current drugs (protease and reverse transcriptase inhibitors).

In the setting of surgical pathology, a role is beginning to be developed for molecular techniques in the pathologic assessment of infection. The most relevant techniques in the setting of tissue diagnosis are in situ microbial detection using nucleic acid probes (in situ hybridization) and PCR using nucleic acids purified from tissue sections. These two techniques can allow for diagnosis when special stains and immunohistochemical stains are insensitive (e.g., low antigen expression), and in some instances, they can allow for speciation when microbes are identified with those techniques. In addition, molecular identification can accelerate definitive diagnosis with organisms that grow slowly or not at all in culture (e.g., fastidious organisms such as mycobacteria).

In Situ Hybridization

In situ hybridization (ISH) is a technique that uses fluorescent or radiolabeled nucleic acid probes to recognize specific microbial sequences in tissue sections. The probes contain RNA or

DNA sequences complementary to the target genetic elements and allow for specific localization of microbes in tissue or within cells. Depending on the sequence, some ISH probes can also bind specifically to nucleic acids from individual species, allowing for differentiation of organisms with variable virulence. Although there is great specificity with many ISH probes, immunohistochemistry is preferred, if possible, because of ease of incorporation into the modern automated pathology laboratory.

Most critical to the surgical pathologist is the identification of human papillomavirus (HPV) infection in cervical cancer screening, and this is most often accomplished with the use of PCR or similar techniques from liquid Pap smear specimens. ISH can also be very effective for definitive detection of high-risk HPV subtypes in cervical biopsy analysis for dysplasia and in defining HPV status of oropharyngeal squamous cell carcinomas.[15] Immunohistochemistry for HPV antigens has not proved sensitive enough (although p16 positivity is a reasonable surrogate marker of HPV infection). The HPV genome is present as episomes in low-grade lesions, so ISH reveals diffuse and intense staining (Fig. 2-22). In high-grade lesions and invasive carcinomas, the HPV genome integrates into the host genome, and ISH reveals a punctate nuclear signal.

ISH is also useful in the detection of Epstein-Barr virus (EBV) in lymphocytes, including in lymphoproliferative disorders, because the EBV-encoded RNAs (EBER1 and EBER2) are expressed at very high levels. Commercial EBER ISH assays have been developed and are automatable.

Recently, a novel chemical variant of DNA called peptide nucleic acids (PNA), consisting of nucleoside bases joined by a peptide backbone rather than a sugar backbone, has been used to detect microbial genetic material. PNA probes offer the advantage of chemical stability and higher sensitivity and specificity. These properties offer the opportunity of developing probes that can differentiate species in situ. Such probes have proved successful in differentiating tuberculous from nontuberculous mycobacterial infections by targeting the 16S ribosomal RNA; others have detected *Staphylococcus aureus*, *Enterococcus faecalis*, and *Candida* species.[16-19]

Polymerase Chain Reaction

PCR amplification to detect infectious agents in surgical pathology specimens is now so common that a basic description of the technique is unnecessary.[20,21] PCR is without a doubt the most sensitive detection method available, and because if can be performed on archived formalin-fixed, paraffin-embedded samples, important diagnoses can be rendered even if cultures were not obtained from tissue biopsies at the time of processing (e.g., lung wedge resections for tumor that later reveal necrotizing granulomas). Common applications of PCR to surgical samples are listed in Table 2-8.

Central to PCR, however, is the requirement the exact RNA or DNA sequences to be amplified must be known. Abundant

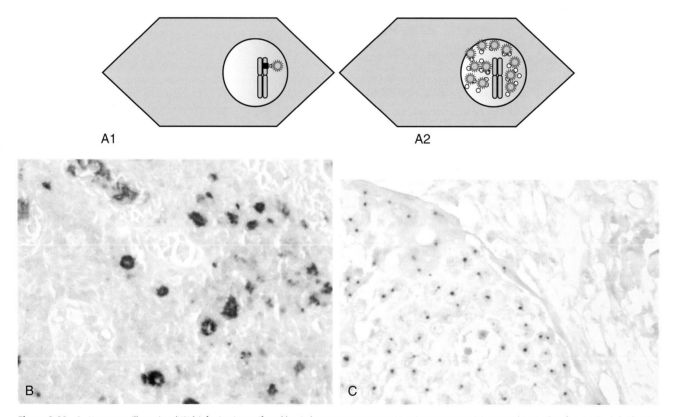

Figure 2-22. A, Human papillomavirus (HPV) infection is manifested by viral genomes present as A1 episomes, or as A2 integrated DNA. Therefore, in situ hybridization (ISH) probes give diffuse (*lower right*) or discrete (*lower left*) staining patterns in HPV-positive tissue. Actual ISH is shown in two oropharyngeal squamous cell carcinomas, with episomal signals **(B)** and integrated virus **(C)**. (Photographs courtesy of Dr. Jennifer Hunt, Cleveland Clinic Department of Pathology) (×250).

Table 2-8 Applications of the Polymerase Chain Reaction to Microbial Detection In Tissues

Organism	Pathologic Process
Aspergillus	Invasive aspergillosis[21]
Human papillomavirus	Cervical HSIL and LSIL, HPV-positive squamous cell carcinoma of the oropharynx
Herpesvirus	Herpes encephalitis (CSF or brain biopsy)
Mycobacteria	Necrotizing granulomatous inflammation
Bartonella	Cat-scratch disease or bacillary angiomatosis
Enterovirus, adenovirus, influenza A virus	Viral myocarditis[20]

CSF, cerebrospinal fluid; HPV, human papillomavirus; HSIL, high-grade squamous intraepithelial lesion; LSIL, low-grade squamous intraepithelial lesion.

microbial sequence data are publicly available, so that any equipped laboratory can analyze the most known pathogens. There are a number of well-conserved genes in microorganisms, such as the ribosomal 16S gene and the heat-shock protein/ chaperonin HSP60/65 (or GroEL), that are excellent targets for PCR. Analysis of the16S ribosomal RNA gene in bacteria by PCR and subsequent sequencing is especially informative, because there are well-conserved sequences that can be used as binding sites for universal PCR primers adjacent to variable sequences and then analyzed and compared to databases of known sequences (Fig. 2-23).

This sensitivity of PCR is not without its problems. Many of the most important infectious agents seen in general practice are found in the environment and can contaminate surgical specimens. For example, *Aspergillus* and mycobacterial species are normal denizens of the clinical laboratory, and if samples are not kept sterile, they may come in contact with these species during tissue processing. Even more vexing, such species also can

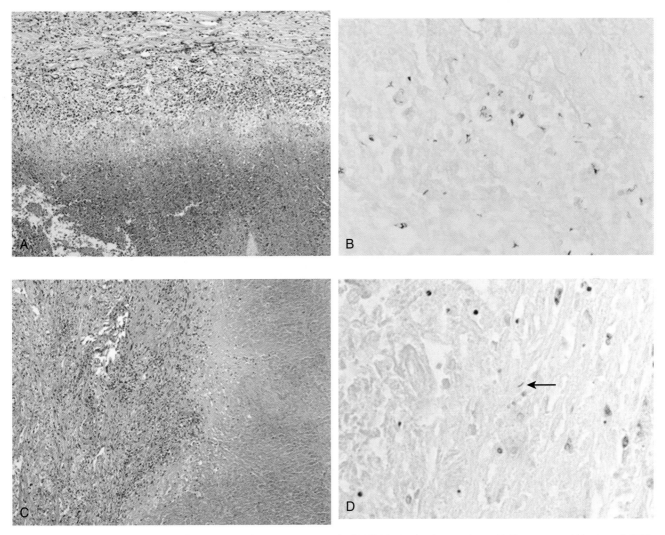

Figure 2-23. Two cases of mycobacterial infection. **A,** *Mycobacterium avium* complex (MAC) infection in a lung specimen with **B,** numerous acid-fast bacteria (AFB). **C,** Lung specimen with *Mycobacterium tuberculosis* complex (MTb) infection with rare AFB (*arrow* in **D**). (×200)

continued

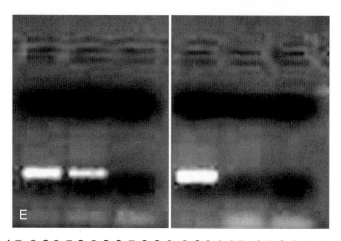

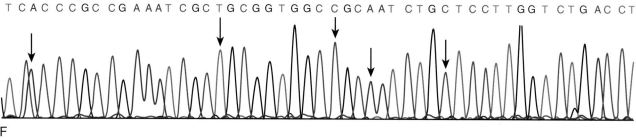

T C A C C C G C C G A A A T C G C T G C G G T G G C C G C A A T C T G C T C C T T G G T C T G A C C T

F

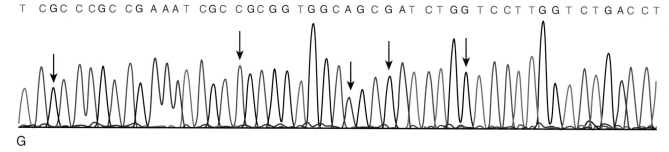

T C G C C C G C C G A A A T C G C C G C G G T G G C A G C G A T C T G G T C C T T G G T C T G A C C T

G

Figure 2-23, cont'd. DNA was isolated from formalin-fixed, paraffin-embedded tissue and amplified with primers to the *HSP65* gene, showing positive bands for the MTb sample (**E,** lane 1) and the MAC sample (**E,** lane 2). An MTb-specific gene polymerase chain reaction assay (*IS6110* gene) reveals a band only with MTb (**E,** lane 4). Water-only control lanes show no band in either reaction (**E,** lanes 3 and 6). The *HSP65* gene products were subject to DNA sequencing with the bacterial sequence from the MTb sample in **F** and from the MAC in **G.** Alignment of the two sequences reveals numerous sequence differences (*arrows*) in the region, which can be used to differentiate the two species.

cause opportunistic infections, and so their identification cannot always be dismissed as clinically irrelevant.

REFERENCES

1. Velez L, Correa LT, Maya MA, et al: Diagnostic accuracy of bronchoalveolar lavage samples in immunosuppressed patients with suspected pneumonia: Analysis of a protocol. Respir Med 2007; 101(10):2160-2167.

2. Dutly F, Altwegg M: Whipple's disease and "*Tropheryma whippelii.*" Clin Microbiol Rev 2001;14(3):561-583.

3. Christie JD, Callihan DR: The laboratory diagnosis of mycobacterial diseases: Challenges and common sense. Clin Lab Med 1995; 15(2):279-306.

4. Procop GW, Wilson M: Infectious disease pathology. Clin Infect Dis 2001;32(11):1589-1601.

5. Weydert JA, Van Natta TL, DeYoung BR: Comparison of fungal culture versus surgical pathology examination in the detection of *Histoplasma* in surgically excised pulmonary granulomas. Arch Pathol Lab Med 2007;131(5):780-783.

6. Niederman MS: The clinical diagnosis of ventilator-associated pneumonia. Respir Care 2005;50(6):788-796; discussion 807-812.

7. Tang YW, Procop GW, Zheng X, et al: Histologic parameters predictive of mycobacterial infection. Am J Clin Pathol 1998;109(3): 331-334.

8. Kradin R, Mark E: Pathology of pulmonary disorders due to *Aspergillus* spp. Arch Pathol Lab Med 2008;132(4):606-614.

9. Chandler FW: Approaches to the pathologic diagnosis of infectious disease. In Connor DH, Chandler RW, Schwartz DA, et al. (eds):

Pathology of Infectious Diseases. Stamford, Conn., Appleton and Lange, 1997.

10. Nilsson K, Lindquist O, Pahlson C: Association of *Rickettsia helvetica* with chronic perimyocarditis in sudden cardiac death. Lancet 1999;354(9185):1169-1173.

11. Lazcano O, Speights VO Jr, Strickler JG, et al: Combined histochemical stains in the differential diagnosis of *Cryptococcus neoformans*. Mod Pathol 1993;6(1):80-84.

12. Lazcano O, Speights VO Jr, Bilbao J, et al: Combined Fontana-Masson-mucin staining of *Cryptococcus neoformans*. Arch Pathol Lab Med 1991;115(11):1145-1149.

13. Eyzaguirre E, Haque AK: Application of immunohistochemistry to infections. Arch Pathol Lab Med 2008;132(3):424-431.

14. Reed JA, Hemann BA, Alexander JL, Brigati DJ: Immunomycology: Rapid and specific immunocytochemical identification of fungi in formalin-fixed, paraffin-embedded material. J Histochem Cytochem 1993;41(8):1217-1221.

15. Nuovo GJ: The surgical and cytopathology of viral infections: Utility of immunohistochemistry, in situ hybridization, and in situ polymerase chain reaction amplification. Ann Diagn Pathol 2006; 10(2):117-131.

16. Lefmann M, Schweickert B, Buchholz P, et al: Evaluation of peptide nucleic acid-fluorescence in situ hybridization for identification of clinically relevant mycobacteria in clinical specimens and tissue sections. J Clin Microbiol 2006;44(10):3760-3767.

17. Peters RP, van Agtmael MA, Simoons-Smit AM, et al: Rapid identification of pathogens in blood cultures with a modified fluorescence in situ hybridization assay. J Clin Microbiol 2006;44(10):4186-4188.

18. Hongmanee P, Stender H, Rasmussen OF: Evaluation of a fluorescence in situ hybridization assay for differentiation between tuberculous and nontuberculous *Mycobacterium* species in smears of Lowenstein-Jensen and Mycobacteria Growth Indicator Tube cultures using peptide nucleic acid probes. J Clin Microbiol 2001;39(3):1032-1035.

19. Reller ME, Mallonee AB, Kwiatkowski NP, Merz WG: Use of peptide nucleic acid-fluorescence in situ hybridization for definitive, rapid identification of five common *Candida* species. J Clin Microbiol 2007;45(11):3802-3803.

20. Guarner J, Bhatnagar J, Shieh WJ, et al: Histopathologic, immunohistochemical, and polymerase chain reaction assays in the study of cases with fatal sporadic myocarditis. Hum Pathol 2007;38(9):1412-1419.

21. Rickerts V, Mousset S, Lambrecht E, et al: Comparison of histopathological analysis, culture, and polymerase chain reaction assays to detect invasive mold infections from biopsy specimens. Clin Infect Dis 2007;44(8):1078-1083.

The Biopsy in the Diagnosis of Infection: Clinical Approach

Jay A. Fishman

Overview: The Biopsy

The practice of clinical infectious disease management has undergone a revolution as a result of the recognition of new clinical syndromes (e.g., acquired immunodeficiency syndrome [AIDS]), the availability of new diagnostic tools, and a wide array of newer antimicrobial agents. The availability of organism-specific molecular or protein-based assays and of anatomically revealing radiologic tests including computed tomography (CT) imaging, magnetic resonance imaging, and positron emission tomography have enhanced the deployment of antimicrobial therapies. Despite these advances, a specific diagnosis is often not achieved to guide therapy. In some conditions, in which the disease process is self-limited or the therapies are broadly active or relatively nontoxic, a specific diagnosis may not be essential. In community-acquired pneumonia, a specific diagnosis is made in fewer than half of the cases, but common therapies (e.g., with an antimicrobial macrolide or fluoroquinolone agent) have an antimicrobial spectrum broad enough to cover the common pathogens, or the patient gets better without therapy (i.e., viral syndrome).

When does the clinical condition of a patient merit invasive testing in the form of a tissue biopsy to achieve a diagnosis? Some common considerations include the following:

- Distinguishing between infectious and noninfectious etiologies (e.g., cancer) for an abnormality discovered by physical or other (endoscopic) examination or radiologic techniques. This is especially important in patients with atypical presentations of diseases.
- Sampling of a likely infection for microbiologic analysis (e.g., culture and susceptibility testing)
- Detection of organisms for which microbiologic culture techniques may be imprecise or unavailable (e.g., parasitic infections)
- Microbiologic evaluation in the patient with a lesion that has failed to respond to presumably appropriate therapy (Fig. 3-1)

- To assess response to antimicrobial therapy or to distinguish infection from the host response to infection
- To help resolve infection (excisional biopsy)
- As an aid to prognostication
- In patients for whom various therapies carry significant or unacceptable toxicities

In general, a biopsy is used in patients for whom a specific diagnosis is critical to optimal management.

The timing of the biopsy procedure is important. Some patients will predictably become sicker or less able to tolerate complications of a biopsy (e.g., bleeding tendency, significant cardiac disease, pneumothorax, infection, bowel perforation) later in the course of their disease process. These include patients undergoing cancer chemotherapy, organ or stem cell transplantation, or planned travel to medically underserved regions. These conditions may lead one to obtain an early definitive diagnosis. Underlying clinical conditions often define the biopsy approach employed. For example, transjugular liver biopsies are used in patients with bleeding tendencies; the patient may bleed, but into the vasculature from which the biopsy was obtained. Transjugular biopsies tend to be adequate for diagnosis less often than percutaneous biopsies (87% versus 69%), but in a retrospective study, the difference was not significant.[1,2] Transjugular biopsies require cardiac monitoring for arrhythmias induced by the catheterization procedure. The samples obtained are often fragmented but are usually adequate for histologic diagnosis.

It is essential that an adequate tissue sample be obtained if a biopsy procedure is performed. This may be limited by the patient's clinical condition and ability to tolerate complications (e.g., low platelet count, mechanical ventilation, encephalitis). However, an inadequate sample often necessitates a repeat biopsy. The specific biopsy procedure selected depends on the urgency for diagnosis, the tissue being sampled, and the likely pathogens in a given host. An example of this decision process is the evaluation of diffuse pulmonary infections. In this setting, a diagnosis may often be made by bronchoalveolar lavage in AIDS patients, whereas transbronchial biopsy is preferred in the non-AIDS immunocompromised host. This reflects the higher organism burden and slower progression of common infectious processes (e.g., *Pneumocystis* pneumonia, mycobacterial infection) in patients with AIDS compared with other immunosuppressed or neutropenic individuals. Similarly, a small tissue sample from fine-needle aspiration may be adequate for diagnosis of a focal process (e.g., abscess), or a small sample obtained from transjugular biopsy may be appropriate for a diffuse process or if molecular amplification techniques can be used (e.g., viral hepatitis). A larger sample (core biopsy) is needed for patchy

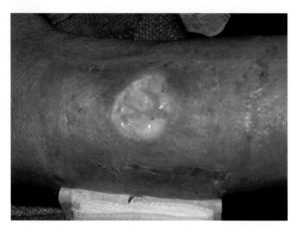

Figure 3-1. Forearm lesion in renal transplant recipient at the site of prior intravenous catheterization. Swab cultures grew methicillin-susceptible *Staphylococcus aureus.* The lesion failed to heal after multiple courses of antibacterial therapy. Biopsy revealed *Cryptococcus neoformans.* Healing occurred on antifungal therapy.

processes (e.g., BK polyomavirus infection of a transplanted kidney). Fine-needle aspiration and percutaneous biopsies may have the disadvantage of tracking of infection or cells along the biopsy path.

We have employed video-assisted thoracoscopic surgical (VATS) or open (thoracotomy) excision of lung lesions in immunocompromised hosts (e.g., for focal *Aspergillus* pneumonia) to provide adequate tissue for microbial diagnosis and, with disease debulking, to allow the initiation of otherwise potentially fatal chemotherapy. Advantages of VATS include larger sample size, better selection of the biopsy site, and direct visualization of the biopsy site, which allows better control of any bleeding encountered. Radiologic techniques are often used to guide the biopsy procedure directly (under ultrasound or CT guidance) or generally, as in patchy processes affecting the lungs.

In general, biopsies should not be obtained if an epidemiologic history suggests the possibility of echinococcal cystic disease, because of the risk of dissemination and anaphylaxis associated with cyst leakage, or if there is suspicion of a perivascular process with a significant bleeding hazard.

Approach to the Patient: General Concepts

The individual with infection often presents in an ambulatory setting. The evaluation of the patient depends on a series of questions that provide clues to management, including the need for hospitalization and the selection of antimicrobial agents. Subsequently, clinical data provide a basis for adjusting antimicrobial therapy. These questions include the following:

1. Is the process life-threatening?
   - What is the time course of the process? Is it rapidly progressive or gradual?
   - Does the patient need to be admitted to the hospital?
   - Is there time to delay therapy or diagnostic procedures?

2. Does the patient have immune deficits?
   - Could the process be underestimated based on the absence of normal inflammatory responses?
   - Will the patient clear infection without specific therapy?

3. Does the history provide clues to a specific etiology of infection or the severity of the illness?
   - Underlying clinical conditions
   - Epidemiologic history (e.g., travel, contacts, exposures, vaccines, medications, prior infections or hospitalizations): Has the patient traveled or does the patient have any hobbies (e.g., gardening, hiking, cooking) that might provide an epidemiologic clue?
   - Symptoms: rate of progression, other systemic signs

4. What can be learned from the physical examination?
   - Skin lesions (e.g., rash attributed to drug allergy versus disseminated fungal infection), lymph nodes (symmetric or regional), retinal examination, perirectal abscess, chest wall or spinous tenderness, neurologic disease (pulmonary-brain syndromes) are often ignored but may provide valuable clinical clues.

5. What can the basic laboratory data tell us?
   - Many systemic processes are reflected in abnormalities of blood counts, urinalysis, and routine blood chemistries.

6. What are the radiologic findings?
   - No radiographic findings are specific enough to define the microbial origin of a given process. One approach can be illustrated best in the evaluation of pulmonary processes using both the rate of symptomatic progression and the radiologic appearance of the lesion (Table 3-1).
   - Define the radiographic pattern as lobar or segmental consolidation, patchy bronchopneumonia, nodules (large, small, or miliary), or an interstitial process. Many large, round pulmonary densities in a renal transplant recipient suggest *Nocardia* infection rather than *Pneumocystis* pneumonia, whereas in a heroin addict with cough, fever, and pleuritic chest pain, such densities suggest acute right-sided endocarditis rather than pneumococcal pneumonia.
   - Compare with prior radiographs: Is the process old or new? Are there multiple processes? Has the patient had surgery in the intervening period? Is the spleen enlarged or absent?
   - Confounding variables: Is it too early in the process to detect radiologic changes (i.e., first 18-24 hours)? Is the patient neutropenic (early viral or fungal pneumonitis) or otherwise immunocompromised? (*Pneumocystis* pneumonia is often with minimal or no findings on plain chest radiographs.) Dehydration is commonly cited as a cause of false-negative radiographs, but, in general, this concept is probably overrated.
   - CT scanning is sensitive to changes unrecognized in plain radiographs and is useful in guiding invasive procedures.

7. Can a provisional diagnosis be made from examination of clinical specimens?
   - Examination of an appropriately stained smear of sputum or pleural fluid, blood buffy coat, skin lesions, or throat swab often provides a provisional diagnosis.
   - Examination of an appropriately stained smear of sputum can provide a shortcut to diagnosis if the findings are

Table 3-1 Differential Diagnosis of Fever and Pulmonary Infiltrates in Organ Transplant Recipients According to Roentgenographic Abnormality and Rate of Progression of Symptoms

Chest Radiographic Abnormality	Etiology According to the Rate of Progression of the Illness	
	Acute*	**Subacute or Chronic***
Consolidation	Bacterial (including Legionnaire disease), thromboembolic, hemorrhage Unusual causes: pulmonary edema	Mold, *Nocardia*, mycobacteria, viral Unusual causes: drug-induced, irradiation, *Pneumocystis*, tumor
Peribronchovascular process	Pulmonary edema Unusual causes: leukoagglutinin, reaction, bacterial	Viral, *Pneumocystis* Unusual causes: fungal, *Nocardia*, tumor, mycobacteria
Nodular infiltrate	Unusual causes: bacterial, pulmonary edema	Mold, *Nocardia*, tuberculous Unusual causes: *Pneumocystis*

*An acute illness develops and requires medical attention in a matter of relatively few hours. A subacute or chronic process develops over several days to weeks.

reasonably definitive. Special staining methods provide additional data, including Kinyoun and modified acid-fast stains for mycobacteria, *Actinomyces*, or *Nocardia* species. Wright-Giemsa or a variant or direct fluorescent antibody staining of induced sputum samples for *Pneumocystis jiroveci* or *Legionella pneumophila* may provide a diagnosis.

- Culture of sputum or blood or other body fluids may provide a specific etiologic diagnosis if evaluation of a sputum smear has not supplied a provisional diagnosis.
- In some patients, an etiologic diagnosis can be made by alternative means, such as urinary antigen tests for *Legionella* or *Histoplasma* infections or antigenemia, molecular, or serologic assays for viral or other less common processes. Such tests may avoid invasive procedures. Screening tests are highly useful for respiratory viruses (urinary antigen or nasal swab coupled with immunofluorescence). Induced sputum examinations have a high yield for *Pneumocystis* and mycobacteria.

8. How can a diagnosis be achieved most expeditiously? Which invasive procedures are done well at my institution?
   - Invasive diagnostic procedures: In patients who are critically ill or unlikely to tolerate invasive infections (e.g., immunocompromise, recent major surgery, heart failure, chronic obstructive pulmonary disease), it is reasonable to consider more invasive diagnostic procedures early in the clinical course. In such patients, only specific etiologic diagnoses can direct appropriate therapy and limit attendant toxicities. However, this observation illustrates the tension between empiric therapies and the risks inherent to invasive tests. Empiric antimicrobial therapies carry the risk of obscuring a specific microbiologic diagnosis as well as the risk of drug-associated toxicities. Invasive diagnostic procedures are used to obtain uncontaminated secretions from the lower respiratory tract or pulmonary tissue for microbiologic and histologic analysis.
   - The selection of such procedures should be based on the nature of the illness and the likelihood of success for each procedure at the institution. Important considerations include the type and location of the lesion, the ability of the patient to cooperate with the required manip-

ulations, the presence of coagulopathies, and the experience at the particular hospital in performing each of the procedures.
- Data from biopsies should be reviewed by the medical teams caring for each patient to optimize the utilization of each specimen (e.g., microbiologic testing, histologic analysis).

Antimicrobial Therapy

In practice, initial therapy is empiric and is based primarily on available clinical clues. The selection of one or more drugs for empiric therapy depends on the clinical setting and on the gravity of the pulmonary process.

Biopsy in the Immunocompromised Host

By the time a biopsy is considered for an infectious lesion, unless time pressure for a diagnosis is critical, noninvasive diagnostic approaches should have been exhausted. The risks of the procedure are balanced against the toxicities, costs, and availability of appropriate empiric therapies. For example, in the case illustrated in Figure 3-2, a woman underwent lung transplantation after years of immunosuppression for dermatomyositis. Immunosuppression was intensified given poor initial lung function. An incidental nasal swab culture grew *Scedosporium prolificans*, which was treated with prophylactic voriconazole and nebulized amphotericin. After extensive rehabilitation, she returned for evaluation of pain with decreased vision in the left eye. Vitreal tap was unrevealing. Retinal biopsy was performed based on the likelihood that this could be a disseminated mold infection of the eye and despite the potential risk of visual loss given multiple areas of retinal detachment. The retinal biopsy revealed invasive fungal infection, and enucleation was performed (see Fig. 3-2). Fungal cultures revealed *S. prolificans* with resistance to voriconazole and susceptibility to a combination of amphotericin, posaconazole, and terbinafine. Although the patient had preexist-

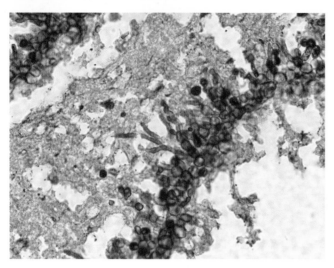

Figure 3-2. Eye enucleation specimen from a patient with disseminated *Scedosporium prolificans* infection. (GMS ×400)

Table 3-2 Factors Affecting the Net State of Immunosuppression

Factor	Examples
Immunosuppressive therapy	Dose, duration, temporal sequence
Underlying immune deficiency	Autoimmune disease, functional immune deficits
Mucocutaneous barrier integrity	Catheters, epithelial surfaces, devitalized tissue, fluid collections
Neutropenia, lymphopenia	
Metabolic conditions	Uremia, malnutrition, diabetes, alcoholism with cirrhosis
Viral coinfection	Cytomegalovirus, Epstein-Barr virus, hepatitis B and C, human immunodeficiency virus

ing renal dysfunction, based on the available data it was considered unlikely that she would survive without therapy that included all potentially effective antimicrobial agents, including liposomal amphotericin B. This decision would not have been possible without the results of the biopsy procedure. Immunosuppression was also reduced. She continues to survive while receiving triple antifungal therapy, despite disseminated infection.

In the normal host, a careful medical history, including epidemiologic exposures and prior procedures, usually indicates the nature of likely pathogens. Unusual infections occur most often in association with anatomic defects, unusual epidemiologic exposures, or unrecognized immune deficits. Immunocompetent individuals mount an inflammatory response that serves to slow disease progression and to indicate, on physical examination or radiology studies, the location of the infectious process.

By contrast, the immunocompromised host has muted signs and symptoms of inflammation, is susceptible to infection by a broad array of pathogens, and is often asymptomatic until infection is quite advanced. Dissemination of infection (e.g., *Nocardia* or *Cryptococcus* species) outside the site of initial infection (the lungs) is common, and morbidity is increased. The key to successful management of the immunocompromised host is the ability to obtain the specimens required for microbiologic diagnosis *before* the initiation of empiric therapies that will obscure subsequent diagnosis.

As for any patient, the risk of infection in an immunocompromised host is determined by the interaction of two factors: the potential pathogens to which the individual is exposed (epidemiologic exposures) and a measure of the individual's susceptibility to infection, termed the "net state of immunosuppression" (Table 3-2). Epidemiologic exposures of importance in the immunocompromised patient can be divided into two general categories: those occurring within the community and those occurring within the hospital. Exposures within the community vary based on such factors as geography and socioeconomic status. Community-acquired opportunistic pathogens include the geographically restricted systemic mycoses (blastomycosis,

coccidioidomycosis, and histoplasmosis), *Mycobacterium tuberculosis*, *Strongyloides stercoralis*, *Leishmania donovani*, *Trypanosoma cruzi*, *Pneumocystis jiroveci*, *Legionella* species, and community-acquired respiratory viral infections (e.g., influenza, respiratory syncytial virus, metapneumovirus, parainfluenza). Common viral agents include herpes simplex virus, cytomegalovirus, varicella-zoster virus, and hepatitis B and C viruses. Within the hospital, excessive environmental exposures can occur on the hospital unit where the patient is housed or from contaminated operating rooms, radiology suites, or catheterization laboratories during procedures. If the air, food, equipment, or potable water supply is contaminated with pathogens such as *Aspergillus* species, *Legionella* species, or vancomycin-resistant enterococci, clustering of cases of infection will be observed.

Specific immune deficits tend to predispose to specific types of infection (Table 3-3). The net state of immunosuppression (see Table 3-2) is a concept that describes all of the host factors that contribute to infectious risk. The additive factors include the dose, duration, and temporal sequence in which immunosuppressive drugs are deployed; injuries to the primary mucocutaneous barrier to infection (e.g., indwelling catheters, gastrointestinal or bronchial anastomoses in organ transplant recipients); neutropenia or lymphopenia; underlying immune deficiency; pulmonary aspiration injury; metabolic problems including protein-calorie malnutrition, uremia, and, perhaps, hyperglycemia; the presence of devitalized tissues and fluid collections (e.g., hematoma, effusions, ascites); and infection with immunomodulating viruses (cytomegalovirus, Epstein-Barr virus, hepatitis B and hepatitis C viruses, and the human immunodeficiency viruses), which predispose to other opportunistic infections as well as to graft rejection or graft-vs-host disease. Generally, more than one factor is present in each host; the identification of the relevant factors, and their correction when possible, is central to the prevention and treatment of infection in these hosts. The spectrum of susceptibility to infection is a continuum ranging from individual deficits (e.g., a viral upper respiratory infection that paves the way for bacterial superinfection) to multiple simultaneous deficits (e.g., in the organ transplant recipient).

Table 3-3 Infections Associated with Specific Immune Defects

Defect	Common Causes	Associated Infections
Granulocytopenia	Leukemia, cytotoxic chemotherapy, AIDS, drug toxicity, Felty syndrome	Enteric GNR, *Pseudomonas, Staphylococcus aureus, Staphylococcus epidermidis*, streptococci, *Aspergillus, Candida,* and other fungi
Neutrophil chemotaxis	Diabetes, alcoholism, uremia, Hodgkin disease, trauma (burns), lazy leukocyte syndrome, CT disease	*S. aureus, Candida*, streptococci
Neutrophil killing	CGD, myeloperoxidase deficiency	*S. aureus, Escherichia coli, Candida, Aspergillus, Torulopsis*
T-cell defects	AIDS, congenital, lymphoma, sarcoidosis, viral infection, organ transplants, steroids	Intracellular bacteria (*Legionella, Listeria,* mycobacteria), HSV, VZV, CMV, EBV, parasites (*Strongyloides, Toxoplasma*), fungi (*Pneumocystis jiroveci, Candida, Cryptococcus*)
B-cell defects	Congenital or acquired agammaglobulinemia, burns, enteropathies, splenic dysfunction, myeloma, ALL	*Streptococcus pneumoniae, Haemophilus influenzae, Salmonella* and *Campylobacter* spp., *Giardia lamblia*
Splenectomy	Surgery, sickle cell disease, cirrhosis	*S. pneumoniae, H. influenzae, Salmonella* spp., *Capnocytophaga*
Complement	Congenital or acquired defects	*S. aureus, Neisseria* spp., *H. influenzae, S. pneumoniae*
Anatomic	Intravenous or Foley catheters, incisions, anastomotic leaks, mucosal ulceration, vascular insufficiency	Colonizing organisms, resistant nosocomial organisms

AIDS, acquired immunodeficiency syndrome; ALL, acute lymphocytic leukemia; CGD, chronic granulomatous disease; CMV, cytomegalovirus; CT, chemotherapy-induced; EBV, Epstein-Barr virus; GNR, gram-negative rods; HSV, herpes simplex virus; VZV, varicella-zoster virus.

Timeline of Infection

In the broad spectrum of immunocompromised hosts, the risk of infection over time can follow several patterns:

- It may be relatively stable over time, as in the diabetic patient with vasculopathy and neuropathy who is prone to skin and soft tissue infections.
- It may be time limited, as in the postsurgical patient without complications or in the autologous bone marrow transplantation recipient with effective engraftment.
- It may be cumulative and progressive, as in the AIDS patient, in whom infection is a function of declining immunity (without therapy), falling CD4-positive T-lymphocyte counts, rising viral loads, and the effects of other persistent infections (e.g., cytomegalovirus). In these individuals, the occurrence of new infections suggests the progression of immune compromise.
- It may be progressive but not cumulative, as in the recipient of an allogeneic stem cell or solid organ transplant. In such patients, the risk changes predictably with time as a function of the evolving condition of the patient: in the early phase, infection is often the result of nosocomial exposures during neutropenia, whereas later, during treatment for acute and chronic graft-versus-host disease, susceptibility to infection is a function of immune suppression and mucosal injuries (possibly from chemotherapy, radiation, or infections such as *Clostridium difficile* colitis).

With standardized immunosuppressive and chemotherapeutic regimens, specific types of infection often occur in a predict-able pattern (timeline) as a reflection of the specific risk factors (e.g., surgery, immune suppression, acute and chronic rejection, reemergence of underlying diseases, viral infections) present at each phase of the post-transplantation course[3] (Fig. 3-3). The patterns have been altered by the availability of a broader range of immunosuppressive and chemotherapeutic agents, the use of stem cells instead of marrow for transplantation, and antimicrobial prophylaxis. However, the general concepts remain the same, and the major determinants of infection are still the exogenous immune suppression or chemotherapy administered, as well as any additional immunosuppressive therapy used to treat graft rejection or graft-versus-host disease. Superimposed viral infection enhances the risk of infection at any point along the timeline.

Because each risk factor renders the patient susceptible to infection by new groups of pathogens, infections that seem to be occurring with the "wrong" pathogen or at the "wrong" time suggest an undiscovered immune deficit (e.g., fluid collection, neutropenia) or an unusual epidemiologic exposure. The occurrence of specific infections can be prevented by the use of antimicrobial prophylaxis, vaccines, and behavioral modifications (e.g., no raw vegetables or digging in gardens without masks). This will result in a shift to the right of the timeline: infections typically observed later in the course of disease or therapy will still be observed at the appropriate time, despite the absence of infections that tend to occur earlier but have been prevented by a variety of preventive measures.

Summary

Invasive diagnostic procedures have been coupled with advanced detection techniques such as immunostaining and molecular

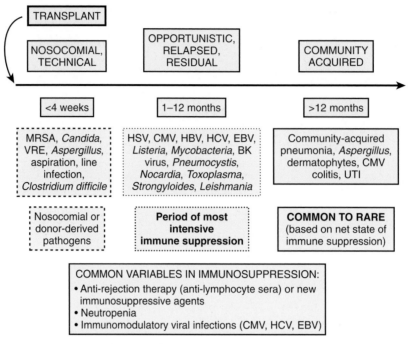

Figure 3-3. The timeline of common infections after solid organ transplantation. CMV, cytomegalovirus; HBV, hepatitis B virus; HCV, hepatitis C virus; EBV, Epstein-Barr virus; HSV, herpes simplex virus; MRSA, methicillin-resistant *Staphylococcus aureus*; UTI, urinary tract infection; VRE, vancomycin-resistant enterococcus.

diagnostics to enhance the specificity of clinical diagnoses. The early and appropriate deployment of invasive procedures often can reduce the exposure of patients to unnecessary antimicrobial agents and associated toxicities. The clinician must be familiar with the available techniques at each institution and work closely with pathologists to exchange clinical information and optimize patient care.

REFERENCES

1. Bravo AA, Sheth SG, Chopra S: Liver biopsy. N Engl J Med 2001;344:495-500.
2. McAfee JH, Keeffe EB, Lee RG, Rosch J: Transjugular liver biopsy. Hepatology 1992;15:726-732.
3. Fishman JA: Infections in solid organ transplantation. N Engl J Med 2007;357:2601-2614.

Cytopathology of Infectious and Inflammatory Diseases

Vicki J. Schnadig

Introduction

Despite its potential benefits to patients, infectious disease cytology is often relegated to the pathology education back burner. This is unfortunate, because accurate diagnosis of infectious and inflammatory diseases (IID) by cytology can be lifesaving and involves noninvasive or minimally invasive procedures. On-site, rapid evaluation of percutaneous fine-needle aspirations (FNA), bronchoscopic brushings, or transbronchial needle aspiration (TBNA) is a decidedly useful procedure that, in the hands of an experienced cytologist, can establish a preliminary diagnosis of IID and exclude neoplasia, guide the procurement of appropriate microbial cultures, and allow for instigation of empiric therapy if needed.

Infectious diseases not infrequently manifest with signs that mimic those of neoplasia, and an experienced cytologist should be as knowledgeable about the clinical and morphologic features of infectious diseases as he or she is familiar with the morphologic patterns of neoplasia. In Figure 4-1, for example, the following gloomy prognostication was rendered on the basis of computed tomography (CT): "Large malignant neoplasm destroys the first rib and sternum and extends and invades the mediastinum and the pectoralis muscles." However, an FNA of the pectoralis mass (Fig. 4-2) led to a presumptive diagnosis of caseating granuloma on the basis of on-site evaluation. An aliquot of aspirated material was then submitted to the microbiology laboratory for bacterial, mycobacterial, and fungal cultures, which identified *Mycobacterium tuberculosis*. Follow-up CT, after appropriate therapy, showed significant improvement with marked decrease in the size of the mass.

In order to accurately diagnose infectious diseases by cytology, one must do the following:

1. First and foremost, think about the possibility of infection
2. Have adequate knowledge of the patient's clinical presentation, immune status, and results of any imaging studies performed
3. Be able to recognize inflammatory patterns by cytology and know what types of infection to suspect based on the type of inflammatory cell reaction combined with the clinical and radiologic findings
4. Be able to appropriately culture and request indicated special stains

Some infections, such as *Strongyloides stercoralis* hyperinfection, are medical emergencies that necessitate immediate action. Others, such as tuberculosis, are communicable diseases that, when suspected, require notification of infection control personnel and the primary caregivers, as well as appropriate cultures or molecular studies to establish or rule out infection by *M. tuberculosis*. FNA and touch or scrape preparations are highly useful, albeit underutilized, stratagems for diagnosing infectious diseases in the autopsy suite.[1-3] Their use obviates the necessity for, and potential contamination of, the cryostat[4,5] and helps to confirm or exclude communicable disease in the preliminary autopsy diagnosis.

We have diagnosed infections and unusual non-neoplastic conditions from all types of samples submitted to the cytopathology laboratory, including sputum, bronchial brushings and washings, body cavity and cerebrospinal fluids, bronchoalveolar lavage (BAL) samples, TBNA, gastrointestinal endoscopic ultrasound, and percutaneous FNA. Most infections can be presumptively diagnosed, or at least suspected, by using a combination of the two workhorse cytology colorants, the Papanicolaou and Romanovski stains. These two stains make an excellent team for diagnosis of IID as well as neoplasia. The advantage of these two dye combinations over the so-called special stains is that they allow one to assess the type of tissue reaction found in the sample

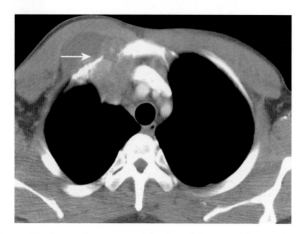

Figure 4-1. Computed tomogram of the chest. A large, partially necrotic mass (*arrow*) involves the right lung, mediastinum, and thoracic soft tissue with destruction of the rib.

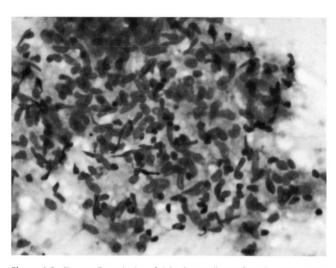

Figure 4-2. Fine-needle aspiration of right chest wall mass from the same patient as in Figure 4-1. An aggregate of epithelioid macrophages admixed with lymphocytes is seen (Romanovski, ×400).

as well as recognize the presence of infectious organisms. The tissue reaction is of great importance and is discussed later in this chapter.

Detailed discussions of the stains used for diagnosis of IID are given in other references.[6-9] Briefly stated, the Papanicolaou stain is similar to the workhorse of histopathology, the hematoxylin and eosin (H&E) stain, with the following exceptions. It is performed on preparations that are wet-fixed in alcohol, most commonly 95% ethanol. This technique coarsens and sharpens nuclear chromatin and produces a translucency to the stained preparation that allows one to examine relatively thick cell preparations at various levels of focus. As with the H&E preparation, the nuclear stain is hematoxylin that has been alkalinized to give a bluish color to the cell nuclei. In contrast to H&E, there are three cytoplasmic stains: eosin, light green or a lead-free equivalent, and Orange G. Moreover, the Papanicolaou stain often colors mucin a purple to red color, which is useful for recognition of *Cryptococcus* and allergic mucin (see later discussion).

The Romanovski stains comprise a number of eosin-thiazide metachromatic stains, including Wright, Giemsa, May-Grünwald, and the rapid variants commercially available as Diff Quik, Quik Dip, and so on. Romanovski stains are usually performed on air-dried slide preparations that are post-fixed in methanol. Because of the air drying, the nuclear and cytoplasmic texture is not as crisp; however, because cells are more thinly spread out over the slide and have more surface area in contact with the slide, there is less cell loss. The Romanovski stain supplements the Papanicolaou by highlighting features that are not well seen with the former. Cell chromatin pattern and cytoplasmic texture are best seen in the Papanicolaou stain, making it advantageous for cancer diagnosis. Certain fungi, nematode larvae, and ova are best seen with the Papanicolaou stain as well. Romanovski is ideal for characterization of leukocytes, and it is an excellent stain for bacteria and certain other fungi, such as *Histoplasma* and *Pneumocystis* (see later discussion). Mucin, colloid, and cytoplasmic granules are best distinguished with this stain.

A small number of ancillary special stains are useful for the diagnosis of infectious agents. In the University of Texas Medical Branch Cytology Laboratory, most of these are performed in the cytopathology rather than the histopathology laboratory. With the exception of the Gomori/Grocott methenamine silver (GMS) stain, the methods used in cytopathology are designed for smear and cytocentrifuge preparations rather than paraffin-embedded sections.

For suspected bacterial infections, Gram staining is performed on air-dried, heat-fixed, very thinly prepared smears or on cytocentrifuge preparations using techniques adapted to the microbiology laboratory.[10] Air drying is preferred for the standard Gram stain, because structures appear larger and are more readily seen. Also, the Gram stain is water-based and is not designed for wet fixation in ethanol.

For suspected *Nocardia* or *Actinomyces* infections, we use a modified Gram technique, the Gram-Weigert stain.[11,12] This was designed as a tissue fibrin stain and is rarely used today, but it is an excellent stain for gram-positive bacteria, especially actinomycetes. The latter are often very faintly colored by the standard Gram stain. In addition, even senescent gram-positive bacteria retain their blue color. As an added bonus, *Pneumocystis* cyst forms, *Candida*, and *Histoplasma capsulatum* blastoconidia are well stained by the Gram-Weigert technique, which substitutes a mixture of aniline and xylene for acetone alcohol as a decolorant. We do use ethanol-fixed slides for this stain. The obvious disadvantage of the Gram-Weigert stain is the necessity to decolorize under a chemical hazard hood. Also, it is not good for the identification of gram-negative bacteria.

For suspected mycobacterial infections, we use a cold Kinyoun stain[12] rather than the standard Ziehl-Neelsen acid-fast stain. The Kinyoun stain does not require heat, uses a stronger carbol-fuscin solution, and colors *M. tuberculosis* in addition to mycobacteria other than tuberculosis (MOTT). It is easily modified for *Nocardia* by shortening of the decolorization time and substitution of a 1% sulfuric or 1% hydrochloric acid solution for acid alcohol.

Fluorochrome stains[10] are typically used in microbiology laboratories and are ideal for large-volume, low-power screening for mycobacteria. Auramine orange has been used to assess FNA for some mycobacteria.[13] A disadvantage of fluorochrome dyes is that they require a fluorescent microscope. In addition, some

MOTT, especially *Mycobacterium fortuitum,* may not be seen with fluorochrome stains.

Nonspecific fluorescent stains, such as Calcofluor white,[10,14-16] have been employed for wet preparation and cytologic identification of *Pneumocystis* and other fungi. Specific immunofluorescent techniques have also been used with varying amounts of enthusiasm.[15-17]

The classic stain for fungi including *Pneumocystis,* the GMS, is much beloved and demanded (by clinicians) and loathed (by histotechnologists).[18] Microwave histotechnology has greatly simplified this rather cumbersome procedure.[19] Automated staining machines are also available for special histologic stains; however, automation may limit one's ability to modify staining techniques to accommodate different types of specimens. We have satisfactorily utilized the manual microwave modification of the GMS technique, with the caveat that a good-quality GMS is a joy to interpret, whereas a poorly performed GMS is nearly useless. In reality, GMS is not always the best choice among the cytologic fungal stains, as discussed in later sections of this chapter. There is no substitute for an experienced technician who understands the characteristics of a good-quality GMS:

1. The methenamine working solution must be made fresh.
2. The chromic acid solution must not be allowed to boil. Our preparation technician has chosen to preheat the chromic acid in the microwave before placing the test slides and control into the solution, thereby avoiding boiling of the chromic acid.

3. Darker is not better. The slides should be removed from the methenamine silver solution and checked under a microscope as soon as the solution begins to turn gray.

An overstained and a correctly stained GMS are illustrated in Figure 4-3. Our protocols for GMS and processing of both BAL samples and induced sputa are provided in the appendix of this chapter.

We use commercial or homemade smear preparations as controls for all of our special stains with the exception of the GMS, for which we use paraffin-embedded section of lung with *Pneumocystis.* The latter is used mainly out of convenience and does not seem to be problematic. Either spit or a buccal scrape makes an excellent control for the Gram or Gram-Weigert stain. Commercial smear preparations containing both acid-fast and non–acid-fast bacteria are used for our Kinyoun and modified Kinyoun stain controls. A blood smear is a good control for the Giemsa (Romanovski) stain.

There are a few histology stains that we occasionally employ for diagnosis. These include:

1. Mayer's mucicarmine, a mucin stain that is useful for confirmation of encapsulated forms of *Cryptococcus*[1,20]
2. Fontana-Masson melanin stain for paucicapsular *Cryptococcus*[21,22] and dematiaceous fungi (pigmented fungi associated with chromoblastomycosis, phaeohyphomycosis, and allergic fungal sinusitis)

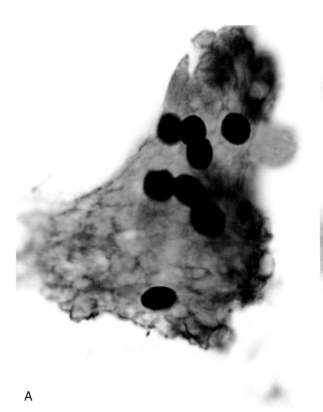

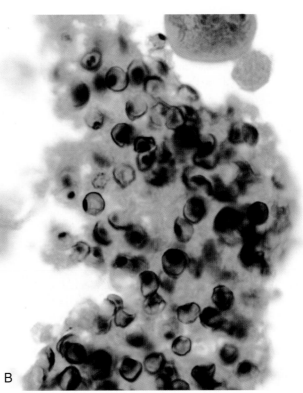

A   B

Figure 4-3. Bronchoalveolar lavage samples with *Pneumocystis.* **A,** Sample is overstained. The cysts appear dense and homogeneously black. **B,** Properly stained sample demonstrates the presence of a small, dot-like thickening in the cyst wall (GMS, ×1000).

3. Periodic acid–Schiff (PAS) with diastase, a nonspecific muco-polysaccharide stain that can be useful in the diagnosis of pulmonary alveolar proteinosis and malakoplakia. As there may be loss of material from the slide during diastase digestion, we prefer to submit material for PAS-diastase staining on charged slides.

Immunohistochemistry techniques for *Pneumocystis* are also available and are as used briefly below.

Processing of Cytologic Samples for Infectious and Inflammatory Diseases

Samples of brushings, washings, lavage fluids, and fine needle aspirates (FNA) are prepared in the same way as for routine cancer diagnosis. For brushing slides, a portion of the slide material can be retained unstained for special staining; however, acid-fast, GMS, and Gram-Weigert stains can be performed over the Papanicolaou after rehydration of the slides back to distilled water. It is not necessary to decolorize the nuclear stain. Restaining is the more effective method if there are only a limited number of slides, because the quality of material present on different slide preparations may vary. We prefer to perform special stains on slide preparations already shown to have inflammatory material suspicious for infection. Cytocentrifuge preparations performed on FNA needle rinses or on centrifuged body fluids are also excellent for staining. The former requires that there be adequate inflammatory material in the rinse fluid. If the cytocentrifuge preparations are paucicellular, restaining of smear preparations is preferable. Cytocentrifuge preparations have the advantage of yielding thin, evenly distributed cellular material. A very thin slide preparation is essential for a good-quality Gram stain.

Induced sputum samples from immunocompromised patients are sometimes submitted to the cytopathology laboratory to be evaluated for *Pneumocystis jiroveci*. We process sputa by first adding a mucolytic agent, 10% dithioreitol, centrifuging the sample, and then preparing four cytocentrifuge preparations: two Papanicolaou, one Romanovski (Giemsa), and one GMS stained. For routine laboratory work, we use a Giemsa stain with a 7.0 pH buffer. For rapid on-site evaluation or when immediate evaluation of sample is needed, a rapid Romanovski technique is employed. Cytocentrifuge preparations of concentrated sputa, fluids, and BAL samples provide well-concentrated, thin, circular sample preparations that can be evaluated for inflammation, fungi (including *Pneumocystis*), and other microorganisms. Figure 4-4 illustrates a cytocentrifuged, Giemsa-stained sputum sample from an AIDS patient that contained both *Strongyloides* larvae and scanty *Pneumocystis*. Note that the intracystic bodies, not the cyst, are stained by the Romanovski method. Our protocol for processing sputa for IID is given in more detail in the appendix to this chapter.

Culturing of Fine-Needle Aspirations for Microorganisms

In general, only FNA material is submitted to the microbiology laboratory by the cytopathologist, so the discussion here is

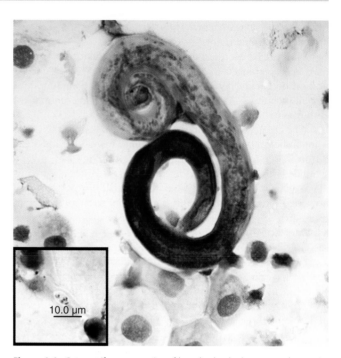

Figure 4-4. Cytocentrifuge preparation of bronchoalveolar lavage sample containing a nematode larva compatible with *Strongyloides stercoralis* (Romanovski stain, ×400). A nonstaining cyst containing tiny intracystic bodies typical of *Pneumocystis* is seen in the inset (Romanovski, ×1000).

limited to methods for submitting FNA samples for microbial cultures.

When FNA yields several milliliters of white-yellow creamy or granular material, one suspects purulent inflammation, caseous necrosis, or coagulative necrosis. Purulent inflammation consists of a mixture of neutrophils, macrophages, and necrotic debris. Caseous necrosis often has a more crumbly dry or granular appearance, and coagulative necrosis, often associated with keratinizing squamous cell carcinoma (SCC) or high-grade lymphoma, may yield material that is grossly indistinguishable from purulent inflammation. Rapid on-site evaluation can help exclude cancer-associated coagulative necrosis and eliminate the need for cultures. Figure 4-5 illustrates the difference between necrosis from a bacterial abscess (*Salmonella enteritidis* was cultured) and coagulative necrosis and apoptosis from a necrotizing large B-cell lymphoma. Compare the neutrophil-rich inflammation with presence of bacilli in Figure 4-5A and B with the presence of cell outlines of coagulative necrosis and apoptotic bodies in Figure 4-5C and D. The former was sent for cultures, and the latter was shown to be predominantly B lymphocytes by immunochemistry and confirmed as large B-cell lymphoma by biopsy. If in doubt, it is best to err on the side of caution and submit an aliquot of FNA from suspected infections for aerobic and anaerobic bacterial, fungal, and mycobacterial cultures. If limited material is procured, one should use rapid on-site evaluation to guide the sample processing. The cytologist should collaborate with the microbiology laboratory personnel. Culture techniques and methods should be discussed and should be mutually acceptable to professionals working in both areas.

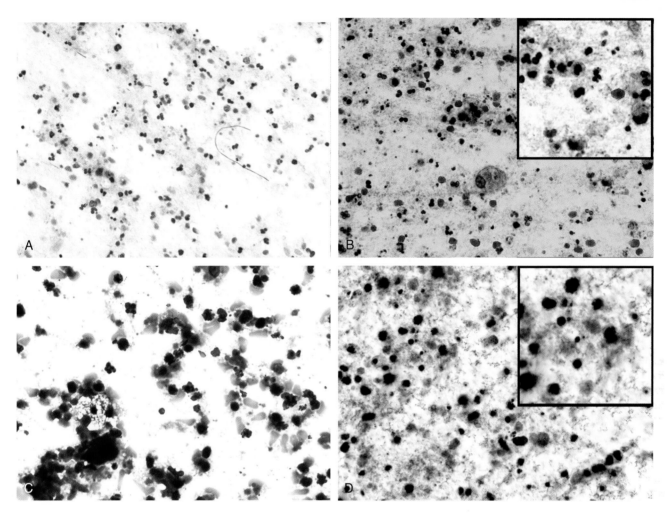

Figure 4-5. Fine needle aspirations of a gram-negative bacterial abscess (**A** and **B**) and a large cell lymphoma (**C** and **D**). **A,** Neutrophil-rich exudate contains some bacilli (×400). **B,** Neutrophils and macrophages are seen (Papanicolaou, ×400, inset ×1000). **C,** Smudgy cells, larger than the neutrophils seen in **A,** represent coagulative necrosis (Romanovski, ×400). **D,** Coagulative necrosis, apoptosis, and degenerated blood (×400, inset ×1000).

The cytopathologists and radiologists who submit material for culture must discipline themselves to provide adequate clinical information to aid the microbiologist. The exact site from whence the specimen came, the types of culture requested, and the pertinent history should be provided on the request form. It is important to notify the laboratory of any specific organisms suspected, because processing of the sample may vary if unusual organisms are suspected. For example, if one sees evidence of *Actinomyces* infection, the laboratory will incubate the anaerobic culture broth longer than usual before reporting the culture as negative. If organisms whose culture forms are potentially hazardous to microbiology personnel, such as *Coccidioides immitis,* are seen, it is considerate and professional to inform the laboratory.

Culture of FNA for bacteria requires either the proper type of transport medium or immediate inoculation of culture broth on-site. If one chooses to use transport medium, various tactics must be employed to submit samples for aerobic and anaerobic cultures. We prefer, whenever possible, to perform or request that the radiologist perform a dedicated pass for microbial cultures. If 5 mL or more of purulent-appearing material is aspi-

rated, several drops of sample should be expelled into a vial of anaerobic transport medium. There are several commercially available types of anaerobic transport kits,[10] and it is best to obtain and use the type that is used by the microbiology laboratory. The remaining material can be expelled from the syringe into a sterile specimen cup and submitted to the laboratory for aerobic, fungal, and mycobacterial cultures. Swab transport kits are also available for submission of material for aerobic culture; however, swabs should not be used to send samples for either mycobacterial or fungal cultures.

If scanty material is aspirated, one can rinse the needle in approximately 5 mL of sterile saline and process as described. For pathologist-performed FNA, however, we do not use swabs or anaerobic transport media for bacterial cultures; we prefer to use a pair of aerobic and anaerobic blood culture bottles for bacterial cultures. Our microbiology laboratory employs the automated Bactec system (BD Diagnostic Systems, Franklin Lakes, NJ). About 0.5 to 1 mL of aspirated pus or needle rinse material is injected into each of the two (aerobic and anaerobic) Bactec bottles using the sterile aspirating needle and syringe. This is an efficient method for immediately placing the sample into nutrient culture media with aerobic and anaerobic environments. Because the cytopathologist will perform a Gram stain on a directly made smear or cytospin of the FNA, it is not important to have this repeated by the microbiology laboratory. We have found the blood culture bottle method to be easy and effective and have successfully cultured *Staphylococcus*, *Streptococcus*, gram-negative bacilli, and anaerobes, including *Actinomyces* spp. from blood culture–bottled FNA samples. Our high correlation of directly observed bacteria with culture results and our success with culture of anaerobic organisms leads us to believe that the blood culture bottle method is effective. (Correlation of culture and cytology results should be just as much a part of cytology quality assurance as histology-cytology correlation.) Two studies that examined the efficiency of the Bactec system for direct culture of body fluids found that it performed as well or better than the conventional methods.[23,24] After an aliquot of material is placed in the blood culture bottles, the remainder of the dedicated IID pass should be submitted in a sterile specimen cup for mycobacterial and fungal cultures.

Recognizing the different types of inflammatory and tissue reaction patterns by cytology and being able to construct a differential diagnosis based on those patterns is essential to cytodiagnosis of IID. An important concept to grasp in understanding the histopathology and cytopathology of infection is that the type of tissue response observed is highly dependent on the host's immune status and the manner in which the microorganism interacts with the host. As knowledge of immunology increases, so does awareness of the complexity and variability of the host reaction to infection. The variety of clinical disorders caused by, and types of host response to, *Aspergillus* spp. alone would be sufficient to fill an entire volume. In an admittedly simplified manner, inflammatory patterns and their differential diagnoses are discussed in the following sections. Formation of a differential diagnosis involves not only recognition of the inflammatory pattern but knowledge of the host's immune status and the clinical and radiologic findings. A summary of inflammatory patterns, organisms, and preferred stains is given in Table 4-1.

Inflammatory Patterns and Associated Pathogens

Purulent Inflammatory Response

If a predominance of neutrophils, macrophages, and fibrin is seen in a sample, one should include the following in the differential diagnosis: pyogenic bacteria (commonly *Staphylococcus aureus*, *Streptococcus* spp., gram-negative bacilli); actinomycetes (*Actinomyces* and *Nocardia* spp.); and some fungi (*Candida*, *Aspergillus*, and zygomycetes). The clinical history and findings narrow the range of suspects, as does the cytopathologist's evaluation of the Papanicolaou- and Romanovski-stained slides. The following two case studies illustrate commonly encountered diagnostic issues.

Case 1: Elicitors of the Not So Laudable Pus

A 59-year-old man presented with sudden onset of a painful swelling in the neck. A tender, soft, fluctuant, and slightly erythematous, 5 × 4 cm mass was palpated in the level II region of the left neck. Two smaller, soft and tender nodules were noted along the cervical lymph node chain. Teeth were in good condition, and no recent dental procedures were reported. The patient was a prison inmate and a smoker, and the clinicians were concerned about tuberculous lymphadenitis and SCC. An FNA was done and yielded approximately 3 mL of creamy, white-gray material. The Romanovski- and Papanicolaou-stained slides are shown in Figure 4-6. Because the mass was aspirated by the cytopathologists, the patient was both interviewed and examined by the team that was to process and interpret the FNA results. Having the opportunity to talk with and examine the patient is optimal for high-quality FNA interpretation. The clinical findings of relatively rapid onset, erythema, and tenderness were suggestive of infection rather than inflammation, and a pyogenic bacterial infection was favored. The rapid Romanovski-stained slide (see Fig. 4-6A) confirmed the presence of a purulent

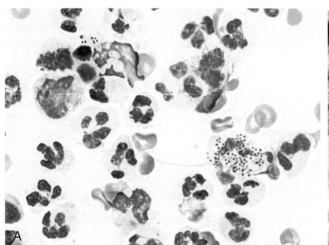
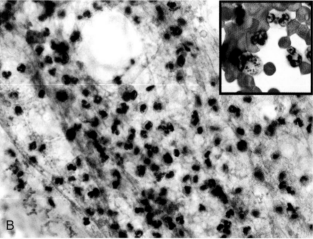

Figure 4-6. Fine-needle aspiration of neck mass. **A,** Exudate composed predominantly of neutrophils with a single macrophage containing blue-colored cocci that are readily distinguished from the more purple-colored cell nuclei (Romanovski, ×1000). **B,** Fibrinopurulent exudate (Papanicolaou, ×400) with neutrophil containing small, dark cocci, also shown in the inset (Papanicolaou, ×1000).

Table 4-1 Summary of Inflammatory Patterns, Likely Organisms, and Stains of Value in Diagnosis

Inflammation	Organisms	Ideal Stains for Microorganism in Cytology	Other Useful Special Stains	Comments
Purulent	1. Pyogenic 2. Actinomycetes 3. *Aspergillus*/Zygomycetes	1. Romanovski or Gram 2. Gram-Weigert/Gram 3. Pap	1. None 2. Modified Kinyoun 3. GMS (*Aspergillus*)	2. Modified Kinyoun is useful for distinguishing between *Nocardia* sp. or *Mycobacterium fortuitum* and *Actinomyces* sp.
Allergic mucin	1. *Aspergillus*/dematiaceous fungi	1. Romanovski or Pap	1. GMS 2. Fontana-Masson (melanin)	
Granuloma	1. Mycobacteria 2. *Histoplasma* 3. *Cryptococcus*	1. Kinyoun or Ziehl-Neelsen 2. GMS 3. GMS	1. Modified Kinyoun	2 & 3. In well-formed granulomas, *Histoplasma* and *Cryptococcus* tend to be scant in number and nonviable (*Histoplasma*) or paucicapsulated (*Cryptococcus*); GMS is the preferred stain in this situation.
Mixed granuloma/purulent	1. *Blastomyces* 2. *Coccidioides* 3. *Paracoccidioides* 4. Chromoblastomycosis and phaeohyphomycosis agents 5. Sporotrichosis	1. Pap 2. Pap 3. Pap 4. Pap 5. GMS	4. Fontana-Masson (melanin)	5. *Sporothrix* is usually very scant in cytologic and histologic samples and poorly stained by Papanicolaou stain unless a Splendore-Hoeppli phenomenon is seen; in GMS, the yeast forms have elongated, cigar-shaped blastoconidia.
Diffuse macrophage	1. Mycobacteria, especially MAC 2. *Histoplasma* 3. *Leishmania*	1. Romanovski and Kinyoun/Ziehl-Neelsen 2. Romanovski 3. Romanovski	2. GMS	1. MAC and other mycobacteria often have a negative stain/refractile red appearance with Romanovski stain.
Scant to none	1. *Pneumocystis* 2. *Cryptococcus* 3. *Aspergillus*/Zygomycetes (neutropenic patients) 4. *Candida* (neutropenic patients)	1. Romanovski/GMS 2. Romanovski 3. Pap 4. Romanovski	2. Mucin 3. GMS (*Aspergillus*) 4. Gram	1. *Pneumocystis* can usually be presumptively diagnosed on Pap-stained slides.

GMS, Gomori/Grocott methenamine silver stain; MAC, *Mycobacterium avium* complex; Pap, Papanicolaou stain.

exudate composed largely of neutrophils and macrophages. Dark blue cocci, both intracellular and extracellular, were seen. Because of these findings, an aliquot of the exudate was submitted for bacterial cultures.

Even if infection with *Staphylococcus* or, possibly, other aerobic pyogenic cocci is suspected, abscesses should always be cultured for both aerobic and anaerobic bacteria. Also, if there is adequate material, we habitually submit material (as described earlier) for fungi and acid-fast bacilli determinations. Although it might be argued that this is not cost-effective, we believe that it is better, especially if the FNA was obtained under image guidance, to err on the side of a relatively inexpensive overkill. Neutrophils may predominate in some fungal infections as well as mycobacterial infections in an immunocompromised host (as discussed later). Culture of the FNA from this patient grew methicillin-resistant *S. aureus* (MRSA). Culture with request for

sensitivity testing of bacterial infections is essential, because often the antibiotic sensitivity spectrum cannot be predicted on the basis of either morphology or speciation of the isolate. Fibrino-purulent exudate is also seen in the Papanicolaou-stained slide (see Fig. 4-6B). Bacteria can often be seen as red- or gray-colored structures in Papanicolaou-stained slides (see Fig. 4-6B, inset); however, the contrast between the organisms and the background is not as great as with Romanovski-stained preparations. By Gram stain—and again we prefer the classic method as utilized by microbiology laboratories over the tissue Gram stains—one can discriminate between gram-positive and gram-negative bacteria, as demonstrated in Figure 4-7.

The differential diagnosis of FNA yielding turbid fluid containing neutrophils includes noninfectious conditions, and the cytopathologist must be aware of these. Two common mimics of infectious lymphadenitis are developmental cysts of the neck

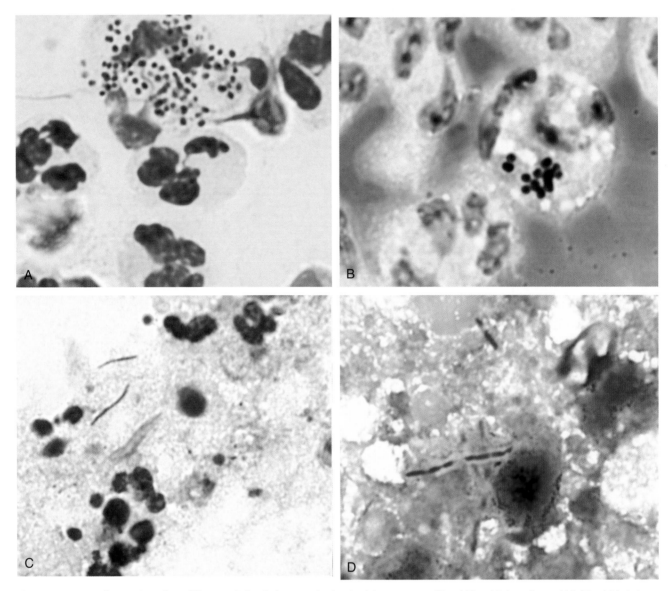

Figure 4-7. Fine-needle aspirations of two different cervical neck abscesses, showing *Staphylococcus aureus* (**A** and **B**) and *Salmonella enteritidis* (**C** and **D**). **A,** Large blue cocci within macrophage (Romanovski stain). **B,** Cocci are gram-positive (Gram stain). **C,** Blue-colored bacilli admixed with degenerating inflammatory cells (Romanovski stain). **D,** Gram-negative bacilli are seen (Gram stain). All magnifications are ×3000.

and cystic degeneration within metastatic SCC. Figure 4-8 illustrates these conditions, from two patients with level II neck masses. In Figure 4-8A, rapid Romanovski-stained FNA, there is inflammation composed of both neutrophils and giant cell macrophages. Focally (*inset*), atypical cells are seen. This process may be misinterpreted as an abscess. In Papanicolaou-stained slides, malignant keratinizing cells were seen, and metastatic SCC was diagnosed. Figure 4-8B shows Papanicolaou-stained FNA from the second neck mass. Neutrophilic inflammation and benign-appearing squamous cells are seen, and the case was interpreted as consistent with an inflamed branchial cleft cyst, which was later confirmed by histology. Although, in our experience, bacterial cultures are typically negative, neutrophils may be abundant in developmental cyst fluid, particularly with branchial cleft cysts. Metastatic SCC, especially from primaries in the tonsil or other parts of Waldeyer's ring, is often cystic in nature,[25]

and neutrophils may be seen in necrotic SCC from any site. A clue to the correct diagnosis is an abundance of coagulative necrosis that should stimulate a search for neoplastic cells. A prominent granulomatous inflammatory reaction, especially in keratinizing SCC, may also be seen, as demonstrated by the giant cell reaction in Figure 4-8A.

Case 2: A More Indolent Fibrinopurulent Infection That Goes Bump in the Neck

A 25-year-old man with no significant past medical history came to the otolaryngology clinic complaining of a swelling in the right jaw. He had undergone extraction of his right third mandibular molar 7 months previously and had noticed progressive swelling in that region thereafter. The patient was a nonsmoker and had recently tested HIV seronegative. A prior CT of the

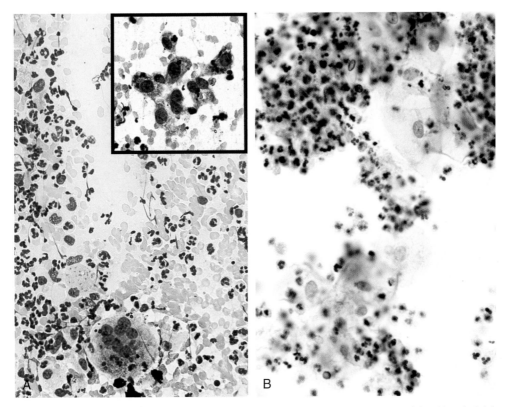

Figure 4-8. Fine-needle aspirations of two different neck masses: metastatic squamous cell carcinoma (**A**) and branchial cleft cyst (**B**). **A,** Purulent exudate is admixed with presence of a giant cell; a cluster of atypical, poorly preserved cells is seen in the inset (both Romanovski, ×400). **B,** Neutrophil-rich inflammatory exudate with presence of benign-appearing squamous cells (Papanicolaou, ×400).

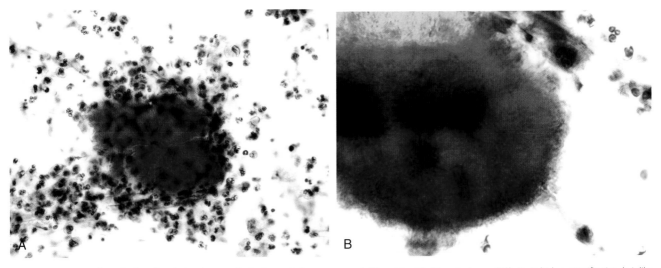

Figure 4-9. Fine-needle aspiration of cervical actinomycosis. **A,** A granule is seen surrounded by neutrophils (Papanicolaou, ×200). **B,** At higher magnification, hair-like filaments and a yellow-colored band are seen at the periphery of the granule (Papanicolaou, ×400).

neck showed a 3 × 2 × 1 cm, necrotic-appearing mass in the left neck in the region of the hyoid bone, and physical examination revealed a 4 × 3, firm, mildly tender, right-sided mass just inferior to the angle of the mandible. Approximately 2 mL of thick, white, creamy material was aspirated. Neutrophils were seen on a rapid Romanovski–stained slide, and material was submitted

for cultures, as described previously. Again, the clinical findings are useful: the patient's age and the lesion's temporal relation to tooth extraction are evidence against neoplasia, and he had no known immunosuppressive disease. Papanicolaou-stained preparations showed a neutrophilic exudate and several interspersed, grain-like structures (Fig. 4-9A). On high-power magnification,

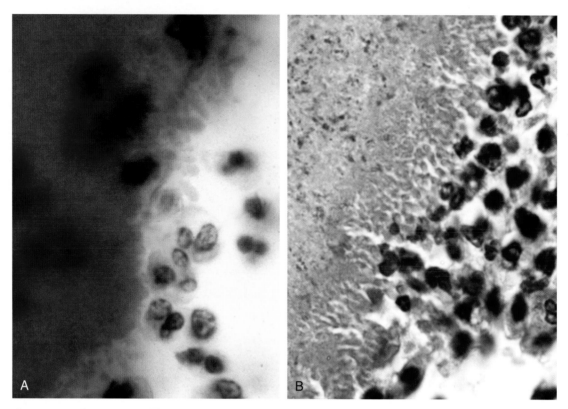

Figure 4-10. High-power images of fine-needle aspiration (FNA) and histologic section of actinomycosis with Splendore-Hoeppli phenomenon. **A,** FNA of neck mass shows club-shaped structures at the interface between the granule and the neutrophilic exudate (Papanicolaou, ×1000). **B,** Autopsy section from fatal pulmonary actinomycosis demonstrates a bright eosinophilic band and clubs at the microbe-exudate interface (hematoxylin and eosin, ×1000).

the grains were found to consist of aggregates of bacteria; individual, filamentous bacilli could be seen extending outward from the granules (see Fig. 4-9B). At the interface between some of the granules and the inflammatory exudate, there was a yellow-colored band surrounding the granule. This band is a Splendore-Hoeppli phenomenon (SHP).[26,27]

The SHP is seen in H&E staining as club-shaped or band-like eosinophilic structures surrounding either microorganisms or foreign bodies. Its composition and etiology have been debated but are thought to represent a host reaction including glycoprotein and, in some instances, antigen-antibody complexes. SHP coats the bacteria at the interface and forms club-shaped structures that appear yellow in Papanicolaou stain and dark pink in H&E (Fig. 4-10). The combination of granules of filamentous bacteria and SHP is highly suggestive of an actinomycotic mycetoma, and anaerobic culture is indicated. In such cases, it is mandatory to communicate this suspicion to the microbiology laboratory personnel, so that the anaerobic culture bottle will be incubated for at least 1 week before being discarded. Mycetomas are infections that manifest as tumor-like masses and are characterized by the presence of grain- or granule-like structures composed of tangled aggregates of microorganisms.[28] Mycetomas can be caused by actinomycetes, other types of bacteria (botryomycosis), or fungi (eumycotic mycetomas).[27,28] Like other types of mycetoma, actinomycotic mycetomas are chronic lesions, and draining sinuses and extensive fibrosis are common.

Two caveats should be considered:

1. Fibrosis may predominate over purulent exudate and may prevent successful diagnosis by FNA.

2. Proliferating fibroblasts and reactive squamous atypia may result in misdiagnosis as malignancy.

In the case of this patient, both *Actinomyces meyeri* and *Actinomyces odontolyticus* were cultured from FNA material placed into an anaerobic blood culture bottle. In our experience, actinomycetes, like mycobacteria, are not as readily recognized in Romanovski-stained preparations. We usually recognize actinomycosis by the granules present in the Papanicolaou-stained material. Gram stain, especially the Gram-Weigert, is important for confirmation that the granule is composed of branching gram-positive bacilli (Fig. 4-11).

The clinical and cytologic findings described in this case are greatly in favor of actinomycosis; however, botryomycosis and nocardiosis are part of the differential diagnosis. Gram staining helps rule out the former, and a modified acid-fast stain, the latter. Although nocardial mycetomas are common in tropical countries, in the United States, nocardiosis typically manifests as a necrotizing pneumonia in an immunosuppressed patient (Fig. 4-12). *M. fortuitum* infections in AIDS patients may manifest as necrotizing, neutrophil-rich cervical neck abscesses, and the morphology of *M. fortuitum* is difficult or impossible to differentiate from that of *Nocardia* species.[29] On Gram stains, both appear as branching, beaded, gram-positive bacilli and are at least weakly acid fast. *M. fortuitum* often does not fluoresce with routine auramine fluorochrome staining,[29] and, like *Nocardia*, sometimes prefers a modified stain to show off its acid-fast qualities (Fig. 4-13).

Neither the pseudoactinomycotic radiating granules (PAMRGs) seen in cervical Papanicolaou (Pap) tests from pregnant women[30,31] nor the cockleburr- or rhomboid-shaped crystals of hematoidin are indicative of actinomycosis, and these should not be confused with mycetomas (Fig. 4-14). Although PAMRGs, like actinomyces, have been described in people with intrauterine devices, our experience of the past 25 years is that these are predominantly seen in pregnant women, as described by Zaharopoulos and colleagues.[30] PAMRGs have features similar to the Splendore-Hoeppli reaction[31]; however, they are not associated with an underlying microorganism. Hematoidin, a golden-brown cockleburr- or rhomboid-shaped structure, has been found to be a byproduct of erythrocyte degradation and consists of golden pigment, akin to bilirubin, and lipid.[32] Hematoidin is distinct from both actinomycosis and PAMRG and is often found in cavities containing old blood. In our experience, aspirates from pancreatic pseudocysts and organizing hematomas are good places to find hematoidin crystals (Fig. 4-15). We have rarely seen them in cervicovaginal smears. PAMRGs are far more common in the latter.

Neutrophils are an important first line of defense against certain fungi,[33] including *Candida*, *Aspergillus*, and zygomycetes (mucormycosis agents). In non-neutropenic patients, invasive infections with these fungi elicit a neutrophil-rich inflammatory cell reaction. Because of the importance of granulocytes as a defense mechanism, invasive candidiasis, zygomycosis, and aspergillosis are potential complications of severe neutropenia. All three have propensities to invade blood vessels, and infarcts with coagulative necrosis are common complications of the invasive forms of these fungal infections. The cytologic features of these fungi are discussed in the sections dealing with cytodiagnosis of infections in immunocompromised patients.

Eosinophils and Allergic Mucin

Inflammatory exudates with a predominance of eosinophils are found in asthma and other allergic conditions including noninvasive, allergic fungal diseases; parasitic infections; and eosinophilic pneumonia and as a nonspecific finding in chronic pleural effusions of varying etiologies. One should remember that where there are Charcot-Leyden crystals, there are eosinophils, and where there are eosinophils, one must look for allergic disease and parasites. Charcot-Leyden crystals are elongated, dipyramidal to rectangular crystals with pointed or raggedy ends, quite variable in size. They are composed of lysolecithin acylhydrolase, which has lysophospholipase, an enzyme important in the antiparasitic, antineoplastic, and immune functions of eosinophils.[34] In Romanovski-stained preparations, they have a light blue color, and in Papanicolaou stain, they may be orange or turquoise. Cases that exemplify eosinophil-rich disease processes diagnosed by cytology, visceral larva migrans–associated eosinophilic hepatic pseudotumor, and allergic fungal disorders are described here.

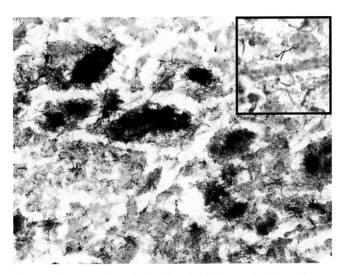

Figure 4-11. Fine-needle aspiration of cervical actinomycosis. Clumps of gram-positive bacilli are seen (Gram-Weigert, ×400), with branching form seen in inset (Gram-Weigert, ×1000).

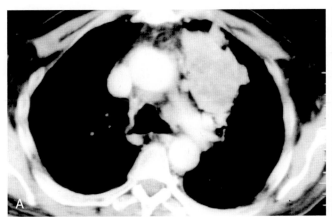
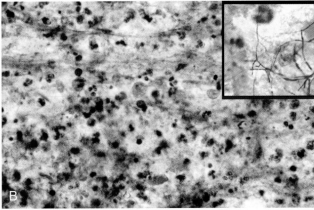

Figure 4-12. Pulmonary nocardiosis in a heart transplant recipient. **A,** Chest computed tomography (CT) shows large left upper lobe infiltrate with areas of necrosis. **B,** CT-guided fine-needle aspiration of infiltrate demonstrates the presence of a necrotizing, fibrinopurulent inflammation (Papanicolaou, ×400). Branching gram-positive filamentous bacilli are revealed by a Gram stain (Gram-Weigert, ×1000).

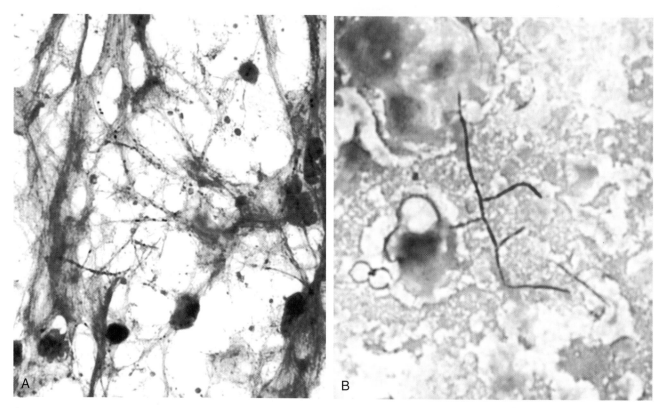

Figure 4-13. *Nocardia* sp. **(A)** and *Mycobacterium fortuitum* **(B)** in modified acid-fast stains. **A,** Branching, beaded filaments. **B,** In this image, *M. fortuitum* appears slightly thicker and has shorter branches than *Nocardia*; however, these features are not adequate for definitive distinction from *Nocardia* sp. (Kinyoun, ×2000).

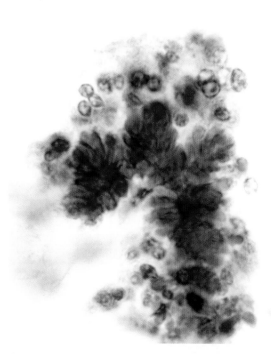

Figure 4-14. Cervical liquid-based Papanicolaou test from pregnant woman with pseudoactinomycotic radiating granules. Note the similarity to actinomycotic Splendore-Hoeppli phenomenon. No bacterial filaments are present, however (Papanicolaou, ×1600).

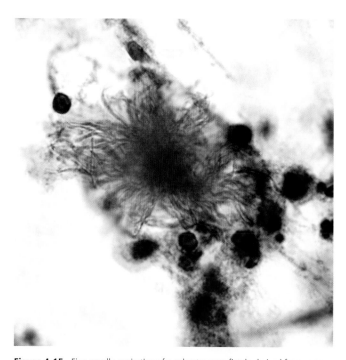

Figure 4-15. Fine-needle aspiration of a subcutaneous fistula derived from pancreatic pseudocyst. A cockleburr-like, golden-yellow crystal typical of hematoidin is seen (Papanicolaou, ×1600).

Case 3: The Hepatocellular Carcinoma that Was Not

CT monitoring for hepatocellular carcinoma in a Cambodian man with hepatitis C disclosed a liver mass that was sampled by FNA. Figure 4-16 illustrates the findings in an on-site rapid Romanovski stain. Note the presence of necrosis and a large number of reddish granules. Abundant Charcot-Leyden crystals are seen, and for this reason, cancer was preliminarily rejected, and suspicion turned to parasites. The preliminary diagnosis was hepatic eosinophilic pseudotumor, and visceral larva migrans needed to be ruled out. Subsequent serotesting for *Toxocara* was positive, and the nodule regressed with therapy.

Necrosis, necrotic eosinophils, and Charcot-Leyden crystals in a solitary liver nodule, especially from a child or from an adult with recent foreign travel, makes one suspect visceral larva migrans.[35] Nonhuman ascarid larvae are the most common culprits; however, the actual nematode larva is rarely seen, even in histologic preparations.[36] A portion of larva surrounded by abundant eosinophils is seen in Figure 4-17. This is a histologic section taken from another case of visceral larva migrans–associated hepatic pseudotumor that was resected without presurgical biopsy or FNA. Nodular collections of eosinophils can also be found in Hodgkin disease and other lymphomas, hypereosinophilic syndrome, and carcinomas, most notably gastric adenocarcinoma.[36-38] Again, careful attention to patients' clinical history and laboratory findings are essential.

Case 4, 5, and 6: If There Is Allergic Mucin, the Fungi Are Not Invasive

Figure 4-18 illustrates the bronchial brush findings from an elderly woman who had a pulmonary infiltrate and a past history of therapy for uterine cancer. Eosinophils and abundant mucin were found, and a GMS stain was performed over one of the slides. Mucin, eosinophils, and fungi are consistent with an allergic fungal mucus plug, the differential of which is discussed in the following paragraphs. Figure 4-19 illustrates an aspiration of

sphenoid sinus contents from a 6-year-old boy with a history of allergic rhinitis and multiple paranasal sinus opacifications and cranial nerve palsies. Note the presence of granular debris, necrotic eosinophils, and Charcot-Leyden crystals. Elsewhere in the preparations, fungal hyphae were found, and the patient proved to have a noninvasive condition known as allergic fungal sinusitis. Figure 4-20 is an aspirate from an ethmoid sinus of another patient with allergic fungal sinusitis. Note the presence of hyaline, cyanophilic hyphae admixed with degenerating eosinophils. Elsewhere in the sample, mucin admixed with relatively

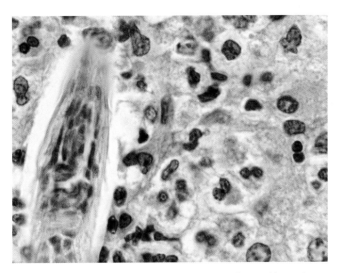

Figure 4-17. Excisional biopsy of liver mass in a case of visceral larva migrans. Abundant eosinophils are seen surrounding a portion of nematode larva. Dot-like internal structures are often seen in cytologic and histologic preparations of nematodes (hematoxylin and eosin, ×1000).

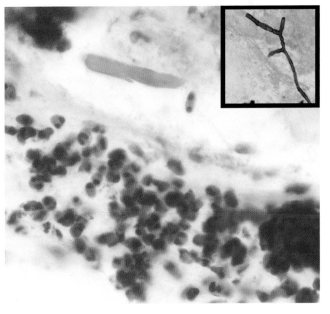

Figure 4-18. Fungal mucus plug in a bronchial brushing slide. Within strands of pale blue-colored mucin, there are sheets of eosinophils in the lower half of image and a Charcot-Leyden crystal in the upper center (Papanicolaou, ×400). In the inset, branching hyphae are seen in silver-stained preparation (GMS, ×400).

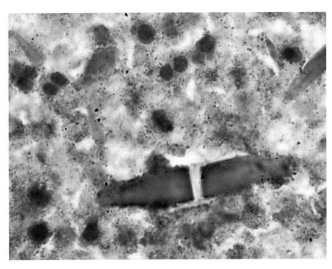

Figure 4-16. Fine-needle aspiration of a hepatic eosinophilic pseudotumor. Abundant degenerating eosinophils, extracellular eosinophilic granules, and blue-colored Charcot-Leyden crystals are seen (Romanovski, ×1000).

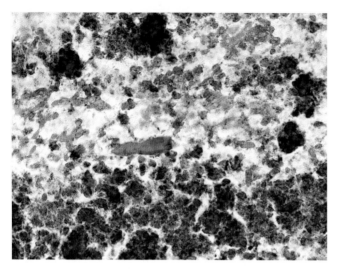

Figure 4-19. Aspiration of sphenoid sinus material from a patient with allergic fungal sinusitis. Aggregates of degenerating eosinophils are seen in lower and upper portions, and a Charcot-Leyden crystal is present in the center (Papanicolaou, ×200).

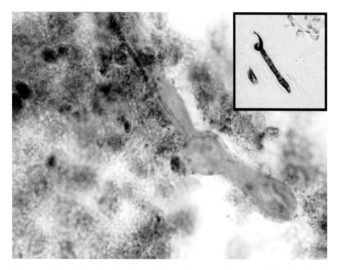

Figure 4-20. Aspiration of ethmoid sinus from another case of allergic fungal sinusitis. There are necrotic eosinophils and a strand of cyanophilic fungal hyphae (Papanicolaou, ×1600). The fungi did not appear brown on Papanicolaou stain; however, they were shown to be dematiaceous by melanin stain of surgical curettage (inset; Fontana-Masson, ×400).

intact eosinophils were seen. The fungi proved to be dematiaceous by melanin stain (see Fig. 4-20, inset).

These three cases illustrate the diagnostic significance of allergic mucin. Allergic mucin, composed of a mixture of mucin, cellular debris, eosinophils, and Charcot-Leyden crystals, is found within the conducting airways in allergic airway diseases. The hallmark of *Aspergillus* (and other fungal-associated) noninvasive allergic disease is allergic mucin.[39,40] If one sees allergic mucin and fungi in an FNA or bronchial brushing (Fig. 4-18), as in the case of the elderly woman, allergic bronchopulmonary aspergillosis (ABPA) must be ruled out, and communication with the clinical team is recommended. ABPA is most often associated with cystic fibrosis and asthma and is defined by clin-

ical parameters that include eosinophilia, immediate cutaneous reactivity to *Aspergillus* antigen, presence of *Aspergillus*-specific precipitins, elevated serum immunoglobulin E, fixed or transient pulmonary infiltrates, and central bronchiectasis.[41]

Bronchial mucoid impaction may also occur that demonstrates the presence of allergic mucin and fungi but lacks the other criteria for ABPA. In the case of the elderly woman, no fungus-specific antibodies were found. Allergic mucin, containing fungal organisms, most commonly dematiaceous fungi, are also seen in allergic fungal sinusitis. This is similar to ABPA in that the fungi are noninvasive and the disease symptoms are caused by massive mucus impaction within the paranasal sinuses. The impaction may cause compression of cranial nerves and symptoms suspicious for neoplasia.[42] Evacuation of contents of involved sinuses typically yields grumous material that has been described as foul-smelling and having the consistency of peanut butter.[43] Cytologists should be familiar with the microscopic features of allergic mucin to help establish the diagnosis of allergic fungal disease and rule out both neoplasia and invasive fungal disease.[44]

Rarely, peripheral blood eosinophilia and eosinophils admixed with granulomatous inflammation can be associated with chronic, disseminated coccidioidomycosis.[45,46] Figures 4-21 and 4-22 demonstrate the FNA and lymph node biopsy findings, respectively, in a young man from Mexico who presented with lower extremity lymphedema, eosinophilia, and a history of an unknown type of fungal infection. Granulomatous inflammation and abundant eosinophils were seen, with very focal fungal spherules (not illustrated) present in the biopsy sample. Cultures of lymph node grew *C. immitis*. Special attention should be paid to the patient's history, to the country of origin or travel, and, always, to the culture results when inflammation is present.

Granulomatous Inflammation

Granulomatous inflammation is a type of chronic inflammation characterized by immunologically modified macrophages that are better suited to containment of organisms and large-particle phagocytosis than to intracellular killing and that tend to occur when there is absence of efficient intracellular killing of microorganisms.[47] The term *granuloma* is used to describe the aggregation of these modified macrophages into nodular aggregates. Lymphocytes and plasma cells are also seen, usually at the periphery of granulomas. In cytologic preparations, the transformed macrophages of granulomas have elongate oval to boomerang-shaped nuclei and abundant, finely granular cytoplasm that is pink in H&E-stained slides and cyanophilic in Papanicolaou. The cytoplasmic borders are not well defined, and adjacent cells blend into one another. The cells bear some resemblance to epithelial cells and are called *epithelioid macrophages*. Multinucleated giant cells are often seen but not essential for the diagnosis of granuloma. Two FNA preparations showing noncaseating granulomatous inflammation are illustrated in Figure 4-23. The Papanicolaou-stained sample derives from a cervical lymph node in a 33-year-old man who had sarcoidosis. The Romanovski-stained preparation was taken from a lymph node FNA in a woman with tuberculosis and widespread lymphadenopathy. Noncaseating granulomas found in a lymph-node or visceral-organ FNA from an asymptomatic young person frequently indicates sarcoidosis; however, one must not be complacent. One

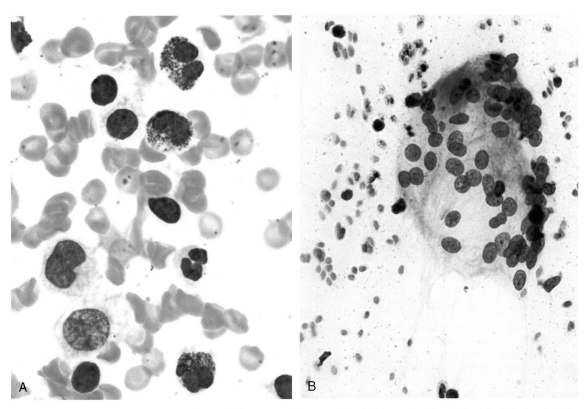

Figure 4-21. Fine-needle aspiration of inguinal lymph node from a case of disseminated coccidioidomycosis with marked peripheral blood eosinophilia. **A,** Mixed inflammatory cell reaction with presence of eosinophils (Romanovski, ×1000). **B,** Giant cell macrophage (Romanovski, ×400).

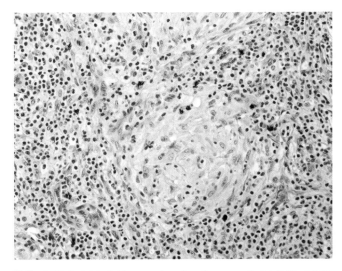

Figure 4-22. Lymph node biopsy specimen from the same patient as in Figure 4-21. Well-formed granulomas are surrounded by an eosinophil-rich inflammatory exudate (hematoxylin and eosin, ×200).

Caseating granuloma refers to the presence of epithelioid macrophages surrounding granular amorphous material that, by gross evaluation, has the appearance of crumbly white cheese. In Papanicolaou-stained cytologic preparations, caseating necrosis has a granular, gray-green appearance (Fig. 4-25). Entrapped, degenerated cells are seen, and, with luck, some epithelioid macrophages may be found. It is very important to recognize caseation in a cytologic preparation, because acid-fast and fungal staining are indicated. In Romanovski-stained preparations, caseous material is more faintly stained, usually rather pink, but the gross appearance of the material expelled from the FNA needle often provides a clue. It is creamy, somewhat granular, and often drier in appearance than pus. If the Romanovski stain (see Fig. 4-25, inset) fails to demonstrate neutrophils and abundant amorphous material is seen in a compatible clinical setting, one should suspect caseation and request mycobacterial and fungal cultures. Epithelioid cell aggregates without caseation may be found in aspirates from chronic coccidioidomycosis, blastomycosis, and histoplasmosis. A presumptive diagnosis of sarcoidosis and therapy with steroids can prove deadly in patients with disseminated tuberculosis or fungal infection.

Cases 7 and 8: A Tale of Two Tubercles

A 73-year-old man had complained of weight loss and cough. By CT, he was found to have a thick-walled cavitary mass in the right upper lung and two smaller masses near the pleura. Clinicians were concerned about cavitary SCC. A bronchial brushing

cannot distinguish between sarcoidosis and infectious causes of noncaseating granulomas on the basis of morphology. Always culture the sample, and be sure that the clinician is aware of the patient's clinical and radiologic findings. Figure 4-24 is taken from a tonsil biopsy of the man with sarcoid. It is easy to see why the term "epithelioid cells" is appropriate!

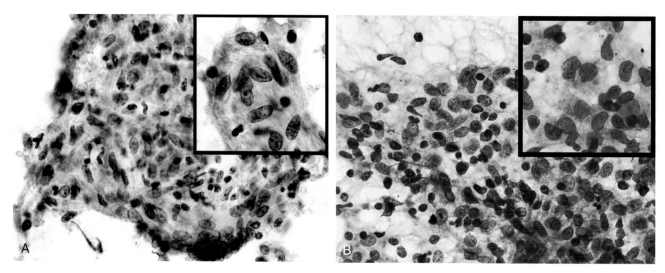

Figure 4-23. Fine-needle aspiration of lymph nodes that had noncaseating granulomas. **A,** Cervical lymph node from a patient with sarcoidosis shows aggregates of epithelioid macrophages (Papanicolaou, ×400). Inset shows poorly defined cytoplasmic cell borders and presence of elongate to boomerang-shaped nuclei (Papanicolaou, ×1000). **B,** Cervical lymph node from a woman with tuberculosis shows similar features (Romanovski, ×400, Inset ×1000).

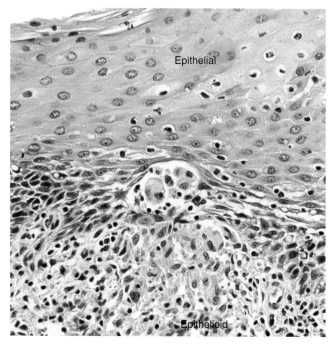

Figure 4-24. Tonsil biopsy from a patient with sarcoidosis. Note the squamous epithelium above and the aggregates of epithelioid macrophages below (hematoxylin and eosin, ×400).

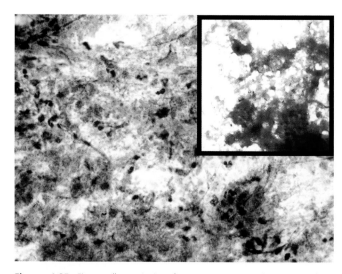

Figure 4-25. Fine-needle aspiration from caseating granuloma. Amorphous granular, green material is admixed with few cell nuclei (Papanicolaou, ×400). The material appears less granular and equally amorphous in Romanovski stain (inset; Romanovski, ×400).

slide contained the findings illustrated in Figure 4-26A. Note the loosely formed epithelioid cells with interspersed granular material, indicative of caseating granuloma. Scanty acid-fast bacilli were seen on a Kinyoun stain performed over a Papanicolaou-stained brushing slide. Culture of the respiratory material from bronchoscopy grew *Mycobacterium avium* complex (MAC), and the cavity wall markedly thinned after therapy; however, 1 year later, a dependent, bulbous mass appeared within the base of the cavity. FNA revealed the presence of branching septate hyphae,

and the diagnosis rendered was fungus ball arising in a preexisting cavity.

A 41-year-old woman also presented with cough and chest CT interpreted as suspicious for bronchogenic carcinoma. Abundant caseous material with reactive squamous metaplasia was seen (see Fig. 4-26B). Acid-fast bacilli were seen on Kinyoun stain performed over Papanicolaou-stained slides of bronchial brushing and bronchial washing samples, but culture of bronchoscopic material was not performed. One must keep in mind that mycobacterial infections can mimic neoplasia and that granular amorphous material in an FNA, bronchial brush, or TBNA sample should lead one to request acid-fast (and fungal) stains as well as cultures.

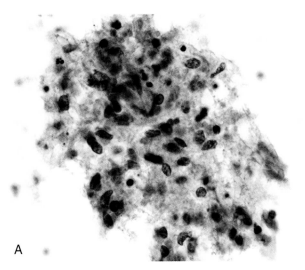
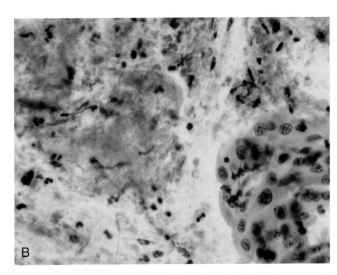

Figure 4-26. Caseating granulomata diagnosed by bronchial brushings. **A,** A loosely formed aggregate of epithelioid macrophages admixed with amorphous granular material is seen (Papanicolaou, ×400). **B,** Amorphous granular material with entrapped nuclei is seen on the left, and reactive squamous metaplasia on the right. The latter can result in misdiagnosis of neoplasia (Papanicolaou, ×400).

Two caveats should be kept in mind:

1. Reactive squamous metaplasia can lead to misdiagnosis of SCC in cases of infections. We have seen markedly atypical squamous metaplasia associated with tuberculosis and actinomycosis.

2. MAC cannot be accurately distinguished from *M. tuberculosis* complex (MTC) by acid-fast stain, and MAC infections are not confined to severely T-cell immunosuppressed patients.[48-51] Culture is required for identification of MOTT, and culture or presumptive identification by molecular methods such as RNA amplification for MTC. *M. kansasii* has a distinct morphology that can allow for presumptive diagnosis in some cases,[52,53] and *M. fortuitum* closely resembles *Nocardia* sp., as mentioned previously. The comparative acid-fast staining features of MTC, MAC, and *M. kansasii* are shown in Figure 4-27. All slides were taken from cytologic samples.

Case 9: Willowy Macrophages and AIDS

Figure 4-28 illustrates the TBNA and transbronchial biopsy findings from a man with AIDS and mediastinal lymphadenopathy. Lymphoma was suspected. Note the presence of spindle-shaped cells that could be misinterpreted as an Epstein-Barr–associated smooth muscle tumor[54] or Kaposi sarcoma.[55] The spindle cells in this type of pseudotumor have immunohistochemical features of macrophages[56]; in an AIDS patient, they are highly suspicious for mycobacterial infection. MTC, MAC, and *M. kansasii* have all been isolated from patients with so-called spindle cell granulomas.[53,57] In this case, very long, coarsely beaded, acid-fast bacilli with curved ends are seen. Their shape has been compared to a shepherd's crook, although a Christmas candy cane might be a better simile. This is the classic appearance of *M. kansasii* and is the only type of mycobacteria that we can usually speciate presumptively on the basis of morphology. *M. fortuitum* also has a relatively unique appearance; however, as previously stated, differentiation from *Nocardia* is problematic.

Case 10: Granulomatous Inflammation with Vesiculose Macrophages

A 37-year-old HIV-seronegative man was referred for evaluation of an abnormal chest radiograph. CT showed multiple bilateral pulmonary opacities 1 to 4 cm in diameter (Fig. 4-29). An atypical infectious process was favored, and a CT-guided FNA was performed. Findings are illustrated in Figure 4-30. This patient was relatively immunocompetent, and epithelioid macrophages, giant cells, lymphocytes, and plasma cells were present, consistent with granulomatous inflammation; however, the macrophage cytoplasm had a vesiculated rather than granular appearance. To best see the intracytoplasmic structures, the substage condenser must be closed. This gives fungi a refractile appearance and makes them much easier to see. On high-power examination, one sees relatively round structures that are clear to slightly pink. The fungi lack abundant capsular material, as is common in infections in immunocompetent or mildly immunosuppressed patients. Note the considerable variation in size, a very important clue to the diagnosis! These organisms typically vary from 5 to 20 μm in diameter. This is well demonstrated in the GMS stain (Fig. 4-31). Also note the thin cell wall and round shape, which are typical of *Cryptococcus. Cryptococcus* infection in T-cell–immunosuppressed patients is discussed in the next section.

One should be aware that cryptococci are easily overlooked in H&E- and Papanicolaou-stained preparations. They may also be mistaken for phagocytized erythrocytes or lipid (Fig. 4-32). Remember to close the substage condenser! Paucicapsular forms of *Cryptococcus* often stain weakly with mucicarmine. Fontana-Masson melanin stain is recommended in these cases.[20-22]

Granulomatous Inflammation Admixed with Neutrophils

A mixture of epithelioid macrophages and neutrophils is the typical inflammatory response to many of the dimorphic fungi,

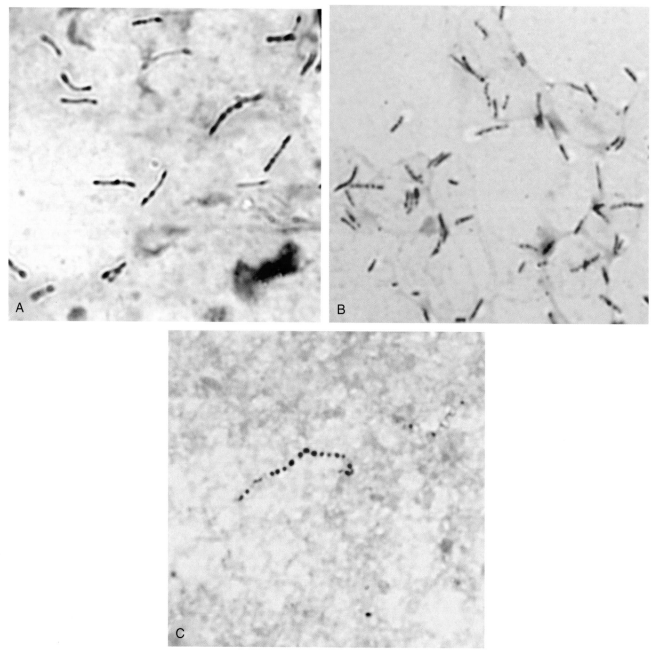

Figure 4-27. Mycobacteria are seen in Kinyoun stain from cytologic preparations. **A,** *Mycobacterium tuberculosis* complex. **B,** *Mycobacterium avium* complex. **C,** *Myco-bacterium kansasii* (Kinyoun, ×2000).

including *C. immitis, Blastomyces dermatitidis, Paracoccidioides brasiliensis, Sporothrix schenckii,* and the dematiaceous fungi associated with chromoblastomycosis and phaeohyphomycosis.[27] Neutrophils are rarely seen in cases of histoplasmosis or cryptococcosis. *H. capsulatum* and *Cryptococcus neoformans* usually elicit either a granulomatous, diffuse macrophage reaction or, in the case of *Cryptococcus,* scant to absent inflammation. Diffuse macrophage infiltration, typically found in patients with deficient Th1 cell-mediated immunity, is discussed in the following section. In dimorphic fungal infections, the proportion of epithelioid macrophages to neutrophils varies with the host's ability to interact with the pathogen. In chronic, indolent infections,

one sees a predominance of granulomatous inflammation. In fulminant infections, neutrophils predominate. In advanced AIDS, abundant necrosis admixed with myriad fungi and varying numbers of neutrophils is typical.

It is important that the cytologist know which stains best demonstrate the features of the dimorphic fungi. Although GMS is often considered the gold standard, it is not the best stain for all fungi. *C. immitis, B. dermatitidis,* and *P. brasiliensis* are best seen on H&E or Papanicolaou stain. These stains allow one to scrutinize the internal features of the organisms, including cell wall, endoplasm, and nuclei. In the case of *C. immitis,* endospore formation can be seen. Agents of chromoblastomycosis and phaeo-

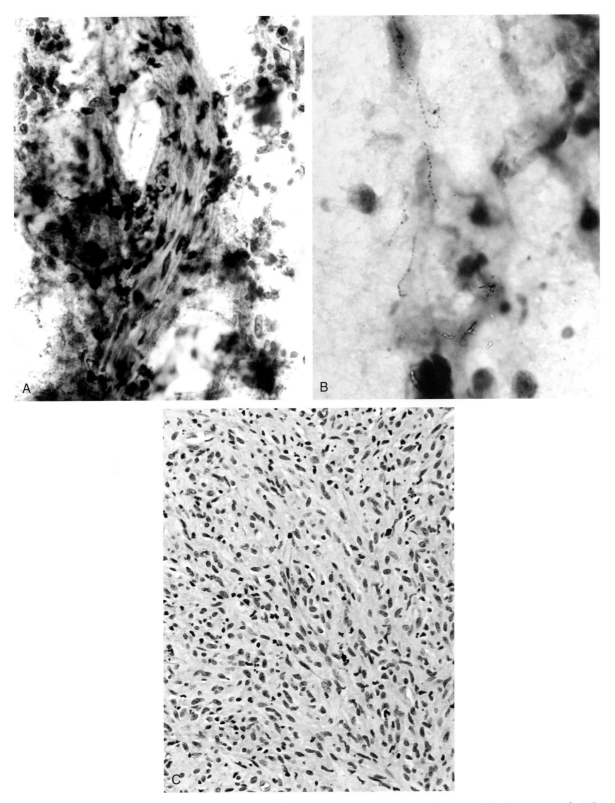

Figure 4-28. *Mycobacterium kansasii* spindle-cell granuloma in an AIDS patient. **A,** Transbronchial fine-needle aspiration (FNA) shows a group of spindly cells (Papanicolaou, ×600). **B,** Long, coarsely beaded bacilli are seen in an acid-fast stain of the FNA sample (Kinyoun, ×1600). **C,** Transbronchial biopsy from the same patient (hematoxylin and eosin, ×600).

hyphomycosis, dematiaceous fungi, are also usually well seen on H&E and Papanicolaou stains. Chromoblastomycosis pertains to infections localized to the epidermis and dermis and is characterized by presence of multiseptate bodies or Medlar bodies. Phaeohyphomycosis pertains to subcutaneous or visceral infections.[58] In phaeohyphomycosis, hyphae and moniliform pseudohyphae usually predominate; however, we have seen multiseptate bodies admixed with hyphae in an FNA in one case of disseminated phaeohyphomycosis caused by *Fonsecaea pedrosoi*.[59] Figure 4-33 shows the comparative features of *B. dermatitidis*, *C. immitis*, and *P. brasiliensis*, which can easily be confused in cytologic or histologic preparations. Note the pseudococcidioidal, nonbudding *Blastomyces* in Figure 4-33D and the paired pseudoblastomycoid *Coccidioides* immature spherules in Figure 4-33E. *Cryptococcus* rarely is confused with these because it lacks a thick, double refractile cell wall, but an image is included (see Fig. 4-33F) to illustrate the contrast between *C. neoformans* and the others. The differential features are discussed in the following sections.

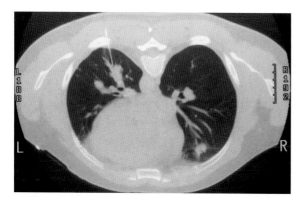

Figure 4-29. Chest computed tomogram showing multiple, bilateral pulmonary opacities, one of which was sampled by percutaneous fine-needle aspiration (see Fig. 4-30).

Case 11: The Community-Acquired Pneumonia That Wasn't

A 21-year-old male student from eastern Louisiana underwent bronchoscopy because of a right lower lung infiltrate, chills, and fever that failed to respond to therapy for community-acquired pneumonia. The man had no history of alcohol or drug abuse and was HIV negative. His bronchial brushing material is illustrated in Figure 4-34. Note the combination of epithelioid macrophage aggregates and neutrophils (see Fig. 4-34A). This type of inflammatory pattern and the clinical history should generate a search for dimorphic fungi. In Figure 4-34B, one sees the characteristic features of *B. dermatitidis*. In tissue, *B. dermatitidis* is seen as blastoconidia (yeast-like forms) that are 15 to 20 μm in length; the cell wall is thick and double-contoured, and the endoplasm is typically retracted so as to leave a clear zone between the cell wall and the internal structures (see Fig. 4-33A and D). Under very high magnification, multiple nuclei can sometimes be seen as tiny dots, but these may be difficult to discern in Papanicolaou and H&E stains. Broad-based budding is typical of *Blastomyces* and is useful if found (see Fig. 4-33A). The main differential includes *P. brasiliensis* and *C. immitis* (see Fig. 4-33). Because these organisms have different geographic distributions,[27] knowing the travel history or region of birth of the patient is extremely helpful. *P. brasiliensis* is thick-walled like *B. dermatitidis*, but it has narrow-necked budding, and multiple buds are common. The characteristic "ship's wheel" budding pattern is lovely and diagnostic if you can find it, but it may be difficult to find. A very useful differentiating feature is the marked variability in size that is found in *P. brasiliensis* compared with *B. dermatitidis*. The greatest diagnostic pitfall is the immature spherule of *C. immitis*, which may closely resemble *B. dermatitidis* and *P. brasiliensis* (see Fig. 4-33). The *Paracoccidioides* yeast forms illustrated here derive from a lung section rather than a cytologic specimen and are shown for the sake of comparison.

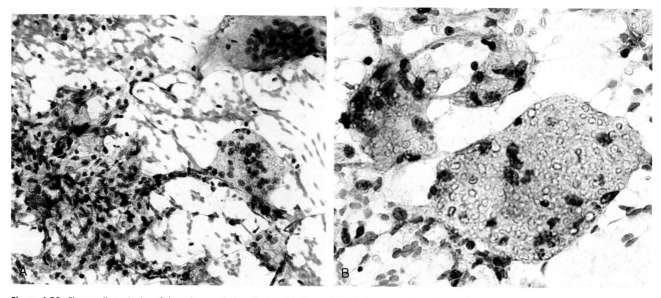

Figure 4-30. Fine-needle aspiration of the pulmonary lesions illustrated in Figure 4-29. **A,** An aggregation of macrophages and several multinucleated giant cells are seen (Papanicolaou, ×200). **B,** Multinucleated cells contain refractile, round yeast forms (Papanicolaou, ×400).

Case 12: Fluctuant and Full of Fungi

A 26-year-old man who had been working in the Texas Rio Grande Valley presented with fever and several fluctuant, subcutaneous masses. Chest radiography revealed diffuse interstitial infiltrates. FNA was done from a 3 × 3 cm subcutaneous mass

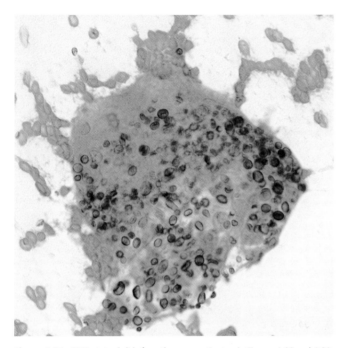

Figure 4-31. GMS-stained slide from the same patient as in Figures 4-29 and 4-30, showing round shape and variability in size of yeast forms (GMS, ×400).

overlying the fifth lumbar vertebra. Several milliliters of gray-colored, thick material was aspirated. A Papanicolaou-stained slide of aspirate is illustrated in Figure 4-35. Spherules of markedly varying sizes are seen in a background of necrosis, giant cells, and neutrophils. Endosporulation is seen within some of the spherules. Note that immature and empty spherules that lack endosporulation can readily be mistaken for pollen grains, *Blastomyces*, or *Paracoccidioides*. Cutaneous and subcutaneous lesions of *Blastomyces*, *Paracoccidioides*, and *Coccidioides* typically represent disseminated pulmonary disease; however, in some cases, pulmonary lesions are not apparent. This was a fulminant case, and neutrophils and necrosis are prominent, although epithelioid macrophages and giant cells are also seen.

This patient tested negative for HIV. In patients with coccidioidomycosis and advanced AIDS, extensive necrosis, myriad organisms, and variable numbers of neutrophils and macrophages are seen. Granulomas are absent (Fig. 4-36). Similar histologic reactions to *Paracoccidioides*, *Blastomyces*, and *Sporothrix* have been reported in AIDS patients.[60-63]

Unusual Host Reactions to Infections in the Immunocompromised Patient

Patients with Neutropenia or Defective Neutrophils

Neutropenic patients are susceptible to a number of infections, including pyogenic bacteria, invasive aspergillosis, candidiasis, and mucormycosis. In these patients, one sees abundant organisms but not the expected purulent inflammatory reaction.

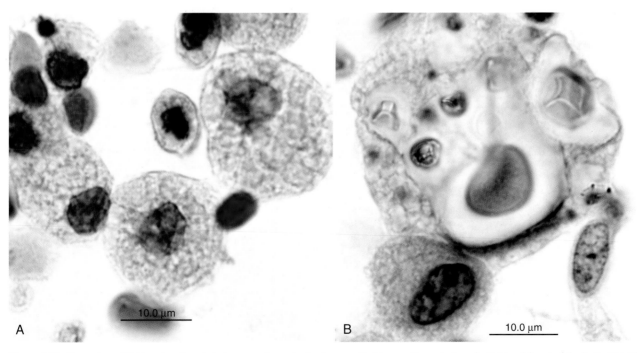

A   B

Figure 4-32. Comparison of lipid- and erythrocyte-laden macrophages to *Cryptococcus*. **A,** Intraoperative aspiration of a Rathke cleft cyst of the brain. Macrophages containing lipid-like vacuoles and degenerating erythrocytes are seen (Papanicolaou, ×2000). **B,** Bronchoalveolar lavage specimen containing macrophages with phagocytized *Cryptococcus neoformans.* Note marked variation in size of yeast forms and the presence of refractile granular material within some yeast (Papanicolaou, ×2000).

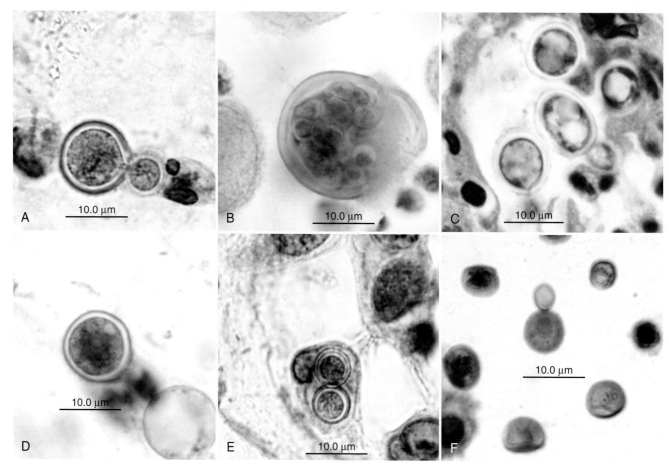

Figure 4-33. Comparison of *Blastomyces dermatitidis, Coccidioides immitis, Paracoccidioides brasiliensis,* and *Cryptococcus neoformans.* **A,** *B. dermatitidis.* The yeast form is about 12 μm in diameter, with a broad-based bud and a thick, refractile cell wall. A narrow clear zone separates the fungal protoplasm from the cell wall. **B,** Mature spherule of *C. immitis.* The spherule has a round shape, is relatively large, has a thick cell wall, and contains multiple round endospores. **C,** Yeast forms of *P. brasiliensis* lack the classic "ship's wheel" budding. Yeasts are more variable in size than *Blastomyces* but are easily confused with both *Blastomyces* and with immature forms of *Coccidioides.* **D,** Nonbudding form of *Blastomyces.* **E,** Two examples of closely apposed immature spherules of *Coccidioides immitis* imitating *Blastomyces.* **F,** Yeast forms of *Cryptococcus neoformans* (Papanicolaou, ×2000).

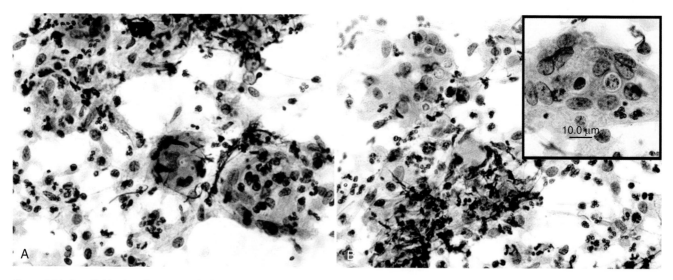

Figure 4-34. Bronchial brushing from a case of pulmonary blastomycosis. **A,** An inflammatory exudate composed of neutrophils, epithelioid cells, and giant cells is seen (Papanicolaou, ×400). **B,** Yeast-like cells are seen within giant cell macrophages (Papanicolaou, ×400). Higher magnification of yeast forms is seen in the inset (Papanicolaou, ×1000).

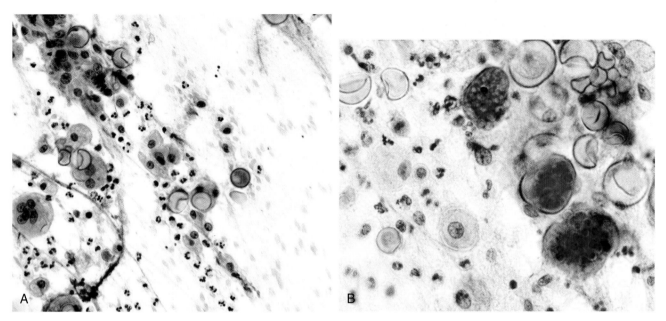

Figure 4-35. Fine-needle aspiration of subcutaneous coccidioidomycosis. **A,** A mixture of neutrophils, epithelioid macrophages, and giant cells is seen, along with empty and collapsing spherules (Papanicolaou, ×200). **B,** Mature endosporulating spherules are seen, along with empty and collapsed forms (Papanicolaou, ×400).

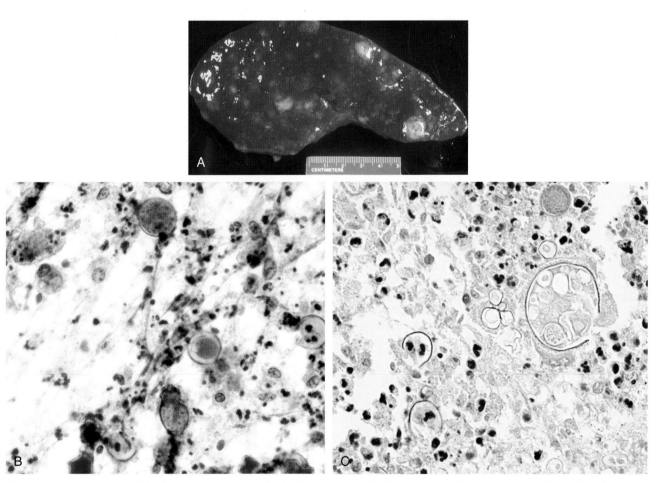

Figure 4-36. Disseminated coccidioidomycosis in a patient with AIDS. **A,** Gross photograph of spleen at autopsy. **B,** Postmortem scraping of one of the splenic lesions shows necrotic debris, scanty macrophages and neutrophils, and abundant spherules (Papanicolaou, ×400). **C,** Postmortem section of spleen shows the presence of abundant necrosis and spherules and relatively scanty inflammation (hematoxylin and eosin, ×400).

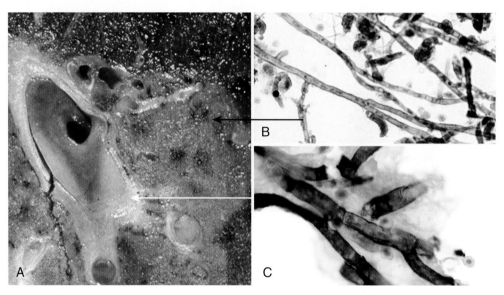

Figure 4-37. Invasive pulmonary aspergillosis in a severely neutropenic patient. **A,** Cross-section of lung taken at autopsy shows the presence of round, pale regions and vascular thromboses. **B,** Scraping of pale round area indicated by black arrow. Fibrin and fungal hyphae with narrow angle branching are seen (Papanicolaou, ×1000). **C,** Scraping of intravascular thrombus indicated by white arrow. Fungal hyphae are present (GMS, ×1500).

Patients with adequate numbers of neutrophils but defective neutrophil function (e.g., in diabetes) also are at risk for invasive infections with these fungi. Vascular invasion is typical of invasive aspergillosis, candidiasis, and mucormycosis, although this phenomenon is usually appreciated on histologic sections rather than in the cytology laboratory. We have, however, demonstrated fungi within rounded infarcts and thrombosed blood vessels by postmortem cytology. Figure 4-37 shows the gross and scrape preparation findings from the autopsy of a severely neutropenic patient with multiple round pulmonary infarcts and vascular thromboses. Fungal hyphae were found within the infarcts and blood vessels by cytology. Examination of sections confirmed the presence of invasive fungal disease. Postmortem cultures grew *Aspergillus glaucus*. Normally, the clinical history and radiologic features are needed to differentiate between aggressive, invasive fungal disease and more indolent invasive disease such as chronic necrotizing aspergillosis[64] or intrabronchial zygomycosis.[65,66] Using the clinical and radiologic information, however, the cytologist can and should discuss the possibilities with the clinician. The variety of diseases associated with *Aspergillus* alone is mind-boggling and includes noninvasive fungus ball, ABPA and mucoid impaction, chronic necrotizing aspergillosis, ulcerative bronchitis, and aggressive invasive aspergillosis, to name a few.[64,67,68] Allergic disease can be diagnosed on the basis of allergic mucin, as discussed previously; however, the other potential diagnoses require careful clinical correlation. By tissue morphology alone, *Aspergillus* cannot be definitively differentiated from other hyalohyphal fungi unless conidia-bearing fruiting heads are seen. Figure 4-38 demonstrates conidiophores and fruiting heads of *Aspergillus fumigatus* found in a bronchial brushing from a patient with endobronchial aspergillosis. This finding so delighted the cytopathologist that the cells deriving from small cell carcinoma, also present in the preparation, were overlooked. Zygomycetes, as a group, can be differentiated from other

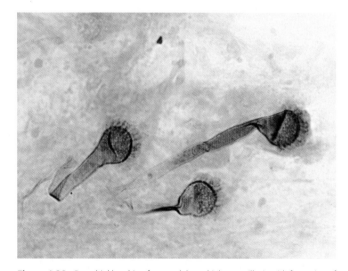

Figure 4-38. Bronchial brushing from endobronchial aspergillosis with formation of fruiting heads. Conidiophores contain the typical fruiting heads of *Aspergillus fumigatus* (GMS, ×1500).

mycelia-producing fungi (Fig. 4-39); however, the genus cannot be identified in the absence of fruiting heads.

Candida infections can be superficial and limited to the epithelium of mucous membranes, as in thrush and vulvovaginitis, or they can be locally invasive or aggressive, with vascular invasion and hematogenous dissemination. *Candida* found in cervical Pap test slides usually derives from a superficial infection, and aggregates or stacks of squamous cells are seen entangled in pseudohyphae with often scanty inflammation. Vaginal candidiasis is discussed elsewhere in this text. *Candida* vaginitis is rarely misdiagnosed as another type of infection, but we have

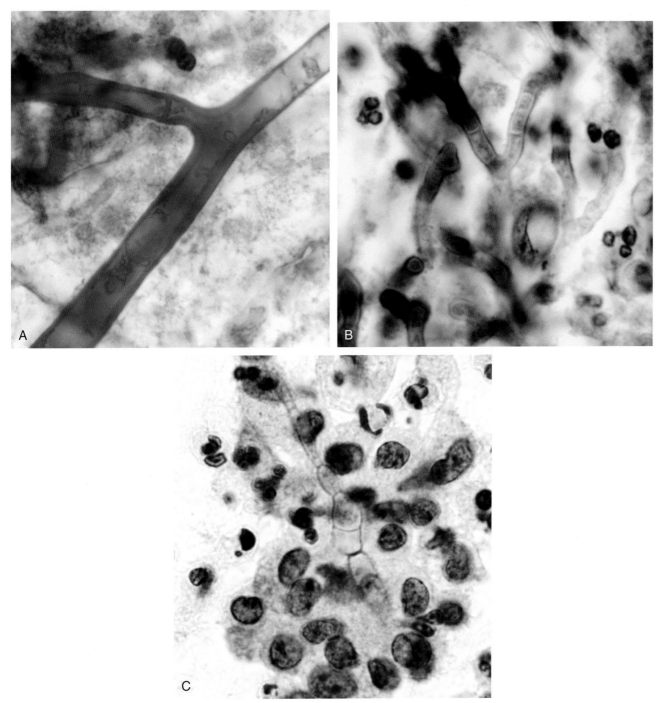

Figure 4-39. Comparison of fungal hyphae in Papanicolaou-stained preparations. **A,** Zygomycete (*Rhizopus* sp. by culture) with easily seen broad hyphae. **B,** Culture-proven *Aspergillus* sp. showing more narrow hyphae. **C,** Dematiaceous fungus (*Phialophora verrucosa* by culture) showing brown cell wall and moniliform pseudohyphae (Papanicolaou, ×2000).

seen a couple of instances of spermatozoa misinterpreted as *Candida* in liquid-based preparations. Invasive candidiasis cannot be distinguished from upper tract contamination or superficial candidiasis on the basis of brushings, washings, or BAL; however, the finding of blastoconidia and pseudohyphae in a visceral organ aspirate or an ulcerative lesion with pseudomembrane formation should suggest invasive fungal infection in the proper clinical

setting. Figure 4-40 illustrates the postmortem scrapings from the rectum of a severely neutropenic patient with ulcerative, pseudomembranous lesions of the esophagus and rectum. In the Papanicolaou-stained sample, note the fibrinous exudate associated with presence of colonic-type columnar epithelium and fungal pseudohyphae. Cytologic evaluation of ulcer scrapings allowed for a preliminary diagnosis of candidiasis and excluded

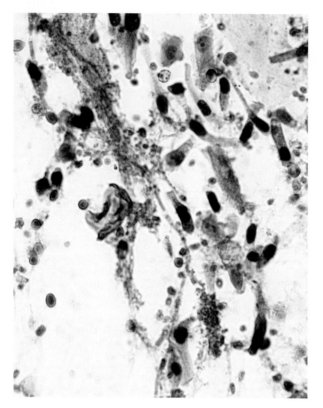

Figure 4-40. Postmortem scrape preparation of pseudomembranous proctitis secondary to *Candida albicans.* Colonic columnar epithelial cells and fungal blastoconidia and pseudohyphae are seen admixed with fibrin (Papanicolaou, ×400).

other causes of ulcerative mucosal lesions (e.g., herpesvirus, cytomegalovirus). On the basis of the gross appearance, at least superficial invasive disease was suspected. Candidiasis was confirmed by histologic sections examined subsequently. The only fungus likely to be confused with *Candida* is *Trichosporon,* which can cause invasive disease in immunosuppressed hosts. Differentiation is by culture and by the slightly larger size, greater pleomorphism, and presence of arthroconidia in GMS-stained preparations of *Trichosporon.*[69]

Case 13: Diabetes and Intrabronchial Zygomycosis with Indolent Course

A 37-year-old diabetic man presented with isolated solitary pulmonary and renal lesions. Sputum, urine, and kidney FNA contained zygomycete fungi. Urine and kidney FNA findings are seen in Figure 4-41. Note the presence of neutrophils and broad, well-stained, ribbon-like hyphae typical of zygomycetes. This patient proved to have locally invasive intrabronchial zygomycosis with an isolated mycotic renal abscess. Cultures of both sites grew *Rhizopus* sp. This case illustrates an unusual, indolent presentation of zygomycosis in a non-neutropenic patient who had diabetes mellitus.[65,66] Cytologic examination could only diagnose zygomycosis. Histologic studies of the resected lung lesion demonstrated chronic, intrabronchial zygomycosis, a condition analogous to chronic necrotizing aspergillosis. The kidney lesion was also resected, and no evidence of other infected sites was found subsequently.

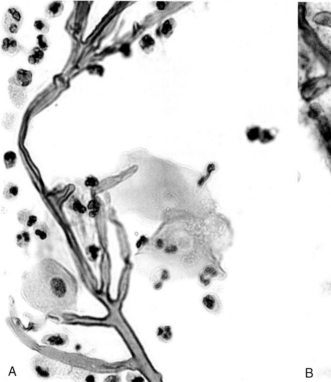
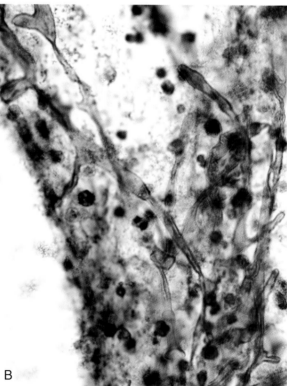

Figure 4-41. Urine (**A**) and (**B**) kidney fine-needle aspirates from a patient with renal and pulmonary zygomycosis. **A,** Large, ribbon-like hyphae are seen admixed with neutrophils. **B,** Necrosis, degenerating inflammatory cells, and broad hyphae are seen (Papanicolaou, ×400).

Severely Impaired Cell-Mediated Immunity and Diffuse Macrophage Infiltration

Patients with severe defects in cell-mediated immunity, such as occurs in HIV infection, have defective T-lymphocyte and macrophage-mediated killing of fungi and *Mycobacteria*. Neither effective killing of microbes nor granuloma formation occurs in these patients. Instead, in some infections, one sees a diffuse infiltration of macrophages containing massive numbers of microorganisms. Several different types of microbes, including *Mycobacteria* (especially MAC), *Leishmania*, and *Histoplasma*, elicit granulomas in immunocompetent patients and diffuse macrophage infiltration in patients with defective cell-mediated immunity. The host reaction to infection with *C. neoformans* varies with the immune status of the individual and the amount of cryptococcal encapsulation.[70,71] Alveolar macrophages and T cell–mediated immunocompetence are of major importance in the defense against this organism.[33,70] Although neutrophils are believed to be important as a second line of defense, they are rarely seen in histologic or cytologic preparations from cases of cryptococcosis. The inflammatory response to *Cryptococcus* varies from well-formed granulomas, as found in chronic, localized infections, to disseminated infection with absence of granuloma formation and minimal inflammation, predominantly macrophages. *Histoplasma* and *Mycobacteria* elicit some interesting inflammatory patterns in T-cell immune-deficient patients, and these are illustrated in the following cases.

Case 14: The Young Lady with the Polka-Dotted Macrophages

A 21-year-old woman presented with chills, fever, weight loss, and an abnormal chest radiograph. CT of the chest (Fig. 4-42) demonstrated anterior mediastinal lymphadenopathy with necrosis, findings suspicious for lymphoma. CT-guided FNA of a mediastinal lymph node was done, and a Papanicolaou-stained sample is seen in Figure 4-43. One sees macrophages containing dark, oval "polka dots" surrounded by narrow halos. These oval structures are about 3 μm in length. Findings are very suggestive

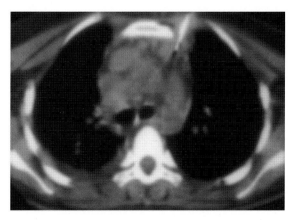

Figure 4-42. Chest computed tomogram demonstrating image-guided fine-needle aspiration of mediastinal lymphadenopathy.

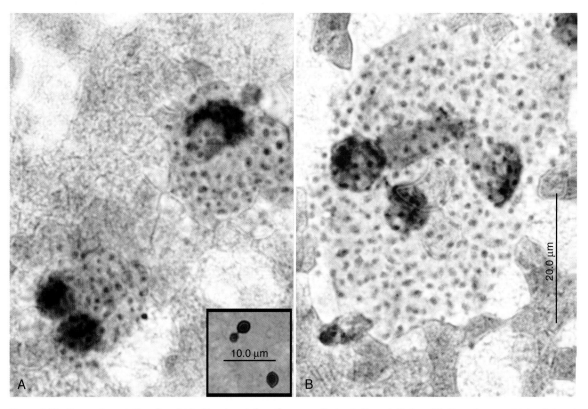

Figure 4-43. Fine-needle aspiration of mediastinal lymph node from the same patient as in Figure 4-42. **A** and **B,** Macrophages containing dark oval structures surrounded by narrow halos are seen (Papanicolaou, ×2000). Budding yeast form is seen in the inset in **A** (GMS, ×1500).

of *H. capsulatum*. The GMS-stained slide contained abundant small yeast with narrow-necked buds, one of which is seen in the inset of Figure 4-43A. Yeast forms are slightly larger in GMS preparations because of precipitation of silver around the organism. Culture confirmed *H. capsulatum*. Based on the cytologic findings of abundant yeast forms and a diffuse macrophage reaction, HIV testing was suggested. HIV serology was positive, and the patient was diagnosed with AIDS. Although the finding of intracellular, small yeast forms of 3 to 5 μm with narrow-necked buds on GMS is suggestive of *H. capsulatum*, the morphology on Romanovski stain is much more specific, as is seen in a BAL sample from a 41-year-old HIV-seropositive man who presented with bilateral, mixed interstitial and alveolar pulmonary infiltrates and air bronchograms on chest radiographs (Fig. 4-44). Abundant, 2- to 3-μm, oval, intracellular yeast forms are seen. These have a characteristic magenta-colored cap of protoplasm, and the remaining internal structure appears light blue or has a clear vacuole. Many yeast forms are surrounded by a narrow halo. This represents retraction of the yeast endoplasm from a very thin cell wall rather than an actual capsule. Nonetheless, the name *H. capsulatum* has persevered. In Romanovski-stained preparations, the organism most resembles the amastigote stages of *Leishmania* sp. and *Trypanosoma cruzi*.

A comparison of *H. capsulatum* and *Leishmania* is seen in Figure 4-45. Another cause of polka-dotted macrophages, albeit rare in Western countries, is *Penicillium marneffei*, a pathogenic dimorphic fungus endemic to southeastern and far eastern Asia (see later discussion). *Candida* blastoconidia also bear some resemblance to *H. capsulatum* in Romanovski-stained preparations, especially *Candida glabrata* that does not form pseudohyphae; however, *Candida* is slightly larger and lacks the

magenta-colored cap. *Candida* also has a pseudocapsule caused by the presence of a thin, nonstaining cell wall. A single dot-like structure consistent with its single nucleus is seen (Fig. 4-46). In this figure, the pathogen is *Candida albicans*, and pseudohyphae are prominent.

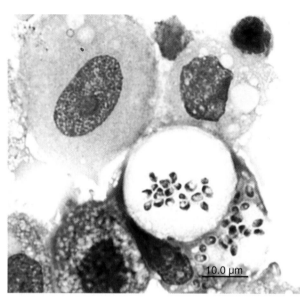

Figure 4-44. Bronchoalveolar lavage sample from a patient with AIDS and histoplasmosis. Alveolar macrophages and small, intracytoplasmic oval yeast forms with a magenta-colored cap are seen. Some contain an intracytoplasmic vacuole (Romanovski, ×1200).

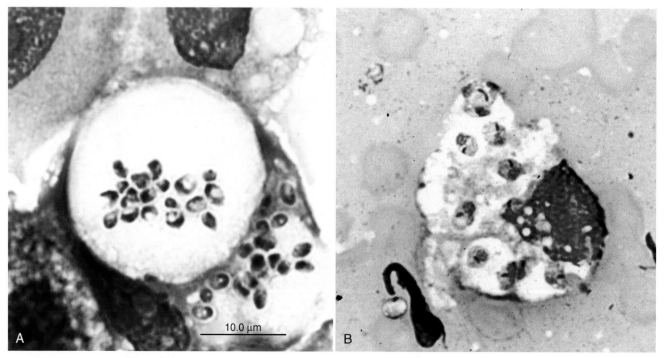

Figure 4-45. Comparison of *Histoplasma capsulatum* and *Leishmania* sp. **A,** *H. capsulatum* with magenta-colored cap and halo. **B,** *Leishmania* sp. with kinetoplast (Romanovski, ×2000).

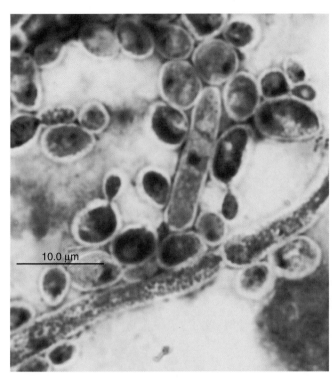

Figure 4-46. Postmortem esophageal brushing demonstrates candidiasis. Budding blastoconidia and pseudohyphae are seen (Romanovski, ×2500).

Case 15: The Macrophage Wore Pinstripes

A 33-year-old man died in hospice. At autopsy, he was found to have hepatosplenomegaly and diffuse subcentimeter nodules throughout his liver and spleen (Fig. 4-47A). During autopsy, touch preparations of spleen were taken. A rapid Romanovski–stained preparation is seen in Figure 4-47B and C. In Figure 4-47B, one can see many white linear structures that represent negatively stained bacilli. Figure 4-47C, taken at a different level of focus, shows refractile reddish-colored bacilli. The macrophages' cytoplasm is not well visualized. This negative staining and refractile appearance is typical of a mycobacterial infection, most commonly MAC.[72] In AIDS patients, the pathogen is usually *Mycobacterium avium-intracellulare*, although other *Mycobacteria* species may be associated with a diffuse macrophage reaction. Although they are reportedly gram-neutral, it has been our experience that some mycobacteria, especially *M. fortuitum* and sometimes MTC, retain the gentian violet dye and appear as beaded, gram-positive bacilli in both the classic Gram and Gram-Weigert stains. In the case presented here, cultures grew MAC. On Papanicolaou stain, intracytoplasmic grayish stripes can sometimes be seen associated with diffuse macrophage infiltration secondary to mycobacteriosis. Pinstriped macrophages lead one to suspect infection and to perform an acid-fast stain, as seen in Figure 4-48, taken from an FNA of an enlarged axillary lymph node in an HIV-positive patient. Note that the

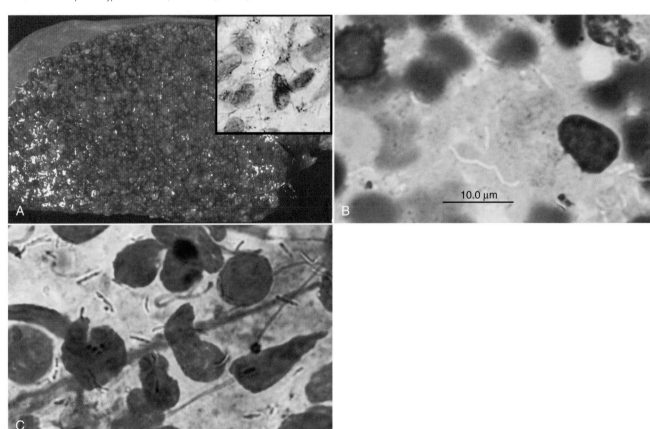

Figure 4-47. Postmortem case of disseminated *Mycobacterium avium* complex in an AIDS patient. **A,** Gross image of spleen at autopsy. Acid-fast bacilli are seen in the inset in **A** (Kinyoun, ×1000). Scrape preparations of spleen demonstrate rod-shaped structures with negative staining **(B)** and refractile, red staining bacilli **(C)** at a different level of focus (Romanovski, ×1200).

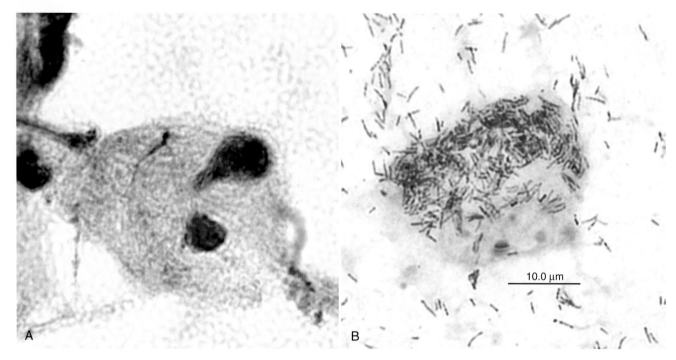

Figure 4-48. Fine-needle aspiration of axillary lymph node from patient with disseminated *Mycobacterium avium* complex. **A,** A macrophage containing intracytoplasmic striations is seen (Papanicolaou, ×2000). **B,** Abundant intracellular and extracellular bacilli are seen (Kinyoun, ×2000).

macrophages are stuffed full of bacilli and have a striated appearance. In acid-fast stained preparations, one might refer to these macrophages as flagellated or flogged. Others have referred to Papanicolaou-stained mycobacteria-laden macrophages as pseudo-Gaucher cells.[73]

An interesting and recently recognized phenomenon associated with AIDS, highly active antiretroviral therapy (HAART), and MAC, as well as other infectious organisms, is immune reconstitution syndrome.[74] In this setting, AIDS patients may have florid granuloma formation. Immune reconstitution syndrome should be considered in patients with marked granuloma formation or other type of inflammatory response, a high CD4 count, and negative cultures despite the presence of visible microorganisms on direct examination.

Case 16: Overstuffed Macrophages with Lysosome Indigestion

A 33-year-old HIV-seropositive man presented with cough. Bilateral pulmonary infiltrates with cavitation in the left upper lobe were found on chest radiography. He had a past medical history of *Rhodococcus* and *M. kansasii* infections. BAL findings are shown in Figures 4-49 and 4-50. The alveolar macrophages appear to be stuffed with globules and vacuoles of varying size (see Fig. 4-49A and B). Focally, vacuoles containing beaded coccobacilli are seen (see Fig. 4-49C); also focally, round, laminated intracytoplasmic inclusions are present (see Fig. 4-49D). Intracytoplasmic, gram-positive coccobacilli can be seen on a Gram-Weigert–stained slide (see Fig. 4-50). There are narrow halos around some of the organisms. The findings are consistent with malakoplakia, and the organisms seen are suggestive of *Rhodococcus* sp.

Pulmonary malakoplakia is a known complication of *Rhodococcus equi* pneumonia in AIDS patients.[75] The bacteria seen here

are morphologically consistent with *Rhodococcus* sp. They are coccoid to diphtheroid and beaded in appearance and can easily be mistaken for streptococci on Gram stain. A narrow halo suggestive of a capsule is seen around some of the bacteria. BAL culture grew *R. equi*. Although its pathogenesis is still controversial, malakoplakia is believed to represent a defect in lysosome-mediated killing of intracellular bacteria and is most commonly found associated with *Escherichia coli* and *Klebsiella* infections of the genitourinary tract.[76] Malakoplakia is characterized by sheets of macrophages containing globules or vacuoles of varying size, some of which may contain bacteria. These globules have been found to be phagosomes, giant lysosomes, and phagolysosomes. Bacteria can often be identified within some of the phagocytic vacuoles.[76,77] Pathognomonic findings are these overstuffed macrophages and the presence of intracytoplasmic, laminated Michaelis-Gutmann bodies that contain traces of iron and calcium. The latter are roughly 3 to 7 μm in diameter and are thought to represent lysosomal calcifications that may form in reaction to undigested bacteria.[78,79]

Descriptions of *Rhodococcus*-associated malakoplakia diagnosed by FNA and BAL have been published.[80,81] We have seen *Rhodococcus* infections in cytologic preparations from FNA of an arm lesion, BAL samples, and in TBNA of a mediastinal lymph node, all in AIDS patients. One BAL sample, illustrated in Figure 4-49D, had typical Michaelis-Gutmann bodies. The TBNA sample contained coccobacilli and macrophages containing large globules; however, Michaelis-Gutmann bodies could not be found.

Figure 4-51 shows PAS-, iron-, and modified acid-fast stains of lung taken at autopsy from a patient who died of *R. equii* pneumonia. The macrophages contain PAS-diastase–resistant globules (see Fig. 4-51A), and iron stain (see Fig. 4-51 inset)

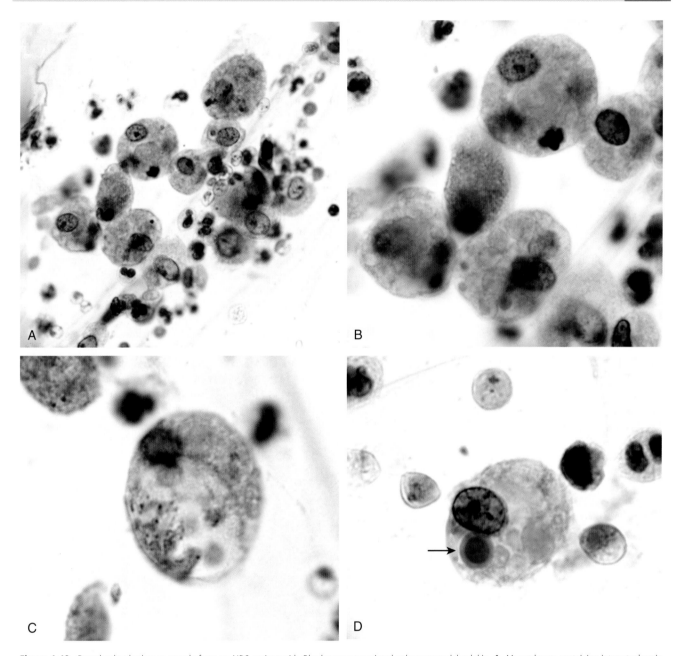

Figure 4-49. Bronchoalveolar lavage sample from an AIDS patient with *Rhodococcus*-associated pulmonary malakoplakia. **A,** Macrophages containing intracytoplasmic globules are seen (Papanicolaou, ×800). Higher magnification illustrates globular cytoplasm **(B)**, intracytoplasmic bacilli **(C)**, and a Michaelis-Gutmann body **(D)** (*arrow*) (Papanicolaou, ×2000).

shows a faintly iron-positive Michaelis-Gutmann body. *Rhodococcus* is sometimes, but not invariably, acid fast when a *Nocardia* modification is used (see Fig. 4-51B). Positive staining of cytologic preparations using Fite stain have been reported.[82]

The overstuffed macrophages of malakoplakia bear some resemblance to the foamy macrophages found in amiodarone therapy; however, the clinical histories and presentations are likely to be quite different. Therapy with amiodarone, an antiarrhythmic agent, is associated with phospholipidosis of the lung and other tissues.[83,84] Some patients develop diffuse alveolar damage secondary to amiodarone toxicity.[84,85] Foamy macro-

phages are only an indication of amiodarone therapy effect, not toxicity; however, absence of foamy macrophages would militate against amiodarone toxicity.[83] It has been debated whether toxicity is directly related to phospholipidosis or a hypersensitivity reaction.[86] Israel-Biet and colleagues found that BAL samples from patients receiving amiodarone, regardless of the presence or absence of toxicity, typically contained macrophages with both clear and dense vacuoles.[86] The dense vacuoles were found to represent phagolysosomes containing phospholipid.

We have also noted two types of vacuoles in BAL from patients receiving amiodarone. Figure 4-52 illustrates BAL find-

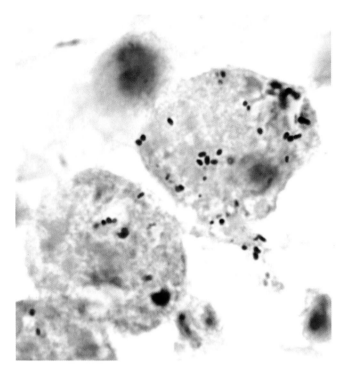

Figure 4-50. Bronchoalveolar lavage sample from the same patient as in Figure 4-49, showing macrophage-containing gram-positive coccoid and bacillary bacteria surrounded by narrow halos (Gram-Weigert, ×2000).

ings in a patient who had been treated with amiodarone. Macrophages containing clear and cyanophilic globules are seen. When we receive a BAL sample with notice of possible amiodarone toxicity, we consider that our main role is to rule out other causes of respiratory failure. One expects to see the foamy macrophages; however, they represent therapy effect, not toxicity, and we usually look for evidence of diffuse alveolar damage. If neutrophils, fibrin, or hyperplastic pneumocytes or fibroblasts are present, we suspect diffuse alveolar damage. This is definitively diagnosed by histologic examination. Figure 4-53 shows an open biopsy from the patient whose BAL result was illustrated in Fig. 4-52. Interstitial fibrosis, lymphoplasmacytic inflammation, and foamy macrophages are seen. Bronchiolitis obliterans (not illustrated) was also noted. No specific infection or other causative agents were found, and the findings were considered consistent with amiodarone toxicity.

Pulmonary alveolar proteinosis (PAP) is, like malakoplakia, a disease related to macrophage dysfunction. The acquired form of PAP appears to be caused by defects in granulocyte-macrophage colony-stimulating factor (GM-CSF)–mediated surfactant catabolism by alveolar macrophages.[87] As with malakoplakia and amiodarone effect, foamy macrophages are present in BAL samples from patients with PAP; however, in PAP, there is generally an abundance of extracellular granular and globular material and a relative paucity of macrophages (Fig. 4-54).[88,89] If this pattern is seen in a BAL sample, one immediately asks to see the centrifuged BAL fluid. The fluid typically has 1 to 2 cm of precipitate in the bottom of the tube. The pulmonologist usually

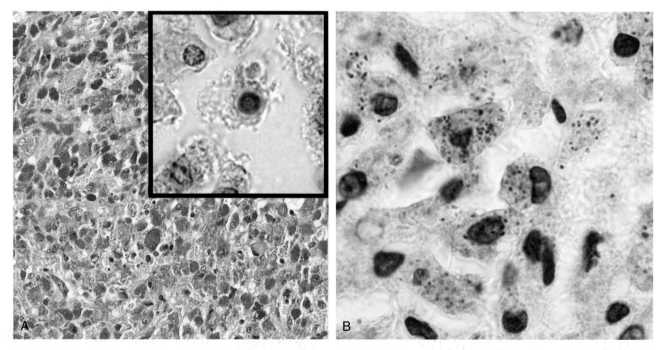

Figure 4-51. Autopsy sections of lung from a patient with *Rhodococcus* pulmonary malakoplakia. **A,** Sheets of macrophages containing pink material (periodic acid–Schiff with diastase, ×400). Inset shows a Michaelis-Gutmann body (Prussian blue stain, ×1000). **B,** Intracellular coccobacilli (Fite, ×1000).

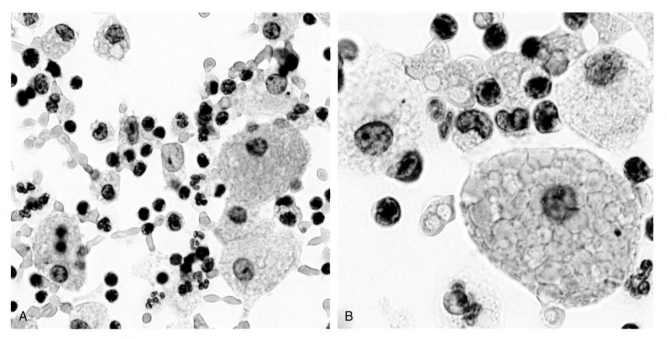

Figure 4-52. Amiodarone effect in bronchoalveolar lavage fluid. **A,** There are some macrophages containing clear vacuoles; others have cyanophilic vacuoles (Papanicolaou, ×600). **B,** High power illustrates the intracytoplasmic vacuoles (Papanicolaou, ×1000).

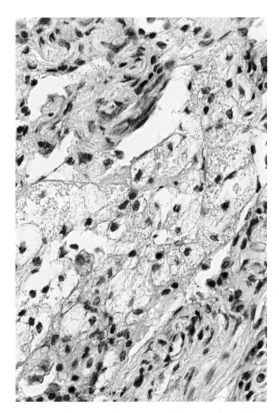

Figure 4-53. Open lung biopsy from patient with suspected amiodarone toxicity showing fibrosis and presence of foamy macrophages (hematoxylin and eosin, ×400).

has noted that the BAL fluid was markedly turbid when extracted from the bronchus. The granular intracellular and extracellular material seen on microscopic examination of the BAL represents abnormal surfactant that has not been degraded by alveolar macrophages. The intra-alveolar material is largely composed of phospholipid and is PAS positive, diastase resistant. Fine granules and larger globules are seen. The gross appearance of the fluid, the clinical and radiologic findings, and the presence of abundant PAS-positive extracellular material are usually sufficient evidence on which to make a presumptive diagnosis of PAP. In acquired PAP, anti–GM-CSF autoantibodies are typically present and can be used to confirm diagnosis.[87] Electron microscopic examination of the BAL precipitate in cases of PAP demonstrates abnormal surfactant accumulation including the presence of multilamellated structures and, occasionally, abnormally formed tubular myelin lattices.[90,91] In a few cases of PAP, we have submitted an aliquot of BAL sediment for transmission electron microscopy. Figure 4-55 is a transmission electron micrograph derived from a case of acquired PAP in a renal transplantation patient, showing concentrically laminated structures and abnormal tubular myelin lattice formation.

Defective GM-CSF signaling also appears to result in defective macrophage immune function,[87] and patients with acquired PAP are susceptible to a number of opportunistic infections, including, among others, MAC, pneumocystosis, and nocardiosis. It is a good idea to culture and perform special stains for these organisms on BAL sediment. Figure 4-56 illustrates a case of PAP in which fungi consistent with *Cryptococcus* were found in BAL fluid, and *C. neoformans* was cultured subsequently.

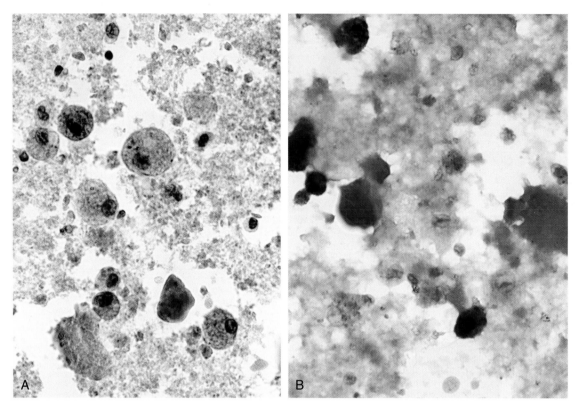

Figure 4-54. Bronchoalveolar lavage sample from a patient with pulmonary alveolar proteinosis. **A,** Abundant granular and globular material with relative paucity of macrophages (Papanicolaou, ×400). **B,** Extracellular and intracellular material is periodic acid–Schiff (PAS) positive, diastase resistant (PAS with diastase, ×400).

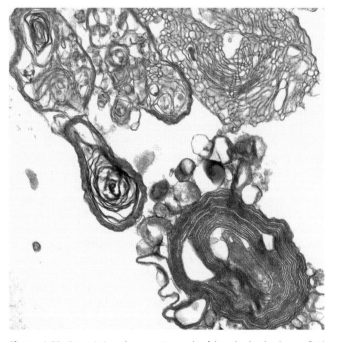

Figure 4-55. Transmission electron micrograph of bronchoalveolar lavage fluid sediment from a case of pulmonary alveolar proteinosis. A typical, concentrically laminated multilamellate body is seen in the lower right, and lattice formation of atypical tubular myelin in the upper right (×15,000). (Electron micrograph image courtesy of Julie Wen.)

Organisms That Elicit Scanty to No Inflammation in Patients with Impaired Cell-Mediated Immunity

Very scanty to no inflammation is seen with *Cryptococcus* and *Pneumocystis* infections in patients with severely impaired cell-mediated immunity. *Cryptococcus*, as mentioned earlier, is associated with granuloma formation in nonimmunocompromised and mildly immunocompromised hosts. *P. jiroveci* (formerly called *Pneumocystis carinii*) was originally described in conjunction with plasma cell pneumonia in malnourished children during and after World War II[92]; today, *P. jiroveci* pneumonia is most commonly seen in patients with AIDS and transplant recipients.[93] In T cell–immunocompromised patients, the inflammatory response to the organism is minimal, usually consisting of macrophages, lymphocytes, and plasma cells.

C. neoformans infection in a severely immunocompromised patient is seen in Figure 4-57. The figure shows Papanicolaou- and mucicarmine-stained cerebrospinal fluid samples from a patient with AIDS. Figure 4-58 shows a sputum sample from another AIDS patient who had both a massive cryptococcal pneumonia and meningitis. Note the absence of inflammatory cells, the round yeast cell shape, and the marked variation in size. The yeast forms often appear purple to red in Papanicolaou stain; however, sometimes they are not well colorized and are difficult to find. Closing the substage condenser helps a lot. Focally, there is crystalline-like material within some of the yeast

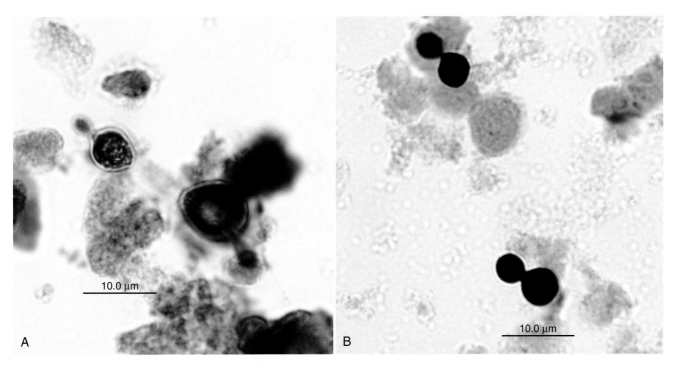

Figure 4-56. Bronchoalveolar lavage sample from a patient with acquired pulmonary alveolar proteinosis and *Cryptococcus* infection. **A,** Budding yeast forms are seen admixed with granular material (Papanicolaou, ×2000). **B,** Budding yeast forms (GMS, ×2000).

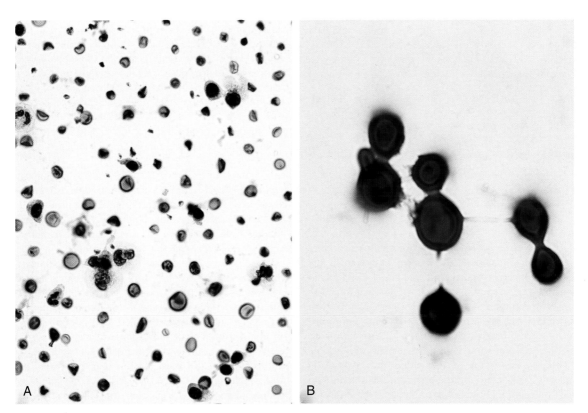

Figure 4-57. Cerebrospinal fluid from patient with AIDS and *Cryptococcus* meningitis. **A,** Round yeast forms of varying size (Papanicolaou, ×400). **B,** Yeast forms are bright red, and blastoconidia are connected to parent yeast by a narrow tube (mucicarmine, ×1000).

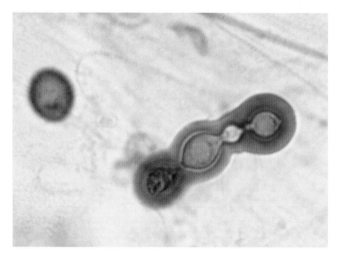

Figure 4-58. *Cryptococcus* forming pseudohyphae in sputum sample from a patient with AIDS. Note thick capsule and crystalline material in the yeast cell in the lower center (Papanicolaou, ×1000).

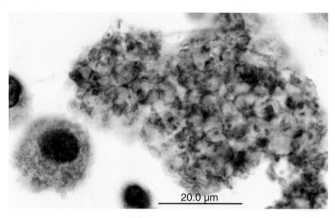

Figure 4-60. Bronchoalveolar lavage sample from an AIDS patient with pneumocystosis. A macrophage is seen on the left and foamy material containing dark dots typical of *Pneumocystis* on the right (Papanicolaou, ×1000).

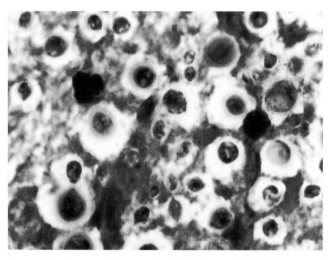

Figure 4-59. Autopsy scrape preparation of spleen from patient with disseminated cryptococcosis (Romanovski, ×1000).

cells. This is typical of *Cryptococcus* in Papanicolaou stain. Note also the abundant capsular material which is best seen in the mucicarmine stain of cerebrospinal fluid (see Fig. 4-57B) and in the Papanicolaou stain of sputum (see Fig. 4-58). Pseudohyphae formation is also common in immunodeficient patients with fulminant infections (see Fig. 4-58). In AIDS patients, symptomatic pulmonary disease is relatively common, and we have seen massive vascular dissemination with involvement of multiple organs at autopsy. Abundant mucin within the cryptococci causes a pink or clear halo around the organism. In Romanovski stains, the cell wall appears bright pink or purple and the capsule clear to pink (Fig. 4-59). Mucicarmine staining is usually not necessary for diagnosis, but it can be done if the identity of the fungus is in doubt. Immunosuppressed patients typically have encapsulated forms of the organism, and mucicarmine is usually strongly positive.

P. jiroveci may be found in cytologic preparations of adequately induced sputum and in BAL fluid. We recommend the addition of a mucolytic agent, followed by centrifugation and cytocentrifugation. This concentrates the sample and provides a small, round area that facilitates examination. Our technique for processing sputum is given in the appendix. Gill and colleagues also recommended use of mucolytic agents and cytocentrifugation for the processing of sputum for *Pneumocystis* diagnosis.[94] This group found peak recovery of organisms by cytocentrifugation at 1200 rpm for 10 minutes. We have found that a combination of Papanicolaou, GMS, and Romanovski stains is usually adequate for evaluation in samples that are concentrated as described. As previously stated, others have touted fluorescent antibody immunostaining and autofluorescence. The take-home message is that laboratory personnel must choose the methods that work best for their individual laboratory. Variations in type of stains used, processing of samples, and expertise of observers with different stain techniques make published studies difficult to compare.

Figure 4-60 shows *P. jiroveci* in a Papanicolaou-stained sample of BAL fluid. Note the bubbly appearance of the "exudate." Also, of great importance, note the small, dark dots within the bubbles. The latter are, in our experience, very characteristic of *P. jiroveci* in Papanicolaou-stained material and possibly represent the dense area in the cyst wall seen on GMS. The so-called foamy exudate is actually not an exudate but rather a massive collection of cysts and extracystic forms of the fungus. With the substage condenser closed, these bubbles appear refractile, as do yeast forms of many other fungi (Fig. 4-61). In a properly performed GMS stain, *P. jiroveci* cysts appear as round structures approximately 6 to 7 µm in diameter with a light gray center containing a black dot representing a thickened area in the cell wall. Under very high power, this area is seen actually to be two small dots (Fig. 4-62). Fibrinous debris, as may be observed in the exudative stage of diffuse alveolar damage or organizing pneumonia, appears stringy and lacks the bubbly appearance of *P. jiroveci*. It should be noted that pneumocystosis may be accompanied by the presence of fibrinous debris and hyperplastic pneumocytes along with clinical findings consistent with acute respiratory distress syndrome.[93,95]

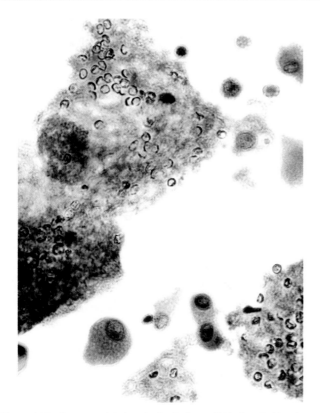

Figure 4-61. *Pneumocystis* in bronchoalveolar lavage fluid, viewed with substage condenser diaphragm closed (Papanicolaou, ×600).

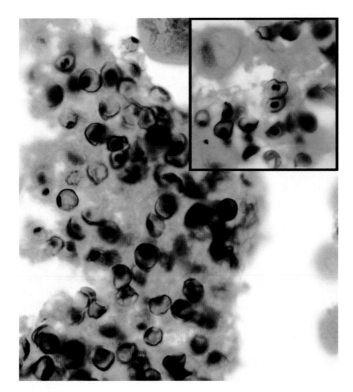

Figure 4-62. *Pneumocystis* in silver-stained bronchoalveolar lavage sample, showing small dots believed to be thickened areas in cyst walls. The inset shows the presence of two small dots within each of two small cysts. (GMS, ×1000).

In Papanicolaou stain, degenerating erythrocytes also appear bubbly and can resemble *P. jiroveci*; however, erythrocytes lack the dots (Fig. 4-63). Romanovski stains color only the intracystic and extracystic bodies; the cyst walls appear clear (Fig. 4-64). The organisms bear a resemblance to malarial trophozoites, although *P. jiroveci* is now classified as a fungus. Evaluation of a Romanovski stain for *Pneumocystis* requires high-power magnification and a good deal of experience, and that may explain its lack of popularity. Nonetheless, in some hands, it is an excellent stain for *P. jiroveci* diagnosis.[16] Individuals who are both accustomed to routine use of Romanovski stain for *P. jiroveci* detection and not reluctant to use high-power magnification are likely to do better than those who are more used to GMS and low power. We have found that, particularly in treated patients, the cysts may stain poorly or not at all with GMS, although one can still see the extracystic stages in Romanovski-stained preparations.

Whereas *P. jiroveci* can potentially be confused with *H. capsulatum*, particularly in overstained GMS preparations, the two organisms appear completely different in Romanovski stains (Fig. 4-65). *P. marneffei* may also be confused with both *H. capsulatum* and *Pneumocystis* in GMS preparations. *P. marneffei* endemicity is limited to southeastern and far eastern Asia and is predominantly an infection of the immunosuppressed, mainly patients with AIDS. The disease caused by *P. marneffei* is remarkably similar to disseminated histoplasmosis.[96,97] *P. marneffei* differs from both *H. capsulatum* and *Pneumocystis* by its division via fission. In GMS stain, the presence of a single transverse septum is characteristic of *P. marneffei*; this feature is not seen in either *Histoplasma* or *Pneumocystis*. In FNA samples, *P. marneffei* organisms appear as intracytoplasmic, yeast-like cells that very closely mimic *H. capsulatum* in Papanicolaou and Romanovski stains. The presence of division by transverse septa, best seen on GMS, and the absence of budding are important differential characteristics. In Romanovski-stained preparations, the transverse septa of *P. marneffei* appear clear.[98] *P. marneffei* is also somewhat larger and more variable in size than *Histoplasma* and more elongate than *Pneumocystis*. In Romanovski-stained material, *Pneumocystis* can be readily distinguished from *Histoplasma* and *P. marneffei*.

Cytodiagnosis of Viral Infections

Cytodiagnosis of viral infections is limited to those viruses that produce a characteristic cytopathic effect (CPE), and identification hinges on recognizing that effect. The accompanying inflammatory pattern, or lack thereof, is generally not useful for diagnosis. Although viral infection can be detected by recognition of the CPE, the clinical relevance of the virus cannot necessarily be predicted on the basis of cytology. The site at which the viral CPE is found and the clinical findings are very important in determining the significance of the infection. The main viruses that are identified by CPE in cytology include human papillomavirus (HPV), herpes simplex virus (HSV)/varicella-zoster (VZ), Cytomegalovirus, adenovirus, molluscum contagiosum (a poxvirus), and human polyomavirus. Formerly known as koilocytosis, the CPE of a productive HPV infection is discussed *ad infinitum* in cytopathology texts and will not be dealt with further here. Respiratory syncytial virus (RSV) and measles also

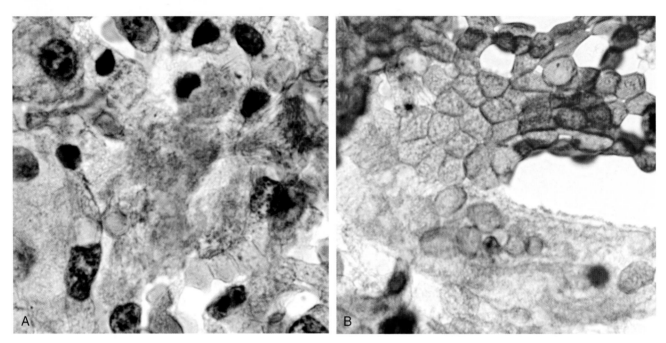

Figure 4-63. Bronchoalveolar lavage samples with fibrin **(A)** and ghosts of erythrocytes **(B)**, findings that could be confused with *Pneumocystis* in Papanicolaou stain (Papanicolaou, ×1500).

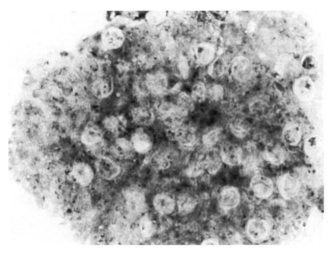

Figure 4-64. Induced sputum containing *Pneumocystis* is seen in Romanovski stain. Cysts are clear, and intracystic and extracystic bodies have bluish cytoplasm and magenta-colored nuclei (Romanovski, ×1000).

cause a CPE that is associated with multinucleated giant cells and with intracytoplasmic inclusions in RSV and both intracytoplasmic and intranuclear inclusions in measles. These CPEs have infrequently been described in cytologic preparations of respiratory samples.[99,100]

The HSV/VZ CPE is best seen in an alcohol wet-fixed, Papanicolaou-stained preparation. Despite the age-old tradition of sending an air-dried smear for Romanovski staining (the Tzanck smear), 95% ethanol wet fixation followed by Papanicolaou staining has unequivocal advantages over an air-dried Romanovski-stained preparation. With the latter, one must look

for multinucleated giant cells with molded nuclei, although these findings are nonspecific. The characteristic feature of HSV/VZ—the complete margination of nuclear chromatin that leaves a clear, glassy nucleoplasm—is not seen in the air-dried Romanovski slide. Neither are intranuclear Cowdry A–type inclusions or intranuclear dispersed particles easily seen in an air-dried preparation. The artifactual chromatin coarsening that occurs with wet ethanol fixation provides much better appreciation of the HSV/VZ CPE.

Case 17: Intensive Care Unit Vocal Cord Lesion

A 62-year-old man died of *S. aureus* endocarditis. He had been intubated and had received prolonged mechanical ventilation. Autopsy revealed the presence of a large mitral valve vegetation, septic emboli, and myocardial abscesses. A 0.5-cm white, roughened area was found on the right vocal cord. An early neoplasm was suspected, and the pathologist made a scraping of the lesion and wet-fixed the slides in 95% ethanol. The cytologic findings in Papanicolaou-stained slides are seen in Figure 4-66. The typical CPE of HSV/VZ is seen. Multinucleation with nuclear molding, complete margination of the nuclear chromatin, dispersed intranuclear viral material, and intranuclear Cowdry A inclusions are seen. The histology of the lesion is seen in Figure 4-67. Sections of lung showed the presence of diffuse alveolar damage. Neither hemorrhagic pneumonitis nor unequivocal viral CPE was found in the lungs. Herpes simplex reactivation is known to occur in patients undergoing prolonged mechanical ventilation; however, the clinical significance of herpesvirus reactivation in tracheobronchial material is still under investigation.[101] The cytopathologist can report the presence of viral CPE, but correlation with the clinical and anatomic pathologic findings is essential for determining its significance.

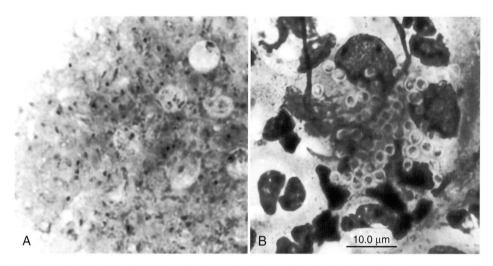

Figure 4-65. Comparison of *Pneumocystis* **(A)** and *Histoplasma* **(B)** in bronchoalveolar lavage fluid (Romanovski, ×1000).

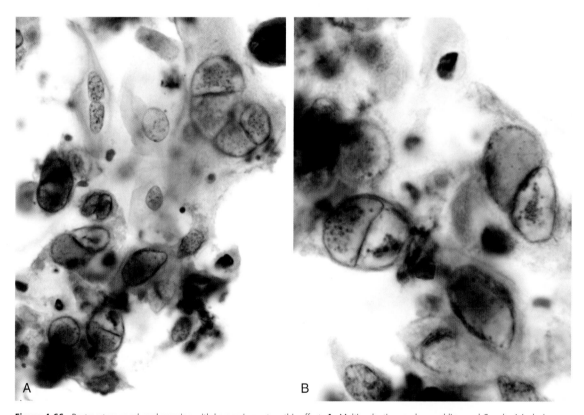

Figure 4-66. Postmortem vocal cord scraping with herpesvirus cytopathic effect. **A,** Multinucleation, nuclear molding, and Cowdry A inclusions are present (Papanicolaou, ×1000). **B,** Dispersed viral material and Cowdry A inclusions are seen (Papanicolaou, ×1500).

When sampling an ulcerative or vesicular lesion for cytologic evaluation for suspected viral infection, it is best to remove the cap of the vesicle and gently scrape the base of the ulcer at the junction of the ulcer crater with the intact epithelium. The CPE is present in the squamous cells at the edge of the ulcer (see Fig. 4-67). If one samples the central portion of the ulcer, there may be no epithelium and no CPE. HSV/VZ CPE must be differentiated from squamous regenerative changes associated with nonspecific ulceration. This can be problematic in the interpretation of cervical Pap tests, as illustrated in Figure 4-68. Note that the intranuclear inclusion of herpesvirus CPE is much larger than the prominent nucleolus found in regenerative changes. Herpes simplex infection of the cervix must also be distinguished from trophoblast and keratinizing SCC, and immunostaining and molecular techniques have been employed.[102]

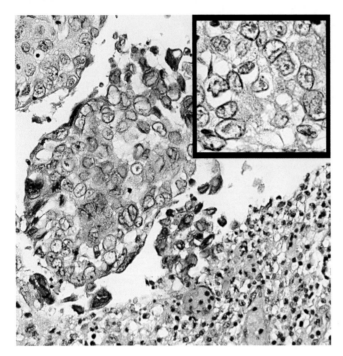

Figure 4-67. Histologic section of ulcerated vocal cord lesion, from the same patient as in Figure 4-66 (hematoxylin and eosin, ×400; inset ×800).

CMV cytopathic effect is beautifully and diagnostically seen in Papanicolaou-stained preparations. As in histologic preparations, the infected cells are enlarged and uninucleated and have single, large, red intranuclear (Cowdry A–type) inclusions that are much larger than a nucleolus. The nuclear chromatin is marginated, leaving a clear space between the inclusion and the nuclear membrane. Intracytoplasmic inclusions are characteristic of CMV CPE; however, these are often not seen in Papanicolaou-stained material, or they appear as fuzzy, blue-gray colored areas. The intracytoplasmic inclusions are much more readily apparent in Romanovski-stained, air-dried preparations, where they appear as multiple, small, round balls, whereas the intranuclear inclusions are less well seen. BAL samples containing CMV CPE in Papanicolaou and Romanovski stains are shown in Figure 4-69. Early infections may lack cells with typical CMV CPE, and immunostaining, in situ hybridization, and other molecular techniques may be useful for documenting infected cells in biopsy or BAL samples if clinically significant infections are suspected.[103] On the other hand, CMV CPE may be found in cytologic preparations from patients lacking clinically significant manifestations of CMV disease, and clinical correlation is mandatory. CMV, like HSV/VZ, may colonize the conducting airways or other organs without causing overt disease. CMV CPE has been reported in cervical Papanicolaou tests,[104,105] but this finding is not necessarily indicative of symptomatic disease.

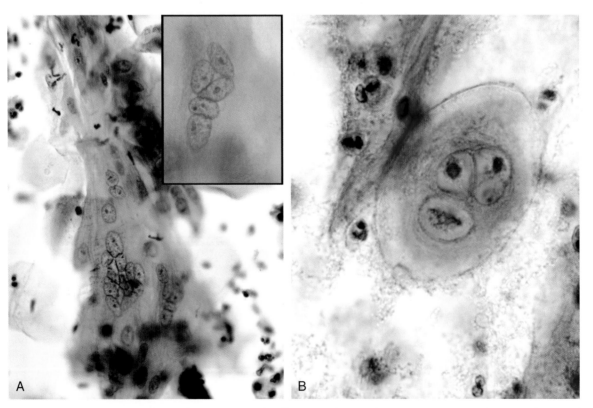

Figure 4-68. Regenerative changes compared with herpes cytopathic effect in cervical Papanicolaou tests. **A,** Regenerative changes are characterized by preservation of fine chromatin and presence of small nucleoli (Papanicolaou, ×400; inset ×1000). **B,** Herpesvirus cytopathic effect features large intranuclear inclusions and margination of chromatin (Papanicolaou, ×1000).

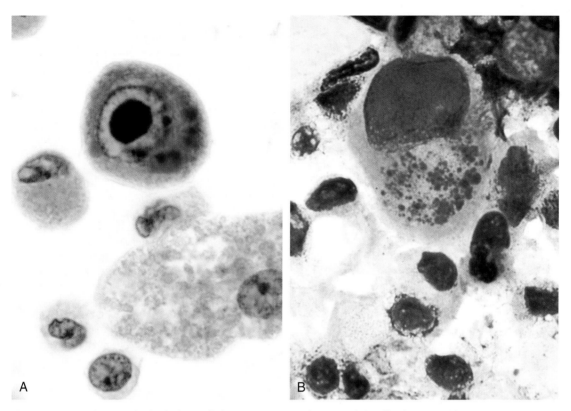

Figure 4-69. A and **B,** Bronchoalveolar lavage fluid containing cytomegalovirus cytopathic effect (**A,** Papanicolaou; **B,** Romanovski, both ×1500).

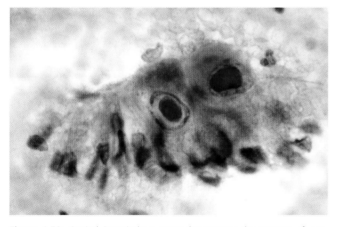

Figure 4-70. Cervical Papanicolaou smear demonstrates the presence of cytomegalovirus cytopathic effect in endocervical columnar cells (Papanicolaou, ×1000).

Although rarely seen in Papanicolaou tests, CMV shedding has been demonstrated by polymerase chain reaction (PCR) in a large number of women infected with HIV-1.[105] We have seen CMV CPE twice in Pap smears, one from a woman with advanced AIDS and disseminated CMV (Fig. 4-70), and the other from a healthy, asymptomatic woman. In cervical Pap tests, CMV CPE is usually found within the endocervical gland cells rather than the squamous cells, where one typically sees HSV CPE.

Case 18: Is It Herpes or Molluscum?

Ethanol-fixed scrapings were prepared from erythematous, roughened, and focally vesicular lesions that followed a dermatome pattern on the chest of a 16-year-old boy with Wiskott-Aldrich syndrome and a history of VZ infection. The pediatric oncologists wanted to know whether the lesions represented recurrent HSV/VZ or molluscum contagiosum. The Papanicolaou stain findings are seen in Figure 4-71. Anucleated keratin and foci of large, smudgy, oval inclusions are seen. The cell nuclei cannot be seen. These smudgy structures are in fact intracytoplasmic inclusions that fill essentially the entire cytoplasm. The cell nuclei are pushed to the side and are not seen in the cytologic preparations. The findings are typical of the CPE caused by the poxvirus responsible for molluscum contagiosum and are not compatible with HSV/VZ. In this case, the vesicular and eczematoid gross appearance of the skin lesions and the past history of VZ necessitated ruling out herpes viral infection.

One should be aware that adenovirus infection may be confused with CMV or herpes. All three viruses can produce severe interstitial pneumonia in immunosuppressed patients. Figure 4-72 illustrates a postmortem lung FNA from a patient with Kartagener syndrome who had undergone lung transplantation and died of fulminant adenovirus pneumonia. Note the lack of cell enlargement and the presence of smudge cells and intranuclear inclusions. Adenovirus was confirmed by culture and immunostaining.

Case 19: To Immunosuppress or Immunoenhance; That Is the Question!

A urine sample was received from a 45-year-old kidney transplant recipient with acute renal failure. Figure 4-73 illustrates a Papanicolaou-stained cytospin slide preparation of a centrifuged urine sample. Note the presence of degenerated cellular debris. The sample is hypercellular and contains atypical, enlarged and pleomorphic epithelial cells that are worrisome for neoplasia; however,

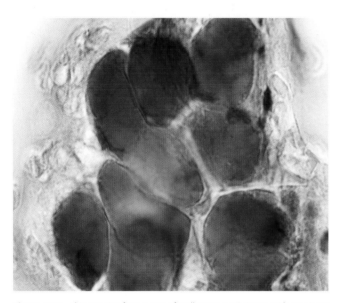

Figure 4-71. Skin scraping from a case of molluscum contagiosum with prominent intracytoplasmic inclusions (Papanicolaou, ×1000).

it should also be noted that many of the cells appear highly degenerated. They have granular cytoplasm and anisonucleosis. In some cells, the nuclei appear smudgy and have margination of the chromatin. Within other images, the chromatin appears grossly and irregularly clumped. Large intranuclear inclusions with clearing of the surrounding nuclear chromatin are seen in some cells, and focally mitotic figures and binucleation are also seen. In this case, there was positive nuclear immunostaining for BK virus large T antigen, and electron microscopy, performed on urine sediment for teaching purposes, demonstrated typical intranuclear polyomavirus particles (Fig. 4-74). Renal biopsy demonstrated the presence of interstitial nephritis and abundant intranuclear inclusions within the renal tubules.

Widely known in the cytology vernacular as decoy cells, courtesy of a senior cytotechnologist at Memorial Hospital during the 1950s,[106] urothelial cells with polyomavirus CPE are notorious mimics of malignancy. The urine cytopathology of BK virus infection has been intricately described.[106,107] Urine cytology has been found to be a sensitive test for detection of BK viral infection; however, it is again important to point out that the presence of viral inclusions in the urine does not necessarily indicate BK virus nephropathy. Distinguishing between polyomavirus-induced renal failure and acute rejection is essential, because the former is treated by decreasing, and the latter by increasing, immunosuppression. Renal biopsy represents the gold standard for confirming polyomavirus nephropathy.[108]

The take-home message for those diagnosing viral infections by cytology is that viral disease may occur without CPE, and CPE indicative of active viral infection may occur without symptomatic disease! Clinical and, in some instances, histologic correlation may be required.

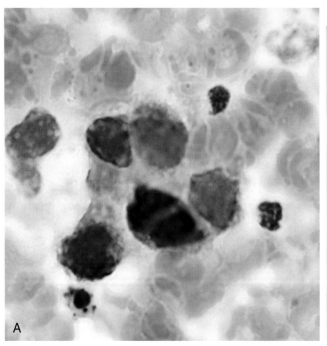
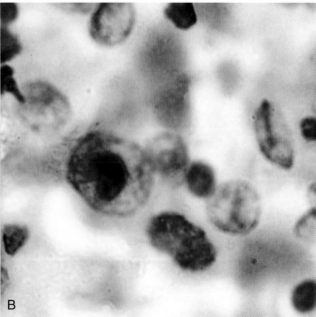

Figure 4-72. Fine-needle aspiration of lung from a case of adenovirus pneumonia. **A,** Smudge cells with focal margination of chromatin. **B,** Intranuclear inclusion (Papanicolaou, ×1500).

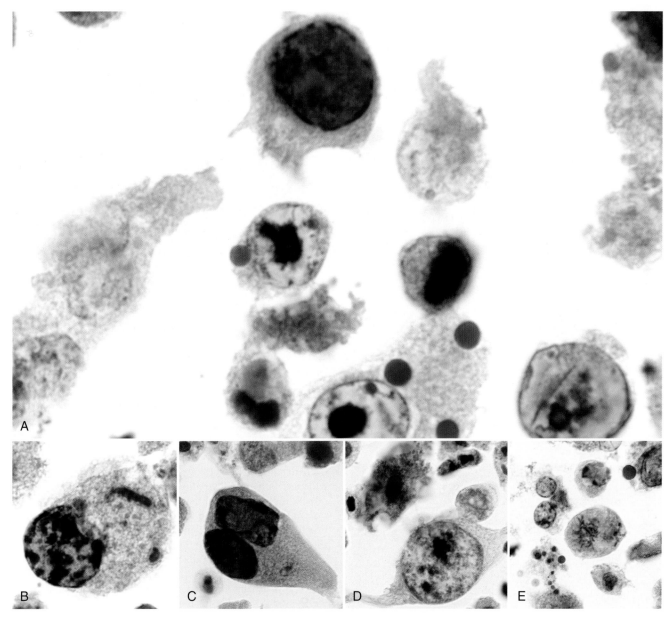

Figure 4-73. Voided urine sample from a case of BK virus nephropathy in a renal transplantation patient. **A,** Hypercellular sample with granular debris and atypical cells. Margination of chromatin and intranuclear inclusions are seen. **B,** Cell with coarsely clumped chromatin. **C,** Smudged chromatin. **D,** Cell with coarsely clumped chromatin. **E,** Mitotic activity (Papanicolaou, ×1500).

Parasitic Disease in Cytology

In parts of the world where protozoan and helminthic diseases are common, parasite infections are more frequently found in cytologic preparations than in northern climates; however, one should never be complacent about diagnosis of parasitic disease by cytology, and knowledge of the basic morphology of some of the more common pathogens is useful. Also, one should always be on the lookout for something new and different. To paraphrase a line from *Forrest Gump*, examination of an FNA is like a box of chocolates: you never know what you are going to get. Figure 4-75 illustrates a portion of a cestode larva—a sparganum,

to be more precise—that emerged from the FNA puncture site of a thigh nodule found in an elderly woman originally from rural Louisiana. It appeared that the newly materialized stuff was gauze or mucus, so the faculty pathologist decided to pull on the structure, and out came approximately 3 cm of cestode larva. This was duly placed in a cell-block preparation and proved, by histologic sections, to be consistent with a sparganum, the larval form of *Spirometra* sp. This adventure resulted in resolution of the thigh nodule and no surgery for the happy patient and disappointed surgeon.

The parasite most commonly seen in cytology in the United States is *Trichomonas vaginalis*; this protozoan is discussed in the chapter on cervical pathology. *Entamoeba histolytica* has also

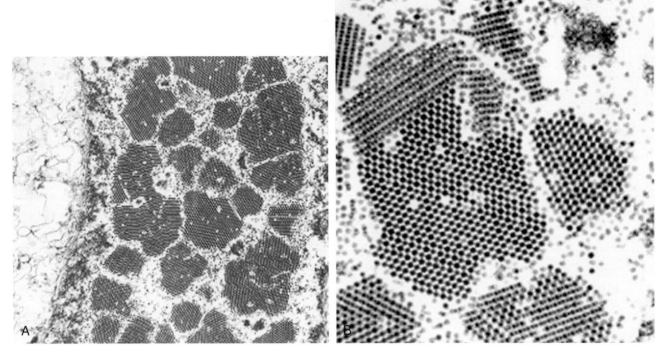

Figure 4-74. Transmission electron micrograph of urine sediment from the same patient as in Figure 4-73, showing intranuclear icosahedral viral capsids. (**A,** ×15,500; **B,** ×39,000). (Electron photomicrographs courtesy of Julie Wen.)

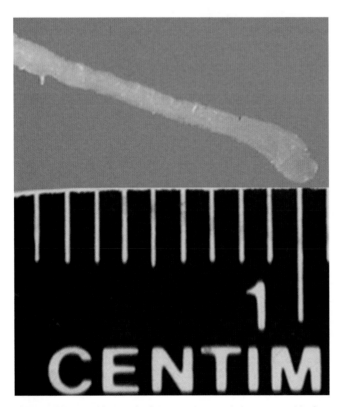

Figure 4-75. Gross photograph of *Sparganus,* a cestode larva extracted by fine-needle aspiration from a thigh mass.

been diagnosed by cytology in areas where the protozoan is endemic.[109] Numerous individual case reports of cytodiagnosis of parasitic infections can be found in the literature, and discussion of them all is beyond the scope of this chapter. Instead, we briefly cover a few of the infections more commonly found in the United States, with a couple of zebras thrown in for fun.

Giardia lamblia is a ubiquitous protozoan that is common in the United States and throughout the world. In the United States, it is usually transmitted via drinking water contaminated with sewage or wild animal excreta.[110] The pear-shaped trophozoite stage of *G. lamblia* has a ventral concave surface and a convex dorsal surface. It is found in the small intestine, where it lies along the surface of the epithelium. *G. lamblia*, therefore, is readily picked up in duodenal brushings (Fig. 4-76); however, because of its small size, roughly 15 μm in length, it can easily be missed. High-power magnification reveals a pear-shaped, flagellated organism with two prominent nuclei that give the trophozoite the appearance of a face or "Mardi Gras mask."

S. stercoralis is an important nematode for the cytology professional to remember. The life cycle of this nematode is reviewed in parasitology texts.[110] However, two aspects of *S. stercoralis* are important to emphasize here:

1. Subclinical infections with *S. stercoralis* may persist for 30 to 40 years or even longer.
2. Immunosuppression (most importantly treatment with corticosteroids) and severe malnutrition can lead to a life-threatening, often fatal, hyperinfection.[110-113]

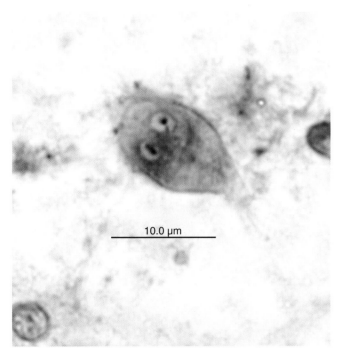

Figure 4-76. Duodenal brushing containing *Giardia lamblia* trophozoite (Papanicolaou, ×3000).

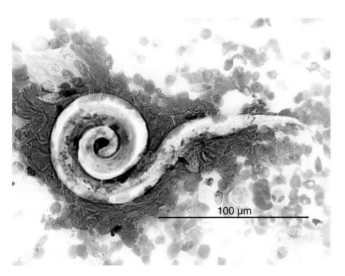

Figure 4-77. Bronchial brushing from patient with *Strongyloides stercoralis* hyperinfection. Larva admixed with blood is seen (Papanicolaou, ×400).

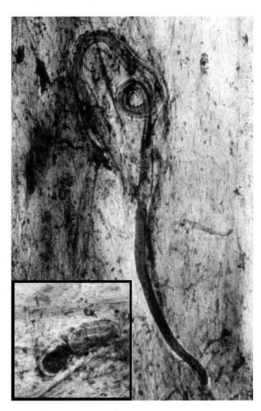

Figure 4-78. Sputum sample from a patient with *Strongyloides* hyperinfection shows adult worm and eggs (*inset*) in respiratory material (Papanicolaou, ×100; inset ×1000).

During hyperinfection, literally millions of worms pass through the lungs. This massive worm migration leads to pulmonary hemorrhage and bronchopneumonia. Infectious-stage (filariform) larvae can be found in sputum, bronchial washings, brushes, and lavage fluid. Figure 4-77 illustrates a *Strongyloides* larva found in a bronchial brushing sample. We regard this finding as a medical emergency and notify the clinician immediately if nematode larvae are found in respiratory samples. The patients at highest risk for life-threatening infections are those receiving corticosteroids, and screening for persons at risk for strongyloidiasis has been recommended for such patients.[112,113] Usually, only the filariform larval stages are found in the lung; rarely, however, adolescents, adults, and eggs have been found. We have seen only one such case, in a patient treated with steroids for chronic obstructive pulmonary disease, who had first-stage larvae, an adult, and eggs in cytologic preparations of his sputum (Fig. 4-78).

Case 20: A Worm with the Wanderlust

A conventional Pap smear is done on a young woman as part of a well-woman examination. The findings are seen in Figure 4-79, in which one sees a portion of nematode with a striated cuticle. Within the worm are oval eggs that have a convex surface and a somewhat more flattened opposing surface. Figure 4-79B, taken from another part of the smear and external to the nematode, shows eggs, roughly 50 μm in length. Some are fully embryonated. The nematode is *Enterobius vermicularis,* also known as pinworm. *E. vermicularis* is an extremely common and ubiquitous parasitic nematode, especially in children who attend school or daycare. The worms dwell in the large intestine, where they mate. The gravid female crawls out onto the perineal skin, usually at night, where she deposits embryonated, and hence infectious, eggs. The female occasionally gets the urge to ramble and can wander into the vaginal canal and even up into the uterus, fal-

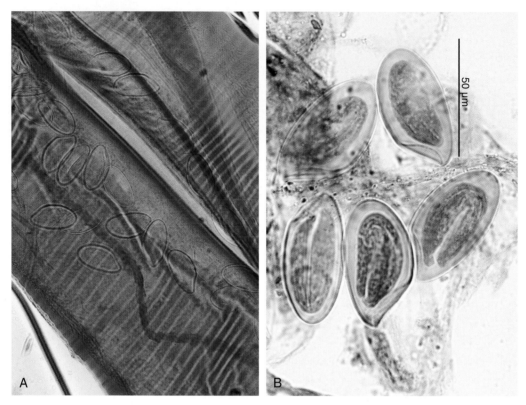

Figure 4-79. Cervical Papanicolaou smear containing portion of *Enterobius vermicularis* female and eggs. **A,** Nematode cuticle and intrauterine eggs (Papanicolaou, ×200). **B,** Embryonated eggs (Papanicolaou, ×400).

lopian tubes, or peritoneal cavity.[114] The adult female is approximately 1 cm in length, and the entire worm or fragments of disintegrating worm can be picked up in Pap smears. The morphology of the egg is characteristic and diagnostic. Usually, this parasite is a harmless, albeit itchy and irritating, nuisance; however, intraperitoneal granulomas and pelvic abscesses have been associated with pinworm infections, with occasional diagnosis by cytology.[115]

As previously stated, it is beyond the capacity of this chapter to cover all parasitic infections that can be or have been diagnosed by cytology. Do not be complacent! One should always be vigilant for interesting and unusual infections and be willing to learn new information about infectious diseases and their diagnosis.

Cases 21 and 22: Parasite Infections Seen in Postmortem Cytology

Smear and FNA preparations taken at autopsy have provided us with some of our most interesting cases, and postmortem cytology has proved excellent for IID diagnosis.[3] The postmortem cytology findings from two interesting parasitic infections found at autopsy are described here.

At autopsy, an enlarged, slate-gray spleen and severe cerebral edema were found in a patient who had died en route home from West Africa. Figure 4-80 shows a Romanovski-stained scrape preparation of spleen. Note the presence of abundant dark golden pigment and a banana-shaped structure containing pigment in the center. In the inset, one sees cuboidal-shaped

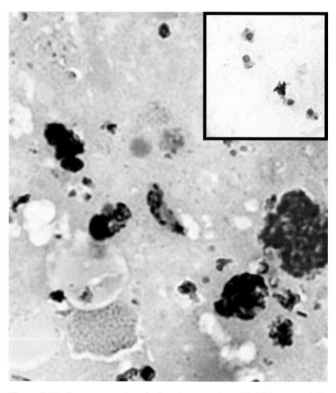

Figure 4-80. Scrape preparation of spleen from a patient with falciparum malaria. Abundant hematin pigment and a gametocyte are present (Romanovski, ×2500). Inset shows asexual forms (Romanovski, ×3000).

asexual forms that have single, eccentrically placed red-dot nuclei and blue-colored cytoplasm. These findings led to a diagnosis of malaria; the clinical findings and banana-shaped structure, morphologically typical of a gametocyte, were consistent with *P. falciparum*. Cerebral malaria was confirmed by histologic sections of brain.

Figure 4-81 illustrates a scraping of brain from an immunosuppressed patient who died with severe pneumonia. Necrotizing bronchopneumonia and hemorrhagic cerebral lesions were found at autopsy. Histologic sections established a diagnosis of free-living amebic pneumonia and encephalitis.[116] The primary diagnosis, in this case, was not made by cytology; however, the cytologic preparations of brain provided useful teaching material. In Figure 4-81A, one sees a small, rounded structure, about 12 µm in diameter. It has a small nucleus containing a large karyosome similar to that seen in *Entolimax nana*. This was a free-living ameba, later identified as a species of *Acanthamoeba*. Compared with the macrophage (see Fig. 4-81B), with which these organisms can be confused, the ameba has a much smaller nucleus, and a vacuole surrounds the cytoplasm. Figure 4-82A

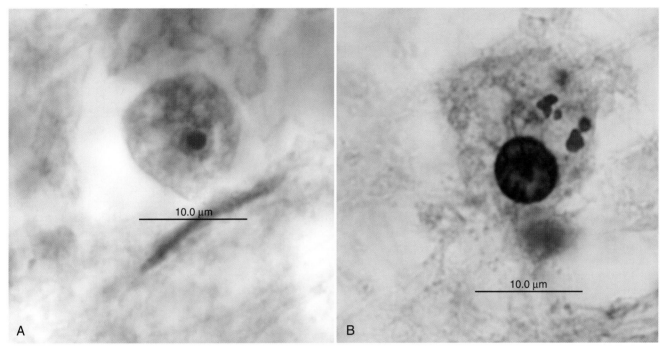

Figure 4-81. Touch preparation of brain from a patient with *Acanthamoeba* pneumonia and encephalitis. **A,** Free-living ameba with large intranuclear karyosome. **B,** Macrophage with larger nucleus and absence of karyosome (Papanicolaou, ×3000).

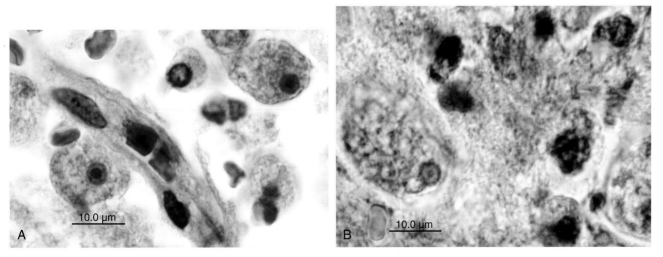

Figure 4-82. Histologic sections of *Acanthamoeba,* from the same patient as in Figure 4-81 **(A)**, and *Entamoeba histolytica* proctitis (hematoxylin and eosin, ×1500).

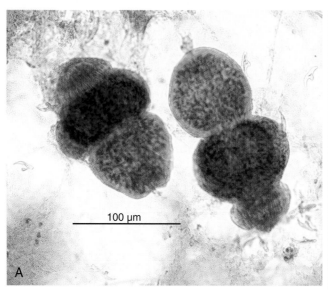

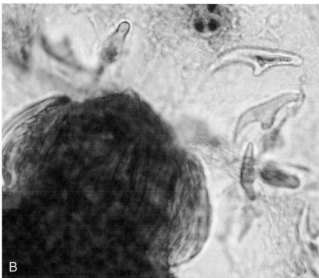

Figure 4-83. Fine-needle aspiration of hepatic echinococcal hydatid cyst. **A,** Two scoleces are present (Papanicolaou, ×400). **B,** Rostellum of scolex with many hooklets is present (Papanicolaou, ×1000). (Glass slide donated courtesy of Dr. A. Joe Saad.)

is an H&E-stained section of the brain showing two free-living amebic trophozoites gathering around a capillary. For comparison, a section of *E. histolytica* from a rectal ulcer biopsy is shown in Figure 4-82B. The sizes are similar; however, the *E. histolytica* karyosome is much smaller and often is difficult to see in sections. Both organisms have a much smaller nucleus-to-cytoplasm ratio than do macrophages. Free-living amebas are well-known causes of keratitis in contact lens wearers and in patients who have sustained ocular trauma.[117] Impression smear cytology has been used to diagnose amebic keratitis in a limited number of cases.[118]

Cestode larvae that are pathogenic for humans include mainly *Echinococcus granulosus* (hydatid cyst), *Echinococcus multiceps,* and *Taenia solium* (cysticercus cellulosae). Cestode larvae have occasionally been aspirated by FNA. Figure 4-83 illustrates the scoleces of a hepatic hydatid cyst. Note the hooklets arranged around the rostella of the scoleces and the free-lying hooklets.

There are certainly other parasites that may be found by cytodiagnosis; here we have only attempted to discuss some of the more common pathogens and a few unusual and interesting cases. For discussions of trematodes (flukes) and ectoparasites, the reader is referred to parasitology textbooks.

Conclusion

One cannot diagnose infectious diseases if one does not think about them. Infections are often treatable and curable, and skillful diagnosis by the cytopathologist can be of enormous benefit to both patient and clinician by providing a rapid and accurate preliminary diagnosis and material for appropriate cultures with minimally invasive techniques. IID should share the front burner of cytopathology education with neoplasia.

APPENDIX
Sample Preparation and Staining for Diagnosis of Infectious and Inflammatory Diseases Including *Pneumocystis*

This section provides a few modifications of sample preparation and staining procedures that have been found useful for diagnosis of IID. The author wishes to acknowledge Steven Burke, BS, for his assistance with composition of the Appendix.

Bronchoalveolar Lavage and Induced Sputum Evaluation for *Pneumocystis*

Staining for *Pneumocystis jiroveci* is performed on induced sputum samples or bronchoalveolar lavage (BAL) samples.

BAL samples usually contain 10 to 20 mL of fluid. The sample is first centrifuged at a relative centrifugal force (RCF) of 600 *g* for 5 minutes. The supernatant is drawn off with a pipette or by decanting, leaving 1 to 2 mL of fluid for resuspension of the sediment. Two to four drops of suspension, depending on the turbidity of the suspension, is placed into each of four cytocentrifuge specimen holders (Shandon Scientific Limited, Cheshire, UK); 2 drops of normal saline are added to the chambers, and the specimens are cytocentrifuged for 2 minutes at 1200 rpm. Three of the slide preparations are fixed in 95% ethanol for Papanicolaou and Gomori/Grocott methenamine silver (GMS) staining, and one is air dried for Giemsa staining.

It is our policy to routinely prepare two additional ethanol-fixed cytospin preparations, one Kinyoun and one Gram-Weigert, for BAL samples from severely immunosuppressed patients, in order to evaluate for bacterial, actinomycete, and mycobacterial infections.

Preparation of Sputum Samples

Sputum samples for detection of *Pneumocystis* should be induced by trained respiratory therapy personnel. In the laboratory, a mucolytic agent is added to make the specimen adequately fluid for centrifugation and cytocentrifugation.

Procedure

Reagents

- Sputum sample, approximately 2 to 10 mL, usually received in clean specimen cup
- Dithiothreitol:Mucolyse (Pro-Lab Diagnostics, Ontario, Canada)
- Normal saline

Technique

1. Approximately 10 mL of distilled water is added to the dithiothreitol powder vial and agitated until the powder is dissolved. The contents of the vial are then added to a container of water to make a final volume of 100 mL.
2. The mucolytic agent solution is then added to the sputum container at a ratio of 1 to 3 times the volume of sputum, placed in a 50-mL conical centrifuge tube, and vortexed for 15 to 30 seconds. The solution is then allowed to stand at room temperature for 1 to 3 hours or until the sputum sample appears liquid and nonviscous. (Fifteen minutes has been recommended by the manufacturer for culture purposes; however, we have found that more than 1 hour is required for optimal cytocentrifuge preparations. Also, Gill and colleagues[94] reduced the mucolysis period to 3 to 5 minutes by incubating in a 37° C waterbath).
3. The sample is then centrifuged at 600 RCF for 5 minutes. The supernatant is decanted, the sediment is resuspended in approximately 5 mL of normal saline.
4. Four cytocentrifuge preparations are made as described earlier. One is allowed to air dry, and the others are wet–fixed in 95% ethanol. Cytocentrifuge preparations are made on clear, ionized (charged) slides to minimize sample loss.

Staining

Standard staining for sputum with request for *P. jiroveci* is as follows:

1. Two ethanol-fixed cytocentrifuge preparations stained by non-gynecologic Papanicolaou method
2. One air-dried cytocentrifuge preparation stained by Giemsa Romanovski method
3. One ethanol-fixed cytocentrifuge preparation stained by microwave modification of GMS stain as described in the following section.

Microwave Modification of Gomori/Grocott Methenamine Silver Stain for Fungi including *Pneumocystis*

Types of Samples

- Formalin—fixed, paraffin-embedded sections, air dried or fixed with 95% ethanol
- Fixed smears
- Cytocentrifuge preparations.

Procedure

Reagents

- 5% CHROMIC ACID*
  Chromic acid..............5 g
  Distilled water.......100 mL
  Chromic acid is an irritant and should be stored in an acid cabinet. Coplin jars with 5% chromic solution are stored under a chemical fume hood.

- 5% SILVER NITRATE SOLUTION*
  Silver nitrate...........................5 g
  Distilled water..................100 mL

- 3% METHENAMINE SOLUTION
  Hexamethenamine USP............3 g
  Distilled water...................100 mL

- 5% BORAX SOLUTION
  Borax....................................5 g
  Distilled water..................100 mL

- STOCK METHENAMINE SILVER NITRATE SOLUTION
  5% Silver nitrate solution........5 mL
  3% Methenamine solution...100 mL

  Note: A white precipitate will form when reagents are first combined. This will dissolve with agitation. Store stock solution in the refrigerator at 5° C to 10° C in a dark or opaque, sealed bottle. Although this is supposed to be fairly stable, it is best not to make up more than stated or more than can be consumed in 2 weeks.

- WORKING METHENAMINE SILVER NITRATE SOLUTION
  5% Borax...2 mL
  Distilled water...25 mL
  Methenamine silver nitrate stock solution......25 mL

*Reagents may be doubled or tripled and water added to make up 200- or 300-mL aliquots, if desired.[5]

Note: *This must be made up fresh with every run.* Make up this solution just before initiation of the staining procedure.

- **1% SODIUM BISULFITE SOLUTION†**
  Sodium bisulfite ....1 g
  Distilled water............100 mL

- **2% SODIUM THIOSULFATE SOLUTION†**
  Sodium thiosulfate............2 g
  Distilled water...........100 mL

- **2% GOLD CHLORIDE**

- **STOCK LIGHT GREEN SOLUTION**
  Light green, S.F.................0.2 g
  Distilled water................100 mL
  Glacial acetic acid..............0.2 ml

- **WORKING LIGHT GREEN COUNTERSTAIN**
  Stock light green solution...10 mL
  Distilled water.................50 mL

General Comments

A *Pneumocystis* control slide should be run whenever this stain is done for detection of *Pneumocystis*. Paraffin sections are used for this purpose. The section should be deparaffinized in xylene for 10 minutes or longer. Some controls can be kept in xylene if the stain is run frequently. The control must then be rehydrated through 100% ethanol and 95% ethanol to distilled water before running the stain. Alcohol-fixed cytocentrifuge preparations are placed in distilled water before running. Preparations for GMS staining over Papanicolaou should be placed in xylene to remove coverslip and mountant, then rehydrated up to distilled water. Decolorization of hematoxylin with dilute hydrochloric acid is not necessary.

Technique

1. Loosely place cap on chromic acid jar without test slides or control, and microwave on high for 30 seconds. Place slides in heated chromic acid jar for 1 minute. Overheating or boiling of chromic acid may result in unsatisfactory staining. Always replace hot acid under the fume hood immediately after removal from the oven.

2. Remove slides from chromic acid and place in a Coplin jar filled with distilled water. Rinse slides with distilled water to remove excess chromic acid.

3. Place slides in 1% sodium metabisulfite for 30 to 60 seconds to clear.

4. Place slides back in Coplin jar and rinse in distilled water.

5. Heat methenamine silver working solution in microwaveable Coplin jar for 33 seconds on high. Immediately place slides in heated methenamine silver solution. Ideally, the solution should be clear to faintly gray when removed from the oven. Watch carefully for control specimen color change. Remove slides to a Coplin jar of distilled water. This may vary with laboratory and characteristics of water and solutions. Sometimes the solution must turn a dark black color before ade-

quate staining has occurred. In other instances, a dark color may be indicative of overstaining. Therefore, slides should be removed before the solution turns an opaque black, rinsed in distilled water, and checked under the microscope for staining of control slide.

6. Rinse the control slide in distilled water and examine microscopically for black staining (or brownish red before clearing in gold chloride) of the *Pneumocystis* cysts.

7. If necessary, the time in silver solution can be extended by replacing slides in the warm methenamine solution. If the sample has turned opaque black but no staining has occurred, there is a problem with the reagents, and additional staining will not help. Usually, the problem is that the working silver nitrate methenamine solution is old and must be made up fresh or that the sample was overheated during the microwaving in chromic acid.

8. If staining of the control is adequate, place slides in gold chloride solution for 30 to 60 seconds. Rinse in distilled water.

9. Place slides in Coplin jar filled with 2% sodium thiosulfate for 2 minutes.

10. Rinse in distilled water.

11. Cover with light green working solution for 2 to 5 minutes. Rinse in 95% alcohol, dehydrate to 100% ethanol. Clear with xylene and coverslip.

Results

The *Pneumocystis* cyst wall should stain black with a gray, more lucent center. Often, one or two dark dots are seen within the cyst, representing a thickening in the cyst wall. If the cysts appear solid black without a lucent center or if the background is black, overstaining has occurred, and slides may be difficult to interpret. This should be avoided. Fungi also stain black. When overstained, leukocyte granules, bacteria, and reticulin may also appear black and can lead to misinterpretation.

Problems

Overheating of chromic acid may result in loss of material or nonstaining of organisms. Also, although stock methenamine is fairly stable, we have found that it should be stored in a dark container and should be made up fresh after a couple of weeks or if nonstaining occurs with no other valid explanation.

REFERENCES

1. Suen KC, Yermakov V, Raudales O: The use of imprint technic for rapid diagnosis in post mortem examinations: A diagnostically rewarding procedure. Am J Clin Pathol 1976;65:201-300.
2. Cina S, Smaialek J: Prospects for utilization of post-mortem cytology. Am J Forensic Med Pathol 1997;18:331-334.
3. Schnadig VJ, Molina CP, Aronson JF: Cytodiagnosis in the autopsy suite: A tool for improving autopsy quality and resident education. Arch Pathol Lab Med 2007;131:1056-1062.
4. Walker E, Going JJ: Cytopathology in the post-mortem room. J Clin Pathol 1994;47:714-717.
5. Dada MA, Ansari NA: Post-mortem cytology: A reappraisal of a little used technique. Cytopathology 1997;8:417-420.

†*Reagent can be made in large quantities, if desired.*

6. Bales CE: Laboratory techniques. In Koss LG, Melamed MR (eds): Koss' Diagnostic Cytopathology and its Histopathologic Bases. Philadelphia, Lippincott Williams & Wilkins, 2006.

7. Woods GL, Walker DH: Detection of infection or infectious agents by use of cytologic and histologic stains. Clin Microbiol Rev 1996;9:382-404.

8. Boon ME, Drijve JS: Routine Cytologic Staining Techniques. New York, Elsevier, 1986.

9. Wittekind D: On the nature of Romanowsky dyes and the Romanowsy-Giemsa effect. Clin Lab Haematol 1979;1:247-262.

10. Winn W Jr, Allen S, Janda W, et al. (eds): Koneman's Color Atlas and Textbook of Diagnostic Microbiology, 6th ed. Philadelphia, Lippincott Williams & Wilkins, 2006.

11. Lillie RD: Histopathologic Technic and Practical Histology. New York, Blakiston, 1954,

12. Lennette EH, Balows A, Hausler WJ, et al (eds): Manual of Clinical Microbiology, 4th ed. Washington DC, American Society of Microbiology, 1985.

13. Cheng AG, Chang A, Farwell DG, Agoff SN: Auramine orange stain with fluorescence microscopy is a rapid and sensitive technique for the detection of cervical lymphadenitis due to mycobacterial infection using fine needle aspiration cytology: A case series. Otolaryngol Head Neck Surg 2005;133:381-385.

14. Monheit JE, Cowan DF, Moore DG: Rapid detection of fungi using calcofluor white and fluorescence microscopy. Arch Pathol Lab Med 1984;108:616-618.

15. Procop GW, Haddad S, Quinn J, et al: Detection of *Pneumocystis jiroveci* in respiratory specimens by four staining methods. J Clin Microbiol 2004;42:3333-3335.

16. Armbruster C, Pokieser L, Hassl A: Diagnosis of *Pneumocystis carinii* pneumonia by bronchoalveolar lavage in AIDS patients: Comparison of Diff Quik, Fungifluor, direct immunofluorescence test and polymerase chain reaction. Acta Cytol 1995;39:1089-1093.

17. Ng VL, Yajko DM, McPhaul LW, et al: Evaluation of an indirect fluorescent-antibody stain for detection of *Pneumocystis carinii* in respiratory specimens. J Clin Microbiol 1990;28:975-979.

18. Grocott RG: A stain for fungi in tissue sections and smears using Gomori's methenamine silver nitrate technic. Am J Clin Pathol 1955;35:975-979.

19. Brinn NT: Rapid metallic histological staining using the microwave oven. J Histotechnol 1983;6:125-129.

20. Lazcano O, Speights VO, Strickler JG, et al: Combined histochemical stains in the differential diagnosis of *Cryptococcus neoformans*. Mod Pathol 1993;6:80-84.

21. Kwon-Chung KJ, Hill WB, Bennett JE: New, special stain for histopathological diagnosis of *Cryptococcus*. J Clin Microbiol 1981;13:383-387.

22. Ro J, Lee SS, Ayala AG: Advantage of Fontana-Masson stain in capsule-deficient cryptococcal infection. Arch Pathol Lab Med 1987;111:53-57.

23. Cetin ES, Kaya S, Demirci M, Aridogan BC: Comparison of the BACTEC blood culture system versus conventional methods from culture of normally sterile body fluids. Adv Ther 2007;24:1271-1277.

24. Akcam FZ, Yayli G, Uskun E, et al: Evaluation of the Bactec microbial detection system for culturing miscellaneous sterile body fluids. Res Microbiol 2006;157:433-436.

25. Goldenberg D, Sciubba J, Koch WM: Cystic metastasis from head and neck squamous cell cancer: A distinct disease variant? Head Neck 2006;28:633-638.

26. Chandler FW, Kaplan W, Ajello L: A Colour Atlas and Textbook of the Histopathology of Mycotic Diseases. Lochem, Netherlands, Wolfe Medical Publications, 1980.

27. Rippon JW: Medical Mycology, 2nd ed. Philadelphia, WB Saunders, 1982.

28. Zaias N, Taplin D, Rebell G: Mycetoma. Arch Dermatol 1969;99:215-225.

29. Smith MB, Schnadig VJ, Boyars MC, Woods GL: Clinical and pathologic features of *Mycobacterium fortuitum* infections: An emerging pathogen in patients with AIDS. Am J Clin Pathol 2001;116:225-232.

30. Zaharopoulos P, Wong JY, Edmonston G, Keagy N: Crystalline bodies in cervicovaginal smears: A cytochemical and immunochemical study. Acta Cytol 1985;29:1035-1042.

31. Bhagavan BS, Ruffier J, Shimm B: Pseudoactinomycotic radiating granules in the lower female genital tract: Relationship to the Splendore-Hoeppli phenomenon. Hum Pathol 1982;13:898-903.

32. Brenner D, Drachenberg CB, Papadimitrious JC: Structural similarities between hematoidin crystals and asteroid bodies: Evidence of lipid composition. Exp Molec Pathol 2001;70:37-42.

33. Harrison TS, Levitz SM: Immunology. In Anaissie EJ, McGinnis MR, Pfaller MA (eds): Clinical Mycology. New York, Churchill Livingstone, 2003.

34. Pantanowitz L: Charcot-Leyden crystals: Pathology and diagnostic utility. Ear Nose Throat J 2004;83:489-490.

35. Jackson G, Kathuria M, Bincy A, Schnadig VJ: Fine needle diagnosis of necrotizing eosinophilic abscess clinically mimicking hepatic neoplasia. Acta Cytol (in press).

36. Kaplan K, Goodman Z, Ishak K: Eosinophilic granuloma of the liver: A characteristic lesion with relationship to visceral larva migrans. Am J Surg Pathol 2001;10:1316-1321.

37. Won JH, Kim MJ, Kim BM, et al: Focal eosinophilic infiltration of the liver: A mimic of metastasis. Abdom Imaging 1999;24:369-372.

38. Yoo SY, Han JK, Kim YH, et al: Focal eosinophilic infiltration of the liver: Radiologic findings and clinical course. Abdom Imaging 2003;28:326-332.

39. Katzenstein AA, Sale SR, Greenberger PA: Pathologic findings in allergic aspergillus sinusitis. Am J Surg Pathol 1983;7:439.

40. Marple BF: Allergic fungal rhinosinusitits: Current theories and management strategies. Laryngoscope 2001;111:1006-1019.

41. Vernig C, Bush RK: Allergic bronchopulmonary aspergillosis: A US perspective. Curr Opin Pulm Med 2007;13:67-71.

42. Kinsella JB, Bradfield JJ, Gourley WK, et al: Allergic fungal sinusitis. Clin Otolaryngol Allied Sci 1996;21:389-392.

43. Goldstein MF: Allergic fungal sinusitis: An underdiagnosed problem. Hosp Pract 1992;27:73-74.

44. Schnadig VJ, Rassekh CH, Gourley WK: Allergic fungal sinusitis: A report of two cases with diagnosis by intraoperative aspiration cytology. Acta Cytol 1999;43:268-272.

45. Echols RM, Palmer DL, Long GW: Tissue eosinophilia in human coccidioidomycosis. Rev Infect Dis 1982;4:656-664.

46. Harley BW, Blaser MJ: Disseminated coccidioidomycosis associated with extreme eosinophilia. Clin Infect Dis 1994;18:627-629.

47. Abbas AK, Lichtman AH: Cellular and Molecular Immunology, 5th ed. Philadelphia, Saunders, 2003.

48. Rotterdam H: *Mycobacterium avium* complex (MAC) infection: In Conner DH, Chandler FW (eds): Pathology of Infectious Diseases. Stamford, Conn., Appleton & Lange, 1997.

49. Rosenwieg DY: Nontuberculous mycobacterial disease in the immunocompetent adult. Semin Respir Dis 1996;11:252-261.

50. Prince DS, Peterson DD, Steiner RM, et al: Infection with *Mycobacterium* complex in patients without predisposing conditions. N Engl J Med 1989;321:863-868.

51. Reich JM, Johnson RE: *Mycobacterium avium* complex pulmonary infection presenting as isolated lingular or middle lobe pattern: The Lady Windermere syndrome. Chest 1992;101:1605-1609.

52. Schnadig VJ, Quadri SF, Boyvat F, Borucki M: *Mycobacterium kansasii* osteomyelitis presenting as a solitary lytic lesion of the ulna: Fine-needle aspiration findings and morphologic comparison with other mycobacteria. Diagn Cytopathol 1998;19:94-97.

53. Smith MB, Molina CP, Schnadig VJ, et al: Pathologic features of *Mycobacterium kansasii* infection in patients with acquired immunodeficiency syndrome. Arch Pathol Lab Med 2003;127:554-560.

54. Weiss S: Smooth muscle tumors of soft tissue. Adv Anat Pathol 2002;9:351-359.

55. Corkill M, Stephens J, Bitter M: Fine needle aspiration of mycobacterial spindle cell pseudotumor: A case report. Acta Cytol 1995;39:125-128.

56. Brandwein M, Choi HS, Strauchen J, et al: Spindle cell reaction to nontuberculous mycobacteriosis in AIDS mimicking spindle cell neoplasm: Evidence for dual histiocytic nad fibroblast-like characteristics of spindle cells. Virchows Archiv A Pathol Anat 1990; 416:281-286.

57. Morrison A, Gyure K, Sonte J, et al: Mycobacterial spindle cell pseudotumor of the brain: A case report and review of the literature. Am J Surg Pathol 1999;23:1294-1299.

58. McGinnis MR: Chromoblastomycosis and phaeophyphomycosis: New concepts, diagnosis and mycology. J Am Acad Dermatol 1983;8:1-16.

59. Zaharopoulos P, Schnadig VJ, Davie KD, et al: Multiseptate bodies in systemic phaeohyphomycosis diagnosed by fine needle aspiration cytology. Acta Cytol 1988;32:885-891.

60. Graham AR, Sobonya RE, Bonnimann DA, Galgiani JN: Quantitative pathology of coccidioidomycosis in acquired immunodeficiency syndrome. Hum Pathol 1988;1:800-806.

61. Harding CV: Blastomycosis and opportunistic infections in patients with acquired immunodeficiency syndrome: An autopsy study. Arch Pathol Lab Med 1991;115:1133-1136.

62. Bernard G, Duarte AJS: Paracoccidioidomycosis: A model for evaluation of the effects of human immunodeficiency virus infection on the natural history of endemic tropical diseases. Clin Infect Dis 2000;31:1032-1039.

63. Ware AJ, Cockerell CJ, Shiest DJ, Kussman HM: Disseminated sporotrichosis with extensive cutaneous involvement in a patient with AIDS. J Am Acad Dermatol 1999;40:350-355.

64. Denning DW, Riniotis K, Dobrashian R, Sambatakou H: Chronic cavitary and fibrosing pulmonary and pleural aspergillosis: Case series, proposed nomenclatures change and review. Clin Infect Dis 2003;37(Suppl 3):S265-S280.

65. Donohue JF, Scott RJ, Walker DH, Bromberg PA: Phycomycosis: A cause of bronchial obstruction. South Med J 1980;73:734-738.

66. Kimura M, Schnadig VJ, McGinnnis MR: Chlamydoconidia formation in zygomycosis due to *Rhizopus* species. Arch Pathol Lab Med 1998;122:1120-1122.

67. Nash G, Irvine R, Kerschmann RL, Herndier B: Pulmonary aspergillosis in acquired immune deficiency syndrome: Autopsy study of an emerging pulmonary complication of human immunodeficiency virus infection. Hum Pathol 1997;28:1268-1275.

68. Al-Alawi A, Ryan CF, Flint JD, Muller NL: Aspergillus-related lung disease. Can Respir J 2005;12:277-287.

69. McGinnis MR, Chandler FW: Trichosporonosis. In Connor DH, Chandler FW, Schwartz DA, Lack EE: Pathology of Infectious Diseases. Stamford, Conn., Appleton & Lange, 1997.

70. Brummer E: Human defenses against *Cryptococcus neoformans*: An update. Mycopathologia 1999;143:121-125.

71. Farmer SG, Komorwski RA: Histologic response to capsule-deficient *Cryptococcus neoformans*. Arch Pathol 1973;96:383-387.

72. Torlakovic E, Clayton F, Ames ED: Refractile mycobacteria in Romanowski-stained bone marrow smears: A comparison of acid fast-stained tissue sections and Romanowski-stained smears. Am J Clin Pathol 1992;97:318-321.

73. Solis OG, Belmonte AH, Ramaswamy G, Tchertkoff V: Pseudogaucher cells in *Mycobacterium avium intracellulare* infections in acquired immune deficiency syndrome (AIDS). Am J Clin Pathol 1986;85:233-235.

74. Stoll M, Schmidt R: Adverse events of desirable gain in immunocompetence: The immune restoration inflammatory syndromes. Autoimmunity Rev 2004;3:243-249.

75. Guerro MF, Remos JM, Gadea I, Alix A: Pulmonary malakoplakia associated with *Rhodococcus equi* infection in patients with AIDS: Case report and review. Clin Infect Dis 1999;28:1334-1336.

76. Abdou NI, NaPomberjara C, Sagawa A: Malakoplakia: Evidence for moncyte lysosomal abnormality correctable by cholinergic agonist in vitro and in vivo. N Engl J Med 1977;297:1413-1419.

77. Damjanov I, Katz SM: Malakoplakia. Pathol Annu 1981;16:103-126.

78. Underwood JCE, Durrant TE, Coup AJ: X-ray microanalysis of the Micahelis Gutmann bodies of malakoplakia. J Pathol 1982;138:41-48.

79. Yuoh G, Hove MG, Wen J, Haque AK: Pulmonary malakoplakia in acquired immunodeficiency syndrome: An ultrastructural study of morphogenesis of Michaelis Gutmann bodies. Mod Pathol 1996;9:476-483.

80. van Hoeven KH, Dookhan DB, Petersen RO: Cytologic features of pulmonary malakoplakia related to *Rhodococcus equi* in an immunocompromised host. Diagn Cytopathol 1996;15:325-328.

81. Sughaver M, Ali SZ, Erozan YS, et al: Pulmonary malacoplakia associated with *Rhodococcus equi* infection in an AIDS patient: Report of a case with diagnosis by fine needle aspiration. Acta Cytol 1997;41:507-512.

82. Echeverri C, Matherne J, Jorgensen JH, Fowler LJ: Fite stain positivity in *Rhodococcus equi*: Yet another acid-fast organism in respiratory cytology. A case report. Diagn Cytopathol 2001;24:244-246.

83. Ohar JA, Farris J, Dettenmeier PA, et al: Bronchoalveolar lavage cell count and differential are not reliable indicators of amiodarone-induced pneumonitis. Chest 1992;102:999-1004.

84. Martin WJ, Rosenow EC: Amiodarone pulmonary toxicity recognition and pathogenesis: Parts 1 and 2. Chest 1988;93:1067-1075, 1242-1248.

85. Dean PJ, Groshart K, Porterfield JG, et al: Amiodarone-associated pulmonary toxicity: A clinical and pathologic study of eleven cases. Am J Clin Pathol 1987;87:7-13.

86. Israel-Biet D, Venet A, Caubarrere I, et al: Bronchoalveolar lavage in amiodarone pneumonitis: Cellular abnormalities and their relevance to pathogenesis. Chest 1987;91:214-221.

87. Trapnell BC, Whitsett JA, Nakata K: Pulmonary alveolar proteinosis. N Engl J Med 2003;349:2527-2539.

88. Maygarden SJ, Iacocca MV, Funkhouser WK, Novotny DB: Pulmonary alveolar proteinosis: A spectrum of cytologic, histochemical and ultrastructural findings in bronchoalveolar lavage fluid. Diagn Cytopathol 2001;24:389-395.

89. Mermolja M, Rott T, Debeljak A: Cytology of bronchoalveolar lavage in some rare pulmonary disorders: Pulmonary alveolar proteinosis and amiodarone pulmonary toxicity. Cytopathology 1994: 5:9-16.

90. Hook GER, Gilmore LB, Talley FA: Multilamellated structures from the lungs of patients with pulmonary alveolar proteinosis. Lab Invest 1984;60:711-725.

91. Takemura T, Fukuda Y, Harrison M, Ferrans VJ: Ultrastructural, histochemical and freeze-fracture evaluation of multilamellated structures in human pulmonary alveolar proteinosis. Am J Anat 1987;179:258-268.

92. Nouza M: *Pneumocystis carinii* pneumonia after 40 years. Infection 1992;20:113.

93. Thomas CF, Limper AH: *Pneumocystis* pneumonia. N Engl J Med 2004;350:2487-2498.

94. Gill VJ, Nelson NA, Stock F, Evans G: Optimal use of the cytocentrifuge for the recovery and diagnosis of *Pneumocystis carinii* in bronchoalveolar lavage and sputum specimens. J Clin Microbiol 1988;26:1641-1644.

95. Benfield TL, Prentø P, Junge J, et al: Alveolar damage in AIDS-related *Pneumocystis carinii* pneumonia. Chest 1997;111:1193-1199.

96. Cooper CR, McGinnis MR: Pathology of *Penicillium marneffei*: An emerging acquired immunodeficiency syndrome-related pathogen. Arch Pathol Lab Med 1997;121:798-804.

97. Mootsikapun P, Srikulbutr S: Histoplasmosis and penicilliosis: Comparison of clinical features, laboratory findings and outcome. Int J Infect Dis 2006;10:66-71.

98. Chaiwun B, Khunamornpong S, Sirivanichai C, et al: Lymphadenopathy due to *Penicillium marnefei* infection: Diagnosis by fine needle aspiration cytology. Mod Pathol 2002;15:939-943.

99. Harboldt SL, Dugan JM, Tronic BS: Cytologic diagnosis of measles pneumonia in bronchoalveolar lavage specimen: A case report. Acta Cytol 1994;38:403-406.

100. Zaman SS, Seykora JT, Hodinka ARl, et al: Cytologic manifestations of respiratory syncytial virus pneumonia in bronchoalveolar lavage fluid: A case report. Acta Cytol 1996;30:546-551.

101. Luyt C-E, Combes A, Deback C, et al: Herpes simplex virus lung infection in patients undedrgoing prolonged mechanical ventilation. Am J Resp Crit Care 2007;175:935-942.

102. Koss LG: Benign disorders of the uterine cervix and vagina. In Koss LG, Melamed MR (eds): Koss' Diagnostic Cytology and its Histopathologic Bases, 5th ed. Philadelphia, Lippincott Williams & Wilkins, 2006, pp 241-281.

103. Azumi N: Immunohistochemistry and in situ hybridization techniques in the detection of infectious organisms. In Connor DH, Chandler FW, Schwartz DA, et al. (eds): Pathology of Infectious Disease. Stamford, Conn, Appleton & Lange, 1997, pp 35-44.

104. Huang JC, Naylor B: Cytomegalovirus infection of the cervix detected by cytology and histology: A report of five cases. Cytopathology 1993;4:237-241.

105. Mostad SB, Kreiss JK, Ryncarz AJ, et al: Cervical shedding of cytomegalovirus in human immunodeficiency virus type I-infected women. J Med Virol 1999;59:469-473.

106. Koss LG: The lower urinary tract in the absence of cancer. In Koss LG, Melamed, MR (eds): Koss' Diagnostic Cytology and its Histopathologic Bases, 5th ed. Philadelphia, Lippincott Williams & Wilkins, 2006.

107. Coleman DV: The cytodiagnosis of human polyomavirus infection. Acta Cytol 1975;19:93-96.

108. Hariharan S: BK virus nephritis after renal transplantation. Kidney Int 2006;69:655-662.

109. Bhambhani S, Kashvap V: Amoebiasis: Diagnosis by aspiration and exfoliative cytology. Cytopathology 2001:12:329-333.

110. John DT, Petri WA: Markell and Voge's Medical Parasitology, 9th ed. St. Louis, Saunders, 2006.

111. Genta RM: Dysregulation of strongyloidiasis: A new hypothesis. Clin Microbiol Rev 1992;5:345-355.

112. Keiser PB, Nutman TB: *Strongyloides stercoralis* in the immunocompromised population. Clin Microbiol Rev 2004;17:208-217.

113. Marcos LA, Terashima A, DuPont HL, Gotuzzo E: *Strongyloides* hyperinfection: An emerging global infectious disease. Trans Royal Soc Trop Med Hygiene 2008;102:314-318.

114. Smolyakov R, Talalay B, Yanai-Inbar I, et al: *Enterobius vermicularis* infection of female genital tract: A report of three cases and review of literature. Eur J Obstet Gynecol Reprod Biol 2003: 107:220-222.

115. Das Dk, Pathan SK, Hira PR, et al: Pelvic abscess from enterobius vermicularis: Report of a case with cytologic detection of eggs and worms. Acta Cytol 2001;45:425-529.

116. Duarte AG, Sattar F, Granwehr B, et al: Disseminated acanthamoebiasis after lung transplantation. J Heart Lung Transplant 2006;25:237-240.

117. Sun X, Zhang Y, Li R, et al: Acanthamoeba keratitis: Clinical characteristics and management. Ophthalmology 2006;113:412-416.

118. Sawada Y, Yuan C, Huang AJ: Impression cytology in the diagnosis of acanthamoeba keratitis with surface involvement. Am J Ophthalmol 2004;137:323-328.

Ultrastructural Diagnosis of Infection

Alton B. Farris III, Martin K. Selig, and G. Petur Nielsen

5

CHAPTER

Introduction

Electron microscopy (EM) can assist in the identification of infectious organisms in surgical and clinical pathology specimens. However, since the advent of immunohistochemical, molecular (e.g., in situ hybridization, polymerase chain reaction), and serologic techniques, EM has been less often used to identify infectious pathogens. EM can still be useful, particularly in the identification of specific infections and the classification of novel organisms. Additionally, EM is advantageous in situations in which most viral particles are present as empty virions devoid of nucleic acid. This chapter is not intended to be an exhaustive compendium of the EM characterization of all infectious diseases; rather, this chapter focuses on those infections in which EM plays a critical role[1-4] (Table 5-1).

Electron Microscopy Technique

EM is best conducted on freshly fixed tissue. Surgical specimens (from biopsies or resections), cytology specimens, fecal samples in the case of gastrointestinal episodes, fluids or smears from skin lesions, cerebrospinal fluid, nasopharyngeal washes, saliva, tears, and urine are examples of samples that may be used for EM. In our laboratory, we typically use a modified Karnovsky's fixative consisting of 2.0% glutaraldehyde, 2.5% formaldehyde, and 0.025% CaCl in a 0.1 M sodium cacodylate buffer pH 7.4. Fixation times vary with tissue type. Skin biopsies require long fixation times, sometimes longer than 3 hours, whereas cell suspensions or tissue-cultured cells can be adequately fixed in as little as 15 minutes. Postfixation with osmium tetroxide is necessary for good ultrastructural preservation, because it preserves lipids which are typically lost in formalin-fixed, paraffin-embedded tissues. For a more comprehensive overview of our tissue processing method, see Table 5-2. Sometimes tissue for conventional light microscopy that has been fixed in conventional buffered formaldehyde or paraffin-embedded tissue is the only material available. This tissue can also be used for EM, although significant artifact is typically present. Tissue remaining in buffered formaldehyde after fixation gives better results than tissue embedded in paraffin or tissue fixed in Bouin, Zenker, or B-5 fixative.[1-4]

Although it is not routinely performed in our laboratory, rapid diagnosis of negatively stained viral particles by EM may be achieved within 10 minutes of receiving a sample. Negative staining methods usually employ staining with a heavy metal aqueous salt solution, such as 2% uranyl acetate, 5% ammonium molybdate, or 1.0% potassium salt of phosphotungstic acid (PTA).[5] Samples are dried onto thin-film carbon-coated grids, washed, stained, air-dried, and taken directly to the microscope. Viral inactivation is usually accomplished through drying and

then irradiation with ultraviolet light. In our laboratory, we create agar cell blocks from samples otherwise too small to process. Briefly, in small Eppendorf tubes, samples (from fine-needle aspiration, bronchial lavage, urine, ascites fluid, or tiny tissue fragments) are fixed in standard fixative, centrifuged at 1000 rpm, resuspended in warm (liquid) 2% agar, and centrifuged again. The agar is then allowed to cool and harden. The centrifuge tube tip containing material is then cut off with a sharp razor blade, and the resulting tissue-containing agar block is processed routinely.[4,6]

Transmission electron microscopy (TEM) is typically the technique used to examine surgical and clinical pathology specimens. With this technique, electrons are passed through samples and then imaged. Samples must be quite thin (80-100 nm) for the electrons to be able to pass through the specimen.[1-3]

Prions

Most research related to diseases thought to be mediated by prions (small proteinaceous infectious particles) indicates that prions are protease-resistant proteins that do not contain nucleic acid. Prions are difficult to isolate and too small to be visualized by standard EM techniques. Typically, only vacuolated nervous tissue and reactive astrocytosis are seen histologically, and EM shows vacuoles in neurons and neuropils, as well as altered plasma membranes.

Table 5-1 Comparative Sizes of Important Pathogens

Pathogen	Approximate Size
Prion	12-230 nm[31]
Virus	0.02-0.22 μm
Bacteria	
Staphylococcus aureus	0.7 μm
Escherichia coli	0.5 μm
Fungal hyphae	
Histoplasma	3 μm
Cryptococcus	20 μm
Red blood cell	7 μm
Parasite	
Worm eggs	16-80 μm
Worms	≥300 μm

Adapted from Hawley LB: High-Yield Microbiology and Infectious Diseases. Philadelphia, Lippincott Williams & Wilkins, 2000.

Table 5-2 Routine Automatic Processor Program for Electron Microscopy*

Vial #	Contents	Time (min)	Temperature (° C)	Agitation?
1	Na cacodylate buffer	5	10	No
2	Na cacodylate buffer	5	10	No
3	1.3% Osmium teroxide, aqueous	90	10	Yes
4	Na cacodylate buffer	10	10	No
5	25% ethanol (aq.)	15	15	No
6	50% Ethanol (aq.)	15	15	No
7	3% Uranyl acetate in 70% ethanol	90	RT	Yes
8	95% Ethanol (aq.)	15	RT	No
9	95% Ethanol (aq.)	15	RT	No
10	100% Ethanol (absolute)	15	RT	No
11	100% Ethanol (absolute)	15	RT	No
12	100% Ethanol (absolute)	15	RT	No
13	Propylene oxide (100%)	10	RT	No
14	Propylene oxide (100%)	10	RT	No
15	PPO/Epoxy resin (70/30)	90	25	Yes
16	PPO/Epoxy resin (30/70)	90	30	Yes
17	Epoxy resin (100%)	180	30	Yes
18	Epoxy resin (100%)	180	30	Yes
19	Empty vial			
20	Empty			

Recent research has focused on using immunologic methods to identify prions such as prion protein (PrP) immunohistochemistry and cryo-immunogold EM. It is hoped that such techniques will yield insights into disorders in which prions are considered to be critical, such as Creutzfeldt-Jakob disease and Gerstmann-Sträussler syndrome in humans and bovine spongiform encephalopathy (BSE) in cattle—and even other neurodegenerative disorders such as Alzheimer, Parkinson, and Huntington diseases.[7-10]

Viral Infections

Viruses can be recognized as organized structures (Fig. 5-1) smaller than cells and may be intracellular or extracellular, ranging from 20 to 300 nm in diameter. Viruses typically have one or more layers surrounding an electron-dense core consisting of DNA or RNA, referred to as the nucleoid (Table 5-3), and are surrounded by a single or multilayer outer coating or shell, the capsid.[1]

Size, shape, and organization of virions are useful characteristics in identifying viruses. Sizes range from small (e.g., papovaviruses) to intermediate (e.g., adenoviruses, herpesviruses) to large (e.g., poxviruses). Virions may be organized into lattice-like arrangements (e.g., adenoviruses), which vary from regular to random (e.g., papovavirus). Although the morphology and size are useful in identifying viruses, there is overlap, and complementary techniques to EM are often needed, including

Icosahedral virus

Enveloped icosahedral virus

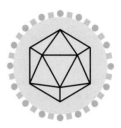

Poxvirus brick-shaped complex

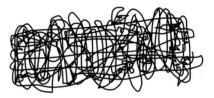

Figure 5-1. Basic structure of viruses.

Table 5-3 Important Viruses Confronted by Electron Microscopy and Their Important Features

Virus Family	Size* (nm)	Nucleic Acid Material	Shape
Parvoviridae	18-26	Naked ss DNA	Icosahedral
Hepadnaviridae	22-27	Enveloped ds circular DNA	Icosahedral
Papovaviridae	45-55	Naked ds circular DNA	Icosahedral
Adenoviridae	80-110	Naked ds DNA	Icosahedral
Herpesviridae	150-200	Enveloped ds circular DNA	Icosahedral
Poxviridae	140-260 × 220-450	Coated ds DNA	Complex
Picornaviridae, Astroviridae, Caliciviridae	27-38	Naked ss RNA	Icosahedral
Reoviridae	60-80	Naked ds segmented RNA	Icosahedral
Togaviridae	50-70	Enveloped ss RNA	Icosahedral
Flaviviridae	45-60	Enveloped ss RNA	Complex
Arenaviridae	50-300	Enveloped ss segmented RNA	Complex
Coronaviridae	80-220	Enveloped ss RNA	Complex
Retroviridae	80-100	Enveloped ss diploid RNA	Complex
Bunyaviridae, Orthomyxoviridae	80-120	Enveloped ss segmented RNA	Helical
Paramyxoviridae	150-300	Enveloped ss RNA	Helical
Rhabdoviridae	60-80 × 130-220	Enveloped ss RNA	Helical, bullet-shaped
Filoviridae	80 × 1000	Enveloped ss RNA	Helical

*Size is expressed as diameter or diameter × length.
DNA, deoxyribonucleic acid; ds, double-stranded; nm, nanometers; RNA, ribonucleic acid; ss, single-stranded.
Data from references 1, 10, 12, and 22.

immunohistochemistry, in situ hybridization, Southern blot analysis, and polymerase chain reaction for viral DNA.[1]

Herpesvirus

Herpesvirus virions (Figs. 5-2 and 5-3) are surrounded by limiting lipid bilayers, giving the virions a "fried egg" look. The envelopes serve both a functional and a structural role. The virions have a hexagonal outline (icosahedral morphology) and are covered with 152 tubular capsomeres. The complete herpes viral structure with envelope is 150 to 180 nm in diameter, and the internal portion of all herpes group viruses is about 100 nm in diameter. Viral inclusion bodies of herpesvirus are composed of lattice arrangements of mature viral particles (virions). Other members of the herpesvirus family (i.e., herpes simplex, cytomegalovirus, and Epstein-Barr virus) have a similar appearance, and all are 100 to 120 nm in size. They all replicate in the nucleus of the host cell.[10,11]

Varicella Virus

Varicella virus, the causative agent of chickenpox (also known as human herpesvirus 3) is usually a benign disease of childhood. Ultrastructurally (Fig. 5-4), viral nucleocapsids can be identified in the nucleus and budding through the nuclear envelope. Virions may be present in cytoplasmic vacuoles and are sometimes abundant. Herpes zoster (shingles) is a reinfection of the varicella virus that commonly manifests in the skin, often as

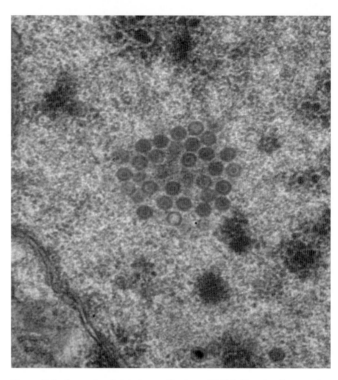

Figure 5-3. Herpesvirus (original magnification, ×44,000). Round to hexagonal or "stop sign"–shaped, targetoid viral particles are seen.

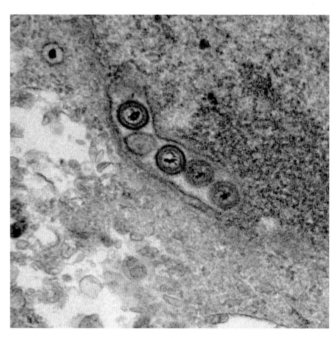

Figure 5-4. Varicella virus (original magnification, ×57,000). Round to hexagonal or "stop sign"–shaped, targetoid viral particles are seen in cell culture. (Epon blocks contributed by William Taylor, M.D., and Lynne A. Farr, B.A., Rhode Island Hospital, Providence, Rhode Island.)

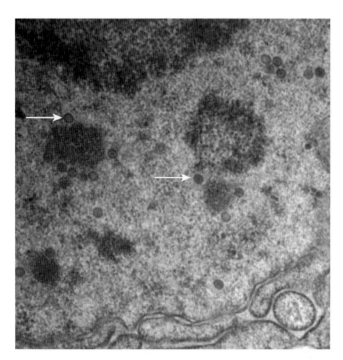

Figure 5-2. Herpesvirus (original magnification, ×28,000). Numerous clusters of intranuclear viral particles *(arrows)* are seen in a sample from the cerebrum of a patient with herpes simplex encephalitis.

vesicular eruptions in a dermatomal distribution along sensory nerves. Virus is produced in lower quantities than in the primary chickenpox infection.[10]

Adenovirus

Adenovirus (Figs. 5-5 and 5-6) commonly infects the respiratory and enteric tracts. Rarely, the liver and pancreas may be involved. Adenovirus is contained as numerous packets of virions in a paracrystalline array, often in the nucleus of cells when newly synthesized, and sometimes in the nucleolus as an inclusion body. In early infection, incoming virus is seen in the cytoplasm. Individual virions have a hexagonal (icosahedral) shape with 20 sides and 12 vertices. Surrounding the core of the virus are 252 pentagonal capsomeres, each with a filamentous projection (fiber). Cells may become large (cytomegaly) with large eosinophilic inclusions appreciable by light microscopy. Granular aggregates in the nuclei of cells infected by adenovirus are made up of various viral-induced proteins.[1,10,12]

Influenza

Influenza virus (Figs. 5-7 and 5-8), an orthomyxovirus, is a pleomorphic virus consisting of round to spherical, kidney-shaped, or elongated virions located at and beneath the cell surface. Virions are 80 to 120 nm in diameter, and filamentous forms may be several micrometers in length. Viruses typically

enter respiratory tract epithelium by attaching to and fusing with the cell membrane, mediated by hemagglutinin binding to sialic acid residues in a ligand-receptor interaction. Hemagglutinin and neuraminidase spikes project 8 to 10 nm from the viral envelope, and the nucleocapsid, 9 to 15 nm in diameter, has helical sym-

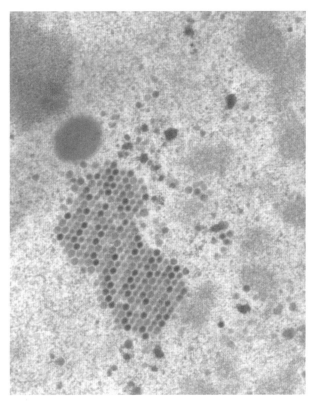

Figure 5-6. Adenovirus (original magnification, ×34,000). Numerous packets of virions in a regular lattice-like arrangement are seen. (Epon blocks contributed by William Taylor, M.D., and Lynne A. Farr, B.A., Rhode Island Hospital, Providence, Rhode Island.)

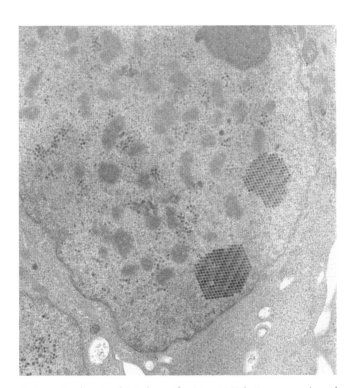

Figure 5-5. Adenovirus (original magnification, ×11,000). Numerous packets of virions in a regular lattice-like arrangement are seen in cell culture. (Epon blocks contributed by William Taylor, M.D., and Lynne A. Farr, B.A., Rhode Island Hospital, Providence, Rhode Island.)

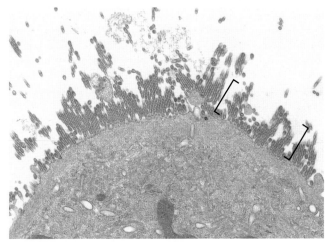

Figure 5-7. Influenza A (original magnification, ×15,000). Round and elongate virions at the cell surface are seen in cell culture *(brackets)*. (Epon blocks contributed by William Taylor, M.D., and Lynne A. Farr, B.A., Rhode Island Hospital, Providence, Rhode Island.)

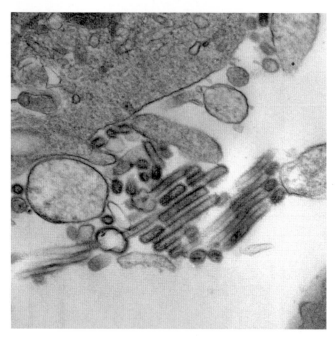

Figure 5-8. Influenza A (original magnification, ×45,000). Round and elongated virions are seen. (Epon blocks contributed by William Taylor, M.D., and Lynne A. Farr, B.A., Rhode Island Hospital, Providence, Rhode Island.)

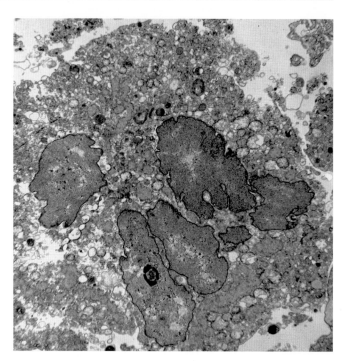

Figure 5-9. Parainfluenza virus (original magnification, ×3400). Multiple nuclei with a ground glass texture are seen in a sample of lung. Measles can have a similar appearance.

metry. Infected cells may have an increased density of nucleoli during active protein synthesis. Hemagglutinin proteins form in the cytoplasm and may be present in excess as long fibers. Dense protein lattices surrounded by small dense ribosomes are present. Virions emerge by budding from the host cell plasma membrane.[1,10,12]

Paramyxovirus

Members of the Paramyxoviridae family measure 120 to 300 nm in size. There are many members of Paramyxoviridae, including mumps, parainfluenza (Figs. 5-9 and 5-10), *Morbillivirus* species (including measles), and *Pneumovirus* species (including respiratory syncytial virus). One common place to identify paramyxovirus is in type II pneumocytes, which may be multinucleated and may have a ground-glass appearance. The virions are diffusely dispersed in the cell and have a filamentous protein nucleocapsid protecting the viral nuclei acid, giving the virus a "herringbone" appearance.[1,10,11]

Smallpox

Variola virus, the agent of smallpox, is often recognized from material collected from skin lesions. The slightly rounded, brickshaped virions measure about 270 by 350 nm. The organisms have a complex surface structure and may be recognized in one of two types: a mulberry form with 10- to 20-nm diameter and a beaded short-tubular surface and a capsular form with a 30-nm membrane.[4,6]

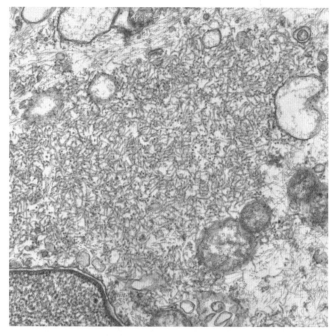

Figure 5-10. Parainfluenza virus (original magnification, ×19,000). Virions are diffusely dispersed in the cytoplasm in a sample of lung. Measles can have a similar appearance.

Hepatitis Viruses

Hepatitis A Virus

Hepatitis A virus (enterovirus 72) is a member of the picornavirus family, 24 to 30 nm in diameter, and roughly spherical. Cytopathic effect leads to an increase in intracellular ribosomes and large polyribosomes.[12]

Hepatitis B Virus

Hepatitis B virus, a hepadnavirus (Figs. 5-11 and 5-12), is 22 to 27 nm in diameter and consists of a central core of double-stranded DNA with nucleocapsid DNA. An envelope containing the hepatitis B surface antigen (HBsAg) is 7 nm wide and contains a 27-nm diameter central core, also referred to as the Dane particle, which contains the hepatitis B core antigen (HBcAg) and e antigen (HBeAg). The viral particles may form spherules and tubules.[1,10,11]

Parvovirus B19

Parvovirus B19 is a small, round, non-enveloped icosahedral virus, 18 to 26 nm in diameter, without distinctive surface features. They may be confused with ribosomes. At high magnification, they have a roughly hexagonal outline. Virus is assembled in the nucleus and appears either "empty" or "full." It may be recognized in blood serum by EM.[11,12]

Enterovirus

Enterovirus (Figs. 5-13 and 5-14) is a member of the picornavirus family, which also includes poliovirus, coxsackievirus, echovirus, hepatitis A, rhinovirus, and aphthovirus (the causative agent of foot-and-mouth disease), among others. The enterovi-

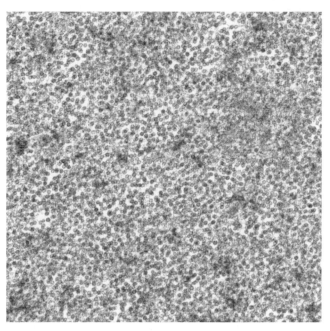

Figure 5-12. Hepatitis B virus (original magnification, ×56,000). Numerous granular viral particles are seen.

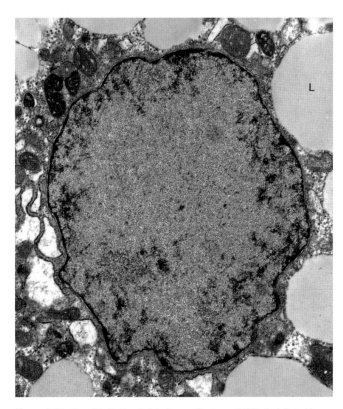

Figure 5-11. Hepatitis B virus (original magnification, ×9100). An infected hepatocyte is seen with numerous intranuclear viral particles and surrounding lipid droplets (*left*).

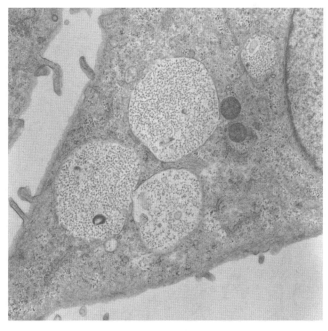

Figure 5-13. Enterovirus: Coxsackie A (original magnification, ×15,000). Membrane-bound vesicles containing numerous virions are seen in a tissue culture sample. (Epon blocks contributed by William Taylor, M.D., and Lynne A. Farr, B.A., Rhode Island Hospital, Providence, Rhode Island.)

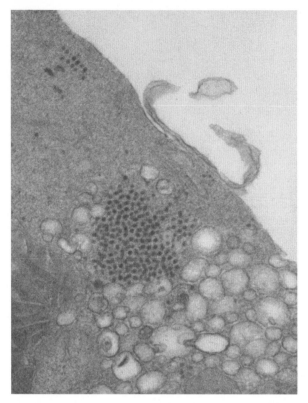

Figure 5-14. Enterovirus: echovirus (original magnification, ×45,000). Numerous round virions can be seen in a tissue sample. (Epon blocks contributed by William Taylor, M.D., and Lynne A. Farr, B.A., Rhode Island Hospital, Providence, Rhode Island.)

rus genus includes poliovirus, coxsackievirus A and B, echovirus, enterovirus, and others. Cells infected by enterovirus have innumerable spherical virions, some of which are enclosed in membrane-bound vesicles. The vesicles may be appreciated on lower magnification. Enterovirus typically infects the gastrointestinal tract but may extend to the brain, where neurons may be infected, producing cell swelling, chromatolysis, and cell death.

Poliovirus replicates in enteric mucosa and is present in large quantities in the feces. It targets the nervous system, infecting vascular endothelium of the brain. Viruses may replicate in circulating leukocytes. Virions are the size of ribosomes and are often difficult to identify. Coxsackieviruses are enteroviruses that can cause enteric, respiratory, meningeal, and cutaneous infections. Infections resemble the EM changes of poliovirus. Infection with echovirus, which derives its name from "enteric cytopathic human orphan," is usually subclinical but can manifest with febrile illness and meningitis, often in newborns, who may develop fatal disseminated infections. The EM findings are similar to those of poliovirus.[1,10]

Viral Gastroenteritis

Enzyme-linked immunosorbent assay (ELISA) kits are available for the detection of rotavirus, but new strains may not be recognized by these kits, which recognize only those strains that have an antigen common to the rotavirus that was used in making the antiserum for the kit. EM may be useful in identifying other rota-

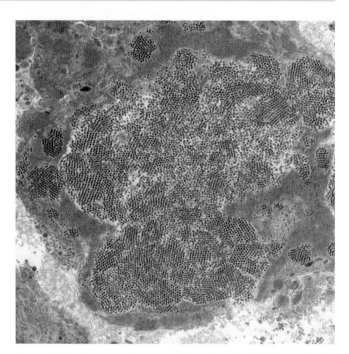

Figure 5-15. Polyomavirus in a case of BK nephropathy (original magnification, ×19,000). Numerous virion packets of polyomavirus can be seen embedded in renal tubular debris.

viruses and causes of viral gastroenteritis, particularly those for which kits are not available. The EM appearance of viruses can be diagnostic in many of these circumstances. For example, rotavirus may be identified on EM of stool specimens as a 70-nm viral particle with three protein layers and a characteristic "wheel" shape (hence, the prefix *rota*, which means "wheel").[6,13,14]

Polyomaviruses

The Papovaviridae (Figs. 5-15 and 5-16) derive their name from the first two letters of the viruses in the papovavirus family: papilloma, polyoma, and vacuolating agents. Virions measuring approximately 50 nm in diameter are present in packets and are found in oligodendrocytes in cases of progressive multifocal leukoencephalopathy (PML). JC polyomavirus, a member of the papovavirus family, is the causative agent of PML. BK polyomavirus is a common inhabitant of the genitourinary tract that may cause a nephropathy in immunocompromised transplant recipients (renal transplant recipients in particular). In cases of human papillomavirus (HPV)–related disease, there may be keratohyaline granules, which are seen by EM as large, dense cytoplasmic granules.[10,12] Recent research has indicated that EM may be useful in the identification of urinary polyomavirus in cases of BK nephropathy.[15]

Rabies Virus

Rabies virus (Figs. 5-17 and 5-18), a member of the Rhabdoviridae family and *Lyssavirus* genus, is a bullet-shaped virus that aggregates around or in electron-dense cytoplasmic material. This correlates to the Negri bodies seen in neurons in rabies virus

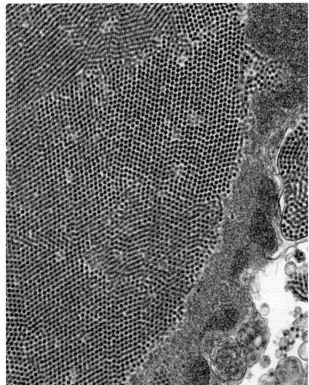

Figure 5-16. Polyomavirus (original magnification, ×25,000). Numerous virion packets of polyomavirus with a relatively regular organization in groups, also referred to as a paracrystalline arrangement, can be seen.

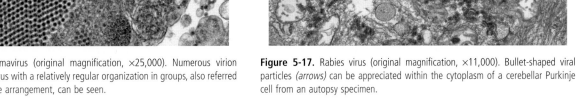

Figure 5-17. Rabies virus (original magnification, ×11,000). Bullet-shaped viral particles *(arrows)* can be appreciated within the cytoplasm of a cerebellar Purkinje cell from an autopsy specimen.

infections, notably in hippocampal pyramidal cells and less frequently in cortical neurons and Purkinje cells of the cerebellum. A process of budding off of membrane-bound organelles leads to formation of individual virions.[1,9]

Eastern Equine Encephalitis Virus

The Eastern (Fig. 5-19) and Western equine encephalitis viruses, members of the Togaviridae family and the *Alphavirus* genus, are transmitted to humans, horses, and other animals. In fatal infections, neuronal degeneration and inflammation are present in the cerebral cortex, basal ganglia, hippocampus, and medullary nuclei, with relative sparing of the cerebellum and spinal cord. Viruses are 55 to 58 nm in diameter and typically have a dense, 28- to 30-nm core surrounded by a spherical translucent layer. There may be projecting subunits. Viruses are seen in the cytoplasm and associated with membranous structures. The outer envelope typically comes from budding from the plasma membrane but may also come from endoplasmic reticulum. Dense particles may be seen in the nucleus late in infection and are thought to be a possible early phase of the viral life cycle.[10,12]

Human Immunodeficiency Virus

Human immunodeficiency virus (HIV) (Figs. 5-20 and 5-21), a retrovirus and member of the *Lentivirus* genus, is recognized by

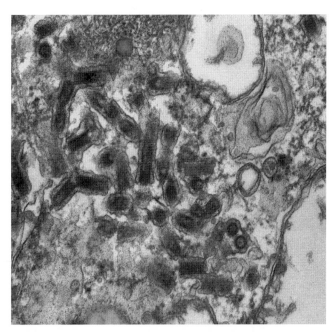

Figure 5-18. Rabies virus from an autopsy specimen of cerebellum (original magnification, ×25,000). Bullet-shaped viral particles are seen.

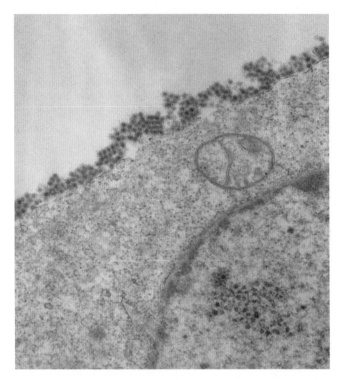

Figure 5-19. Eastern equine encephalitis virus in a cell culture sample (higher magnification, ×25,000). Many virions can be appreciated at the cell surface and within the nucleus. (Epon blocks contributed by William Taylor, M.D., and Lynne A. Farr, B.A., Rhode Island Hospital, Providence, Rhode Island.)

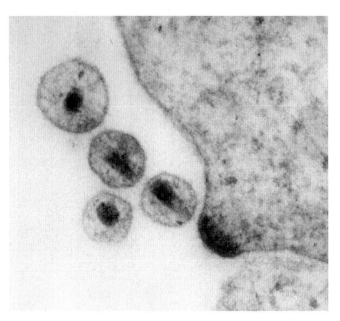

Figure 5-21. Human immunodeficiency virus: virions bud from the plasma membrane (from cell culture, ×10,000). (Photographs contributed by Jan M. Orenstein, M.D., Department of Pathology, George Washington University Medical Center.)

its conical dense nucleoid, which forms from cytoplasmic membrane and vacuolar membrane of lymphocytes and cells in the monocyte-macrophage lineage. Host cell membranes form the outer membrane of the virus, and the immature virus forms surface spikes during budding.[1]

Bacterial Infections

As prokaryotic single-celled organisms, bacteria (Fig. 5-22) have a simple internal structure without a membrane-bound nucleus, membrane-bound organelles, endoplasmic reticulum, or mitochondria. Bacteria have an outer cell wall (except for *Mycoplasma*), an inner cell membrane, dense cytoplasm composed primarily of ribosomes, and vesicles formed from the inner cell membranes (known as mesosomes), storage vacuoles, and endospores. They may have a loose, fuzzy extracellular capsule (glycocalyx), flagella, pili (fimbria), and a non–membrane-bound nucleus. Gram-positive bacteria have a thicker outer wall compared with gram-negative bacteria. Although bacteria may be visible by light microscopy, smaller bacteria are much more readily visualized with EM, particularly *Legionella pneumophila*. Bacteria have a variety of shapes, including cocci; coccobacilli; and straight, curved, or branched rods. The size of bacteria ranges from less than 1 μm in diameter and up to 1 to 6 μm long.[1]

Gram-Positive Bacteria

Gram-positive bacteria (Figs. 5-23 and 5-24) are characterized by their thick walls, which are composed of peptidoglycans and mucocomplexes containing muramic acid and stain prominently with osmium as 20- to 50-nm thick, electron-dense layers surrounding the plasma membrane. Gram positivity is due to the thick peptidoglycan layer, which gives shape, strength, and rigid-

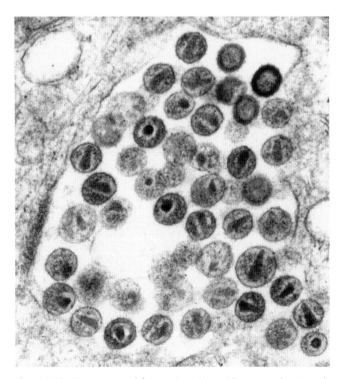

Figure 5-20. Human immunodeficiency virus: virions within a macrophage vacuole (from cell culture). Virions are ring-shaped, and some have conical nucleoids (×7500). (Photographs contributed by Jan M. Orenstein, M.D., Department of Pathology, George Washington University Medical Center.)

GRAM POSITIVE

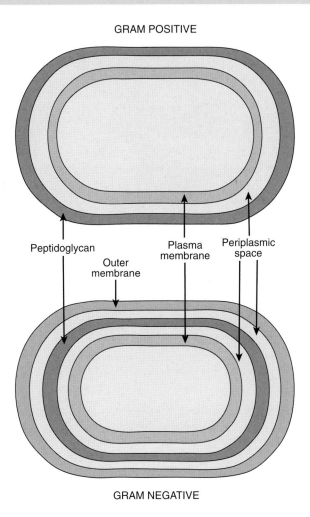

Peptidoglycan

Outer
membrane

Plasma
membrane

Periplasmic
space

GRAM NEGATIVE

Figure 5-22. Basic structure of bacteria.

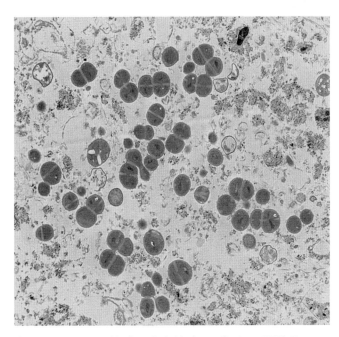

Figure 5-23. Gram-positive bacteria (original magnification, ×5700). Numerous gram-positive bacteria are appreciable at relatively low electron microscopic magnification after retrieval from a paraffin block.

ity to the cell wall. An ultrastructural Gram technique replaces the crystal violet–iodide complex with a complex platinum salt–containing compound.[10,16-18]

Gram-Negative Bacteria

Gram-negative bacteria have a rigid peptidoglycan layer that separates outer and inner membranes. The outer membrane is often undulant. Gram-negative bacteria also may have outer membranes made of phospholipids, glycolipids, lipopolysaccharides (LPS), and proteins. A periplasmic space separates the outer membrane from the cell membrane. LPS may be visualized as long, tubular complexes or as spherical disks. LPS, along with other membrane components such as proteins and phospholipids help to form endotoxin.[10,18]

Mycobacteria

Mycobacteria (Figs. 5-25 and 5-26) are coccobacillary or filamentous, acid-fast bacterial organisms that may be present as straight or curved rods and aggregate in branching forms,

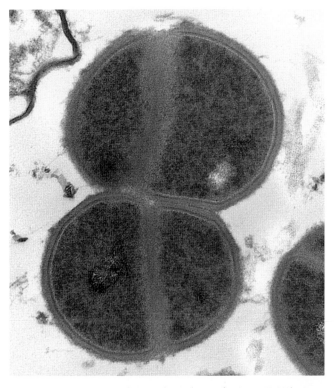

Figure 5-24. Gram-positive bacteria (original magnification, ×71,000). Gram-positive bacteria have a plasma membrane and a thick peptidoglycan layer. By contrast, gram-negative bacteria have an additional, undulant outer membrane, a plasma membrane (inner membrane), and a narrow, irregular peptidoglycan layer.

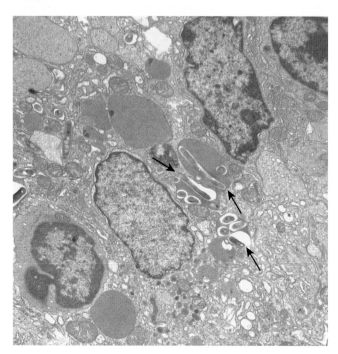

Figure 5-25. *Mycobacterium avium-intracellulare* (original magnification, ×3400). Mycobacteria can be seen *(arrows)* in the lamina propria of the duodenum with surrounding chronic inflammatory cells.

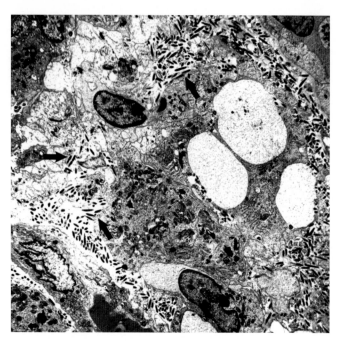

Figure 5-27. Whipple's disease (original magnification, ×1900). Whipple's disease of the jejunum in which extracellular bacilli *(arrows)* can be seen.

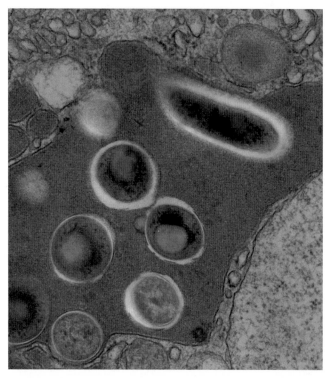

Figure 5-26. *Mycobacterium avium-intracellulare* (original magnification ×25,000). Mycobacteria are seen within histiocytic secondary lysosomes in a sample of duodenum.

approximately 0.3 to 0.6 μm wide and 1 to 4 μm long. They have special cell wall lipids that form a waxy coating, together with polysaccharides, glycerides, and high-molecular-weight alcohols, and they are present in macrophages as facultative intracellular organisms. There is a variable-thickness capsule in close contact with a cell wall. The cell wall can be identified as having a high-density outer portion surrounding an inner, electron-opaque, fibrillar portion (containing mycosides) and nuclear region; the cytoplasm has lipid storage bodies and polyphosphates present as dense granules. *Mycobacterium tuberculosis* may be present in lysosomes of macrophages, and these macrophages typically aggregate, forming a tubercle.[10]

Other Important Bacteria

Tropheryma whippelii

Tropheryma whippelii (Figs. 5-27, 5-28, 5-29), the causative organism of Whipple's disease, is a small (1-2 μm long, 0.25 μm in diameter) organism in which the rods are typically found free within macrophages of the intestine. The bacilli have a thick (approximately 20 nm) outer cell wall with a trilaminar membrane. Bacteria replicate extracellularly but are typically ingested by macrophages and digested into intracellular myelin figures, in which case histiocytes are seen distended with lysosomes that are filled with serpiginous membranes (see Fig. 5-27).[1,11]

Chlamydia trachomatis

Chlamydia trachomatis (Figs. 5-30 and 5-31), formerly thought to be a virus until it was determined to be a bacterium, has an outer membrane and is present within cytoplasmic inclusion vacuoles, which contain numerous chlamydia in infected host cells. It is present as elementary and reticulate bodies with inter-

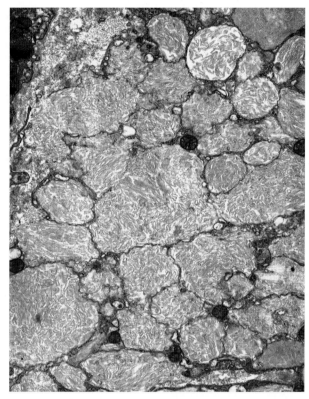

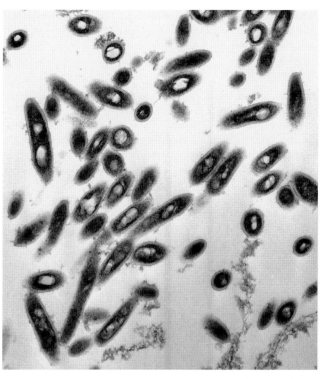

Figure 5-28. Whipple's disease (original magnification, ×7100). Serpiginous bodies in a case of Whipple's disease of the cardiac ventricle in which only the confluent bacterial membrane remnants can be seen (material retrieved from paraffin).

Figure 5-29. Whipple's disease (original magnification, ×19,000). Whipple's disease of the jejunum in which extracellular bacilli with cytoplasmic vacuoles can be seen.

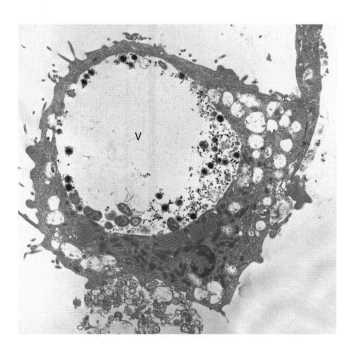

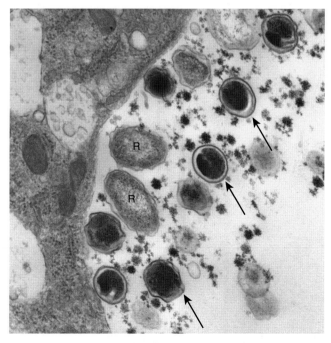

Figure 5-30. *Chlamydia trachomatis* (original magnification, ×3400). Chlamydial organisms in various stages can be seen in a large cytoplasmic inclusion vacuole (V) from cell culture. (Epon blocks contributed by William Taylor, M.D., and Lynne A. Farr, B.A., Rhode Island Hospital, Providence, Rhode Island.)

Figure 5-31. *Chlamydia trachomatis* (original magnification, ×19,000). Higher-power image of chlamydia showing elementary *(arrows)* and reticulate (R) bodies. (Epon blocks contributed by William Taylor, M.D., and Lynne A. Farr, B.A., Rhode Island Hospital, Providence, Rhode Island.)

mediate forms. Elementary bodies enter the host cell by endocytosis and phagocytosis. Inclusion bodies undergo lysis and exit the cell through endocytosis.[1]

Helicobacter pylori

Helicobacter pylori is a 2- to 6-μm long, 0.5-μm wide, gram-negative organism that has a surface flagellar sheath; the sheath is thought to provide acid resistance in its typical acidic gastric environment, along with the ureases the organism produces. *H. pylori* attaches to the gastric mucus layer and cell surface microvilli and is the causative agent of many cases of gastritis and gastric ulcers. Numerous *Helicobacter* organisms have been identified. One example is *Helicobacter felis,* a tightly spiraled bacterium that colonizes cats and dogs and has characteristic periplasmic fibrils.[10,11]

Legionella pneumophila

Legionella pneumophila (Figs. 5-32 and 5-33) is a gram-negative coccobacillus and a facultative intracellular pathogen that replicates in pulmonary macrophages and causes acute fibrinopurulent bronchopneumonia. Large numbers can be found in phagolysosomes and rough endoplasmic reticulum of macrophages or free in cellular debris. Pseudopodia may be found surrounding bacterial cells, leading to rapid macrophage ingestion of bacteria, a process called "coiling phagocytosis."[10,19-21]

Fungal Infections

Histoplasma capsulatum

Histoplasma capsulatum (Figs. 5-34 and 5-35) consists of both intracellular and extracellular oval yeast forms, 2 to 4 μm in diam-

eter, with no true capsule, a thin cell wall, and a single nucleus. Intracellularly, they are found in the cytoplasm of histiocytes. The yeast form may have heavier wall components composed of chitin. There is typically a clear cytoplasmic halo at the periphery of the organisms, which may be appreciated on histologic sections, particularly when stained with silver impregnation or periodic acid–Schiff (PAS) stains. Histiocytes typically contain several organisms, lipid droplets, and organelles within a copious amount of cytoplasm. Breakdown of organism cell walls occurs in macrophage phagolysosomes containing lysosomal acid hydrolases. After the organisms have been killed in chronic infections, cell walls and electron-dense material may remain.[1,10]

Pneumocystis jiroveci

Pneumocystis jiroveci (Figs. 5-36, 5-37, 5-38, 5-39, 5-40), once thought to be a protozoan and formerly named *Pneumocystis carinii*, is now believed to be a fungus with a close relationship to ascomycetes based on molecular biologic studies.[22] *P. jiroveci* consists of thick-walled, spherical intact cysts and crescentic collapsed cysts surrounded by trophozoite processes and vacuoles. The cysts are 4 μm in diameter and have an outer dense layer and an inner less dense layer. They may be empty or may enclose sporozoites. Trophozoites are 1.5 to 12 μm long, pleomorphic, intracystic or extracystic, and have a nucleus, cytoplasm, and extensively folded plasmalemmas.[1]

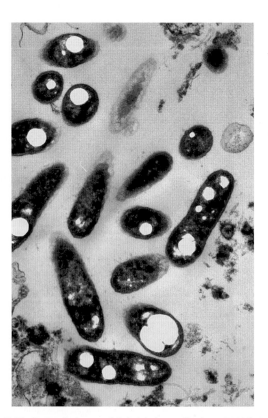

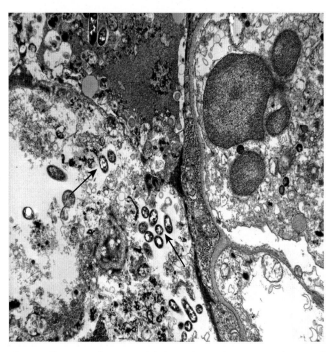

Figure 5-32. *Legionella pneumophila* (original magnification, ×1900). Bacterial rods *(arrows)* are seen in alveolar exudate.

Figure 5-33. *Legionella pneumophila* (original magnification, ×34,000). Bacterial rods that are largely degenerative are seen. The outer cell membrane and cytoplasmic vacuoles can be appreciated (retrieved from paraffin).

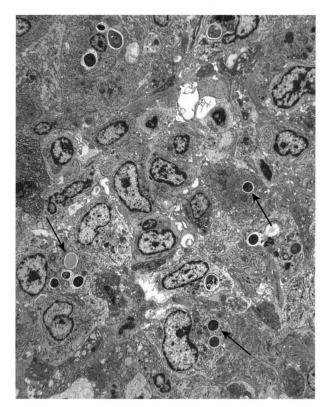

Figure 5-34. *Histoplasma* yeast from supraclavicular regional lymph node (original magnification, ×1900). Numerous round yeast forms *(arrows)* can be seen within the cytoplasm of histiocytes. Clear halos surround the organisms underneath their cell membrane.

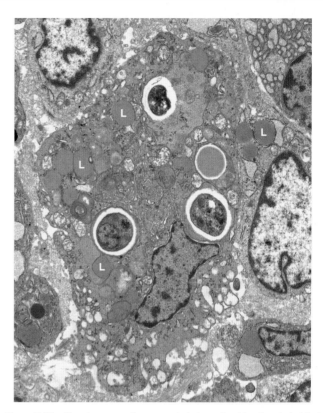

Figure 5-35. *Histoplasma* yeast from supraclavicular regional lymph node (original magnification, ×3400). Clear halos surround the organisms underneath their cell membrane. The histiocyte containing the organism has numerous lipid vacuoles (L).

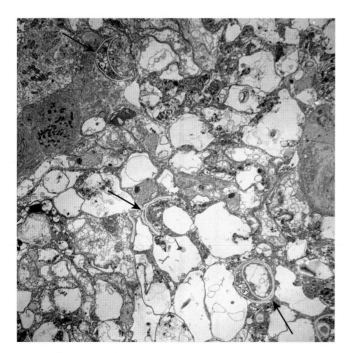

Figure 5-36. *Pneumocystis jiroveci* (original magnification, ×1900). Crescent-shaped cysts *(arrow)* of the *Pneumocystis* organism can be seen in a pulmonary alveolar exudate.

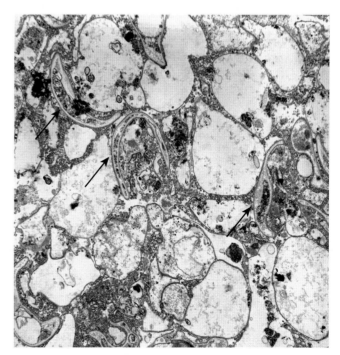

Figure 5-37. *Pneumocystis jiroveci* (original magnification, ×3400). Crescent-shaped cysts of the *Pneumocystis* organism *(arrow)* can be seen in a pulmonary alveolar exudate.

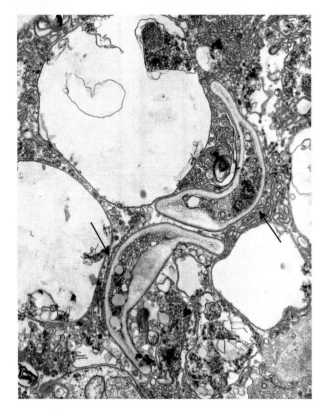

Figure 5-38. *Pneumocystis jiroveci* (original magnification, ×7100). Two collapsed crescent-shaped cysts of the *Pneumocystis* organism *(arrows)* can be appreciated.

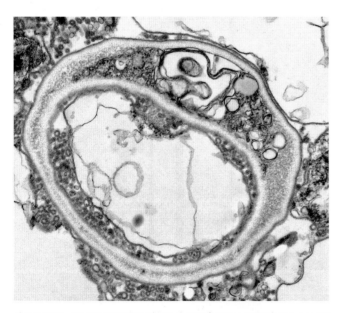

Figure 5-39. *Pneumocystis jiroveci* (original magnification, ×15,000). *Pneumocystis* organism is seen in a pulmonary alveolar exudate with outer dense and inner less dense layers.

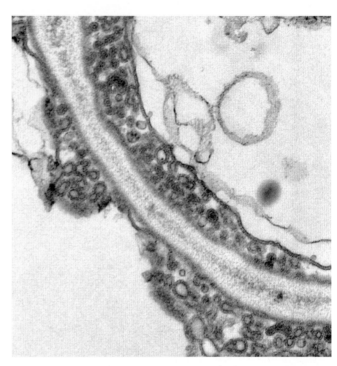

Figure 5-40. *Pneumocystis jiroveci* (higher magnification). Higher power reveals the ultrastructural characteristics of the elaborately folded, whorled organismal membrane.

Parasitic Infections

Acanthamoeba

Acanthamoeba (Fig. 5-41) is a pathogenic protozoan that is classified as an ameboflagellate, like *Naegleria fowleri*. *Acanthamoeba* is most commonly seen in humans as the causative agent of keratitis. *Acanthamoeba* may also cause chronic granulomatous lesions, notably chronic amebic encephalitis, in which the organisms typically enter the brain through the cribriform plate. Infections of the respiratory tract and skin may also occur and particularly affect the immunosuppressed. Healthy individuals may be affected by *Acanthamoeba* keratitis, particularly after trauma to the cornea or exposure to contaminated water, contact lenses, or contact lens solutions. The trophozoite, measuring 15 to 30 μm, is the invasive, infective form.[10,23,24]

Toxoplasma gondii

Toxoplasma gondii (Figs. 5-42, 5-43, 5-44) consists of ovoid, elliptical, or teardrop-shaped parasites (approximately 3 × 2 μm) within vacuoles in macrophages. *Toxoplasma* has a single posterior nucleus, a triple-layered cell membrane, and organelles that are considered specific and nonspecific. At the anterior end of the organism, there are organelles that have a conoid (conical opening) and 30 to 50 micronemes (secretory tubules in convoluted groups). At the anterior end are rhoptries (club-shaped storage sacs), which empty by ducts into the conoid. EM is useful for helping distinguish *Toxoplasma* from other sporozoites in the *Apicomplexa* genera, such as *Trypanosoma cruzi*. *Trypanosoma cruzi* have kinetoplasts, and *Toxoplasma* does not. *Toxoplasma*

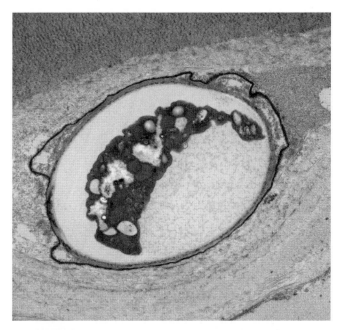

Figure 5-41. *Acanthamoeba* in acanthamoeba keratitis (original magnification, ×7900). A double-walled cyst with intracystic structures is seen. (Courtesy of Norman Michaud at the Massachusetts Eye and Ear Infirmary.)

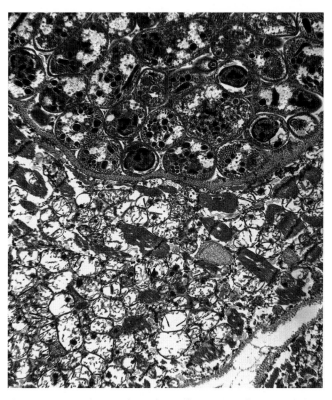

Figure 5-42. Toxoplasmosis (original magnification, ×3400). Numerous *Toxoplasma gondii* sporozoites are seen within parasitophorous vacuoles in heart muscle in an autopsy specimen from a patient with human immunodeficiency virus infection.

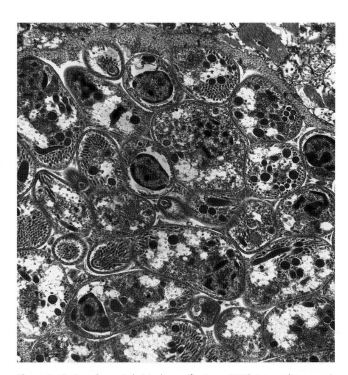

Figure 5-43. Toxoplasmosis (original magnification, ×7100). Intermediate magnification of heart muscle from the same case as in Figure 5-42 shows numerous *Toxoplasma gondii* sporozoites.

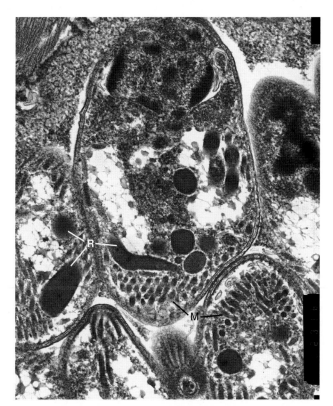

Figure 5-44. Toxoplasmosis (original magnification, ×25,000). *Toxoplasma gondii* sporozoites are seen within heart muscle with characteristic rhoptries (R) and micronemes (M).

has conoids and endogenous division (internal budding of daughter cells), and trypanosomes do not.[1]

Cryptosporidium parvum

Cryptosporidium parvum (Figs. 5-45, 5-46, 5-47), consists of 3- to 4-μm, spherical structures, referred to as cryptosporidia, that are located along the gastrointestinal epithelium, specifically the small intestine. At light microscopic levels, the spherical structures are often seen attached to the epithelial cell surface. The attachment site usually lacks microvilli and is dense and raised. The parasites have different morphologies based on the phase of their life cycle (i.e., microgamete, merozoite, schizont, trophozoite). Secondary lysosomes (phagosomes) are frequently seen in the apical cytoplasm of epithelial attachment sites.[1]

Giardia lamblia

Giardia lamblia (Figs. 5-48 and 5-49) consists of pear-shaped trophozoites, alternatively convex dorsally and concave ventrally, measuring 9.5 to 21 μm long and 5 to 15 μm wide, that are normally present free in the small intestine and in cysts in the large intestine. *Giardia* is binucleate, with symmetrically spaced nuclei and a prominent karyosome, and has four pairs of flagella adjacent to an adhesion disc. *Giardia* has a rigid cytoskeleton with evenly spaced microtubules linked by microribbons. It does not have mitochondria, peroxisomes, endoplasmic reticulum, or nucleoli. Morphologic types of *Giardia* can be distinguished ultrastructurally, as can the stage of the life cycle (i.e., free trophozoites in the small bowel and cysts in the large bowel and

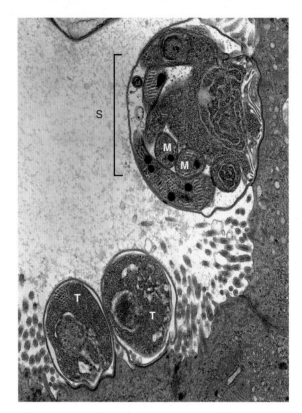

Figure 5-46. Cryptosporidia (original magnification, ×11,000). Numerous spherical microorganisms are located along the mucosal surface, attached to the mucosal epithelium with trophozoites (T) and an appreciable schizont (S) containing merozoites (M).

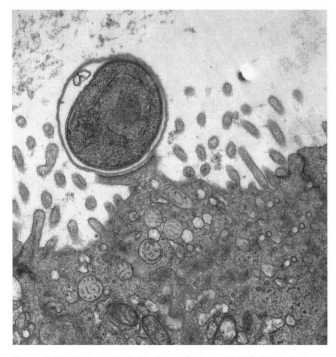

Figure 5-45. Cryptosporidia (original magnification, ×11,000). Spherical microorganism is located along the mucosal surface, attached to the mucosal epithelium.

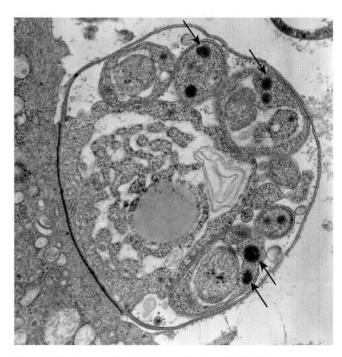

Figure 5-47. Cryptosporidia (original magnification, ×19,000). Higher-power image of a gamete shows dense granules *(arrows).*

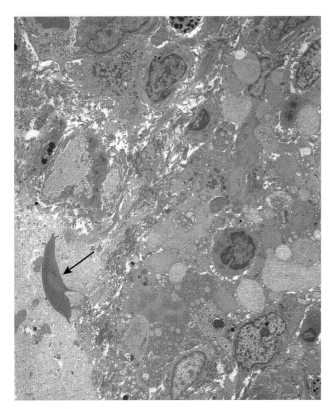

Figure 5-48. *Giardia* (original magnification, ×1900). Convex trophozoite *(arrow)* is seen at relatively low electron microscopic magnification. (Epon blocks contributed by William Taylor, M.D., and Lynne A. Farr, B.A., Rhode Island Hospital, Providence, Rhode Island.)

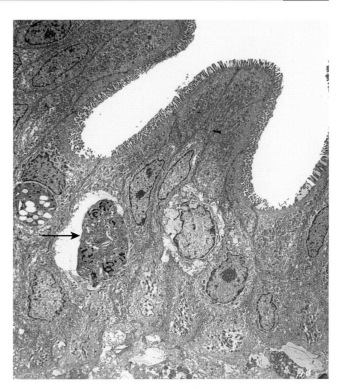

Figure 5-50. *Isospora belli* (original magnification, ×2500). *Arrow* indicates *I. belli* organism with lobated nuclei in the intestinal lamina propria (retrieved from paraffin).

feces). Mature cysts are 8 to 12 μm long and 7 to 10 μm wide and have four nuclei, a dense wall, dense cytoplasm with ribosomes and glycogen granules, and peripheral vacuoles or tubules.[1]

Isospora belli

Isospora belli (Figs. 5-50 and 5-51) belongs to a genus of the pathogenic coccidia that includes other organisms such as *Cyclospora* and *Eimeria*; and the morphology of *Isospora* is quite similar to *Eimeria*. Coccidiosis caused by these organisms involves invasion of intestinal epithelial cells by sporozoites, which form through sporogony from oocysts (the organismal zygotes). In the schizony or growth phase, sporozoites form blastophores, which rupture at the cell surface, releasing merozoites; the merozoites infect more cells and form microgametes in the sexual phase. These then form more oocysts, completing the cycle. In human isosporiasis, the condition may be chronic, with villous atrophy and a lymphoplasmacytic reaction in the lamina propria. The organism may be recognized in all life cycle phases. Unsporulated oocysts are shed in the feces. Encysted zoites may be identified in the lamina propria of the intestinal villi and, rarely, in lymph nodes.[10]

Microsporidia

Microsporidia (Figs. 5-52, 5-53, 5-54, 5-55, 5-56) are obligate intracellular parasites in the phylum Microspora.[3] The spores of this organism are 0.5 to 5 μm in diameter. The most common

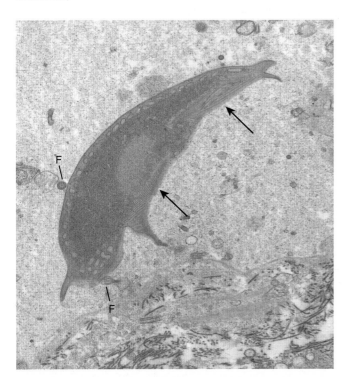

Figure 5-49. *Giardia* (original magnification, ×9100). Convex trophozoite with visible intracellular structures including flagellum (F) and adhesion disc *(arrows)*. (Epon blocks contributed by William Taylor, M.D., and Lynne A. Farr, B.A., Rhode Island Hospital, Providence, Rhode Island.)

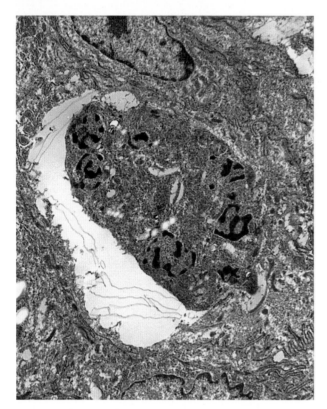

Figure 5-51. *Isospora belli* (original magnification, ×5700). Higher magnification shows the lobated nuclei of *I. belli* organism (retrieved from paraffin).

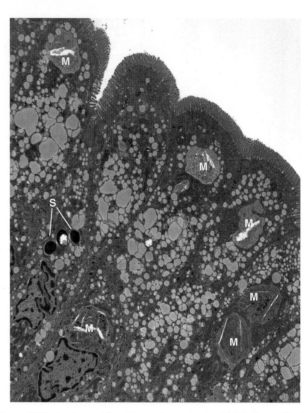

Figure 5-52. A microsporidian, *Enterocytozoon bieneusi* (original magnification, ×1900). Enterocytes filled with numerous microsporidia spores (S) and meronts (M) are seen in a sample of duodenum.

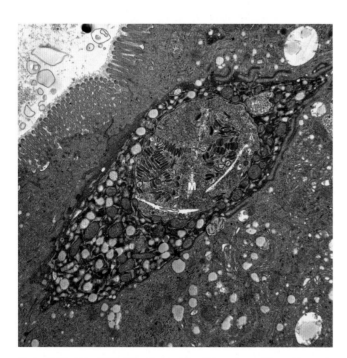

Figure 5-53. Meront (M) of the microsporidian, *Enterocytozoon bieneusi*, in sample of duodenum (original magnification, ×5700).

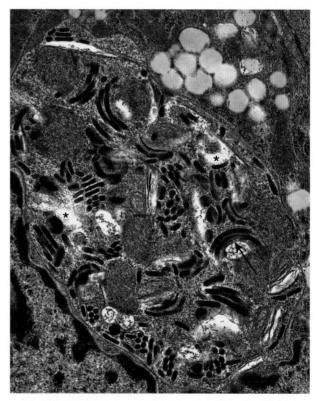

Figure 5-54. The microsporidian, *Enterocytozoon bieneusi* (original magnification, ×19,000). High magnification of a meront in a sample of duodenum shows clear clefts (*) and electron-dense discs *(arrow)*.

species in humans is *Enterocytozoon bieneusi*. Organisms are identified in fecal material or in routinely processed tissue biopsies. The major ultrastructural features used for typing microsporidia are the characteristic size and shape, the characteristic nuclei in spores and developmental stages, the host-parasite interface, and the number of coils in the tubular extrusion apparatus (sometimes present as single-coiled polar tubes in the spores). In *E. bieneusi*, cross-sections of the coiled polar tube are seen as a double row in the posterior half of the spore, whereas in the microsporidian *Septata intestinalis* there is a single row. *E. bieneusi* may be seen as spores in direct contact with enterocytes. Enterocytes may be seen infected with microsporidia spores and meronts. In *S. intestinalis*, spores are grouped with septae surrounding individual spores in parasitophorous vacuoles in the supranuclear cytoplasm of enterocytes.[11,25-31]

Trypanosoma cruzi

Trypanosoma cruzi (Fig. 5-57) consists of oval and elliptical organisms, 10 to 30 μm in diameter, with a characteristic kinetoplast and flagellum in addition to the usual nucleus and cytoplasmic organelles. At the base of the basal body of the flagellum is a kinetoplast, which consists of a curved, electron-dense structure containing DNA. *T. cruzi* has a single, long mitochondrion just underneath the cell membrane, extending from the kinetoplast to the posterior compartment of the cytoplasm, and there may also be a free flagellum outside the cell membrane. The kineto-

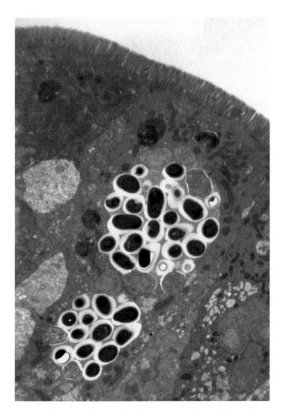

Figure 5-55. A microsporidian, *Septata intestinalis*, in a sample of duodenum (original magnification, ×25,000). Organismal spores are present in the supranuclear cytoplasm of an enterocyte within parasitophorous vacuoles with vaguely defined septae surrounding individual spores.

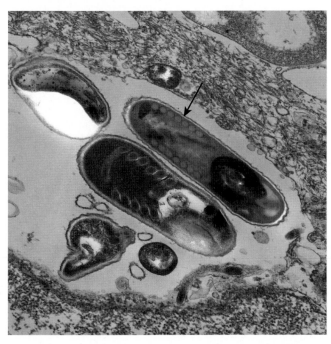

Figure 5-56. Microsporidian *Septata intestinalis* spores in urine (original magnification, ×27,300). A double row of cross-sections of coiled polar filament *(arrow)* is seen. (From Case records of the Massachusetts General Hospital: Weekly clinicopathological exercises. Case 51-1993: A 36-year-old man with AIDS, increase in chronic diarrhea, and intermittent fever and chills. N Engl J Med 1993;329:1946-1954.© Massachusetts Medical Society, 1993; used with permission.)

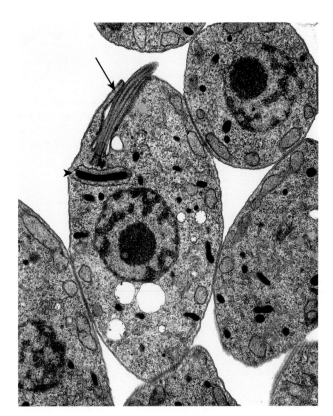

Figure 5-57. *Trypanosoma cruzi* from a tissue culture sample. Oval/elliptical trypanosomes are seen with a nucleus and numerous cytoplasmic organelles and a portion of the kinetoplast *(arrowhead)* and flagellum *(arrow)* structures.

plast position and the flagellum position and length vary based on the life cycle stage of the organism (e.g., promastigote, trypomastigote, amastigote, epimastigote).[1]

REFERENCES

1. Dickersin GR: Infectious agents. In Dickersin GR (ed): Diagnostic Electron Microscopy: A Text/Atlas, 2nd ed. New York, Springer-Verlag, 2000, p 648.
2. Rosai J: Special techniques in surgical pathology. In Rosai J (ed): Rosai and Ackerman's Surgical Pathology, vol 1, 9th ed. Philadelphia, Mosby/Elsevier Health Sciences, 2004, p 37.
3. Woods AE, Stirling JW: Electron microscopy. In Bancroft JD, Gamble M (eds): Theory and Practice of Histological Techniques, 6th ed. Philadelphia, Churchill Livingstone Elsevier, 2008, p 601.
4. Hazelton PR, Gelderblom HR: Electron microscopy for rapid diagnosis of infectious agents in emergent situations. Emerg Infect Dis 2003;9:294-303.
5. Hajibagheri MAN (ed): Electron Microscopy Methods and Protocols. Totowa, N.J., Humana Press, 1999.
6. Fong CK: Electron microscopy for the rapid detection and identification of viruses from clinical specimens. Yale J Biol Med 1989; 62:115-130.
7. Fournier JG: Cellular prion protein electron microscopy: Attempts/limits and clues to a synaptic trait. implications in neurodegeneration process. Cell Tissue Res 2008;332:1-11.
8. Godsave SF, Wille H, Kujala P, et al: Cryo-immunogold electron microscopy for prions: Toward identification of a conversion site. J Neurosci 2008;28:12489-12499.
9. Mandell GL, Bennett JE, Dolin R, eds: Mandell, Douglas, and Bennett's Principles and Practice of Infectious Diseases, 6th ed. Philadelphia, Elsevier; 2005.
10. Cheville NF: Ultrastructural pathology: An introduction to interpretation. Hoboken, N.J., Wiley-Blackwell, 1994.
11. Curry A, Appleton H, Dowsett B: Application of transmission electron microscopy to the clinical study of viral and bacterial infections: Present and future. Micron 2006;37:91-106.
12. Doane FW, Anderson N: Electron Microscopy in Diagnostic Virology: A Practical Guide and Atlas. Cambridge, UK, Cambridge University Press, 1987.
13. Kisielius JJ, Ueda M, Rácz M: Virus-rotavirus electron microscopy. Available at http://www.microbelibrary.org/Virus/details.asp?id=590&Lang= (accessed July 7, 2009).
14. Parashar UD, Glass RI: Rotavirus vaccines: Early success, remaining questions. N Engl J Med 2009;360:1063-1065.
15. Singh HK, Andreoni KA, Madden V, et al: Presence of urinary haufen accurately predicts polyomavirus nephropathy. J Am Soc Nephrol 2009;20:416-427.
16. Beveridge TJ: Mechanism of gram variability in select bacteria. J Bacteriol 1990;172:1609-1620.
17. Hobot JA: New aspects of bacterial ultrastructure as revealed by modern acrylics for electron microscopy. J Struct Biol 1990;104:169-177.
18. Cabeen MT, Jacobs-Wagner C: Bacterial cell shape. Nat Rev Microbiol 2005;3:601-610.
19. Horwitz MA: Phagocytosis of the legionnaires' disease bacterium (*Legionella pneumophila*) occurs by a novel mechanism: Engulfment within a pseudopod coil. Cell 1984;36:27-33.
20. Horwitz MA: The legionnaires' disease bacterium (*Legionella pneumophila*) inhibits phagosome-lysosome fusion in human monocytes. J Exp Med 1983;158:2108-2126.
21. Horwitz MA: Formation of a novel phagosome by the legionnaires' disease bacterium (*Legionella pneumophila*) in human monocytes. J Exp Med 1983;158:1319-1331.
22. Brooks GF, Butel JF, Morse SA: Jawetz, Melnick, and Adelberg's Medical Microbiology, 22nd ed. New York, Appleton & Lange/Lange Medical Books/McGraw-Hill, 2001.
23. Ebrahimi KB, Green WR, Grebe R, Jun AS: Acanthamoeba sclerokeratitis. Graefes Arch Clin Exp Ophthalmol 2009;247:283-286.
24. Marciano-Cabral F, Cabral G: *Acanthamoeba* spp. as agents of disease in humans. Clin Microbiol Rev 2003;16:273-307.
25. Wasson K, Peper RL: Mammalian microsporidiosis. Vet Pathol 2000;37:113-128.
26. Canning EU, Curry A, Vavra J, Bonshek RE: Some ultrastructural data on *Microsporidium ceylonensis,* a cause of corneal microsporidiosis. Parasite 1998;5:247-254.
27. Curry A, Smith HV: Emerging pathogens: Isospora, cyclospora and microsporidia. Parasitology 1998;117(Suppl):S143-S159.
28. Kyaw T, Curry A, Edwards-Jones V, et al: The prevalence of *Enterocytozoon bieneusi* in acquired immunodeficiency syndrome (AIDS) patients from the north west of england: 1992-1995. Br J Biomed Sci 1997;54:186-191.
29. Curry A: Electron microscopy and the investigation of new infectious diseases. Int J Infect Dis 2003;7:251-257.
30. Curry A: Electron microscopy as a tool for identifying new pathogens. J Infect 2000;40:107-115.
31. Silveira JR, Raymond GJ, Hughson AG, et al: The most infectious prion protein particles. Nature 2005;437:257-261.

6

Ear, Nose, and Throat Infections

Matthew M. Johnson

The head and neck area is arguably the most complex area of the human body; with its many physical connections to the outside environment, it plays host to a myriad of infectious processes. The aim of this chapter is to provide the surgical pathologist with important information that will aid in establishing an accurate diagnosis of infection. Because many of the infectious processes affecting the head and neck involve multiple sites, the chapter is organized around causative organisms rather than specific locations in the head and neck.

Bacterial Rhinosinusitis

Acute bacterial rhinosinusitis is an uncommon complication of acute viral rhinosinusitis, and it is caused by a variety of organisms, including *Streptococcus pneumoniae*, *Haemophilus influenzae*, *Moraxella catarrhalis*, *Staphylococcus aureus*, streptococci, and various anaerobes. Signs and symptoms include purulent nasal discharge, unilateral facial pain and tenderness, and worsening symptoms, often after an initial improvement.[1] The rare surgical specimen from a patient with acute bacterial rhinosinusitis demonstrates nonspecific findings including congestion, edema, and subepithelial mixed inflammation showing mainly neutrophils, with chronic inflammation and fibrosis being absent.

By definition, chronic rhinosinusitis persists for at least 12 weeks despite therapy and manifests with mucopurulent drainage, nasal obstruction, facial pain or pressure, and decreased sense of smell.[2] Chronic rhinosinusitis can be divided into three clinicopathologic syndromes: chronic rhinosinusitis with polyposis or without polyposis, and allergic fungal rhinosinusitis.[3] The pathophysiology of chronic rhinosinusitis is complex and incompletely understood, but bacteria contribute to all forms of chronic rhinosinusitis through failed resolution of acute infection, by the formation of biofilms on the sinus mucosa, or by the stimulation of enterotoxin-specific immunoglobulin E (IgE) antibodies, as in chronic rhinosinusitis with nasal polyposis and *S. aureus* colonization.[4,5] In contrast to acute bacterial rhinosinusitis, surgical specimens from patients with chronic rhinosinusitis are commonly seen, and histologic evaluation reveals a wide range of pathologic changes.

Gross examination may show polypoid sinonasal mucosa with varying amounts of mucus and fragments of swollen or scarred sinonasal mucosa admixed with bone fragments. The inflammatory response includes predominantly lymphocytes and plasma cells, with smaller numbers of eosinophils and neutrophils (Fig. 6-1). A predominance of eosinophils should prompt consideration of allergic fungal rhinosinusitis, although this may also be seen as a component of chronic rhinosinusitis with or without polyposis. Depending on chronicity, stromal fibrosis may be sparse or marked, with hyperplasia of seromucinous glands. The respiratory mucosa varies from attenuated to hyperplastic, particularly in polypoid fragments, which typically show stromal edema, basement membrane thickening, inflammation, and fibrosis. Bone fragments may appear reactive and sclerotic or unremarkable.

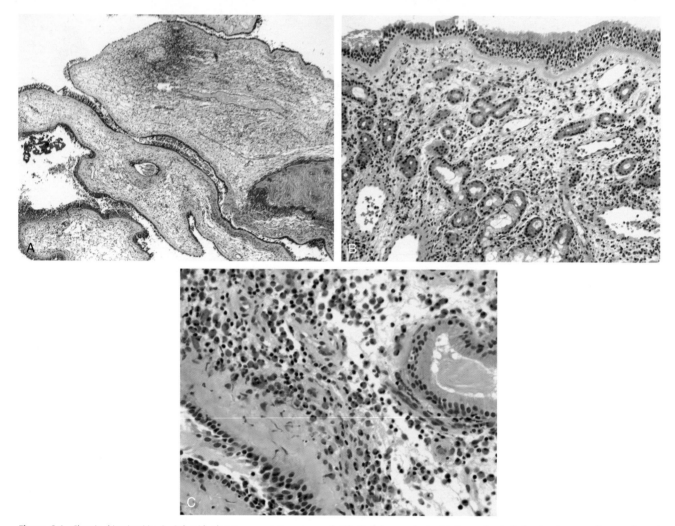

Figure 6-1. Chronic rhinosinusitis. **A,** Polypoid edematous respiratory mucosa (×40). **B,** Submucosal mixed inflammation including lymphocytes, plasma cells, and eosinophils (×200). **C,** Prominent eosinophils should prompt consideration of fungal rhinosinusitis. GMS stain was negative in this case. Note thickened basement of respiratory epithelium (×400).

Otitis Media

Otitis media, infection of the middle ear, may be acute or chronic. Acute otitis media is the most common disease of childhood and is usually caused by bacteria such as *S. pneumoniae*, *H. influenzae*, and *M. catarrhalis*.[6] The most common presenting symptom is earache, although patients may also demonstrate sore throat, night restlessness, or fever.[7] Examination typically reveals a bulging opaque tympanic membrane with decreased mobility. Recurrent infections lead to chronic otitis media, which may eventually result in myringotomy and tympanostomy tube placement.[8]

The histologic findings in acute and chronic otitis media are nonspecific, and pathologists do not generally evaluate specimens from patients with acute otitis media. In patients with chronic otitis media, specimens from corrective surgery may reveal connective tissue with a mixed chronic inflammatory infiltrate, granulation tissue, metaplastic glands, and fibrosis, as well as evidence of tympanosclerosis in the form of hyalinization, calcification, or ossification of the fibrous tissues (Fig. 6-2). Polypoid granulation

tissue with mixed chronic inflammation and a respiratory-type or metaplastic squamous surface lining is often seen, constituting the otic or aural polyp. A giant cell reaction to cholesterol (cholesterol granuloma) is a common feature of chronic otitis. Occasionally, an associated cholesteatoma is present, characterized by a cyst lined by keratinizing squamous epithelium, containing abundant acellular keratin debris, and surrounded by fibrosis, granulation tissue, and a mixed inflammatory infiltrate, often with giant cells.

Tonsillitis

Tonsillitis is a common disease of the head and neck, and it can be acute or chronic, with a variety of bacteria and viruses as the usual etiologic culprits. Acute pharyngotonsillitis is not usually treated with surgery. It is most often attributable to infection with a respiratory virus, such as adenovirus, influenza virus, parainfluenza virus, rhinovirus, or respiratory syncytial virus, but in 30% to 40% of cases, a bacterial infection is the cause, most com-

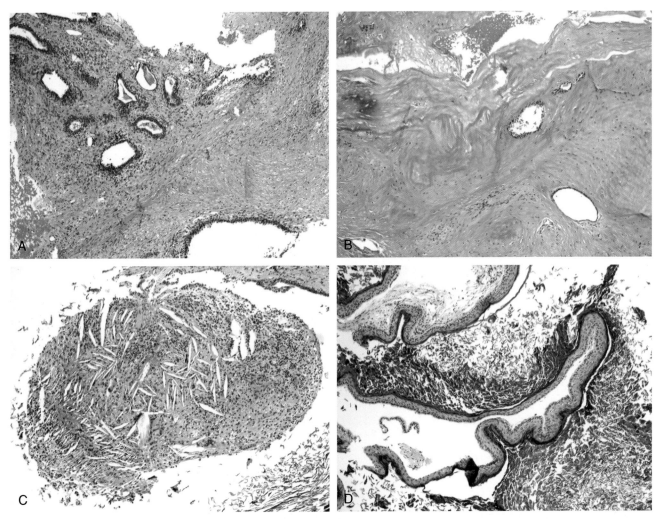

Figure 6-2. Chronic otitis media. **A,** Fibrosis, chronic inflammation, and scattered respiratory-type mucosa-lined tubular glands (×100). **B,** Tympanosclerosis, characterized by hyalinized fibrous tissue with focal calcification and several adjacent metaplastic glandular structures with surrounding fibrosis (×100). **C,** Cholesterol granuloma, with lymphoplasmacytic and granulomatous inflammation surrounding cholesterol clefts (×100). **D,** Cholesteatoma, demonstrating abundant keratin debris, keratinizing squamous epithelium, and subjacent fibrosis (×100).

monly group A β-hemolytic streptococci.[9] Recurrent infection results in chronic tonsillitis, often with tonsillar enlargement that can cause obstruction. One study identified *S. aureus* (30.3%), *H. influenzae* (15.5%), and *Streptococcus pyogenes* (14.4%) as the most common isolates in chronic tonsillitis, and *H. influenzae* (31.4%), *S. pyogenes* (24.2%), *S. aureus* (22.9%), and *S. pneumoniae* (12.6%) as the most common isolates in tonsillar hypertrophy.[10]

For the most part, unless there is clinical concern for malignancy, adenoids and tonsils removed for chronic tonsillitis or hypertrophy are not processed for histologic examination.[11] Microscopically, one sees reactive lymphoid hyperplasia, often with associated fibrosis, accentuating the interlobular fibrous septae (Fig. 6-3).[12] Acute inflammation is usually absent, and occasionally the commensal "sulfur granules" of *Actinomyces* can be identified between crypts.[13] Epstein-Barr virus (EBV) and herpes simplex virus (HSV) can manifest particular histologic findings in the tonsil that are identical to those seen in lymph nodes, as discussed later in this chapter and described in detail in Chapter 11.

Peritonsillar Abscess

Peritonsillar abscess, or quinsy, is the most common deep infection of the head and neck. It occurs as a complication of tonsillitis and cellulitis and is a polymicrobial infection associated with a wide variety of bacteria, both aerobic and anaerobic (most commonly *S. pyogenes* and *Fusobacterium* spp., respectively).[14] The disease affects mainly young adults during November to December and April to May, when streptococcal pharyngitis and exudative tonsillitis are at their highest incidence. Abscess forms in the area between the palatine tonsil and its capsule, causing such signs and symptoms as fever, malaise, sore throat, dysphagia, otalgia, trismus, drooling, swelling, muffled "hot potato" voice, rancid breath, and lymphadenopathy.[15]

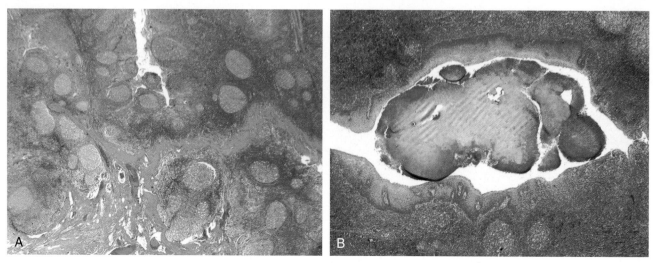

Figure 6-3. Chronic tonsillitis. **A,** Reactive lymphoid follicular hyperplasia with fibrotic accentuation of interlobular septae (×20). **B,** Commensal "sulfur granule" of *Actinomyces* (×40).

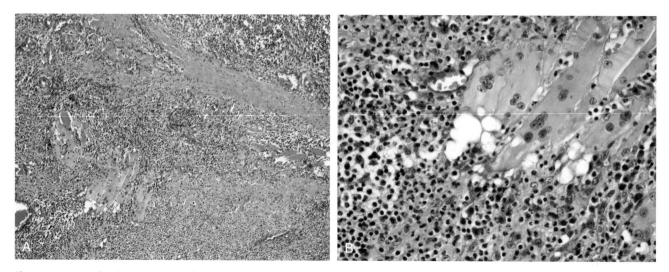

Figure 6-4. Peritonsillar abscess. **A,** Abscess formation is seen at the bottom of the image, adjacent to the peritonsillar skeletal muscle (×100). **B,** Neutrophils infiltrating degenerate-appearing peritonsillar skeletal muscle (×400).

Lemierre syndrome (postanginal sepsis, necrobacillosis), a rare but severe complication of peritonsillar abscess most often associated with *Fusobacterium necrophorum*, consists of the development of internal jugular vein suppurative thrombophlebitis which leads to septicemia and metastatic infection in the lungs and joints.[16]

Diagnosis of peritonsillar abscess is usually made on clinical grounds with or without imaging or needle aspiration for direct examination and culture, and treatment includes antibiotic therapy and drainage.[14] Surgical specimens demonstrate abscess formation and acute inflammation of peritonsillar connective tissues (Fig. 6-4).

Rhinoscleroma

Previously referred to as "scrofulous lupus," rhinoscleroma (scleroma) is a chronic, indolent disease that primarily affects the upper aerodigestive tract and is caused by the gram-negative coccobacillus, *Klebsiella rhinoscleromatis*. Rare in the United States, the disease is not uncommon in endemic areas including Central and South America, Egypt, India, and central and eastern Europe, where it affects patients in the third and fourth decades and is related to poor hygiene, overcrowding, and malnutrition, with human leukocyte antigen (HLA) research suggesting a genetic predisposition.

The disease is characterized by three distinct phases: a catarrhal (also called atrophic or rhinitic) phase, consisting of mucopurulent rhinitis lasting months to years; a proliferative or granulomatous phase, with formation of multiple firm nodules that obstruct and deform the nasal passages; and a cicatricial phase, characterized by mucosal sclerosis.[17,18] Diagnosis is usually established in the proliferative phase. Microscopic findings in this phase include a submucosal mixed inflammatory infiltrate of lymphocytes and plasma cells with scattered Russell bodies, a prominent granulomatous component, and numerous clusters of

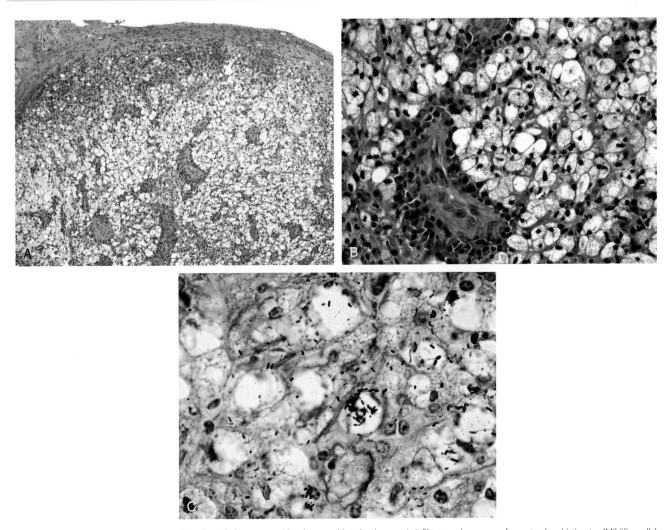

Figure 6-5. Rhinoscleroma. **A,** Attenuated nasal vestibule mucosa with submucosal lymphoplasmacytic infiltrate and numerous foamy to clear histiocytes (Mikülicz cells) (×100). **B,** Perivascular accentuation of lymphoplasmacytic infiltrate and adjacent cluster of Mikülicz cells (×600). **C,** Warthin-Starry stain, highlighting intracytoplasmic coccobacilli (×1000).

foamy histiocytes known as Mikülicz cells that contain bacterial organisms. The organisms can at times be seen on hematoxylin and eosin (H&E) stain but are more readily visualized with silver impregnation stain (e.g., Warthin-Starry) (Fig. 6-5). Immunohistochemical methods for bacterial detection have also been developed.[19] The overlying respiratory mucosa may demonstrate hyperplasia, squamous metaplasia, or ulceration. The cicatricial phase is marked by extensive submucosal fibrosis with a paucity of Mikülicz cells.

Actinomycosis

Actinomycosis is a polymicrobial bacterial infection of the orocervicofacial region caused by gram-positive anaerobic or microaerophilic filamentous oral flora of the genus *Actinomyces*, most commonly *Actinomyces israelii*.[20] Infection follows mucosal injury, often related to dental manipulation, caries, or trauma, and usually manifests as a chronic, progressively enlarging, fluctuant purple mass at the border of the mandible, although it may

also manifest as a mass or ulcer affecting the tongue, larynx, paranasal sinuses, salivary glands, or buccal mucosa, with lymph node involvement developing late in the disease course.[21-23] In chronic lesions, central necrosis and abscess formation occur, and sinus tracts and fistulas may eventually develop and drain foulsmelling, purulent material containing characteristic yellow granular colonies of bacteria known as sulfur granules[24]

Histologic evaluation reveals mixed granulomatous and purulent inflammation with abscess formation and clusters of bacteria with central basophilia and a peripheral rim of eosinophilic, club-like projections composed of immunoglobulin, fibrin, and tissue debris; this is known as the Splendore-Hoeppli phenomenon (Fig. 6-6).[25] Organisms are highlighted on Gomori methenamine silver (GMS) and tissue Gram stains and are often seen in the crypts of routine tonsillectomy specimens removed for hypertrophy, where they most likely exist as saprophytes (see Fig. 6-3).[26] *Actinomyces* may be confused histologically with *Nocardia*, which, in contrast to the former, affects predominantly immunocompromised patients, is weakly acid fast, and is only rarely associated with orocervicofacial disease.[27,28]

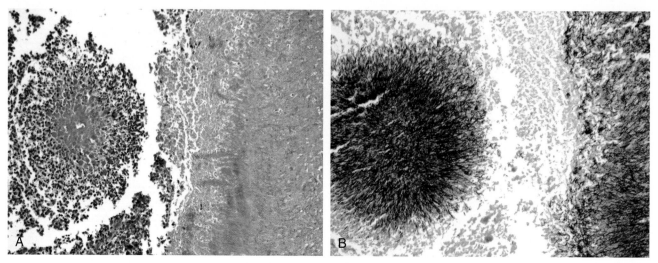

Figure 6-6. Actinomycosis. **A,** Small cluster of *Actinomyces* with surrounding mixed inflammation and Splendore-Hoeppli phenomenon, with a larger cluster of organisms at right (×200). **B,** GMS stain of the same field, highlighting the filamentous forms (×200).

Besides routine histology, other diagnostic methods include fine-needle aspiration and molecular methods, in addition to culture, which is typically of low yield.[29,30] Treatment generally consists of prolonged antibiotic therapy, usually with penicillin.[31]

The two other main forms of actinomycosis, pulmonary and abdominal disease, are covered in other chapters. Additionally, whereas past literature suggested a role for *Actinomyces* in the pathogenesis of osteoradionecrosis and bisphosphonate-related osteonecrosis of the jaw, it is currently held that the bacteria identified in such cases represent a secondary infection of necrotic bone.[32]

Botryomycosis

Botryomycosis is caused by a chronic bacterial infection and is analogous to mycetoma but unrelated to fungi or *Actinomyces* spp. It most commonly involves the subcutis but can also affect mucosal or visceral sites in rare cases.[33] Cutaneous infections are caused most commonly by *S. aureus*, with *Pseudomonas aeruginosa* as the second most common pathogen, although reported cases suggest that *P. aeruginosa* may be the most common pathogen at sinonasal sites.[34,35] Although the pathophysiology is incompletely understood, the disease is most commonly seen in patients with some degree of immunosuppression.[36]

In general, botryomycosis manifests as a firm nodule or mass associated with a sinus draining granular material. Microscopic examination reveals the botryomycotic granules consisting of bacterial aggregates best appreciated with tissue Gram or silver stains, with club-like projections of amorphous eosinophilic material radiating from them (Splendore-Hoeppli phenomenon). The botryomycotic granule is surrounded by a polymorphic infiltrate of neutrophils, lymphocytes, and histiocytes. Well-formed granulomas with central necrosis may be seen, together with edema and fibrosis.[37] Surgical management is usually necessary, because these infections are resistant to medical therapy.

Syphilis

Since reaching an all-time nadir in 2000, the incidence of primary and secondary syphilis in the United States has increased, largely driven by cases among men who have sex with men.[38,39] It remains a significant cause of morbidity in this country. The oral cavity is the most common extragenital site of infection,[40] and the disease may affect virtually any region of the head and neck, with clinical manifestations in the primary, secondary, and tertiary stages, as well as in congenital infections.

After an incubation period of 9 to 90 days, primary syphilis manifests as one or more painless ulcers or chancres at the inoculation site, which can include the oral mucosa and tongue, associated with painless lymphadenopathy.[41] Additionally, primary infection may manifest as painless tonsillar enlargement.[42] Histologic examination of the chancre reveals a diffuse inflammatory infiltrate of lymphocytes and plasma cells, with scattered histiocytes, neutrophils, and eosinophils (Fig. 6-7). The inflammatory infiltrate shows a tendency to surround small blood vessels, producing endothelial proliferation and obliterative endarteritis; poorly formed granulomas, plasma cell neuritis, and focal necrosis can also be seen.[43] Lymph node findings are discussed in Chapter 11.

Secondary syphilis manifests 6 to 8 weeks after spontaneous recovery from the primary infection, producing flu-like symptoms and a rash that often affects the palms and soles. Tonsils may be affected by highly infectious, gray-white, necrotic mucous patches with surrounding erythema, which may extend to the buccal mucosa, tongue, uvula, and soft palate. Maculopapular lesions, moist ulcers, and irregular linear "snail track" erosions can be seen, histologically characterized by dense subepithelial inflammation composed predominantly of plasma cells.[44]

"Lues maligna," or ulceronodular syphilis, is a rare aggressive form of secondary syphilis that most commonly affects individuals coinfected with human immunodeficiency virus (HIV). It is characterized by papulopustular skin lesions that rapidly enlarge and evolve into sharply demarcated ulcers with a central

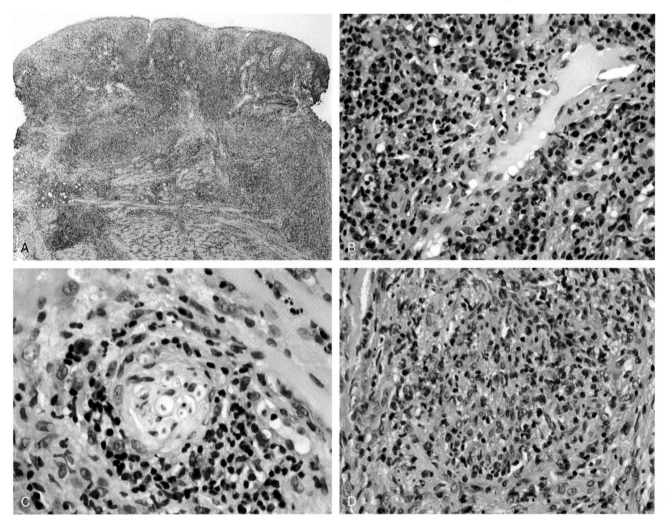

Figure 6-7. Primary syphilis. **A,** Tongue biopsy from a patient with an indurated and ulcerated lesion of the tongue, showing dense deep inflammation involving the skeletal muscle fibers (×40). **B,** Perivascular accentuation of plasma cells and reactive-appearing endothelial cells (×400). **C,** Neurotropism of mixed inflammatory infiltrate (×600). **D,** Vaguely granulomatous inflammatory component (×400).

rupioid crust with associated constitutional symptoms, and it may show involvement of the mucous membranes of the mouth and nose.[45] The histopathology is similar to that of other lesions of secondary syphilis. If untreated, patients pass into the asymptomatic latent phase of disease and lose infectivity before developing signs and symptoms of tertiary disease 4 to 8 years later.

Tertiary syphilis is characterized by multiorgan involvement and is sometimes referred to as "the great imitator" because of its protean manifestations. The gumma is the hallmark lesion of tertiary syphilis. It manifests as a painless swelling of the palate or tongue or, less commonly, the alveolus or parotid gland. Lesions swell and coalesce, eventually forming areas of ulceration, with possible bone destruction, palatal perforation, or oronasal fistula formation.[46] Histologically, gummas are characterized by obliterative endarteritis with necrosis and mixed inflammation consisting of plasma cells (which may be scarce), lymphocytes, epithelioid histiocytes that often form loose granulomas, and giant cells. Syphilitic leukoplakia of the tongue may also be seen and may predispose to the development of

squamous cell carcinoma.[47] The lesions appear as homogeneous white plaques on the dorsum of the tongue; histologically, they show psoriasiform hyperplasia and parakeratosis of the mucosa with infiltrates of lymphocytes, plasma cells, and histiocytes. Interstitial glossitis also occurs.[48] Spirochetal sensorineural hearing loss is an infrequent late consequence of acquired syphilis.[49]

Congenital syphilis occurs after transplacental spread during pregnancy and can result in numerous abnormalities in surviving affected progeny. Early signs of congenital infection typically occur between 1 month and 2 years of age and include rhinitis ("snuffles"), vesiculobullous eruptions of the mucous membranes, and radial perioral skin lesions ("rhagades"). Late signs occur after 2 years and include keratitis (often leading to blindness) and eighth nerve deafness, as well as more typical signs of tertiary syphilis. Such patients are additionally affected by typical orofacial stigmata, including tooth abnormalities (Hutchinson incisors, Fournier "mulberry" molars, and Moon molars), saddle-nose deformity (caused by destruction of the vomer), frontoparietal bossing, and maxillary hypoplasia ("bulldog jaw").[50,51]

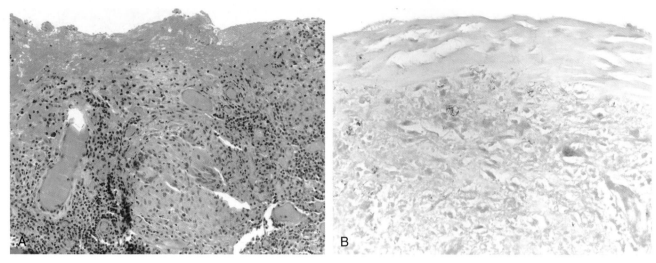

Figure 6-8. Tuberculous otitis. **A,** Well-formed granuloma with surrounding granulation tissue and mixed inflammatory infiltrate (×200). **B,** Acid-fast stain, highlighting scattered bacilli within degenerate connective tissue (×400).

The diagnosis of syphilis may be accomplished in several ways. In the primary and secondary stages, as well as in early congenital disease, lesions contain numerous spiral-shaped treponemal organisms, often within the surface epithelium, surrounding small vessels and within macrophages, and they can be visualized with the Warthin-Starry stain, immunohistochemistry, or dark-field microscopy. However, microscopic findings should be interpreted with caution, because spirochetes are part of the normal flora of the oral cavity. Serologic techniques are currently the mainstay of diagnosis and include both treponemal (specific) and nontreponemal (nonspecific) antibody tests. Nonspecific tests include the Venereal Disease Research Laboratory (VDRL) and the rapid plasma reagin (RPR) tests, which are rapid and inexpensive and traditionally have served as screening tests. Specific tests such as the fluorescent treponemal antibody-absorbed assay (FTA-ABS) should be performed for confirmation of the diagnosis. No single test should be used alone in making a diagnosis of syphilis.[42]

Tuberculosis

Tuberculosis, one of the most important global infectious causes of morbidity and mortality, is most commonly caused by the acid-fast aerobic bacterium, *Mycobacterium tuberculosis*, which is estimated to infect one third of the world's population, and less commonly by the other members of the *M. tuberculosis* complex, which includes *Mycobacterium bovis*, *Mycobacterium africanum*, *Mycobacterium canetti*, and *Mycobacterium microti*.[52,53] Although it most commonly manifests as pulmonary disease, tuberculosis is a systemic infection and can affect virtually any part of the body, including the head and neck. Extrapulmonic manifestations are more common in immunosuppressed patients, particularly those with HIV.[54,55]

Tuberculosis of the head and neck most commonly manifests as cervical lymphadenopathy, although many other sites may be involved, either with and without pulmonary involvement, including the larynx, pharynx, middle ear, salivary glands, tongue, sinonasal region, thyroid gland, and oral cavity.[56-70] Lesions take on a variety of clinical appearances depending on site of involvement, and patient may present with a parotid mass, a mouth ulcer, a soft tissue abscess, a retropharyngeal space swelling, otorrhea, or many other signs and symptoms.[71-81] Material for pathologic examination is vital and may be obtained by incisional biopsy or fine-needle aspiration.

Histologic evaluation reveals caseating granulomatous inflammation, including well-formed granulomas with scattered Langhans-type giant cells and surrounding lymphocytes and fibroblasts (Fig. 6-8). Organisms are typically sparse, and acid-fast staining techniques are required for visualization of the bacilli. In addition to traditional diagnostic tests, such as sputum smear and tuberculin skin testing, newer methods have become available, including nucleic acid amplification and interferon-release assays.[82]

Leprosy

Leprosy is an infection caused by *Mycobacterium leprae*, also known as Hansen's bacillus, which produces a chronic systemic granulomatous disease that may affect the skin, mucous membranes, peripheral nerves, skeleton, and viscera. Although it is infrequently encountered in the United States, leprosy continues to be a significant health problem worldwide. Transmission of the disease is incompletely understood, but current research suggests that contacts of untreated affected individuals are at risk for infection through respiratory exposure to organisms shed into the environment from skin and nasal mucosa, with salivary anti-*M. leprae* IgA levels correlating with protection.[83,84] Recent research has identified *Mycobacterium lepromatosis sp. nov.* as a second species responsible for clinical leprosy.[85]

The two main clinical forms are tuberculoid leprosy (the paucibacillary form, representing intact cell-mediated immunity) and lepromatous leprosy (the multibacillary form, representing relative anergy); there are additional intermediate clinical forms depending on the degree of cell-mediated immunity.[86] Mucosal lesions usually are present in the chronic lepromatous form, and they consist of multiple nodules (lepromas) or ulcers affecting

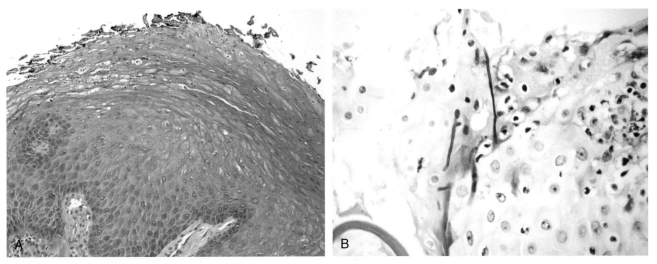

Figure 6-9. Oral candidosis. **A,** Biopsy of a tongue lesion, showing mucosal hyperplasia, hyperparakeratosis, spongiosis, several intraepithelial neutrophils, and fungal elements consisting of superficial spheroid yeast forms and scattered pseudohyphal forms present within the parakeratotic layer (×200). **B,** PAS stain with diastase digestion, highlighting the intraepithelial pseudohyphae (×600).

the palate and nasal mucosa, and, less commonly, the tongue, lips, and gums, with destruction of the anterior maxilla and loss of teeth.[87,88] Histologic analysis of nasal and palatal lesions reveals mucosal hyperplasia or ulceration with a dense submucosal inflammatory infiltrate consisting of lymphocytes as well as foamy histiocytes containing numerous acid-fast bacilli (lepra cells). However, histologic findings, particularly in oral lesions, may consist of nonspecific chronic inflammation without associated organisms. Well-formed granulomas and giant cells are infrequent but may be seen in intermediate forms of the disease as well as in clinically normal mucosa of patients with lepromatous leprosy.[89] In contrast, in the tuberculoid form, well-formed granulomas are often identified in the skin, but the mucosa remains relatively unaffected by disease, both clinically and histologically. Because mucosal lesions of lepromatous disease often show nonspecific inflammatory changes, the diagnosis is usually based on smear or biopsy of cutaneous lesions in conjunction with clinical findings. Molecular methods of diagnosis are also available.[90]

Oral Candidosis

Candida albicans is a dimorphic fungus that frequently colonizes the oral cavity, and it is also the most common fungal pathogen isolated from this location, causing opportunistic infection in the immunosuppressed, the elderly, and the very young.[91] Other *Candida* species, including *Candida glabrata* and *Candida tropicalis*, are less commonly isolated. Oral infection is classified as primary or secondary. Primary oral candidosis includes acute forms such as pseudomembranous candidosis (thrush) and erythematous candidosis, chronic forms such as erythematous candidosis and hyperplastic candidosis, and several *Candida*-associated lesions (denture stomatitis, angular cheilitis, and median rhomboid glossitis). Secondary oral candidosis includes oral disease associated with systemic infection, usually as a result of congenital or acquired immunodeficiency.[92] Patients may be

asymptomatic, or they may report burning or dysgeusia, and on clinical examination they demonstrate a variety of lesions depending on the form of disease.

The histologic appearance of lesions also varies but often demonstrates epithelial hyperplasia with hyperparakeratosis, spongiosis, and scattered intraepithelial neutrophils, as well as a submucosal mononuclear cell infiltrate (Fig. 6-9). Fungal pseudohyphae are seen within the superficial parakeratotic layer, and ovoid yeast forms may also be present more superficially. GMS stain and periodic acid–Schiff (PAS) with diastase can aid in the identification of organisms, which are gram positive on tissue Gram stain. Exfoliative cytology is a useful diagnostic tool, and immunohistochemical and molecular methods are also available.[93,94]

Fungal Rhinosinusitis

Sinonasal mycotic disease is classified based on clinical, radiologic, and histologic findings and includes both tissue invasive and noninvasive processes. The invasive forms of disease are acute fulminant invasive fungal sinusitis, chronic invasive fungal sinusitis, and granulomatous invasive fungal sinusitis; the noninvasive forms are sinus fungal ball, allergic fungal rhinosinusitis, and saprophytic fungal infestation (Table 6-1).[95]

Acute fulminant invasive fungal sinusitis occurs almost exclusively in immunocompromised patients and constitutes a medical emergency. It is referred to as mucormycosis, zygomycosis, or fulminant invasive sinusitis, depending on the pathogen, but as the clinical syndromes are virtually identical, the term *acute fulminant invasive fungal sinusitis* is currently favored.[96] This disease is most commonly caused by molds of the class Zygomycetes, including *Mucor, Rhizopus,* and *Absidia* spp. among others, but can also result from infection with *Aspergillus* spp., *Fusarium* spp., and *Pseudallescheria boydii*.[97] Clinical signs and symptoms include fever, headache, cough, epistaxis, nasal discharge or crusting, facial swelling, and mental status

Table 6-1 Classification of Sinonasal Fungal Disease

Classification	Immune Status	Causative Organisms	Clinical Presentation	Microscopic Findings	Management
Invasive Disease					
Acute fulminant invasive fungal sinusitis	Compromised	Class Zygomycetes, *Aspergillus* spp., *Fusarium* spp.	Fever, headache, discharge, epistaxis, mental status changes	Necrosis, hemorrhage, acute and chronic inflammation, fungal tissue and angioinvasion	Emergent débridement, antibiotic therapy
Chronic invasive fungal sinusitis	Compromised (usually diabetics)	*Aspergillus fumigatus*	Fever, headache, discharge, epistaxis, mental status changes	Necrosis, chronic inflammation, fungal invasion, abundant organisms resembling fungal ball	Emergent débridement, antibiotic therapy
Granulomatous invasive fungal sinusitis	Competent	*Aspergillus flavus*	Slowly progressive sinusitis, headache, unilateral proptosis	Granulomatous inflammation, fungal tissue invasion	Débridement, aeration, antibiotic therapy
Noninvasive Disease					
Sinus fungal ball	Competent	*A. fumigatus*	Facial pain, headache, nasal obstruction and discharge, cacosmia, visual changes	Matted fungal hyphae, mixed sinus inflammation, absence of tissue invasion	Débridement, aeration
Allergic fungal rhinosinusitis	Competent	*Aspergillus, Fusarium, Curvularia, Bipolaris,* and *Pseudallescheria* spp.	Chronic pansinusitis, nasal polyps, history of atopy	Polypoid sinus mucosa with stromal edema and mixed inflammation with many eosinophils, allergic mucin, sparse fungal forms	Débridement, aeration, corticosteroid therapy
Saprophytic fungal infestation	Competent	Various	Asymptomatic	Fungal spores within mucus crusts	Crust removal, irrigation

changes. The presence of orbital or cranial nerve symptoms at presentation is more often related to *Mucor* than to *Aspergillus* species.[98]

Examination may reveal a palatal ulcer or eschar, as well as necrosis of nasal mucosa. Gross surgical débridement specimens typically consist of necrotic, hemorrhagic soft tissue, and occasionally bone fragments. Microscopic evaluation reveals hemorrhage, necrosis, and mixed acute and chronic inflammation that may have a granulomatous component (Fig. 6-10). Fungal hyphal forms are usually evident on routine H&E staining but are best appreciated with GMS. Tissue invasion occurs with striking angiotropism and angioinvasion, often occluding vessel lumens and resulting in thrombosis with surrounding necrosis. *Mucor* also has a propensity for perineural involvement.[99] Hyphal forms of *Aspergillus* spp. are septate with acute-angle branching, whereas *Mucor, Rhizopus,* and similar species produce pauciseptate, ribbon-like hyphae that tend to branch at right angles. Immunohistochemistry for mucin 5B (MUC5B) expression is positive in most cases of *Aspergillus* infection and generally absent in order Mucorales sinusitis.[100] Given the urgent nature of acute fulminant invasive fungal sinusitis, intraoperative evaluation of frozen sections may be requested, and antibiotic therapy should be initiated before culture results are available.

Chronic invasive fungal sinusitis, a rare disease, is usually seen in diabetic patients and is defined as sinusitis of at least 4 weeks' duration with compatible radiologic findings and histologic evidence of tissue invasion by fungal hyphal forms.[101] Patients may develop the orbital apex syndrome, which consists of ocular immobility and loss of vision owing to the presence of a mass in the superior part of the orbit, caused by fungal spread from the ethmoid sinus. Histologically, chronic invasive fungal sinusitis is characterized by vascular, bone, and soft tissue invasion by fungal hyphae, most commonly *Aspergillus fumigatus,* with necrosis and a mild associated chronic inflammatory infiltrate. Fungal organisms are abundant and resemble a sinus fungal ball, a finding that has led some to postulate that the two diseases exist along a spectrum.[97] Like acute fulminant invasive fungal sinusitis, chronic invasive fungal sinusitis has a poor prognosis, requiring aggressive management.

Granulomatous invasive fungal sinusitis is a subtype of chronic invasive fungal sinusitis that shows a few key differences. The disease is most commonly reported in northern Africa, where it affects apparently immunocompetent individuals and is caused almost invariably by *Aspergillus flavus.*[96] Also known as indolent fungal sinusitis or primary paranasal granuloma, granulomatous invasive fungal sinusitis is characterized clinically by

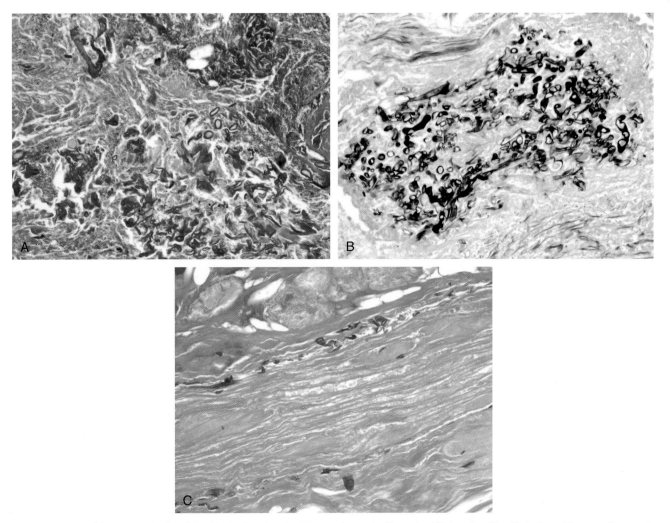

Figure 6-10. Acute fulminant invasive fungal sinusitis. **A,** Tissue invasive *Mucor* sp. characterized by eosinophilic irregular, ribbon-like hyphae with surrounding necrotic fibrous tissue (×400). **B,** GMS stain highlighting angioinvasive *Mucor* sp. (×400). **C,** Scattered hyphae of *Mucor* sp. surrounding a necrotic nerve (×400).

slowly progressive sinusitis with headache and unilateral proptosis.[102] Pathologically, it shows florid granulomatous inflammation with tissue invasion by fungal hyphae. Noncaseating granulomata with giant cells and occasional central eosinophilic microgranulomata, as well as fibrinoid necrosis, vasculitis, vascular proliferation, and perivascular fibrosis, have also been described.[103,104] Fungal forms may be sparse and within giant cells or profuse and mass-forming.[97,105] Prognosis is better than in other invasive fungal sinus infections, and patients tend to respond to débridement, aeration, and antifungal therapy, with recurrence being common.

Sinus fungal ball, frequently (and inappropriately) referred to as mycetoma or aspergilloma, is a dense conglomeration of fungal hyphae that forms a mass within a sinus cavity without invading the surrounding host tissue.[106] Patients are immunocompetent and usually present with facial pain because the maxillary sinus is most commonly involved, but they may also experience headache, nasal obstruction and discharge, cacosmia, and visual disturbances.[107] Radiologic findings include unilateral sinus opacification, often with associated flocculent calcifications owing to calcium oxalate deposition by the fungus. Examination

of sinus contents reveals mucopurulent, caseous, or clay-like material.[108] The most common fungus recovered is *A. fumigatus*, although culture is often negative.[109]

Histologic examination of sinus contents reveals matted fungal hyphae that are evident on H&E stain but best delineated with GMS (Fig. 6-11). Intact hyphae are identified at the periphery of the mass but are often densely packed and difficult to recognize centrally. Tissue invasion is absent, but fragments of sinus mucosa may demonstrate mixed inflammation consisting of neutrophils, lymphocytes, plasma cells, mast cells, and eosinophils. Neither the presence of allergic mucin nor a predominance of eosinophils is a feature of sinus fungal ball, and these findings suggest a concomitant allergic fungal rhinosinusitis.[108,110]

Therapy consists of débridement and aeration, and antifungal medication is not required. It has been proposed that another form of noninvasive fungal sinusitis exists, so-called chronic erosive sinusitis, that is characterized by radiologic evidence of bony erosion without histologic evidence of tissue invasion; however, it is presently unclear whether this represents a separate entity or more extensive involvement by sinus fungal ball. Pos-

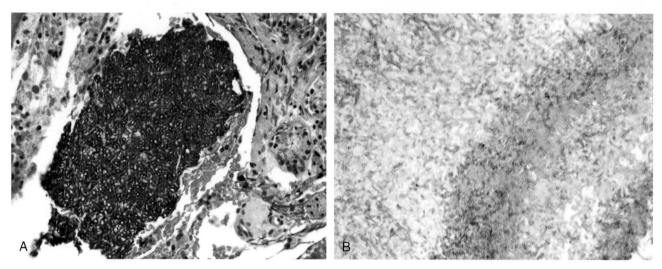

Figure 6-11. Sinus fungal ball. **A,** Matted hyphae of *Aspergillus* sp. removed during endoscopic sinus surgery with adjacent submucosal glands (×400). **B,** GMS stain highlighting the matted hyphae (×400).

sibly it represents an intermediary form of disease between sinus fungal ball and chronic invasive fungal sinusitis.[106,111]

Allergic fungal rhinosinusitis is currently thought to represent a hypersensitivity reaction to fungus within the sinus cavity, and the proposed diagnostic criteria include the presence of allergic mucin and fungal hyphae within a sinus, radiographic findings confirming sinusitis, absence of tissue invasion by the fungus, and absence of predisposing immunodeficiency or immunosuppression.[112] Hyaline molds such as *Aspergillus* and *Fusarium*, as well as pigmented dematiaceous fungi such as *Curvularia*, *Bipolaris*, and *Pseudallescheria*, are commonly implicated.[105] With regard to identification of the fungus, it has been suggested that histologic evidence is preferable to culture isolation, because research has revealed the frequent presence of fungus in cultured nasal lavage specimens of normal individuals, and culture carries an inherent risk of contamination.[113,114] However, speciation by histology is not possible. Because fungus is ubiquitous in the environment and is present in the nasal passages of apparently normal individuals, it is believed that disease manifestation is caused not by the fungus per se but rather by an exaggerated immune response against it. Allergic fungal sinusitis is an area of intense study, and, although the pathology is incompletely understood, there is evidence to support both IgE- and cell-mediated processes.[115-118] Current terminology reflects this uncertainty and includes such terms as eosinophilic fungal rhinosinusitis (a term used to stress the eosinophil-mediated nature of the disease) and eosinophilic mucin rhinosinusitis (proposed to represent a disease unrelated to fungus).[119-121]

The typical patient with allergic fungal sinusitis presents with chronic, often intractable, pansinusitis and associated nasal polyposis, with a history of atopy and multiple sinus operations.[97] Examination of surgical specimens of allergic mucin reveals chalky gray to black or brown tenacious mucus that microscopically appears as thick, gray-green to pink, lamellated material containing mucin, serum, abundant eosinophils with scattered neutrophils and Charcot-Leyden crystals, cellular debris, and sparse, often fragmented, fungal hyphae, usually visualized only with special stains such as GMS (Fig. 6-12). Sinonasal mucosa is often polypoid and usually demonstrates underlying mixed inflammation consisting primarily of eosinophils with admixed lymphocytes, plasma cells, mast cells, and scattered neutrophils, together with associated stromal edema. Although tissue invasion is not a feature of allergic fungal sinusitis, the collection of allergic mucin may be large enough to cause adjacent bony erosion, cranial nerve palsies, sinus perforation, and disease extension into the orbit or anterior skull base, sometimes mimicking neoplasia; however, despite this potentially aggressive behavior, most patients respond to débridement, aeration, and corticosteroid therapy.[122-125]

Saprophytic fungal infestation is the finding of fungal spores on mucous crusts of respiratory passages. Its natural history and role in sinonasal pathology are uncertain, but the condition is considered distinct from that of asymptomatic individuals with positive fungal cultures alone.[95] Patients typically respond to crust removal and home irrigation,[95] and, because crusts are usually removed in a clinic setting, specimens are not typically submitted for histologic evaluation.

Paracoccidioidomycosis

Paracoccidioidomycosis (also known as South American blastomycosis or Lutz-Splendore-Almeida disease) is a systemic granulomatous disease caused by the dimorphic fungus *Paracoccidioides brasiliensis*, which is endemic to Latin America, where about 10 million people are infected, 2% of whom manifest disease.[126] Primary infection typically occurs in the second decade of life but can occur at any age, with a lower female incidence in pubertal years owing to the inhibitory effect of estrogen against fungal transition from mycelia to yeast form.[127,128] Infection is thought to occur through inhalation of conidia, with the two main clinical forms of disease being the acute/subacute (juvenile) form and the more common chronic (adult) form; these affect primarily the reticuloendothelial system and the lungs, respectively, although any organ may be involved.[129]

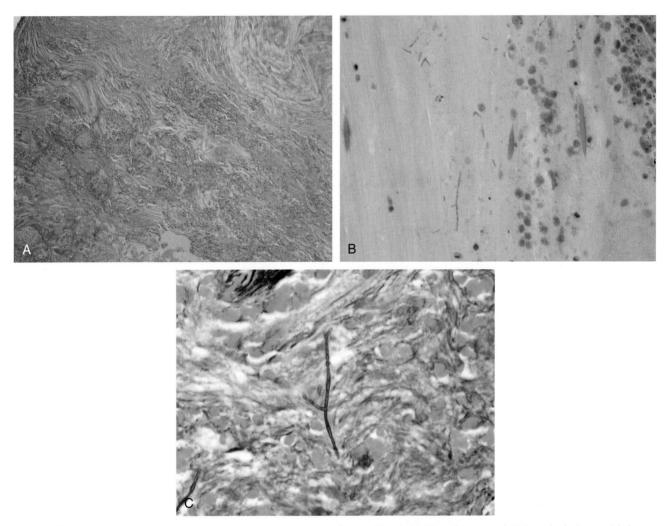

Figure 6-12. Allergic fungal sinusitis. **A,** Allergic mucin, characterized by clusters of eosinophils imbedded in acellular mucus (×100). **B,** Slender bipyramidal Charcot-Leyden crystals and several sparse hyphal forms, here identifiable on routine H&E stain (×400). **C,** GMS stain, highlighting a septate hyphal form with acute-angle branching, surrounded by allergic mucin. (×600).

Head and neck manifestations commonly occur in the chronic form of the disease, usually in oral sites, including the alveolar process, gingiva, tongue, lip, buccal mucosa, palate, and floor of mouth, as well as the larynx and, uncommonly, the nasal mucosa.[130-135] Patients present with stomatodynia, hoarseness, odynophagia, sore throat, and dyspnea. On examination, they may exhibit characteristic muriform lesions, which are reminiscent of a mulberry and are characterized by a fine granular surface, as well as ulcers, plaques, tooth loss, thickening of the lips, and, rarely, palatal perforation.[136-139] Infection may mimic carcinoma both clinically and histologically, with chronic and progressive lesions that histologically demonstrate pseudoepitheliomatous hyperplasia.[140]

Microscopic examination reveals intraepithelial abscesses and subepithelial granulomatous inflammation with scattered multinucleate giant cells, as well as admixed neutrophils, lymphocytes, plasma cells, and eosinophils (Fig. 6-13).[141] Well-formed granulomas are composed mainly of macrophages and CD4-positive T lymphocytes and contain fewer yeast particles

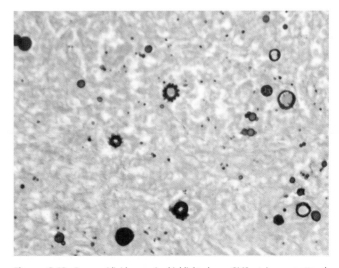

Figure 6-13. Paracoccidioidomycosis, highlighted on GMS stain as scattered, double-contoured yeast forms with multiple surrounding budding forms (×400).

than poorly formed granulomatous areas, possibly reflecting a more effective host immune response.[142] The characteristic polygemulating yeast forms appear as double-contoured structures 6 to 30 μm or more in diameter with multiple surrounding budding forms, often likened to a captain's wheel (although single budding may also be seen), as well as smaller yeast forms that may cause confusion with *Histoplasma capsulatum*.[143] Organisms are usually visible on routine H&E staining, although they are better appreciated by GMS staining. Exfoliative cytology has proved to be a useful rapid diagnostic tool, and immunohistochemical and molecular methods of identification have also been developed.[144-150] Antifungal therapy with sulfonamides or azoles is effective in treating infection, with fibrotic sequelae being a common and sometimes disfiguring complication in healed lesions.[129,151]

Sporotrichosis

Sporotrichosis is caused by *Sporothrix schenckii*, a dimorphic fungus with worldwide distribution that thrives in tropical and temperate climates, where it exists as a common saprophyte found in plant materials, soil, and a variety of animals.[152] The disease usually manifests as lymphocutaneous or fixed cutaneous disease or, uncommonly, as disseminated disease.[153] There are several case reports of sporotrichosis involving the nasal passages, paranasal sinuses, or oral cavity, and it appears that many of the affected patients suffered from some form of immunocompromise.[154-161] The histologic findings are identical to those seen in cutaneous disease.

Blastomycosis

Blastomycosis (sometimes referred to as North American blastomycosis) is a chronic granulomatous and suppurative disease caused by *Blastomyces dermatitidis*, a dimorphic fungus endemic to the south-central and midwestern United States.[162] There are five categories of blastomycosis occurring in humans: primary pulmonary disease, single organ system disease, generalized multiorgan disease, chronic cutaneous disease, and inoculation blastomycosis.[163] It is generally accepted that most cases of cutaneous disease occur after lymphohematogenous spread from a primary pulmonary infection, even in the absence of clinical pulmonary disease.[164] Blastomycosis has been reported in the nasal passages, paranasal sinuses, mouth, and parotid gland, often manifesting as a mass and mimicking a neoplasm.[165-179] The histologic findings are identical to those seen in cutaneous disease.

Coccidioidomycosis

Coccidioidomycosis, commonly referred to as valley fever, is caused by *Coccidioides immitis* and *Coccidioides posadasii*, two morphologically identical but genetically distinct dimorphic fungi endemic to the southwestern United States and Mexico as well as parts of Central and South America.[180-182] The five main clinical manifestations of coccidioidal infection are acute pneumonia, chronic progressive pneumonia, pulmonary nodules and cavities, extrapulmonary nonmeningeal disease, and meningi-

tis.[183] Head and neck manifestations are rare and are usually associated with disseminated disease.[184] Reported sites of involvement include the tongue, retropharyngeal space, deep neck, temporal bone, and thyroglossal duct cyst.[185-187]

Cryptococcosis

Cryptococcosis is caused by the ubiquitous yeast of the *Cryptococcus* species complex, which includes *Cryptococcus neoformans* (further divided into var. *neoformans* and var. *grubii*) and *Cryptococcus gattii*.[188] *Cryptococcus* can cause disease in any organ of the body but most commonly affects the lungs and central nervous system, particularly in immunocompromised patients.[189] Involvement of various head and neck sites, including the oral cavity, thyroid gland, paranasal sinuses, and salivary glands, has rarely been reported and typically occurs in the setting of immunocompromise with disseminated disease.[190-199]

Histoplasmosis

Histoplasmosis, also known as Darling's disease, is caused by *Histoplasma capsulatum* var. *capsulatum*, a dimorphic fungus that is found worldwide and is highly endemic to the Ohio and Mississippi River valleys.[200-202] Clinical manifestations include pulmonary, mediastinal, inflammatory, and disseminated syndromes and are dependent on the size of the inoculum as well as the underlying health and immune status of the patient.[203] Involvement of head and neck sites is uncommon and usually occurs in the setting of disseminated disease in HIV/AIDS.[204-235]

Rhinosporidiosis

Rhinosporidiosis is a rare chronic granulomatous disease that most commonly affects the nasal and nasopharyngeal mucosa but also can involve various other sites, including the oropharynx, conjunctiva, skin, trachea, and urethra, occasionally manifesting as disseminated disease.[236-238] The causative agent is generally believed to be *Rhinosporidium seeberi*, which was once thought to be a fungus but is currently categorized as a protist of class Mesomycetozoea, which comprises mostly uncultivable aquatic microbes at the animal-fungal boundary.[239] It has also been suggested that the causative organism is a cyanobacterium.[240] The disease is encountered in the Americas, Europe, Africa, and Asia and has its highest incidence in Sri Lanka and southern India, usually affecting but not restricted to adult men.[241] The mode of transmission is unknown, but water and soil are believed to be reservoirs for infection, and the incidence of disease is higher among sandworkers, paddy cultivators, and people bathing in stagnant waters.[242]

Presenting symptoms include nasal obstruction, epistaxis, and viscid nasal discharge. Examination reveals a friable vascular polyp studded with tiny white dots, giving the characteristic "strawberry" appearance.[243] Histologic examination reveals hyperplastic mucosa with an underlying dense lymphoplasmacytic infiltrate and scattered intraepithelial and subepithelial, large (up to 350 μm or larger), thick-walled (up to 5 μm), cystic structures called sporangia, which contain multiple small

(2-10 μm), round endospores, both of which stain with H&E, GMS, mucicarmine, and PAS (Fig. 6-14).[242,244] In addition to the lymphoplasmacytic infiltrate, neutrophils, histiocytes, and occasional giant cells may be seen, as well as submucosal hyper-vascularity and foci of necrosis.[245] Fine-needle aspiration cytology has proved useful in diagnosis.[246] The histologic differential diag-nosis includes *C. immitis*, which is smaller and negative for mucicarmine, and myospherulosis, a foreign body response to petroleum-based material. The mainstay of treatment is surgical removal of lesions, occasionally with dapsone as adjunct therapy, and recurrence is a known complication.[247,248]

Mucocutaneous Leishmaniasis

Leishmaniasis is a vector-borne parasitic disease caused by any of more than 25 species of the hemoflagellate *Leishmania*. It is transmitted by the bite of an infected sandfly and is prevalent in

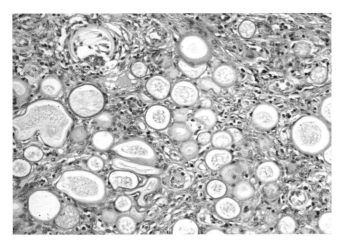

Figure 6-14. Rhinosporidiosis, characterized by multiple, thick-walled sporangia of variable diameter containing multiple endospores, with surrounding lymphoplasma-cytic inflammation (×200).

at least 88 countries worldwide.[249] The four forms of disease generally recognized are localized cutaneous leishmaniasis, diffuse cutaneous leishmaniasis, mucocutaneous leishmaniasis (also known as espundia), and visceral leishmaniasis (also known as kala-azar). The mucocutaneous form is most commonly observed in South America, where *Leishmania brasiliensis* is the major cause.[250-252]

Mucocutaneous leishmaniasis predominates in adults, with mucosal lesions occurring concomitantly with, or years after, cutaneous manifestations and involving the nose, lips, mouth, pharynx, and larynx in the form of progressively enlarging swell-ings or nodules with associated granulation tissue that can result in severe disfigurement if left untreated.[253] Histologically, lesions may show pseudoepitheliomatous hyperplasia or ulceration and associated granulation tissue, with an underlying mixed inflam-matory infiltrate consisting of lymphocytes, plasma cells, and histiocytes, as well as occasional giant cells containing amasti-gotes, which are visible on routine H&E, Giemsa, or immuno-histochemistry staining as 2- to 4-μm, round to oval, intracytoplasmic bodies (Fig. 6-15).[254-256] In addition to biopsy, lesional smear preparation is a routine method of amastigote identification, but because lesions may contain few organisms, other diagnostic methods, including culture and molecular anal-ysis, should also be considered.[257,258] Treatment options include meglumine, amphotericin B, and pentamidine, with a cure rate of about 88%.[259]

Epstein-Barr Virus

EBV is an enveloped DNA herpesvirus that infects more than 90% of people worldwide and is associated with a variety of head and neck infections, notably infectious mononucleosis and oral hairy leukoplakia, as well as numerous neoplastic processes, both epithelial and hematogenous, including nasopharyngeal carci-noma, Hodgkin lymphoma, nasal type NK/T-cell lymphoma, Burkitt lymphoma, and lymphoepithelial carcinoma of the sali-vary glands.[260-262]

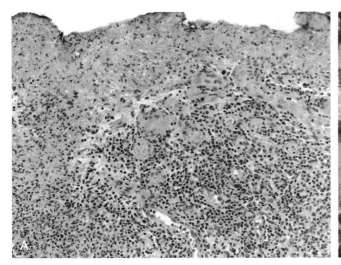
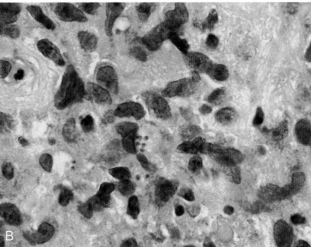

Figure 6-15. Leishmaniasis. **A,** Nasal septal biopsy specimen from a patient with chronic infection, showing surface ulceration, underlying granulation tissue, and mixed inflammation (×200). **B,** Organisms appear as intracytoplasmic bodies within histiocytes (×1000).

Infectious mononucleosis, commonly referred to as the "kissing disease," is one of the most common diseases of adolescence. It is transmitted primarily through saliva and typically produces fever, malaise, pharyngitis, lymphadenopathy, and an atypical lymphocytosis that reflects the virus's infection of B lymphocytes.[263] Diagnosis relies on a combination of clinical findings and serologic studies, the most common being heterophile antibody detection (as in the Monospot test), which is used to identify the presence of EBV-induced antibodies that cross-react with horse, sheep, and bovine erythrocytes.[264] Other organisms associated with an infectious mononucleosis–like syndrome (heterophile-negative infectious mononucleosis) include cytomegalovirus, HIV, HSV, human herpesvirus 6 (HHV-6), *S. pyogenes*, adenovirus, and *Toxoplasma gondii*.[265] Additional serologic evaluation of antibodies to various viral protein complexes, including early antigen (EA), viral capsid antigen (VCA), and nuclear antigen (EBNA), is useful for patients in whom a falsely heterophile-negative infection (common in young children and older adults) is suspected or to document prior EBV infection.[266] Tissue diagnosis is not usually required except in cases with atypical or incomplete presentations (e.g., asymptomatic tonsillitis).[267,268]

Histologic findings in tonsillar tissue mirror those seen in the lymph nodes and are described in detail in Chapter 11. Infectious mononucleosis usually follows a benign, self-limited course, although some patients may develop chronic active infection characterized by recurrent bouts of infectious mononucleosis–like symptoms, hepatosplenomegaly (rarely encountered in acute infection), and an abnormal pattern of anti-EBV antibodies.[269]

Oral hairy leukoplakia is a benign condition seen almost exclusively in immunocompromised patients, particularly HIV patients, but also in the setting of transplantation, leukemia, and chemotherapy; it manifests on the lateral and dorsolateral tongue as white vertical folds or ridges that cannot be scraped off.[270] The histologic features include ballooning degeneration of keratinocytes of the upper stratum spinosum (sometimes with Cowdry type A inclusions or peripheral chromatin beading), epithelial hyperplasia with hyperparakeratosis, and mild to absent submucosal chronic inflammation (Fig. 6-16).[271,272]

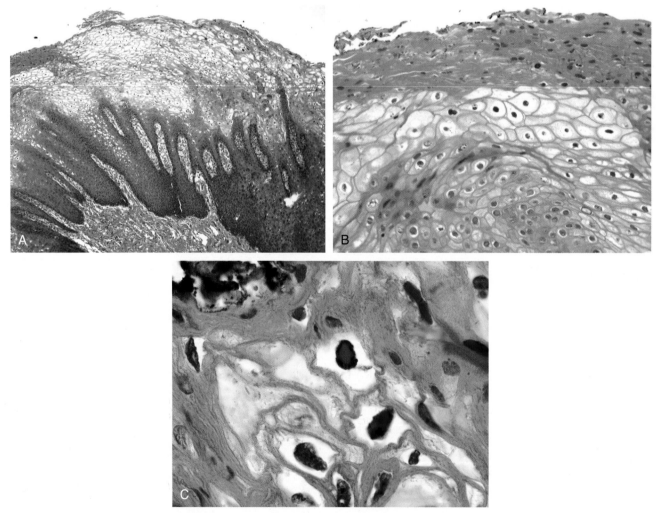

Figure 6-16. Oral hairy leukoplakia. **A,** Irregular hyperplasia with parakeratosis and superficial cytoplasmic clearing (ballooning degeneration) (×100). **B,** Ballooning degeneration in the upper spinous layer in a patient with a concomitant candidal infection (×400). **C,** Balloon cell with a Cowdry type A inclusion, characterized by a glassy intranuclear inclusion and peripheral chromatin margination (×1000).

Immunohistochemistry, in situ hybridization, and PCR are all available as diagnostic aids.[273] Therapy is not necessary unless lesions are symptomatic, and antiviral therapy is generally effective treatment.[274]

Herpes Simplex Virus

HSV types 1 and 2 are closely related neurotropic, double-stranded DNA viruses of the Herpesviridae family that gain entry to the body through the skin and mucous membranes, producing chronic recurrent mucocutaneous disease during the active "lytic" infectious phase and lying dormant in sensory neurons during the "latent" phase.[275] Although HSV types 1 and 2 are considered to be "oral" and "genital" types, respectively, they are not restricted to these sites with regard to causing disease.[276] Primary infection is usually subclinical, although rare infected individuals may present with acute herpetic gingivostomatitis or pharyngotonsillitis.[277]

The most common head and neck manifestation of HSV infection is recurrent herpes labialis, commonly referred to as a cold sore or fever blister, which represents reactivation of dormant virus and is characterized by burning or tingling in the affected site, followed several hours later by the formation of vesicles that rupture and coalesce to form larger, irregular, crusted erosions.[278] Recurrent herpes stomatitis is much less common than recurrent herpes labialis and may be mistaken clinically for recurrent aphthous stomatitis or shingles. In immunocompromised patients, recurrent herpes stomatitis can be extensive and severe.[279]

Diagnosis is usually made clinically, although a number of laboratory methods are available for use when the diagnosis is not straightforward, including cytology (Tzanck smear), biopsy, culture, serology, and viral DNA detection.[280] The Tzanck method involves direct examination of lesional material for the presence of the Tzanck cell, an epithelial cell containing numerous nuclei demonstrating nuclear molding and viral inclusions that give the nuclei a homogeneous, glassy appearance and can be seen in HSV, herpes zoster, varicella, and the pemphigus

group of autoimmune blistering diseases.[281,282] Although biopsy is not usually performed, it reveals intraepithelial vesicles with epithelial ballooning degeneration, acantholysis, intranuclear inclusions, and multinucleate giant cells with characteristic nuclear molding and positive staining by immunohistochemistry (Fig. 6-17). Treatment is aimed at reducing symptom duration, as well as the frequency and severity of attacks, and consists of antiviral therapy.[283]

Human Papillomavirus

The human papillomavirus (HPV) family comprises a heterogeneous group of epitheliotropic, double-stranded DNA viruses that cause verrucae and cervical cancer as well as a variety of reactive and neoplastic processes affecting the head and neck, including 25% to 33% of oropharyngeal cancers, which are attributable to infection with the high-risk anogenital subtypes 16 and 18.[284] Oral squamous papillomas, oral verruca vulgaris, oral condyloma acuminatum, focal epithelial hyperplasia (also known as Heck's disease), and fungiform sinonasal Schneiderian papillomas are all associated with HPV infection to some degree, and they share the common histologic feature of epithelial koilocytosis, characterized histologically by a nucleus that appears shrunken, dense, and irregular (often referred to as "raisinoid") surrounded by a sharp rim of perinuclear clearing (the "halo") (Fig. 6-18).[285-287] Verruca vulgaris and condyloma acuminatum are described in detail in Chapter 19.

Focal epithelial hyperplasia is an uncommon benign, contagious HPV infection (usually caused by HPV type 13 or 32) that affects mainly Native Central and South American children, particularly those who express HLA-DR4. It causes multiple, asymptomatic, 1- to 10-μm exophytic papules or nodules on the oral mucosa, gingiva, tongue, lip, and palate.[288,289] Biopsy reveals abrupt exophytic acanthosis and hyperparakeratosis of the mucosa with confluent, widened, club-shaped rete ridges that extend to the same depth as adjacent normal rete, with scattered koilocytes and mitosoid bodies (irregular nuclei resembling mitotic figures) (Fig. 6-19).[290] Immunohistochemistry and hybridization tech-

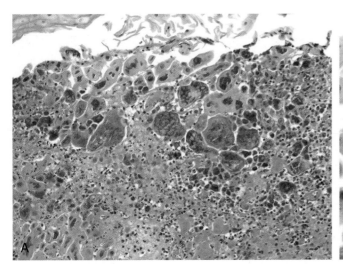
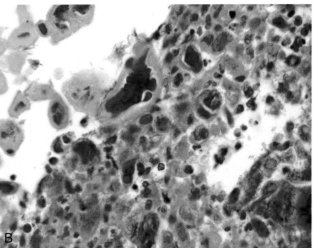

Figure 6-17. Herpes labialis. **A,** Severe infection characterized by necrosis, acantholysis, and numerous intracellular inclusions (×100). **B,** Typical herpes simplex virus inclusion, demonstrating multinucleation and molding (×600).

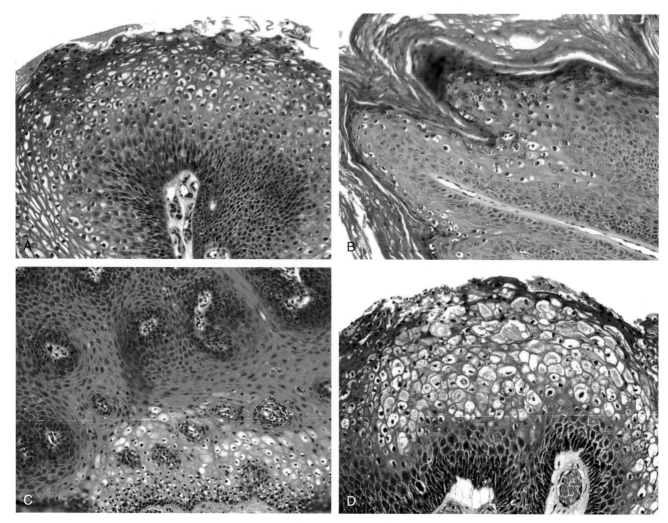

Figure 6-18. Human papillomavirus effect (koilocytosis). **A,** Oral squamous papilloma (×200). **B,** Nasal vestibular verruca vulgaris (×200). **C,** Oral condyloma acuminatum (×200). **D,** Fungiform sinonasal Schneiderian papilloma (×200).

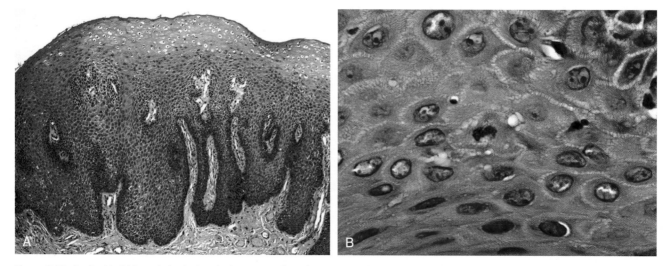

Figure 6-19. Focal epithelial hyperplasia. **A,** Acanthotic mucosa with parakeratosis, irregular rete, and superficial koilocytes (×100). **B,** Characteristic mitosoid body (×1000).

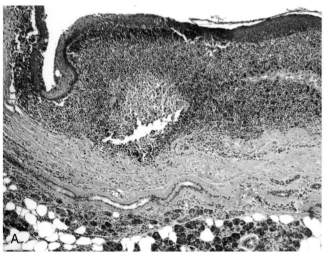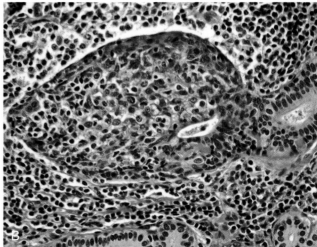

Figure 6-20. Human immunodeficiency virus–associated lymphoepithelial cyst. **A,** Squamous-lined cyst with surrounding follicular lymphoid infiltrate and fibrosis (×100). **B,** Characteristic lymphoepithelial lesion, showing squamous metaplasia of the affected duct (×400).

niques are available to confirm the presence of HPV; in cases in which lesions do not regress spontaneously, topical interferon, cryosurgery, or laser treatment may be beneficial.[291,292]

Human Immunodeficiency Virus

HIV is a lentivirus that is responsible for the clinical syndrome of acquired immunodeficiency syndrome (AIDS); it infects CD4-positive T-lymphocytes and other cells in the human body and results in disease manifestations relating directly to the virus as well as a variety of opportunistic infectious agents.[293] Specific head and neck manifestations (excluding opportunistic infections) include acute retroviral syndrome, infection of extranodal lymphoid tissues, and HIV salivary gland disease. Acute retroviral syndrome manifests 2 to 6 weeks after exposure, with nonspecific symptoms and laboratory findings that can include fever, fatigue, pharyngitis, weight loss, night sweats, lymphadenopathy, myalgias, headache, nausea, diarrhea, leukopenia, thrombocytopenia, and mild transaminitis, as well as an infectious mononucleosis–like syndrome that may provide an important clue to the diagnosis.[294]

Infection of the extranodal lymphoid tissues of Waldeyer's ring results in tonsillar enlargement with histologic changes identical to those seen in nodal tissue, with the additional finding of virus-harboring Langhans-type multinucleate giant cells that concentrate at the lymphoepithelial junction and have also been identified in HIV-associated lymphoepithelial cysts of salivary gland tissue.[295] Such cysts affect the parotid gland, with infection of periparotid nodal tissue causing gland enlargement and histologic findings similar to those seen in affected lymph nodes, along with cystic dilation of squamous-lined ductal structures that demonstrate infiltration by lymphoid cells and a variety of metaplastic changes (lymphoepithelial lesions) (Fig. 6-20).[296] Lymphoepithelial cysts of the salivary gland are not limited to HIV patients, and there is evidence to suggest that, at least in some cases, they arise not from lymphoid hyperplasia but from chronic sialadenitis.[297]

Mumps

Mumps is caused by a single-stranded RNA virus of the paramyxovirus family that is transmitted through respiratory droplets and commonly affects the salivary glands of unvaccinated children.[298] In recent years, several outbreaks have led to reconsideration of current vaccination practices to account for waning immunity.[299] After an incubation period of 16 to 18 days, patients experience a prodrome of headache, anorexia, malaise, myalgias, and fevers followed by unilateral or bilateral parotid swelling and tenderness, sometimes with associated otalgia, difficulty speaking, or trismus.[298] Although the diagnosis is usually made on clinical findings, histologic features of the affected gland include hemorrhage, necrosis, and a chronic inflammatory infiltrate composed of lymphocytes and plasma cells. Therapy is generally not required, because the infection is self-limited.

REFERENCES

1. Scheid DC, Hamm RM: Acute bacterial rhinosinusitis in adults: Part I. Evaluation. Am Fam Physician 2004;70:1685-1692.
2. Benninger MS: Adult chronic rhinosinusitis: Definitions, diagnosis, epidemiology, and pathophysiology. Otolaryngol Head Neck Surg 2003;129(3 Suppl):S1-S32.
3. Hamilos DL: Chronic rhinosinusitis patterns of illness. Clin Allergy Immunol 2007;20:1-13.
4. Van Zele T, et al: *Staphylococcus aureus* colonization and IgE antibody formation to enterotoxins is increased in nasal polyposis. J Allergy Clin Immunol 2004;114:981-983.
5. Ramadan HH: Chronic rhinosinusitis and bacterial biofilms. Curr Opin Otolaryngol Head Neck Surg 2006;14:183-186.
6. Yamanaka N, Hotomi M, Billal DS: Clinical bacteriology and immunology in acute otitis media in children. J Infect Chemother 2008;14:180-187.
7. Kontiokari T, et al: Symptoms of acute otitis media. Pediatr Infect Dis J 1998;17:676-679.
8. Schraff SA: Contemporary indications for ventilation tube placement. Curr Opin Otolaryngol Head Neck Surg 2008;16:406-411.

9. Brook I, Dohar JE: Management of group A beta-hemolytic strep-tococcal pharyngotonsillitis in children. J Fam Pract 2006;55:S1-S11; quiz S12.

10. Jeong JH, et al: Bacteriologic comparison of tonsil core in recurrent tonsillitis and tonsillar hypertrophy. Laryngoscope 2007;117:2146-2151.

11. Randall DA, Martin PJ, Thompson LD: Routine histologic exami-nation is unnecessary for tonsillectomy or adenoidectomy. Laryn-goscope 2007;117:1600-1604.

12. Mogoanta CA, et al: Chronic tonsillitis: Histological and immuno-histochemical aspects. Rom J Morphol Embryol 2008;49:381-386.

13. Dell'Aringa AR, et al: Histological analysis of tonsillectomy and adenoidectomy specimens—January 2001 to May 2003. Braz J Otorhinolaryngol 2005;71:18-22.

14. Steyer TE: Peritonsillar abscess: Diagnosis and treatment. Am Fam Physician 2002;65:93-96.

15. Galioto NJ: Peritonsillar abscess. Am Fam Physician 2008;77:199-202.

16. Dool H, et al: Lemierre's syndrome: three cases and a review. Eur Arch Otorhinolaryngol 2005;262:651-654.

17. Chan TV, Spiegel JH: *Klebsiella rhinoscleromatis* of the membra-nous nasal septum. J Laryngol Otol 2007;121:998-1002.

18. Sanchez-Marin LA, et al: Association of HLA-DQA1*03011-DQB1*0301 haplotype with the development of respiratory scle-roma. Otolaryngol Head Neck Surg 2007;136:481-483.

19. Lenis A, et al: Rhinoscleroma. South Med J 1988;81:1580-1582.

20. Hansen T, et al: Actinomycosis of the jaws: Histopathological study of 45 patients shows significant involvement in bisphosphonate-associated osteonecrosis and infected osteoradionecrosis. Virchows Arch 2007;451:1009-1017.

21. Belmont MJ, Behar PM, Wax MK: Atypical presentations of acti-nomycosis. Head Neck 1999;21:264-268.

22. Ozcan C, et al: Actinomycosis of the middle turbinate: An unusual cause of nasal obstruction. Eur Arch Otorhinolaryngol 2005;262:412-415.

23. Ermis I, et al: Actinomycosis of the frontal and parotid regions. Ann Plast Surg 2001;46:55-58.

24. Lahoz Zamarro MT, et al: [Base tongue actinomycosis]. Acta Otor-rinolaringol Esp 2005;56:222-225.

25. Hussein MR: Mucocutaneous Splendore-Hoeppli phenomenon. J Cutan Pathol 2008;35:979-988.

26. Samant S, et al: Actinomycosis mimicking a tonsillar neoplasm in an elderly diabetic patient. Br J Oral Maxillofac Surg 2009;47:417-418.

27. Agterof MJ, et al: Nocardiosis: A case series and a mini review of clinical and microbiological features. Neth J Med 2007;65:199-202.

28. Mootsikapun P, Intarapoka B, Liawnoraset W: Nocardiosis in Sri-nagarind Hospital, Thailand: Review of 70 cases from 1996-2001. Int J Infect Dis 2005;9:154-158.

29. Custal-Teixidor M, et al: Fine-needle aspiration cytology in the diagnosis of cervicofacial actinomycosis: Report of 15 cases. Med Oral Patol Oral Cir Bucal 2004;9:467-470; 464-467.

30. Yeung MK: Molecular and genetic analyses of *Actinomyces* spp. Crit Rev Oral Biol Med 1999;10:120-138.

31. Brook I: Actinomycosis: Diagnosis and management. South Med J 2008;101:1019-1023.

32. Saussez S, et al: Bisphosphonate-related osteonecrosis of the jaw and its associated risk factors: A Belgian case series. Laryngoscope 2009;119:323-329.

33. Saadat P, et al: Botryomycosis caused by *Staphylococcus aureus* and *Pneumocystis carinii* in a patient with acquired immunodeficiency disease. Clin Exp Dermatol 2008;33:266-269.

34. Pruitt JW, et al: Botryomycosis with orbital invasion: Case report and literature review. J Oral Maxillofac Surg 1995;53:599-605.

35. Wenig BM, Smirniotopoulos JG, Heffner DK: Botryomycosis ("bacterial ball") of the sinonasal tract caused by *Pseudomonas aeruginosa*. Arch Pathol Lab Med 1996;120:1123-1128.

36. Gupta K, et al: Cardiac botryomycosis: An autopsy report. J Clin Pathol 2008;61:972-974.

37. Wada R, et al: Granulomatous colitis associated with botryomyco-sis of *Propionibacterium acnes*. Arch Pathol Lab Med 2001;125:1491-1493.

38. HIV prevention through early detection and treatment of other sexually transmitted diseases—United States recommendations of the Advisory Committee for HIV and STD Prevention. MMWR Recomm Rep, July 31, 1998. Available at http://www.cdc.gov/mmwr/Preview/mmwrhtml/00054174.htm (accessed July 7, 2009).

39. Eccleston K, Collins L, Higgins SP: Primary syphilis. Int J STD AIDS 2008;19:145-151.

40. Siegel MA: Syphilis and gonorrhea. Dent Clin North Am 1996;40:369-383.

41. Veraldi S, et al: Multiple aphthoid syphilitic chancres of the oral cavity. Int J STD AIDS 2008;19:486-487.

42. Scott CM. Flint SR: Oral syphilis: Re-emergence of an old disease with oral manifestations. Int J Oral Maxillofac Surg 2005;34:58-63.

43. Barrett AW, et al: The histopathology of syphilis of the oral mucosa. J Oral Pathol Med 2004;33:286-291.

44. Lu SY, Eng HL: Secondary syphilis-related oral ulcers: Report of four cases. Chang Gung Med J 2002;25:683-688.

45. Passoni LF, et al: Lues maligna in an HIV-infected patient. Rev Soc Bras Med Trop 2005;38:181-184.

46. Leao JC, Gueiros LA, Porter SR: Oral manifestations of syphilis. Clinics 2006;61:161-166.

47. Dickenson AJ, Currie WJ, Avery BS: Screening for syphilis in patients with carcinoma of the tongue. Br J Oral Maxillofac Surg 1995;33:319-320.

48. Aquilina C, Viraben R, Denis P: Secondary syphilis simulating oral hairy leukoplakia. J Am Acad Dermatol 2003;49:749-751.

49. Abuzeid WM, Ruckenstein MJ: Spirochetes in otology: Are we testing for the right pathogens? Otolaryngol Head Neck Surg 2008;138:107-109.

50. Little JW: Syphilis: An update. Oral Surg Oral Med Oral Pathol Oral Radiol Endod 2005;100:3-9.

51. Hillson S, Grigson C, Bond S: Dental defects of congenital syphilis. Am J Phys Anthropol 1998;107:25-40.

52. Arnold C, et al: Single-nucleotide polymorphism-based differentia-tion and drug resistance detection in *Mycobacterium tuberculosis* from isolates or directly from sputum. Clin Microbiol Infect 2005;11:122-130.

53. Arentz M, Hawn TR: Tuberculosis infection: Insight from immu-nogenomics. Drug Discov Today Dis Mech 2007;4:231-236.

54. Hale RG, Tucker DI: Head and neck manifestations of tuberculo-sis. Oral Maxillofac Surg Clin North Am 2008;20:635-642.

55. Hanley ME, Welsh CH: Current Diagnosis and Treatment in Pul-monary Medicine. New York, Lange Medical Books/McGraw-Hill, 2003.

56. Swart JG, de Flamingh DQ, Hamersma T: Histologically detected extrapulmonary tuberculosis in the head and neck region: A review of 222 cases. S Afr Med J 1987;71:700-702.

57. Manolidis S: Mycobacterial infections of the head and neck. Oto-laryngol Head Neck Surg 1993;109(3 Pt 1):427-433.

58. Penfold CN, Revington PJ: A review of 23 patients with tubercu-losis of the head and neck. Br J Oral Maxillofac Surg 1996;34:508-510.

59. Konishi K, et al: Study of tuberculosis in the field of otorhinolar-yngology in the past 10 years. Acta Otolaryngol Suppl 1998;538:244-249.

60. Perlman DC, D'Amico R, Salomon N: Mycobacterial infections of the head and neck. Curr Infect Dis Rep 2001;3:233-241.

61. Al-Serhani AM: Mycobacterial infection of the head and neck: Presentation and diagnosis. Laryngoscope 2001;111(11 Pt 1):2012-2016.

62. Munck K, Mandpe AH: Mycobacterial infections of the head and neck. Otolaryngol Clin North Am 2003;36:569-576.

63. Nalini B, Vinayak S: Tuberculosis in ear, nose, and throat practice: Its presentation and diagnosis. Am J Otolaryngol 2006;27:39-45.

64. Menon K, et al: A clinical review of 128 cases of head and neck tuberculosis presenting over a 10-year period in Bradford, UK. J Laryngol Otol 2007;121:362-368.

65. Prasad KC, et al: Tuberculosis in the head and neck: Experience in India. J Laryngol Otol 2007;121:979-985.

66. Cho YS, et al: Tuberculous otitis media: A clinical and radiologic analysis of 52 patients. Laryngoscope 2006;116:921-927.

67. Wang WC, et al: Tuberculosis of the head and neck: A review of 20 cases. Oral Surg Oral Med Oral Pathol Oral Radiol Endod 2009;107:381-386.

68. Kim YH, et al: Diagnosis of major salivary gland tuberculosis: Experience of eight cases and review of the literature. Acta Otolaryngol 2005;125:1318-1322.

69. Sierra C, et al: Extra-laryngeal head and neck tuberculosis. Clin Microbiol Infect 2000;6:644-648.

70. Choudhury N, et al: 4 Years' experience of head and neck tuberculosis in a south London hospital. J R Soc Med 2005;98:267-269.

71. Sethi A, et al: Primary parotid tuberculosis: Varied clinical presentations. Oral Dis 2006;12:213-215.

72. Sareen D, Sethi A, Agarwal AK: Primary tuberculosis of the tongue: A rare nodular presentation. Br Dent J 2006;200:321-322.

73. Nawaz G, Khan MR: Primary sinonasal tuberculosis in north-west Pakistan. J Coll Physicians Surg Pak 2004;14:221-224.

74. Ito FA, et al: Primary tuberculosis of the oral cavity. Oral Dis 2005;11:50-53.

75. Sezer B, et al: Oral mucosal ulceration: A manifestation of previously undiagnosed pulmonary tuberculosis. J Am Dent Assoc 2004;135:336-340.

76. Smolka W, et al: Primary tuberculosis of the oral cavity in an elderly nonimmunosuppressed patient: Case report and review of the literature. Arch Otolaryngol Head Neck Surg 2008;134:1107-1109.

77. Chou YH, et al: Tuberculosis of the parotid gland: Sonographic manifestations and sonographically guided aspiration. J Ultrasound Med 2004;23:1275-1281.

78. Kim CW, Jin JW, Rho YS: Tuberculous otitis media developing as a complication of tympanostomy tube insertion. Eur Arch Otorhinolaryngol 2007;264:227-230.

79. Birkent H, et al: Primary parotid tuberculosis mimicking parotid neoplasm: A case report. J Med Case Rep 2008;2:62.

80. Mascarenhas S, Tuffin JR, Hassan I: Tuberculous submasseteric abscess: Case report. Br J Oral Maxillofac Surg 2008, Dec 5 [Epub ahead of print].

81. Lin CJ, Kang BH, Wang HW: Laryngeal tuberculosis masquerading as carcinoma. Eur Arch Otorhinolaryngol 2002;259:521-523.

82. Davies PD, Pai M: The diagnosis and misdiagnosis of tuberculosis. Int J Tuberc Lung Dis 2008;12:1226-1234.

83. Job CK, et al: Transmission of leprosy: A study of skin and nasal secretions of household contacts of leprosy patients using PCR. Am J Trop Med Hyg 2008;78:518-521.

84. Ramaprasad P, et al: Transmission and protection in leprosy: Indications of the role of mucosal immunity. Lepr Rev 1997;68:301-315.

85. Han XY, et al: A new *Mycobacterium* species causing diffuse lepromatous leprosy. Am J Clin Pathol 2008;130:856-864.

86. de Abreu MA, et al: The oral mucosa in paucibacillary leprosy: A clinical and histopathological study. Oral Surg Oral Med Oral Pathol Oral Radiol Endod 2007;103:e48-e52.

87. Chimenos Kustner E, et al: Lepromatous leprosy: A review and case report. Med Oral Patol Oral Cir Bucal 2006;11:E474-E479.

88. Motta AC, et al: Leprosy-specific oral lesions: A report of three cases. Med Oral Patol Oral Cir Bucal 2008;13:E479-E482.

89. de Abreu MA, et al: The oral mucosa in leprosy: A clinical and histopathological study. Braz J Otorhinolaryngol 2006;72:312-316.

90. Moschella SL: An update on the diagnosis and treatment of leprosy. J Am Acad Dermatol 2004;51:417-426.

91. Scully C, el-Kabir M, Samaranayake LP: Candida and oral candidosis: A review. Crit Rev Oral Biol Med 1994;5:125-157.

92. Sitheeque MA, Samaranayake LP: Chronic hyperplastic candidosis/candidiasis (candidal leukoplakia). Crit Rev Oral Biol Med 2003;14:253-267.

93. De Marco D, et al: Development and validation of a molecular method for the diagnosis of medically important fungal infections. New Microbiol 2007;30:308-312.

94. Jarvensivu A, et al: Specificity of the monoclonal antibody 3H8 in the immunohistochemical identification of *Candida* species. Oral Dis 2006;12:428-433.

95. Stammberger H, Kountakis SE, Senior BA, Draf W (ed): The Frontal Sinus. New York, Springer, 2005.

96. Deshazo RD: Syndromes of invasive fungal sinusitis. Med Mycol 2009;47(Suppl 1):S309-S314.

97. deShazo RD, Chapin K, Swain RE: Fungal sinusitis. N Engl J Med 1997;337:254-259.

98. Ingley AP, Parikh SL, DelGaudio JM: Orbital and cranial nerve presentations and sequelae are hallmarks of invasive fungal sinusitis caused by *Mucor* in contrast to *Aspergillus*. Am J Rhinol 2008;22:155-158.

99. Ghadiali MT, et al: Frozen-section biopsy analysis for acute invasive fungal rhinosinusitis. Otolaryngol Head Neck Surg 2007;136:714-719.

100. Piao YS, et al: The use of MUC5B antibody in identifying the fungal type of fungal sinusitis. Hum Pathol 2008;39:650-656.

101. Michael RC, et al: Mycological profile of fungal sinusitis: An audit of specimens over a 7-year period in a tertiary care hospital in Tamil Nadu. Indian J Pathol Microbiol 2008;51:493-496.

102. Hedayati MT, et al: *Aspergillus flavus:* Human pathogen, allergen and mycotoxin producer. Microbiology 2007;153(Pt 6):1677-1692.

103. Veress B, et al: Further observations on the primary paranasal aspergillus granuloma in the Sudan: A morphological study of 46 cases. Am J Trop Med Hyg 1973;22:765-772.

104. Chakrabarti A, Sharma SC: Paranasal sinus mycoses. Indian J Chest Dis Allied Sci 2000;42:293-304.

105. Chakrabarti A, Das A, Panda NK: Overview of fungal rhinosinusitis. Indian J Otolaryngol Head Neck Surg 2004;56:251-258.

106. Grosjean P, Weber R: Fungus balls of the paranasal sinuses: A review. Eur Arch Otorhinolaryngol 2007;264:461-470.

107. Pagella F, et al: Paranasal sinus fungus ball: Diagnosis and management. Mycoses 2007;50:451-456.

108. deShazo RD, et al: Criteria for the diagnosis of sinus mycetoma. J Allergy Clin Immunol, 1997;99:475-485.

109. Dufour X, et al: Paranasal sinus fungus ball: Epidemiology, clinical features and diagnosis. A retrospective analysis of 173 cases from a single medical center in France, 1989-2002. Med Mycol 2006;44:61-67.

110. Taxy JB: Paranasal fungal sinusitis: Contributions of histopathology to diagnosis. A report of 60 cases and literature review. Am J Surg Pathol 2006;30:713-720.

111. Uri N, et al: Classification of fungal sinusitis in immunocompetent patients. Otolaryngol Head Neck Surg 2003;129:372-378.

112. deShazo RD, Swain RE: Diagnostic criteria for allergic fungal sinusitis. J Allergy Clin Immunol 1995;96:24-35.

113. Saravanan K, et al: Allergic fungal rhinosinusitis: An attempt to resolve the diagnostic dilemma. Arch Otolaryngol Head Neck Surg 2006;132:173-178.

114. Lackner A, et al: Fungi: A normal content of human nasal mucus. Am J Rhinol 2005;19:125-129.

115. Ponikau JU, et al: The diagnosis and incidence of allergic fungal sinusitis. Mayo Clin Proc 1999;74:877-884.

116. Wise SK, et al: Antigen-specific IgE in sinus mucosa of allergic fungal rhinosinusitis patients. Am J Rhinol 2008;22:451-456.

117. Chang YT, Fang SY: Tissue-specific immunoglobulin E in maxillary sinus mucosa of allergic fungal sinusitis. Rhinology 2008;46:226-230.

118. Sasama J, et al: New paradigm for the roles of fungi and eosinophils in chronic rhinosinusitis. Curr Opin Otolaryngol Head Neck Surg 2005;13:2-8.

119. Braun H, et al: "Eosinophilic fungal rhinosinusitis": A common disorder in Europe? Laryngoscope 2003;113:264-269.

120. Ferguson BJ: Eosinophilic mucin rhinosinusitis: A distinct clinicopathological entity. Laryngoscope 2000;110(5 Pt 1):799-813.

121. Aeumjaturapat S, et al: Eosinophilic mucin rhinosinusitis: Terminology and clinicopathological presentation. J Med Assoc Thai 2003;86:420-424.

122. Reitzen SD, Lebowitz RA, Jacobs JB: Allergic fungal sinusitis with extensive bone erosion of the clivus presenting with diplopia. J Laryngol Otol 2009;123:817-819.

123. Liu JK, et al: Neurosurgical implications of allergic fungal sinusitis. J Neurosurg 2004;100:883-890.

124. Aribandi M, Bazan C 3rd: CT and MRI features in *Bipolaris* fungal sinusitis. Australas Radiol 2007;51:127-132.

125. Rassekh CH, et al: Skull base allergic fungal sinusitis with abducens palsy in the third trimester. Skull Base Surg 1996;6:253-258.

126. Ramos ESM, Saraiva Ldo E: Paracoccidioidomycosis. Dermatol Clin 2008;26:257-269, vii.

127. Peres LC, et al: Infectious diseases in paediatric pathology: Experience from a developing country. Pathology 2008;40:161-175.

128. Felipe MS, et al: Functional genome of the human pathogenic fungus *Paracoccidioides brasiliensis*. FEMS Immunol Med Microbiol 2005;45:369-381.

129. Borges-Walmsley MI, et al: The pathobiology of *Paracoccidioides brasiliensis*. Trends Microbiol 2002;10:80-87.

130. Bicalho RN, et al: Oral paracoccidioidomycosis: A retrospective study of 62 Brazilian patients. Oral Dis 2001;7:56-60.

131. Silva CO, et al: Gingival involvement in oral paracoccidioidomycosis. J Periodontol 2007;78:1229-1234.

132. Sposto MR, et al: Oral paracoccidioidomycosis: A study of 36 South American patients. Oral Surg Oral Med Oral Pathol 1993;75:461-465.

133. de Almeida OP, et al: Oral manifestations of paracoccidioidomycosis (South American blastomycosis). Oral Surg Oral Med Oral Pathol 1991;72:430-435.

134. Weber SA, et al: Dysphonia and laryngeal sequelae in paracoccidioidomycosis patients: A morphological and phoniatric study. Med Mycol 2006;44:219-225.

135. de Freitas MR, Nascimento OJ, Chimelli L: Tapia's syndrome caused by *Paracoccidioidis brasiliensis*. J Neurol Sci 1991;103:179-181.

136. de Castro CC, et al: MRI of head and neck paracoccidioidomycosis. Br J Radiol 1999;72:717-722.

137. Deps PD, Neves MB, Pinto Neto LF: Paracoccidioidomycosis: An unusual presentation with a rapid progression. Rev Soc Bras Med Trop 2004;37:425-426.

138. Castro LG, et al: Hard palate perforation: An unusual finding in paracoccidioidomycosis. Int J Dermatol 2001;40:281-283.

139. Bisinelli JC, et al: Manifestações estomatológicas da paracoccidioidomicose. Revista Bras Otorrinolaringol 2001;67:683-687.

140. Meneses-Garcia A, et al: Paracoccidioidomycosis: Report of 2 cases mimicking squamous cell carcinoma. Oral Surg Oral Med Oral Pathol Oral Radiol Endod 2002;94:609-613.

141. Almeida OP, Jacks J Jr, Scully C: Paracoccidioidomycosis of the mouth: An emerging deep mycosis. Crit Rev Oral Biol Med 2003;14:377-383.

142. Kaminagakura E, et al: Characterization of inflammatory cells in oral paracoccidioidomycosis. Oral Dis 2007;13:434-439.

143. Londero AT, Severo LC, Ramos CD: Small forms and hyphae of paracoccidioides brasiliensis in human tissue. Mycopathologia 1980;72:17-19.

144. de Araujo MS, et al: Oral exfoliative cytology in the diagnosis of paracoccidioidomycosis. Acta Cytol 2001;45:360-364.

145. Cardoso SV, et al: Exfoliative cytology: A helpful tool for the diagnosis of paracoccidioidomycosis. Oral Dis 2001;7:217-220.

146. Talhari C, et al: Oral exfoliative cytology as a rapid diagnostic tool for paracoccidioidomycosis. Mycoses 2008;51:177-178.

147. Jensen HE, et al: Diagnosis of systemic mycoses by specific immunohistochemical tests. Apmis 1996;104:241-258.

148. De Brito T, et al: In situ hybridization in paracoccidioidomycosis. Med Mycol 1999;37:207-211.

149. Lindsley MD, et al: Rapid identification of dimorphic and yeast-like fungal pathogens using specific DNA probes. J Clin Microbiol 2001;39:3505-3511.

150. Ricci G, et al: Genotyping of *Paracoccidioides brasiliensis* directly from paraffin embedded tissue. Med Mycol 2008;46:31-34.

151. Menezes VM, Soares BG, Fontes CJ: Drugs for treating paracoccidioidomycosis. Cochrane Database Syst Rev 2006(2):CD004967.

152. Criseo G, Zungri D, Romeo O: Stable yeast-like form of sporothrix schenckii: Lack of dimorphic stage. J Clin Microbiol 2008;46:3870-3871.

153. Morris-Jones R: Sporotrichosis. Clin Exp Dermatol 2002;27:427-431.

154. Theissing G, Schmidt W: [Sporotrichosis of the paranasal sinuses and the mouth, with skin involvement, a rare syndrome.] Z Laryngol Rhinol Otol 1957;36:141-149.

155. Clay BM, Anand VK: Sporotrichosis: Nasal obstruction in an infant. Am J Otolaryngol 1996;17:75-77.

156. Morgan M, Reves R: Invasive sinusitis due to *Sporothrix schenckii* in a patient with AIDS. Clin Infect Dis 1996;23:1319-1320.

157. Aarestrup FM, et al: Oral manifestation of sporotrichosis in AIDS patients. Oral Dis 2001;7:134-136.

158. Kumar R, et al: Pansinusitis due to *Sporothrix schenckii*. Mycoses 2005;48:85-88.

159. da Rosa AC, et al: Epidemiology of sporotrichosis: A study of 304 cases in Brazil. J Am Acad Dermatol 2005;52(3 Pt 1):451-459.

160. Fonseca-Reyes S, et al: Extracutaneous sporotrichosis in a patient with liver cirrhosis. Rev Iberoam Micol 2007;24:41-43.

161. Fontes PC, et al: Sporotrichosis in an HIV-positive man with oral lesions: A case report. Acta Cytol 2007;51:648-650.

162. Bradsher RW: Blastomycosis. Clin Infect Dis 1992;14(Suppl 1):S82-S90.

163. Rippon JW: Medical mycology: The Pathogenic Fungi and the Pathogenic Actinomycetes. 3rd ed. Philadelphia, Saunders, 1988, pp ix, 797.

164. Mason AR, et al: Cutaneous blastomycosis: A diagnostic challenge. Int J Dermatol 2008;47:824-830.

165. Ling FT, Wang D, Gerin-Lajoie J: Blastomycosis presenting as a locally invasive intranasal mass: Case report and literature review. J Otolaryngol 2003;32:405-409.

166. Damm DD, Fantasia JE: Exophytic mass of buccal mucosa: Blastomycosis. Gen Dent 2002;50:561, 564.

167. Witzig RS, et al: *Blastomyces dermatitidis* infection of the paranasal sinuses. Clin Infect Dis 1994;18:267-268.

168. Day TA, Stucker FJ: Blastomycosis of the paranasal sinuses. Otolaryngol Head Neck Surg 1994;110:437-440.

169. Reder PA, Neel HB 3rd: Blastomycosis in otolaryngology: Review of a large series. Laryngoscope 1993;103(1 Pt 1):53-58.

170. Macfarland FM, Cotelingam JD: Blastomycosis presenting as a chronic facial sinus: Case report. Mil Med 1982;147:676-678.

171. Rose HD, Gingrass DJ: Localized oral blastomycosis mimicking actinomycosis. Oral Surg Oral Med Oral Pathol 1982;54:12-14.

172. Gerwin JM, Myer CM 3rd: Intranasal blastomycosis. Am J Otolaryngol 1981;2:267-273.

173. Siebert WT, Williams TW Jr: Blastomycosis of paranasal sinuses. South Med J 1978;71:981.

174. Simon GB, Berson SD, Young CN: Blastomycosis of the tongue: A case report. S Afr Med J 1977;52:82-83.

175. Green R Jr: Blastomycosis of the lung and parotid gland: Case report. Mil Med 1976;141:100-103.

176. Bell WA, Gamble J, Garrington GE: North American blastomycosis with oral lesions. Oral Surg Oral Med Oral Pathol 1969;28:914-923.

177. Pavlov S, et al: [A rare case of blastomycosis of the nasal mucosa with particular allergic manifestations.] Otorinolaringologie 1966;11:169-172.

178. Mincer HH, Oglesby RJ Jr: Intraoral North American blastomycosis. Oral Surg Oral Med Oral Pathol 1966;22:36-41.

179. Greer AE: North American blastomycosis of a nasal sinus: Report of a case. Dis Chest 1960;38:454-458.

180. Saubolle MA: Laboratory aspects in the diagnosis of coccidioidomycosis. Ann N Y Acad Sci 2007;1111:301-314.

181. Afshar K, Boydking A, Sharma OP: Exudative pleurisy of coccidioidomycosis: A case report and review of the literature. J Med Case Rep 2008;2:291.

182. Tintelnot K, et al: Taxonomic and diagnostic markers for identification of *Coccidioides immitis* and *Coccidioides posadasii*. Med Mycol 2007;45:385-393.

183. Parish JM, Blair JE: Coccidioidomycosis. Mayo Clin Proc 2008;83:343-348; quiz 348-349.

184. Arnold MG, et al: Head and neck manifestations of disseminated coccidioidomycosis. Laryngoscope 2004;114:747-752.

185. Rodriguez RA, Konia T: Coccidioidomycosis of the tongue. Arch Pathol Lab Med 2005;129:e4-e6.

186. Sipp JA, et al: *Coccidioides immitis*: An unexpected fungal pathogen causing retropharyngeal abscess. Otolaryngol Head Neck Surg 2007;136:500-501.

187. Nelson JJ, et al: An unusual thyroglossal duct cyst infection with coccidioidomycosis. J Otolaryngol 2007;36:69-71.

188. Lin X, Heitman J: The biology of the *Cryptococcus neoformans* species complex. Annu Rev Microbiol 2006;60:69-105.

189. Chayakulkeeree M, Perfect JR: Cryptococcosis. Infect Dis Clin North Am 2006;20:507-544, v-vi.

190. Casadevall A, Perfect JR: Cryptococcus neoformans. Washington, DC, ASM Press, 1998.

191. Avram AM, et al: Cryptococcal thyroiditis and hyperthyroidism. Thyroid 2004;14:471-474.

192. Vaidya KP, Lomvardias S: Cryptococcal thyroiditis: Report of a case diagnosed by fine-needle aspiration cytology. Diagn Cytopathol 1991;7:415-416.

193. Szporn AH, Tepper S, Watson CW: Disseminated cryptococcosis presenting as thyroiditis: Fine needle aspiration and autopsy findings. Acta Cytol 1985;29:449-453.

194. Isaacson JE, Frable MA: Cryptococcosis of the larynx. Otolaryngol Head Neck Surg 1996;114:106-109.

195. Schmidt-Westhausen A, et al: Oral cryptococcosis in a patient with AIDS: A case report. Oral Dis 1995;1:77-79.

196. Lucatorto F, Eversole FR: Deep mycoses and palatal perforation with granulomatous pansinusitis in acquired immunodeficiency syndrome: Case reports. Quintessence Int 1993;24:743-748.

197. Tzerbos F, Kabani S, Booth D: Cryptococcosis as an exclusive oral presentation. J Oral Maxillofac Surg 1992;50:759-760.

198. Monteil RA, et al: Oral cryptococcosis: Case report of salivary gland involvement in an AIDS patient. J Oral Pathol Med 1997;26:53-56.

199. Vargas PA, et al: Parotid gland involvement in advanced AIDS. Oral Dis 2003;9:55-61.

200. Jelliffe DB: Histoplasmosis of Darling. J Trop Med Hyg 1949;52:177-182.

201. Kurowski R, Ostapchuk M: Overview of histoplasmosis. Am Fam Physician 2002;66:2247-2252.

202. Gugnani HC, Muotoe-Okafor F: African histoplasmosis: A review. Rev Iberoam Micol 1997;14:155-159.

203. Wheat LJ: Histoplasmosis: A review for clinicians from non-endemic areas. Mycoses 2006;49:274-282.

204. Valle AC, et al: Chronic disseminated histoplasmosis with lesions restricted to the mouth: Case report. Rev Inst Med Trop Sao Paulo 2006;48:113-116.

205. Epifanio RN, Brannon RB, Muzyka BC: Disseminated histoplasmosis with oral manifestation. Spec Care Dentist 2007;27:236-239.

206. Chinn H, et al: Oral histoplasmosis in HIV-infected patients: A report of two cases. Oral Surg Oral Med Oral Pathol Oral Radiol Endod 1995;79:710-714.

207. Swindells S, et al: Oral histoplasmosis in a patient infected with HIV: A case report. Oral Surg Oral Med Oral Pathol 1994;77:126-130.

208. Economopoulou P, Laskaris G, Kittas C: Oral histoplasmosis as an indicator of HIV infection. Oral Surg Oral Med Oral Pathol Oral Radiol Endod 1998;86:203-206.

209. Gomes Ferreira O, et al: Orofacial manifestations of histoplasmosis in HIV-positive patients: A case report. Med Oral 2001;6:101-105.

210. Solari R, et al: Disseminated histoplasmosis with lesions restricted to the larynx in a patient with AIDS: Report of a case and review of the literature. Rev Iberoam Micol 2007;24:164-166.

211. Casariego Z, et al: Disseminated histoplasmosis with orofacial involvement in HIV-I-infected patients with AIDS: Manifestations and treatment. Oral Dis 1997;3:184-187.

212. Narayana N, et al: Oral histoplasmosis: An unusual presentation. Head Neck 2009;31:274-277.

213. White J, et al: Oral histoplasmosis as the initial indication of HIV infection: A case report. SADJ 2007;62:452, 454-455.

214. Coiffier T, et al: Pharyngo-laryngeal histoplasmosis: One case in an immunocompetent child. Int J Pediatr Otorhinolaryngol 1998;45:177-181.

215. Chee L: Histoplasmosis in the head and neck. Ann Acad Med Singapore 1997;26:510-513.

216. Gerber ME, et al: Histoplasmosis: The otolaryngologist's perspective. Laryngoscope 1995;105(9 Pt 1):919-923.

217. Hiltbrand JB, McGuirt WF: Oropharyngeal histoplasmosis. South Med J 1990;83:227-231.

218. Cole MC, Grossman ME: Disseminated histoplasmosis presenting as tongue nodules in a patient infected with human immunodeficiency virus. Cutis 1995;55:104-106.

219. Cobb CM, et al: Chronic pulmonary histoplasmosis with an oral lesion. Oral Surg Oral Med Oral Pathol 1989;67:73-76.

220. Felix F, et al: Nasal histoplasmosis in the acquired immunodeficiency syndrome. J Laryngol Otol 2006;120:67-69.

221. Machado AA, et al: Histoplasmosis in individuals with acquired immunodeficiency syndrome (AIDS): Report of six cases with cutaneous-mucosal involvement. Mycopathologia 1991;115:13-18.

222. Vijayan C, et al: Primary mucocutaneous histoplasmosis presents as oral ulcer. Indian J Dermatol Venereol Leprol 2007;73:209.

223. Cunha VS, et al: Mucocutaneous manifestations of disseminated histoplasmosis in patients with acquired immunodeficiency syndrome: Particular aspects in a Latin-American population. Clin Exp Dermatol 2007;32:250-255.

224. Ezzedine K, Accoceberry I, Malvy D: Oral histoplasmosis after radiation therapy for laryngeal squamous cell carcinoma. J Am Acad Dermatol 2007;56:871-873.

225. Alcure ML, et al: Oral histoplasmosis in an HIV-negative patient. Oral Surg Oral Med Oral Pathol Oral Radiol Endod 2006;101:e33-e36.

226. Ferreira OG, et al: Oral histoplasmosis in Brazil. Oral Surg Oral Med Oral Pathol Oral Radiol Endod 2002;93:654-659.

227. Hernandez SL, et al: Oral histoplasmosis associated with HIV infection: A comparative study. J Oral Pathol Med 2004;33:445-450.

228. Scheepers A, Lemmer J: Disseminated histoplasmosis: Aspects of oral diagnosis. J Dent Assoc S Afr 1992;47:441-443.

229. Loubiere R, et al: [Buccal histoplasmosis: Apropos of a case with a difficult histopathologic diagnosis.] Ann Pathol 1988;8(4-5):328-331.

230. Thiago Pde T, dos Santos JI, Steindel M: [Histoplasmosis in the region of the hard palate simulating a lesion caused by *Leishmania*.] Rev Soc Bras Med Trop 1998;31:225-229.

231. Padhye AA, et al: Oral histoplasmosis in India: A case report and an overview of cases reported during 1968-1992. J Med Vet Mycol 1994;32:93-103.

232. Sood N, et al: Mucocutaneous nasal histoplasmosis in an immunocompetent young adult. Indian J Dermatol Venereol Leprol 2007;73:182-184.

233. Butt AA, Carreon J: *Histoplasma capsulatum* sinusitis. J Clin Microbiol 1997;35:2649-2650.

234. Motta AC, et al: Unusual orofacial manifestations of histoplasmosis in renal transplanted patient. Mycopathologia 2006;161:161-165.

235. Pochini Sobrinho F, et al: Histoplasmosis of the larynx. Braz J Otorhinolaryngol 2007;73:857-861.

236. Sudarshan V, et al: Rhinosporidiosis in Raipur, Chhattisgarh: A report of 462 cases. Indian J Pathol Microbiol 2007;50:718-721.

237. Echejoh GO, et al: Nasal rhinosporidiosis. J Natl Med Assoc 2008;100:713-715.

238. Arora R, Gupta R, Dinda AK: Rhinosporidiosis of trachea: A clinical cause for concern. J Laryngol Otol 2008;122:e13.

239. Silva V, et al: Molecular evidence for multiple host-specific strains in the genus *Rhinosporidium*. J Clin Microbiol 2005;43:1865-1868.

240. Dhaulakhandi DB, et al: Detection of 16S rRNA gene in round bodies isolated from polyps of rhinosporidiosis. Infect Genet Evol 2006;6:331-336.

241. Rekha P, et al: Tracheal rhinosporidiosis. J Thorac Cardiovasc Surg 2006;132:718-719.

242. Morelli L, et al: Human nasal rhinosporidiosis: An Italian case report. Diagn Pathol 2006;1:25.

243. Chao SS, Loh KS: Rhinosporidiosis: An unusual cause of nasal masses gains prominence. Singapore Med J 2004;45:224-226.

244. Ali A, et al: Rhinosporidiosis: An unusual affliction. Arch Pathol Lab Med 2001;125:1392-1393.

245. Hussein MR, Rashad UM: Rhinosporidiosis in Egypt: A case report and review of literature. Mycopathologia 2005;159:205-207.

246. Mahapatra S, et al: Rhinosporidiosis of parotid duct: A rare case report. Indian J Pathol Microbiol 2007;50:320-322.

247. Kumar BV, Osmani M, Mudhar HS: Rhinosporidiosis: An unusual presentation. Int Ophthalmol 2005;26:243-245.

248. Agirdir BV, et al: Cutaneous rhinosporidiosis presents with recurrent nasal philtrum mass in southern Turkey. Int J Dermatol 2008;47:700-703.

249. Singh S, Sivakumar R: Challenges and new discoveries in the treatment of leishmaniasis. J Infect Chemother 2004;10:307-315.

250. Chaudhary RG, Bilimoria FE, Katare SK: Diffuse cutaneous leishmaniasis: Co-infection with human immunodeficiency virus (HIV). Indian J Dermatol Venereol Leprol 2008;74:641-643.

251. Milian MA, et al: Oral leishmaniasis in a HIV-positive patient: Report of a case involving the palate. Oral Dis 2002;8:59-61.

252. Neuber H: Leishmaniasis. J Dtsch Dermatol Ges 2008;6:754-765.

253. Lessa MM, et al: Mucosal leishmaniasis: Epidemiological and clinical aspects. Braz J Otorhinolaryngol 2007;73:843-847.

254. Cobo F, et al: The histological spectrum of non-granulomatous localized mucosal leishmaniasis caused by *Leishmania infantum*. Ann Trop Med Parasitol 2007;101:689-694.

255. Ahluwalia S, et al: Mucocutaneous leishmaniasis: An imported infection among travellers to central and South America. BMJ 2004;329:842-844.

256. el-Hassan AM, Zijlstra EE: Leishmaniasis in Sudan: Mucosal leishmaniasis. Trans R Soc Trop Med Hyg 2001;95(Suppl 1):S19-S26.

257. Culha G, et al: Comparison of conventional and polymerase chain reaction diagnostic techniques for leishmaniasis in the endemic region of Adana, Turkey. Int J Dermatol 2006;45:569-572.

258. Lawn SD, et al: New world mucosal and cutaneous leishmaniasis: An emerging health problem among British travellers. QJM 2004;97:781-788.

259. Amato VS, et al: Treatment of mucosal leishmaniasis in Latin America: Systematic review. Am J Trop Med Hyg 2007;77:266-274.

260. Sckolnick J, Murphy J, Hunt JL: Microsatellite instability in nasopharyngeal and lymphoepithelial carcinomas of the head and neck. Am J Surg Pathol 2006;30:1250-1253.

261. Greenspan JS, et al: Replication of Epstein-Barr virus within the epithelial cells of oral "hairy" leukoplakia, an AIDS-associated lesion. N Engl J Med 1985;313:1564-1571.

262. Tyan YS, et al: Detection of Epstein-Barr virus and human papillomavirus in head and neck tumors. J Clin Microbiol 1993;31:53-56.

263. Ebell MH: Epstein-Barr virus infectious mononucleosis. Am Fam Physician 2004;70:1279-1287.

264. Ventura KC, Hudnall SD: Hematologic differences in heterophile-positive and heterophile-negative infectious mononucleosis. Am J Hematol 2004;76:315-318.

265. Hurt C, Tammaro D: Diagnostic evaluation of mononucleosis-like illnesses. Am J Med 2007;120:911, e1-e8.

266. Gulley ML, Tang W: Laboratory assays for Epstein-Barr virus-related disease. J Mol Diagn 2008;10:279-292.

267. Malik UR, et al: Atypical clonal T-cell proliferation in infectious mononucleosis. Med Oncol 1996;13:207-213.

268. Sari I, Birlik M, Servet A, et al: Atypical infectious mononucleosis in a patient receiving tumor necrosis factor alpha inhibitory treatment. Rheumatol Int 2009;29:825-826.

269. Lu G, et al: Clinical analysis and follow-up study of chronic active Epstein-Barr virus infection in 53 pediatric cases. Chin Med J (Engl) 2009;122:262-266.

270. Slots J, et al: Epstein-Barr virus in oral diseases. J Periodontal Res 2006;41:235-244.

271. Dias EP, et al: Prevalence of oral hairy leukoplakia in 120 pediatric patients infected with HIV-1. Braz Oral Res 2006;20:103-107.

272. Guccion JG, Redman RS: Oral hairy leukoplakia: An ultrastructural study and review of the literature. Ultrastruct Pathol 1999;23(3):181-187.

273. Komatsu TL, et al: Epstein-Barr virus in oral hairy leukoplakia scrapes: Identification by PCR. Braz Oral Res 2005;19:317-321.

274. Walling DM, Flaitz CM, Nichols CM: Epstein-Barr virus replication in oral hairy leukoplakia: Response, persistence, and resistance to treatment with valacyclovir. J Infect Dis 2003;188:883-890.

275. Ryan DA, Federoff HJ: Immune responses to herpes viral vectors. Hum Gene Ther 2009, Feb 13 [Epub ahead of print].

276. Gupta R, Warren T, Wald A: Genital herpes. Lancet 2007;370:2127-2137.

277. Chauvin PJ, Ajar AH: Acute herpetic gingivostomatitis in adults: A review of 13 cases, including diagnosis and management. J Can Dent Assoc 2002;68:247-251.

278. Siegel MA: Diagnosis and management of recurrent herpes simplex infections. J Am Dent Assoc 2002;133:1245-1249.

279. Fatahzadeh M, Schwartz RA: Human herpes simplex labialis. Clin Exp Dermatol 2007;32:625-630.

280. Arduino PG, Porter SR: Herpes simplex virus type 1 infection: Overview on relevant clinico-pathological features. J Oral Pathol Med 2008;37:107-121.

281. Durdu M, Baba M, Seckin D: The value of Tzanck smear test in diagnosis of erosive, vesicular, bullous, and pustular skin lesions. J Am Acad Dermatol 2008;59:958-964.

282. Cohen LM: Images in clinical medicine: Positive Tzanck smear. N Engl J Med 1997;337:535.

283. Arduino PG, Porter SR: Oral and perioral herpes simplex virus type 1 (HSV-1) infection: Review of its management. Oral Dis 2006;12:254-270.

284. zur Hausen H: Papillomaviruses in the causation of human cancers: A brief historical account. Virology 2009;384:260-265.

285. Syrjanen S: Human papillomavirus infections and oral tumors. Med Microbiol Immunol 2003;192:123-128.

286. Weiner JS, et al: Relationship of human papillomavirus to Schneiderian papillomas. Laryngoscope 1999;109:21-26.

287. Gaffey MJ, et al: Human papillomavirus and Epstein-Barr virus in sinonasal Schneiderian papillomas: An in situ hybridization and polymerase chain reaction study. Am J Clin Pathol 1996;106:475-482.

288. Bennett LK, Hinshaw M: Heck's disease: Diagnosis and susceptibility. Pediatr Dermatol 2009;26:87-89.

289. Borborema-Santos CM, et al: Oral focal epithelial hyperplasia: Report of five cases. Braz Dent J 2006;17:79-82.

290. Jayasooriya PR, et al: Focal epithelial hyperplasia (Heck's disease): Report of two cases with PCR detection of human papillomavirus DNA. Oral Dis 2004;10:240-243.

291. Castro TP, Bussoloti Filho I: Prevalence of human papillomavirus (HPV) in oral cavity and oropharynx. Braz J Otorhinolaryngol 2006;72:272-282.

292. Steinhoff M, et al: Successful topical treatment of focal epithelial hyperplasia (Heck's disease) with interferon-beta. Br J Dermatol 2001;144:1067-1069.

293. Levy JA: HIV pathogenesis: Knowledge gained after two decades of research. Adv Dent Res 2006;19:10-16.

294. Kassutto S, Rosenberg ES: Primary HIV type 1 infection. Clin Infect Dis 2004;38:1447-1453.

295. Dargent JL, et al: HIV-associated multinucleated giant cells in lymphoid tissue of the Waldeyer's ring: A detailed study. Mod Pathol 2000;13:1293-1299.

296. Dave SP, Pernas FG, Roy S: The benign lymphoepithelial cyst and a classification system for lymphocytic parotid gland enlargement in the pediatric HIV population. Laryngoscope 2007;117:106-113.

297. Wu L, et al: Lymphoepithelial cyst of the parotid gland: Its possible histopathogenesis based on clinicopathologic analysis of 64 cases. Hum Pathol 2009;40:683.

298. Senanayake SN: Mumps: A resurgent disease with protean manifestations. Med J Aust 2008;189:456-459.

299. Shanley JD: The resurgence of mumps in young adults and adolescents. Cleve Clin J Med 2007;74:42-44, 47-48.

Pulmonary Infections

Richard L. Kradin and Eugene J. Mark

Introduction

In its role as a portal between the ambient environment and the internal milieu, the lung is the most frequent site of serious infection. A variety of factors predispose to pulmonary infection, including distortions in lung anatomy, decreased mucociliary clearance, and abnormal cellular and humoral immunity. Iatrogenic immunosuppression and that resulting from human immunodeficiency virus (HIV-1) infection have led to the emergence of opportunistic infections that can present diagnostic challenges for the surgical pathologist.

Because a variety of microbes can potentially infect the lung, and because the histopathology of noninfectious conditions frequently mimics that of infection, the differential diagnosis of pulmonary infection is broad. In many cases, the clinical history, radiographic findings, and the noninvasive sampling of secretions can establish the cause of infection, but, at times, lung biopsy is required. Deciding how to approach the sampling of the lung in infection is an area of some complexity, and it is incumbent on both clinicians and pathologists to recognize the advantages and limitations of the current available methods.

Approach to Sampling for Infection

The optimal approach to sampling the lung for infection depends primarily on whether disease is localized or diffuse (Table 7-1). In immunosuppressed patients, diffuse pulmonary infiltrates resulting from infection can often be diagnosed by sputum induction or bronchoalveolar lavage (BAL). This is particularly the case when the microbial burden is also large. But noninvasive approaches are less sensitive than biopsy for diagnosis of localized infections, and they cannot distinguish a colonizing commensal from an invasive pathogen.[1] In addition, the lung biopsy affords an opportunity to evaluate host immunity in detail that cannot be achieved by noninvasive or minimally invasive methods. Lung biopsy may also be required to exclude infection definitively and to establish noninfective diagnoses such as acute lung injury due to chemotherapy.

Pathologists prefer to examine generous samplings of lung, because, as already noted, diagnoses based on such biopsies are more accurate, yield a greater degree of information with respect to host immunity, and can reveal other potentially treatable disorders.[2] Based on the specific details of a case, the diagnostic pathologist should be prepared to educate clinicians with respect to the limits of minimally invasive lung sampling, thereby sparing patients the unnecessary discomforts and delays of having one or more nondiagnostic procedures.

Transbronchial Biopsy

The lung has roughly the surface area of a tennis court, so sampling error is an unavoidable pitfall in diagnostic pulmonary pathology. The transbronchial biopsy preferentially samples peribronchiolar lung tissue, yielding tissue fragments of 1 to 3 mm in diameter.[3] However, peripherally located lung lesions often cannot be accessed by this approach.

Transbronchial biopsy is generally adequate for diagnosing diffuse pulmonary infections and peribronchiolar granulomatous diseases, such as sarcoidosis and lymphangitic spread of tumor or tuberculosis. At times, however, the findings can be nonspe-

Table 7-1 Approach to the Isolation of Pulmonary Microorganisms

Expectorated sputum

Induced sputum

Bronchoalveolar lavage

Fine-needle aspirate (1 mm)

Bronchial biopsy (1-3 mm)

Transbronchial biopsy (1-3 mm)

Transbronchial needle biopsy (1 mm)

Video-assisted thoracoscopic biopsy (2-3 cm)

Open-lung biopsy (2-3 cm)

Surgical lobectomy

Autopsy

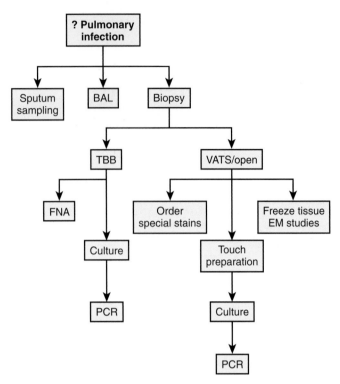

Figure 7-1. Approach to the handling of lung biopsies. BAL, bronchoalveolar lavage; EM, electron microscopy; FNA, fine-needle aspiration; PCR, polymerase chain reaction; TBB, transbronchial biopsy; VATS, video-assisted thoracoscopic biopsy.

cific and misleading. For example, "organizing pneumonia" in a transbronchial biopsy specimen may represent a nonspecific reaction adjacent to a focus of infection or malignancy, a nonspecific manifestation of chemotherapy effect, aspiration, or cryptogenic disease. For this reason, the findings gleaned from a transbronchial biopsy must always be thoughtfully correlated with clinical and radiographic findings.[4]

Fine-Needle Aspiration Biopsy

Computed tomography–guided fine-needle aspiration biopsies have a high yield in the diagnosis of peripheral nodular infiltrates.[5] Biopsies can be semiliquid, or they can include a 1-mm core of tissue. When they are performed with the assistance of a cytotechnologist, rapid diagnoses can be proffered by examination of stained smears directly at the bedside. Fine-needle aspirates are useful in diagnosing localized infections, and cytopathologists can also suggest the pattern of inflammation based on the types of inflammatory cell subsets in the sample and the presence or absence of necrosis.

Transbronchial Needle Aspiration Biopsy

Transbronchial needle aspiration biopsy of regional lymph node groups is often a low-yield procedure, because nonspecific reactive regional lymphadenitis is common in the presence of pulmonary infection.[6] The procedure is prone to artifacts that may present diagnostic difficulties for the surgical pathologist. However, when adopted judiciously, this approach may be adequate for the diagnosis of infection. In one series, approximately 50% of cases of tuberculous lymphadenitis were accurately diagnosed.

Video-Assisted and Open Thoracoscopic Biopsy

Video-assisted thoracoscopic lung biopsy has largely replaced open thoracotomy biopsy as the optimal approach for obtaining large samples of lung.[7] The procedure is associated with modest and acceptable morbidity, has the advantage of allowing direct access to widely separated lung segments, and provides generously sized wedge biopsies of 2 to 3 cm. Consequently, this procedure should be considered a first-line approach when a timely, accurate diagnosis is essential.

Handling Lung Biopsy Specimens

Appropriate handling of the lung biopsy specimen is essential for obtaining the highest diagnostic yield (Fig. 7-1).[8] Sampling of the lung for microbiologic culture should ideally take place under sterile conditions in the operating room, but the pathologist processing the biopsy specimen should try to ascertain that all necessary diagnostic tests have been ordered and be prepared to harvest additional samples for testing that may have been overlooked. When tissue is prepared for microbiologic isolation, the lung should be minced rather than crushed, because hyphate fungi (e.g., zygomycetes) may fail to grow in culture after maceration.[9] A pathologist should not place a lung biopsy sample directly into fixative without first considering a diagnosis of infection. If questions arise as to which tests to order or how best to transport the specimen to the laboratory, discussions with the hospital microbiology laboratory staff or a hospital infectious disease specialist will be of assistance.

The examination of touch imprints of lung tissue is a simple and rapid way of identifying pathogens. Touch imprints can be prepared from foci of pulmonary consolidation, necrosis, or suppuration and rapidly stained for bacteria, mycobacteria, and fungi in the surgical pathology suite or the microbiology laboratory. Concomitantly, biopsy specimens may be harvested for ultrastructural analysis, polymerase chain reaction (PCR) assays, or research purposes. For large biopsy samples, it may be possible to inflate the lung tissue with 5% formalin via a small (23-25 gauge) needle in order to optimize subsequent histologic examination.

Pulmonary Injury in Infection

Pulmonary Host Response

The diagnosis of infection requires both an interpretation of the morphologic changes evoked by the pathogen and identification of a pathogen in situ. The pattern of pulmonary inflammation often suggests the route of entry of an infectious agent and may help to narrow the diagnostic possibilities. It is necessary to be familiar with the multiplicity of response patterns evoked by infection and to recognize that these can vary depending on the route of entry, pathogen load, and competence of host defenses. For example, whereas *Human herpesvirus 1* can produce a miliary pattern of fibrinoid necrosis in an immunosuppressed patient with viremia, it can also cause ulceration of the tracheobronchial mucosa in a chronically intubated patient.

Microbes are rarely identified randomly or diffusely in infections; rather, they tend to be compartmentalized, so that substantial effort may be wasted in searching for them where they are not likely to be found. Mycobacteria and fungi are usually localized in areas of necrosis; *Rickettsia* and *Bartonella* species largely target the microvasculature; and viruses tend to attack the airways. The surgical pathologist must be acquainted with the pulmonary microanatomy and also with the preferential localization of microbes in pulmonary tissues.

Anatomy of Pulmonary Defense

The lung is an elastic organ composed of dichotomously branching conducting airways that terminate in alveolated surfaces.[10]

It has a dual blood supply: the pulmonary circulation arises from the cardiac right ventricle and carries deoxygenated blood at low arterial pressures to the alveolar surfaces, and the bronchial circulation arises from branches of the aorta and nourishes both the airways and the connective tissue stroma with oxygenated blood. All new growths within the lung, including regions of infective bronchiectasis, lung abscess, and tuberculous cavities, evoke neo-angiogenesis from the bronchial microcirculation.

Two systems of pulmonary lymphatic channels drain the lung, either centrifugally toward the hilum or centripetally along the convexities of the pleural surfaces before coursing to the hilar lymph nodes. From the lymph nodes, organisms can enter the systemic circulation and spread widely throughout the body. Group A streptococci, for example, rapidly invade pulmonary lymphatics and course to the pleura to produce an empyema.

Pulmonary Defenses

Most microbes are small (<5 μm) and can penetrate to the distal gas-exchanging surfaces of the lung, although the majority are excluded by the defenses of the upper airways or are deposited along the conducting airways to be cleared by the mucociliary escalator. Humoral factors, including secretory immunoglobulin A (sIgA) and defensins released by airway cells, limit microbial penetration into tissues. Airway mucosal dendritic cells trap microbial antigens and transport them to regional lymph nodes, where they are processed and presented to both T- and B-lymphocytes, evoking adaptive immunity (Fig. 7-2).[11]

Ulceration or thickening of the gas-exchange surface limits diffusion of oxygen and carbon dioxide. For this reason, the alveolus, under normal conditions, is maintained sterile by resident macrophages that scavenge inhaled particulates and secrete monokines, including interleukin 10 and transforming growth

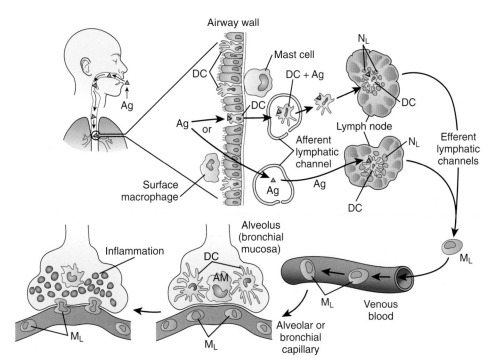

Figure 7-2. Pulmonary immune anatomy. Ag, antigen; AM, alveolar macrophage; DC, dendritic cells; M_L, mucosal lymphatic vessel; N_L, lymph node lymphatic vessel.

factor-β, that locally suppress inflammation and promote immunotolerance.

If the alveolar lining is injured, or if the number of invading organisms exceeds the phagocytotic capacities of resident macrophages, neutrophils and exudate monocytes are recruited to sites of lung infection.[12] Even small numbers of virulent pathogens can greatly amplify inflammation through the release of chemokines, cytokines, and complement by host immune cells. These defenses promote the clearance of infection but can also damage the lung. Lung biopsies afford the pathologist a unique opportunity to assess these dynamic responses directly, in addition to identifying a causative pathogen.

Patterns of Lung Injury Due to Infection

A number of generic patterns of inflammation may be evoked by infection, but how they are distributed is often specific to the involved tissue (Table 7-2). Clinicians and radiologists have developed classification systems with respect to pulmonary infection that are distinct from those of pathologists. For example, a variety of infectious agents yield a picture that clinicians generically term "atypical" interstitial pneumonia, in order to differentiate these infections from "typical" bacterial pneumonias,[13] but the histopathology of an "atypical pneumonia" may be centered on the lung interstitium, the small airways, or the alveolar spaces. Because this text is aimed primarily at surgical pathologists, pathologic schemas of classification are used, with reference to their clinical counterparts when appropriate.

Tracheobronchitis, Bronchiolitis, and Miliary Infection

Many pathogens target the conducting airways to produce tracheobronchitis and bronchiolitis. Pathologic changes range from superficial erosion of the lining respiratory epithelium to ulceration and repair. The type of inflammation varies from intraluminal neutrophilic exudates (Fig. 7-3A) to airway cuffing by lymphocytes and histiocytes (see Fig. 7-3B), depending on the offending pathogen.

Diffuse Alveolar Damage

Disease of the gas-exchange alveolar surfaces can show a spectrum of changes, including acute ulceration and septal infiltration by chronic inflammatory cells.[14] Diffuse alveolar damage (DAD) represents a global injury to the gas-exchange surfaces that is caused by disruption of the blood-air barrier leading to exudative edema and fibrosis, and resulting in severely impaired blood and tissue oxygenation (Fig. 7-4). The *sine qua non* of DAD is the hyaline membrane; it is composed of necrotic alveolar lining cell debris and an extravascular fibrin coagulum apposed to an ulcerated alveolar wall, which yields a gel that entraps lung water (Fig. 7-5). Although DAD is the most frequent pathologic cause of the clinical entity known as adult respiratory distress syndrome (ARDS), other diseases, including extensive bronchopneumonia and acute pulmonary hemorrhage, can also lead to ARDS (Table 7-3). The pathology of the exudative phase of DAD can focally

Table 7-2 Injury Patterns Seen in Lung Infection

Tracheobronchitis
Bronchiolitis (acute, chronic, necrotizing)
Bronchiectasis
Bronchopneumonia (acute, chronic, necrotizing)
Eosinophilic pneumonia
Pulmonary hemorrhage
Pulmonary edema
Diffuse alveolar damage
Pulmonary nodules and micronodules
Cavitary pneumonia
Vasculitis
Capillary dissemination
Lymphatic dissemination
Pulmonary hypertension
Pleuritis

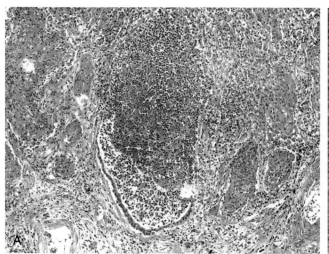
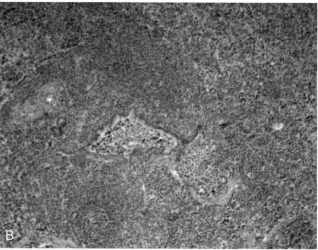

Figure 7-3. **A,** Acute bronchiolitis showing neutrophilic exudate in the lumen of a small airway (×200). **B,** Chronic lymphocytic bronchiolitis (×150).

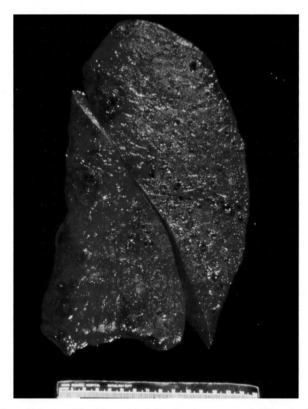

Figure 7-4. Consolidated lung with the beefy-red appearance of diffuse alveolar damage in a patient who died of influenzal pneumonia.

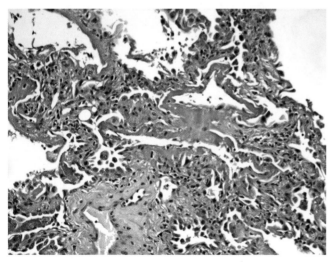

Figure 7-5. Hyaline membrane lining an alveolar duct in diffuse alveolar damage (×400).

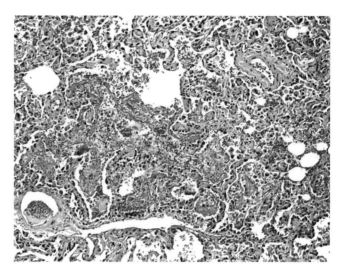

Figure 7-6. Lung in exudative phase of diffuse alveolar damage with hemorrhage and inflammation. This finding should not be overinterpreted as evidence of infection (×250).

Table 7-3 Causes of Diffuse Alveolar Damage

Pulmonary infection

Systemic infection with sepsis

Vasodilatory shock

Aspiration

Drugs

Radiation

Trauma

Accelerated phase of chronic interstitial pneumonia

Idiopathic

mimic acute bacterial infection, and one must maintain a high threshold of suspicion for making the diagnosis of acute infection in this setting (Fig. 7-6).

Viruses are the most common infectious cause of DAD, although bacteria, fungi, and parasites also produce diffuse lung injury. DAD can result from sepsis that complicates pulmonary or extrapulmonary infection. Whenever DAD is present, the surgical pathologist must examine the lung for evidence of viral-induced cytopathic changes. These vary with the type of viral infection, and some viruses do not produce cytopathic changes, so that viral infection is always in the differential diagnosis of DAD (Table 7-4). A common pitfall in diagnosis is to mistake the hyperplastic reparative alveolar type II cells of DAD, which can exhibit prominent nucleoli, for virus-infected cells, particularly when examining rapidly frozen sections, in which these changes may be especially prominent (Fig. 7-7).

RNA Viruses

Influenza

Influenza is a rod-shaped RNA virus that can cause either bronchiolitis or DAD without apparent cytopathic changes. Influenza infection recurs each year due to a high incidence of mutation of its hemagglutinin (H) and neuraminidase (N) antigens, and these determine its virulence. When mutations occur concomitantly in both the H and N antigens, pandemics with potentially high degrees of morbidity may ensue because of the lack of immunity in the population (Fig. 7-8).[15] Currently, epidemiologists are carefully monitoring the evolution of an avian influenza in Southeast Asia for evidence of spread to humans.

Influenza is the most common cause of viral pneumonia, although most cases are subclinical. The virus most commonly causes a diffuse tracheobronchitis/bronchiolitis in which the normal ciliated respiratory epithelium is sloughed.[16] If DAD develops, however, it can carry a high mortality even in the absence of acute bacterial superinfection (Fig. 7-9).[17] The lungs in DAD caused by influenza in patients with prolonged survival often develop prominent squamous metaplasia of the bronchial and alveolar lining cells (Fig. 7-10A). Although these findings are characteristic, they are also nonspecific, so that immunostains, in situ hybridization, electron microscopy, or viral antigen detection may be required to establish the diagnosis (see Fig. 7-10B). Superinfection by pyogenic bacteria, including *Haemophilus influenzae*, group A *Streptococcus*, and *Staphylococcus*, is a well-recognized complication and may mask evidence of a healing influenza infection.

Novel H1N1 Influenza (Swine Flu)

Novel influenza A (H1N1) is a new emerging flu virus that first caused illness in Mexico in the spring of 2009. The virus is of swine origin and spreads, like seasonal influenza, by aerosol transport but can also spread via fomites. Symptoms include fever, cough, sore throat, headache, myalgias, chills, and fatigue; gastrointestinal symptoms have also been reported. In April 2009, the United States Government declared a public health emergency, and in June 2009, the World Health Organization raised the worldwide pandemic alert level to phase 6, indicating that a global pandemic was underway.

The disease spread rapidly, with all 50 states in the United States reporting cases. The infection can be rapidly diagnosed by PCR methods that are currently available in all state testing facilities. Despite reports of excess mortality in the herald cases

Table 7-4 Changes Seen in Virus-Infected Lung Cells

Organism	Cytopathic Change
Influenza	No cytopathic change
SARS (coronavirus)	No cytopathic change
Respiratory syncytial virus	Polykaryons, inconspicuous cytoplasmic inclusions
Parainfluenza	Polykaryons, intracytoplasmic inclusions
Measles	Polykaryons, intranuclear inclusions
Adenovirus	Intranuclear inclusions (smudge cells)
Herpesvirus	Intranuclear inclusions, polykaryons
Cytomegalovirus	Intranuclear and cytoplasmic inclusions
Varicella-zoster	Intranuclear inclusions
Epstein-Barr virus	No cytopathic change

SARS, severe acute respiratory syndrome.

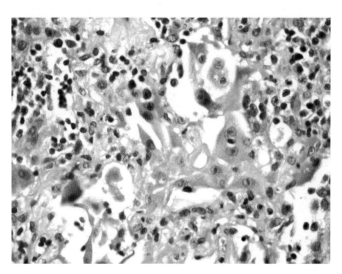

Figure 7-7. Lung in reparative phase of acute lung injury showing highly atypical alveolar lining cells with changes that mimic viral infection (×400).

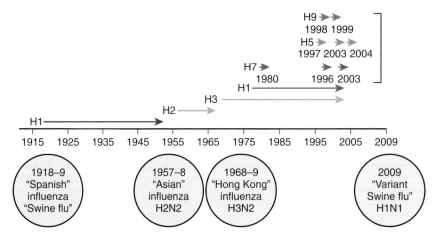

EMERGENCE OF NEW INFLUENZA A VIRUS
SUBTYPES IN HUMANS

Figure 7-8. Emergence of new influenza A virus subtypes in humans. Neuraminidase and hemagglutinin expression of influenza correlates with epidemic outbreaks.

in Mexico, at the current time, the incidence of lethal cases in the United States has not exceeded that observed for other types of influenza, and most patients recover completely without treatment. Nevertheless, there is prudent concern for increased virulence secondary to mutation and the lack of acquired immunity in most patients. For these reasons, efforts to develop a vaccine before "flu season" returns in the fall of 2009 are aggressively being pursued.

When deaths have occurred, the cause has been acute respiratory distress, with DAD as the underlying pathology. Like other forms of influenza, the virus produces no diagnostic cytopathic changes. The risk of bacterial superinfection appears to be comparable to that observed with seasonal influenza.

Severe Acute Respiratory Syndrome

The recent epidemic of the zoonotic coronavirus infection termed severe acute respiratory syndrome (SARS) has not recurred. Infection with the virus led to acute respiratory distress

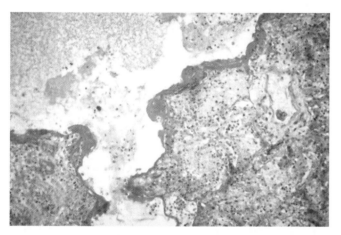

Figure 7-9. Lung from patient who died in the 1918 influenza epidemic showing diffuse alveolar damage with no cytopathic changes (×400).

with high mortality. The lungs at autopsy showed DAD with scattered multinucleated giant cells of uncertain diagnostic significance. Otherwise, the virus produced no cytopathic changes and was essentially histologically indistinguishable from DAD due to influenza.[18]

Respiratory Syncytial Virus

Respiratory syncytial virus (RSV) causes a benign respiratory infection in older children and has been recognized as a cause of adult community-acquired pneumonia, acute bronchiolitis, and DAD in the immunosuppressed host.[19] The infection targets the respiratory lining epithelium, producing syncytial giant cells with nonprominent eosinophilic inclusions (Fig. 7-11). Human metapneumovirus produces changes comparable to RSV and must be included in its differential diagnosis.

Parainfluenza

Parainfluenza causes a benign upper respiratory infection in children that rarely progresses to DAD, although severe disease may develop in the immunosuppressed host. Like RSV, parainfluenza produces bronchiolitis and DAD with syncytial giant cells and epithelial cell intracytoplasmic inclusions.[20] However, the latter are both more frequent and larger than those seen in RSV (Fig. 7-12).

Measles

Measles pneumonia is a rare and serious complication of the childhood viral exanthem. The pathology of pulmonary measles infection ranges from bronchiolitis (Fig. 7-13A) to DAD. The virus produces multikaryons with prominent glassy eosinophilic nuclear Cowdry type A inclusions (see Fig. 7-13B).[21] The differential diagnosis of giant cell pneumonia includes RSV and hard-metal pneumoconiosis; however, the giant cells in the latter disorders lack intranuclear inclusions, and hard-metal pneumoconiosis specifically lacks the exudative features of an acute infection.

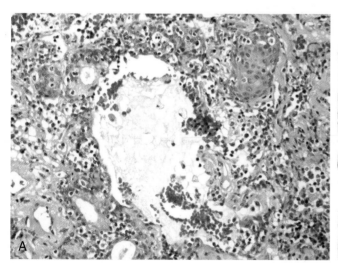

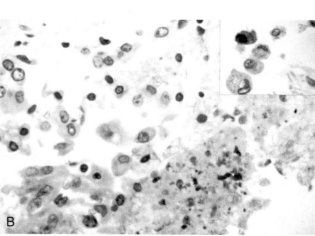

Figure 7-10. A, Lung in patient with diffuse alveolar damage due to influenza showing prominent squamous metaplasia of terminal airways (×250). **B,** Immunostain confirms the presence of influenza A (×400).

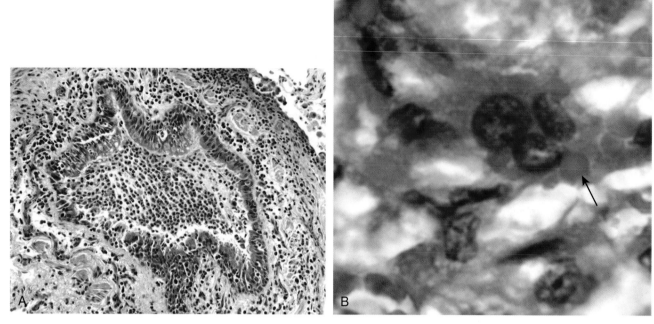

Figure 7-11. A, Acute bronchiolitis in a patient with respiratory syncytial virus (RSV) infection (×400). **B,** Multinucleated epithelial cells in RSV contain inconspicuous eosinophilic cytoplasmic inclusions *(arrow)* (×1000).

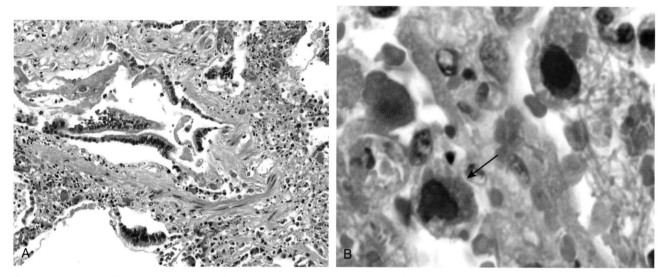

Figure 7-12. A, Bronchiolitis in a patient with parainfluenza infection (×250). **B,** Epithelial cell showing eosinophilic inclusions that are both larger and more frequent than in respiratory syncytial virus infection *(arrow)* (×600).

DNA Viruses

Adenovirus

Adenovirus primarily affects the immunosuppressed host but can produce outbreaks in healthy subjects living at close quarters (e.g., military recruits). Adenovirus typically produces (1) ulcerative bronchiolitis with karyorrhexis (Fig. 7-14A); (2) neutrophilic pneumonia (see Fig. 7-14B); (3) acute intrapulmonary necrosis with hemorrhage (see Fig. 7-14C); or (4) DAD. Infected cells can exhibit amphophilic intranuclear inclusions with peri-

nuclear clearing that mimic herpesvirus infection, but they more characteristically produce "smudge cells" (see Fig. 7-14D), which show hyperchromatic nuclei extruding beyond the confines of their nuclear membranes.[22]

The appearance of smudge cells can be mimicked by pulmonary cytotoxic drug injury or by epithelial repair in the early proliferative phase of DAD. For this reason and because of the potential overlap with herpesvirus-induced cytopathic changes, the diagnosis of Adenovirus infection should always be confirmed by immunohistochemical staining, ultrastructural examination, or viral isolation.

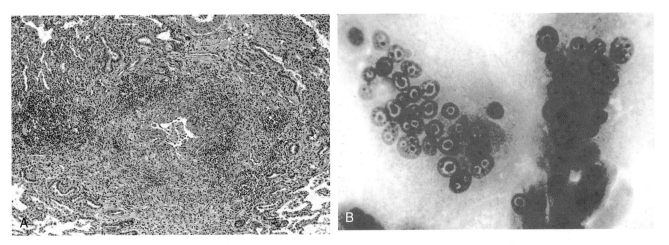

Figure 7-13. A, Chronic inflammation involving a small airway in a patient with measles (×150). **B,** Multinucleated cell showing glassy nuclear Cowdry type A inclusions (×1000).

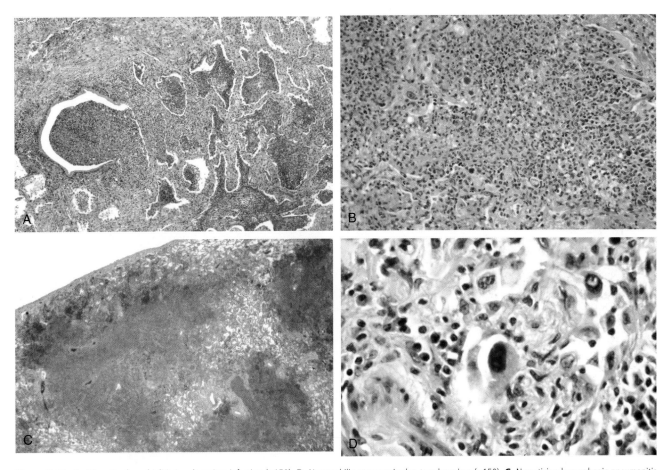

Figure 7-14. A, Ulcerative bronchiolitis in adenovirus infection (×150). **B,** Neutrophilic pneumonia due to adenovirus (×150). **C,** Necrotizing hemorrhagic pneumonitis (×100). **D,** Smudge cell showing extrusion of nuclear contents beyond the confines of the nuclear membrane (×400).

Cytomegalovirus

Cytomegalovirus (CMV) occurs at the extremes of age or as a result of immunosuppression, and it is a common infection in patients with HIV/AIDS.[23] The number of cells showing cytopathic changes can vary considerably and parallels the severity of infection. CMV primarily targets pulmonary macrophages and endothelial cells, but virtually any cell can show cytopathic features. The most common distribution is bloodborne miliary disease (Fig. 7-15), but bronchiolitis and DAD also occur. The diagnostic features of infection are (1) cytomegaly; (2) intranuclear inclusions with characteristic Cowdry Type B inclusions

(Fig. 7-16A); and (3) ill-defined amphophilic intracytoplasmic inclusions that are seen with H&E, PAS, and GMS stains (see Fig. 7-16B). In patients receiving prophylactic treatment with antiviral agents, CMV infection may fail to exhibit cytopathic changes. However, immunostains and in situ hybridization continue to identify intracellular CMV antigens (see Fig. 7-16C).[24]

CMV is a frequent copathogen in the immunosuppressed patient and a cause of immunosuppression in its own right. CMV infection can be seen together with other viral infections, *Pneumocystis jiroveci*, or opportunistic fungal infections (Fig. 7-17).

Herpesvirus

Herpesvirus types 1 and 2 both infect the lung.[25] The incidence of herpesvirus infection increases with immunosuppression and when mucosal barrier defenses have been breached. Herpesvirus characteristically elicits a prominent neutrophilic response that mimics pyogenic bacterial infection, but foci of necrosis, cell karyorrhexis, and piled-up viral infected cells with amphophilic nuclei confirm the diagnosis (Fig. 7-18). Diagnostic cytopathic changes include type A or type B Cowdry nuclear inclusions showing molding of adjacent cells with multikaryon formation (Fig. 7-19). Immunosuppressed patients with herpesvirus viremia develop miliary foci of hemorrhagic necrosis with prominent fibrinous exudates (Fig. 7-20).[26]

Herpesvirus pulmonary infections also develop in patients with structural abnormalities of the airways or as a complication of primary infections of the oropharynx and esophagus. Intubated patients receiving chronic ventilatory support are at increased risk due to local barotrauma from inflated endotracheal tubes. The respiratory mucosa is the primary target (Fig. 7-21). At times, extensive necrosis of an ulcerated airway suggests the diagnosis, but immunostaining for herpes viral antigen can demonstrate high background staining, obscuring the diagnosis.[24] If this is the case, examination of paraffin-embedded tissues by electron microscopy can reveal diagnostic virions (Fig. 7-22).

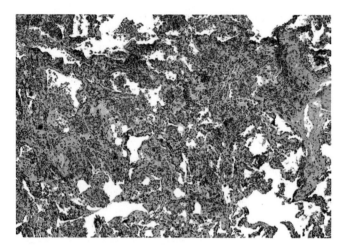

Figure 7-15. Focus of miliary infection in a patient with cytomegalovirus infection (×100).

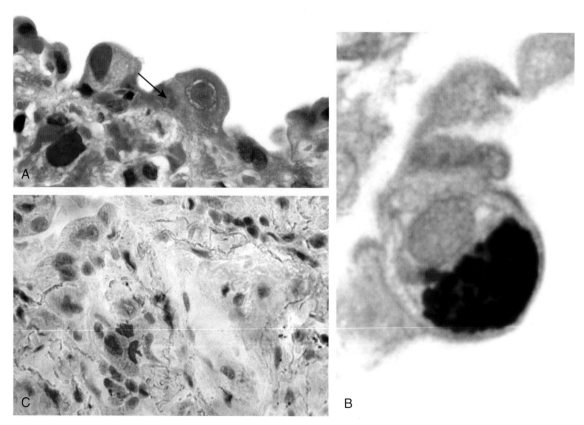

Figure 7-16. A, Alveolar type II lining cells with prominent cytomegaly, Cowdry type B inclusions, and cytoplasmic inclusions *(arrow)* (×400). **B,** Cytoplasmic inclusions stain positive with GMS (×1000). **C,** Immunostain demonstrates cytomegalovirus antigen in patient treated with ganciclovir (×400).

Varicella-Zoster

Varicella-zoster pneumonia is a rare complication of childhood chickenpox but is more commonly encountered as the consequence of reactivated virus in the immunocompromised host. After nonlethal pulmonary infection in childhood, the lung

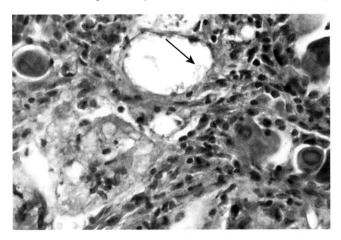

Figure 7-17. Cytomegalovirus infection and cryptococcal pneumonia *(arrow)* complicating HIV/AIDS (×250).

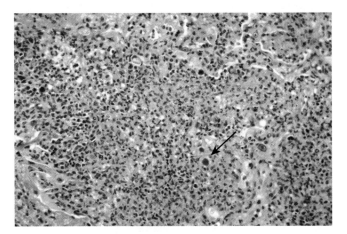

Figure 7-18. Neutrophilic bronchopneumonia caused by Human herpesvirus 1 *(arrow)* (×200).

shows multiple calcified miliary lesions. Cases coming to biopsy or autopsy show miliary nodules of hemorrhagic necrosis in lung and pleura or DAD (Fig. 7-23).[27] Infected cells with primarily Cowdry type A inclusions may be seen at the edges of the lesion, but they are harder to identify than in herpesvirus pneumonia.

Hantavirus

Hantavirus was the cause of an epidemic in the Four Corners region of the southwestern United States in 1993.[28] The infection is a zoonosis transmitted by infected rodent feces. The most common radiographic presentation is diffuse pulmonary edema with pleural effusions mimicking congestive heart failure. Histologically, the lung shows pulmonary edema with scant, poorly formed hyaline membranes (Fig. 7-24A) and atypical lymphocytes circulating within the pulmonary vasculature (see Fig. 7-24B).[29] Confirmation of the diagnosis requires specific immunohistochemistry, serologic evidence of *Hantavirus*-specific IgM, PCR, or ultrastructural identification of the causative virions.

Other Atypical Pneumonias

Mycoplasma *Pneumonia*
Mycoplasma are the smallest (0.2-0.8 μm) free-living bacteria, but they lack a true cell wall. They are facultative anaerobes,

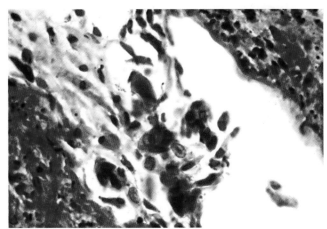

Figure 7-19. Nuclear inclusions in herpetic pneumonia (×400).

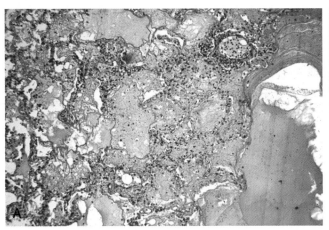
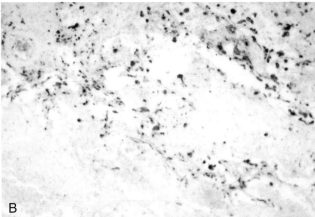

Figure 7-20. A, Hemorrhagic necrotizing pneumonia in immunosuppressed patient with Human herpesvirus 1 (HHV-1) viremia (×150). **B,** Multiple infected cells immunostaining for HHV-1 (×250).

except for *Mycoplasma pneumoniae*, the most common pulmonary pathogen, which is a strict aerobe. *Mycoplasma* pneumonia occurs worldwide with no increased seasonal activity, but epidemics predictably occur every 4 to 8 years. Although it is primarily an infection of young adults, it can attack the elderly. The most common clinical syndrome is tracheobronchitis, with one third of patients developing a mild but persistent pneumonia.

Mycoplasma pneumonia is rarely biopsied, because positive cold agglutinin and specific complement fixation antigen assays establish the diagnosis. Biopsied cases show lymphocytic or neutrophilic bronchiolitis with alveolar wall inflammation and fibrinous exudates (Fig. 7-25).[30] Similar changes are seen in both *Chlamydia* (Fig. 7-26) and *Coxiella* pneumonia.

Epstein-Barr Virus

Epstein-Barr virus (EBV) has been implicated in disorders ranging from the mononucleosis syndrome to malignant lymphoid neoplasia.[31] The mononucleosis syndrome includes pharyngitis, lymphadenitis, and hepatosplenomegaly. Pulmonary involvement can occur as part of the syndrome, but it is unusual and is rarely biopsied. EBV pneumonia shows patchy peribronchiolar and interstitial polyclonal lymphoid infiltrates with scant

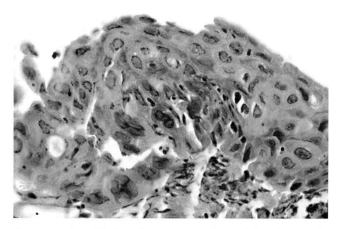

Figure 7-21. Herpetic inclusions in squamous respiratory epithelium of a chronically intubated patient (×200).

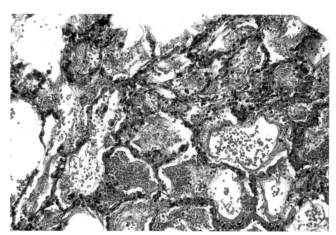

Figure 7-23. Hemorrhagic pneumonia caused by varicella-zoster virus (×250).

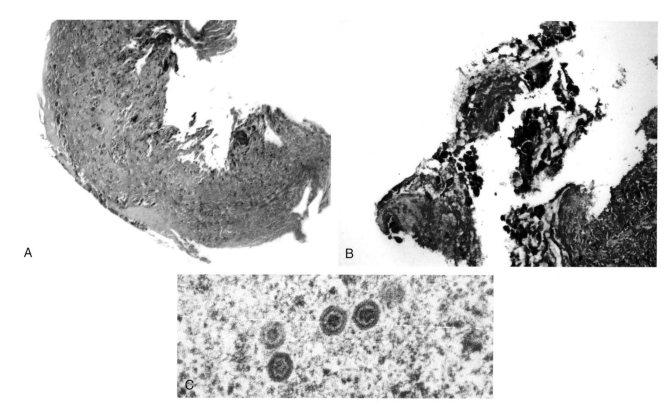

Figure 7-22. Ulcerated tracheal lesion (×100) **(A)**, showing intense immunostaining for Human herpesvirus 1 (×250) **(B)**, and confirmed by ultrastructural examination demonstrating diagnostic virions **(C)** (×8000).

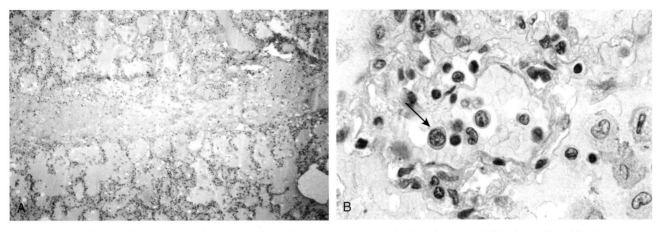

Figure 7-24. A, Pulmonary edema in patient with *Hantavirus* infection (×100). **B,** Pulmonary vessel with intraluminal atypical lymphocytes *(arrow)* (×400).

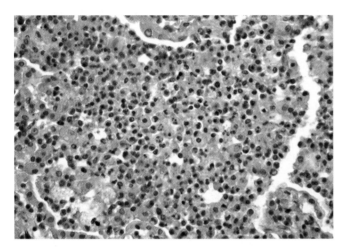

Figure 7-25. Histiocytic and fibrinous exudates in a patient with *Mycoplasma* pneumonia (×25).

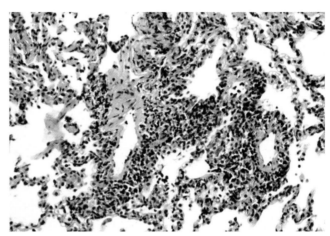

Figure 7-27. Dense lymphoid infiltrate in patient with Epstein-Barr virus pneumonia (×150).

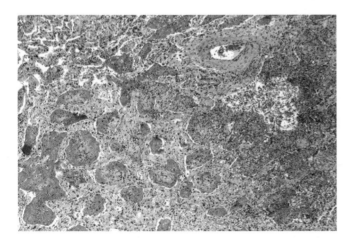

Figure 7-26. Prominent fibrinous and histiocytic exudate due to *Chlamydia* sp. (×100).

interstitial and intra-alveolar fibrin exudates (Fig. 7-27). The diagnosis is usually established serologically by EBV antigen titers but can be confirmed by in situ hybridization.

Pneumocystis jiroveci

For years, the organism formerly known as *Pneumocystis carinii* was thought to be a protozoon; however, it is now confidently classified as a fungus. Originally described as causing a plasma-cell interstitial pneumonia in malnourished children, it was subsequently seen in patients with hematologic malignancies and in those receiving chemotherapy or chronic corticosteroid therapy. In the 1980s, *Pneumocystis* pneumonia (PCP) became a signal infection in establishing the diagnosis of AIDS. It was encountered in epidemic proportions, until prophylactic use of trimethoprim-sulfamethoxazole (Bactrim) became a routine aspect of HIV/AIDS management. *P. jiroveci* is currently most often diagnosed by sputum induction, and lung biopsy is reserved for diagnostic challenges.[32]

Although the disease manifests radiographically as an atypical interstitial pneumonia, interstitial inflammation is not its most striking pathologic feature. In PCP, the alveoli are filled with a frothy eosinophilic exudate that mimics exudative pulmonary edema or alveolar lipoproteinosis (Fig. 7-28A). The pulmonary interstitium shows a mild, plasma cell–rich pneumonitis and prominent alveolar type II cell hyperplasia.

The diagnosis is confirmed by the presence of oval, helmet- or crescenteric-shaped GMS-positive "cysts," 4 to 6 μm in greatest dimension, within the alveolar froth (see Fig. 7-28B).[33] Pneumocysts are distinguished from GMS-positive fungal yeast forms by the absence of budding, pericapsular accentuation, and a so-called intracytoplasmic dot in the former. However, when these features are absent and the organism load in the biopsy is low, it may be difficult to confidently exclude *Histoplasma* or

Cryptococcus. In such cases, specific immunohistochemistry can confirm the diagnosis.

Multiple patterns of unusual host reactions to *P. jiroveci* have been recognized.[34] These include DAD (Fig. 7-29A), solitary necrotizing granulomas (see Fig. 7-29B), miliary infection, lymphoid interstitial pneumonia, and regional lymphadenitis. Microcalcifications may be seen in areas of infection, and thin-walled cyst formation may develop.

Bronchiectasis

Bronchiectasis is one of the major manifestations of pulmonary infection. Dilatation and anatomic distortion of conducting

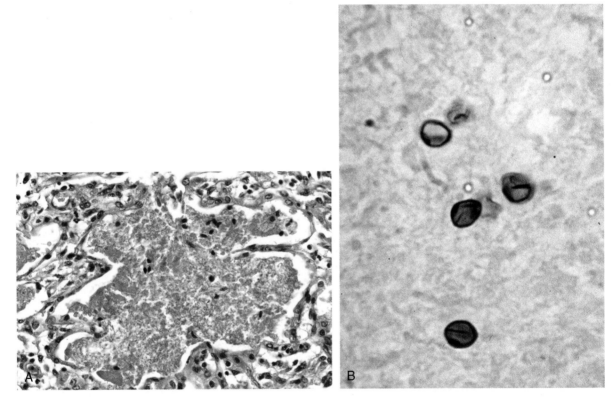

Figure 7-28. Alveolar eosinophilic exudate in *Pneumocystis* pneumonia **(A)** (×400), showing GMS-positive cyst forms with pericapsular accentuation **(B)** (×600).

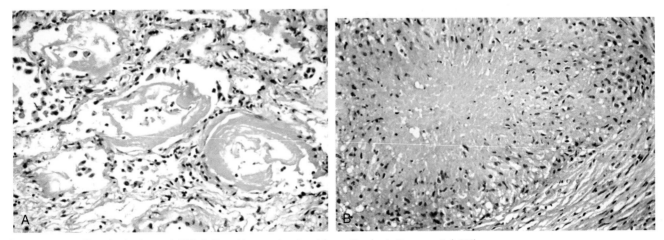

Figure 7-29. A, Diffuse alveolar damage (×250). **B,** Necrotizing granulomatous inflammation due to *Pneumocystis* (×250).

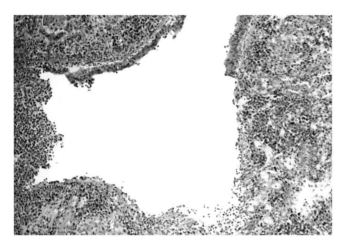

Figure 7-30. Bronchiolitis secondary to *Bordetella pertussis* infection, once a common cause of bronchiectasis (×250).

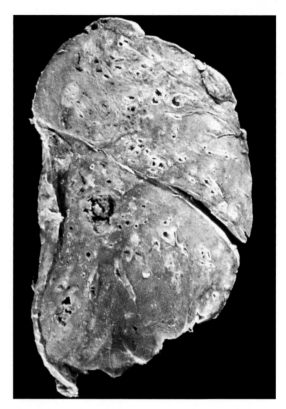

Figure 7-31. The lung in cystic fibrosis, showing bronchiectasis and a cavitary abscess.

airways can result from acute and chronic airway injury due to airway infection (wet bronchiectasis) or adjacent parenchymal scarring (dry or traction bronchiectasis). A number of infections can damage the large airways and lead to bronchiectasis. Reversible cylindrical bronchiectasis may appear radiographically after an acute bacterial pneumonia. Because this change often resolves, biopsies of suspicious bronchiectatic regions should be deferred until a period of weeks has elapsed after an acute infection. Because regions of chronic bronchiectasis are fed by varicose bronchial arteries that often course directly beneath the airways surface, endoscopic biopsies of bronchiectatic areas are generally contraindicated.

Before the development of childhood vaccination, viral exanthems and *Bordetella pertussis* were common causes of bronchiectasis (Fig. 7-30). Cystic fibrosis, a genetic disorder of chloride transport, is currently a leading cause of severe bronchiectasis in young adults, as advances in management have resulted in survival of these patients beyond childhood (Fig. 7-31).

In bronchiectasis, the airways lose their cartilaginous support due to chronic inflammation, and they become dilated and prone to repeated bouts of mucoid impaction and infection.[35] The airways develop a spectrum of gross changes ranging from cystic, to varicose, to cylindrical dilatation, associated with distal peribronchiolar inflammation (Fig. 7-32A) and increasing degrees of parenchymal scarring with loss of gas-exchanging alveoli (see Fig. 7-32B). Although the large airways are invariably ectatic, the distal airways in bronchiectasis are generally narrowed by constrictive bronchiolitis.

Recurrent polymicrobial infections with necrotizing bronchopneumonia and abscess formation complicate bronchiectasis. Patients are also prone to develop infections due to antibiotic-resistant mucoid forms of *Pseudomonas*, *Burkholderia* spp., *Stenotrophomonas maltophilia*, *Achromobacter xylosoxidans* (see Fig. 7-32C), or *Staphylococcal* spp.[36] Some patients with infective bronchiectasis develop allergic bronchopulmonary aspergillosis (ABPA) and superinfection with atypical mycobacteria.[37]

Acute Bronchopneumonia

Acute bronchopneumonia is the most common distribution of pulmonary infection. Gram-positive and gram-negative bacteria, as well some viruses, including herpesvirus and adenovirus, elicit primarily an exudation of neutrophils, whereas the cellular response to other viruses, fungi, mycoplasma, and chlamydia are primarily lymphohistiocytic. Bronchopneumonia generally results from microaspiration of pathogens that have colonized the oropharynx (Fig. 7-33A). At times, the aspiration of colonized food particles can carry bacteria and fungi into the lung (see Fig. 7-33B). Terminal episodes of aspiration often show colonies of gram-positive aerococci, previously referred to as the genus *Gaffkya* (see Fig. 7-33C), and their appearance is both common and characteristic in lung specimens obtained at autopsy.[38]

Bacterial Infections

The pyogenic bacteria are distinguished by their propensity to evoke acute neutrophilic inflammation and pus. Pyogenic infections and other acute necrotizing bronchopneumonias progress to organizing pneumonia, which is characterized by a fibrohistiocytic response that obliterates small airways along with inflammation of the surrounding alveolar interstitium (Fig. 7-34). This reaction is nonspecific, and "organizing pneumonia" or "bronchiolitis-obliterans–organizing pneumonia" is a rubric for the generic lesion that may result from infection, noninfective inflammatory disorders, or idiopathic causes.[39] It is important for the surgical pathologist to convey clearly to the treating clinicians that a diagnosis of "organizing pneumonia" does not indicate a specific etiology.

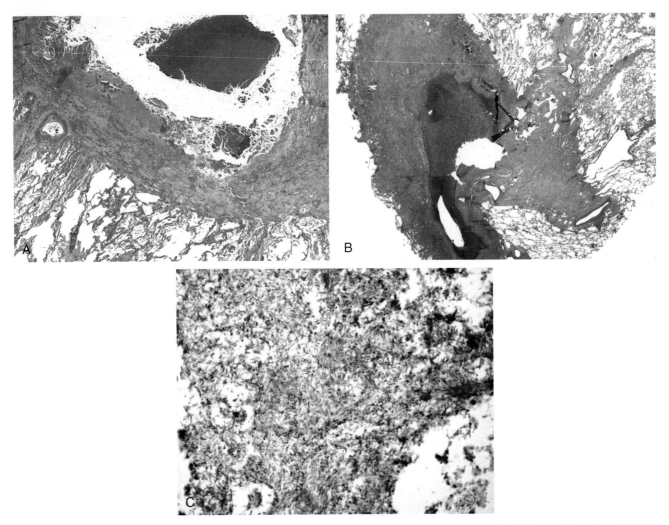

Figure 7-32. A, Bronchiectasis in cystic fibrosis, showing dilatation and destruction of airway wall (×200). **B,** Dense peribronchiolar scar in bronchiectasis (×150). **C,** Bronchiectatic airway with colonies of gram-negative bacilli identified by culture as *Burkholderia cepacia* (×400).

Pneumococcal Pneumonia

Streptococcus pneumoniae pneumonia (pneumococcal pneumonia) is a community-acquired pneumonia that classically produces a lobar pneumonia that heals by resolution (i.e., without necrosis or scarring).[40] In some cases, pneumococcal pneumonia complicates a resolving viral tracheobronchitis or influenza. In the age of antibiotic treatment, most cases do not progress to lobar involvement and are limited to acute, non-necrotizing bronchopneumonia. A large number of serotypes of *S. pneumoniae* have been isolated, and certain ones (e.g., type 3), can be virulent, producing necrotizing pneumonia, bacteremia, and death, despite prompt antibiotic treatment.

Although it is rarely biopsied, lobar pneumococcal pneumonia is still seen at autopsy. The early phase of the disease, known as the red hepatization, shows exudation of edema fluid with the diapedesis of red blood cells (Fig. 7-35A). The exudate spreads to fill an entire lung lobe via the pores of Kohn, interalveolar potential channels within the normal lung (see Fig. 7-35B). The acute cellular response is neutrophilic, but this is followed within days by filling of the alveoli with macrophages that ingest the infected exudate, known as the gray hepatization (see Fig. 7-35C). Despite the extensive inflammatory changes, alveolar necrosis is absent (a finding best assessed by elastic stains), and the lung heals by resolution with minimal sequelae. The offending organisms are gram-positive, lancet-shaped cocci growing in pairs (diplococci) and in short chains, and they can be identified by tissue Gram stain and GMS stains (see Fig. 7-35D).

Group A Streptococcal Pneumonia

Group A streptococcal pneumonia occurs at the extremes of life or as a complication of resolving influenza infection.[41] It produces a rapidly progressing and life-threatening pneumonia with edema, hemorrhage, abscess formation, empyema, and septicemia. Group A streptococci evoke a brisk increase in pulmonary capillary permeability, yielding what can be mistaken for cardiogenic pulmonary edema on low-power microscopic examination (Fig. 7-36A). Further scrutiny reveals necrotic macrophages and innumerable gram-positive bacteria in chains (see Fig. 7-36B). Pulmonary hemorrhage and abscess formation are frequently seen. Streptococci have a predilection to course along pulmonary

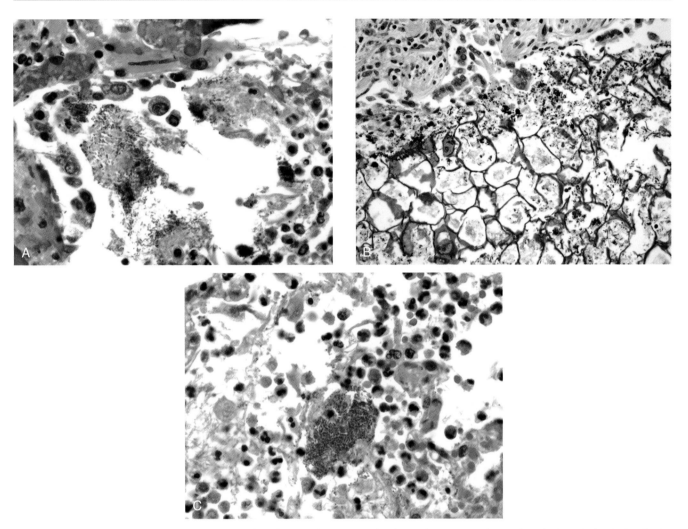

Figure 7-33. A, Acute bronchiolitis due to *Staphylococcus* (×400). **B,** Lentil aspiration with colonies of gram-positive bacteria (×400). **C,** Terminal aspiration showing intraluminal colony of gram-positive *Aerococcus* (*Gaffkya*) sp. (×400).

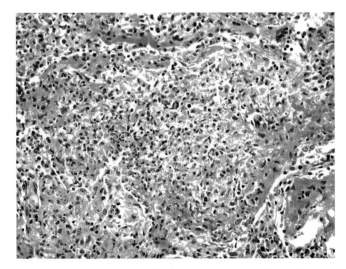

Figure 7-34. Organizing pneumonia showing macrophages and early fibrosis in respiratory bronchioles and alveoli (×250).

lymphatic channels, recapitulating erysipeloid spread in the skin, to produce an early empyema (Fig. 7-37).

Staphylococcus aureus

Staphylococcus aureus has emerged as a frequently encountered, life-threatening pulmonary pathogen. Previously seen as a community-acquired complication of influenza, staphylococcal infection is now a primary cause of nosocomial pneumonia, and its evolving drug resistance accounts for methicillin-resistant *S. aureus* (MRSA) strains that are of particular concern for hospital infection control epidemiologists.[42]

S. aureus produces a necrotizing pyogenic pneumonia with abscess formation (Fig. 7-38A). The organisms grow in clusters as gram-positive microcolonies (see Fig. 7-38B). Infection heals by organization with scarring, and cystic pneumatoceles may develop. Some phage-infected strains of the organism produce an exotoxin that can activate the CD3 receptor to promote the release of the T lymphocyte's complement of lymphokines, leading to a toxic-shock syndrome with sepsis physiology, DAD,

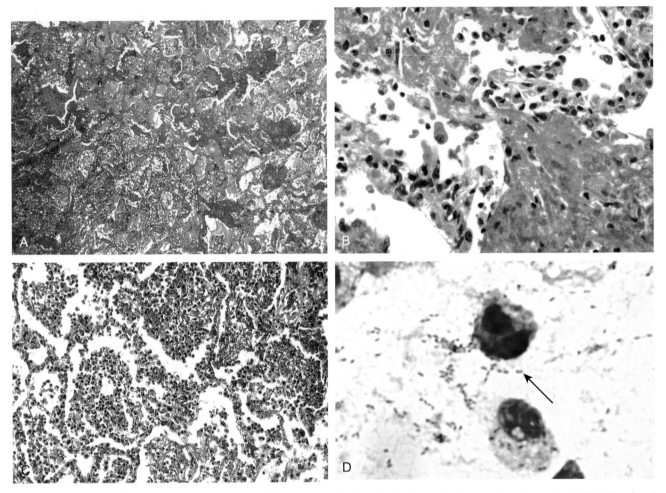

Figure 7-35. A, In the red hepatization phase of pneumococcal lobar pneumonia, alveoli are filled by fibrin with diapedesis of red blood cells (×100). **B,** The infected exudate extends throughout the lobe via the pores of Kohn, potential channels between adjacent alveoli (×250). **C,** In the gray hepatization phase, alveoli are filled by leukocytes that scavenge bacteria and detritus before resolution of the infection (×200). **D,** The pneumococcus is a lancet-shaped, gram-positive coccus that grows in pairs (diplococci) *(arrow)* and chains (×600).

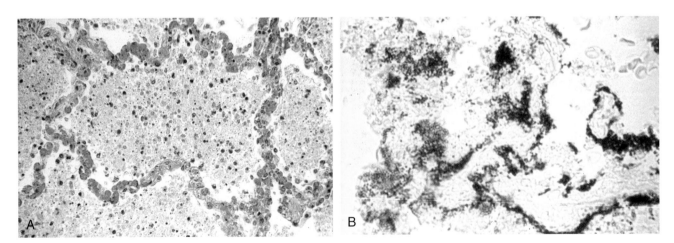

Figure 7-36. A, The alveolar spaces in streptococcal pneumonia show an eosinophilic exudate that mimics proteinaceous pulmonary edema at low power (×250). **B,** Innumerable gram-positive cocci in chains are seen in the exudates and tend to invade lymphatics (×250).

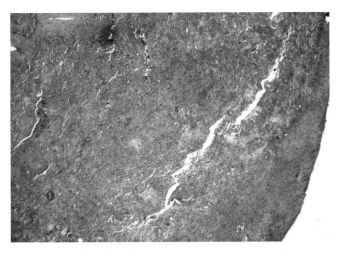

Figure 7-37. Abscess formation and empyema occur early in streptococcal pneumonia (×100).

and disseminated intravascular coagulation that is fatal if not treated promptly.

Gram-Negative Bacteria

Most gram-negative bacilli produce a necrotizing bronchopneumonia with hemorrhage and abscess formation. Certain virulent gram-negative species, including *Klebsiella, Pseudomonas, Acinetobacter*, and *Burkholderia* spp., have a propensity to infect the pulmonary microvasculature, leading to necrosis, bacteremia, and septic shock.[43] The lung shows fibrinoid necrosis with colonies of gram-negative bacilli streaming along the vessel walls, where they create an ill-defined purplish hue in H&E-stained sections (Fig. 7-39A, B).

Klebsiella

Klebsiella pneumonia typically occurs in patients who are immunocompromised due to age, ethanol abuse, or diabetes mellitus.

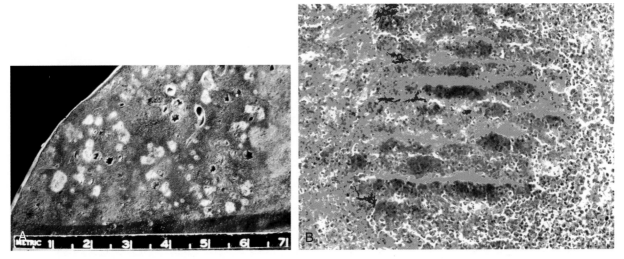

Figure 7-38. A, Lung sample from a patient with staphylococcal pneumonia showing bronchopneumonia with abscess formation. **B,** Microabscess with gram-positive *Staphylococcus aureus* in clusters (×400).

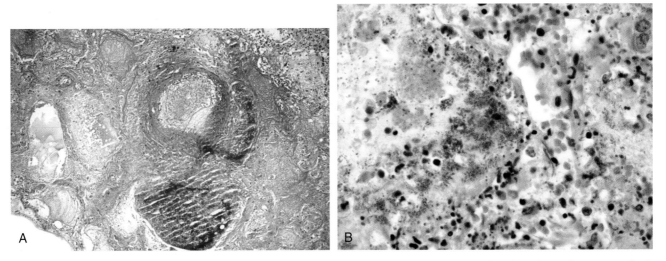

Figure 7-39. A, Fibrinoid necrosis with dense bacterial growth visible in H&E-stained sections in *Pseudomonas* pneumonia (×250). **B,** Clusters of gram-negative bacilli are identified (×600).

It is a common ventilator-associated pneumonia.[44] Like the pneumococcus, *Klebsiella* spp. classically produce a lobar pneumonia with a slimy "mucoid" appearance and an unexplained predilection for the upper lobes (Fig. 7-40A). Infection produces hemorrhagic necrosis, microabscesses, and cavity formation. The organisms are short, gram-negative bacilli that can be demonstrated with both tissue Gram stain (see Fig. 7-40B) and GMS by virtue of their capsules. Less commonly, *Klebsiella* spp. produce a chronic necrotizing pneumonia with scarring and distortion of the pulmonary anatomy (see Fig. 7-40C).

Lung Abscess Due to Oropharyngeal Aspiration

Lung abscess complicates the aspiration of polymicrobial oropharyngeal bacteria. The organisms isolated from a lung abscess include mixed gram-positive and gram-negative aerobic flora as well as anaerobes. Patients with poor oral hygiene due to dental caries, those with gingival or tonsillar disease, and those with disorders that impair consciousness or interfere with normal swallowing (e.g., ethanolism, seizure disorder, cerebrovascular accident) are at increased risk for aspiration pneumonia and

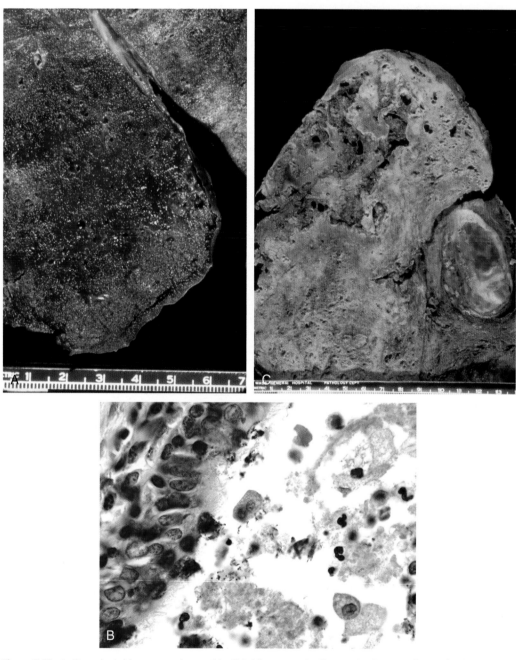

Figure 7-40. A, Hemorrhagic lobar pneumonia caused by *Klebsiella pneumoniae.* The organism has a predilection for the upper lung lobes. **B,** *Klebsiella* is a small, non-motile, gram-negative rod that also stains with GMS. **C,** Chronic necrotizing pneumonia due to *Klebsiella* sp. with extensive scarification of necrotic lung (×600).

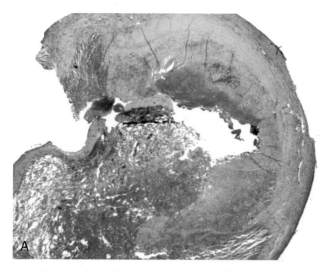

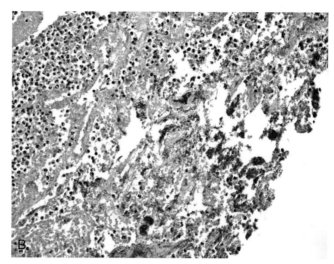

Figure 7-41. A, Shaggy fibrinous exudate lining wall of lung abscess caused by aspiration of oropharyngeal mixed flora (×100). **B,** Necrosis and bacteria in lung abscess (×250).

lung abscess.[45] The disorder begins as a necrotizing bronchopneumonia in a dependent segment of the lung and progresses to produce a cavitary abscess communicating with a feeding adjacent airway. Most lung abscesses are diagnosed and treated noninvasively; however, poor drainage and closure may lead to failure to respond to medical treatment, prompting surgical excision.

Microscopically, the wall of the lung abscess is irregular, with a shaggy fibrinous lining (Fig. 7-41A) that can be difficult to distinguish from a necrobiotic rheumatoid nodule or Wegener granulomatosis. However, palisading granulomatous inflammation is not a prominent finding in lung abscess. The area around the cavity shows acute and organizing bronchopneumonia (see Fig. 7-41B). The activity of a lung abscess may be determined microscopically by examining its lining: actively infected cavities show a squamous epithelium which indicates complete healing and may be mistaken for a region of primary bronchiectasis.

Actinomycosis

Actinomyces spp. are gram-positive, filamentous bacteria that cause a chronic distal necrotizing pneumonia with a proclivity for penetration into the adjacent soft tissues of the chest wall.[46] *Actinomyces* spp. are aspirated from the oropharynx, where they are commonly part of the tonsillar flora in younger patients or a pathogen related to poor oral hygiene and gingivitis in the elderly. The risk factors for actinomycosis are similar to those for lung abscess. The infection extends into the pleura and then forms sinuses within the soft tissues of the chest wall that ultimately exit at the skin surface. The indurated pulmonary lesion may be mistaken clinically for an aggressive peripheral lung malignancy, but its gross appearance at surgery is usually distinct (Fig. 7-42).

The histologic response evoked by actinomycosis is variegate, with microabscesses, polymorphous infiltrates of lymphocytes, histiocytes, plasma cells, giant cells, and fibrosis. At times, the extent of the fibroinflammatory response can lead one to consider a diagnosis of "inflammatory pseudotumor." The correct diagnosis is established by the presence of so-called sulfur

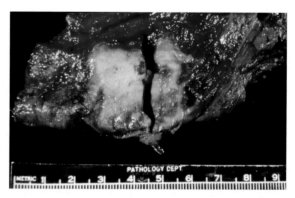

Figure 7-42. Subpleural nodule of actinomycosis resected for suspicion of carcinoma. Note the yellow-tan appearance that suggests inflammation rather than malignancy.

granules (Fig. 7-43A)—bright yellow specks seen with the naked eye or with the aid of a hand lens that microscopically represent colonies of tangled gram-positive, GMS-positive, beaded filamentous bacilli (see Fig. 7-43B, C) coated by an eosinophilic matrix of exudate plasma proteins termed the Splendore-Hoeppli reaction. Treatment includes long-term antibiotic therapy and surgical resection.

The differential diagnosis of sulfur granules in the lung includes botryomycosis, a term used to describe a variety of infections by colonies of gram-positive cocci, either *Streptococcus* or *Staphylococcus,* that grossly appear comparable to the sulfur granules caused by *Actinomyces.*[47] Distinguishing these entities depends on the morphology of the bacteria in the granules (i.e., cocci in botryomycosis versus filamentous bacteria in actinomycosis) (Fig. 7-44).

Nocardia

Nocardia produces pneumonia primarily in the immunosuppressed host.[48] The organism shares morphologic and histochemical staining features with *Actinomyces,* but its clinical and

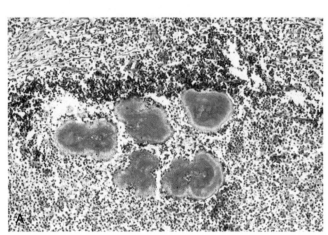

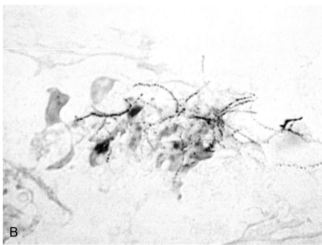

Figure 7-43. A, Multiple actinomycotic sulfur granules within granulohistiocytic inflammatory response (×100). **B,** Gram stain shows irregularly beaded filaments of *Actinomyces* sp. that also stain with GMS. GMS stains all gram-positive organisms with no specificity for actinomycosis (×1000).

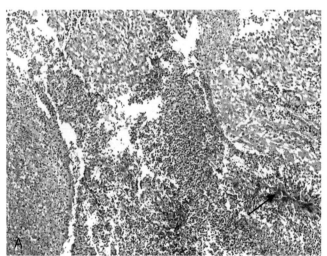

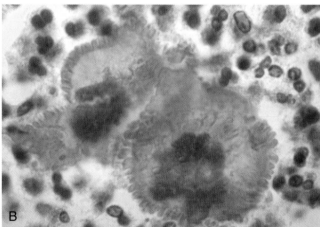

Figure 7-44. A, Low-power view of botryomycosis in an infected airway (×25). **B,** High-power view of botryomycotic granule caused by *Staphylococcus aureus* (×600).

histologic responses are usually easily distinguished. *Nocardia* produces a necrotizing pneumonia with granulohistiocytic inflammation (Fig. 7-45A), and special stains highlight tangles of gram-positive, GMS-positive filamentous organisms that show less beading than *Actinomyces* (see Fig. 7-45B). Sulfur granules are rarely seen in pulmonary infections. As distinct from *Actinomyces*, *Nocardia* spp. are weakly acid-fast and can be highlighted with modified Ziehl-Neelsen stains (e.g., Fite-Ferraco) (see Fig. 7-45C). Nocardiosis is a recognized complication of pulmonary alveolar lipoproteinosis and has recently been observed in patients receiving therapies that interfere with the activities of tumor necrosis factor-α.

Legionella

Legionella spp. produce pulmonary infections ranging in severity from a mild respiratory illness to life-threatening pneumonia. Patients may suffer from a modest degree of immunosuppression

due to diabetes or ethanolism. The organism can be inhaled from contaminated water and air-conditioning sources, and these have led to point outbreaks of infection.

The diagnosis of *Legionella* infection is currently established noninvasively by immunoassays; however, the disease may be identified histologically in biopsy or autopsy tissues. The infected lung characteristically shows a fibrinohistiocytic response with alveolar filling by fibrin and necrotic macrophages with a sparse neutrophilic component, (Fig. 7-46A), although its histology may also be indistinguishable from that of pyogenic infections.[49] It can be mimicked by acute fibrinous organizing pneumonia (AFOP), a recently recognized noninfective pattern of pulmonary injury (see Fig. 7-46B). Although *Legionella* is a gram-negative coccobacillus, it stains weakly with Gram stains, and silver impregnation stains are required to blacken the organisms, which are often abundant in situ in the absence of prior treatment (Fig. 7-47A). *Legionella micdadei* is distinguished by its staining with modified Ziehl-Neelsen stains (see Fig. 7-47B).

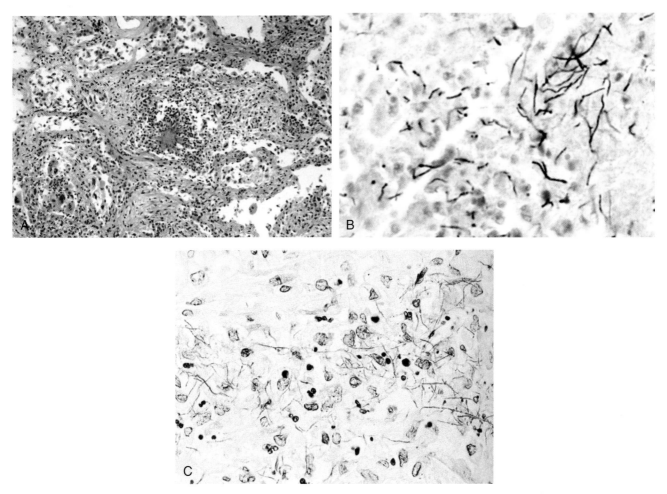

Figure 7-45. A, Necrotizing pneumonia due to *Nocardia asteroides* shows granulohistiocytic response (×250). **B,** Like *Actinomyces*, *Nocardia* is a gram-positive, filamentous, bacillary actinomycete that also stains with GMS (×600). **C,** Unlike *Actinomyces*, *Nocardia* is weakly acid-fast and can be demonstrated with the Fite-Ferraco stain (×400).

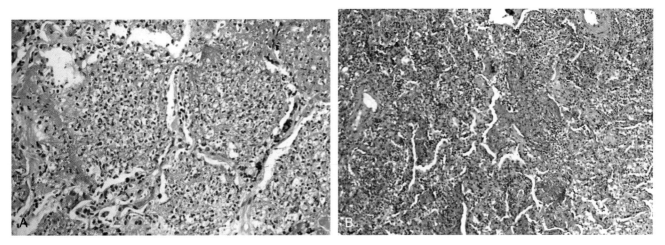

Figure 7-46. A, *Legionella* spp. characteristically produce a necrotizing bronchopneumonia with alveolar filling by fibrin and histiocytes. This appearance must be distinguished from acute fibrinous organizing pneumonia (×25). **(B)**, in which the alveolar spaces are filled with fibrin but the disorder is not caused by infection (×250).

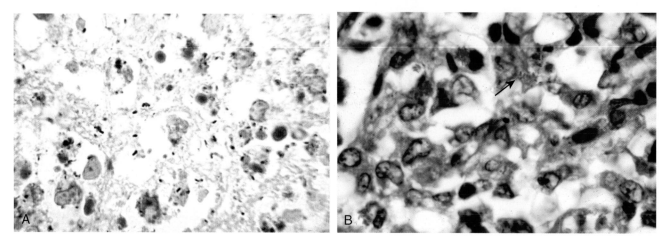

Figure 7-47. A, *Legionella* spp. are gram-negative coccobacilli but must be demonstrated by silver impregnation (×400). **B,** *Legionella micdadei*, the Pittsburgh pneumonia agent, also stains with modified AFB stains (×1000).

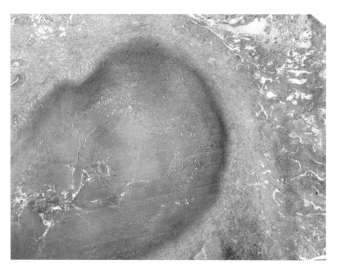

Figure 7-48. *Rhodococcus equi* causes a cavitary nodular pneumonia (×150).

Rhodococcus equi

Rhodococcus pneumonia is a zoonotic infection that causes a nodular histiocytic and cavitary pneumonia in immunosuppressed patients, most commonly in patients with HIV/AIDS (Fig. 7-48).[50] The causative gram-positive cocci are easily identified (Fig. 7-49A) and also stain positive with the modified Ziehl-Neelsen stain (see Fig. 7-49B). The inflammatory response shows malakoplakia (Fig. 7-50A) with formation of intracellular calcific concretions termed Michaelis-Gutman bodies that, although nonspecific, are characteristically seen in the infection and can be highlighted by both PAS and iron stains (see Fig. 7-50B).[51]

Tropheryma whippelii (Whipple Disease)

Whipple disease is a rare disorder caused by the actinomycete *Tropheryma whippelii*. It most commonly causes intestinal malabsorption, but pulmonary and neurologic disease also occurs. In the lung, Whipple disease can manifest as interstitial infiltrates, pleural effusions, or pulmonary hypertension.[52] The characteristic change in the disorder is the accumulation of foamy macrophages that show intense staining with PAS (Fig. 7-51). In some cases, microgranulomas that are histologically comparable to those seen in sarcoidosis may confuse the diagnosis (Fig. 7-52), and the PAS staining in these granulomas may be equivocal as well. It is uncertain whether sarcoidosis is associated with Whipple disease or whether the sarcoidal granulomas are evidence of early infection. In these cases, a small-bowel biopsy usually establishes the diagnosis. Further confirmation can be achieved by ultrastructural examination demonstrating the bacillary organisms (Fig. 7-53) or by specific PCR.

Granulomatous Pneumonia

Pathologists apply the term *granuloma* to a variety of histologic responses, including micronodular collections of tightly knit epithelioid macrophages (tuberculoid granulomas), necrotizing histiocytic reactions (necrotizing granuloma), and diffuse polymorphic infiltrates composed of lymphocytes, histiocytes, and plasma cells (granulomatous inflammation). The organisms that evoke these cellular responses are limited and include the actinomycetes, mycobacteria, fungi, and helminths.

Mycobacterial Infections

Pulmonary necrotizing granulomatous inflammation is most commonly caused by mycobacterial or fungal infection. Tuberculosis is caused by a gram-positive soil actinomycete. The disease was recognized in antiquity, and it continues to represent a major source of global morbidity and mortality, largely because of its recrudescence in the settings of poverty and HIV/AIDS.[53] The term *tuberculosis* is properly limited to infections caused by *Mycobacterium tuberculosis* and its genetically related congeners (e.g., *Mycobacterium bovis*) and is not the appropriate appellation for infections caused by nontuberculous or atypical mycobacteria.

M. tuberculosis can affect the pulmonary airways, parenchyma, or pleura. Inhaled mycobacteria proliferate in the alveolar spaces and are then transported via lymphatics to regional

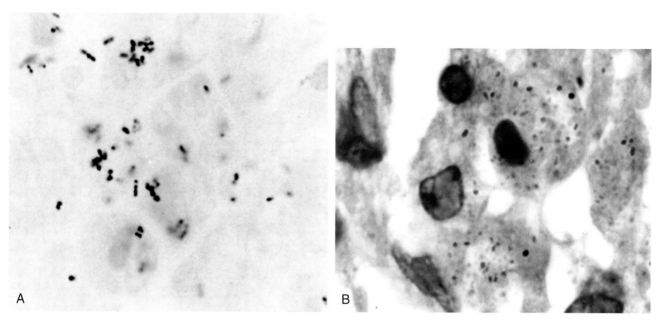

Figure 7-49. A, The causative gram-positive cocci (*Rhodococcus equi*) (×1000). **B,** Stain with modified AFB preparations (×1000).

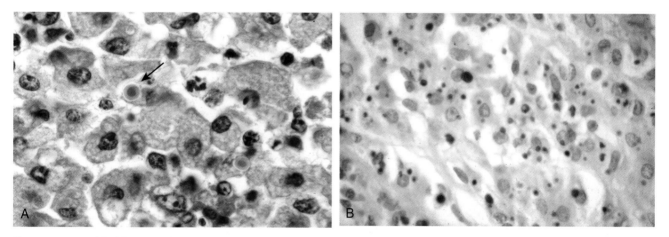

Figure 7-50. A, Malakoplakia with Michaelis-Gutman bodies (×600), calcific concretions that are also positive in PAS and iron-stained sections (×600) **(B)**.

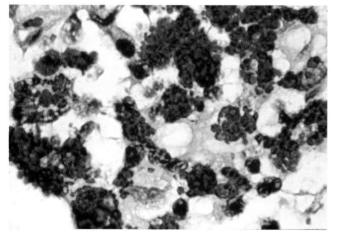

Figure 7-51. Macrophages staining intensely PAS positive in Whipple disease (×600).

hilar lymph nodes, from which they can enter the systemic circulation to spread to other organs. Progression of infection is limited by the acquisition of effective cell-mediated immunity.[54] The initial pulmonary focus of infection (Ghon focus) heals by fibrosis and may show dystrophic calcification. This Ghon focus and the accompanying calcified site of infection in a hilar lymph node are termed the Ranke complex (Fig. 7-54), and the foci of primary disseminated infection are termed Simon foci. At all sites, the cellular response to *M. tuberculosis* is characterized by nodular collections of epithelioid macrophages with multinucleated giant cells, known as the tuberculoid granuloma or tubercle. These can undergo central necrosis due to a cell-mediated hypersensitivity response. Sites of tuberculous infection may also show neutrophilic and eosinophilic exudates, but these are generally not prominent features.

The mature tuberculoid granuloma is surrounded by a rim of T lymphocytes and contained by an outer zone of fibrosis (Fig.

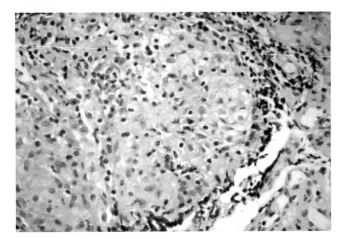

Figure 7-52. Non-necrotizing granulomas mimicking sarcoidosis in Whipple disease (×250).

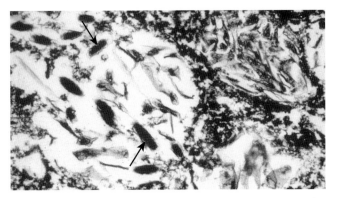

Figure 7-53. Ultrastructural image (×5000) demonstrates bacilli of *Tropheryma whippelii (arrow).*

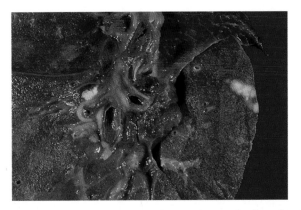

Figure 7-54. The Ranke complex includes the intrapulmonary Ghon focus of initial infection and the calcified hilar lymph node.

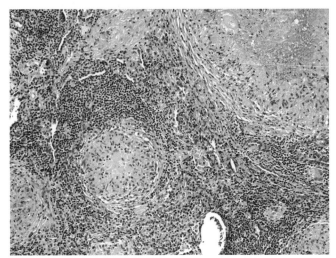

Figure 7-55. The tuberculoid granuloma is a collection of epithelioid histiocytes, often with giant cells, surrounded by a lymphocytic infiltrate and fibrosis (×200).

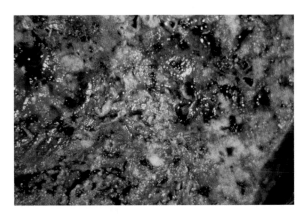

Figure 7-56. The cheesy gross appearance of a focus of caseous necrosis.

7-55). The presence of tuberculoid granulomas can be a distinguishing clue in differentiating tuberculosis from other forms of necrotizing granulomatous inflammation (e.g., Wegener granulomatosis), in which tuberculoid granulomas are infrequent.

The term *caseous necrosis* properly refers to the "cheesy" appearance of the necrotic lesion on gross inspection. The his-

tologic correlate is destruction of lung tissue (Fig. 7-56) with loss of the underlying reticulin stroma. But the latter finding is not apparent in H&E-stained sections, so it is best, in practice, to refer to tuberculous lesions as either "necrotizing" or "non-necrotizing" and to avoid the terms "caseating" and "noncaseating."

Because the response to mycobacterial infection reflects a component of immune hypersensitivity, even small numbers of organisms can evoke substantial lung injury, and this complicates the task of identifying mycobacteria in situ. The organisms are best identified by their red color in AFB-stained sections (i.e., Ziehl-Neelsen stain or one of its modifications, such as Fite-Ferraco stain). Mycobacteria can show substantial morphologic variability. They are curvilinear, vary in length, and exhibit a characteristic beaded appearance attributable to nonhomogeneous uptake of the AFB stain (Fig. 7-57A).

However, there is no reliable way to distinguish *M. tuberculosis* from atypical mycobacteria by histochemical staining. Because mycobacteria are weakly gram positive, they can also be demonstrated in GMS-stained sections, a finding that is nonspecific but can at times aid in identification of the inconspicuous bacilli (see Fig. 7-57B). Nonmycobacterial organisms can also be

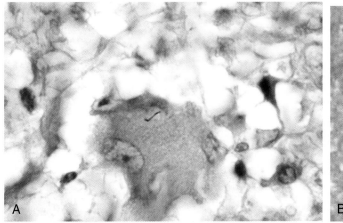
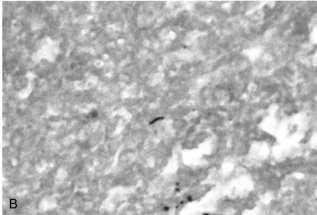

Figure 7-57. A, Mycobacterial tuberculosis, the "red snapper," is a short, beaded bacillus that can be equally well demonstrated with the Ziehl-Neelsen stain or its weakly acid-fast modifications (×600). **B,** Mycobacteria are apparent in GMS-stained sections, but this finding is less specific than with AFB staining (×1000).

Table 7-5 Acid-Fast Bacteria
Mycobacteria
Nocardia
Rhodococcus
Legionella micdadei

Table 7-6 Pulmonary Manifestations of Tuberculosis
Exposures with no disease (Ranke complex)
Caseating pneumonia
Acinar-nodose pneumonia
Nodular disease (tuberculoma)
Cavitary pneumonia
Tracheobronchitis
Miliary disease
Lymphadenitis and calcification
Pleuritis
Fibrothorax (late)

AFB positive, so differential staining and culture results may be required to establish an accurate diagnosis (Table 7-5).

In practice, the identification of *M. tuberculosis* by Ziehl-Neelsen staining is relatively insensitive, identifying mycobacteria in roughly 60% of culture-positive cases, so the diagnosis may depend on isolating organisms in culture. In one study of more than 300 biopsy specimens, mycobacteria were cultured from the specimens that contained necrotizing granulomas (38.2%), non-necrotizing granulomas (32.4%), poorly formed granulomas (30.0%), or acute inflammation (15.8%). Tissues with fibrotic or hyalinized granulomas, nonspecific chronic inflammation, nonspecific reactive or reparative changes, no significant histologic abnormality, or malignancy failed to yield positive cultures. This study concluded that biopsy specimens with the latter diagnoses were inappropriate samples for either mycobacterial culture and histochemical staining.

Mycobacteria grow slowly in culture, and it can take weeks before they are eventually isolated. Consequently, ancillary methods have been developed with the aim of increasing the likelihood of establishing a diagnosis in a timely fashion. Sensitive fluorescent staining techniques, including the auramine-rhodamine stain, are used routinely in some laboratories to examine smears and tissues. PCR methods have been developed that can identify *M. tuberculosis* and distinguish this organism from atypical mycobacteria in fresh tissues and in paraffin-embedded sections.

Spectrum of Pulmonary Tuberculous Infection
Tuberculosis has protean manifestations in the lung (Table 7-6). After most exposures, the primary infection is limited by the host's cellular immune system, and the host remains asymptom-

atic, the only evidence of previous limited infection being a positive tuberculin skin test. However, small numbers of mycobacteria can remain potentially viable, and active infection may ensue if cell-mediated immunity is diminished by age, use of corticosteroids, diabetes, ethanolism, or chronic infection. There is a marked increase in tuberculosis among patients with pulmonary silicosis, and establishing the presence of mycobacterial infection in a patient with progressive massive fibrosis due to silicosis can be difficult.

As previously noted, histologic examination can provide an estimation of the adequacy of host immunity. The morphology of giant cells may be an indicator of whether host cell-mediated immunity is adequate in containing tuberculous infection. Before the development of effective cell-mediated immunity, many giant cells in the lesions show nuclei that have aggregated toward one pole of the multikaryon (Fig. 7-58A); after infection is effectively contained, Langhans giant cells with peripheral nuclei or giant cells with centrally placed nuclei predominate (see Fig. 7-58B). If cell-mediated immunity is profoundly diminished, granulomas may be poorly formed or absent.

Failure to contain the primary infection leads to its progression. Primary tuberculosis may show necrotizing pneumonia (Fig. 7-59), regionally involved lymph nodes, and a granulomatous pleuritis with lymphocytic effusion. Dissemination of organ-

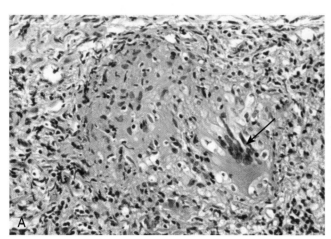
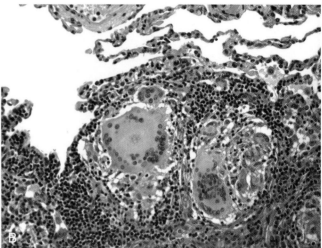

Figure 7-58. A, Polarized giant cells (×400) in early infection with *Mycobacterium tuberculosis (arrow).* These cells may reflect host difficulties in containing the infection. **B,** Mature infection shows Langhans giant cells and giant cells with central nuclei (×400).

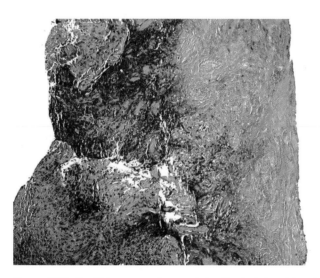

Figure 7-59. Necrotizing pneumonia caused by *Mycobacterium tuberculosis* (×250).

isms via the bloodstream can yield miliary disease, in which innumerable foci of active infection with poorly formed granulomas are seen (Fig. 7-60).[55]

Tuberculous acinar-nodose bronchopneumonia results from mycobacterial infection that extends along the pulmonary acinus (Fig. 7-61). Tuberculomas are defined foci of nodular tuberculous infection (Fig. 7-62). Cavitation of a tuberculoma into an adjacent bronchus can lead to the discharge of numerous bacilli with cough or expectoration (Fig. 7-63A). Although bacillary counts in cavitary lesions are typically high, even large cavities at times fail to show a single identifiable organism by histochemical staining, and the diagnosis must be made presumptively based on histologic appearance and empiric response to anti-tuberculosis medications.[56] The extension of cavitary disease to involve an accompanying pulmonary artery may produce a Rasmussen aneurysm and risk of vascular rupture leading to fatal hemoptysis (see Fig. 7-63B).

Mycobacteria can spread along the mucosal surfaces of the airways to produce ulcerated lesions in the larynx and tracheo-bronchial tree that can mimic Wegener granulomatosis (Fig. 7-64). However, as previously noted, the latter disorder rarely includes well-formed tuberculoid granulomas, and their presence favors the diagnosis of infection.

Reactivation Tuberculosis

Most clinically encountered cases of tuberculosis occurring previously asymptomatic individuals with positive cutaneous responses to purified protein derivative (PPD) represent either reactivation or reinfection. Reactivation indicates an acquired defect in cell-mediated immunity. Tuberculosis tends to reactivate in the upper lobes of the lung, where ventilation/perfusion ratios are high. Histologically, the lung shows necrotizing granulomas in areas of scarring and traction bronchiectasis (Fig. 7-65) resulting from the initial mycobacterial infection. In addition to reactivation of tuberculosis, the differential diagnosis of necrotizing granulomatous inflammation in this setting includes fungal infection and atypical mycobacterial infection, because both have a predilection to develop in areas of old pulmonary apical scarring. The distinction may be difficult in the case of atypical mycobacterial infection, because special stains cannot distinguish these possibilities, and culture or ancillary diagnostic tests are necessary (Fig. 7-66).

Atypical Mycobacteria

A number of mycobacteria that are genetically distinct from *M. tuberculosis* can produce pulmonary infection.[57] These organisms vary in virulence, and this fact is often reflected in the histologic appearance of the infection (Table 7-7). *Mycobacterium-avium intracellulare,* also called *Mycobacterium-avium* complex (MAC), can attack the lung in a variety of clinical settings.[58] Patients immunosuppressed by HIV/AIDS can develop virulent infections with features that mimic tuberculosis. If adaptive T cell-mediated immunity is severely compromised, the host response may be limited to foamy histiocytes that have ingested large numbers of mycobacteria.[59] MAC can be demon-

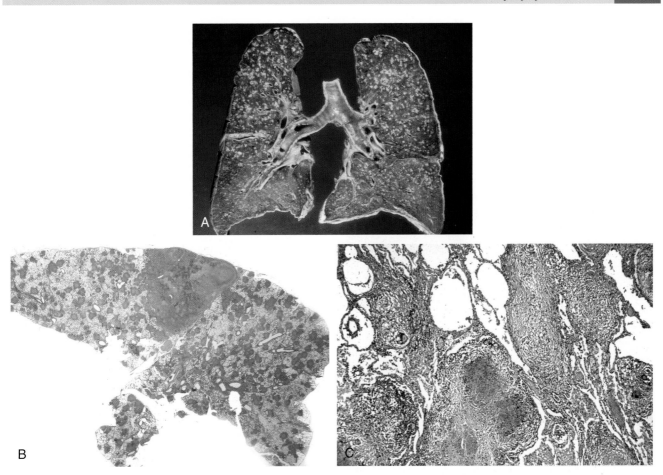

Figure 7-60. **A,** Miliary tuberculosis in lung reflects the failure of the host to contain either primary or reactivation infection. **B,** Innumerable millet-sized nodules are seen in lung with focus of necrotizing pneumonia (×50). **C,** The response in miliary tuberculosis includes poorly formed granulomas. With profound immunodeficiency, granulomatous changes may be absent (×250).

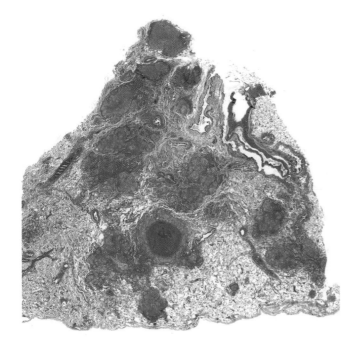

Table 7-7 Classification of Mycobacteria

Group	Species
MTB complex	*Mycobacterium tuberculosis* (MTB)
	Mycobacterium bovis
Runyon Classification	
Group I	*Mycobacterium kansasii*
	Mycobacterium marinum
Group II	*Mycobacterium gordonae*
	Mycobacterium scrofulaceum
Group III	*Mycobacterium intracellulare*
	Mycobacterium avium
	Mycobacterium xenopi
Group IV	*Mycobacterium fortuitum*
	Mycobacterium chelonei
	Mycobacterium abscessus

Figure 7-61. Geographic infiltrates of necrotizing acinar-nodose tuberculosis (×50).

strated by both AFB and PAS stains, and clinical signs of either tuberculosis or MAC disease may be recognized only after treatment with antivirals—the so-called immune reconstitution syndrome.

In the immunocompetent host, MAC tends to affect elderly women (Lady Windermere disease) and patients with bronchiectasis or bullous emphysema. It is commonly seen in the right-middle lobe syndrome caused by bronchiectasis and chronic

atelectasis. The lesions of MAC infection are detected radiographically as "tree-in-bud" opacities, reflecting terminal bronchiolar infection (Fig. 7-67A), together with nodules that may be solid or cavitary. Histologically, the pathology often shows extensive areas of non-necrotizing epithelioid histiocytes and is highly characteristic (see Fig. 7-67B). The causative mycobacteria are indistinguishable from *M. tuberculosis,* and only culture or PCR can accurately establish the diagnosis.

A recently described variant of MAC infection is known as "hot tub lung." The lung shows a microgranulomatous hypersensitivity pneumonitis that may be accompanied by necrotizing granulomatous inflammation. The pathology appears to represent primarily a cell-mediated hypersensitivity response to mycobacterial antigens, with a possible element of direct infection as well (Fig. 7-68).

An unusual presentation of MAC infection in the immunosuppressed host is the pseudosarcomatous nodule.[60] This can

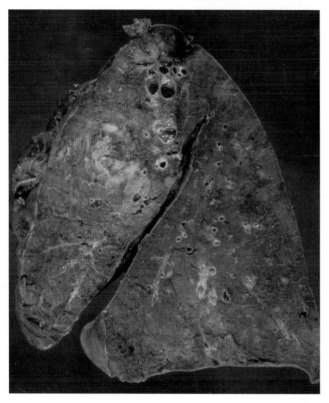

Figure 7-62. Localized tuberculoma.

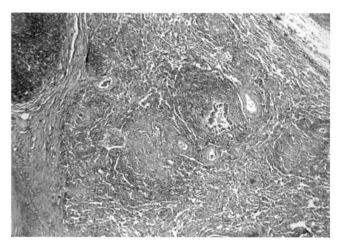

Figure 7-64. Tracheobronchial tuberculosis (×250). These lesions can mimic Wegener's granulomatosis, but the presence of tuberculoid granulomas is a distinguishing diagnostic feature, because they are rarely seen in Wegener's.

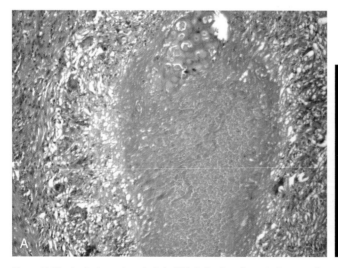

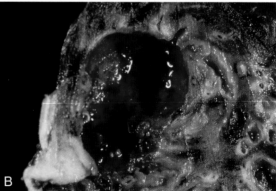

Figure 7-63. A, Cavitary tuberculosis (×400). **B,** Erosion of a cavity into an adjacent pulmonary artery can produce a Rasmussen aneurysm and lead to fatal pulmonary hemorrhage.

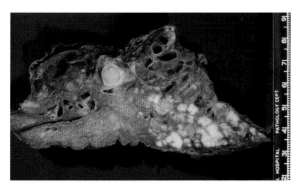

Figure 7-65. Bronchiectasis in tuberculosis.

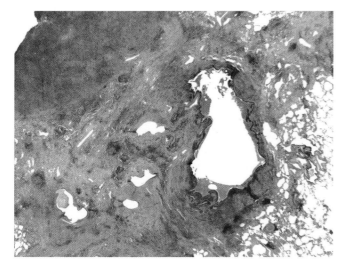

Figure 7-66. Necrotizing granulomas in area of old calcified focus of bronchiectasis were caused by atypical mycobacterial infection (×200).

develop in the lung or in soft tissues and hematopoietic tissues. The nodules are composed of spindle cells and may be mistaken for a low-grade spindle-cell neoplasm (Fig. 7-69A). However, examination reveals the foamy appearance of the spindle cells, which proves to be CD68-positive macrophages containing large numbers of ingested mycobacteria (see Fig. 7-69B), and the absence of mitotic activity. Within the spectrum of unusual mesenchymal reactions seen in the immunocompromised, one must consider inflammatory myofibroblastic tumors that may include foamy histiocytes (Fig. 7-70A) associated with *Human herpesvirus* 8 (HHV-8) infection (see Fig. 7-70B).

Other mycobacteria also cause pulmonary infection. *Mycobacterium kansasii* is a virulent species of atypical mycobacteria that produces necrotizing infection indistinguishable from tuberculosis. The organism often shows a prominent pattern of "cross-linking" on mycobacterial stains in situ that is characteristic but not diagnostic (Fig. 7-71). Other rapidly growing mycobacteria, including *Mycobacterium abscessus,* infect preexisting areas of active bronchiectasis, particularly in cystic fibrosis (Fig. 7-72). *Mycobacterium fortuitum* produces limited infection in patients with diabetes, HIV/AIDS, or chronic upper gastrointestinal disease; and all of the rapid growing nontuberculous mycobacteria, including *Mycobacterium smegmatis,* can complicate pneumonia caused by aspiration of lipid-based substances such as nose drops.[61]

Melioidosis

Rarely seen outside of Southeast Asia where it is endemic, chronic infections due to *Pseudomonas pseudomallei* developed in veterans of the Vietnam War many years after they had left the region.[62] Acute melioidosis is a systemic infection that produces widespread coalescent microabscesses; it may resolve without being recognized, only to recur many years later in lung, lymph nodes, and bone. The lung shows necrotizing granulomatous lesions surrounded by a zone of fibrosis (Fig. 7-73), and regional lymph nodes show stellate necrosis that can mimic that of so-called cat-scratch disease (*Bartonella henselae*). The offending

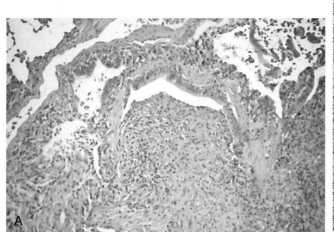

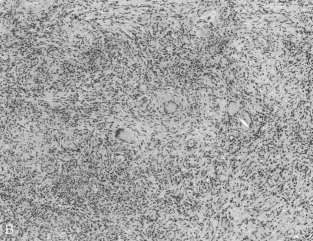

Figure 7-67. A, Non-necrotizing granulomatous inflammation ulcerates a small airway in a patient with *Mycobacterium avium* complex infection (×200). **B,** Sheets of epithelioid histiocytes are characteristically seen in MAC infection in nonimmunosuppressed patients with chronic airways disease (×200).

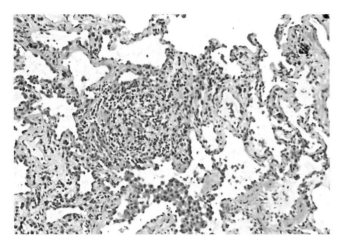

Figure 7-68. Micronodular granulomatous inflammation in "hot tub lung," a hypersensitivity reaction to *Mycobacterium avium* complex (×250).

organism is a gram-negative, motile bacillus that shows bipolar staining that can be difficult to demonstrate in situ.

Fungal Infection Due to Yeasts

Fungi produce a spectrum of changes in the lung, ranging from benign colonization of airways to malignant angioinvasive infections. Some fungi grow as yeast at body temperatures, whereas others are hyphate molds (Table 7-8). Most fungal yeasts are soil organisms that are topographically distributed in the United States. Whereas *Histoplasma capsulatum* may be encountered virtually anywhere that soil and water coexist, most cases in this country are endemic to the Mississippi and Ohio River valleys. *Blastomyces dermatitidis* predominantly affects individuals living in the Great Lakes region and in the southeastern United States, whereas *Coccidioides immitis* is primarily encountered in the San Joaquin

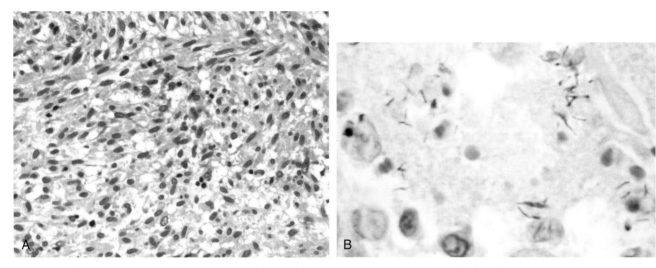

Figure 7-69. A, A pseudosarcomatous nodule in a patient with HIV/AIDS, caused by *Mycobacterium avium* complex (×400). **B,** Large numbers of AFB/PAS-positive mycobacteria are generally seen in this response (×1000).

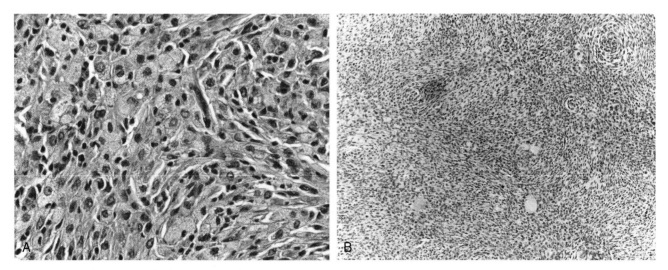

Figure 7-70. A, Inflammatory myofibroblastic tumor with foamy histiocytes; associated with *Human herpesvirus 8* infection (×400). **(B)** in a patient with AIDS, can mimic *Mycobacterium avium* complex infection (×200).

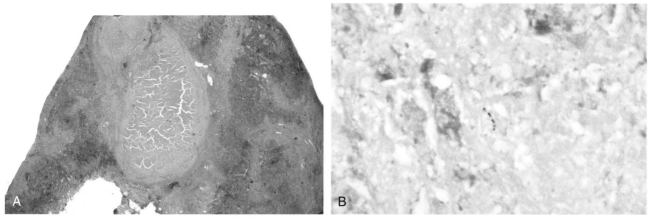

Figure 7-71. A, *Mycobacterium kansasii* is a virulent organism that produces necrotizing granulomatous inflammation comparable to *M. tuberculosis* (×100). **B,** The elongate bacilli exhibit irregularity in their uptake of AFB stain, producing a characteristic pattern of "cross-linking" (×600).

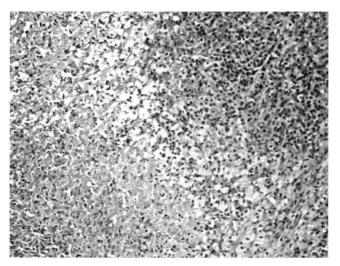

Figure 7-72. *Mycobacterium abscessus* complicates areas of bronchiectasis and may be exceedingly difficult to eradicate fully with antimycobacterial agents (×250).

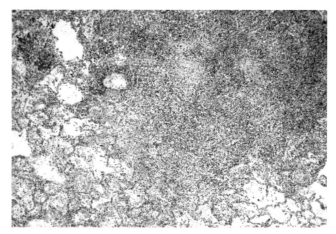

Figure 7-73. *Pseudomonas pseudomallei*, the cause of melioidosis, may reactivate many years after initial exposure to produce a necrotizing granulomatous pneumonia that resembles tuberculosis (×200).

Valley of the Southwest. But despite their usual distribution, modern air travel and a highly mobile population have resulted in the possibility of encountering these infections almost anywhere, and pathologists must be acquainted with their characteristic histologic appearances. However, it is always prudent to inquire into possible travel before diagnosing an exotic fungal infection, because substantial overlap can exist in fungal morphologies.

Histoplasmosis

Primary *Histoplasma* infection produces a viral-like illness that typically resolves spontaneously.[63] However, if there is a defect in cell-mediated immunity, or if the yeast burden is large, progression of infection may ensue.[64] Chronic histoplasmosis tends to develop in the lung apices in areas of bullous emphysema or bronchiectasis. Although most yeasts can be identified in H&E-stained sections, *Histoplasma* spp. require special histochemical staining due to their small size. GMS is the stain of choice, because PAS at times fails to decorate the yeast.

Necrotizing granulomas caused by *Histoplasma* spp. show central necrosis often surrounded by regions of mummefactive necrosis in which the "ghost outlines" of the underlying framework of the lung can still be distinguished in H&E- and reticulin-stained sections (Fig. 7-74A, B). The lining of the necrotic granuloma includes epithelioid histiocytes and giant cells, but, unlike tuberculosis, does not show extensive tubercle granuloma formation, and the wall of the lesion characteristically exhibits paucicellular hyalinized fibrosis (Fig. 7-75).

Although they are facultative intracellular pathogens, *Histoplasma* spp. cluster in areas of necrosis and are often seen outside of histiocytes.[65] The 2- to 4-μm yeast forms are teardrop-shaped and reproduce by single narrow-neck buds whose presence is diagnostic. Despite their name, no capsule is present (Fig. 7-76A). At times, pseudohyphae may be seen, and this should not dissuade the pathologist from making the correct diagnosis (see Fig. 7-76B) if all other diagnostic criteria are met. The differential diagnosis includes microforms of *Cryptococcus* or *Blastomyces*, *P. jiroveci*, and *Candida glabrata*. The presence of larger yeast forms eliminates the possibility of *H. capsulatum*

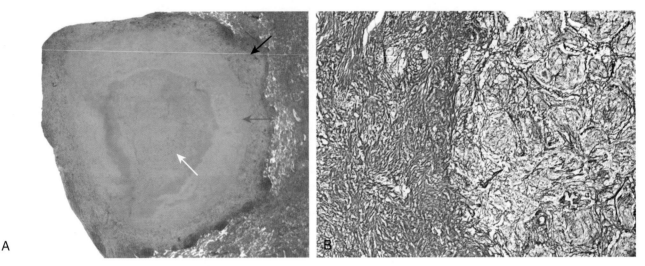

Figure 7-74. A, Nodular pneumonia due to *Histoplasma capsulatum* (×100) often shows necrotizing granulomatous inflammation with three zones. The outer capsule *(black arrow)* encloses an area of mummefactive necrosis *(red arrow)*, which in turn surrounds an area of caseating necrosis *(white arrow)*. **B,** Findings confirmed by reticulin stains (×250).

Table 7-8 Fungal Identification in Tissue

Organism	Size (Width, μm)	Defining Morphologic Characteristics
Histoplasma capsulatum	2-5	Narrow-neck bud
Cryptococcus neoformans	5-20	Narrow-neck bud
Blastomyces dermatitidis	15-30	Broad-based bud
Candida glabrata	3-5	Budding, no pseudohyphae
Candida spp.	2-3	Yeast, pseudohyphae, hyphae
Aspergillus spp.	3-5	Acute-angle branching, septate, conidial head
Zygomycetes	5-8	Right-angle branching, ribbons, pauciseptate
Pseudallescheria spp.	3-4	Acute-angle branching, septate, terminal chlamydospore, pigmented conidia
Fusarium spp.	4-5	Acute- and right-angle branching, septate, narrowed branch points
Coccidioides immitis	20-200	Endosporulation

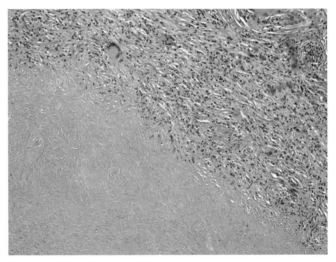

Figure 7-75. The wall of the necrotizing granuloma shows poorly formed granulomas and giant cells with a highly characteristic hyalinized basket-weave fibrosis (×250).

infection. *P. jiroveci* shows irregularly shaped cysts with pericapsular accentuation on GMS stain, and the organisms do not bud; *C. glabrata* can closely mimic the infection in GMS-stained sections, but, unlike *Histoplasma*, they also stain amphophilic with H&E and are strongly gram positive (Fig. 7-77A, B).

However, the most common and greatest difficulties in diagnosis arise in distinguishing small, regular microcalcifications in GMS-stained sections, because they can closely resemble degenerate yeast (Fig. 7-78). The presence of irregular calci-

fications is a clue to their actual nature, but ultrastructural examination may be required to exclude infection. In the immunosuppressed host, disseminated infection is primarily distributed within interstitial and alveolar macrophages (Fig. 7-79).[66]

Extension of infection from a peribronchial lymph node can produce mediastinal granuloma, a lesion characterized by dense, whorled hyaline fibrosis with aggregates of plasma cells (Fig. 7-80A). Organisms are rarely identified in the areas of paucicellular scarring, and this form of the disease appears to be immunologically mediated. At times, necrotizing granulomatous inflammation is concomitantly present and confirms the diagnosis (see Fig. 7-80B). The lesion can entrap the large vessels of the mediastinum, leading to the superior vena caval syndrome and death. Surgical excision is required but may not always be technically possible.

Remotely infected, calcified peribronchial lymph nodes caused by histoplasmosis can erode into adjacent airways to be

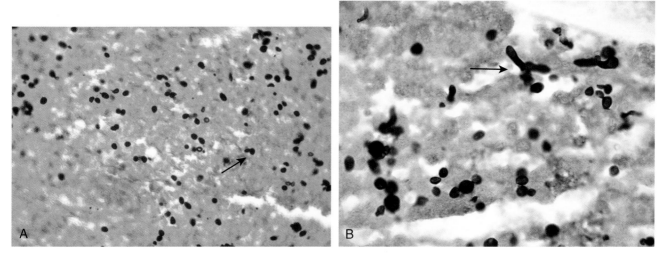

Figure 7-76. A, Narrow-necked budding *(arrow)* in 2- to 4-μm yeast of *Histoplasma capsulatum* in GMS-stained section (×400). PAS is not reliable for demonstrating this yeast. **B,** *H. capsulatum* infection with irregular yeast forms (×600) and pseudohyphae *(arrow).*

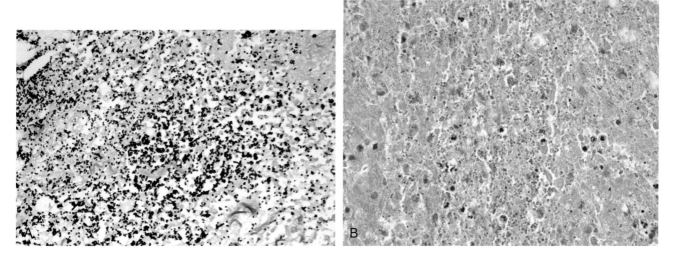

Figure 7-77. A, *Candida glabrata* can easily be mistaken for *Histoplasma capsulatum* on GMS stain (×200). **B,** The yeast are amphophilic in H&E-stained sections and are easily differentiated on this basis (×200).

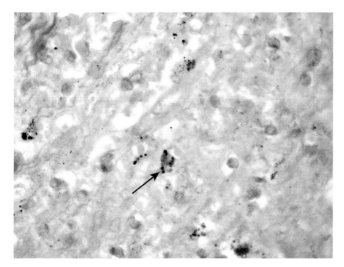

Figure 7-78. Microcalcifications *(arrow)* can closely resemble *Histoplasma capsulatum.* At times, ultrastructural examination may be required to exclude infection (×400).

either expectorated or aspirated as broncholiths. Surprisingly, these may show persistently viable yeast forms and colonization by aspirated oropharyngeal bacteria (Fig. 7-81).

Old, calcified granulomas are commonly encountered in surgical resection of lungs for neoplasia.[67] Most of these are the result of healed tuberculosis or histoplasmosis, depending on exposure. In most cases, no organism is identified, but occasionally nonviable degenerate *Histoplasma* organisms may be seen, although distinguishing them with confidence from microcalcifications can be difficult, and a high threshold of suspicion for the diagnosis of histoplasmosis should be maintained in this setting.

Blastomyces

B. dermatitidis shows a propensity to infect lung, skin, and bone.[68] The spectrum of pulmonary presentations includes consolidative pneumonia, DAD, and pulmonary nodules that radiographically may mimic pulmonary carcinoma (Fig. 7-82). The

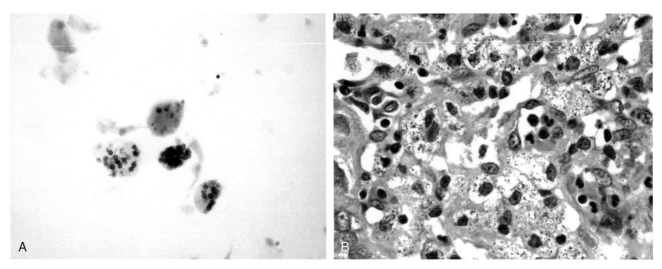

Figure 7-79. A, Intracytoplasmic *Histoplasma capsulatum* in macrophages in bronchoalveolar lavage sample from a patient with disseminated infection and HIV/AIDS (×400). **B,** Debris within macrophage phagolysosomes can resemble intracellular yeast (×400).

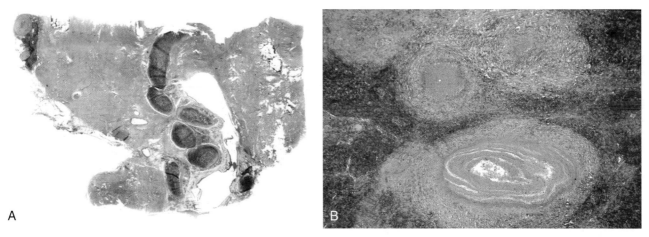

Figure 7-80. A, Mediastinal granuloma is a serious complication of pulmonary histoplasmosis. The mediastinum shows paucicellular hyaline scarring (×100). **B,** It also may include foci of necrotizing granulomatous infection (×200).

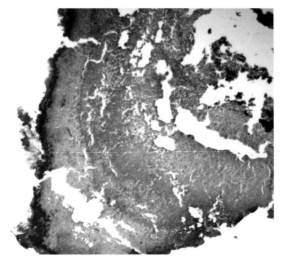

Figure 7-81. Expectorated broncholith from a patient with histoplasmosis (×150).

Figure 7-82. Pulmonary nodule excised as carcinoma due to blastomycosis.

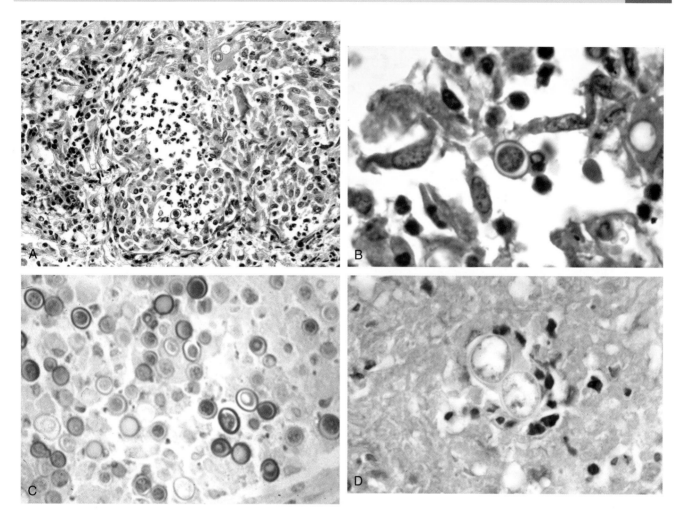

Figure 7-83. A, Granulohistiocytic response to *Blastomyces dermatitidis* (×250). **B,** Yeast of *B. dermatitidis* with refractile cell wall (×600). **C,** *B. dermatitidis* with multinucleation (×1000). **D,** *B. dermatitidis* showing broad-based budding (×600).

pulmonary lesion characteristically shows a granulohistiocytic response (Fig. 7-83A). The yeast are large (15-30 μm) and are easily identified in H&E-stained sections, where they are distinguished by their thick, refractile cell wall (see Fig. 7-83B). The organism is also multinucleate (see Fig. 7-83C) and proliferates via single broad-based budding (see Fig. 7-83D). Microforms may be present and should not be confused with coinfection by *H. capsulatum*.[69] Giant yeast forms can also occur and may be confused with *C. immitis*.[70]

Cryptococcus

Cryptococcus neoformans infects immunocompromised patients but can also be seen in apparently normal hosts.[71] Meningoencephalitis is the most common clinical presentation, and it represents a complication of subclinical pulmonary infection. *C. neoformans* can produce localized necrotizing cryptococcomas (Fig. 7-84A), confluent bronchopneumonia (see Fig. 7-84B), granulomatous pneumonia (see Fig. 7-84D), or a null response characterized by "yeast lakes" with minimal inflammation (see Fig. 7-84E). Grossly, the infected lesions are glistening and "slimy."

The organism shows substantial variability in size (2-15 μm) and in shape (Fig. 7-85A), and innumerable microforms can occasionally be seen that must be distinguished from histoplasmosis (see Fig. 7-85B). The yeast proliferate via single narrow-necked buds; they secrete a capsule that is optimally visualized with mucicarmine in situ (Fig. 7-86A). With GMS, the yeast body stains gray-black, and the capsule is not decorated (see Fig. 7-86C). In capsule-deficient organisms, the Fontana-Masson stain reacts with a melanin precursor in the yeast wall, highlighting the organisms (Fig. 7-87A), although a careful examination of the mucicarmine stain invariably reveals a poorly developed rim of capsular staining (see Fig. 7-87B).[72]

Coccidioides immitis

Generally affecting patients from the southwestern United States, *C. immitis* is distinct from other yeast by virtue of its size (20-200 μm) and its endosporulating mode of reproduction.[73] *C. immitis* produces a spectrum of changes that includes fibrocaseous granulomas (Fig. 7-88), granulomatous pneumonia, and miliary disease, often accompanied by tissue eosinophilia. The endospores are contained within a spherular capsule, and both

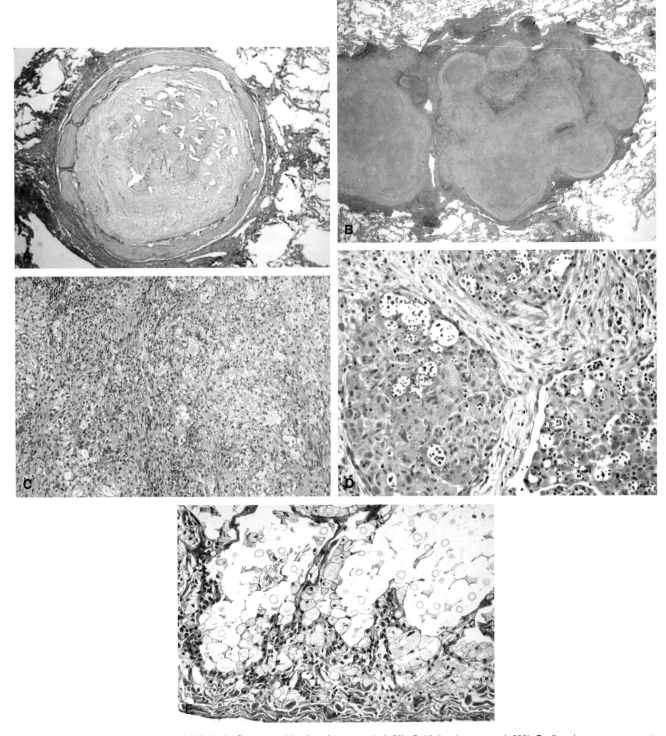

Figure 7-84. A, Nodular cryptococcoma (×50). **B,** Confluent necrotizing bronchopneumonia (×50). **C,** Histiocytic response (×250). **D,** Granulomatous response to *Cryptococcus neoformans* (×400). **E,** Yeast lake (×400).

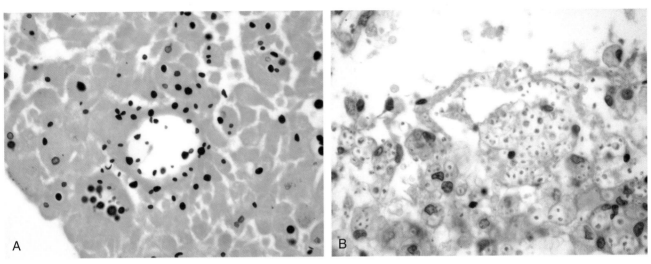

Figure 7-85. A, Narrow-necked budding of *Cryptococcus neoformans* showing variability in size and shape. Microforms of *C. neoformans* within histiocytes (×400). **(B)** must be distinguished from intracellular *Histoplasma capsulatum* (×400).

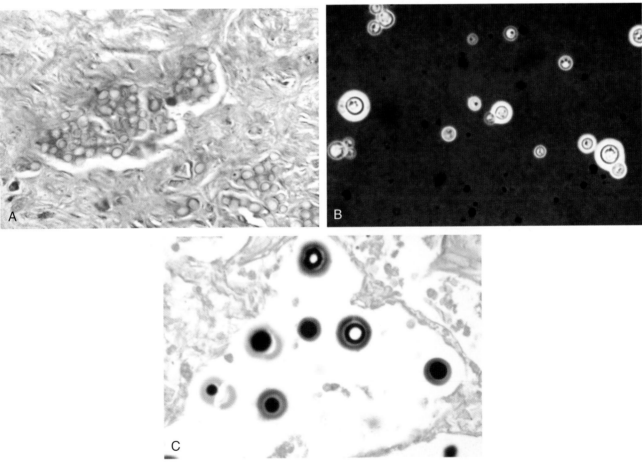

Figure 7-86. A, Mucicarmine stains capsule of *Cryptococcus neoformans* (×600). **B,** India ink preparation shows capsule of yeast. Both GMS **(C)** and PAS stain the body of yeast but not its capsule (×1000).

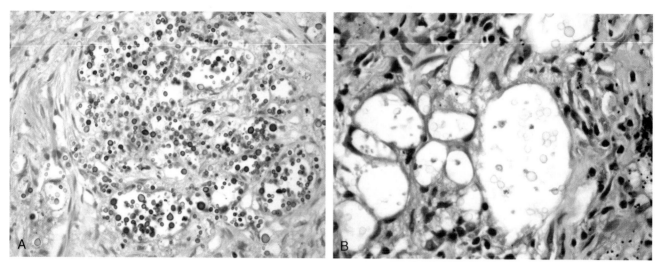

Figure 7-87. A, "Capsule-deficient" organisms stain with Fontana-Masson stain (×400). **B,** "Capsule-deficient" yeasts invariably show a faint rim of mucicarminophilic staining (×400).

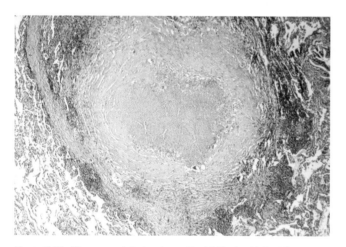

Figure 7-88. Fibrocaseous infection due to *Coccidioides immitis* (×150).

stain well with GMS (Fig. 7-89A), whereas spherules are variably stained by PAS. The cysts of *C. immitis* have a characteristic tendency to collapse after having discharged their endospores in situ (see Fig. 7-89B).

In endemic areas, *C. immitis* can form fungus balls within preexisting pulmonary cavities (Fig. 7-90A). The organism is dimorphic, and the presence of the infective hyphal arthroconidia should not be confused with a concomitant mold infection (see Fig. 7-90B).[74]

Paracoccidioides

Paracoccidioides brasiliensis infection is endemic in South America, where it produces a range of pulmonary findings comparable to those of blastomycosis; but cases are rare in the United States. The organism is large (10-60 µm) and replicates by multiple narrow-necked buds which produce a "ship's wheel" appearance that is pathognomonic (Fig. 7-91).[75] However, if this feature is absent, the infection can be confused with other fungi.

Candida

Superficial colonization of the upper airways by *Candida* spp. is common in patients treated with inhaled corticosteroids and in chronically ill and diabetic patients (Fig. 7-92). Foci of aspiration pneumonia and abscess cavities may show colonization, but deep pulmonary infection is rarely seen in the absence of fungemia (Fig. 7-93A, B).[76]

Candida can have a pleomorphic morphology that includes yeast (blastoconidia), pseudohyphae, and true hyphae, although in some cases only yeast forms may be present.[77] The organisms can be highlighted by either GMS or PAS, and they are strongly gram positive (Fig. 7-94A) At times, blastoconidia of *Candida* spp. can be large and mimic other fungal infections (see Fig. 7-94B). *C. glabrata* (*Torula glabrata*) shows multiple, 2- to 5-µm, budding yeast that are amphophilic in H&E-stained sections; they are distinct from other *Candida* species, because pseudohyphae and hyphae are never present.[78]

Hyphate Fungi

Hyphate fungi ("molds") are responsible for pulmonary disorders ranging from colonization of pulmonary airways to angio-invasive, life-threatening infections. *Aspergillus* spp. account for the majority of pulmonary mold infections, but other organisms, including the zygomycetes, *Pseudallescheria*, and *Fusarium*, also produce pulmonary disease.

Aspergillus

The hyphae of *Aspergillus* spp. range in diameter from 2.5 to 4.5 µm and show frequent septation. *Aspergillus* spp. branch progressively, primarily at acute angles of approximately 45 degrees, mimicking an arborizing tree branch (Fig. 7-95A); when cut in cross-section, however, they may be mistaken for yeast, although the absence of budding suggests the correct diagnosis. In areas of mycelial growth, organisms become tangled, bulbous, and distorted, and it may be impossible to confirm the diagnosis with accuracy based on morphology (see Fig. 7-95B).

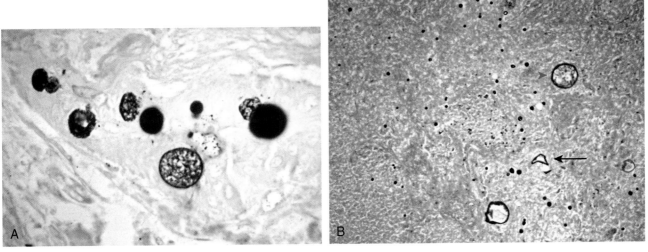

Figure 7-89. A, Endospores are variably present within PAS-positive cysts (×600). **B,** Cysts (*arrow*) of *Coccidioides immitis* have a characteristic tendency to collapse after discharging their contents (×400).

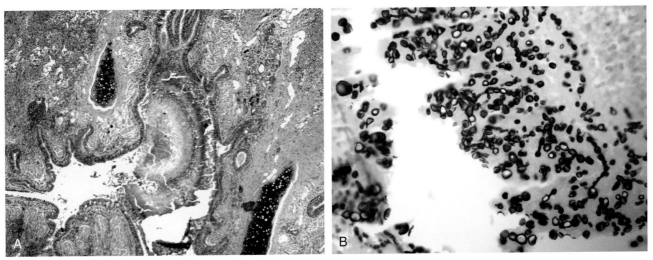

Figure 7-90. A, Fungus ball due to *Coccidioides immitis* (×150). **B,** Yeast and arthroconidia must not be confused with a concomitant mold infection (×400).

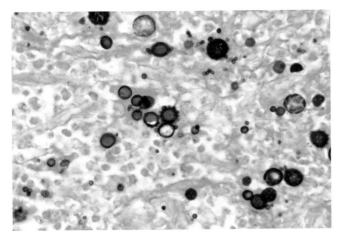

Figure 7-91. *Paracoccidioides brasiliensis* (×600) shows multiple narrow buds that resemble a ship's wheel, but this diagnostic feature is not always present.

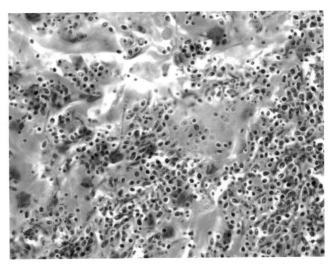

Figure 7-92. Dense colonization of airway with *Candida albicans* in intubated patient (×400).

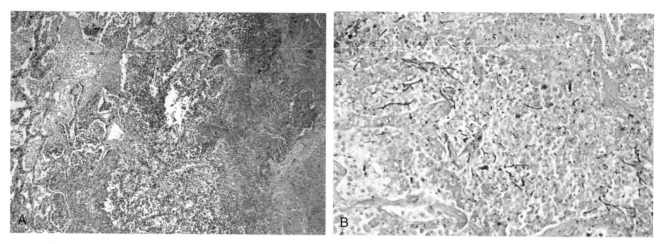

Figure 7-93. A, Sample from the same patient as in Figure 7-92 shows necrotizing pneumonia due to *Candida albicans* (×250). **B,** PAS stain highlights the organism (×400).

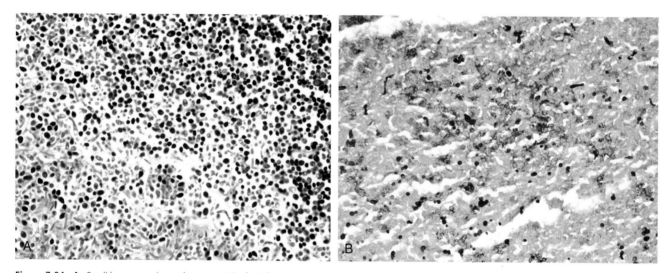

Figure 7-94. A, Candida yeast are intensely gram positive (×400). **B,** Large yeast and pseudohyphae proved to be *Candida tropicalis* (×400).

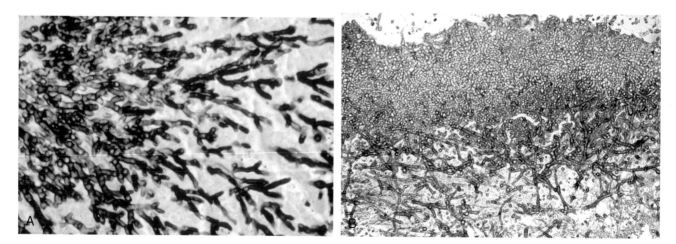

Figure 7-95. A, *Aspergillus* spp. characteristically branch dichotomously and progressively at acute angles (×600). **B,** Tangled and distorted mycelial growth. It is impossible to speciate fungi based on this morphology (×400).

The aspergil, a ritual implement used in the Roman Catholic mass, resembles the fruiting body of *Aspergillus* and gives the fungus its name (Fig. 7-96). Fruiting bodies develop from mycelia in areas of high oxygen tension, such as lung or sinus cavities, but do not develop in tissues. They are composed of a vesicle with one or two layers of phialides that produce the infective conidial spores, and the morphology of the fruiting body allows for accurate speciation in situ. In general, the specific diagnosis of "aspergillosis" should be avoided unless the aspergil is identified, because other fungi can be morphologically almost indistinguishable in tissue. Diagnoses are therefore optimally phrased as "acute-angle branching hyphae consistent with aspergillus."

Immune Disorders Due to *Aspergillus* Infection
Aspergillus spp. give rise to a spectrum of disorders, some reflecting hypersensitivity responses to the organisms, and others as the consequence of invasive infection (Fig. 7-97). Distinguishing among these disorders is critical for proper management.

Allergic Bronchopulmonary Aspergillosis
Allergic bronchopulmonary aspergillosis (ABPA) shows a range of findings, including intractable asthma, proximal bronchiectasis,[79] and peripheral blood eosinophilia. It is not certain whether the fungus plays an opportunistic role in exacerbating an atopic response or is primary in its pathogenesis.[80] Patients develop intractable bronchospasm, with elevated serum IgE levels specific for *Aspergillus* spp. The pathology includes central cystic bronchiectasis with mucoid impaction (Fig. 7-98A). The impacted mucus is viscid and forms a cast of the airways, a disorder termed plastic bronchitis. Microscopically, the mucus plugs show layers of degenerating eosinophils interspersed within the mucin (see Fig. 7-98B), and the surrounding lung may show patchy eosinophilic pneumonia. The fragmented fungal hyphae can at times be difficult to identify (see Fig. 7-98C), so silver stains should be applied routinely in the evaluation of allergic mucus plugs. Whereas the clinical and histologic features of this disorder are most frequently caused by hypersensitivity to *Aspergillus* spp., other fungi, such as *Candida* spp., can yield a comparable syndrome. A subset of patients with cystic fibrosis develop concomitant ABPA, and establishing the diagnosis in this setting can be difficult.[37]

Bronchocentric Granulomatosis
Bronchocentric granulomatosis appears to reflect an abnormal cell-mediated response to *Aspergillus* spp. or, less commonly, other fungi (e.g., *Candida* spp., and *C. immitis*), in which small-

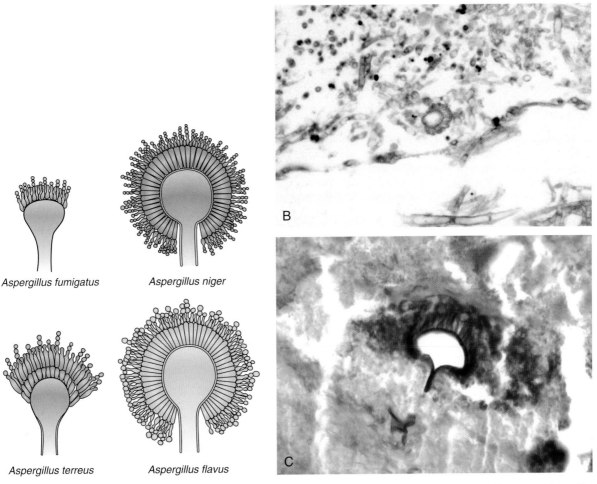

Aspergillus fumigatus

Aspergillus niger

Aspergillus terreus

Aspergillus flavus

Figure 7-96. A, Morphology of aspergil fruiting body. **B,** Gram stain shows fruiting body of *Aspergillus fumigatus* with innumerable gram-positive conidia (×250). **C,** *Aspergillus niger* with innumerable pigmented conidia (×600).

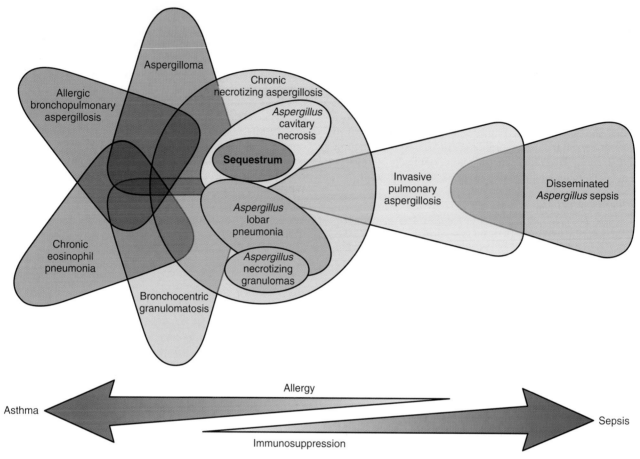

Figure 7-97. Spectrum of disease caused by *Aspergillus* spp.

caliber airways develop circumferential granulomatous inflammation, loss of the normal lining respiratory epithelium, and impaction of the airway lumen by granular basophilic mucin admixed with cellular debris (Fig. 7-99). The disorder may be first noted radiographically as isolated or multiple airway-centered nodules.[81] Bronchocentric granulomatosis may be seen as part of the spectrum of findings in ABPA or as an isolated disorder. As in ABPA, fragmented hyphae may be difficult to identify, and surrounding areas of eosinophilic pneumonitis are common. If the disease is suspected clinically, it can be treated noninvasively with corticosteroids; however, definitive resection may be undertaken to exclude neoplasia.

Hypersensitivity Pneumonitis
Hypersensitivity pneumonitis reflects a combined abnormality of humoral and cell-mediated immunologic responses to organic antigens. Most cases are caused by thermophilic actinomycetes, but hypersensitivity to *Aspergillus* spp. is well documented. Upper lobe predominance is the rule, and this can be a helpful feature in establishing the diagnosis.

The diagnosis of hypersensitivity pneumonitis is based primarily on establishing an historical link between antigen exposures and the clinical findings, but lung biopsies can establish the diagnosis. Microscopically, the lung shows bronchiolocentric lymphohistiocytic interstitial infiltrates with poorly formed microgranulomas (Fig. 7-100) and giant cells that may contain

birefringent crystals and cholesterol crystals. Whereas CD8-positive lymphocytes characteristically predominate in BAL fluid specimens, immunostains reveal dominance of either CD4- or CD8-positive lymphocytes in situ. In addition, other histopathologies, including nonspecific cellular interstitial pneumonitis (NSIP), organizing pneumonia, lymphoid interstitial pneumonitis (LIP), and non-necrotizing granulomatous inflammation resembling sarcoidosis, can be caused by hypersensitivity pneumonitis. The presence of interstitial and alveolar eosinophils is characteristically seen in hypersensitivity pneumonitis due to *Aspergillus* antigens and is less common in response to other antigens.

Aspergillus *Bronchitis and Chronic Necrotizing Aspergillosis*
The presence of primary airway infection by *Aspergillus* spp. is a poorly recognized entity. It is usually seen in the setting of modest immunosuppression accompanying disorders such as diabetes mellitus or the use of aerosolized steroids in asthmatics. In some cases, it is a precursor lesion for invasive disease. Fungal hyphae can be seen filling the lumen of airways (Fig. 7-101A), without evidence of frank tissue invasion. Elastic stains are helpful in determining whether organisms have begun to transgress normal tissue barriers (see Fig. 7-101B). Centrally necrotic lesions (Fig. 7-102A) of chronic necrotizing aspergillosis can resemble those caused by mycobacteria or other fungi (see Fig. 7-102B).

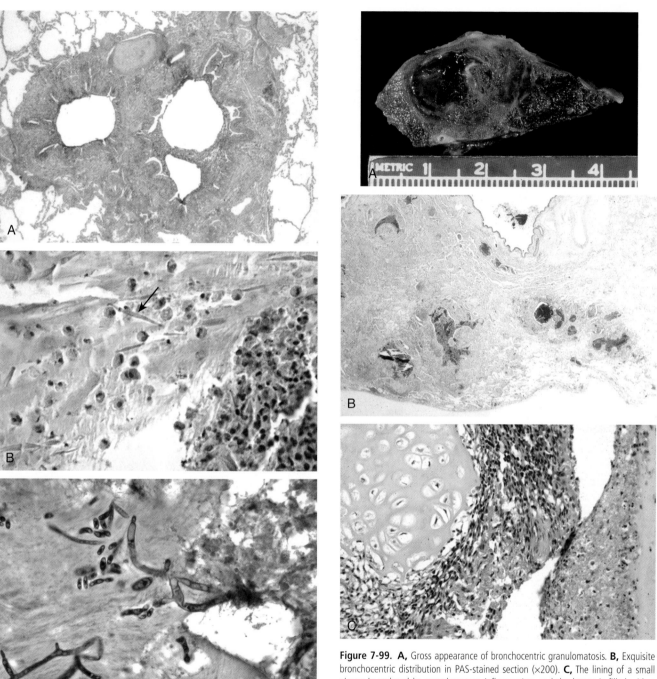

Figure 7-98. A, Central bronchiectasis with dense peribronchiolar scarring in patient with allergic bronchopulmonary aspergillosis (×100). **B,** Expectorated "allergic" mucus plug with eosinophils and Charcot-Leyden crystals (×400). **C,** *Aspergillus* hyphae in mucus plug (×600).

Figure 7-99. A, Gross appearance of bronchocentric granulomatosis. **B,** Exquisite bronchocentric distribution in PAS-stained section (×200). **C,** The lining of a small airway is replaced by granulomatous inflammation, and the lumen is filled with a granular basophilic exudate (×400).

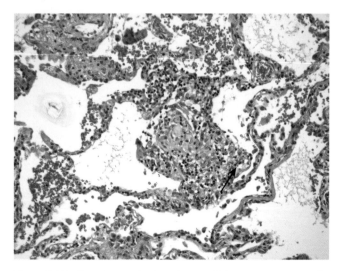

Figure 7-100. The microgranulomatous hypersensitivity response to *Aspergillus* often includes tissue eosinophils (×200).

Fungus Balls

The colonization of old fibrocavitary disease (e.g., areas of bronchiectasis due to healed tuberculosis or sarcoidosis, emphysematous bullae) by *Aspergillus* is the most common cause of a pulmonary fungus ball (Fig. 7-103A,B).[82] The term *mycetoma* should not be applied to intracavitary fungal mycelial growth, because it accurately applies only to soft tissue infections. Patients may be asymptomatic, or they may present with episodes of hemoptysis, at times massive and requiring emergent bronchial arterial embolization or definitive resection.

The morphology of the hyphae in a fungus ball is frequently distorted, and it can be impossible to identify the diagnostic septate, acute-angle branching forms. *Aspergillus* fungus balls show heterogeneous staining intensity on H&E stain (see Fig. 7-103C), giving the impression of alternating zones of growth. The wall of the fungus ball frequently shows increased numbers of tissue eosinophils (see Fig. 7-103D). The Splendore-Hoeppli phenomenon is often present and is reassuring evidence that angioinvasion is unlikely, unless there has been a recent super-

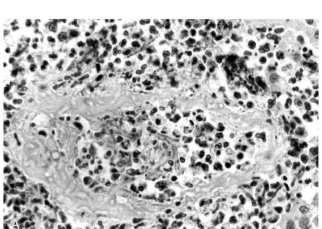

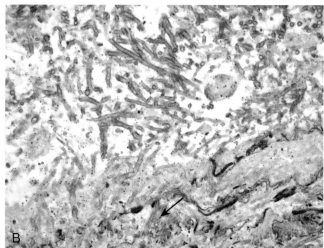

Figure 7-101. **A,** *Aspergillus* bronchitis/bronchiolitis is a precursor to invasive disease (×400). **B,** Elastic stains (×600) can determine whether tissue invasion has occurred *(arrow)*.

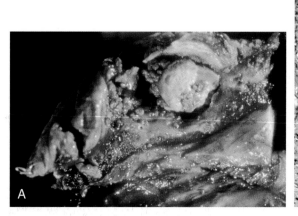

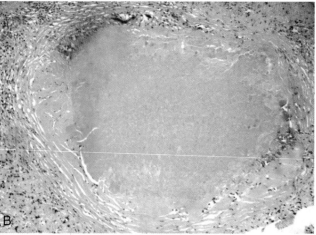

Figure 7-102. **A,** Necrotizing lesions due to *Aspergillus*. **B,** These lesions can resemble mycobacterial or yeast infection (×200).

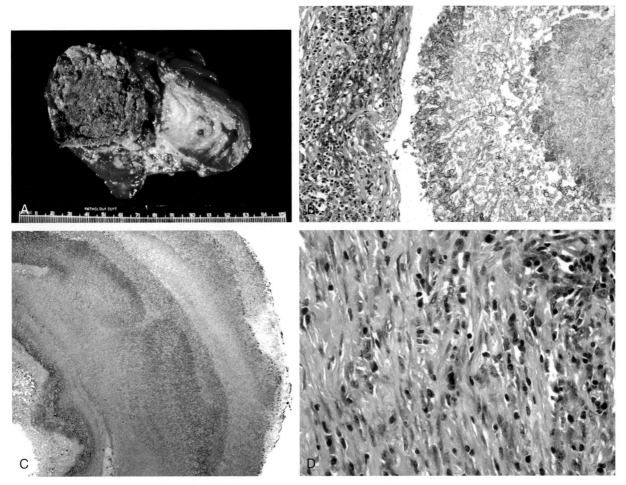

Figure 7-103. A, Fungus ball growing in an old bronchiectatic cavity resulting from sarcoidosis. **B,** Histology shows tangled mass of hyphae and the Splendore-Hoeppli phenomenon (×250). **C,** Fungus balls often show alternating "zones" of staining intensity with H&E (and GMS) stain (×250). **D,** Fungus balls frequently contain eosinophils in their wall (×400).

vening cause of immunosuppression or neutropenia. The walls of the cavity are lined with granulation tissue, granulomatous inflammation, or metaplastic squamous epithelium, depending on the activity of the disease. The occasional presence of germinative fruiting bodies of *Aspergillus* spp. with characteristic phialides and conidial forms allows definitive speciation.

One may rarely see rapid expansion of a cavity due to vascular thrombosis induced by calcium oxalate crystal deposition, a disorder termed chronic pulmonary oxalosis.[83] Oxalic acid is produced by a variety of *Aspergillus* spp. but is most commonly a feature of *Aspergillus niger* infection (Fig. 7-104A). Diffusion of oxalate into surrounding blood vessels is prothrombotic and can lead to extensive ischemic necrosis (see Fig. 7-104B, C). Oxalate crystal deposition in the renal tubules may also be seen. Emergency resection of the fungus ball is the only effective treatment.

Angioinvasive Aspergillosis
This life-threatening infection is seen in patients who have been chronically immunosuppressed or neutropenic. It is a complication of bone marrow or solid organ transplantation and of antileukemic chemotherapies. Angioinvasive aspergillosis is an uncommon complication of HIV/AIDS, despite the associated

profound immune deficiency. Grossly, the lung shows targetoid lesions with central thrombosed vessels secondary to angioinvasion, surrounded by a rim of consolidated lung, confluent bronchopneumonia, or lobar consolidation (Fig. 7-105A); microscopically, a necrotizing pneumonia (see Fig. 7-105B), at times featuring giant cells (see Fig. 7-105C), may be present.[84] Angioinvasion is identified microscopically and may be enhanced with silver and elastic stains (Fig. 7-106). Rarely, foci of infarcted lung can produce an infected, nonviable pulmonary sequestrum (Fig. 7-107).

The fungal hyphae tend to invade blood vessels and to "metastasize" to other organs. The presence of sunburst vasculocentric hyphal growth is diagnostic of a metastatic focus of infection (Fig. 7-108), and virtually any organ can be secondarily involved. Circulating *Aspergillus* spp. can also seed abnormal cardiac valves to produce endocarditis, with fatal embolic hemorrhagic infarctions to brain and other vital organs.

Other Aspergillus *Species*
Aspergillus terreus is an opportunistic fungus that infects patients with chronic granulomatous disease, as well as other immunocompromised hosts.[84] Its hyphae are pyriform with orthogonal

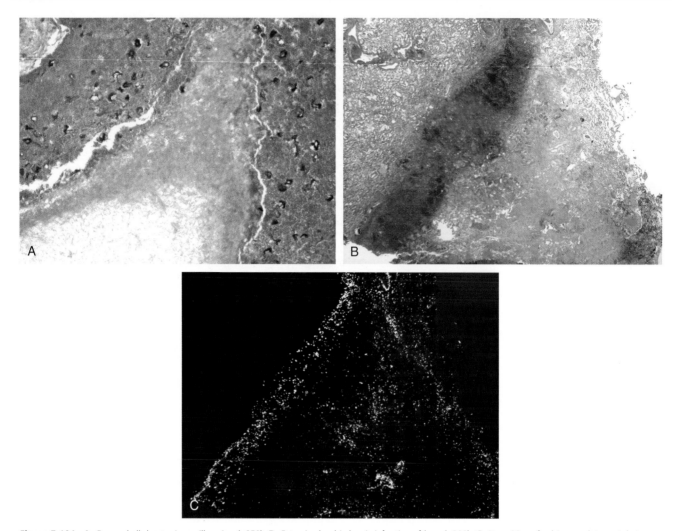

Figure 7-104. A, Fungus ball due to *Aspergillus niger* (×250). **B,** Extensive local ischemic infarction of lung (×200). **C,** Deposition of calcium oxalate crystals is seen with polarized light (×200).

branches (Fig. 7-109). Fungus balls produced by *Aspergillus nidulans* have a propensity to produce pale-staining, enlarged fungal forms or Hulle cells, that show Maltese-cross birefringence when examined under polarized light (Fig. 7-110).[85]

Other Hyphate Fungi

Although the majority of acute-angle branching septate hyphae encountered in medical practice prove to be *Aspergillus* spp., exceptions do occur and can be difficult to distinguish in situ. Organisms that closely mimic *Aspergillus* include the zygomycetes, *Pseudallescheria boydii (Scedosporium)*, and *Fusarium* spp. Pulmonary infection with zygomycetes is caused by organisms of the order Mucorales, including *Mucor, Rhizopus, Absidia, Rhizomucor,* and *Apophysomyces*.[86] Infection generally occurs in immunosuppressed hosts and in patients with diabetic ketoacidosis or disorders of iron metabolism. Because treatment invariably includes surgical resection, establishing an accurate diagnosis is critical.

The histologic responses to infection are comparable to those produced by angioinvasive aspergillosis. The hyphae of the zygomycetes are broad (5-25 μm), pauciseptate, and tend to branch at right angles (Fig. 7-111A), although acute-angle

branching does occur, and its presence should not dissuade one from the correct diagnosis. The hyphae of the zygomycetes are well stained by hematoxylin, and they have a proclivity to produce ribbon-like structures (see Fig. 7-111B), but caution in diagnosis is required, because treated *Aspergillus* can assume this appearance as well. The fungus rapidly invades vessels, perineural lymphatics, and cartilage and tends not to respect tissue boundaries. Zygomycetes and all other hyphate fungi can rarely form noninvasive fungus balls in the lung.

Pseudallescheria (Scedosporium)

The hyphae *of Pseudallescheria* are smaller (2-4 μm) than those of *Aspergillus* spp.; the fungus branches predominantly at acute angles, but, unlike *Aspergillus*, tends to branch haphazardly rather than progressively, and terminal chlamydospores mimicking a "tennis racket" may be apparent (Fig. 7-112). Although it is a hyaline fungus, the conidia produced by *Pseudallescheria* in fungus balls are ovoid and pigmented.[10]

Fusarium

Fusarium causes an opportunistic infection of lung that is seen in patients who are severely immunosuppressed. The septate

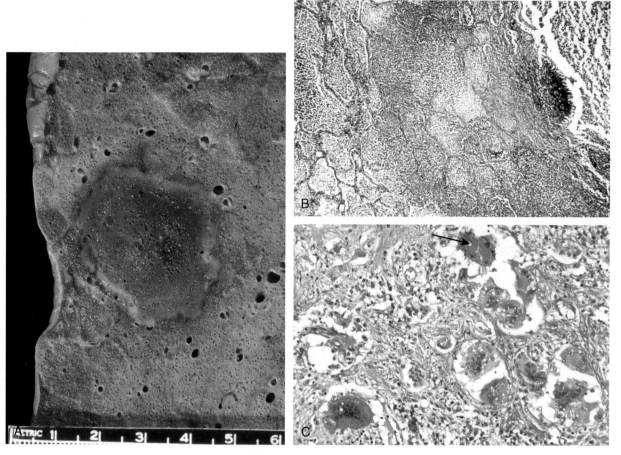

Figure 7-105. A, Angioinvasive aspergillosis with targetoid lesion caused by vascular thrombosis, ischemic infarction, and fungal invasion into surrounding tissues. **B,** Necrotizing pneumonia due to angioinvasive aspergillosis with mycelial fungal growth developing at the surface of a cavitary lesion (×250). **C,** Giant cells in pneumonia caused by *Aspergillus fumigatus* (×400).

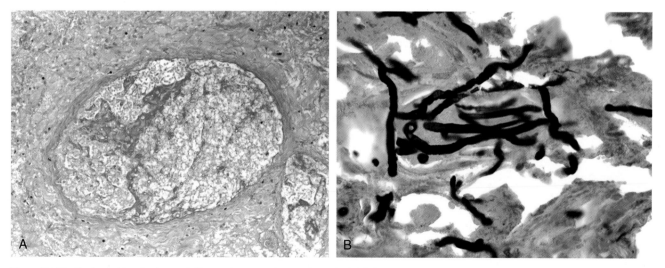

Figure 7-106. Blood vessel invasion by *Aspergillus* may be seen with H&E staining (×250) **(A)** and is seen to better advantage in section costained with GMS and H&E (×600) **(B)**.

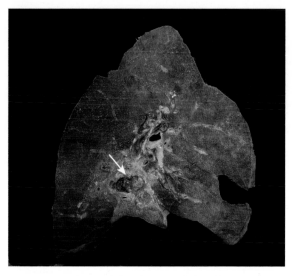

Figure 7-107. Area of nonviable lung (sequestrum) caused by angioinvasive aspergillosis *(arrow).*

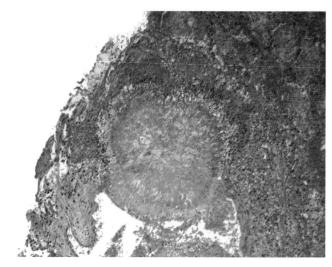

Figure 7-108. Focus of "metastatic" fungal infection showing sunburst pattern of growth out of blood vessel (×200).

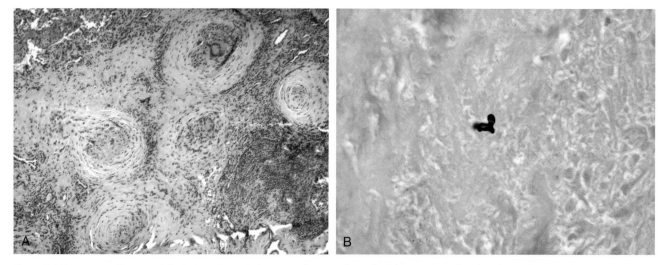

Figure 7-109. A, *Aspergillus terreus* infection in patient with chronic granulomatous disease (×200). **B,** Fragmented pyriform hyphae branching at right angle (×1000).

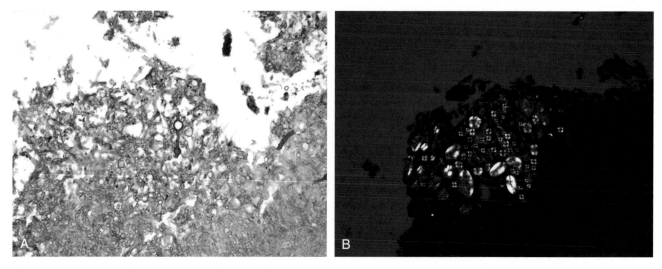

Figure 7-110. A, Fungus ball due to *Aspergillus nidulans* with Hulle cells (×400). **B,** Maltese cross configuration (×250) is visible when the specimen is examined with polarized light.

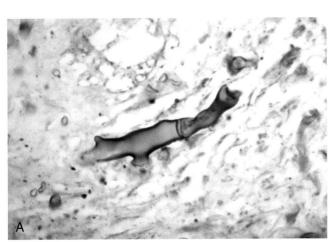

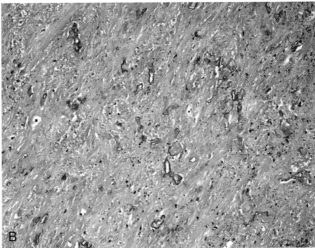

Figure 7-111. A, Zygomycete hyphae are broad and pauciseptate and tend to branch at right angles (×1000). **B,** Area of necrotizing angioinvasive disease with ribbon-like hyphae that stain well with hematoxylin (×200).

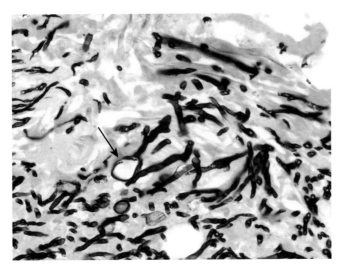

Figure 7-112. *Pseudallescheria boydii* are slightly smaller than *Aspergillus* spp. and tend to grow randomly, with prominent terminal chlamydospores *(arrow)*. Definitive diagnosis is usually not possible based solely on morphology in tissue sections (×600).

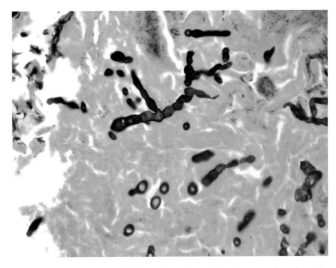

Figure 7-113. *Fusarium* tend to branch at right angles with narrow-branch points, but definitive classification is usually not achieved in tissue sections (×600).

hyphae of *Fusarium* spp. branch irregularly and at right angles, showing constrictions at branch points (Fig. 7-113).[10]

Differential Diagnosis

Although distinguishing hyphate fungal pathogens from one another in tissue can be exceedingly difficult, it is important, because the efficacy of available fungal antibiotics depends on the diagnosis. For example, whereas both *Aspergillus* spp. and *Pseudallescheria* are sensitive to voriconazole, *Pseudallescheria* are resistant to amphotericin. The sensitivity of *Fusarium* spp. to most antifungal antibiotics appears to be both unpredictable and limited. In all cases, culture remains the gold standard for diagnosis. Immunohistochemical reagents that can distinguish between hyphate fungi exist but are not commercially widely

available, and all reagents must be carefully tested with appropriate controls. The PCR assay is presently not an effective diagnostic approach.

Dematiaceous (Pigmented) Fungi

Pigmented fungi can be divided into those forming yeast (chromoblastomycosis) and those due to hyphate fungi (phaeohyphomycosis).[87] The specific organisms producing disease cannot be diagnosed morphologically, and isolation in culture is required. The Fontana-Masson stain can be applied if questions exist as to whether a fungus seen in H&E-stained sections is pigmented. *Bipolaris, Curvularia, Alternaria,* and other pigmented hyphate fungi cause allergic pulmonary disorders mimicking those of *Aspergillus* spp. (Fig. 7-114). The correct diagnosis is suggested

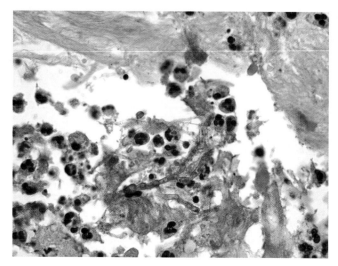

Figure 7-114. Phaeohyphomycosis shows pigmented fungal hyphae (×600). Sub-classification requires microbiologic culture.

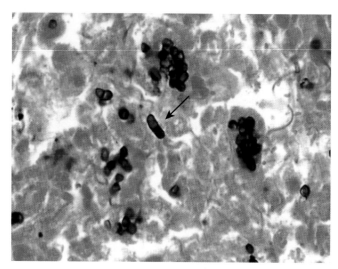

Figure 7-116. *Penicillium marneffei* (×600) is a dimorphic fungus that is often seen within histiocytes and has a sausage shape with characteristic septation *(arrow)*.

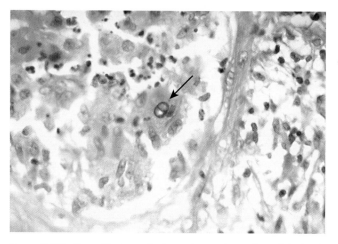

Figure 7-115. Chromoblastomycosis shows pigmented yeast forms (×600) with characteristic "sclerotic" Medlar bodies with multiaxial septation *(arrow)*.

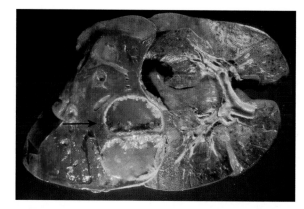

Figure 7-117. Amebic abscess with anchovy paste gross appearance.

Parasites

The lung can be host to a variety of parasitic infections. Many are seen primarily in tropical climates, but others occur in temperate climes or as a result of immunosuppression. As previously noted, the current ease of global travel has greatly increased encounters with tropical diseases.

Protozoa

Amebas

Several species of protozoa can produce pulmonary infection. *Entamoeba histolytica* affects the lung secondary to the transdiaphragmatic extension of a hepatic amebic abscess or, less commonly, as the result of bloodborne spread from an intestinal source.[89] A pulmonary amebic abscess may extend to the pleura or rupture into an airway, leading to intrapulmonic dissemination. The amebic abscess shows liquefactive necrosis that grossly resembles anchovy paste (Fig. 7-117). The histologic response in areas of necrosis primarily includes neutrophils, but the margins of the lesion show a polymorphous infiltrate of macro-

by the presence of pigmented hyphae within allergic mucus or within fungus balls. Chromoblastomycosis is appreciated by the presence of sclerotic (Medlar) bodies. These are clusters of pigmented yeast that show characteristic multiaxial septae (Fig. 7-115).

Penicillium marneffei

Pulmonary infection due to *Penicillium marneffei* is rarely seen except in patients from Southeast Asia with HIV/AIDS, but it is a significant cause of necrotizing bronchopneumonia in that region. The organism is a small (2-5 μm), dimorphic fungus with an elongate sausage shape showing a characteristic septum. The organisms can be identified free within areas of necrosis or within foamy histiocytes (Fig. 7-116). The infection may also disseminate, commonly to involve the skin. Other fungi, including *Geotrichum* and *Sporothrix*, are rare causes of pulmonary infection.[88]

phages, lymphocytes, and plasma cells; tissue eosinophilia is uncommon (Fig. 7-118A) Amebas can be distinguished from macrophages by their larger size, amphophilic bubbly cytoplasm, a sharply defined nuclear karyosome (see Fig. 7-118B), and, in the case of *E. histolytica*, the ingestion of erythrocytes.

Free-living amebas, including *Acanthamoeba, Balamuthia*, and *Naegleria*, rarely affect the lung and primarily cause meningoencephalitis. However, in immunosuppressed patients, infection may spread beyond the confines of the nervous system to include the lung.

Toxoplasma

Toxoplasma gondii produces pneumonia in patients who are immunosuppressed, most often with HIV/AIDS.[90] Whereas *Toxoplasma* is a common infection of the central nervous system and retina in HIV/AIDS, pulmonary infection is rare. When present, it includes a fibrinopurulent pneumonitis with areas of necrosis (Fig. 7-119A). The organisms are obligate intracellular parasites and are identified as engorged pseudocysts containing crescent-shaped tachyzoites or GMS- and PAS-positive true cysts containing bradyzoites (see Fig. 7-119B).

Cryptosporidium

Cryptosporidium parvum is a water-borne opportunistic infection that affects patients with HIV/AIDS but has also been seen as outbreaks among children in daycare centers.[91] The disease primarily affects the small bowel, leading to a cholera-like watery diarrhea. In patients with HIV/AIDS, the infection can spread to the hepatobiliary tree and to the pulmonary airways.

The diagnosis is made by identifying the amphophilic spores (3-5 μm) of *Cryptosporidium* along the surface of infected respiratory epithelium (Fig. 7-120). Although the cysts are apparently extracellular by light microscopic determination, ultrastructural analysis demonstrates that they are actually intracytoplasmic and invested by apical cytoplasm. The underlying mucosa shows a mild lymphocytic infiltrate. Although the cysts are well seen with H&E stain, they are also stained by GMS, modified AFB, and Giemsa. The diagnosis is obvious, once considered, but can easily go unnoticed unless the differential diagnosis includes this organism.

Microsporidia

Microsporidia are spore-forming protozoa that, like *Cryptosporidium*, infect immunosuppressed patients to produce a watery

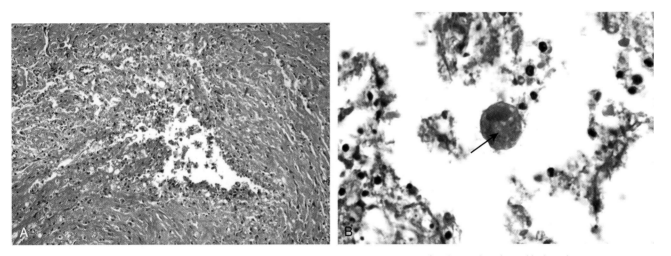

Figure 7-118. A, Liquefactive necrosis in lung abscess due to *Entamoeba histolytica* (×250). **B,** Ingestion of erythrocyte (×600) is visible *(arrow)*.

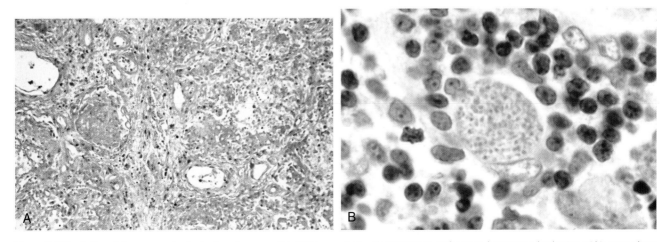

Figure 7-119. A, Necrotizing pneumonia due to *Toxoplasma gondii* (×200) in a patient with HIV/AIDS. **B,** High power demonstrates bradyzoites within macrophage (×600).

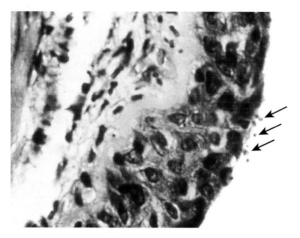

Figure 7-120. *Cryptosporidium parvum* (×400) is seen along the surface of ciliated pulmonary epithelium *(arrows)*. The cysts are actually invested by apical cytoplasm.

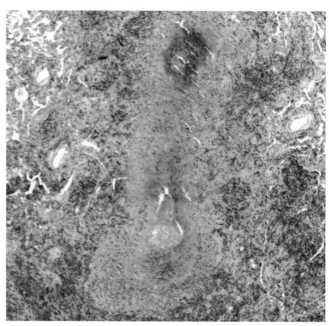

Figure 7-122. Necrotizing granulomatous and eosinophilic inflammation due to *Sparganum mansoni* (×200).

Table 7-9 Nematodes with a Pulmonary Larval Phase
Ascaris lumbricoides
Strongyloides stercoralis
Necator americanus
Ancylostoma duodenale

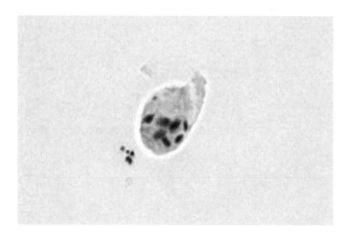

Figure 7-121. Macrophage from bronchoalveolar lavage sample (×600) contains *Microsporidium* sp., demonstrated by Brown-Hopps stain.

diarrheal illness. Extraintestinal disease, including bronchial involvement, is uncommon but has been observed. The organisms are intracytoplasmic and generally located within the apical cytoplasm.[92] Because of their small size (1-2 μm), they can be exceedingly difficult to detect, especially if the organism load is low. Special stains, including tissue Gram stain, trichrome, Warthin-Starry, and GMS, can assist in their identification (Fig. 7-121). Further speciation requires ultrastructural examination.

Nematodes (Roundworms)

Several nematodes (roundworms) have a larval developmental phase in the lung (Table 7-9).[93] The larvae of *Ascaris, Necator, Ancylostoma,* and *Strongyloides* migrate through the airways toward the mouth, where they are swallowed or expectorated. This process can evoke wheezing, migratory pneumonia, and blood eosinophilia, a complex termed *Loeffler syndrome*. The presence of track-like necrotizing granulomatous bronchitis and bronchopneumonia with prominent eosinophilic infiltrates should alert the pathologist to the presence of a migratory parasitic pulmonary infection (Fig. 7-122).

Strongyloides stercoralis is most often seen in the tropics, but is also endemic to the southeastern United States. Patients receiving high doses of corticosteroids are susceptible to infection and what is termed "hyperinfection." In hyperinfection, filariform organisms exit the gut and migrate to the lungs, where they may be found in airways, alveoli, and blood vessels, and produce a hemorrhagic and eosinophilic pneumonia. If normal pathways of maturation are inhibited, the filariform larvae mature to egg-laying adults that give rise to rhabditiform larvae, and the presence of expectorated ova indicates hyperinfection (Fig. 7-123A). Parasitemia predisposes to gram-negative sepsis that can lead to concomitant DAD (see Fig. 7-123B).

Dirofilaria
In temperate climates, *Dirofilaria immitis* is a zoonosis that causes canine heartworm disease. Mosquitoes transfer microfilariae into subcutaneous tissues, where they mature silently and enter the systemic venous circulation. From there, they travel to the right side of the heart, but in humans they do not mature further. Pulmonary disease reflects embolism of a nonviable helminth from the heart into the pulmonary circulation, where it typically lodges in a small, muscular artery to produce an area of localized, rounded infarction with a chronic immunologic reaction to the dead worm.[94] The embolic event itself may be clinically silent or associated with chest pain, fever, chills, hemoptysis,

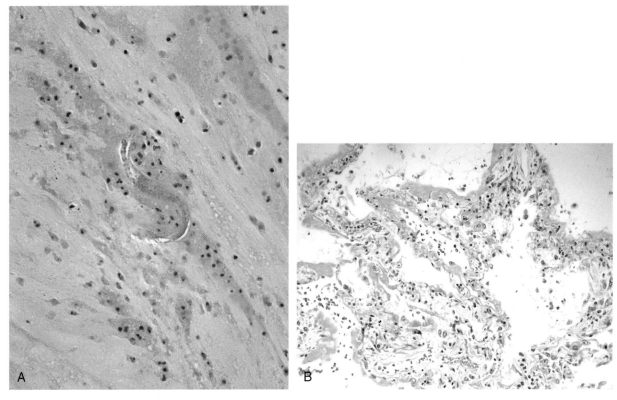

Figure 7-123. A, Rhabditiform larval form of *Strongyloides stercoralis* (×400) in patient with hyperinfection. **B,** Patient died from diffuse alveolar damage due to superimposed gram-negative sepsis (×250).

and peripheral blood eosinophilia. The disease is often first recognized as a solitary pulmonary nodule that is resected to exclude neoplasia.

Microscopically, one sees a rounded area of pulmonary infarction (Fig. 7-124A). The diagnosis is facilitated by identification of the coiled nematode within an occluded muscular pulmonary artery. The area of surrounding necrosis is enclosed by a zone of granulomatous inflammation with lymphocytes, plasma cells, and variable degrees of tissue eosinophilia, all contained within a dense fibrous capsule. Trichrome, elastic, and reticulin stains highlight the features of the helminth and help to localize it in a vessel (see Fig. 7-124B and C). *Dirofilaria* are distinguished from other nematodes by their prominent, muscular lateral cords and a striated cuticle that bulges inward in the region of the lateral cords, yielding a "bat wing" appearance.

Trematodes (Flukes)

A number of trematodes produce pulmonary disease that can manifest as solitary pulmonary nodules, pulmonary infarctions, necrotizing granulomas, or eosinophilic pneumonia. The most frequent fluke infection in the United States is schistosomiasis, which has a wide distribution in both the Eastern and Western hemispheres.

Pulmonary involvement reflects aberrant migration of adult worms into the lung, where they are found within pulmonary vessels (Fig. 7-125A). The helminth evokes an intense granulomatous and eosinophilic response; extravascular refractile ova

may be present and, like the helminth, can evoke granulomatous and eosinophilic reactions.

The ova are large, 70 to 170 μm, depending on the species. The ova of *Schistosome mansoni*, which produces most cases of pulmonary disease, show a prominent lateral spine that can be seen with H&E staining and is highlighted by modified acid-fast bacteria (AFB) stains, although the latter finding is inconstant (see Fig. 7-125B). Other species, including *Schistosoma hematobium* and *Schistosoma japonicum*, rarely cause pulmonary disease, and their ova show, respectively, a prominent or an inconspicuous terminal spine.

Schistosomiasis can also produce a granulomatous pulmonary hypertensive arteriopathy due to the presence of ova or migrating schistosomules within small-caliber pulmonary arteries and arterioles (Fig. 7-126).[95] The thickened vascular walls show epithelioid histiocytes and giant cells with adventitial fibrosis and eosinophils. This disorder usually arises from infection by *S. mansoni* or, less commonly, *S. japonicum*, that has already produced pipestem hepatic fibrosis and presinusoidal portal hypertension, leading to shunting of portal blood into the systemic venous circulation; ova are swept into the pulmonary arterial bed, where they evoke the pathologic response.

Paragonimiasis
Paragonimus, often referred to as lung fluke, is a globally distributed trematode, with human disease limited to endemic regions.[96] Most cases in Asia are due to *Paragonimus westermani*, but other species are responsible for disease in Africa and Central

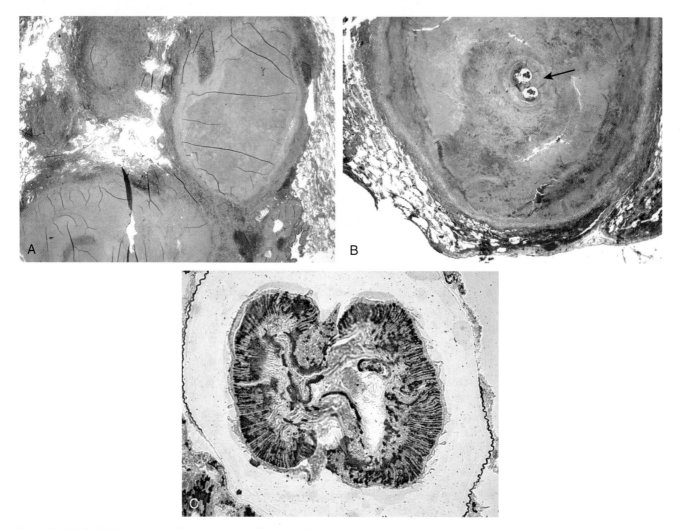

Figure 7-124. A, Nodular pulmonary infarction due to *Dirofilaria immitis* (×150). **B,** Trichrome stain showing *Dirofilaria* (×100) within thrombus (*arrow*). **C,** Reticulin stain. Nematode shows muscular lateral chords with invagination of overlying cuticle (×200).

and South America. Zoonotic forms of human infection occur rarely in North America, secondary to *Paragonimus kellicotti* infections of rodents and cats.

The organism is a freshwater species that infects crabs and crayfish as intermediate hosts; the disease is transmitted to humans through ingestion of these crustaceans, although cases may be seen that are caused by ingestion of contaminated seaweed or watercress. The larvae mature in the bowel and migrate through the diaphragm to infect the lung. Patients present with pulmonary infiltrates, fever, weight loss, and malaise. Hemoptysis is common. Pleural involvement is present in roughly half of the patients. Peripherally located cystic lesions develop in the lung, together with areas of pneumonic consolidation, and concomitant bacterial and mycobacterial infections may be present.

Grossly, *Paragonimus* is a large (10 mm), reddish fluke. Its wall consists of a tegument with prominent spiny projections best seen on high-power examination of trichrome-stained sections (Fig. 7-127A). It exhibits prominent oral and ventral suckers and a loose internal stroma. The worm evokes a cystic necrotizing granulomatous and fibrotic response with tissue eosinophilia.

The ova of *Paragonimus* are approximately 80 μm in size and show a flattened operculum (see Fig. 7-127B). They are also intensely birefringent under polarized light, and this is an important factor distinguishing *Paragonimus* from schistosome ova (see Fig. 7-127C).

Cestodes (Tapeworms)

The most common cestode pathogen in the lung is *Echinococcus*, although other tapeworm larvae, including cysticerci and spargana, can rarely infect the lung (Fig. 7-128).[97] The adult tapeworm lives attached to the wall of the small intestine of carnivorous canids. Intermediate hosts are the grazing ungulates, including sheep, goats, deer, and bison. In the continental United States, the disease is endemic to midwestern and western states.

Pulmonary disease is generally the result of preexisting hepatic involvement by *Echinococcus granulosus*, although other species, including *Echinococcus vogeli* and *Echinococcus multilocularis*, are also pathogenic.[98] The appearance of the disease is characteristic on chest radiographs, which show single or mul-

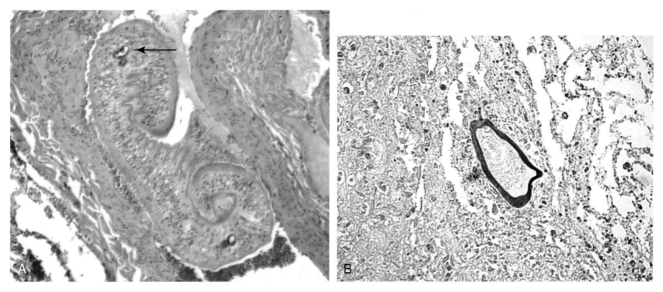

Figure 7-125. A, Coiled tuberculated schistosome (×150) with pigmented inclusions (*arrow*) within pulmonary artery. **B,** Large lateral spine and cortex of *Sparganum mansoni* ovum is decorated by modified AFB stain (×400).

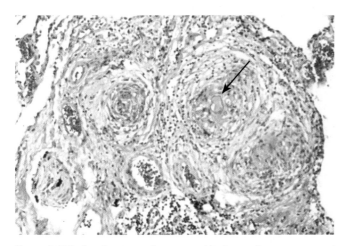

Figure 7-126. Granulomatous pulmonary arteritis due to *Sparganum mansoni* (×250). Both eggs *(arrow)* and schistosomules can be found in vessels, although their demonstration may require the examination of multiple sections.

tiple large, fluid-filled cysts (Fig. 7-129). These cysts can be asymptomatic, or they can cause symptoms due to compression of the surrounding airways and lung. Rupture into an airway can lead to suppurative pneumonia, with the proliferation of new cysts, and can generate a fatal anaphylactic reaction.

The cyst wall shows contributions from the cestode as well as from the host. The inner germinative layer of the lamellar cyst wall is the matrix for protoscolices, which detach to form secondary brood capsules (Fig. 7-130A). The rostellum of the attachment apparatus of the protoscolex contains rows of hooklets that are refractile and stain with modified AFB stain (see Fig. 7-130B). The cestode component is acellular chitinous lamellar wall that is apparent with H&E stain and is further highlighted with GMS; within the cyst wall, detritus and hooklets give rise to so-called hydatid sand (Fig. 7-131).

Microbes Associated with Bioterrorism

Recent world events have prompted interest in biologic agents that can potentially be used as weapons of mass destruction. Several of these produce pneumonia and depend on dissemination via aerosolized secretions to achieve their ignominious goal. Whereas most of these infections are naturally virulent, they tend to occur under situations that are no longer commonly encountered in modern societies. Their adoption by bioterrorists may include a need to bioengineer the organisms so as to increase their attack rate.

Anthrax

Bacillus anthracis, a toxin-producing gram-positive bacillus, was first isolated by Robert Koch as the cause of anthrax, a disease that primarily involved sheep and other farm animals. However, transmission to humans from infected animals has been recognized from antiquity as a complication of wool sorting (wool sorter's disease). An epidemic of inhalational anthrax occurred in 1979 at a biofacility in Sverdlovsk, in the former U.S.S.R, and in 2001 there was a limited epidemic of anthrax due to contaminated letters sent through the U.S. mail service by an unidentified terrorist.[99]

Cutaneous penetration by the bacillus produces a necrotic eschar with rapid extension to blood vessels resulting in bacteremia, sepsis, meningitis, and death. However, the most deadly form of infection is pulmonary. In these cases, the bacilli are inhaled and proliferate rapidly in the lung, where they produce a localized hemorrhagic pneumonia with associated pleural effusion and scant neutrophilic reaction (Fig. 7-132). They then spread via the pulmonary lymphatics to the regional lymph nodes to produce hemorrhagic mediastinitis, followed by bacteremia,

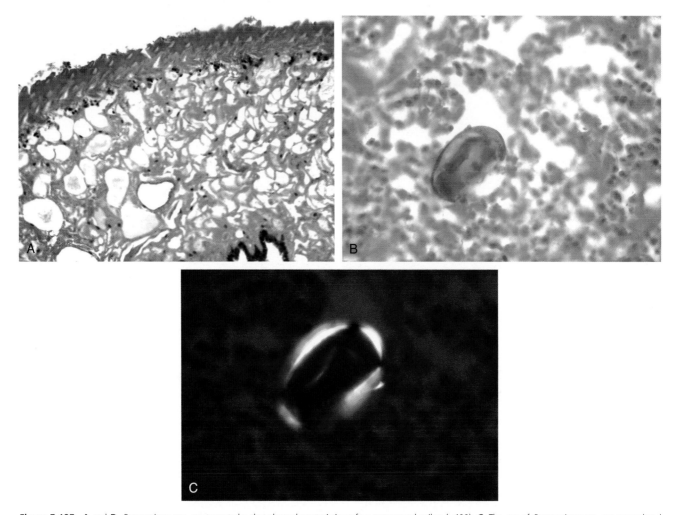

Figure 7-127. **A** and **B,** *Paragonimus* spp. are trematodes that show characteristic surface tegumental spikes (×400). **C,** The ova of *Paragonimus* spp. are operculated and refractile and show diagnostic birefringence with polarized light (×600).

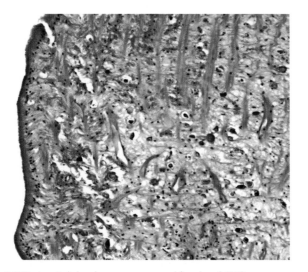

Figure 7-128. A cestode larval sparganum removed from lung (×250).

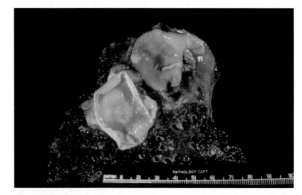

Figure 7-129. Pulmonary cyst due to *Echinococcus granulosus*.

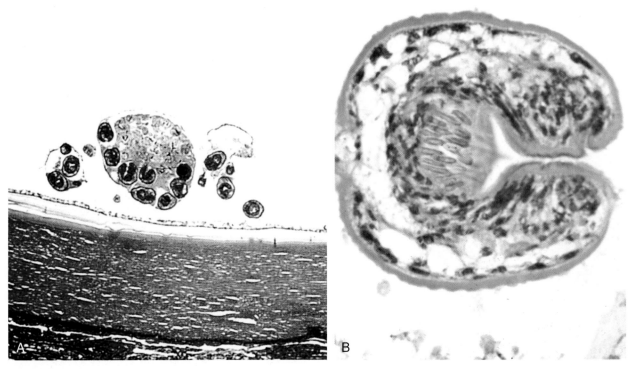

Figure 7-130. A, Germinative layer of echinococcal cyst giving rise to protoscolices (×200). **B,** Rostellum and hooklets of a protoscolex stained with modified AFB stain (×600).

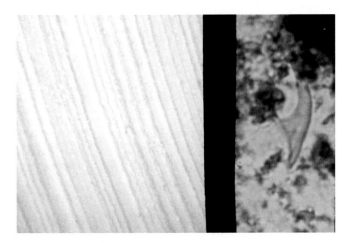

Figure 7-131. Chitinous cyst wall (*left panel*, ×200) and refractile hooklet (*right panel*, ×1000) of *Echinococcus granulosus*.

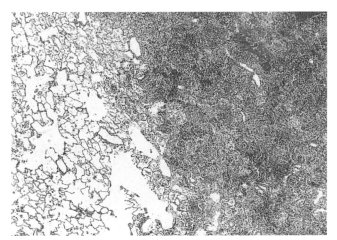

Figure 7-132. Hemorrhagic pneumonia due to anthrax (×50).

toxic shock, and death in a high percentage of cases. The diagnosis must be suspected and treated early to effect a cure. However, the disease has most often first been recognized at autopsy, where tissues prove to be teeming with bacteria.

Yersinia pestis (Plague Pneumonia)

Plague has played an important role in world history. The causative agent is *Yersinia pestis,* a gram-negative rod that is carried by animal fleas.[100] Infection occurs from contact with infected

animals, with transmission occurring via aerosol or direct contact with infected secretions. Throughout history, the black rat, *Rattus rattus,* has been most responsible worldwide for the persistence and spread of plague in urban epidemics, but any rodent can mechanically transmit infected fleas. Although *Y. pestis* has not yet been seen as a bioterrorist agent, it has received attention as a potential weapon of mass destruction, because as few as 1 to 10 bacilli are sufficient to cause infection when introduced via the oral, intradermal, subcutaneous, or intravenous route.

Yersinia produces a necrotizing hemorrhagic pneumonia and large numbers of extracellular organisms that can be seen

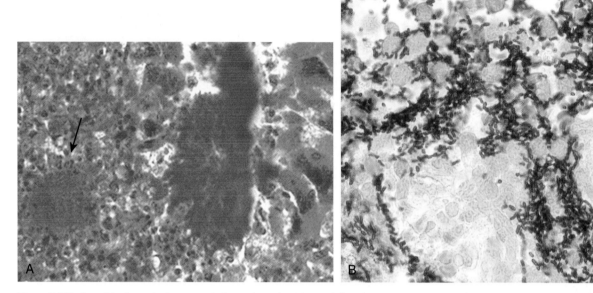

Figure 7-133. Necrotizing hemorrhagic pneumonia due to plague (*Yersinia pestis*), (×400). **A,** Organisms are seen *(arrow)* in H&E-stained section and in silver-stained section (×1000) **(B)**.

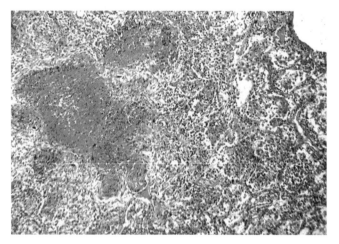

Figure 7-134. Granulomatous pneumonia caused by tularemia (*Francisella tularensis*, ×250).

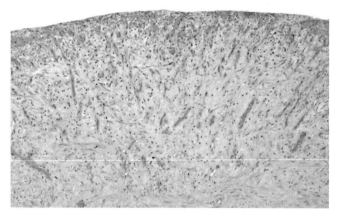

Figure 7-135. Organizing fibrinous pleuritis caused by pneumococcal pneumonia. The patient had parapneumonic effusion (×150).

with H&E staining (Fig. 7-133). Pulmonary infection leads rapidly to bacteremia and to death by sepsis.

Francisella tularensis (Tularemia Pneumonia)

Francisella tularensis causes tularemia, a necrotizing bronchopneumonia that leads to sepsis and death. However, the gram-negative bacillus is less virulent than either anthrax or plague, and it produces a relatively slow progression of disease, a fact that limits its potential role as an agent of bioterrorism.[101] The histologic response in the lung is polymorphic and includes an early hemorrhagic granulohistiocytic response with microabscess formation (Fig. 7-134), followed by granulomatous inflammation. When these coexist, the appearance of this infection is characteristic. The short coccobacillary forms require silver impregnation to be visualized in tissues.

Pleural Infections

Parapneumonic effusions can complicate bacterial pneumonias, but they are rarely biopsied unless they lead to a restrictive rind around the lung that requires decortication (Fig. 7-135). Both gram-positive and gram-negative bacteria can produce empyema (i.e., abscess in the pleural space) (Fig. 7-136). Mycobacteria (Fig. 7-137), actinomyces (Fig. 7-138), fungi (Fig. 7-139), and parasites can all produce pleural disease, and the nature of the inflammatory response substantially assists in narrowing the differential diagnosis, even when organisms cannot be identified. Tuberculosis can result years later in a fibrothorax, often with dystrophic calcification, but with no residual granulomatous response. Pleural eosinophilia can be a clue to the presence of an underlying parasitic infection (Fig. 7-140), but it can also be seen in fungal and mycobacterial infections, in response to drugs and pleural metastases, and after pneumothorax.

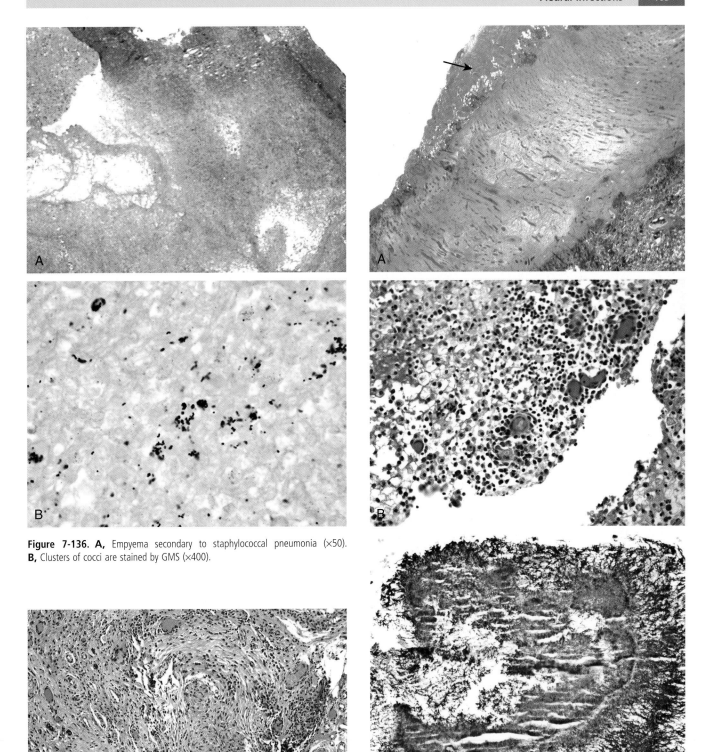

Figure 7-136. A, Empyema secondary to staphylococcal pneumonia (×50). **B,** Clusters of cocci are stained by GMS (×400).

Figure 7-137. Granulomatous pleuritis in tuberculosis (×250).

Figure 7-138. A, Dense pleural adhesion transgressing diaphragm (*arrow*, ×150). **B,** Abscess cavity with granulohistiocytic inflammation (×250). **C,** Steiner stain shows filamentous bacteria in sulfur granule (×400). Organisms were also positive with tissue Gram stain and GMS.

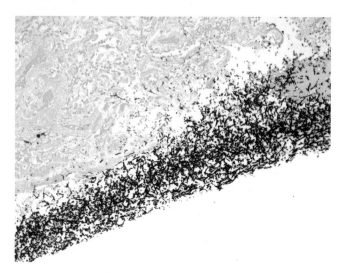

Figure 7-139. Aspergillus pleuritis (×250).

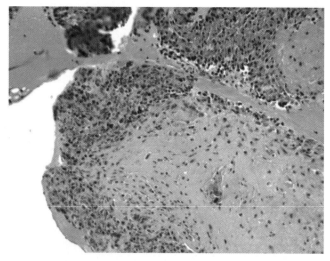

Figure 7-140. Eosinophilic calcifying pleuritis in a patient with underlying *Trichuris* infection (×250).

REFERENCES

1. Marr K, Patterson T, Denning D: Aspergillosis: Pathogenesis, clinical manifestations, and therapy. Infect Dis Clin North Am 2002;16:875-891.
2. Toledo-Pereyra L: Benefit of open lung biopsy in patients with previous non-diagnostic transbronchial lung biopsy: A guide to appropriate treatment. Chest 1980;77:647-650.
3. Velez L, Correa LT, Maya MA, et al: Diagnostic accuracy of bronchoalveolar lavage samples in immunosuppressed patients with suspected pneumonia: Analysis of a protocol. Respir Med 2007; 101:2160-2167.
4. Jaffe J, Maki D: Lung biopsy in immunocompromised patients: One institution's experience and an approach to management of pulmonary disease in the compromised host. Cancer 1981;48:1144-1153.
5. Nasuti J, Gupta P, Baloch Z: Diagnostic value and cost-effectiveness of on-site evaluation of fine needle aspiration specimens: Review of 5,688 cases. Diagn Cytopathol 2002;27:1-4.
6. Harkin TJ, Ciotoli C, Addrizzo-Harris DJ, et al: Transbronchial needle aspiration in patients infected with HIV. Am J Respir Crit Care Med 1998;157:1913-1919.
7. McKenna R, Mountain C, McMurtey M: Open lung biopsy in immunocompromised patients. Chest 1984;86:671-674.
8. Leslie K, Will M: Practical Pulmonary Pathology. Philadelphia, Churchill Livingstone, 2005.
9. Koneman E, Gade W: Mycology at a distance. Clin Lab Sci 2002;15:131-135.
10. Kradin R, Mark E: Pathology of pulmonary disorders due to *Aspergillus* spp. Arch Pathol Lab Med 2008;132:606-614.
11. Kradin R: Pulmonary immune response. In Kradin R, Robinson B (eds): Immunopathology of the Lung. Boston, Butterworth-Heinemann, 1996, pp 1-13.
12. MacLean JA, Xia W, Pinto CE, et al: Sequestration of inhaled particulate antigens by lung phagocytes: A mechanism for the effective inhibition of pulmonary cell-mediated immunity. Am J Pathol 1996;148:657-666.
13. O'Donnell WJ, Kradin RL, Evins AE, Wittram C: Case records of the Massachusetts General Hospital: Weekly clinicopathological exercises. Case 39-2004: A 52-year-old woman with recurrent episodes of atypical pneumonia. N Engl J Med 2004;351:2741-2749.
14. Mandal RV, Mark EJ, Kradin RL: Organizing pneumonia and pulmonary lymphatic architecture in diffuse alveolar damage. Hum Pathol 2008;39:1234-1238.
15. Gerberding JL, Morgan JG, Shepard JA, Kradin RL: Case records of the Massachusetts General Hospital: Weekly clinicopathological exercises. Case 9-2004: An 18-year-old man with respiratory symptoms and shock. N Engl J Med 2004;350:1236-1247.
16. Yeldandi AV, Colby TV: Pathologic features of lung biopsy specimens from influenza pneumonia cases. Hum Pathol 1994;25:47-53.
17. Oseasohn R, Adelson L, Kaji M: Clinicopathologic study of the thirty-three fatal cases of Asian influenza. N Engl J Med 1959;260:509-518.
18. Franks TJ, Chong PY, Chui P, et al: Lung pathology of severe acute respiratory distress syndrome (SARS): A study of 8 autopsy cases. Hum Pathol 2003;34:743-748.
19. Groothuis JR, Gutierrez KM, Lauer BZ: Respiratory syncytial virus infection in children with bronchopulmonary dysplasia. Pediatrics 1988;82:199-203.
20. Ding Y, Wang H, Shen Z, et al: Lung pathology of fatal severe acute respiratory syndrome. Lancet 2003;361:1773-1778.
21. Kipps A, Kaschula R: Virus pneumonia following measles: A virological and histological study of autopsy material. S Afr Med J 1976;50:1083-1088.
22. Ohori N, Michaels M, Jaffe R, et al: Adenovirus pneumonia in lung transplant recipients. Hum Pathol 1995;26:1073-1079.
23. Drew WL: Cytomegalovirus infection in patients with AIDS. Clin Infect Dis 1992;14:608-615.
24. Strickler JG, Manivel JC, Copenhaver CM, Kubic VL: Comparison of in situ hybridization and immunohistochemistry for detection of cytomegalovirus and herpes simplex virus. Hum Pathol 1990; 21:443-448.
25. Ramsey PG, Fife KH, Hackman RC, et al: Herpes simplex virus pneumonia: Clinical, virologic, and pathologic features in 20 patients. Ann Intern Med 1982;97:813-820.
26. Graham BS, Snell JD Jr: Herpes simplex virus infection of the adult lower respiratory tract. Medicine (Baltimore) 1983;62:384-393.
27. Sargent EN, Carson MJ, Reilly ED: Roentgenographic manifestation of varicella pneumonia with post-mortem correlation. AJR Am J Roentgenol 1967;98:305-317.
28. Duchin JD, Koster FT, Peters CJ, et al: Hantavirus pulmonary syndrome: A clinical description of 17 patients with a newly recognized disease. N Engl J Med 1994;330:949-955.

29. Nolte KB, Feddersen RM, Foucar K, et al: Hantavirus pulmonary syndrome in the United States: A pathological description of a disease caused by a new agent. Hum Pathol 1995;26:110-120.

30. Rollins S, Colby T, Clayton F: Open lung biopsy in *Mycoplasma pneumoniae* pneumonia. Arch Pathol Lab Med 1986;110:34-41.

31. Marzouk K, Corate L, Saleh S, Sharma OP: Epstein-Barr-virus-induced interstitial lung disease. Curr Opin Pulm Med 2005;11:456-460.

32. Weber WR, Askin FB, Dehner LP: Lung biopsy in *Pneumocystis carinii* pneumonia: A histopathologic study of typical and atypical features. Am J Clin Pathol 1977;67:11-19.

33. Amin MB, Mezger E, Zarbo RJ: Detection of *Pneumocystis carinii*: Comparative study of monoclonal antibody and silver staining. Am J Clin Pathol 1992;98:13-18.

34. Travis WD, Pittaluga S, Lipschik GY, et al: Atypical pathologic manifestations of *Pneumocystis carinii* pneumonia in the acquired immune deficiency syndrome: Review of 123 lung biopsies from 76 patients with emphasis on cysts, vascular invasion, vasculitis, and granulomas. Am J Surg Pathol 1990;14:615-625.

35. Vawter GG, Shwachman H: Cytic fibrosis in adults: An autopsy study. Pathol Annu 1979;14:357-382.

36. Polosa R, Cacciola RR, Prosperini G, et al: Endothelial-coagulative activation during chronic obstructive pulmonary disease exacerbations. Haematologica 2008;93:1275-1276.

37. Stevens DA, Moss RB, Kurup VP, et al: Allergic bronchopulmonary aspergillosis in cystic fibrosis: State of the art. Cystic Fibrosis Foundation Consensus Conference. Clin Infect Dis 2003;37(Suppl 3):S225-S264.

38. Branson D: Identification of Micrococcaceae in clinical bacteriology. Appl Environ Microbiol 1968;16:906-911.

39. Yousem SA: The historical spectrum of chronic necrotizing forms of pulmonary aspergillosis. Hum Pathol 1997;28:650656.

40. Tuomanen E, Austrian R, Masure H: Pathogenesis of pneumococcal pneumonia. N Engl J Med 1995;332:1280-1284.

41. Barnham M: Rapidly fatal group B and G streptococcal infections in adults. J Infect 1980;2:279-281.

42. Gilet Y, Issartel B, Vanheims P: Association between strains carrying gene for Panton-Valentine leukocidin and highly lethal necrotising pneumonia in young immunocompetent patients. Lancet 2002;359:753-759.

43. Pierce AK, Edmonson EB, McGee G, et al: An analysis of factors predisposing to gram-negative bacillary necrotizing pneumonia. Am Rev Respir Dis 1966;94:309-315.

44. Kirtland SH, Corley DE, Winterbauer RH: The diagnosis of ventilator-associated pneumonia. Chest 1997;112:445-457.

45. le Roux B, Mohlala M, Odell J, Whitton I: Suppurative diseases of the lung and pleural space. Part I: Empyema thoracis and lung abscess. Curr Probl Surg 1986;23:1-89.

46. Brown JR: Human actinomycosis: A study of 181 subjects. Hum Pathol 1973;4:319330.

47. Winslow DJ: Botryomycosis. Am J Pathol 1959;35:153-167.

48. Beaman BL, Burnside J, Edwards B, Causey W: Nocardial infections in the United States, 1972-1974. J Infect Dis 1976;134:286-289.

49. Winn WC, Myerowitz RL: The pathology of the *Legionella* pneumonias: A review of 74 cases and literature. Hum Pathol 1981;12:401-422.

50. Harvey RL, Sunstrum JC: *Rhodococcus equi* infection in patients with and without human immunodeficiency virus infection. Rev Infect Dis 1991;13:139-145.

51. Kwon KY, Colby TV: *Rhodococcus equi* pneumonia and pulmonary malakoplakia in acquired immunodeficiency syndrome: Pathologic features. Arch Pathol Lab Med 1994;118:744-748.

52. Dobbins W: Diagnosis of Whipple's disease. N Engl J Med 1995;332:390-392.

53. Sepkowitz KA, Raffalli J, Riley L: Tuberculosis in the AIDS era. Clin Microbiol Rev 1995;8:180-199.

54. Dannenberg AM Jr: Delayed-type hypersensitivity and cell-mediated immunity in the pathogenesis of tuberculosis. Immunol Today 1991;12:228-233.

55. Kim JH, Langston AA, Gallis HA: Miliary tuberculosis: Epidemiology, clinical manifestations, diagnosis, and outcome. Rev Infect Dis 1990;12:583-590.

56. Lupatkin H, Brau N, Flomenberg P, Simberkoff MS: Tuberculosis abscess in patients with AIDS. Clin Infect Dis 1992;14:1040-1044.

57. Woods GL, Washington JA II: Mycobacteria other than *Mycobacterium tuberculosis*: Review of microbiologic and clinical aspects. Rev Infect Dis 1987;9:275-294.

58. Inderlied CB, Kemper CA, Bermudez LEM: The *Mycobacterium avium* complex. Clin Microbiol Rev 1993;6:266-310.

59. Strom RL, Gruninger RP: AIDS with *Mycobacterium avium-intracellulare* lesions resembling those of Whipple's disease. N Engl J Med 1983;309:1323-1325.

60. Klatt EC, Jensen DF, Meyer PR: Pathology of *Mycobacterium avium-intracellulare* infection in acquired immunodeficiency syndrome. Hum Pathol 1987;18:709-714.

61. Greenberger PA, Katzenstein AL: Lipid pneumonia with atypical mycobacterial colonization: Association with allergic bronchopulmonary aspergillosis. Arch Intern Med 1983;143:2003-2005.

62. Piggott J, Hocholzer L: Human melioidosis. Arch Pathol 1970;90:101-111.

63. Goodwin RA Jr, Des Prez RM: State of the art: Histoplasmosis. Am Rev Respir Dis 1978;117:929-956.

64. Wheat LJ, Slama TG, Zeckel ML: Histoplasmosis in the acquired immune deficiency syndrome. Am J Med 1985;78:203-210.

65. Goodwin RA Jr, Des Prez RM: Pathogenesis and clinical spectrum of histoplasmosis. South Med J 1973;66:13-25.

66. Sarosi GA, Johnson PC: Disseminated histoplasmosis in patients infected with human immunodeficiency virus. Clin Infect Dis 1992;14(Suppl 1):S60-S67.

67. Gottridge JA, Meyer BR, Schwartz NS, Lesser RS: The nonutility of chest roentgenographic examination in asymptomatic patients with positive tuberculin test results. Arch Intern Med 1989;149:1660-1662.

68. Tenenbaum MJ, Greenspan J, Kerkering TM: Blastomycosis. Crit Rev Microbiol 1982;9(3):139-163.

69. Tuttle JG, Lichtwardt HE, Altshuler CH: Systemic North American blastomycosis: Report of a case with small forms of blastomycetes. Am J Clin Pathol 1953;23:890-897.

70. Watts JC, Chandler FW, Mihalov ML, et al: Giant forms of *Blastomyces dermatitidis* in the pulmonary lesions of blastomycosis: Potential confusion with *Coccidiodes immitis*. Am J Clin Pathol 1990;93:575-578.

71. Mitchell TG, Perfect JR: Cryptococcosis in the era of AIDS: 100 Years after the discovery of *Cryptococcus neoformans*. Clin Microbiol Rev 1995;8:515-548.

72. Lazcano O, Speights VO Jr, Strickler JG, et al: Combined histochemical stains in the differential diagnosis of *Cryptococcus neoformans*. Mod Pathol 1993;6:80-84.

73. Stevens DA: Coccidioidomycosis. N Engl J Med 1995;332:1077-1082.

74. Singh VR, Smith DK, Lawrence J, et al: Coccidioidomycosis in patients infected with human immunodeficiency virus: Review of 91 cases at a single institution. Clin Infect Dis 1996;23:563-568.

75. Drut R: Paracoccidioidomycosis: Diagnosis by fine-needle aspiration cytology. Diagn Cytopathol 1995;13:52-53.

76. Rose HD, Sheth NK: Pulmonary candidiasis: A clinical and pathological correlation. Arch Intern Med 1978;138:964-965.

77. Okudaira M, Kurata H, Sakabe F: Studies on the fungal flora in the lung of human necropsy cases: A critical survey in connection with

the pathogenesis of opportunistic fungus infections. Mycopathologia 1977;61:3-18.

78. Fishman JA, Kubak BM: Clinical cases in transplantation. Transpl Infect Dis 2002;4(Suppl 3):62-66.

79. McCarthy DS, Pepys J: Allergic broncho-pulmonary aspergillosis. Clinical immunology: 2. Skin, nasal and bronchial tests. Clin Allergy 1971;1:415-432.

80. Basich JE, Graves TS, Nasir Baz M, et al: Allergic bronchopulmonary aspergillosis in corticosteroid-dependent asthmatics. J Allergy Clin Immunol 1981;68:98-102.

81. Gefter WB: The spectrum of pulmonary aspergillosis. J Thorac Imaging 1972;7:56-74.

82. Smith FB, Beneck D: Localized *Aspergillus* infestation in primary lung carcinoma: Clinical and pathological contrasts with post-tuberculous intracavitary aspergilloma. Chest 1991;100:554-556.

83. Roehrl MH, Croft WJ, Liao Q, et al: Hemorrhagic pulmonary oxalosis secondary to a noninvasive *Aspergillus niger* fungus ball. Virchows Arch 2007;451:1067-1073.

84. Stergiopoulou T, Meletiadis J, Roilides E, et al: Host-dependent patterns of tissue injury in invasive pulmonary aspergillosis. Am J Clin Pathol 2007;127:349-355.

85. Segal BH, DeCarlo ES, Kwon-Chung KJ, et al: *Aspergillus nidulans* infection in chronic granulomatous disease. Medicine (Baltimore) 1998;77:345-354.

86. Sugar AM: Mucormycosis. Clin Infect Dis 1992;14(Suppl 1):S126-S129

87. Fader RC, McGinnis MR: Infections caused by dematiaceous fungi: Chromoblastomycosis and phaeohyphomycosis. Infect Dis Clin North Am 1988;2:925-938.

88. Sekhon AS, Stein L, Garg AK, et al: Pulmonary penicillosis marneffei: Report of the first imported case in Canada. Mycopathologia 1994;128:3-7.

89. Gutierrez Y: The Intestinal Amebae. Philadelphia, Lea & Febiger; 1990.

90. Bertoli F, Espino M, Arosemena JR, et al: A spectrum in the pathology of toxoplasmosis in patients with acquired immunodeficiency syndrome. Arch Pathol Lab Med 1995;119:214-224.

91. Current WL, Garcia LS: Cryptosporidiosis. Clin Lab Med 1991;11:873-897.

92. Giang TT, Kotler DP, Garro ML, Orenstein JM: Tissue diagnosis of intestinal microsporidiosis using the chromotrope-2R modified trichrome stain. Arch Pathol Lab Med 1993;117:1249-1251.

93. Gutierrez Y: *Rhabditis strongyloides* and Other Free Living Nematodes. Philadelphia, Lea & Febiger, 1990.

94. Echeverii A, Long R, Check W, Burnett C: Pulmonary dirofilariasis. Ann Thorac Surg 1999;67:201-202.

95. Sadigursky M, Andrade Z: Pulmonary changes in schistosomal cor pulmonale. Am J Trop Med Hyg 1982;31:779-784.

96. Bercovitz Z: Clinical studies on human lung fluke disease (endemic hemoptysis) caused by *Paragonimus westermani* infestation. Am J Trop Med 1937;1937:101-122.

97. Iwatani K, Kubota I, Hirotsu Y, et al: *Sparganum mansoni* parasitic infection in the lung showing a nodule. Pathol Int 2006;56:674-677.

98. Katz AM, Pam CT: Echinococcus disease in the United States. Am J Med 1958;25:759-770.

99. Abramova F, Grinberg L, Yampolskaya O, Walker D: Pathology of inhalational anthrax in 42 cases from the Sverdlovsk outbreak of 1979. Proc Natl Acad Sci U S A 1993;90:2291-2294.

100. Pollitzer R: Plague. Geneva, World Health Organization, 1954.

101. Guarner J, Jennigan J, Shieh W, et al: Pathology and pathogenesis of bioterrorism-related inhalational anthrax. Am J Pathol 2003;163:701-709.

Cardiac Infections

H. Thomas Aretz and Richard L. Kradin

Introduction

Infections can involve all three layers of the heart, and virtually all classes of organisms infect cardiac tissues. Because the entire cardiac output is delivered to the lungs and other vital organs by the cardiac ventricles with each cardiac cycle, the propensity for bloodborne infections to be carried to and from the heart is substantial.

This chapter is divided according to the layers involved, in the order of frequency seen by the surgical pathologist: *infective endocarditis* involving the valves (and, rarely, the endocardium lining the chambers); *myocarditis* involving the myocardium; and *pericarditis* involving the pericardium.

The Pathology of Infective Endocarditis

The true incidence of infective endocarditis (IE) is uncertain, but it has been estimated to account for 1 of every 1000 hospital admissions.[1] The morbidity of this disorder is substantial, because it can cause cardiac valvular insufficiency, congestive heart failure, and cardiac conduction system abnormalities. Embolization of infected vegetations can damage vital organs, including brain, kidney, and lung. Circulating immune complexes that develop in response to endovascular infection can result in microvascular injury, arthritis, and renal failure.

Revised diagnostic criteria for IE have improved diagnosis,[2] although cases of IE continue to be discovered at the time of valve surgery and at autopsy. The emergence of fastidious microorganisms has led to increased recognition of the microbiologic spectrum of this disease. The widespread use of endovascular prosthetic devices and bioprosthetic grafts has expanded the scope of IE and complicated its management.[3] Finally, research into bacterial interactions with vascular endothelium and recognition of the importance of bacterial biofilms promises to change how IE is treated in the future.

The pathology of IE is complex; it reflects the virulence of the organism, host immunity, the biology of the endocardial surface, and the topography of infection. For example, infection of a cardiac valve by *Staphylococcus aureus* in a patient with acquired immunodeficiency syndrome (AIDS) is more likely to produce a rapidly progressive syndrome of valvular incompetence and acute heart failure than is endocarditis due to an organism of low virulence in a normal host. Whereas IE can affect an ostensibly normal endocardial surface, it far more commonly targets anatomically distorted valves (Table 8-1).[4] The site of infection is critical with respect to the spectrum of possible complications; for example, IE on the left side of the heart is more likely to result in acutely life-threatening embolic events, including cerebral and myocardial emboli, than is right-heart endocarditis. Extension of aortic valve infection into the heart can produce myocardial abscess and complete heart block. Infected fistulous tracts forming between cardiac chambers can lead to intracardiac shunting of blood, depending on the anatomy of the involved valve. For these reasons, IE must always be approached nongenerically, because the specific pathology determines both potential complications and the optimal therapeutic approach in each case.

The Cardiac Valves

Most cases of IE involve the cardiac valves. The normal atrioventricular mitral and tricuspid valves of the cardiac inflow tracts and the semilunar aortic and pulmonary valves of the outflow tracts share a common structure. They consist of a dense, avascular, collagenous core, termed the valvular fibrosa, which is

Table 8-1 Conditions Associated with Infective Endocarditis

Rheumatic valvular disease	Mechanical prosthetic valves
Bioprosthetic valve	Swan-Ganz catheter
Post-traumatic valvulitis	Pacemaker leads
Annular calcifications	Internal defibrillators
Atherosclerotic degeneration	Left ventricular assist devices
Mural thrombi	Intravenous catheters
Hypertrophic cardiomyopathy	Intravenous hyperalimentation
	Hemodialysis shunts

contiguous with the fibrous skeleton of the heart, surrounded by a spongiosa that consists of a loose matrix of collagen, elastic fibers, and glycosaminoglycans. The valve surfaces are lined by endothelium. This topographic arrangement is critical to the normal function of the valves during the cardiac cycle. The cardiac ventricles fill with blood that passes through the open leaflets of atrioventricular valves during diastole, and the valves must remain tightly apposed during systole. Conversely, the semilunar valves must open during systole and remain competently closed during diastole. This is achieved by the elastic and deformable properties of the valves. Because the normal cardiac valve is normally avascular, stromal cells that contribute to the valvular fibrosa and spongiosa must dynamically maintain valvular structure.

With the mechanical wear and tear that accompanies age—valves must open and close almost 3 million times in the course of a 75-year lifetime—the normal configuration of the valve changes. Fibrosis is the most common complication of aging, whereas myxomatous change can result from altered hemodynamics (e.g., the functional insufficiency that follows dilatation of a valve ring) or genetically encoded defects (e.g., Marfan syndrome).

Mechanical degeneration leads to increased collagen deposition by valvular mesenchymal cells and to a relative decrease in the size of the spongiosa. In addition, shear forces produce focal endothelial denudation of the valvular surface, leading to the deposition of a platelet-fibrin coagulum that signals subendothelial fibrogenesis.

Valvular calcifications complicate both age-related fibrosis and postinflammatory valvulitis. The structural distortions produced by scarring are further enhanced by calcifications that grow by accretion to be nodular and bulky, leading to valvular stenosis and insufficiency.[5] In some cases, concomitant foci of ossification also develop.

Rheumatic fever, an immunologic complication of group A *Streptococcus* infection, is the most common cause of valvulitis. Rheumatic fever causes a pancarditis that affects the cardiac valves, myocardium, and pericardium. Histiocytic inflammation is accompanied by neovascularization and fibrosis. In the case of the atrioventricular valves, the chordae tendineae become scarred and foreshortened, promoting the late hemodynamic consequences of valvular distortion. The end result is a scarred valve that is predisposed to further deformation by dystrophic calcification and functionally to both stenosis and insufficiency.[6]

Infective Endocarditis

IE results from the growth of microorganisms on the endocardial surfaces of the cardiac valves or vascular endothelium. Most infections are caused by bacteria that have been entrapped in a mesh of fibrin and platelets previously deposited along an injured endocardial surface. These deposits are termed vegetations. They are friable and grow by accretion to be potentially bulky, depending on the cause, location, and duration of the infection. In the absence of antimicrobial treatment, effective healing of vegetations does not occur, and the risk of infected platelet-thrombi dislodging and traveling into the circulation is substantial.

In the past, IE was termed "bacterial endocarditis," but with increased recognition that nonbacterial species, including fungi and rickettsia, can also cause endocarditis, the term *infective endocarditis* is currently preferred. Modifiers such as acute, subacute, or chronic refer to the clinical course of the disease; however, they are imprecise and do not correlate well with the underlying pathology. Instead, IE should be considered a spectral disorder that can exhibit either an aggressive or an indolent course, depending on the circumstances of infection.

The once-universal mortality associated with IE has been substantially reduced by improved diagnosis, antimicrobial treatment, and aggressive surgical intervention. The current mortality rate ranges from 10% to 30%.[7] In the first half of the 20th century, most cases of IE were complications of rheumatic mitral valvular disease. However, with decreased prevalence of rheumatic valvular disease and increased aging of the population, the senile fibrocalcific aortic valve has become an increasingly common presentation.[8] New sources of infection include intravenous drug use and the widespread iatrogenic use of intravenous catheterization.[9] Host immunosuppression in patients receiving corticosteroids and other immunosuppressant agents, human immunodeficiency virus (HIV-1) infection,[10] diabetes, renal failure, alcoholism, and cirrhosis all substantially increase the risk for development of IE.[11]

Cardiac and vascular prostheses are potential nidi for infection and present a continued risk for IE after implantation.[12] Right-heart pacemaker implantation can lead to infection along the pacemaker leads and the tricuspid valve. *S. aureus* and *Staphylococcus epidermidis* are the most common pathogens in the early (first 60 days) and late periods, respectively, after implantation.[13] Left-ventricular assist devices are currently used in the treatment of intractable left ventricular failure and as a bridge to cardiac transplantation. The prevalence of IE associated with these devices ranges from 15% to 44%, and the diagnosis can be difficult to establish noninvasively. *Enterococcus* and *Staphylococcus* species are the most common infective agents, but fungi and low-virulence organisms also cause disease.[14]

Pathogenesis of Infective Endocarditis

Experimental models have demonstrated that a catheter introduced into the right side of the heart of a rabbit or a rat can cause endothelial injury to the tricuspid valve.[15] Endocardial injury greatly increases the risk of developing IE when coupled with subsequent exposure to circulating bacteria (Fig. 8-1). Endothelial injury exposes basement membrane proteins, including laminin, fibronectin, and vitronectin, which serve as adhesion molecules for bacteria. Activation of platelets and thrombus

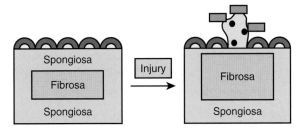

Figure 8-1. Pathogenesis of infective endocarditis. The diagram shows the sequence of events leading from the configuration of a normal cardiac valve to a scarred valve with increased valvular fibrosa, endothelial *(red)* denudation, and the deposition of fibrin *(pink)* with platelets *(black)* and bacteria *(purple)*.

Table 8-2 Organisms That Cause Infective Endocarditis

Organism	% of Cases
Streptococci*	6-80
Enterococci	5-18
Staphylococci†	20-35
Gram-negative bacilli	2-13
Fungi	2-4
Culture negative	5-24

*Includes *Streptococcus viridans* and other *Streptococcus* species.
†Includes coagulase-positive and coagulase-negative organisms.
From Fowler VG, Scheld WM, Bayer AS: Endocarditis and intravascular infections. In Mandell GL, Bennett GE, Dolin R (eds): Principles and Practice of Infectious Diseases, 6th ed. Philadelphia, Elsevier, 2005.

formation further promote bacterial adhesion. Bacterial binding to thrombus is followed by a lag period of several hours before bacterial proliferation is detected.[16]

The risk of developing experimental disease is a function of the virulence and size of the bacterial inoculum and whether the injurious catheter is left in place or removed. For bacterial inocula introduced after catheter removal, the risk of developing IE decreases progressively with time. The histopathology of the valve shows healing of the catheter-induced lesion by re-endothelialization, which appears to protect against subsequent bacterial colonization.

Other animal models of IE that do not require an indwelling catheter have been developed. In the guinea pig, electrocoagulation of the aortic valve followed by inoculation with *S. aureus* or *Coxiella burnetii* yields IE. In addition, electrical stimulation of the cervical vagus nerve can result in injury of the mitral valve and predisposes to IE with subsequent bacterial challenge.

Specific microbial factors have been examined in the pathogenesis of IE.[17] Resistance by an *S. aureus* to a thrombin-induced microbiocidal protein promotes IE. Fibronectin-binding proteins expressed by *S. aureus* facilitate binding to fibronectin and act as invasins. Organisms that do not bind fibronectin show decreased propensity to cause IE. Gelatinase/type IV collagenase enhances the virulence of *Streptococcus gordonii*, and an aggregation substance expressed by *Enterococcus* (formerly *Streptococcus*) *faecalis* increases virulence in the catheter-injury model.

Biofilm formation plays a critical role in the pathogenesis of IE and has important consequences with respect to its treatment.[18] Bacteria can survive as isolated, free-living planktonic organisms or as stationary colonies associated with a substratum. Four criteria have been proposed for the biofilm origin of infection: adherence of pathogenetic bacteria to a substratum; presence of bacteria in clusters or colonies associated with either an endogenous or a host-derived matrix; localized infection; and resistance to antibiotic therapy despite sensitivity of the planktonic organism. Most, if not all, cases of IE associated with prosthetic surfaces meet these criteria. Bacteria within biofilms produce extracellular polymeric substances (EPS)—slime-producing glycocalices that limit the accessibility of host humoral and cellular defenses, as well as antibiotics, to the organisms that are embedded in the matrix. Biofilms confer other advantages to the bacterial colonies as well. If the availability of growth requirements is limited, biofilm bacteria can convert to a slow-growing, stationary state, so-called persisters. Water channels form within the biomass and serve as a circulatory system through which nutrients are shared and waste products released.

The activities of the biofilm are coordinated by redundant interbacterial genetic signals. The properties of the biofilm make it virtually impossible to eradicate infection as long as the stationary phase persists. Organisms can spread along surfaces by means of a ripple effect or, alternatively, as detached clumps of organisms that can break free of the substratum matrix and travel to distant sites in the circulating blood. These mechanisms explain the local and distant spread of infection in IE.

Hemodynamic Factors That Predispose to the Development of Infectious Endocarditis

Structural deformation of a cardiac valve can lead to local shear stresses and injury.[16] Jet lesions produced by critically stenotic valves or shunts from the systemic to the pulmonary circulation increase the risk of IE. Bicuspid aortic valves are at risk because of their propensity to develop both stenosis and insufficiency.[19] Insufficiency of the aortic valve also increases the risk of mitral valve endocarditis, because regurgitant flow through an incompetent aortic valve causes fluttering and superficial injury to the anterior mitral leaflet. A comparable mechanism accounts for mural endocarditis along the ventricular septum in aortic insufficiency. In mitral insufficiency, vegetations may develop along jet lesions formed in the left atrium.[20]

In the absence of primary involvement of the cardiac valve, other conditions, including mitral annular calcification and mural thrombi, become important sites of infection in IE. Left-to-right shunts due to congenital heart disease show a propensity to cause endocarditis at the maximum site of the jet stream. Ventricular septal defects are at high risk, whereas secundum atrial septal defects rarely develop IE. However, endocardial cushion or septum primum defects that involve the mitral apparatus and patent ductus lesions are at risk. Approximately 5% of patients with hypertrophic cardiomyopathy and asymmetric septal thickening develop IE.[21]

The Microbiology of Infective Endocarditis

Virtually all bacterial and fungal pathogens have been reported to cause IE (Table 8-2). The most common cause of IE continues to be *Streptococcus viridans*, a low-virulence organism that is part of the normal oral flora.[22] The classic clinical scenario for the development of IE is transient bacteremia caused by dental manipulation in a patient with rheumatic valvular disease. However, any site of active infection with access to the bloodstream can yield IE. These include cellulitis, puncture wounds, sinus disease, bronchiectasis, pneumonia, surgery within an unsterile field, and urogenital instrumentation.[23] Other oral flora β-hemolytic streptococci, including *Streptococcus sanguis*, *Streptococcus mitis*, *Streptococcus mutans*, and *Streptococcus milleri*, account for approximately half of the cases of IE in the community. *Streptococcus pneumoniae* endocarditis is an unusual complication of a pyogenic pneumonia, otitis media, or meningitis.[24] Patients with defects of opsonization, splenic insufficiency, or diminished phagocytotic capacity are at increased risk. IE due to group D streptococcal enterococci—*Streptococcus bovis*, *Enterococcus* (formerly *Streptococcus*) *faecalis*, and *Enterococcus* (formerly *Streptococcus*) *faecium*—complicates bowel pathologies, including colon carcinoma and diverticulitis, as well as urogenital instrumentation. These organisms account for approximately 20% of cases of IE, and *S. aureus*, *S. epidermidis*, gram-negative bacilli,[25] culture-negative organisms, and fungi roughly account for the remainder.

IE of prosthetic valves is associated with a high rate of complications, including valvular incompetence, obstruction to blood flow, and embolic phenomena.[26] In bioprosthetic valves, IE usually affects the valve cusps, whereas mechanical prosthetic valves develop infections primarily along their sewing rings. Most cases of endocarditis occur within the first 6 months after implantation, but there is a steady annual rate of infection of 2% to 4%.[12] Early infection (≤60 days) is caused by *S. aureus*; by gram-negative bacteria, including *Klebsiella* spp. and coliforms; or by fungi, most often *Candida* spp. Coagulase-negative *S. aureus* accounts for approximately half of the late cases of IE, and non-virulent organisms, including *S. epidermidis* and *S. albus*, account for most of the remainder.

Intravenous drug users have a high incidence of IE.[26] The organisms isolated from blood in these patients tend to be virulent and include *S. aureus* and *Pseudomonas* spp. *Candida albicans* and other fungi account for 10% of cases. Involvement of the tricuspid valve is most common, but mutivalvular disease also occurs. Embolic complications may involve both the lungs and the left side of the circulation.

Blood culture–negative endocarditis accounts for approximately 10% of cases at most major medical centers.[27] Slow-growing gram-negative bacilli can require several weeks before they are detected in culture, and it is optimal laboratory practice to retain blood cultures for at least 3 weeks before discarding them as negative. This group of bacteria has collectively been referred to by the acronym HACEK (*Hemophilus* spp., *Actinobacillus* spp., *Cardiobacterium hominis*, *Eikenella corrodens*, and *Kingella kingii*).

C. burnetii, the cause of Q-fever endocarditis, often eludes diagnose.[28] Blood cultures may be negative and vegetations difficult to detect. The noninvasive diagnosis rests on serologic and polymerase chain reaction results. Other uncommon culture-negative organisms must be considered in the differential diagnosis as well. *Tropheryma whippelii* (Whipple's bacillus) can cause culture-negative endocarditis, and the noninvasive diagnosis centers on PCR, because cross-reactivity with *C. burnetii* con-

founds serologic testing.[29] The diagnosis may require ultrastructural examination to detect the characteristic Whipple bodies. Cases of IE due to *Chlamydia* spp. are uncommon, and their clinical and pathologic features mimic those of *C. burnetii*.

Gross Pathology of Infective Endocarditis

The *sine qua non* of IE is the vegetation. Vegetations are friable, fibrinous excrescences that develop along the endocardial surface. Most vegetations in IE are polypoid, but they can be sessile. Vegetations vary in size, in part depending on the causative organism, the duration of infection, and whether they affect the right or left side of the heart. In Q fever, vegetations may be inconspicuous, exhibiting only a thin coating of fibrin along the valve surface. Bulky vegetations occur on the tricuspid valve, reflecting the virulence of the organisms that tend to attack that valve in intravenous drug users and the lower systolic pressures of the right ventricle. They are white or yellow, as opposed to the usually dark red vegetations that are occur in the left side of the heart. Tricuspid vegetations have a propensity to involve the anterior leaflet of the valve and to produce obstruction of the right ventricular outflow tract.

Vegetations along the mitral valve are dark tan or red (Fig. 8-2). They are distributed primarily along the atrial endocardial surfaces of the valve but do not respect lines of closure. They can extend from the valve surface to involve the adjacent atrial endocardium or inferiorly to infect the chordae tendineae. The continuity of the fibrous skeleton of the mitral and aortic valves allows extension of infection by direct contiguity. Because the anterior leaflet of the mitral valve normally moves toward the aortic outflow tract during systole, infection can spread directly from one valve surface to the other by streaming of organisms at the surface of a biofilm. Infection may also extend directly into the adjacent valve annulus and from there into the subjacent myocardium to produce a myocardial abscess and fistulous tracts to other cardiac chambers.

Vegetations of the aortic valve are generally smaller than those seen along the atrioventricular valves (Fig. 8-3). Infection weakens the valve cusps, leading to aneurysmal dilatation of the sinuses of Valsalva or to tears and ruptures. Rupture of the chordal attachments of an atrioventricular valve can cause a

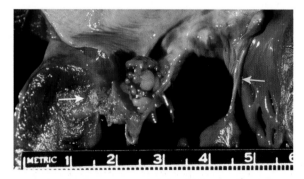

Figure 8-2. Vegetations along the mitral valve. The anterior leaflet of the mitral valve shows large polypoid vegetations caused by *Staphylococcus aureus* infection. Note the predominant involvement of the atrial surface of the leaflet. The valve was distorted by rheumatic valvular disease, as evidenced by the thickened and shortened chordae tendineae *(yellow arrow)*. Calcification of the mitral annulus is present *(white arrow)*.

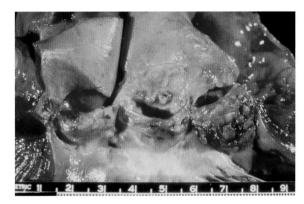

Figure 8-3. Aortic valve endocarditis. All three cusps of the aortic valve are involved by vegetations, with the left coronary cusp *(right)* showing the most severe disease. Note the relatively small size of the vegetations and the involvement of the ventricular surfaces of the cusps.

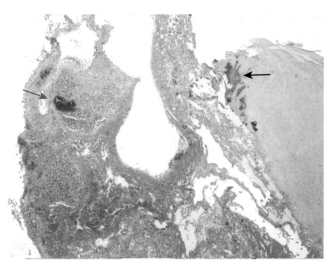

Figure 8-5. Histopathology of vegetation. A fibrotic and calcified aortic valve cusp *(red arrow)* shows vegetation composed of fibrin, platelets, neutrophils, and a colony of *Streptococcus viridans (black arrow)* (×100).

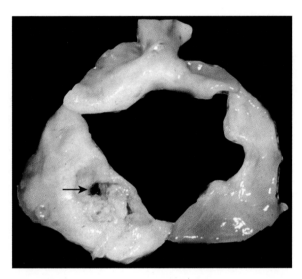

Figure 8-4. Healed aortic endocarditis. A healed vegetation is seen adjacent to a perforation of the noncoronary cusp *(arrow)*. The left coronary cusp is also eroded along its free margin. The valve was resected because of aortic insufficiency after antibiotic treatment.

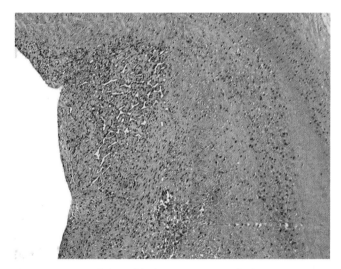

Figure 8-6. Histopathology of healing vegetation. Mitral valve in *Streptococcus viridans* endocarditis shows prominent neoangiogenesis and fibroplasia (×200).

sudden increase in valvular insufficiency and acute pulmonary edema or hepatic centrilobular necrosis and peripheral congestion. If the disease is treated and arrested, healing of the valve takes place, but deformations can result in late hemodynamic complications. Local fibrosis or calcification may mark an area of healed endocarditis, and foci of limited rupture may persist as re-endothelialized fenestrations (Fig. 8-4).

Microscopic Pathology of Infective Endocarditis

The microscopic appearance of IE can vary from subtle to exuberant. In all cases of active IE, it is possible to discern fibrin deposition along the disrupted endocardial surface. Large polypoid excrescences of fibrin and platelets containing colonies of bacteria or fungi may be evident (Fig. 8-5). The vegetations may be paucicellular or acutely inflamed with areas of valvular and leukocyte necrosis. The valve cusp is edematous and commonly

shows a heterogeneous infiltration of neutrophils and histiocytes. The extent and type of inflammation vary with the offending organism. Virulent pyogenic infections, such as those caused by *S. aureus* or *C. albicans,* show substantial acute neutrophilic inflammation, whereas less virulent organisms may show subtle leukocyte infiltration. Early inflammation is rapidly followed by neoangiogenesis and active fibroplasia (Fig. 8-6). In IE caused by *C. burnetii, Chlamydia* spp., or *T. whippelii,* fibrinous vegetations are scant and the pathology primarily exhibits foamy histiocytes in areas of scarring (Fig. 8-7).

Demonstrating Microorganisms in Situ

The demonstration of microorganisms in situ is an essential part of the pathologic evaluation of IE. In most cases of IE that come to surgery, the diagnosis has previously been established by

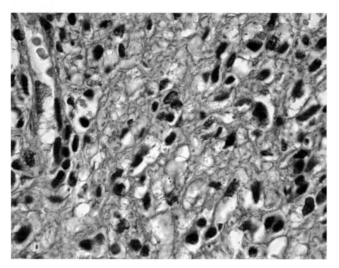

Figure 8-7. Histiocytic inflammation in *Coxiella burnetii* endocarditis. An area of scarring is seen adjacent to an infected prosthetic aortic valve sewing ring with foamy histiocytic inflammation (×400).

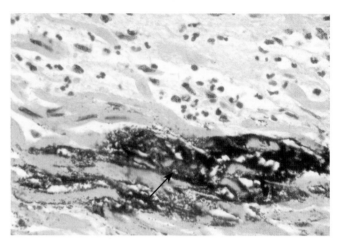

Figure 8-8. Tissue Gram stain of mitral vegetation. Brown-Hopps stain shows a colony of gram-positive cocci consistent with *Staphylococcus aureus*. Note the area of gram-variable staining *(arrow)* that could be mistaken for polymicrobial (mixed gram-positive and gram-negative) infection (×250).

blood culture and weeks of antibiotics have been administered before valve resection. It is incumbent on the surgical pathologist to be certain that the surgeon has properly cultured the infected tissue at the time of surgical excision. Rapid diagnosis may be enhanced by direct touch preparations of the vegetations and appropriate histochemical or immunohistochemical staining of organisms.

Microscopic examination of the valve must include an assessment of inflammatory activity and whether there are local structural complications, including tears, perforations, and myocardial extension. The minimal battery of histochemical stains includes a tissue Gram stain and a silver stain, such as Gomori methenamine silver (GMS). The tissue Gram stain demonstrates most gram-positive and gram-negative organisms, but some gram-negative organisms (e.g., *Legionella* spp.) require silver impregnation techniques. In addition, the phenomenon of variable staining of gram-positive organisms must not be mistakenly diagnosed as polymicrobial infection (Fig. 8-8). In cases that have been treated, and where the underlying valvular pathology includes dystrophic calcifications, it may be difficult to distinguish microcalcifications from bacteria, because both can stain positive on Gram and GMS stains. A positive von Kossa stain for calcium phosphate can help to exclude infection.

The GMS stain detects all gram-positive bacteria and some encapsulated gram-negatives (e.g., *Klebsiella*). In cases that have received antibiotic treatment, residual organisms may fail to stain with the tissue Gram stain but retain their GMS positivity. In those few cases in which it is impossible to decide whether the putative organisms are real or artifactual, the area of interest can be removed from the paraffin block and processed for ultrastructural examination. Most fungi are well visualized with hematoxylin and eosin (H&E) stain, but they are seen to better advantage with GMS. Screening for fungi should routinely include the GMS, because some fungal organisms (e.g., *Histoplasma capsulatum*) are not optimally visualized with periodic acid–Schiff (PAS) stain.

If a diagnosis of IE is clinically suspected but an organism has not been cultured, the pathologist must be prepared to

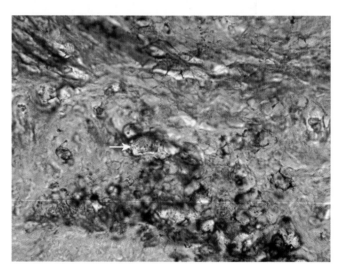

Figure 8-9. Silver impregnation (Warthin-Starry) stain in a case of *Coxiella burnetii* endocarditis. Warthin-Starry stain demonstrates small intracellular organisms *(arrow)* that proved to be *C. burnetii* by polymerase chain reaction assay (×250).

demonstrate the presence of organisms by other methods. Mycobacteria can be demonstrated with routine or modified Ziehl-Neelsen stains. The modified acid-fast stain (Fite or Putts) also detects *Nocardia* spp., *Rhodococcus equi*, and *Legionella micdadei.*

Silver impregnation techniques, including the Warthin-Starry, Steiner, and Dieterle stains, decorate all eubacteria, including mycobacteria and actinomycetes. However, the high background in these stains can preclude a confident diagnosis. All culture-negative cases of endocarditis should be examined by silver impregnation (Fig. 8-9). Other special stains, such as the Gimenez stain, have been used to demonstrate *C. burnetii*, and the Macchiavello stain can assist in detection of *Rickettsia* and *Chlamydia* species.

Ultrastructural examination is useful if there is morphologic suspicion of infection by light microscopic examination. Most microbes withstand processing for routine paraffin sections and

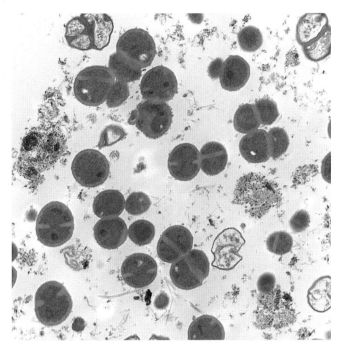

Figure 8-10. Ultrastructural appearance of gram-positive cocci from aortic valve endocarditis. The histologic appearance of a calcified infected valve was suspicious for bacteria, but a definitive diagnosis could not be established by light microscopy. Ultrastructural examination of a section of the paraffin block revealed diagnostic cocci (×7500).

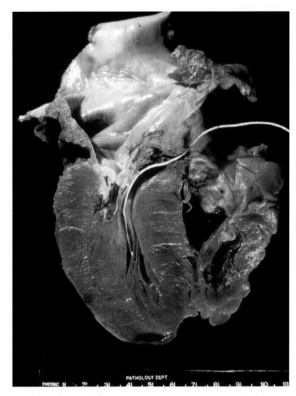

Figure 8-11. Fistulous tract complicating mitral valve endocarditis. Extension of infection from a vegetation of the mitral valve led to fistula formation between the left ventricle and right atrium. The patient died from acute right ventricular failure due to a large left-to-right shunt. A small thread illustrates the fistula.

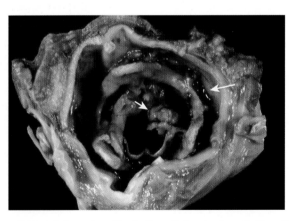

Figure 8-12. Infective endocarditis of a bioprosthetic valve. An aortic bioprosthesis shows vegetations bridging the cusps *(small arrow)* as well as involvement of the sewing ring that led to paravalvular insufficiency *(long arrow).*

can be identified with the electron microscope from the paraffin block (Fig. 8-10). Specific identification of microorganisms in situ can be achieved only by immunohistochemical or peptide nuclear agglutination techniques. Although antibodies to a wide variety of microbial agents have been developed, many are not commercially or widely available. In difficult cases, referrals to regional reference laboratories or to the Pathology Branch of the Centers for Disease Control and Prevention in Atlanta, Georgia, can help to establish the presence of an unusual pathogen.

Complications of Infective Endocarditis

Congestive heart failure is a major complication of IE. There are multiple pathways that lead to heart failure in IE, including valvular insufficiency, valvular stenosis, rupture of an infected fistulous tract, and conduction system abnormalities.

Valvular insufficiency is the most common complication of IE. It reflects either destruction of the valve by tears or penetrations, or loss of structural support by tethering of the chordae or the valve ring. In mechanical prosthetic valves, direct involvement of Silastic balls or metal discs and rings is unusual, but paravalvular leaks secondary to dehiscence of the sewing ring are common (Fig. 8-11). Vegetations may interfere with the mechanics of the valve during the cardiac cycle, leading to both stenosis and regurgitation.

Abscesses of the mitral valve can form fistulous tracts between the left ventricle and the right side of the heart (Fig. 8-12). Abscesses of the aortic sinuses of Valsalva can lead to fistulous tracts that communicate with the right atrium or right ventricle, leading to acute right heart failure due to massive

left-to-right shunting (Fig. 8-13). Periaortic valvular abscesses can extend directly into the adjacent atrioventricular node, causing conduction abnormalities of the atrioventricular node and fascicular block (Fig. 8-14).

Embolic Complications

Embolic complications are common in IE. Involvement of the tricuspid valve by virulent organisms such as *S. aureus* or *Candida* spp. is associated with bulky vegetations that fragment and travel

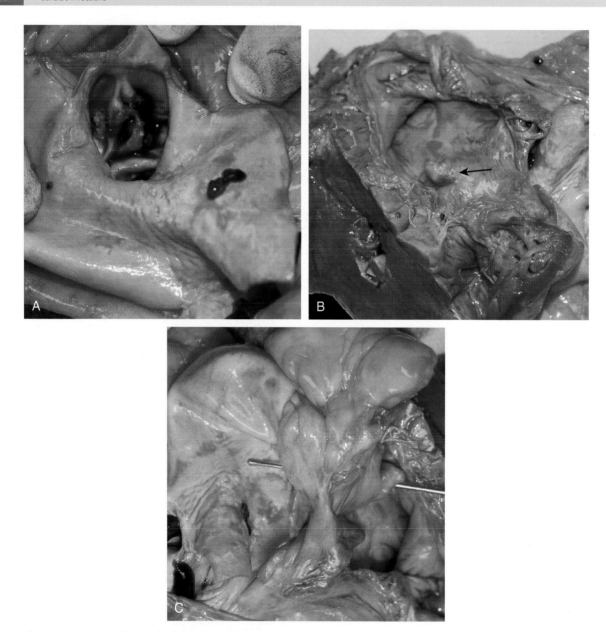

Figure 8-13. Rupture of sinus of Valsalva aneurysm (posterior noncoronary cusp) in a patient with methicillin-resistant *Staphylococcus aureus.* **A,** Aortic valve endocarditis led to an aneurysm of the noncoronary sinus of Valsalva, which ruptured acutely into the right atrium. **B,** The area of rupture appears as a small nubbin on the right atrial surface *(arrow).* **C,** The path of the fistulous tract is demonstrated by a probe.

to the lungs. Because vegetations are composed of both infected and bland fibrin-platelet excrescences, the result is potentially a mixture of bland pulmonary infarctions and septic pulmonary abscesses. Microthrombi can also travel through a patent foramen ovale to produce embolic complications on the left side of the circulation (Fig. 8-15).

Emboli on the left side can affect virtually any organ, but cerebral emboli are of greatest clinical concern (Fig. 8-16). Approximately 20% of patients with IE develop cerebral emboli, with an associated mortality rate of approximately 40%.[8] Hemorrhages and cotton-wool Roth spots reflect septic emboli to the microcirculation of the retina. Splenic emboli (Fig. 8-17) can cause flank pain or diaphragmatic irritation but may also be symptomatically silent. Renal microemboli produce a classic flea-

bitten appearance of the cortex with focal segmental necrosis of the glomerular tuft. Janeway lesions are caused by microemboli to skin, whereas Osler nodes are caused by arteriolar injury due to immune complex deposition. Septic emboli to the skin must be distinguished from other immune-mediated dermatoses such as Sweet syndrome (Fig. 8-18). Coronary artery emboli are uncommon and are most often a complication of prosthetic aortic valve endocarditis (Fig. 8-19). Microemboli to the myocardium can produce patchy areas of necrosis (Bracht-Wächter bodies), leading to myocardial dysfunction and congestive heart failure.

Immune Complex Disease
Circulating immune complexes are detected in the vast majority of patients with IE. Rheumatoid factor can be demonstrated in

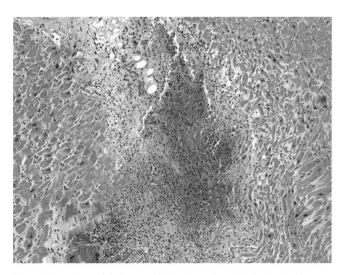

Figure 8-14. Myocardial abscess. Aortic valve endocarditis due to *Streptococcus pneumoniae* extended into the adjacent myocardium, leading to complete blockade of the atrioventricular node. Disrupted myocardial muscle cells surround a central abscess (×150).

50% of patients with endocarditis after 6 weeks of infection.[30] These circulating immune complexes include immunoglobulin, complement, and bacterial antigens.[31] Immune complexes cause arthritis, subungual splinter hemorrhages, and skin lesions.[32] In addition, the deposition of immune complexes leads to proliferative glomerulonephritis (Fig. 8-20) and renal failure. Mycotic aneurysms develop late in the course of IE and most likely reflect a combination of infective emboli and immune complex deposition that predisposes to aneurysmal dilatation and rupture of the affected vessel.

Lesions That Mimic Infective Endocarditis

Other disorders can mimic both the clinical and the pathologic findings of IE. Noninfective (bacterial) thrombotic endocarditis (NBTE) is caused by the presence of bland fibrin thrombi localized along the aortic and mitral valves. As opposed to the vegetations of IE that tend to involve any aspect of the valve cusp or ring, the lesions of NBTE are limited to the valve's lines of closure. On average, the vegetations of IE are larger than those

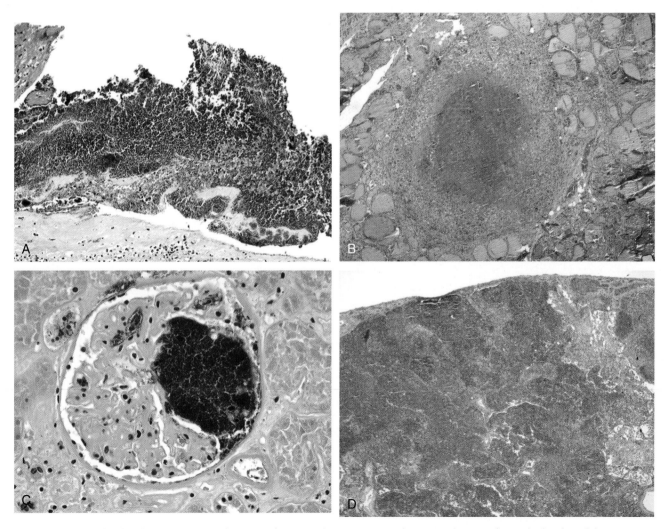

Figure 8-15. Tricuspid endocarditis in a patient with a patent foramen ovale. An intravenous drug user with HIV-1 infection developed *Staphylococcus aureus* endocarditis of the tricuspid valve (×250) **(A)**. At autopsy, infected lesions were found in thyroid (×200) **(B)**, kidney (×250) **(C)**, and lung (×150) **(D)**.

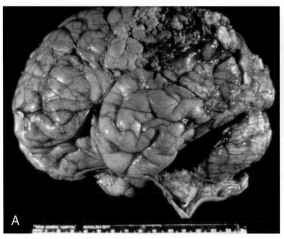
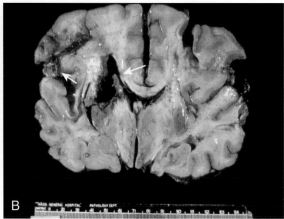

Figure 8-16. Bilateral acute cerebral embolic infarctions. A patient with *Staphylococcus aureus* aortic valve endocarditis developed acute hemiplegia and then rapidly lapsed into coma and died. **A,** The left cerebral hemisphere shows hemorrhagic infarction of the parietal, temporal, and occipital lobes. **B,** Coronal section shows hemorrhage in the left hemisphere *(black arrow)* with distortion of the lateral ventricle *(white arrow)* and dien cephalic displacement.

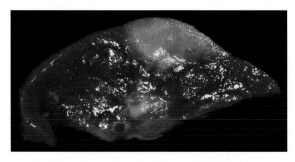

Figure 8-17. Splenic infarction. A pale subcapsular splenic infarction in a patient with *Streptococcus viridans* mitral endocarditis.

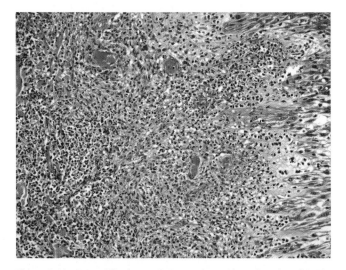

Figure 8-18. Neutrophilic dermatosis in a patient with aortic endocarditis. The patient was treated for *Staphylococcus aureus* aortic valve endocarditis for several weeks with clearance of bacteria from the blood and decreasing size of valvular vegetations by echocardiography. Subsequently, raised purpuric lesions developed on the extremities, with hematuria and increased serum creatinine. Skin biopsy shows a neutrophilic infiltrate with no organisms, consistent with Sweet syndrome. A kidney biopsy showed immunoglobulin A nephropathy attributed to antibiotics (not shown) (×250).

seen in NBTE, but these conditions cannot be distinguished based on size alone. NBTE represents a pathologic syndrome that is associated with carcinomatosis due to mucin-secreting malignancies, chronic infection, or the late stages of other wasting diseases (marantic endocarditis). The pathogenesis appears to reflect a hypercoagulable state in the absence of bacteremia.[33] The embolic complications of NBTE are comparable to those seen in IE (Fig. 8-21).

Other disorders, including rheumatic fever, Libman-Sacks endocarditis, and carcinoid syndrome can produce lesions on the cardiac valves that mimic IE. Libman-Sacks endocarditis affects the mitral valve and is seen in 50% of fatal cases of systemic lupus erythematosus (SLE). The vegetations are flat, cover both surfaces of the valve cusp, and often extend to the adjacent atrial and ventricular myocardium. Histologically, the valve shows fibrinoid necrosis (Fig. 8-22). The pulmonic and tricuspid valves may scar in response to a serotonin-secreting peripheral carcinoid. In the carcinoid syndrome, the pulmonic valve is either stenotic or incompetent, whereas insufficiency dominates with respect to the tricuspid valve. These findings are easily distinguished from vegetations but can be difficult to distinguish from previously treated IE.

Infectious Aneurysms

IE can complicate atherosclerotic aneurysms, and the outcome in the absence of aggressive medical and surgical intervention is invariably fatal. Infrarenal abdominal aortic aneurysms are most often affected, but any site is susceptible. Patients can present with the signs and symptoms of IE, or the disease can be clinically silent. Pain in the region of the aneurysm is an ominous sign, because it often heralds imminent rupture. Efforts should be made to sterilize the lesion with antibiotics, but the definitive treatment is surgical excision and must not be unduly delayed.

Pathologically, the lesions show infection at the base of a mural thrombus, with bacteria and acute inflammation that extends through the wall of the aneurysm (Fig. 8-23A). *Salmonella typhimurium* has an increased propensity to infect atherosclerotic plaques and produces a characteristic lesion with

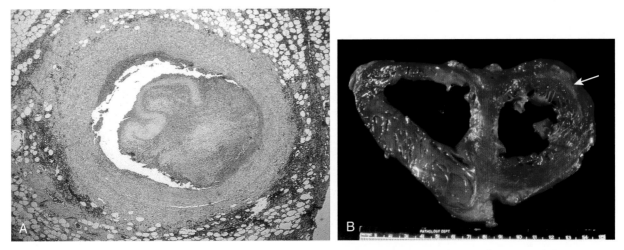

Figure 8-19. Coronary artery embolus resulting from vegetation of aortic valve. **A,** An infected embolus is seen in the circumflex artery. **B,** The heart at autopsy shows an acute myocardial infarction of the lateral wall of the left ventricle *(arrow)*, caused by the embolus.

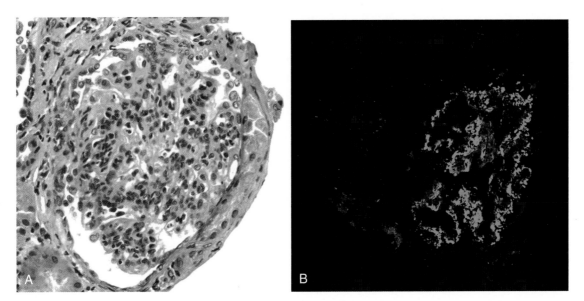

Figure 8-20. Immune-complex glomerulonephritis. A patient with *Streptococcus viridans* mitral endocarditis developed acute renal failure (×150). **A,** Kidney biopsy showed diffuse proliferative glomerulonephritis (×250). Direct immunofluorescence revealed granular deposition of immunoglobulin G **(B)** and complement C3 (not shown) (×250).

aggregates of histiocytes that may include bacilli, best demonstrated by silver impregnation (see Fig. 8-23B and C) Pseudoaneurysms may form in response to blood leakage from the vessel wall. Involvement of vascular grafts by IE mimics the features of prosthetic devices, with infection primarily targeting the areas of graft anastomoses. Pseudoaneurysm and graft rupture are dreaded complications. Septic emboli may lodge at sites distal to the graft, leading to infarction and abscess formation.

Treponema pallidum is the cause of syphilitic aortitis, which accounted for 1% of deaths in the United States between 1950 and 1965. Late syphilitic infections (tertiary syphilis) tend to involve the aortic valve and its ostia, as well as the ascending and transverse thoracic aortic arch. This results in aortic regurgitation and, rarely, aortic rupture.

Infection results from a characteristic spirochetal lymphoplasmacytic endarteritis that targets the vasa vasorum, yielding a thickened aortic wall with a gross "tree-bark" appearance. Microgummas with focal areas of acute necrosis can include viable spirochetes, best demonstrated with the Warthin-Starry silver impregnation stain. Clinically, the diagnosis is most often established by positive nontreponemal (Venereal Disease Research Laboratory [VDRL] test) or treponemal (fluorescent treponemal antibody [FTA] test) serology results; however, elderly patients may lack positive results on serologic studies.

Other infectious causes of aortitis are rare. Tuberculosis can involve both the thoracic and the abdominal aorta and usually results from contiguous spread of infection from the lung, a periaortic lymph node, or tuberculous osteomyelitis (Pott's disease). The pathology is that of necrotizing granulomatous inflammation and must be distinguished from other noninfective causes of granulomatous aortitis, including giant cell aortitis, sarcoidosis, and Wegener granulomatosis.

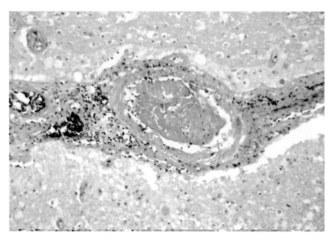

Figure 8-21. Cerebral embolus caused by noninfective thrombotic endocarditis of aortic valve. A patient with advanced carcinoma of the colon developed a lethal cerebral infarction. At autopsy, noninfective vegetations were seen along the lines of closure of the aortic valve, and a bland embolus was seen in the left carotid artery (×250).

Table 8-3 Etiologic Categories of Myocarditis
Infectious
Viral
Bacterial (including *Rickettsia* and *Chlamydia*)
Protozoal
Fungal
Parasitic
Noninfectious
Idiopathic
Giant cell myocarditis
Necrotizing eosinophilic myocarditis
Drug-induced myocarditis
Myocarditis associated with systemic disorders

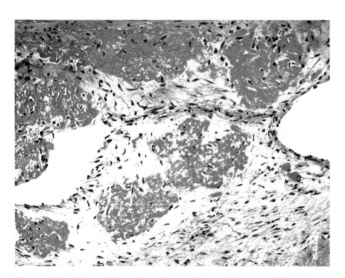

Figure 8-22. Libman-Sacks endocarditis. A 27-year-old woman died during an acute exacerbation of systemic lupus erythematosus. At autopsy, the mitral valve and surrounding endocardium showed small vegetations. Histologic examination showed the fibrinoid necrosis of the valve cusp that is characteristic of Libman-Sacks endocarditis (×250).

The Pathology of Myocarditis

Myocarditis can be simply defined as inflammation involving the myocardium. It is not surprising that there are numerous causes of myocarditis, both infectious and noninfectious. Although the definition seems rather clear and simple, the incidence, the diagnostic criteria, the pathogenesis, and the treatment of myocarditis continue to be debated. The clinical presentation of myocarditis is quite variable, ranging from nonspecific systemic symptoms to arrhythmias, restrictive cardiac physiology, and severe cardiac failure and sudden death, making a clear-cut clinical diagnosis difficult.[34]

The introduction of the endomyocardial biopsy should have made definitive pathologic diagnosis possible and reliable, but this promise was never realized because of a combination of sampling error and lack of agreement on diagnostic criteria (see later discussion). The variability of the clinical presentation, coupled with the difficulty of making the diagnosis, make the determination of the true incidence of myocarditis almost impossible. In selected populations studied prospectively, the incidence has been reported to be 8.6% to 12% in young adults with sudden death,[35,36] and it was identified as the cause of dilated cardiomyopathy in 9% to 16% of cases studied.[37-39] In an autopsy study of 12,000 people who died as a result of violence or accidents, the incidence of myocarditis was approximately 1%.[40] The true incidence in the general population is not known, but cardiac symptoms are frequently associated with viral infections; whether they represent evidence of myocardial inflammation is a matter of conjecture. With the use of molecular techniques, viral genomes have been identified in patients with left ventricular dysfunction [41,42] or other cardiac conditions,[43] lending further credence to the assumption that many cases of myocarditis are subclinical.

Etiology of Myocarditis

Table 8-3 summarizes the major causes of myocarditis. The following sections discuss the infectious causes in greater detail but also touch on the noninfectious ones, especially as they need to be considered in the differential diagnosis of infectious myocarditis. Before proceeding to the pathology of the specific diseases, it is necessary to discuss general criteria for the diagnosis of myocarditis, because they remain a source of controversy.

The Diagnosis of Myocarditis

Until the advent of the endomyocardial bioptome, myocarditis could be diagnosed with certainty only at autopsy. The gross appearance can be quite variable, including completely normal-appearing heart tissue; the presence of fibrinous pericarditis as part of a myo-pericarditis syndrome; an edematous and "stiff"

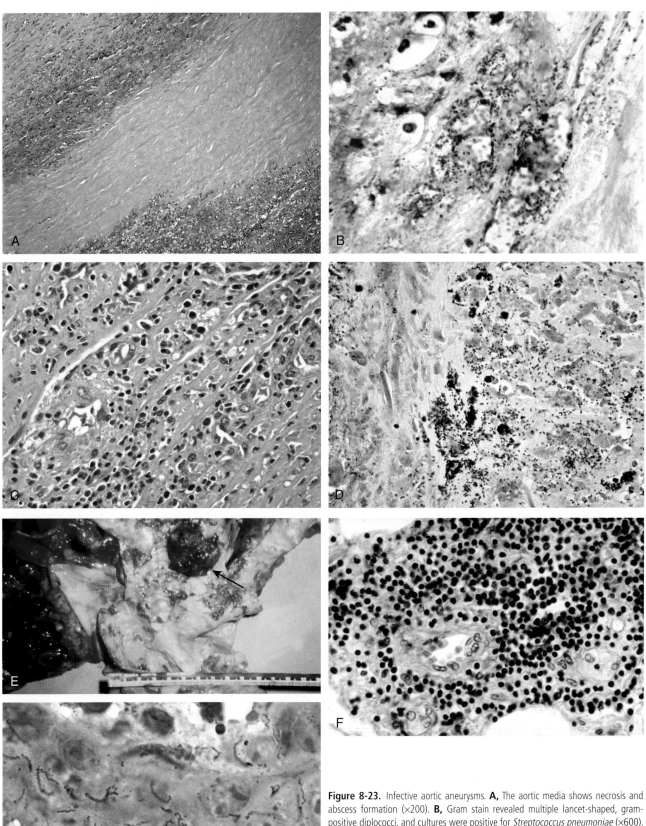

Figure 8-23. Infective aortic aneurysms. **A,** The aortic media shows necrosis and abscess formation (×200). **B,** Gram stain revealed multiple lancet-shaped, gram-positive diplococci, and cultures were positive for *Streptococcus pneumoniae* (×600). **C,** An aneurysm caused by *Salmonella typhimurium* showing characteristic histiocytic inflammation; bacilli were demonstrated **(D)** by silver impregnation (Steiner stain). **E,** Syphilitic aortitis grossly shows aneurysmal dilatation and thickening of the ascending aorta. Focal area of rupture *(arrow)* occurred secondary to superimposed *Escherichia coli* endocarditis, lymphoplasmacytic endarteritis **(F)** (×400), and focal persistence of *Treponema pallidum* spirochetes in aortic wall (×600) **(G).**

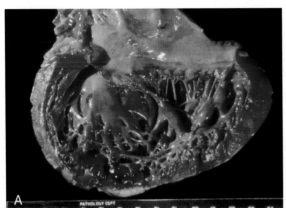
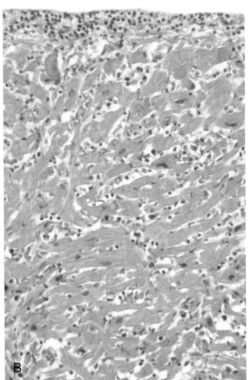

Figure 8-24. Lymphocytic (viral) myocarditis. This 11-year old boy died suddenly at home while at rest after having developed a viral syndrome 2 weeks earlier. The heart **(A)** was dilated and contained interventricular thrombi in both ventricles. Microscopic examination **(B)** revealed a diffuse lymphocytic myocarditis. The photomicrograph shows the prominent endocardial involvement typical of myocarditis, allowing it to be distinguished from ischemic injury, in which the endocardium does not show an inflammatory infiltrate (×250).

myocardium; and a "flabby," dilated heart with thin chamber walls and mural thrombi (Fig. 8-24).

The microscopic criteria for diagnosis of myocarditis in endomyocardial biopsies were established in 1986 at a cardiology meeting in Dallas, and they have been known since then as the Dallas criteria.[44,45] The Dallas criteria essentially divided myocarditis into two forms. An "active" form is characterized by an inflammatory infiltrate associated with myocyte damage not characteristic of ischemic injury. In the absence of myocyte injury, the diagnosis of "borderline" myocarditis should be made. The classification further suggested that pathologists semiquantify the inflammatory infiltrate (e.g., diffuse, multifocal, focal), describe the nature of the inflammatory infiltrate (e.g., lymphocytic, giant cell, eosinophilic, mixed), and remark on the absence or presence of fibrosis and its location (e.g., perivascular, interstitial, replacement).

Figure 8-25 illustrates examples of myocarditis in endomyocardial biopsy specimens. If repeat biopsies were performed, the Dallas classification called for the designation of the myocarditis as ongoing (persistent), resolving (healing), or resolved (healed). The classification served its purpose, to provide diagnostic consensus for a large multicenter myocarditis treatment trial,[46] but it has since been challenged by many authors as not being accurate enough based on sampling error,[47] interobserver variability,[48] or insufficient diagnostic criteria.[49,50] Suffice it to say that none of the proposed alternative classifications is in use, but molecular[43] and immunohistochemical techniques (Fig. 8-26) have clearly shown that the Dallas criteria may indeed underestimate the presence of myocarditis. Viral genome can be present

in myocardial tissue in the absence of histopathologic myocarditis in accordance with the Dallas criteria.

The recommended four to six biopsy specimens result in an unacceptable level of sampling error with standard histopathologic approaches[47]; probes directed at more generalized indicators of inflammatory myocardial disease have therefore been employed in the diagnosis of myocarditis. Immunologic markers for the induction of intercellular adhesion molecule 1 (ICAM1) have been shown to be positive in endomyocardial biopsy specimens from patients with suspected myocarditis when no inflammatory infiltrates were found.[51] However, such findings are not accepted as standard diagnostic criteria, despite the declaration of the demise of the Dallas criteria by some.[52]

The inflammatory infiltrate itself can be quite variable. In one single-institution study of 112 consecutive myocardial biopsies, lymphocytic myocarditis was diagnosed in 55% of the cases, granulomatous myocarditis in 10%, giant cell myocarditis in 6%, and eosinophilic myocarditis in 6%, whereas 22% of the biopsies showed borderline myocarditis.[53] Although the correlation is not perfect, the nature of the infiltrate can serve as a general guide to the cause of myocarditis.[54] Whereas all forms of myocarditis can be idiopathic,

- Lymphocytic infiltrates suggest viral, rickettsial, spirochetal, toxic, or immunologic causes;
- Neutrophils are more often seen in myocardial injury associated with ischemia, bacteria, catecholamine toxicity, or the early stages of viral infections;

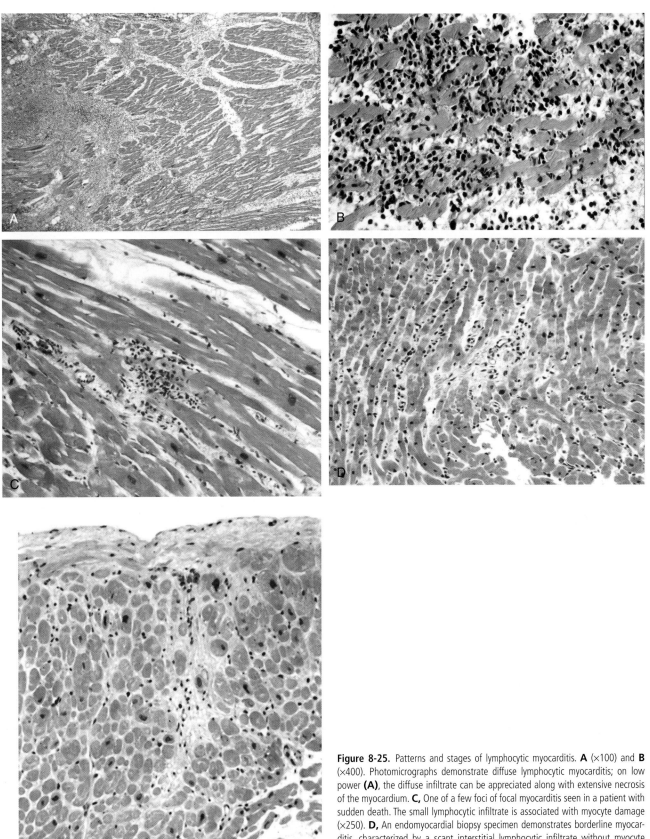

Figure 8-25. Patterns and stages of lymphocytic myocarditis. **A** (×100) and **B** (×400). Photomicrographs demonstrate diffuse lymphocytic myocarditis; on low power **(A)**, the diffuse infiltrate can be appreciated along with extensive necrosis of the myocardium. **C,** One of a few foci of focal myocarditis seen in a patient with sudden death. The small lymphocytic infiltrate is associated with myocyte damage (×250). **D,** An endomyocardial biopsy specimen demonstrates borderline myocarditis, characterized by a scant interstitial lymphocytic infiltrate without myocyte damage (see also Fig. 8-3) (×200). **E,** Resolved myocarditis in an endomyocardial biopsy specimen taken from a patient with a prior biopsy showing myocarditis. There is a small scar with rare remaining chronic inflammatory cells (×250).

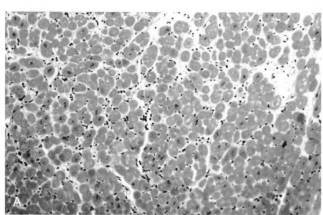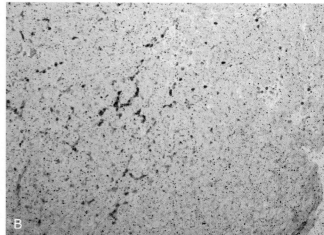

Figure 8-26. Borderline myocarditis. These photomicrographs show sections from the same endomyocardial biopsy specimen demonstrating borderline myocarditis (lymphocytic infiltrate without myocyte damage). Whereas the infiltrate can be appreciated in the H&E-stained section (×100) **(A)**, the section stained by the immunoperoxidase method using a reagent against CD3-positive cells **(B)** shows this infiltrate much more clearly (×100).

- Eosinophils are most frequently associated with eosinophilic myocarditis, hypersensitivity reactions, parasitic diseases, and general states of hypereosinophilia;
- Giant cells are seen in giant cell myocarditis, sarcoidosis, hypersensitivity myocarditis, rheumatic fever, and rheumatoid diseases.

The following is a description of the pathologic findings in the various causes of myocarditis, along with short discussions of the pathogenesis, where appropriate.

Viral Myocarditis

Virtually all classes of microorganisms have been shown to cause myocarditis.[55] Most of what we know about viral myocarditis comes from numerous experimental studies, the detailed discussion of which is beyond the scope of this chapter. Viruses that have been implicated in myocarditis include adenovirus, enteroviruses (e.g., Cocksackie B virus), hepatitis C virus, cytomegalovirus, varicella, and HIV. Although varicella and cytomegalovirus infections can show the characteristic cytopathic effects, the inflammatory infiltrate in viral myocarditis is typically lymphocytic. On the other hand, with molecular techniques, a viral etiology cannot be proved in most cases of lymphocytic myocarditis.[42]

Pathogenesis of Viral Myocarditis

Studies of the pathogenesis of viral myocarditis are ongoing, but experimental studies have shown several mechanisms ranging from direct cell damage to immunologically mediated effects. Numerous experimental studies have identified the role of CD4- and CD8-positive T cells, B cells, and cytokines (interleukin-1, interleukin-2, tumor necrosis factor, and interferon-γ) in initiation and continuation of the process of myocarditis. Recent studies have also shown the activation of inducible nitric oxide synthetase, which has mitigating effects in experimental viral

myocarditis.[56] Summarizing these studies, there are at least three stages and five mechanisms that can explain myocardial damage and inflammation in viral myocarditis[34,57]:

1. Direct invasion of myocytes by cardiotropic viruses, such as Cocksackie B virus, leading to myocyte damage and dysfunction and persistence of the viral genome in the myocardium

2. Cellular immune response directed at virus-associated antigens on the cell surface, resulting in a cellular infiltrate that includes natural killer cells and macrophages, followed by cytokine activation. CD8+ cells directed at virus-associated antigens on the myocyte surface are an additional constituent of the inflammatory infiltrate. Subsequent activation of CD4+ cells initiates the clonal expansion of B cells, leading to further cell damage, increased inflammation, and the production of anticardiac antibodies.

3. Autoimmunity (circulating antibodies and/or cellular mechanisms) directed at myocardial constituents has been shown to be present in many animal models and in human studies (Fig. 8-27).[58] The circulating antibodies that have been found are directed against myocyte constituents responsible for signal transduction, ion transport (calcium), and energy metabolism. The autoimmune mechanisms can be explained by three possible mechanisms[57]:
   a. Presence of self-antigens on infected cells
   b. Molecular mimicry (i.e., presence of self-antigens that cross-react with antigens on infected or noninfected cells)
   c. Epitope spreading (i.e., the expression of self-antigens in response to the infection on noninfected cells).

All those mechanisms could be present in one host, and they could in theory result in the development of chronic myocarditis. However, only mechanisms 1 through 3a require the persistence of virus in the cell; mechanisms 3b and 3c are independent of the presence of virus. These studies may explain why viral genome cannot be demonstrated in many cases of presumed viral myocarditis, and they may also explain why the response to viral and immunosuppressive treatments has been difficult to predict.

Several studies have shown[59-61] that patients with anticardiac antibodies responded better to immunosuppressive treatment than those without antibodies, whereas patients with demonstrable viral genetic materials responded worse than those without.

Bacterial Myocarditis

The majority of direct infections of the myocardium by bacteria occur in the setting of sepsis or septic emboli secondary to bacterial endocarditis. A common form of myocarditis caused by a bacterium is acute rheumatic fever, which represents an immunologic response to an infection by *Streptococcus pyogenes*, rather than direct infection of the myocardium. Although rheumatic fever declined significantly in the United States before 1977, there has been an increase in the incidence of the disease since then. Grossly, the presence of pericarditis and fibrinous vegeta-

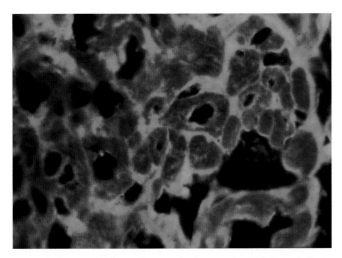

Figure 8-27. Anticardiac antibodies. In a frozen section of human myocardium stained by indirect immunofluorescence using the serum of a patient with biopsy-proved myocarditis, the presence of antibodies against sarcolemmal constituents is shown (×250).

tions on the line of closure of the valves may point one to the pancarditis of acute rheumatic fever, but the myocardium itself shows no gross features distinct from other forms of myocarditis. Microscopically, there is a multifocal granulomatous interstitial inflammatory infiltrate consisting of lymphocytes and giant cells arranged in characteristic Aschoff bodies (Fig. 8-28). Rarely, this pathology can be seen in endomyocardial biopsy samples, but atrial appendages removed at cardiac surgery more frequently show these lesions. The pathogenetic mechanisms relate to the cross-reactivity (autoimmunity) with cardiac antigens including myosin peptides, and the topic has been reviewed in detail in recent years.[62]

Borrelia burgdorferi, the agent responsible for Lyme disease in the United States, can cause a myocarditis characterized by a plasma cell infiltrate; the infectious agents can be demonstrated in the myocardium by silver stain.[63-65] Lymphocytic myocarditis is associated with rickettsial diseases such as Rocky Mountain spotted fever,[66] and chlamydial diseases such as psittacosis[67] have also been associated with acute myocarditis. The production of bacterial toxins (e.g., in diphtheria) may lead to a toxic myocarditis.

Parasitic Infections

In endemic areas of the world, *Trypanosoma cruzi*, the etiologic agent of Chagas disease, is one of the major causes of cardiac dysfunction, and its true incidence in the United States may be underestimated.[68] Grossly, Chagas disease is characterized by dilated ventricles, sometimes associated with apical aneurysms, and, not surprisingly, intracavitary thrombi leading to embolic complications. Microscopically, there is a diffuse lymphocytic myocarditis, associated with fibrosis and myocyte damage. In many patients, the conduction system is involved. Intracellular parasites (Fig. 8-29) can be demonstrated in myocardial biopsy samples but are often absent.

The pathogenesis of Chagas disease, not unlike that of viral myocarditis, is quite complex. Although cellular destruction due to invasion by the parasite and the associated inflammation is clearly the first step in Chagas disease, occasionally leading to

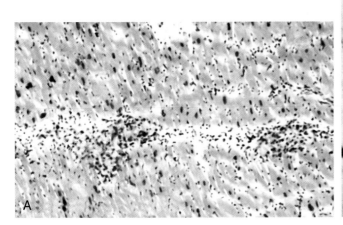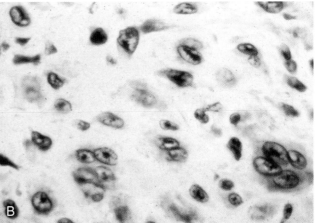

Figure 8-28. Acute rheumatic fever. The low-power photomicrograph **(A)** (×200) shows an interstitial inflammatory infiltrate with two ill-formed granulomas typical of Aschoff bodies. On high power **(B)**, the typical Aschoff cells can be seen, characterized by ample basophilic cytoplasm and ragged cell borders with open, often multiple nuclei (×400).

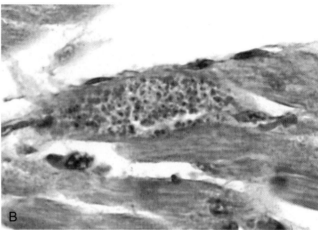
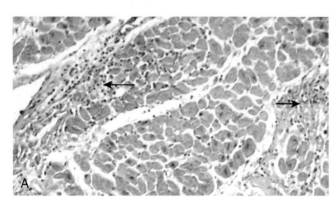

Figure 8-29. Myocarditis of Chagas disease. The low-power photomicrograph (×100) **(A)** shows multifocal myocarditis with areas of myocyte necrosis *(arrows)*. The intracellular *Trypanosoma cruzi* organisms can clearly be seen on high power **(B)**. Note that there is no inflammation surrounding the cell containing the organisms; the inflammatory infiltrate often does not correlate with foci of intracellular organisms (×400).

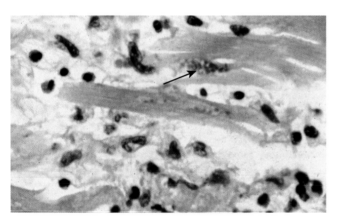

Figure 8-30. *Toxoplasma gondii* myocarditis. The intracellular organisms *(arrow)* are present in this endomyocardial biopsy from an immunosuppressed patient. The inflammatory infiltrate shows a prominent eosinophilic component (×400).

death during the acute phase, the development of the chronic form involves many more mechanisms,[69] including

1. Myocytolysis caused by the parasite
2. Secretion of a toxin by the parasite
3. Microvascular damage induced by the parasite, which leads to small infarcts and myocyte damage
4. T-cell response to persisting parasite antigens, which results in delayed hypersensitivity reaction, causing further damage
5. Polyclonal B-cell activation, which leads to immunosuppression or autoimmune mechanisms. Autoantibodies against myosin, actin, and laminin have been found in humans with Chagas disease.

As in viral myocarditis, a combination of these mechanisms may be active in myocardial damage and in the development of the chronic disease.

Other parasitic infections of the myocardium can be found in patients who are immunosuppressed, including those undergoing transplantation and patients with AIDS. *Toxoplasma gondii* is an intracellular organism (Fig. 8-30), whereas *Pneumocystis*

jiroveci organisms are present in the interstitium and characterized by a typical foamy exudate.[70,71] In many parts of the world, parasitic infestations are common and cause a generalized hypereosinophilic state, which can cause eosinophil-associated cardiomyopathy.

Fungal Myocarditis

Fungal myocarditis is almost always secondary to septicemia and septic emboli, and *Aspergillus*, *Candida*, and *Cryptococcus* species (Fig. 8-31) have all been demonstrated in the myocardium by the usual staining techniques.

Noninfectious Causes of Myocarditis

Idiopathic myocarditis is still the most common form of myocarditis, but there are other forms of noninfectious myocarditis that merit mention, including giant cell myocarditis, necrotizing eosinophilic myocarditis, drug-induced myocarditis, and myocarditis associated with systemic disorders.

Giant Cell Myocarditis

Giant cell myocarditis is a rare but fulminant and aggressive form of myocarditis, which occurs in young people and results in death or need for cardiac transplantation in 70% of cases.[72] Unlike in other forms of myocarditis, the diagnostic accuracy of endomyocardial biopsy in giant cell myocarditis is about 80%, presumably due to the extensive involvement of the heart. The infiltrate is composed of lymphocytes, eosinophils, and giant cells, and there is extensive myocyte destruction (see Fig. 8-34) It is most likely T cell–mediated, and the lymphocytic infiltrate consists of mostly CD8-positive cells.[73,74] Studies have shown that immunosuppressive treatments aimed at T-cell function (e.g., muromonab-CD3, cyclosporine, steroids) prolong survival.[75] The disease recurs in transplanted donor hearts in about one quarter of the cases, but the 5-year survival rate is still about 70%.

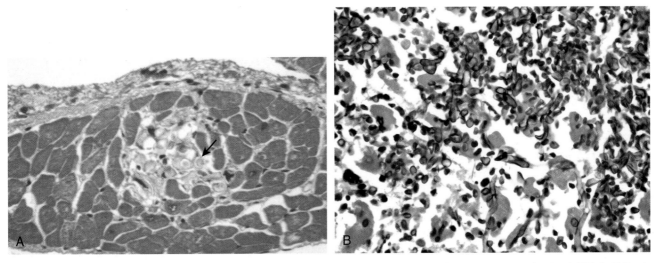

Figure 8-31. Fungal myocarditis. **A,** Cryptococcal yeast forms are present *(arrow)* in histiocytes in myocardium of an immunosuppressed patient (×200). **B,** GMS stain shows abundant yeast and pseudohyphae in patient with *Candida tropicalis* fungemia (×400).

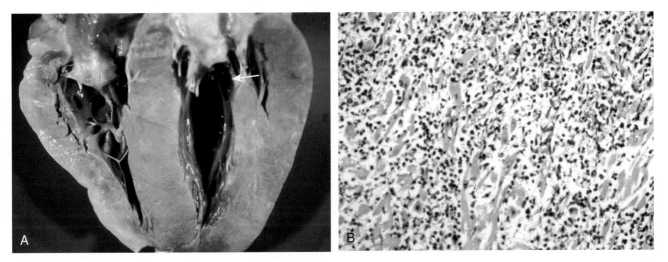

Figure 8-32. Necrotizing eosinophilic myocarditis. The gross photograph **(A)** shows the heart of a 26-year-old patient treated with antibiotics for endocarditis who died suddenly; residual vegetation is present on the mitral valve *(arrow).* The ventricular walls were stiff and thickened, and on microscopic examination **(B),** there was a diffuse myocarditis characterized by a prominent eosinophilic component and extensive myocyte necrosis (×250).

Necrotizing Eosinophilic Myocarditis

Necrotizing eosinophilic myocarditis is another rare but aggressive, often lethal, form of acute myocarditis that frequently occurs in young adults. It is often preceded by a viral syndrome but may occur as an aggressive form of hypersensitivity myocarditis at any age (see later discussion). The presenting symptoms are nonspecific, and patients often die of sudden death or rapidly deteriorating cardiac function, but occasionally they present with cardiac tamponade.[76] Grossly, the myocardium may be quite thickened due to extensive edema (Fig. 8-32A). Microscopically, the myocardium is infiltrated extensively by a mixed inflammatory infiltrate with a prominent eosinophilic component, extensive myocyte necrosis, and interstitial edema (see Fig. 8-32B). If the condition is diagnosed in time by biopsy, successful treatment with steroids is possible.[77]

Drug-Induced Myocarditis

Many drugs have been shown to cause various forms of myocarditis, and the list grows continuously. Many pathologic forms mimic infectious conditions, so a thorough drug history must be taken when determining the etiology of myocarditis. Table 8-4 summarizes the major cardiac effects, both inflammatory and noninflammatory, associated with drugs; a listing of the most common drugs can be found in recent publications.[34,54] The inflammatory forms are discussed in the following paragraphs.

Hypersensitivity Myocarditis

Many drugs have been implicated in the development of hypersensitivity myocarditis, the most common form of drug-induced myocarditis. It is characterized microscopically by a predominantly interstitial, mixed inflammatory infiltrate, with an exten-

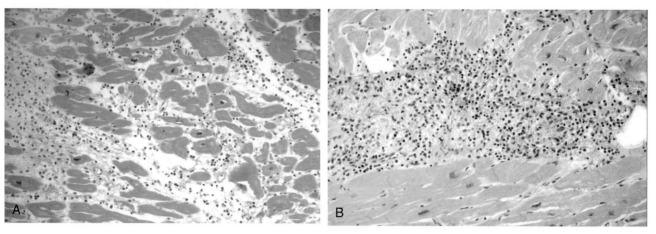

Figure 8-33. Hypersensitivity myocarditis. **A,** A diffuse interstitial inflammatory infiltrate consisting of mostly eosinophils associated with extensive interstitial edema (×250). **B,** A photomicrograph (×200) taken from a myocardial apex specimen removed at the time of placement of a left ventricular assist device. The patient had been receiving intravenous dobutamine, and the photograph shows a mixed interstitial infiltrate with histiocytes surrounding degenerating collagen fibers. Myocyte necrosis is absent in both specimens.

Table 8-4 Cardiac Effects Associated with Drugs

Inflammatory Forms

Inflammatory myocarditis
   Hypersensitivity myocarditis
   Toxic myocarditis
Vasculitis involving the myocardium
   Necrotizing
   Non-necrotizing
Lupus-like reactions
"Pressor lesions" (e.g., catecholamine effect; cocaine)

Noninflammatory Forms

Cardiomyopathy (e.g., Adriamycin)
Intracellular inclusions
Endocardial fibrosis

sive eosinophilic component, sometimes with giant cells and granulomas (Fig. 8-33) Originally, it was thought that myocyte necrosis needed to be absent to make the diagnosis of hypersensitivity myocarditis, but more recent studies and case reports[78] have shown that necrosis may be present and in some cases is quite extensive, resembling necrotizing eosinophilic myocarditis (see earlier discussion). Explanted recipient hearts have shown a high incidence of hypersensitivity myocarditis, and a particular preservative in intravenous dobutamine solutions was identified as the possible cause.[79] This lesion is associated with degenerating collagen bundles on microscopic examination.

Toxic Myocarditis
In contrast to hypersensitivity myocarditis, the lesions in toxic myocarditis are always associated with myocyte damage. The infiltrate is predominantly lymphocytic, admixed with neutrophils. With longer exposure to the toxic drug or toxin, new lesions are formed and older lesions heal. Therefore, the lesions in toxic myocarditis are of varying stages of development, with

active healing and healed (scarred) lesions being present in the same specimen.[80]

Other Inflammatory Forms of Drug-Related Myocarditis
Certain drugs can cause vasculitis syndromes, which can be either necrotizing or of the hypersensitivity type associated with a perivascular inflammatory infiltrate. These lesions may be found in the myocardium and may be confused with primary myocarditis.[81] Drugs that can cause lupus-like syndromes may also give rise to lupus-like lesions in the myocardium (see later discussion).

The cardiac effects of cocaine deserve special mention. Cocaine affects the heart in various ways. Its catecholamine-like effect can lead to microvascular spasm and platelet aggregation. Both mechanisms may lead to small foci of myocyte damage, associated with scant inflammatory infiltrates containing neutrophils and lymphocytes. Myocyte contraction bands are often seen in these lesions. Occasionally, cocaine can cause hypersensitivity myocarditis, with the inflammatory infiltrate containing eosinophils.[82,83]

Myocarditis Associated with Systemic Disorders

Sarcoidosis
Sarcoidosis is an idiopathic disorder that can mimic mycobacterial or fungal infection. Cardiac lesions are found in 25% to 50% of sarcoidosis patients at autopsy.[84,85] This may be an overestimation of cardiac involvement, because congestive failure and sudden death caused by cardiac sarcoidosis may lead to bias in an autopsy population. The hearts of patients with long-standing sarcoidosis show extensive scarring, particularly in the apices of both ventricles, the papillary muscles, and the upper portion of the interventricular septum. The latter often leads to abnormalities in cardiac conduction, because the atrioventricular node and the major branches of the conduction system are located in that region. Dilation of both ventricles is also found, because sarcoidosis can lead to congestive cardiomyopathy.

The hallmark of sarcoidosis on microscopic examination is the presence of noncaseating granulomas associated with a lymphocytic infiltrate and fibrosis. Early lesions of sarcoidosis may show very few giant cells and consist almost exclusively of lym-

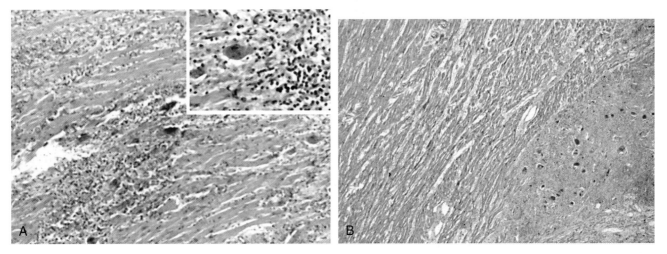

Figure 8-34. Giant cell myocarditis and sarcoidosis. Giant cell myocarditis (×250) **(A)** and sarcoidosis **(B)** can be distinguished by the more ill-defined and diffuse infiltration in giant cell myocarditis, compared with the more circumscribed lesions in sarcoidosis (×200). Myocyte necrosis is also much more extensive in giant cell myocarditis. Both lesions contain giant cells, and the inflammatory infiltrate of giant cell myocarditis is shown at higher power in the inset.

phocytes with little fibrosis. As lesions mature, fibrosis increases and lymphocytes decrease. Sarcoidosis may be diagnosed by endomyocardial biopsy, which has been shown to be useful in the treatment of patients with the disease.[86]

Because the natural history and treatment of sarcoidosis and giant cell myocarditis are quite different, it is important to outline and contrast the histopathologic features of these two conditions (Fig. 8-34).[73,74]

- The lesions of sarcoidosis are often rounded and have relatively sharp borders, whereas the inflammatory infiltrate of giant cell myocarditis is more infiltrative and quite diffuse.
- The predominant population of lymphocytes in sarcoidosis is made up of CD4-positive cells, whereas the lymphocyte population in giant cell myocarditis consists of mostly CD8-positive cells.
- Eosinophils are absent in sarcoidosis but are a prominent feature in giant cell myocarditis.
- Necrosis is extensive in giant cell myocarditis but is not prominent in sarcoidosis, whereas prominent fibrosis is a major feature of sarcoidosis.

Other Systemic Disorders

Many of the collagen vascular diseases can involve various parts of the cardiovascular system: pericardium, myocardium, valves, endocardium, and large and small vessels.[87] The discussion here highlights those that may manifest with myocarditis.

All layers of the heart may be involved in SLE. Fibrinous pericarditis is common, and valves may be involved by verrucous Libman-Sacks lesions. The myocardium may be involved in several ways. SLE causes a lymphocytic, presumably autoimmune, myocarditis; perivascular fibrinoid necrosis, when present, is characteristic of SLE myocarditis.[88,89] Because SLE can cause coronary arteritis, myocardial ischemia can result, which can be confused with myocarditis on pathologic examination. The development of anticardiolipin antibody is associated with SLE and causes microvascular thrombosis, which in turn can cause ischemic damage to the myocardium.[90]

Similar changes may be seen in thrombotic thrombocytopenic purpura (Fig. 8-35). Dermatomyositis/polymyositis can

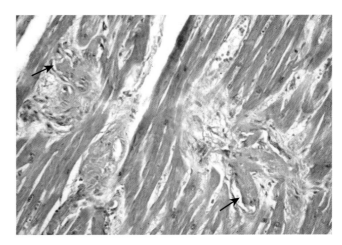

Figure 8-35. Thrombotic thrombocytopenic purpura. Multiple fibrin-platelet thrombi *(arrows)* are seen in small myocardial vessels. Although absent in this field, myocyte necrosis with inflammation is often present in these specimens secondary to small vessel occlusions (×250).

cause a lymphoplasmacytic myocarditis, and the inflammatory infiltrate of the myocarditis seen in Churg-Strauss syndrome contains CD83-positive cells.[91]

Kawasaki disease can involve all layers of the heart. Coronary arteritis is the best-known cardiac manifestation, occurring in 15% to 20% of untreated children. Although Kawasaki disease is most often not life-threatening, it is often associated with myocarditis. Early in the disease, the lesions are characterized by edema and lymphocytic infiltrates, but with time there is increasing development of fibrosis, especially concentric perivascular fibrosis, and abnormal configurations of myocytes (Fig. 8-36).[92]

Complications and Natural History of Myocarditis

Acute complications of myocarditis are sudden death, arrhythmias, and acute dilated cardiomyopathy. Large pericardial

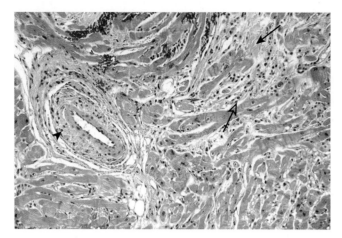

Figure 8-36. Myocarditis associated with Kawasaki disease. This endomyocardial biopsy (×250) from a young patient with a history of Kawasaki disease shows an inflammatory infiltrate associated with interstitial *(open arrow)*, perivascular *(arrowhead)*, and replacement *(solid arrow)* fibrosis.

effusions and pericarditis can be prominent features of the presentation.[93] Chronic sequelae relate to the development of congestive cardiomyopathy. Most patients recover completely or have mildly depressed cardiac function, but a small cohort of patients develop severe cardiac failure requiring transplantation. To date, there are no good clinical or histologic markers that allow reliable prediction of clinical outcome (except for giant cell myocarditis and necrotizing eosinophilic myocarditis). Five-year mortality rates in two series of patients presenting with cardiac dysfunction were about 50%[46,94]; the figure for giant cell myocarditis was less than 20%,[95] and the prognosis for HIV-associated myocarditis is equally dismal.[96] Despite multiple trials using a variety of immunosuppressive regimens, treatment remains mostly supportive.[34]

The Pathology of Pericarditis

Normal Pericardium

The normal pericardium is a fibroelastic sac surrounding the heart that consists of the visceral and parietal pericardium. The visceral pericardium is a simple layer of mesothelial cells covering the pericardium, and the parietal pericardium is a sac made of fibrous and elastic tissue, typically no more than 2 mm thick. It is very well innervated. The potential space between the two layers contains no more than 50 mL of serous fluid under normal circumstances. The pericardium restrains acute dilation of the cardiac chambers, but it accommodates to chronic dilation and fluid accumulation. Pericardial specimens are typically received as part of pericardiectomies to treat cardiac constriction.

Etiology of Pericarditis

More than 90% of cases of acute pericarditis are idiopathic or viral in origin. The remainder may have many causes, the majority of which are summarized in Table 8-5,[54,97,98] that require clinical correlation.[99] Microscopically, viral pericarditis, uremic

Table 8-5 Causes of Pericarditis

Infectious
Viral
Bacterial (including *Rickettsia* and *Chlamydia*)
Fungal
Noninfectious
Idiopathic
Uremia
Acute myocardial infarction (Dressler's syndrome)
Post-cardiac injury syndrome
Autoimmune diseases (e.g., rheumatoid arthritis, systemic lupus erythematosus, mixed connective tissue disease, Sjögren syndrome, Whipple disease, scleroderma)
Irradiation

Adapted from Aretz HT: The heart. In Mills SE, Carter D, Greenson JK, et al. (eds): Sternberg's Diagnostic Surgical Pathology, 4th ed. New York, Raven Press, 2003; and Bonfiglio T, Atwater E: Heart disease in patients with seropositive rheumatoid arthritis: A controlled autopsy study and review. Arch Intern Med 1969;124:714-719.

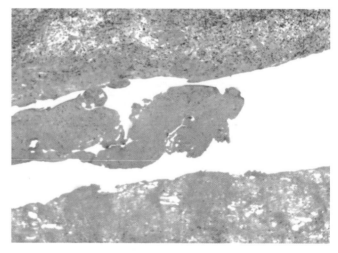

Figure 8-37. Exudative pericarditis. Pericardium shows fibrinous exudate with chronic inflammation and mesothelial hyperplasia (×150).

pericarditis, and the pericarditis associated with collagen vascular diseases are characterized by mesothelial hyperplasia, sometimes with extensive atypia, and a fibrinous exudate (Fig. 8-37). The cellular infiltrate consists of chronic inflammatory cells. Rheumatoid pericarditis rarely shows rheumatoid nodules.[100]

Bacterial pericarditis is caused by a variety of organisms, the most common of which are *Haemophilus influenzae*, meningococci, pneumococci, staphylococci, and streptococci. Microscopically, a purulent exudate and severe acute inflammation are seen. Bacterial pericarditis can be a result of bacteremia, but may also be caused by contiguous spread (e.g., pneumonia). The mortality rate is high, and pericardial drainage may be required in the acute phase.[101]

Tuberculous pericarditis accounts for fewer than 5% of cases of infectious pericarditis in the developed world, but it

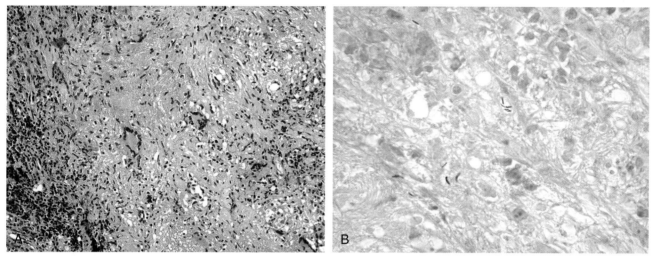

Figure 8-38. Tuberculous pericarditis. **A,** Pericardium showing granulomatous inflammation with multinucleated giant cells (×250). **B,** Mycobacteria are decorated by Ziehl-Neelsen stain (×400).

accounts for 50% to 70% of cases in sub-Saharan Africa.[102,103] It is much more common in HIV-infected patients in both settings. It can manifest as constrictive, constrictive-effusive, or effusive pericarditis.[104] The hallmarks of tuberculous pericarditis are the presence of caseating granulomas and demonstration of the tubercle bacillus (Fig. 8-38). If left untreated, it is fatal in more than half of patients and it leads to constrictive pericarditis in 30% to 50% of patients. Fungal pericarditis[105] occurs mostly in immune-compromised hosts or as part of endemic fungal infections (e.g., *Histoplasma, Coccidioides*); its lesions mimic those elsewhere.

Constrictive Chronic Pericarditis

The cause of constrictive pericarditis cannot be determined in most cases.[106] Except for the pericarditis associated with rheumatic fever and that associated with acute myocardial infarction, almost all forms of acute pericarditis can evolve into constrictive pericarditis. Fibrosis, often associated with calcifications and firm adhesions, can lead to significant constriction, as can loculated effusions.

REFERENCES

1. Harris S: Definitions and demographic characteristics. In Kaye D (ed): Infective Endocarditis. New York, Raven, 1990.
2. Durack D, Lukes A, Bright D: New criteria for diagnosis of infective endocarditis. Am J Med 1994;96:200-209.
3. Romano G, Carozza A, Della Corte A, et al. Native versus primary prosthetic valve endocarditis: Comparison of clinical features and long-term outcome in 353 patients. J Heart Valve Dis 2004;13:200-208.
4. Davis W, Gargusi VF: Human *Aeromonas* infection: A review of the literature and a case report of endocarditis. Medicine (Baltimore) 1978;57:267-277.
5. Pomerance A: Pathological and clinical study of calcification of the mitral valve ring. J Clin Pathol 1970;23:354-361.
6. Roberts W, Perloff J: Mitral valvular disease: A clinicopathological survey of the conditions causing the mitral valve to function abnormally. Ann Intern Med 1972;77:939-975.
7. Malquarti V, Saradarian W, Etienne J, et al: Prognosis of native valve infective endocarditis: A review of 253 cases. Eur Heart J 1984;5:11-20.
8. Chuangsuwanich T, Warnnissorn M, Leksrisakul P, et al: Pathology and etiology of 110 consecutively removed aortic valves. J Med Assoc Thai 2004;87:921-934.
9. Reisberg B: Infective endocarditis in the narcotic addict. Prog Cardiovasc Dis 1979;22:193-204.
10. Bruno R, Sacchi P, Filice G: Overview on the incidence and the characteristics of HIV-related opportunistic infections and neoplasms of the heart: Impact of highly active antiretroviral therapy. AIDS 2003;17(Suppl 1):S83-S87.
11. Devlin R, Andrews MM, Fordham von Reyn C: Recent trends in infective endocarditis: Influence of case definitions. Curr Opin Cardiol 2004;19:134-139.
12. Watanakunakorn C: Prosthetic valve endocarditis. Prog Cardiovasc Dis 1979;22:181-192.
13. Cacoub P, Leprince P, Nataf P, et al: Pacemaker infective endocarditis. Am J Cardiol 1998;82:480-484.
14. Herrmann M, Weyand M, Greshake B, et al: Left ventricular assist device infection is associated with increased mortality but is not a contraindication to transplantation. Circulation 1997;95:814-817.
15. Freedman L, Valone J: Experimental infective endocarditis. Prog Cardiovasc Dis 1979;22:169-180.
16. Durack D, Beeson P: Experimental bacterial endocarditis: I. Colonisation of a sterile vegetation: Survival of bacteria in endocardial vegetations. Br J Exp Pathol 1972;53:44-53.
17. Moreillon P, Que Y: Infective endocarditis. Lancet 2004;363:139-149.
18. Hall-Stoodley L, Costerton JW, Stoodley P: Bacterial biofilms: From the natural environment to infectious disease. Nat Rev 2004;2:95-105.
19. Sabet H, Edwards WD, Tazelaar HD, Daly RC: Congenitally bicuspid aortic valves: A surgical pathology study of 542 cases (1991 through 1996) and a literature review of 2,715 additional cases. Mayo Clin Proc 1999;74:14-26.
20. MacMahon S, Hickey AJ, Wilcken DE, et al: Risk of infective endocarditis in mitral valve prolapse with and without precordial systolic murmurs. Am J Cardiol 1987;59:105-108.
21. Fowler VG, Scheld WM, Bayer AS: Endocarditis and intravascular infections. In Mandell GL, Bennett GE, Dolin R (eds): Principles and Practice of Infectious Diseases, 6th ed. Philadelphia, Elsevier, 2005.

22. Bayliss R, et al: The microbiology and pathogenesis of infective endocarditis. Br Heart J 1983;50:513-519.

23. Sullivan N, Sutter VL, Mims MM, et al: Clinical aspects of bacteraemia after manipulation of the genitourinary tract. J Infect Dis 1973;127:49-55.

24. Wolff F, Regnier B, Witchitz S, et al: Pneumococcal endocarditis. Eur Heart J 1984;5:77-80.

25. Cohen P, Maguire J, Weinstein L: Infective endocarditis caused by gram-negative bacteria: A review of the literature, 1945-1977. Prog Cardiovasc Dis 1980;22:205-242.

26. Nahaas R, Weinstein MP, Bartels J, Gocke DJ: Infective endocarditis in intravenous drug users: A comparison of human immunodeficiency virus type 1-negative and -positive patients. J Infect Dis 1990;162:967-970.

27. Bruneval P, Choucair J, Paraf F, et al: Detection of fastidious bacteria in cardiac valves in cases of blood culture negative endocarditis. J Clin Pathol 2001;54:238-240.

28. Baca O: Pathogenesis of rickettsial infections: Emphasis on Q fever. Eur J Epidemiol 1991;7:222-228.

29. Bouvet A, Acar J: New bacteriological aspects of infective endocarditis. Eur Heart J 1984;5:45-48.

30. Williams RC, Kunkel HG: Rheumatoid factors and their disappearance following therapy in patients with SBE. Arthritis Rheum 1965;5:126-132.

31. Inman R, Redecha PB, Knechtle SJ, et al: Identification of bacterial antigens in circulating immune complexes of infective endocarditis. J Clin Invest 1982;70:271-280.

32. Bayer A, Theofilopoulos A: Immunopathogenetic aspects of infective endocarditis. Chest 1990;97:204-212.

33. Kim H, Suzuki M, Lie JT, Titus JL: Nonbacterial thrombotic endocarditis (NBTE) and disseminated intravascular coagulation (DIC): Autpsy study of 36 patients. Arch Pathol Lab Med 1977;101:65-68.

34. Magnani JW, Dec GW: Myocarditis: Current trends in diagnosis and treatment. Circulation 2006;113:876-890.

35. Fabre A, Sheppard MN: Sudden adult death syndrome and other non-ischaemic causes of sudden cardiac death. Heart 2006;92:316-320.

36. Doolan A, Langlois N, Semsarian C: Causes of sudden cardiac death in young Australians. Med J Aust 2004;180:110-112.

37. Felker GM, Hu W, Hare JM, et al: The spectrum of dilated cardiomyopathy: The Johns Hopkins experience with 1,278 patients. Medicine (Baltimore) 1999;79:270-283.

38. Felker GM, Thompson RE, Hare JM, et al: Underlying causes and long-term survival in patients with initially unexplained cardiomyopathy. N Engl J Med 2000;342:1077-1084.

39. Herskowitz A, Campbell S, Deckers J, et al: Demographic features and prevalence of idiopathic myocarditis in patients undergoing endomyocardial biopsy. Am J Cardiol 1993;71:982-986.

40. Gravanis MB, Sternby NH: Incidence of myocarditis: A 10-year autopsy study from Malmo, Sweden. Arch Pathol Lab Med 1991;115:390-392.

41. Pauschinger M, Bowles NE, Fuentes-Garcia FJ, et al: Detection of adenoviral genome in the myocardium of adult patients with idiopathic left ventricular dysfunction. Circulation 1999;99:1348-1354.

42. Bowles NE, Ni J, Kearney DL, et al: Detection of virus in myocardial tissues by polymerase chain reaction: Evidence of adenovirus as a common cause of myocarditis in children and adults. J Am Coll Cardiol 2003;42:466-472.

43. Baboonian C, Treasure T: Meta-analysis of the association of enteroviruses with human heart disease. Heart 1997;78:539-543.

44. Aretz HT, Billingham ME, Edwards WD, et al: Myocarditis: A histopathologic definition and classification. Am J Cardiovascular Pathol 1986;1:3-14.

45. Aretz HT: Myocarditis: The Dallas criteria. Hum Pathol 1987;19:619-624.

46. Mason JW, O'Connell JB, Herskowitz A, et al; for the Myocarditis Treatment Trial Investigators: A clinical trial of immunosuppressive therapy for myocarditis. N Engl J Med 1995;333:269-275.

47. Hauck AJ, Kearney DL, Edwards WD: Evaluation of postmortem endomyocardial biopsy specimens from 38 patients with lymphocytic myocarditis: Implications for role of sampling error. Mayo Clin Proc 1989;64:1235-1245.

48. Shanes JG, Ghali J, Billingham ME, et al: Interobserver variability in the pathologic interpretation of endomyocardial biopsy results. Circulation 1987;75:401-405.

49. Parrillo JE: Inflammatory cardiomyopathy (myocarditis): Which patients should be treated with anti-inflammatory therapy? Circulation 2001;104:4-6.

50. Lieberman EB, Hutchins GM, Herskowitz A, et al: Clinicopathologic description of myocarditis. J Am Cardiol 1991;18:1617-1626.

51. Wojnicz R, Nowalany-Kozielska E, Wodniecki J, et al: Immunohistological diagnosis of myocarditis: Potential role of sarcolemmal induction of the MHC and ICAM-1 in the detection of autoimmune mediated myocyte injury. Eur Heart J 1998;19:1564-1572.

52. Baughman KL: Diagnosis of myocarditis: Death of Dallas criteria. Circulation 2006;113:593-595.

53. Magnani JW, Danik HJ, Dec GW Jr, DiSalvo TG: Survival in biospy-proven myocarditis: A long-term retrospective analysis of the histopathological, clinical, and hemodynamic predictors. Am Heart J 2006;151:463-470.

54. Aretz HT: The heart. In Mills SE, Carter D, Greenson JK, et al. (eds): Sternberg's Diagnostic Surgical Pathology, 4th ed. New York, Raven, 2003.

55. Abelmann WH: Classification and natural history of primary myocardial disease. Progr Cardiovasc Dis 1984;27:73-94.

56. Zaragoza C, Ocampo C, Saura M, et al: The role of inducible nitric oxide synthase in the host response to cocksackievirus myocarditis. Proc Natl Acad Sci U S A 1998;95:2469-2474.

57. Fujinami RS, von Herrath MG, Christen U, Whitton JL: Molecular mimicry, bystander activation, or viral persistence: Infections and autoimmune disease. Clin Microbiol Rev 2006;19:80-94.

58. Pankuweit S, Portig I, Lottspeich F, Maisch B: Autoantibodies in sera of patients with myocarditis: Characterization of the corresponding proteins by isoelectric focusing and N-terminal sequence analysis. J Moll Cell Cardiol 1997;29:77-84.

59. Martino TA, Liu P, Petric M, Sole MJ: Enteroviral myocarditis and dilated cardiomyopathy: A review of clinical and experimental studies. In Rotbart HA (ed): Human Enteroviral Infections. Washington, DC, ASM Press, 1995.

60. Why HJ, Meany BT, Richardson PJ, et al: Clinical and prognostic significance of detection of enteroviral RNA in the myocardium of patients with myocarditis or dilated cardiomyopathy. Circulation 1994;89:2582-2589.

61. Frustaci A, Chimenti C, Calabrese F, et al: Immunosuppressive therapy for active lymphocytic myocarditis: Virological and immunologic profile of responders versus nonresponders. Circulation 2003;107:857-863.

62. Guilherme L, Kalil J: Rheumatic fever: From innate to acquired response. Ann N Y Acad Sci 2007;1107:426-433.

63. Steere AC, Batsford WP, Weinberg M, et al: Lyme carditis: Cardiac abnormalities of Lyme disease. Ann Intern Med 1980;93:8-16.

64. Marcus LC, Steere AC, Duray PH, et al: Fatal pancarditis in a patient with coexistent Lyme disease and babesiosis: Demonstration of spirochetes in the myocardium. Ann Intern Med 1985;103:374-376.

65. Olson LJ, Okafor EC, Clements IP: Cardiac involvement in Lyme disease: Manifestations and management. Mayo Clin Proc 1986;61:745-749.

66. Walker DH, Paletta CE, Cain BG: Pathogenesis of myocarditis in Rocky Mountain spotted fever. Arch Pathol Lab Med 1980;104:171-174.

67. Coll R, Horner I: Cardiac involvement in psittacosis. BMJ 1967;4:35-36.

68. Hagar JM, Rahimtoola SH: Chagas' heart disease in the United States. N Engl J Med 1991;325:763-768.

69. Engman DM, Leon JS: Pathogenesis of Chagas heart disease: Role of autoimmunity. Acta Tropica 2002;81:123-132.

70. Acierno LJ: Cardiac complications in acquired immunodeficiency syndrome (AIDS): A review. J Am Coll Cardiol 1989;13:1144-1154.

71. Lewis W, Grody WW: AIDS and the heart: Review and consideration of pathogenetic mechanisms. Cardiovasc Pathol 1992;1:53-64.

72. Giant cell myocarditis. Web site. Available at http://www.gcminfo.org/index.htm (accessed July 15, 2009).

73. Okura Y, Dec GW, Hare JM, et al: A clinical and histopathologic comparison of cardiac sarcoidosis and idiopathic giant cell myocarditis. J Am Coll Cardiol 2003;41:322-329.

74. Litovky SH, Burke AP, Virmani R: Giant cell myocarditis: An entity distinct from sarcoidosis characterized by multiphasic myocyte destruction by cytotoxic T-cells and histiocytic giant cells. Mod Pathol 1996;9:1126-1134.

75. Cooper LT: Giant cell myocarditis: Diagnosis and treatment. Herz 2000;25:291-298.

76. Kazama R, Okura Y, Hoyano M, et al: Therapeutic role of pericardiocentesis for acute necrotizing eosinophilic myocarditis with cardiac tamponade. Mayo Clin Proc 2003;78:901-907.

77. Watanabe N, Nakagawa S, Fukunaga T, et al: Acute necrotizing eosinophilic myocarditis successfully treated by high dose methylprednisolone. Jpn Circ J 2001;65:923-926.

78. Burke AP, Saenger J, Mullick F, Virmani R: Hypersensitivity myocarditis. Arch Pathol Lab Med 1991;115:764-769.

79. Spears GS: Eosinophilic explant carditis with eosinophilic hypersensitivity to dobutamine infusion. J Heart Lung Transplant 1995;14:755-760.

80. Billingham ME: Morphologic changes in drug-induced heart disease. In BristowMR (ed): Drug-Induced Heart Disease. Amsterdam, Elsevier/North-Holland Biomedical Press, 1980.

81. Mullick FG, McAllister HA Jr, Wagner BM, Fenoglio JJ Jr: Drug related vasculitis: Clinicopathologic correlations in 30 patients. Hum Pathol 1979;10:313-325.

82. Virmani R: Cocaine associated cardiovascular disease: Clinical and pathological aspects. NIDA Res Monogr 1991;108:220-229.

83. Kloner RA, Hale S, Alker K, Rezkalla S: The effects of acute and chronic cocaine use on the heart. Circulation 1992;85:407-419.

84. Ratner S, Fenoglio JJ Jr, Ursell PC: Utility of endomyocardial biopsy in the diagnosis of cardiac sarcoidosis. Chest 1986;90:528-533.

85. Perry A, Vuitel F: Causes of death in patients with sarcoidosis: A morphologic study of 28 autopsies with clinicopathologic correlation. Arch Pathol Lab Med 1995;119:167-172.

86. Lemery R, McGoon MD, Edwards WD: Cardiac sarcoidosis: A potentially treatable form of myocarditis. Mayo Clin Proc 1985;60:549-554.

87. Ferrans VJ, Rodriguez ER: Cardiovascular lesions in collagen-vascular diseases. Heart Vessels Suppl 1985;1:256-261.

88. Ansari A, Larson PH, Bates HD: Cardiovascular manifestations of systemic lupus erythematosus: Current perspective. Progr Cardiovasc Dis 1985;26:421-434.

89. Wijetunga M, Rockson S: Myocarditis in systemic lupus erythematosus. Am J Med 2002;113:419-423.

90. Greisman SG, Thayaparan RS, Goodwin TA, Lockshin MD: Occlusive vasculopathy in systemic lupus erythematosus: Association with anticardiolipin antibody. Arch Intern Med 1991;151:389-392.

91. Schoppet M, Pankuweit S, Maisch B: CD83+ dendritic cells in inflammatory infiltrates of Churg-Strauss myocarditis. Arch Pathol Lab Med 2003;127:98-101.

92. Takahashi M: Myocarditis in Kawasaki syndrome: A minor villain? Circulation 1989;79:1398-1400.

93. Abelmann WH, Aretz HT: Case records of the Massachusetts General Hospital: Case 20-1982. N Engl J Med 1982;306:1215-1223.

94. Grogan M, Redfield MM, Bailey KR, et al: Long-term outcome of patients with biopsy-proved myocarditis: Comparison with idiopathic dilated cardiomyopathy. J Am Coll Cardiol 1995;26:80-84.

95. Cooper LT, Berry GJ, Shabetai R; for the Multicenter Giant Cell Myocarditis Study Group Investigators: Idiopathic giant-cell myocarditis: Natural history and treatment. N Engl J Med 1997; 336:1860-1866.

96. Pulerwitz TC, Cappola TP, Felker GM, et al: Mortality in primary and secondary myocarditis. Am Heart J 2004;147:746-750.

97. Waller BF, Taliercio CP, Howard J, et al: Morphologic aspects of pericardial disease. Clin Cardiol 1992;15:203-209, 291-298.

98. Little WC, Freeman GL: Pericardial disease. Circulation 2006;113:1622-1632.

99. Oh KY, Shimizu M, Edwards WD, et al: Surgical pathology of the parietal pericardium: A study of 344 cases (1993-1999). Cardiovasc Pathol 2001;10:157-168.

100. Bonfiglio T, Atwater E: Heart disease in patients with seropositive rheumatoid arthritis: A controlled autopsy study and review. Arch Intern Med 1969;124:714-719.

101. Rubin RH, Moellering RC: Clinical, microbiological and therapeutic aspects of purulent pericarditis. Am J Med 1975;59:68-78.

102. Reuter H, Burgess LJ, Doubell AF: Epidemiology of pericardial effusions at a large academic hospital in South Africa. Epidemiol Infect 2005;133:393-399.

103. Cegielski JP, Lwakatare J, Dukes CS, et al: Tuberculous pericarditis in Tanzanian patients with and without HIV infection. Tuber Lung Dis 1994;75:429-434.

104. Mayosi BM, Burgess LJ, Doubell AF: Tuberculous pericarditis. Circulation 2005;112:3608-3616.

105. Maisch B, Seferovic PM, Ristic AD, et al: Guidelines on the diagnosis and management of pericardial diseases. The Task Force on the Diagnosis and Management of Pericardial Diseases of the European Society of Cardiology. European Society of Cardiology, 2004, 28 p. National Guideline Clearinghouse. Available at http://www.guideline.gov/summary/summary.aspx?doc_id=4960&nbr=3524&ss=6&xl=999 (accessed July 15, 2009).

106. Mambo NC: Diseases of the pericardium: Morphologic study of surgical specimens from 35 patients. Hum Pathol 1981;12:978-987.

Infections of the Gastrointestinal Tract

Gregory Lauwers, Mari-Mino-Kenudson, and Richard L. Kradin

Introduction

The surgical pathologist plays a key role in the diagnosis of gastrointestinal infection. Virtually all types of pathogenic microbes can cause gastrointestinal infection, so the diagnostic pathologist must be cognizant of their varied histologic manifestations and acquainted with the complex morphologic features of viruses, bacteria, fungi, and parasites. Because certain noninfectious inflammatory conditions can mimic infection, recognizing their at times subtle distinctions is a critical aspect of the surgical pathologist's charge.

Infections of the Esophagus

Bacteria

Bacterial infection of the esophagus is uncommon; it is usually seen in neutropenic patients or as infection extending from the lung. Most cases occur after epithelial injury by acid reflux or previous viral infection. Neutropenia secondary to hematologic malignancy, intensive chemotherapy, or bone marrow transplantation predisposes to bacterial esophagitis.[1,2] Approximately 15% of infectious esophagitis is seen in immunocompromised patients, but it is less common in patients with the acquired immunodeficiency syndrome (AIDS) than in the oncology setting because of the relative sparing of granulocyte counts in AIDS.[3]

Clinical symptoms include odynophagia, dysphagia, and retrosternal pain. Fever is reported in a minority of cases.[2,4] Endoscopic findings are nonspecific and include mucosal friability, pseudomembranes, plaques, and ulcerations. Significant complications include perforation, fistula formation, and sepsis.[5]

The most common bacterial agents involved in gastrointestinal infection belong to the normal flora of the mouth and upper respiratory tract, including *Staphylococcus aureus*, *Staphylococcus epidermidis*, *Streptococcus viridans*, and *Bacillus* species. Polymicrobial infection is common.

Bacterial infection evokes a marked neutrophilic exudate, cellular necrosis, and degeneration (Fig. 9-1). In severely neutropenic patients, ulcers and pseudomembranes without substantial acute inflammation can be seen. Most bacteria can be identified in tissue sections by light microscopy with tissue Gram stain and oil immersion optics. The diagnosis of bacterial esophagitis is based on the presence of confluent bacteria invading subepithelial tissues (see Fig. 9-1B).[2] Bacterial cultures of endoscopic biopsy samples are usually of little value due to bacterial contamination by the endoscope.

Mycobacterium tuberculosis

Esophageal tuberculosis is usually caused by extension of infection from contiguous organs or from miliary spread.

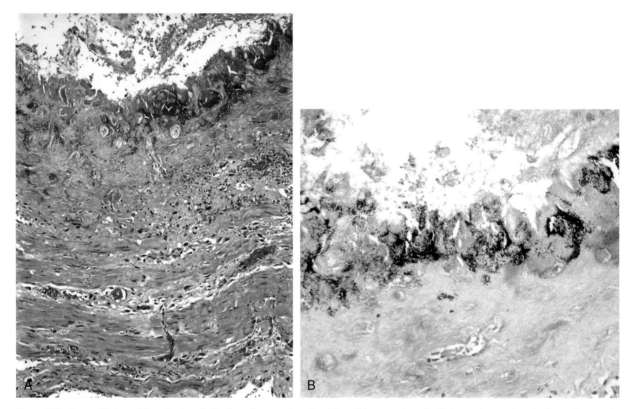

Figure 9-1. Nonspecific bacterial esophagitis. **A,** Esophageal mucosa is replaced by cellular necrosis and a fibrinopurulent exudate. **B,** Brown-Hopps stain highlights bacteria in subepithelial tissues. (Courtesy of Dr. Laura Lamps.)

Autopsy studies show esophageal involvement in 0.15% of patients dying with tuberculosis. Primary esophageal tuberculosis is extremely rare.[6-8] The most common symptoms of esophageal tuberculosis are dysphagia, weight loss, and retrosternal pain.[9] Imaging modalities may show extrinsic compression by involved lymph nodes in the mediastinum, traction diverticula, stricture, kinking of the esophagus, sinus or fistulous tract, and pseudotumoral masses.[10] Chest computed tomography and endoscopic ultrasonography reveal extrinsic nodular masses, consistent with mediastinal lymphadenopathy showing central hypodensity, rim enhancement, and calcification.[6,11] Endoscopic examination shows shallow ulcers with smooth border, a gray purulent base, and irregularly infiltrated edges.[12,13]

The differential diagnosis includes carcinoma, fungal infection, syphilis, and Crohn disease.[14] In some cases, no preoperative diagnosis is established before esophagectomy[15,16]; however, even if a developed stricture has formed, antimycobacterial treatment can successfully save the patient from a complex surgical intervention.[17]

The characteristic histologic features of esophageal tuberculosis include necrotizing, often confluent granulomas, which can be present at any level of the esophagus (Fig. 9-2). A rim of lymphocytes may be present at the periphery. In some cases, granulomas are sparse, or hyalinized and calcified. Acid-fast stains may demonstrate the organisms, but culture confirmation is often required.[18] Polymerase chain reaction (PCR) for *Mycobacterium tuberculosis* can be a rewarding diagnostic approach.[19-22]

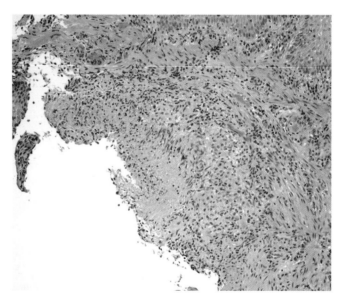

Figure 9-2. *Mycobacterium tuberculosis.* Caseating granuloma involving esophageal wall.

Other granulomatous conditions, including mycobacterial infection due to *Mycobacterium kansasii* or *Mycobacterium bovis*, fungal infection, and Crohn disease, should be excluded. Features favoring Crohn disease include the presence of transmural lymphoid aggregates with deep fistulas and fissures.

Table 9-1 Comparative Morphology of *Candida, Aspergillus,* and *Histoplasma* Species

Organisms	Morphologic Features
Candida albicans *Candida tropicalis*	Mixture of budding yeast and nonbranching pseudohyphae; occasional septate (true) hyphae
Candida glabrata	Budding yeast No hyphae No halo effect
Aspergillus species	Septate hyphae in uniform width True dichotomous branching with regular, acute angles
Histoplasma capsulatum	Intracellular Oval budding yeast with narrow-based buds Halo effect around organisms on H&E stain

H&E, hematoxylin and eosin.

Fungi

Fungal esophagitis is most frequently caused by *Candida* spp., but other pathogens, including *Histoplasma, Aspergillus, Cryptococcus, Coccidioides, Paracoccidioides, Trichosporon, Blastomyces,* and *Mucor,* can cause disease (Table 9-1). Fungal infection is often superimposed on other infections, and efforts at identifying all possible pathogens are mandatory to design optimal treatment. Debilitated and immunocompromised individuals are susceptible to fungal infections, and irradiation, chemotherapy, and chronic motility disorders are predisposing factors. Esophageal candidiasis is the most common cause of esophagitis in HIV-infected patients.[23,24]

Candidiasis

Candida albicans is a constituent of normal flora. Whereas it primarily affects patients with predisposing conditions, *Candida* esophagitis can occur in apparently normal hosts. A variety of *Candida* species are pathogenic, including *Candida glabrata, Candida parapsilosis, Candida tropicalis, Candida stellatoidea,* and *Candida krusei.* Of those, *C. tropicalis* tends to be more virulent, showing a propensity to invade submucosal blood vessels.[25] Patients with intact immunity usually develop inflammation at the infected site that limits penetration by the microorganisms.

Acute candidal esophagitis is the most common manifestation. Presenting symptoms are nonspecific and include odynophagia, dysphagia, and retrosternal chest pain. Esophageal bleeding, perforation, stricture, sinus formation (with secondary pulmonary abscess), extensive necrosis, and systemic invasion are rare.[26] Subacute candidal esophagitis is an uncommon disease that usually affects asymptomatic and immunocompetent patients, but it can cause esophageal strictures and pseudodiverticula. It typically follows an indolent course. Chronic candidal esophagitis is also rare and is usually seen as a feature of chronic mucocutaneous candidiasis. These patients usually have other

gastrointestinal manifestations, including malabsorption and loss of parietal cell function.[27]

Candidal infections can result in significant morbidity and death, especially in high-risk patients. Patients who receive radiation therapy to the thorax for lung or esophageal cancer or inhaled corticosteroid for asthma or chronic obstructive pulmonary disease are predisposed to candidal esophagitis.

Candidal infections yield small, yellow-white, raised plaques with surrounding erythema in mild disease—and confluent linear and nodular plaques or membranes covering a friable, erythematous, ulcerated mucosa in extensive disease—particularly in the middle and distal esophagus.[26] Erosion, ulcers, and strictures can develop. Fungi are densely adherent to the inflamed mucosa. In advanced disease, the esophagus may become stenotic and show mucosal irregularities. In chronic cases, umbilicated, wartlike lesions may develop. The gross features are easily confused with pseudodiverticulosis, varices, or carcinoma. Rarely, fungal esophagitis leads to a botryoid appearance resembling clusters of grapes projecting from the mucosa, and. mucosal bridges may form. In severe candidiasis, necrosis of the entire esophageal mucosa may be seen.[28]

Candida species are characterized by a mixture of blastoconidial spores, 3 to 4 µm in diameter, and nonbranching pseudohyphae that may become quite large, up to 2 µm in diameter. True septate hyphae can also be seen. These structures are best seen with Grocott methenamine silver (GMS) or periodic acid–Schiff (PAS) stain, and the presence of all of these structures is diagnostic of *Candida* infection (Fig. 9-3). Isolated budding yeasts without pseudohyphae or evidence of tissue invasion are often seen in inflammatory exudates at the ulcer bed; however, pseudohyphae or true hyphae are required for accurate diagnosis. Superficial colonization, particularly of nonviable tissue, does not necessarily indicate clinically significant disease. Whereas cytologic brushings from the plaques are more sensitive for fungal detection, biopsies are required to ascertain whether the fungus has invaded tissue. For this reason, it is important to indicate in the pathology report the types of fungal forms that are present (yeast, pseudohyphae, or both) and whether they are only seen in exudates or actually invade tissue.

Candida infections also mimic other fungal infections, such as aspergillosis and histoplasmosis. *Candida* spp. can be differentiated from *Aspergillus* based on the width of hyphae, the presence of acute-angle dichotomous branching by *Aspergillus* spp., and the presence of blastoconidia in *Candida* infection. The presence of pseudohyphae in *Candida* generally differentiates it from *Histoplasma capsulatum.* But if only yeast forms are identified, the differentiation of *Candida* from *Histoplasma* may be difficult. However, tissue Gram stain almost always decorates the gram-positive yeast forms of *Candida.*

Aspergillosis

Aspergillus, which is a ubiquitous fungus, rarely causes esophagitis.[29-32] Several species can infect the esophagus, including *Aspergillus fumigatus, Aspergillus niger,* and *Aspergillus flavus. Aspergillus* commonly colonizes immunocompromised patients[33-35] but can invade tissues and disseminate via the bloodstream, posing a life-threatening condition. Patients with esophageal aspergillosis present with painful or difficult swallowing and weight loss. Concurrent mucosal candidiasis may be present.

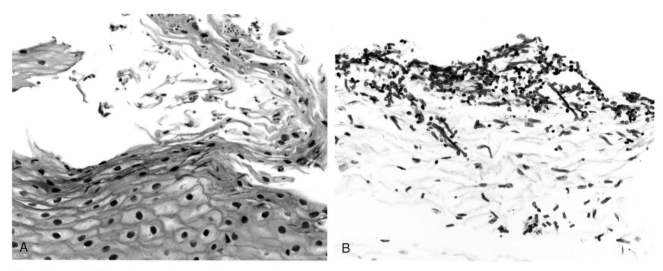

Figure 9-3. A, Candidal esophagitis is characterized by a mixture of spores and nonbranching pseudohyphae that invade the superficial layer of squamous epithelium. **B,** A PAS stain highlights the fungal elements.

Esophageal aspergillosis typically involves the mucosa and extends into the muscularis propria. When vascular invasion occurs, thrombosis and subsequent infarction may lead to perforation. Cytologically, *Aspergillus* is characterized by the presence of acute-angle branching septate hyphae with smooth, parallel walls, ranging in size from 2 to 4 mm in diameter. Characteristic conidiophores are rarely seen in this setting. *Aspergillus* can be differentiated from *Mucor* by its uniform thickness, mode of branching, and presence of frequent septation.

Other Fungal Infections

Blastomyces, Histoplasma, Mucor, and *Cryptococcus* species rarely involve the esophagus,[36] and usually only in patients with disseminated disease, but esophageal infection can arise from infections in contiguous structures, such as the lungs or mediastinum.[30] Patients with histoplasmosis can present with dysphagia resulting from esophageal compression by infected mediastinal lymph nodes or as a complication of mediastinal granuloma or sclerosing mediastinitis. Mediastinal granulomas can cause traction esophageal diverticuli.[36]

Viruses

Herpes Simplex Virus Types 1 and 2

Herpes infection may be seen throughout the gastrointestinal tract but is usually limited to squamous epithelium–lined structures (e.g., esophagus, anorectum). Herpes esophagitis has been reported with both herpes simplex virus type 1 (HSV-1) and HSV-2,[37,38] and it affects 0.5% to 6% of patients, primarily those who are immunocompromised due to AIDS, transplantation, or chemotherapy. However, immunocompetent adults and neonates also develop herpetic esophagitis.

Primary infections are common in neonates with disseminated HSV.[39] In adults, the disease typically manifests as a reactivation of latent disease. Usually, a previously healthy,

immunocompetent patient with a history of recurrent "cold sores" (i.e., nasolabial herpetic lesions) who presents with concurrent esophageal symptoms most likely has HSV esophagitis. In this setting, infections are self-limited. However, immunocompromised individuals may experience severe prolonged infections, and they are at risk for serious complications, including mucosal necrosis, hemorrhage, strictures, tracheobronchial fistula, and disseminated infection.[40]

The endoscopic appearance of HSV esophagitis varies with the time of infection. Early lesions consist of rounded, 1- to 3-mm, clear vesicles seen predominantly in the middle to distal esophagus. Subsequently, the epithelial roof is eroded to leave small, 1- to 3-mm ulcers. After most of the HSV-infected squamous cells have sloughed off, characteristic sharply demarcated ulcers with raised margins and a yellow-gray base are seen (Fig. 9-4). The uninvolved mucosa usually appears normal. If infection progresses, the ulcers may coalesce to produce inflammatory exudates that grossly resemble *Candida* esophagitis.[41-44]

Typical histologic findings include focal ulceration, neutrophils in the lamina propria, and an inflammatory exudate with sloughed necrotic squamous cells. Aggregates of macrophages near the ulcer are characteristic of the inflammatory response.[45] Diagnostic cytopathic changes include nuclear molding, multinucleated giant cells, ballooning degeneration, and eosinophilic type A intranuclear inclusions showing margination of chromatin (Fig. 9-5). Cowdry type B inclusions are more frequently seen than type A inclusions. The edge of the ulcer and the sloughed squamous cells are the best places to sample for identification of the characteristic cytopathic changes. Viral culture is more sensitive than microscopic examination for diagnosis of HSV infection, and the combination of directed brushings and biopsy specimens submitted for culture and histology improves the sensitivity of endoscopic diagnosis compared with biopsy alone.[46,47] Accurate diagnosis can be confirmed in situ by immunostaining with commercially available specific monoclonal antibodies.

The differential diagnosis of HSV esophagitis includes other viral infections such as cytomegalovirus (CMV) and varicella-zoster virus (VZV) infection. Their histologic features overlap, so immunostains and in situ hybridization are required to accurately distinguish them. It is important to distinguish HSV from other infections, because specific antimicrobial agents are required for effective treatment.

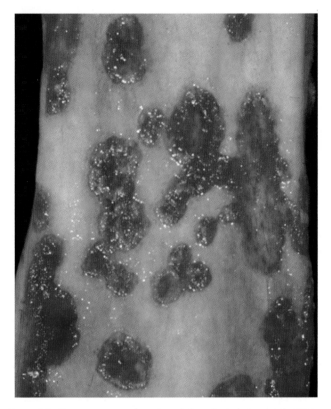

Figure 9-4. Gross appearance of esophageal ulcers due to herpes esophagitis in a patient with HIV infection. Numerous punched-out ulcers are present. (Courtesy of Dr. Rhonda Yantiss.)

Multinucleated squamous epithelial giant cells that are located predominantly in the proliferative basal and suprabasal zones of the preserved squamous epithelium have also been reported in the setting of reflux esophagitis, radiation therapy, and drug esophagitis. The epithelial giant cells may be confused with herpetic infection; however, the former typically lacks ground glass nuclear inclusions and peripheral condensation of chromatin at the nuclear membrane. The multinucleated cells in herpes esophagitis are generally more prominent in the superficial aspects of the epithelium and in luminal inflammatory debris. An immunostain for herpes virus antigen can help to exclude HSV infection.[48]

Cytomegalovirus

Because CMV infection is a systemic infection that involves multiple organs in addition to the esophagus, the clinical presentation of CMV esophagitis is often distinct. The onset of symptoms is more gradual than that of HSV esophagitis and includes fever, epigastric pain, nausea, vomiting, diarrhea, and weight loss, as opposed to the painful difficulties in swallowing and retrosternal pain commonly seen in HSV infection.[1,49,50] Endoscopically, CMV infection manifests as multiple, discrete, small, superficial ulcers in the middle or distal esophagus, but it may yield one or more large, flat, and elongated ulcers. Because HSV esophageal ulcers are rarely several centimeters in diameter, the presence of giant ulcers is suggestive of CMV esophagitis in patients with AIDS (Fig. 9-6A), although HIV-associated idiopathic ulcers may also become large.[51] Penetrating giant ulcers causing fistulas and pseudotumoral lesions may be seen in AIDS patients.[5] CMV esophagitis may coexist with both HSV and *Candida* infection in transplant recipients and in AIDS patients.[1,52]

CMV cytopathic effects typically develop in glandular epithelium, endothelial cells, and fibroblasts rather than in squamous cells (see Fig. 9-6). Therefore, superficial biopsy specimens that contain only squamous epithelium or brushings for cytology

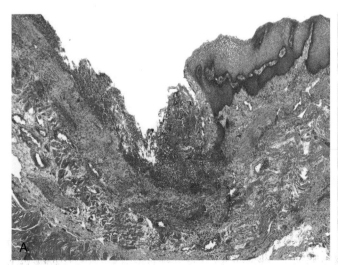

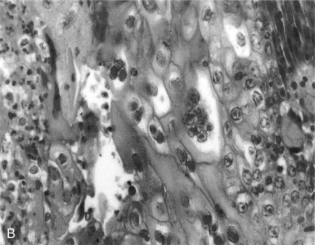

Figure 9-5. Herpes simplex virus (HSV) esophagitis. **A,** A resection specimen shows a sharply demarcated ulcer with raised margins. The ulcer bed is partially covered by inflammatory exudate that contains sloughed squamous cells. **B,** HSV cytopathic changes consist of nuclear molding, multinucleated giant cells, and type A intranuclear inclusions with margination of chromatin.

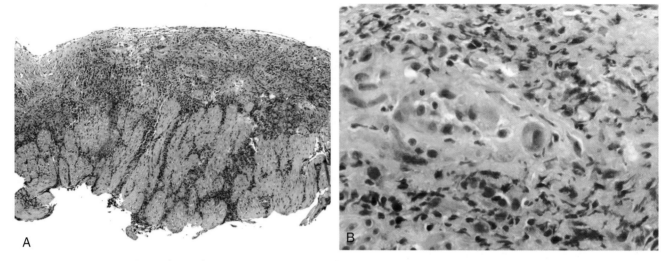

Figure 9-6. Cytomegalovirus (CMV) infection of esophagus. **A,** A mucosal biopsy from a large ulcer in a patient with AIDS demonstrates granulation tissue replacing lamina propria, as well as thickened and inflamed muscularis mucosae. **B,** High-power magnification reveals an endothelial cell with CMV cytopathic changes.

are usually insufficient for the evaluation of CMV infection, and it is recommended that biopsy include the granulation tissue of the ulcer bed. Classic cytopathic effects of CMV include intra-nuclear eosinophilic inclusions surrounded by a halo with margination of the chromatin to the nuclear membrane. In contrast to HSV and VZV, multiple small cytoplasmic inclusions may be seen with hematoxylin and eosin (H&E) stain, and to advantage with PAS and GMS. CMV can superinfect the ulcerations caused by HSV, and mixed infections are common in severely immuno-compromised individuals (Fig. 9-7). Immunohistochemistry with specific antibodies or genetic probing for virus may be necessary to establish the diagnosis, especially if the patient has received antiviral agents prophylactically, because such agents can inhibit nuclear cytopathic changes.

Other Viral Infections

Primary VZV infection (chickenpox) in immunocompromised children is often associated with severe visceral dissemination and has a mortality rate of 7% to 30%.[53,54] VZV esophagitis is rare and occurs in severely ill patients, but not in AIDS patients.[3] VZV cytopathic changes are seen in epithelium, endothelium, and stroma cells and are indistinguishable from those of HSV.[55] Cytoplasmic rarefaction and vacuolization of the infected cells, as well as dissociation of the basal layer from the lamina propria, may be observed. To differentiate VZV infection from HSV infection, immunohistochemical staining with specific monoclo-nal antibodies is required.

Esophageal infections with human papillomavirus (HPV) may manifest as erythematous macules, white plaques, nodules, exuberant frondlike lesions, or even ulcerations.[56-59] Large lesions can be mistaken for malignancy on endoscopic examination, and small lesions may be confused with glycogen acanthosis.[60] Koilo-cytotic changes in squamous epithelium are characteristic. As in the cervix and anus, HPV infection is associated with well-defined papillomas (condylomas) and with mucosal hyperplasia.

Epstein-Barr virus (EBV) esophagitis is infrequently reported but can be seen in otherwise healthy patients with infectious mononucleosis. These patients present with odynophagia and hematemesis and develop multiple small (3-5 mm) midesopha-geal ulcerations that are deep and linear, with erythematous rims and a gelatinous base.[61] Histologically, EBV-infected esophageal mucosa is comparable to oral hairy leukoplakia seen in AIDS patients; it is characterized by epithelial hyperplasia, parakerato-sis, and koilocytosis.[62,63] EBV infections confirmed by in situ hybridization are also seen in AIDS.[63]

Human Immunodeficiency Virus

Esophageal ulceration is an important cause of morbidity in patients with HIV/AIDS and may result from a variety of factors. A prospective study reported that 50% of esophageal ulcers in HIV-infected patients were caused by CMV infection, and about 40% were classified as idiopathic ulcers. Other causes included HSV infection, gastroesophageal reflux disease, and *Candida* infection. In 10% of patients, more than one etiology was dis-covered during long-term follow-up.[64] Acute seroconversion to HIV can produce multiple small esophageal ulcers with an intense inflammatory infiltrate. Based on the ultrastructural detection of viral-like particles in biopsy samples, it was hypoth-esized that HIV was responsible for the ulcerations in these individuals.[65,66]

Large idiopathic esophageal ulcerations have been docu-mented in 4% to 12% of HIV-infected patients with esophageal symptoms, especially those in late stages of AIDS.[52,67] A thor-ough evaluation for other infectious agents was unrevealing.[68] Some have suggested that HIV is causative, based on demonstra-tion of HIV by in situ hybridization[69] and positive immunohis-tochemistry and enzyme-linked immunosorbent assay (ELISA) for HIV p24 core protein in macrophages lining the ulcer-ations.[70,71] However, HIV PCR was also positive in the majority of the examined patients with CMV esophagitis, and HIV can be cultured in about 50% of esophageal specimens from other-wise asymptomatic HIV-infected patients,[72] raising doubt as to whether HIV is the cause of giant ulcerations. These patients may respond to systemic corticosteroid therapy,[69,71,73,74] but

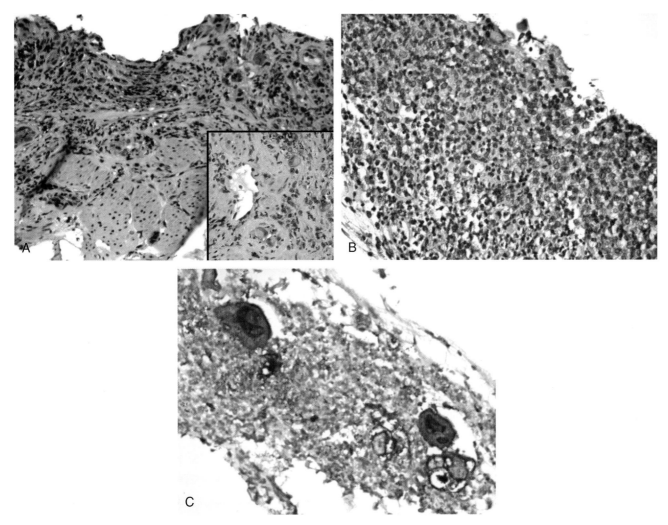

Figure 9-7. Mixed infection in a severely immunocompromised patient. The esophageal biopsy consisted of granulation tissue **(A),** with endothelial cells demonstrating characteristic cytomegalovirus cytopathic changes *(inset),* and detached fragment of fibrinopurulent exudate **(B). C,** Immunostain for herpes simplex virus (HSV) performed on deeper sections also revealed positive multinucleated cells consistent with HSV cytopathic changes.

treatment also predisposes patients to infectious complications (Table 9-2).

Infections of the Stomach

Given the protective mechanism of low ambient gastric pH, only a limited number of infectious agents can thrive in the stomach, usually as a result of a high infectious burden or specific evolved protective mechanisms. Not surprisingly, patients in immunodeficient states are at greater risk for infectious gastritis. Although *Helicobacter pylori* is the most common cause of infectious gastritis, other agents also cause disease (Table 9-3).

Viruses

Cytomegalovirus

Although CMV infection may occur in immunocompetent patients,[75] gastrointestinal CMV usually occurs in immunocom-

promised individuals due to malignant disease, iatrogenic immunosuppression, or AIDS.[76] In these settings, CMV infection can be life-threatening.

Clinical symptoms include epigastric pain, fever, and atypical lymphocytosis. Endoscopically, the gastric mucosa is congested and edematous, with multiple erosions and ulcerations.[77] A pattern of hypertrophic gastritis resembling Ménétrièr disease and associated with protein-losing gastropathy has been described.[78]

The biopsy specimens demonstrate mixed inflammatory infiltrates with characteristically enlarged endothelial, stromal, or epithelial cells showing diagnostic owl's-eye intranuclear inclusions. However, cytopathic changes can be difficult to identify, and multiple granular basophilic cytoplasmic inclusions may be seen instead.[79] It has been noted that inclusions are usually observed in the endothelial cells if the mucosa is not ulcerated. Alternatively, they are commonly seen in endothelial and stromal cells when the mucosa is ulcerated.[80]

Gastric involvement with HSV or VZV is rare. Reactivation of infection acquired at an early age is often the result of radiation therapy, chemotherapy, or malignancies in immunocompro-

Table 9-2 Viral Pathogens of Esophagus

Virus	Location	Macroscopic Features	Histology
HSV, VZV	Middle to distal esophagus not extending to stomach (usually involves squamous mucosa)	Multiple small, sharply demarcated and shallow ulcers	Epithelial ballooning and inclusions at ulcer edge; only inflamed granulation tissue in ulcer bed
CMV	Part of multiple organ involvement (stomach, intestine > esophagus)	Resembles HSV; occasionally one or more giant ulcers	Cytopathic effects involving endothelium, stromal cells, and/or submucosal glands; infection of squamous cells rarely seen
HPV	Esophagus occasionally involved	Normal, elevated lesions, or papillomas	Koilocytosis in squamous epithelium; condyloma, epithelial hyperplasia, or normal-appearing mucosa
EBV	Middle esophagus	Multiple small, deep, and linear ulcers	Similar to oral hairy leukoplakia; epithelial hyperplasia, parakeratosis, and koilocytosis
HIV	Esophageal involvement hard to document	Large ulcers or small ulcers resembling HSV	No specific changes

CMV, cytomegalovirus; EBV, Epstein-Barr virus; HIV, human immunodeficiency virus; HPV, human papillomavirus; HSV, herpes simplex virus; VSV, varicella-zoster virus.

mised patients.[81] Symptoms include nausea, vomiting, fever, chills, and fatigue. Gastroscopic examination shows multiple small ulcers, at times yielding a cobblestone appearance, with ulcerated plaques or linear superficial ulcers. Microscopic examination reveals epithelial cells with ground glass nuclei and eosinophilic intranuclear inclusions surrounded by a clear halo. Acute gastritis due to EBV has been reported but is rarely biopsied. The pathology is characterized by prominent lymphoid hyperplasia. Rare cases of acute measles gastric infection with giant cells of Warthin-Finkeldey type have been described.[82]

Bacteria

Acute Suppurative Gastritis and Emphysematous Gastritis

Acute suppurative gastritis is a rare disorder caused by bacterial infection of the submucosa and muscularis propria. In severe cases, necrotizing gastritis may result.[83] It is associated with ethanol abuse, upper respiratory tract infection, AIDS and other immunocompromised states, and infected peritoneal-jugular venous shunts; it rarely occurs as a complication of surgical biopsy.[84,85]

Patients are acutely ill with acute upper abdominal pain, peritonitis, purulent ascitic fluid, fever, and hypotension. Ultrasonography and CT may establish the diagnosis.[86] Gastroscopic examination reveals a thick and edematous gastric wall. The mucosa may be granular with a dark green exudate. The diagnosis is commonly delayed, and the mortality rate is high. Gastric resection combined with broad antibiotic therapy directed against the most common organisms is the treatment of choice.

Microscopic examination reveals an edematous submucosa with a brisk polymorphonuclear infiltrate and numerous gram-positive and gram-negative organisms. Offending organisms include streptococci as well as *S. aureus*, *Escherichia coli*, Enterobacteriaceae, and other gram-negative bacilli.[87] Intravascular thrombosis is common, and extensive mucosal and mural necrosis can be seen.

Emphysematous gastritis is a rare variant resulting from infection by gas-forming organisms, most commonly *Clostrid-*

ium perfringens, *E. coli*, *Streptococcus*, *Enterobacter*, and *Pseudomonas aeruginosa*. Predisposing factors include gastroduodenal surgery, ingestion of corrosive material, gastroenteritis, and gastrointestinal infarction. In most cases, radiographic studies show gas bubbles conforming to the contours of the stomach.

Mycobacterium tuberculosis

Since the introduction of pasteurization, gastric infection due to *M. tuberculosis* has been rare; it is currently associated with pulmonary tuberculosis. The patient commonly presents with abdominal pain, nausea and vomiting, fever, and weight loss.

Endoscopic examination may demonstrate multiple bleeding ulcers or erosions; a narrowed, deformed antrum; and possibly gastric outlet obstruction due to a thickened wall. Microscopic examination may show an ulcerated mucosa, but the presence of necrotizing granulomas is diagnostic. The presence of acid-fast bacilli (AFB) can be confirmed on acid-fast staining,[88] but PCR for *M. tuberculosis* can also be a contributory tool.

Although *Mycobacterium avium* complex (MAC) infection is common in AIDS patients, the stomach is rarely involved. Gastric MAC may be associated with refractory chronic ulcers. Presenting symptoms include fever, night sweats, anorexia, weight loss, diarrhea, and abdominal pain. Abdominal CT scans may show mesenteric lymphadenopathy.[89] Microscopic examination shows a lamina propria expanded by numerous foamy histiocytes. These aggregate in ill-formed, non-necrotizing granulomas. AFB, often numerous, can be highlighted by Ziehl-Neelsen or Fite stain.

Actinomycosis

Primary gastric actinomycosis is a rare, chronic, suppurative disease. Symptoms include fever, epigastric pain, and bleeding. The stomach reveals a large, ill-defined ulcerative mass that mimics malignancy. Histologically, collections of neutrophils and sinuses are seen. *Actinomyces,* a gram-positive, filamentous,

Table 9-3 Pathogens Associated with Infectious Gastritis

Etiology	Clinical Setting	Histology
Viruses		
Cytomegalovirus Herpes simplex virus Varicella-zoster virus	Immunocompromised patients • AIDS • Cancer • Immunosuppressive therapies	Erosive gastritis
Bacteria		
Streptococcus	• Large intake of alcohol • Upper respiratory tract infection, AIDS, and other immunocompromised states	Necrotizing gastritis
Escherichia coli Enterobacteriaceae *Staphylococcus aureus* *Mycobacterium tuberculosis*	Endemic area	Erosive and fibrosing gastritis with necrotizing granulomas
Helicobacter pylori *Helicobacter heilmannii*	General population	Chronic active gastritis
Mycobacterium avium Actinomyces Syphilis *Clostridium perfringens, E. coli, Streptococcus, Enterobacter, Pseudomonas aeruginosa*	AIDS Sexually transmitted disease • Gastroduodenal surgery • Corrosive material • Gastrointestinal infarction	Ill-formed granulomas Suppurative and mass-forming gastritis Diffuse inflammatory gastritis Emphysematous gastritis
Fungi		
Candida	• Cancer • Immunocompromised patient • Severe alcoholism • Corrosive gastritis	Aphthous, or linear ulcerations or even larger ulcers.
Histoplasma capsulatum Phycomycosis	• Cancer • Immunocompromised patient • Corrosive gastritis	Inflammatory mass. Ulceration and hemorrhagic necrosis
Parasites		
Cryptosporidiosis *Strongyloides stercoralis* Anisakiasis *Ascaris lumbricoides*	AIDS Immunosuppressed patient (e.g., AIDS, diabetes) Consumption of raw shellfish	Minimal inflammation Diffuse mucosal involvement Eosinophilic and granulomatous gastritis Gastric outlet obstruction

anaerobic bacterium, is best observed with a silver stain. The finding of sulfur granules containing long, filamentous, gram-positive bacilli is diagnostic.[90]

Syphilis

Syphilitic infection of the stomach is currently rare. Given the protean manifestations of this disease, gastric involvement in secondary or tertiary syphilis remains a diagnostic challenge. Endoscopic examination may show numerous shallow ulcerations with surrounding erythema, or a nodular mucosa with enlarged, thickened folds, suggestive of adenocarcinoma or lymphoma. Microscopic examination reveals severe gastritis with dense plasma cell infiltrates and varying numbers of neutrophils and lymphocytes. Gland destruction, vasculitis with endothelialitis, and ill-formed granulomas are seen. Warthin-Starry silver stain or modified Steiner stain may reveal numerous spirochetes.

However, in many cases, immunofluorescence studies and PCR are required to establish a definitive diagnosis (Figs. 9-8 and 9-9).[91]

Fungi

Fungal colonization of the stomach may be seen in patients with underlying malignancy or in immunocompromised patients treated with antibiotics or corticosteroids. *Candida* infection also occurs in alcoholic patients and in those who have ingested corrosive chemicals. The organisms can be found on H&E-stained sections but are more readily seen with PAS with diastase or silver stains. The mucosa shows multiple, aphthous, and linear ulcerations, or single or multiple larger ulcers. Microscopically, the superficially necrotic, fibrinopurulent mucosa is infiltrated by yeast and pseudohyphae.

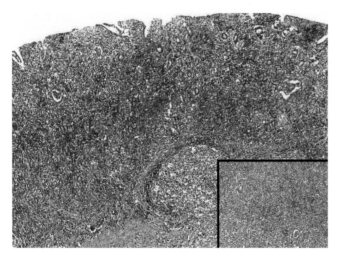

Figure 9-8. Syphilitic involvement of stomach. The mucosa is markedly thickened, and the normal architecture is effaced by a lymphoplasmacytic infiltrate *(inset)*.

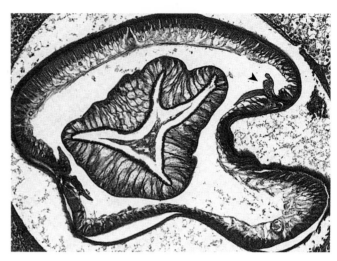

Figure 9-10. Anisakiasis. The helminth displays characteristic Y-shaped lateral cords *(arrowhead)*.

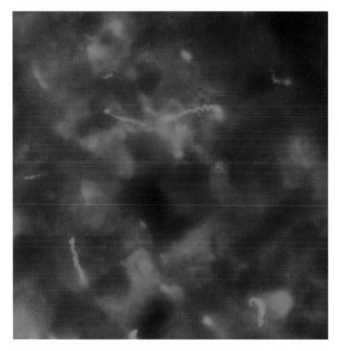

Figure 9-9. Syphilitic involvement of stomach. Immunofluorescence demonstrates numerous *Treponema pallidum*.

Fungal contamination of peptic gastric ulcer with *Candida* species is not uncommon and is likely of limited clinical significance, although it remains a matter of debate. These ulcers tend to be larger and are more often suspected of being malignant.[92]

Gastric histoplasmosis is a rare condition that manifests with hypertrophic gastric folds or masses mimicking adenocarcinoma. Biopsy shows intense infiltration by macrophages containing *H. capsulatum*. Fatal hemorrhage from gastric ulcer has been reported.[93]

Gastric phycomycosis is rare and highly lethal. It is classified as either invasive or noninvasive. The former type is characterized by deep invasion of the gastric wall and blood vessels. Ulceration and hemorrhagic necrosis of the mucosa and wall, with infiltrating pigmented nonseptate hyphae, are seen.[94]

Parasites

Gastric parasitic infections are rare and are reported in specific clinical settings. Cryptosporidiosis, for example, has been reported in AIDS patients.[95,96] The stomach is rarely affected by *Strongyloides stercoralis*, although colonization of peptic ulcers has been reported, and diffuse mucosal involvement may be seen in immunosuppressed patients. On biopsy, the parasite is easily identified infiltrating the mucosa.[97]

Gastric invasive anisakiasis is commonly acquired after ingestion of raw shellfish containing the nematode larvae of *Anisakis*, although cases caused by *Pseudoterranova* spp. have also been reported in the United States. Typically, patients present with epigastric pain as the parasite migrates into the gastric wall. Mild peripheral blood eosinophilia is not universal. Small hemorrhagic erosions are detected endoscopically, and microscopic examination shows either a phlegmonous reaction or an eosinophilic abscess with granulomatous features. The offending nematode larvae of *Anisakis* can be identified based on the presence of characteristic Y-shaped lateral cords and a Y-shaped intestinal lumen at midsection (Fig. 9-10).[98] The lateral cords of *Pseudoterranova* are characteristically butterfly-shaped. Both lack the lateral alae of *Ascaris* larvae.

Rare examples of gastric infection by *Ascaris lumbricoides* have been reported in association with outlet obstruction caused by adult worms.[99]

Helicobacter pylori–associated Chronic Gastritis

H. pylori is a gram-negative rod that has a propensity to infect the gastric mucosa. *H. pylori* are 3.5-μm long and generally comma-shaped or slightly spiral in form.[100] The infection is usually acquired in childhood and causes chronic gastritis if the organisms are not eradicated. The majority of infected patients carry and transmit *H. pylori* without any symptoms. The prevalence of the infection varies worldwide, ranging from less than 15% in some cohorts to almost 100% in underdeveloped countries.[101,102] Currently, despite a decrease of infection worldwide, at least 50% of the world's population is actively infected. The infection is transmitted by close personal contact.

H. pylori produces active and chronic gastritis. The lamina propria is expanded by a mononuclear cellular infiltrate, lymphocytes, and plasma cells, and lymphoid aggregates and follicles can also be seen (Figs. 9-11 and 9-12). If lymphoid inflammation is prominent, the term *follicular gastritis* has been adopted.[103] Normally, lymphocytes rarely enter the epithelium. Various degrees of neutrophilic infiltrate, reported as evidence of activity, may be seen. There are significant variations among infected individuals, based on host factors and the strain of infection.[104,105] *H. pylori* swim freely within the gastric mucus layer that overlays the apical side of the gastric surface cells, as well as in the foveolae.[105] In patients taking proton pump inhibitors, the organism translocates deep into the gastric glands (Fig. 9-13). Whereas *H. pylori*–induced damage is related to humoral and cell-mediated immune mechanisms, the morphologic activity varies significantly, from mild, with rare neutrophils seen, to severe, with glandular microabscesses.

H. pylori–associated chronic gastritis includes a heterogeneous group of clinical and pathologic changes. The most common phenotype observed at our institution is a mild antral gastritis or pangastritis with limited disruption of gastric acid secretion and usually no symptoms. A second syndrome, the duodenal ulcer phenotype, shows a marked antral gastritis with

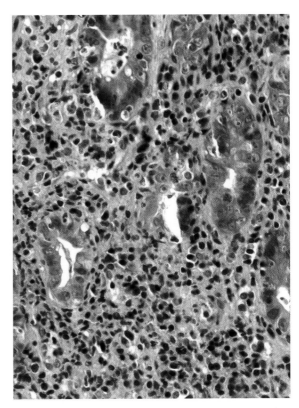

Figure 9-12. *Helicobacter pylori* gastritis. A dense lymphoplasmacytic infiltrate is seen around the foveolae, together with scattered neutrophils.

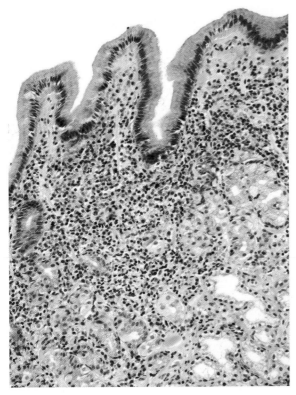

Figure 9-11. *Helicobacter pylori* infection. Low magnification of antral mucosa reveals a superficial band of dense chronic inflammation that is characteristic.

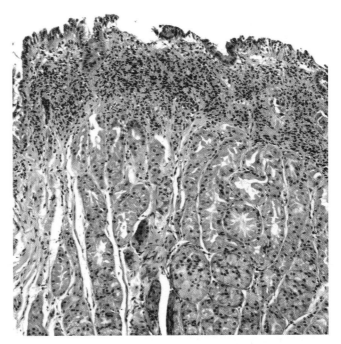

Figure 9-13. *Helicobacter pylori* infection of fundic mucosa. This is the characteristic appearance in a patient receiving proton pump inhibitor therapy without eradication of the bacteria.

high gastric secretion and preserved fundic mucosa. The patients commonly experience symptoms of duodenal ulceration.

Although about 10% of infected patients experience spontaneous regression,[106-108] in most cases gastritis progresses with time, yielding the gastric cancer phenotype. In this stage, the gastric mucosa typically undergoes changes that include glandular atrophy and intestinal metaplasia of the body fundus mucosa, accompanied by hypochlorhydria or achlorhydria. These changes increase the risk of gastric dysplasia and carcinoma. It has been calculated that patients with chronic atrophic gastritis have up to a 16-fold increased risk of developing gastric cancer. They are also at risk for development of mucosa-associated lymphoid tissue (MALT) lymphoma (extranodal marginal zone B-cell lymphoma).

In most cases, *H. pylori* can be identified in H&E-stained sections, although special stains (e.g., Giemsa, silver stains) and specific immunohistochemistry can aid in the detection of bacteria (Fig. 9-14).

Helicobacter heilmannii is a rare cause of diffuse, antral-predominant gastritis. The organism, in the past reported as *Gastrospirillum hominis*, is larger than *H. pylori* and shows corkscrew-like spirals. *H. heilmannii* infection has been associated with the development of MALT lymphoma but not with gastric cancer. Special stains used for *H. pylori* also highlight this organism (Fig. 9-15).[109-111]

Infections of the Small Bowel

Bacteria

Escherichia coli

Although most *E. coli* strains are harmless, some can cause serious food poisoning. The harmless strains belong to the

normal intestinal flora and benefit the host by producing vitamin K_2[112] or by preventing the establishment of pathogenic bacteria within the intestine.[113,114] Virulent strains of *E. coli* that can cause gastroenteritis are classified on the basis of serologic characteristics and virulence properties. These are enterotoxigenic *E. coli* (ETEC), enteropathogenic *E. coli* (EPEC), enteroaggregative *E. coli* (EAggEC), enteroadherent *E. coli* (EAEC), enteroinvasive *E. coli* (EIEC), and enterohemorrhagic *E. coli* (EHEC). Of these, ETEC and EAggEC are noninvasive and induce diarrhea by

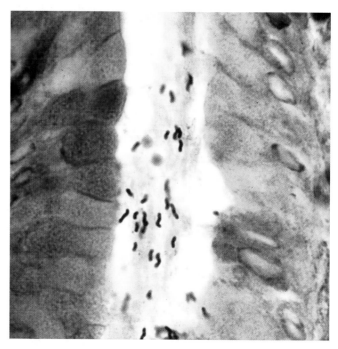

Figure 9-14. Silver stain demonstrating numerous curved *Helicobacter pylori*.

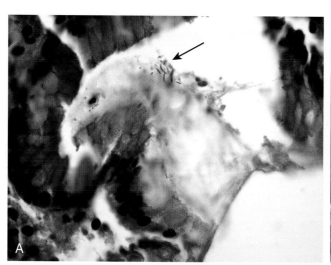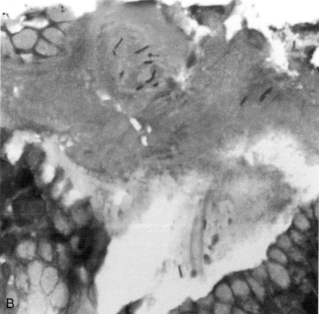

Figure 9-15. *Helicobacter heilmannii*. The thick, elongate, corkscrew bacteria are demonstrated in H&E-stained section (**A,** *arrow*) and with thiazine stain (**B**).

producing enterotoxins or a hemolysin or both. EAEC are non toxigenic and noninvasive[115]; they avidly adhere to the epithelial brush border by means of specific receptors. Therefore, the histology of the intestine in infected individuals is often normal. Conversely, EPEC, EIEC, and EHEC are invasive. ETEC, EPEC, EAggEC, and EAEC colonize the small intestine. EIEC and EHEC preferentially colonize the large intestine before causing diarrhea. In this section, only the histology of EPEC is described.

Enteropathogenic Escherichia coli

EPEC is a leading cause of infantile diarrhea in developing countries, and some types of EPEC are also an important cause of traveler's diarrhea. The mucosal biopsy reveals moderate to severe damage with irregular atrophy of surface epithelium and subnuclear vacuolization of crypt epithelium. Ultrastructural study reveals bacteria adherent to mucosal cells with flattening of microvilli, loss of the cellular terminal web, and cupping of the plasma membrane around individual bacteria—characteristic attachment–effacement lesions.[116]

Salmonella

Salmonella typhi usually causes a mild, self-limited illness, but the elderly, infants, and immunocompromised patients may develop a serious course with sepsis and death. Nontyphoid species (*Salmonella paratyphi*, *Salmonella enteritidis*, *Salmonella typhimurium*, *Salmonella muenchen*, *Salmonella anatum*, and *Salmonella give*) infections result in milder, self-limited gastroenteritis.

Based on a study that examined intestinal function and jejunal biopsy specimens obtained soon after the recovery phase from acute disease in 29 patients with *Salmonella* infection, normal or near-normal small-intestinal histology was seen in more than 90% of cases, despite defective absorption, which was transiently observed in 50%. The remaining patients developed partial villous blunting with increased inflammation in the lamina propria and surface epithelium associated with reactive epithelium.[117] If the disease manifests with severe gastrointestinal bleeding that requires surgical intervention, *Salmonella* spp. commonly involve the ileum and cecum. In these cases, the bowel wall is thickened, and the mucosa displays erosions and ulcers that can be aphthous, linear, discoid, or full thickness in nature (Fig. 9-16A). Perforation with or without fistula formation may be seen.[118]

Microscopically, there is ileal and cecal mucosal thickening resulting from a predominantly monocytic infiltrate. Low-power examination shows nodular and diffuse areas of infiltration, with the latter present predominantly at the center of the lesion (see Fig. 9-16B). The nodules are of two types. The first is a germinal center rimmed by a ragged and compressed mantle zone. The second and predominant type of nodule consists of uniform sheets of monocyte-macrophages with numerous apoptotic bodies and cellular debris, surrounded by small lymphocytes. The centers of these monocytic-rich foci consist of amorphous eosinophilic debris and degenerating cells.

The interfollicular and diffuse areas are replaced by phagocytic monocytes showing round to irregularly shaped nuclei and intermingled with small mature lymphocytes. Neutrophils are rare, even in the areas of mucosal ulceration. The inflammatory process breaches the muscularis propria and may extend into the serosa. Small mucosal erosions in uninvolved portions of the ileum reveal a predominantly lymphoid infiltrate with germinal center formation and clusters of monocyte-macrophages, most likely representing early lesions.[118]

The regional lymph nodes show a necrotizing lymphadenitis and marked sinusoidal and paracortical expansion due to a

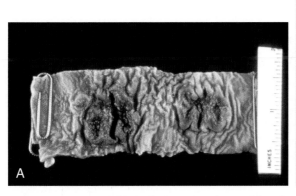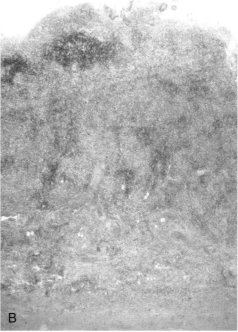

Figure 9-16. A, Opened, formalin-fixed specimen of terminal ileum from a patient with typhoid fever, showing ulceration of the Peyer patches. **B,** Low-power magnification of the ileum reveals diffuse inflammatory infiltrate transmurally involving the intestinal wall with surface ulceration, as well as nodular lymphoid aggregates.

proliferation of monocyte-macrophages identical to those seen in the intestine. Subcapsular sinuses are distended by monocytes but may be compressed or obliterated. Actively phagocytic macrophages are seen, many containing intracellular apoptotic bodies and cell fragments. The necrotic foci tend to be rounded and rimmed by foamy macrophages that blend smoothly with the reminder of the node.[118]

The closest mimic of *S. typhi* enterocolitis is *Yersinia* infection.[119-121] In both lesions, the terminal ileal mucosa and mesenteric lymph nodes are distorted by lymphoid and histiocytic hyperplasia; however, deep, penetrating ulcers and abundant epithelioid granulomas are characteristic features of *Yersinia* infections and not of *S. typhi* enterocolitis.

Also in the differential diagnosis, especially of the nodal involvement, are histiocytic necrotizing lymphadenitis (Kikuchi-Fujimoto disease) and sinus histiocytosis with massive lymphadenopathy (Rosai-Dorfman disease). These entities; however, rarely involve the intestine in a primary fashion.[118]

Vibrio

Eleven *Vibrio* species are recognized to cause human infection.[122-127] Infection with *Vibrio cholerae* results in cholera, an important cause of watery diarrhea and dysentery that may lead to significant dehydration and death. Although the disease is widespread, the role of intestinal biopsy is limited, because *V. cholerae* is a noninvasive, toxin-producing organism that causes minimal or no histologic changes. The intestinal mucosa appears to be intact, with mucin-depleted, dilated crypts in a background of edematous lamina propria with vascular dilatation and no significant inflammation. Ultrastructural examination reveals widening of the intercellular spaces and alteration of apical junctional complexes prominently in the villus epithelium, whereas blebbing of the microvillus border and mitochondrial changes occur in the crypt epithelium. The extent of the changes correlates with clinical severity.[128]

Clostridium

Clostridial infections are discussed more extensively in the infectious colitis section. Only a unique form of clostridial infection of the small intestine, enteritis necroticans, is discussed here.

Enteritis necroticans is a life-threatening infectious disease caused by *C. perfringens*, type C, a β-toxin–producing strain. It is characterized by segmental necrosis of the proximal jejunum and a high mortality rate if not diagnosed early and appropriately treated. In addition to antibiotics, advanced cases require surgical resection of necrotic bowel. The disease was first reported as Darmbrand (burnt bowels) in Northern Germany after World War II, where starved children and adults developed it after ingestion of large meals of meats and vegetables. It was prevalent between 1944 and 1948 but then disappeared in Europe as the nutritional status of its population improved. In 1963, a similar disease was reported from the Highlands of Papua New Guinea, where predominantly male children and young adults presented with severe abdominal pain after ceremonial feasting on large amounts of sweet potatoes and inadequately cooked pork contaminated with pig intestine. It was termed "pigbel," a pidgin English term for abdominal pain following a pig feast. Nowadays, enteritis necroticans is rarely seen in developed countries,

and the majority of affected subjects are diabetics.[129,130] An impaired ability to degrade exogenous toxins due to decreased secretion of pancreatic protease in diabetics and individuals on low-protein diets, or the presence of natural protease inhibitors in sweet potato or soybean flour, together with delayed transit through the small intestine, may contribute to this unique form of clostridial infection.[129]

Histopathologically, the lesion starts abruptly in the proximal jejunum and usually extends distally to the ileum and cecum. Affected bowel segments are dilated, edematous, markedly congested, and thickened. Unaffected skip segments may be seen. Sloughing of the necrotic mucosa leaves severely ulcerated lesions, and transmural inflammation may be seen in severe cases.

The pathology varies depending on the severity and duration of disease, but common findings include severe mucosal necrosis with or without pseudomembrane formation, marked submucosal edema and hemorrhage, and fibrinous or fibrous serosal exudate (Fig. 9-17). Pneumatosis may be observed. The necrosis tends to be more prominent at the crown of plicae circulares, whereas the mucosa may appear normal at the vale of plicae circulares.[130] The necrotic mucosa is often covered by large numbers of club-shaped, gram-positive rods, ranging in length from 0.5 to 1.2 μm. Immunohistochemistry or PCR for the α and β toxins of *C. perfringens*, type C (designated *cpa* and *cpb*, respectively) confirms the diagnosis.[129,130]

Yersinia

The genus of *Yersinia* includes three species that are pathogenic for humans and rodents: *Yersinia pestis* (the causative agent of plague), *Yersinia enterocolitica*, and *Yersinia pseudotuberculosis*. These enteropathogens most often cause self-limited enterocolitis and mesenteric lymphadenitis in humans.[131] An acute abdomen presentation due to acute gastroenteritis, colitis, or pseudoappendicitis resulting from acute terminal ileitis is the most characteristic manifestation of the disease. Patents with iron overload,[132-134] those receiving desferrioxamine,[135-137] those with liver disease,[133] and those who are immunocompromised or debilitated[138] are at increased risk for severe disease. *Yersinia* can occasionally cause extraintestinal manifestations such as arthritis and erythema nodosum,[135-137] as well as fulminate septicemia and peritonitis.[132-134,139]

Enteropathogenic *Yersinia* strains have a tropism for lymphoid tissue.[140] Bacteria bind to and invade M cells within the epithelium overlying the lymphoid follicles of Peyer patches.[141,142] Following their entry into the Peyer patches, the bacteria induce a host immune response characterized by infiltration of neutrophils and macrophages.[143] Because of its lymphoid tropism, *Yersinia* infections preferentially involve the ileocecal and appendiceal regions, although any segment of the small or large intestine can be affected.[144] The intestinal wall is congested and edematous. Diffuse or focal aphthous mucosal ulcers can develop. The serosa appears dull and hyperemic. Enlarged lymph nodes contain yellowish microabscesses that may become matted.

Microscopically, severe active enteritis with cryptitis, crypt abscesses, and ulceration can be seen in both *Y. enterocolitica* and *Y. pseudotuberculosis* infections. Crypt hyperplasia occurs throughout the small intestine, with villous atrophy.[120] Sharply demarcated areas of lymphoid hyperplasia contain prominent

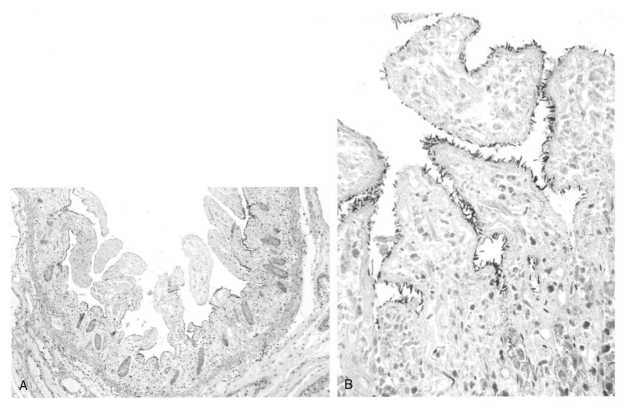

Figure 9-17. *Enteritis necroticans.* **A,** Severe mucosal necrosis. **B,** The necrotic mucosa is covered by numerous club-shaped, gram-positive rods. (Courtesy of Dr. Elena Brachtel.)

germinal centers. The follicular ileitis may persist for months. Notably, the mucosa overlying the follicles develops small, punctate, aphthoid ulcers resembling the early mucosal lesions of Crohn disease.[120] The ulcers are covered by fibrinopurulent exudates and large numbers of gram-positive coccobacilli. Epithelioid granulomas with central necrosis and prominent lymphoid cuffing are usually present in the mucosa, submucosa, and lymph nodes but can be seen on the serosa and lymph nodes as well (Fig. 9-18). The muscularis propria and serosa may be infiltrated by mixed inflammatory cells including eosinophils. Acute vasculitis as well as intussusception has been reported to cause segmental bowel ischemia.

The differential diagnosis includes Crohn disease, and this can be difficult to distinguish on histologic grounds alone. Cultures requiring special media,[144] serologic titers, and PCR assays must be considered in the evaluation of a patient for inflammatory bowel disease (e.g., Crohn disease), or a patient with suspected inflammatory bowel disease for whom steroid therapy has failed, before more aggressive immunosuppressive therapy is elected.[144] Features favoring a diagnosis of Crohn disease include crypt distortion, hyperplasia of the muscularis mucosa, and prominent neural hyperplasia; these features are evidence of chronic changes.

Mycobacterium tuberculosis

In accord with the distribution of lymphoid tissue, the ileocecal region is affected in 90% of patients infected by *M. tuberculosis* who present with gastrointestinal involvement. Grossly, intesti-

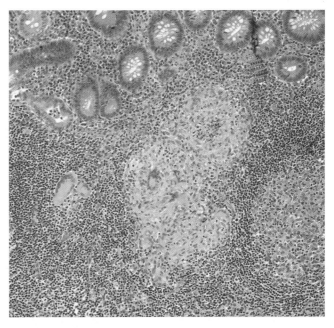

Figure 9-18. *Yersinia* infection. Epithelioid granulomas surrounded by prominent lymphoid infiltrate are seen in the deep mucosa and submucosa. (Courtesy of Dr. Laura Lamps.)

nal tuberculosis displays an ulcerative, hypertrophic, or mixed pattern. The ulcerative form is present in most cases and exhibits multiple superficial ulcers. Patients with this morphology tend to have a virulent clinical course with high mortality. The hypertrophic form is least common and mimics Crohn disease because of its scarring, fibrosis, and heaped-up mass lesions.[145] In the ulcerohypertrophic form, the intestinal wall becomes thickened and ulcerated by an inflammatory mass centered on the ileocecal valve.[146] In this form, the ileocecal valve is frequently obscured by a mass consisting of mesenteric fat, fibrotic tissue, and inflamed lymph nodes.

Tubercles begin in the Peyer patches or lymphoid follicles, giving the mucosa a cobblestone appearance. As disease progresses, they involve the entire intestinal wall with multiple nodules that may also produce serosal and mesenteric "studs." The ulcerative form of the disease begins as ragged ulcers that are varied in number and size. In contrast to Crohn disease, tuberculous ulcers are circumferential, with a long axis perpendicular to the lumen; fissure formation that extends into the muscularis propria may be seen.[145] The ulcers may contain AFB, even in the absence of granulomas. The mucosa appears edematous and hemorrhagic.

Hypertrophic lesions are caused by pronounced intramural thickening with ulceration and obstruction. Ulcers heal with fibrosis, strictures, and stenosis that may be broad, at times several centimeters in length. Epithelioid granulomas with obvious caseation (Fig. 9-19) occur more frequently in ulcerative than in hyperplastic lesions and are distributed throughout the entire thickness of the intestinal wall. Regional mesenteric lymph nodes become enlarged and contain areas of caseous necrosis as well.

Isolated organisms can be visualized in the granulomas and lymph nodes with the use of special stains and are recoverable in tissue culture. However, it is often difficult to detect the bacteria in suspected cases of tuberculosis, even with AFB-stained sections, due to the scarcity of the organisms. In this setting, the detection of mycobacterial DNA in formalin-fixed paraffin-embedded tissue by duplex PCR reactions can confirm the diagnosis. Other mycobacteria (e.g., *M. kansasii*, *M. bovis*) can produce similar pathologic features.

Although tuberculosis classically produces granulomas, other causes include fungal disease and Crohn disease. The latter may be difficult to distinguish from tuberculosis; transmural lymphoid aggregates, deep fistulas, and fissures favor Crohn disease (Table 9-4).

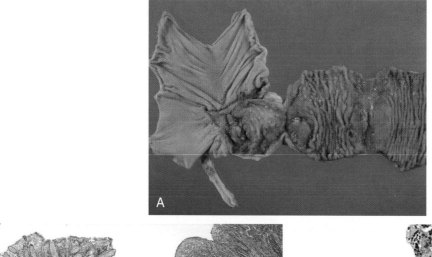

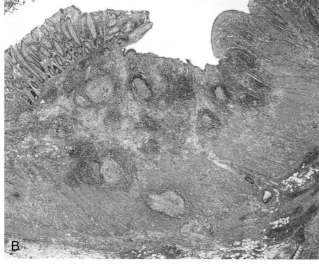

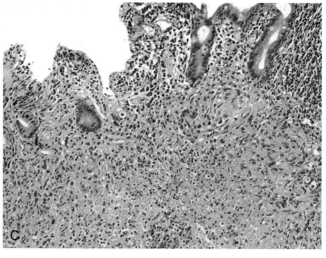

Figure 9-19. *Mycobacterium tuberculosis* of terminal ileum and ileocecal valve demonstrating ulcers that are circumferential, with their long axis perpendicular to the lumen **(A)**. **B,** The intestinal wall is thickened by epithelioid granulomas, lymphoid aggregates, and fibrosis. **C,** High power reveals caseous necrosis and epithelioid histiocytes. (Courtesy of Dr. Sachiko Minmiguchi.)

Table 9-4 Causes of Granulomas in Small Intestine

Crohn disease
Sarcoidosis
Infections
  Mycobacterium tuberculosis, Mycobacterium avium-intracellulare,
    Mycobacterium bovis
  Yersinia
  Histoplasma
  Schistosoma
  Strongyloides
  Actinomyces
  Salmonella
  Campylobacter
  Brucella
Foreign material: sutures, barium, talc, feces due to fistula or
  perforation
Pneumatosis intestinalis
Malacoplakia
Langerhans cell histiocytosis

Mycobacterium avium-intracellulare Complex

MAC is an AIDS-defining opportunistic infection. Disseminated MAC infection is usually seen in patients with advanced HIV infection, generally those with CD4-positive T-lymphocyte counts lower than 50 cells/μL, and is associated with significant morbidity and mortality.[147,148] Since the induction of antimicrobial prophylaxis and highly active antiretroviral therapy (HAART), the incidence of disseminated MAC infection has dramatically declined, leading to improved survival.[149]

Disseminated MAC infection results from a primary infection, and a common portal of entry for MAC infection in AIDS patients appears to be the gastrointestinal tract.[150] The mycobacteria penetrate the gastrointestinal mucosa by yet undetermined mechanisms. This occurs rapidly, and solitary organisms can be seen in the lamina propria without apparent mucosal abnormality. Mycobacteria within the lamina propria are phagocytosed by macrophages, but intracellular killing does not occur. Instead, the macrophages become stuffed with organisms as they multiply intracellularly. With continued bacterial replication, the host cell ruptures. This process leads to the presence of sheets of macrophages laden with AFB. Unimpaired replication of mycobacteria results in massive thickening of the intestinal wall,[151] and infection spreads via mural lymphatics to involve lymph nodes. Mycobacteria replicate in the lymph nodes as well, and eventually the normal histology of the lymph nodes is effaced. Hematogenous dissemination occurs concurrently. Reticuloendothelial organs such as the liver, spleen, and bone marrow are the most frequent distant sites.[150]

The common presenting symptoms include diarrhea, fever, weight loss, and abdominal pain. Gastric ulcer, enterocolitis, enteric fistulas, intra-abdominal abscesses, and hemorrhage can also be seen as gastrointestinal manifestations.[152] Intussusception secondary to hyperplasia of Peyer patches can occur, and clinical and radiologic pictures resembling ileal Crohn disease may also be observed. The duodenum is most frequently involved, followed by the rectum, ileum, colon, esophagus, jejunum, and stomach, for reasons that are uncertain. On endoscopic examination, multiple raised, yellow-white nodules are seen in the duo-

denum, but the mucosa may appear normal. Other endoscopic findings include, in descending order, ulceration, erythema, edema, friability, confluent nodules, and strictures.[152]

Biopsy of nodular lesions reveals atrophic mucosa with villous blunting, as well as widening of lamina propria by an infiltrate of plump macrophages exhibiting granular foamy cytoplasm (Fig. 9-20). However, the overall architecture of the intestine is usually preserved. Other inflammatory cells, such as lymphocytes, plasma cells, and neutrophils, are sparse, if present. Regional lymph nodes display comparable infiltrates. Epithelioid granulomas are rarely seen[151]; if present, they are poorly circumscribed and rarely contain multinucleated giant cells. Small areas of necrosis are present in up to 30% of cases.[153] If necrosis is marked, the infiltrates are easily recognized on H&E stain even on low-power magnification. However, detection of focal involvement may require special stains. In addition to Ziehl-Neelsen and Fite stains, the PAS stain highlights mycobacteria. In contrast to *M. tuberculosis* infection, mycobacteria are usually present within macrophages, and not in giant cells or areas of caseous necrosis.

Whipple Disease (*Tropheryma whippelii*)

Whipple disease is a multisystem disease that results from infection with a gram-positive rod-shaped bacterium, *Tropheryma whippelii*. It is a rare disorder, and only about 1000 cases have been reported to date. Although it occurs in people of all ages, the typical patient is a middle-aged white man.[154] *T. whippelii* appears to be present in the general environment, although neither its source nor its mode of transmission is well established. Since an association between Whipple disease and *Giardia lamblia* infection has been reported, it is plausible that both microorganisms occupy the same ecologic niche.[155] Considering that many people may be exposed to *T. whippelii* but the disease develops in only some of them, it is likely that undefined predisposing immune factors exist.[156]

Several studies have demonstrated defective function of macrophages, with inability to degrade bacterial antigens efficiently, most likely due to inadequate production of interleukin-12 (IL-12),[157] which may lead to diminished production of interferon-γ by T cells and defective macrophage activation. A decrease in IL-12 production may prevent the development of an effective type 1 helper T-cell immune response and favor a shift toward a type 2 helper T-cell response. Replication of *T. whippelii* in macrophages is associated with apoptosis of the host cell that correlates with the expression and release of IL-16.[158]

Whipple disease is characterized by two stages: a prodromal stage and steady-state stage. The prodromal stage is marked by protean symptoms, along with chronic nonspecific findings, mainly arthralgia and arthritis. The steady-state stage is characterized by weight loss, diarrhea, or both, and occasionally by other manifestations affecting the many organs frequently involved.[159] The average time between the prodromal and the steady-state stage is 6 years. Patients on immunosuppressive therapy, such as corticosteroids or tumor necrosis factor antagonists, may experience more rapid clinical progression.[160,161]

Whipple disease frequently involves the small intestine, and jejunum and ileum more often than duodenum.[162] On endoscopic examination, pale yellow, shaggy mucosal changes, attrib-

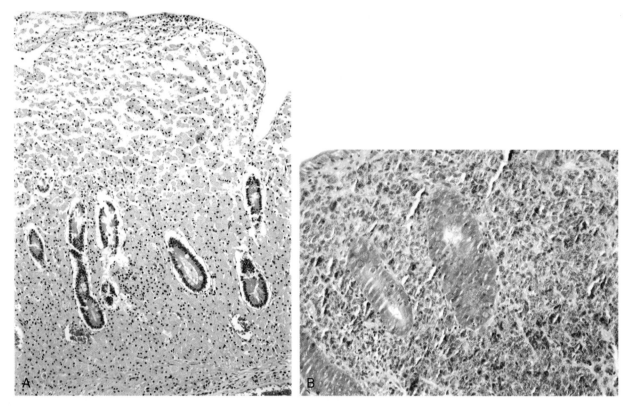

Figure 9-20. *Mycobacterium avium-intracellulare* complex infection. **A,** Intestinal villi are obliterated by infiltration of numerous plump macrophages with foamy cytoplasm in the lamina propria. **B,** The lamina propria macrophages are filled with PAS-positive mycobacteria.

uted to lipid deposits, alternating with eroded, erythematous, or mildly friable mucosal patches, are often seen in the distal aspect of the duodenum and jejunum.[163,164]

The histologic hallmark of Whipple disease is the presence of macrophages with cytoplasmic PAS-positive, diastase-resistant granules or sickle-form particles; these are known as sickle-form particle-containing cells, or SPC cells. Bacilli may also be seen within and between epithelial cells, especially before the initiation of antimicrobial therapy.[164] The intestinal villi are blunted and distorted by the collections of macrophage. In severe cases, subtotal or total villous atrophy can be seen. Conversely, the villous architecture is relatively normal in about one fifth of the cases.[164]

The majority of macrophages accumulate in the lamina propria of the villi, just beneath the luminal epithelial basement membrane (Fig. 9-21). A small number of macrophages may also be seen in the pericryptal lamina propria or submucosa or both.[164] Lymphocytes, neutrophils, eosinophils, and plasma cells can be seen infiltrating among the macrophages. Although rare, nonnecrotizing granulomas composed of epithelioid cells, which are PAS-negative in 40%, may be present in the mucosa, lymph nodes, and other organs, resembling sarcoidosis.[163,165,166] Lymphatic obstruction can cause dilatation of lacteals and can produce lipid deposits in the mucosa.

Antimicrobial treatment may affect the histology of the disease. With a decrease in the number of PAS-positive macrophages, a change occurs in the pattern of mucosal involvement. It may go from diffuse to patchy; the distribution of macrophages may shift from the villous interstitium to the pericryptal interstitium; and the intensity of PAS-positive staining may diminish.[163]

Other entities can yield PAS-positive macrophage collections in the intestinal lamina propria. These include *M. avium-intracellulare* infection, histoplasmosis, chronic granulomatous disease, xanthomas, storage disease, and common variable immunodeficiency. Although the macrophages may appear similar in these conditions, lipid deposits are seen only in Whipple disease. As for differentiating Whipple disease from MAC infection, acid-fast staining occurs only with MAC. Because characteristic histologic features are seen in only 90% of patients,[163] PCR assay is required to confirm the diagnosis in clinically suspicious cases that show nondiagnostic histologic changes (Table 9-5).

Tropical Sprue

Tropical sprue is an intestinal malabsorption syndrome that affects residents and visitors to the tropics, including Puerto Rico, the Caribbean, northern South America, West Africa, India, and southeast Asia.[167] Although its etiology and pathogenesis remain unclear, an infectious cause is strongly suspected because of the occurrence of tropical sprue particularly in rural areas with poor hygiene, susceptibility of visitors from developed countries in endemic regions,[168] and a favorable response to antibiotic therapy.[169] Patients also have been shown to have aerobic bacterial contamination of the small bowel, although no specific microorganisms are common to all patients.[170] In addition, preexisting prolonged orocecal transit time may contribute

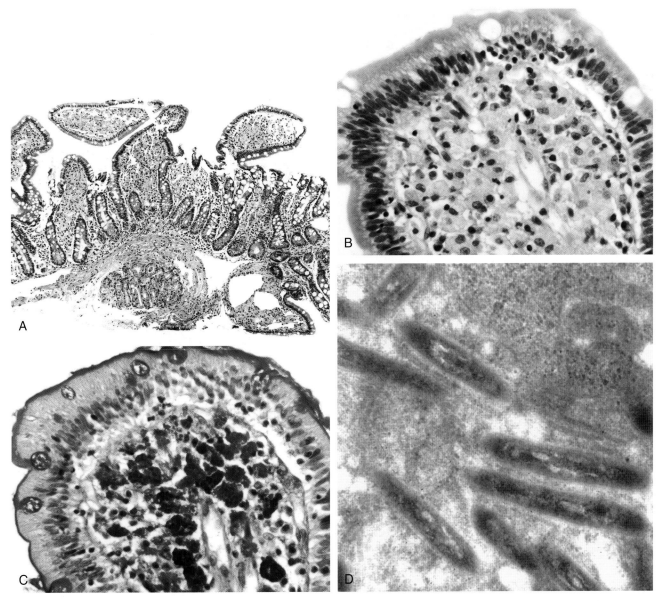

Figure 9-21. Whipple disease involving duodenum. **A,** A mucosal biopsy demonstrates partial villous blunting by collections of macrophages in the lamina propria. **B,** A large number of macrophages have accumulated in the lamina propria beneath the luminal epithelial basement membrane. **C,** PAS stain highlights intracytoplasmic granular particles that are resistant to diastase. **D,** Electron micrograph shows intact bacilli with characteristic thick walls and intracytoplasmic vacuoles.

to the disease process in some patients.[170] Diagnostic evaluation of tropical sprue requires its differentiation from infectious etiologies, especially parasitic diarrheal diseases and Whipple disease, and from other malabsorption syndromes such as celiac disease. Jejunal biopsies are necessary to establish the presence of characteristic histologic features and to exclude other diseases.

Histologic features of tropical sprue consist of villous atrophy, crypt hyperplasia, chronic inflammatory cell infiltration (particularly plasma cells, lymphocytes, eosinophils, and histiocytes), and increased numbers of intraepithelial lymphocytes. Nuclear-cytoplasmic maturational dissociation (i.e., nuclear enlargement and decreased mitotic figures) may be observed in the enterocytes.[171,172] The histologic findings, although similar to those of celiac disease, are not identical, and total villous atrophy is rare (<10%) in tropical sprue.[173-175]

The disease first involves the jejunum, then spreads distally to the ileum. In the early stage, the mucosa may appear normal or may show only increased numbers of intraepithelial lymphocytes. In well-established disease, the pathologic changes become equally prominent in the ileum.[175] Conversely, celiac disease commonly shows prominent mucosal changes in the proximal small intestine. This difference in disease distribution explains the more common association of tropical sprue with megaloblastic anemia caused by deficiencies of vitamin B_{12} and folate.

Fungi

Candida and *Aspergillus* species account for the majority of fungal infections of the small bowel. In comparison to *Candida,*

Aspergillus hyphae are often seen in submucosal vessels spreading within the bowel wall in a radiating pattern.[176] Other fungi that can involve the small bowel include *Histoplasma*, *Mucor*, *Paracoccidioides*, and *Penicillium marneffei*.

Of these, *H. capsulatum* is the most common endemic systemic mycosis in the United States; it occurs primarily, but not exclusively, in the central regions of the country. Gastrointestinal involvement occurs in 40% of patients with disseminated disease, and involvement of the small intestine is seen in 27%[177]; however, in contrast to other forms of disseminated histoplasmosis, fever and pulmonary involvement are unusual in gastrointestinal histoplasmosis.[178] Terminal ileal involvement is commonly seen. Deep ulcerative lesions with undercut margins are characteristic of *H. capsulatum* involvement,[178] but masses mimicking carcinoma, pseudopolyps, and lesions resembling

xanthomas may also be seen.[179] Histologically, yeast forms ranging from 2 to 4 μm in size lie within well-formed granulomas or macrophages scattered in the lamina propria in a pattern resembling Whipple disease or early enteritis caused by *Mycobacterium avium-intracellulare* (Fig. 9-22).

Candida

Small intestinal candidal infections are rare in immunocompetent individuals with intact mucosal integrity, but they can be seen in up to 20% of autopsied patients with disseminated infection.[180] All *Candida* species can infect immunocompromised patients, but there is a higher frequency of disseminated *C. tropicalis*.[25] The gross appearance is variable; it includes mucosal flecks, sloughed membranes, ulcers of varying configuration, and nodular masses. Most invasive *Candida* infections are superficial[176] and must be carefully differentiated from benign colonization. In colonization, *Candida* spp. may be identified embedded in the fibrinopurulent exudate that covers blind loops or in devitalized tissues without invasion of viable tissue. In immunocompromised or chronically debilitated patients, *Candida* can also invade deep into the intestinal wall and gain entry to the microvasculature, leading to ischemia and sepsis.

Viruses

Enteric Virus Infections

Numerous viruses, including rotavirus, enteric adenovirus, Norwalk virus, coronavirus, echovirus, enterovirus, calicivirus, and astrovirus,[181-183] can cause gastroenteritis. Diagnosis is made based on viral culture, electron microscopy, ELISA of stool specimens, or genetic probes. Pathologists rarely obtain biopsies from patients with viral enteritis, but if they do, the bowel displays nonspecific findings such as reactive and degenerative changes of the epithelium and a mononuclear cell infiltrate in the lamina propria. Architectural changes of microvilli may also be seen.

Table 9-5 Comparison of *Mycobacterium avium-intracellulare* Infection and Whipple Disease

	M. avium-intracellulare	**Whipple Disease**
Distribution in small intestine	Duodenum > ileum > jejunum	Jejunum and ileum > duodenum
Macroscopic features	Yellow-white nodules or normal	Erythema alternating with pale yellow, shaggy mucosal changes
Villous architecture	Blunted or normal	Blunted
Lacteals	Not dilated	Dilated
Lipid deposits	−	+
PAS stain	+	+
AFB stain	+	−

AFB, acid-fast bacilli; PAS, periodic acid–Schiff.

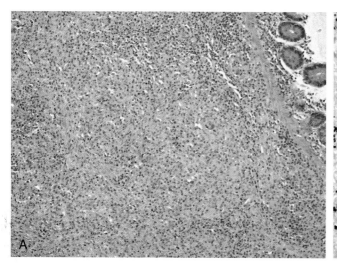

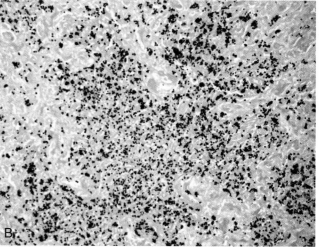

Figure 9-22. A, *Histoplasma capsulatum* infection of the small intestine shows ulceration of the mucosa with non-necrotizing granulomas in the bowel wall. **B,** GMS stain reveals innumerable budding yeast forms.

Cytomegalovirus

CMV infection of the small intestine accounts for only 4% of all CMV infections, and CMV infection of the duodenum accounts for 22% of all CMV infections of the gastrointestinal tract.[184] Immunosuppressed patients, including not only those with HIV infection but also those who undergo small bowel transplantation for short bowel syndrome, are prone to CMV infection. The latter group of patients show a high incidence of recurrence due to the heavy immunosuppression required to manage the graft.[185,186] In this setting, PCR analysis of small-intestinal biopsy specimens may be a sensitive method for early detection of CMV and can be useful for preemptive therapy.[187] The clinical manifestations of CMV infection include a wide spectrum of symptoms such as malaise, anorexia, fever, nausea, diarrhea, abdominal pain, ileus, gastrointestinal bleeding, and perforation. Severe complications such as hemorrhage and perforation are often preceded by vague symptoms for up to 2 weeks.[188,189] The mortality associated with CMV enteritis is related to older age (>65 years) and delay in instituting therapy but not to the anatomic site of the infection.[190]

CMV enteritis tends to involve only a single region, rather than causing a panenteric infection.[191] The pathologic changes range from few stromal or endothelial cells exhibiting CMV viral inclusions with no tissue reaction to frank ulceration and perforation. Almost any cell type may be infected, although CMV most frequently involves vascular endothelial or stromal cells (Fig. 9-23). The infected and swollen endothelial cells lead to luminal compromise, with fibrin thrombi formation that results in ischemic mucosal injury and, subsequently, ulceration.[188]

Human Immunodeficiency Virus–related Enteropathy

HIV enteropathy is a poorly defined clinical entity that represents pathogen-negative diarrhea in an HIV-infected individual. The possibility that it is related directly to local HIV infection is

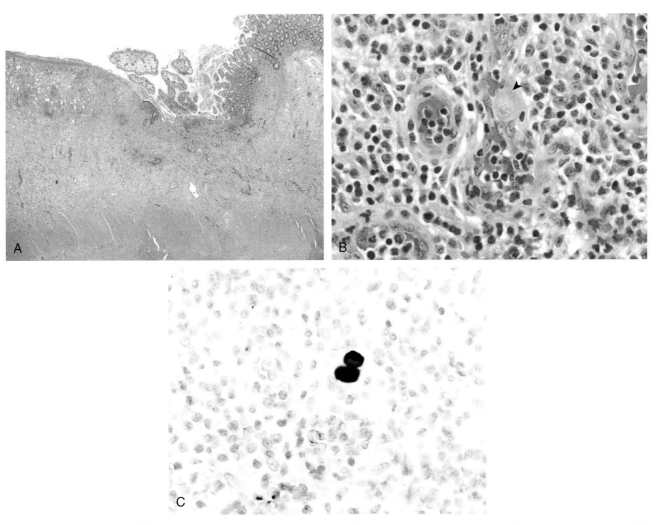

Figure 9-23. *Cytomegalovirus* (CMV) infection superimposed on chronic ischemia of small intestine. The resection specimen of small intestine from a patient with HIV infection who presented with small-bowel obstruction reveals chronic enteritis with ulceration and mural fibrosis (**A**). Proliferating capillaries in the submucosa contain endothelial cells exhibiting atypical CMV cytopathic changes, i.e., cytomegaly with multiple small eosinophilic granules in the cytoplasm (*arrowhead*) (**B**) that react with CMV immunostain (**C**).

supported by the detection of HIV proteins and nuclear acids in various cell types of the intestine (i.e., epithelial cells, lymphocytes, and macrophages). Furthermore, combination antiretroviral therapy has led to improvement of gastrointestinal symptoms in these individuals.[192]

Two competing hypotheses have been advanced to explain the diarrheal disease of mucosal HIV infection. It has been suggested that HIV enteropathy is a pathophysiologic consequence of exposure to gp120, which arises from mononuclear cells of the lamina propria, and therefore is independent of epithelial HIV infection.[193-195] Others have argued that the diarrhea is driven by cytokines (tumor necrosis factor and related moieties) released from infected lymphoid cells that can inhibit mucosal ion flux,[196,197] resulting in malabsorption, diarrhea, and weight loss.[198-200]

Vacuolated enterocytes may show conversion from columnar to cuboidal morphology, with cellular apoptosis, seen in a background of either villus and crypt atrophy or hyperplasia (Fig. 9-24). These epithelial changes are associated with mild mucosal inflammation, intraepithelial lymphocytosis, and dilated lacteals. The histologic changes are often mild and disproportionate to the symptoms.[201,202]

Protozoa

Flagellates

Giardia intestinalis (*Giardia lamblia*) is the most prevalent human protozoan pathogen and the leading cause of waterborne diarrheal outbreaks in North America. *G. intestinalis* infection is associated with a broad spectrum of manifestations. Serious diarrhea illness with intestinal malabsorption and marked weight loss can be seen in young children and in previously unexposed adults, particularly travelers from low- to high-prevalence parts of the world. Infants and young children may suffer impairment of growth and development. However, in the vast majority of individuals world wide, the parasite is apparently carried without significant morbidity.[203]

The life cycle of *Giardia* includes two stages: cyst and trophozoite. The former is the infectious form; it is both relatively inert and environmentally resistant. After ingestion, excystation occurs in the duodenum as a result of exposure to gastric juice and pancreatic enzymes, yielding two trophozoites from each cyst.[204,205] These trophozoites replicate in duodenal crypts and in the upper jejunum, reproducing asexually by binary fission.[203]

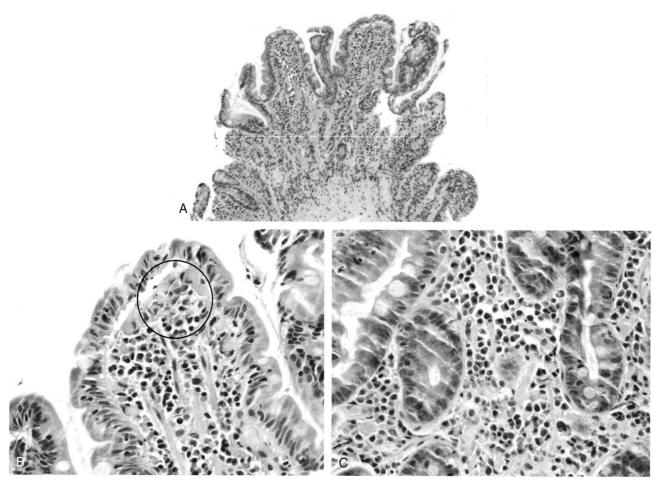

Figure 9-24. Human immunodeficiency virus (HIV) enteropathy. **A,** Small-intestinal mucosa with partial villous blunting demonstrates apoptosis within the epithelium as well as in the lamina propria mononuclear cells. **B,** A region of apoptosis is seen *(within circle)*. **C,** The lamina propria shows increased plasma cells.

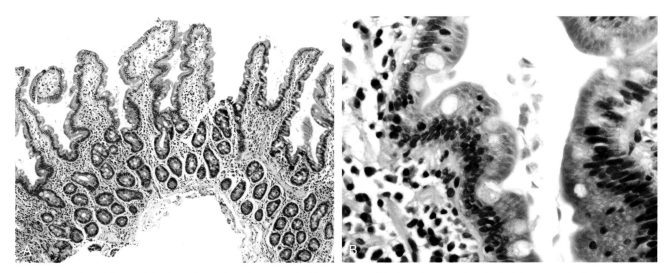

Figure 9-25. *Giardia* infection of duodenum in a patient who presented with acute onset of diarrhea after a camping trip. **A,** At low power, the duodenal mucosa is unremarkable and without significant inflammation or villous architectural distortion. **B,** High power reveals characteristic teardrop-shaped trophozoites between villi.

The cysts may be round or oval and measure 11×10 μm. They each have four nuclei, axonemes, and two median bodies. The trophozoites are 10 to 20 μm in length and 5 to 15 μm in width and have the shape of a teardrop when viewed from the dorsal or ventral aspect. They exhibit two identical nuclei and a ventral concave sucking disk with four pairs of flagella, two axonemes, and two median bodies.[203] Disruption and distortion of the intestinal microvilli occurs at the site where the ventral disk interfaces with the microvillus membrane.[206]

The duodenal and/or jejunal biopsies from infected patients with normal absorption demonstrate preserved villous architecture with or without signs of epithelial damage, and intraepithelial lymphocytes are not increased (Fig. 9-25). Conversely, infected patients with proven intestinal malabsorption are likely to show mild to marked villous blunting, inflammatory expansion of the lamina propria, and increased intraepithelial lymphocytes.[207-210] A flattened mucosa is rarely seen. Even without apparent histologic abnormalities, trophozoites are usually found if at least two biopsy specimens are obtained from the duodenum.[207] The organisms can be detected in gastric or ileal biopsies, and rarely in the colonic biopsies as well.[208] Nodular lymphoid hyperplasia of the small intestine may also be seen.[207] Patients whose biopsies lack lamina propria plasma cells usually have coexisting hypogammaglobulinemia.

If normal or relatively preserved villous architecture is present, the differential diagnosis includes celiac sprue (Marsh I classification), other infectious agents (e.g., postviral enteritis, cryptosporidia, bacterial overgrowth), non-gluten food sensitivity (especially in children), use of nonsteroidal anti-inflammatory drugs (NSAIDs), autoimmune disorders, immunodeficiency, and inflammatory bowel disease, among others. If the mucosa is flat, the most important differential diagnosis is celiac sprue (Marsh III), given that both conditions are often associated with intestinal malabsorption. Other diseases to consider would include tropical sprue, autoimmune enteropathy, immunodeficiency, non-gluten food sensitivity, and infectious enteritis or protracted infection of the small intestine. However, with careful review of the small-intestinal biopsies, the offending trophozoites can usually be identified.

Table 9-6 Comparison of Coccidians

Coccidians	Morphology
Cryptosporidium parvum	2-5 μm basophilic spherical bodies protruding from the apex of the enterocytes GMS negative
Cyclospora cayetanensis	8-10 μm crescent or ovoid microorganisms normally located in enterocytes but can be present at the cell surface At some stages of infection, surrounded by a parasitophorous vacuole (EM) GMS negative
Isospora belli	20-μm oval, blue enterocyte inclusions, both perinuclear and subnuclear Rarely present in the lamina propria or in macrophages At some stages of infection, surrounded by a parasitophorous vacuole (EM)
Microsporidia (*Enterocytozoon bieneusi* and *Encephalitozoon intestinalis*)	Difficult to detect in H&E-stained sections 2-3 μm apical inclusions in the enterocytes

EM, electron microscopy; GMS, Grocott methenamine silver stain; H&E, hematoxylin and eosin stain.

Coccidians

Cryptosporidium, *Microsporidium*, *Isospora*, and *Cyclospora* have all been identified in the small intestine of AIDS patients but are also important pathogens in otherwise healthy persons, including infants and children in developing countries (Table 9-6).[211,212] Of these, microsporidia are single-celled, obligate intracellular parasites that have recently been reclassified from protozoa to fungi but will nevertheless be discussed in this section.[213] Transmission is via the fecal-oral route, either by direct contact or through contaminated water or food.[212]

In immunocompetent individuals, infection is usually self-limited and typically lasts for a few days but may persist for up to 4 weeks. Symptoms often consist of diarrhea, abdominal pain, and malaise. Nausea, vomiting, and fever may be reported. Conversely, immunocompromised patients are at risk for severe and chronic diarrhea that may be life-threatening. Weight loss and cramping abdominal pain are proportional to the severity of the diarrhea.

Other enteric opportunistic pathogens may infect profoundly immunocompromised patients.[212] Patients with isosporiasis are likely to have peripheral eosinophilia. Endoscopic examination often shows normal intestinal mucosa or mild erythema, mucosal granularity, atrophy, and superficial erosions. Although all four coccidians primarily involve the mucosa of the small intestine, especially in the distal segment, the colonic mucosa and biliary tract can also be involved in the setting of heavy infection.[212]

Diagnosis is usually based on the examination of stool specimens. Less frequently, examination of duodenal/jejunal aspirates with special stains can establish the diagnosis. Evaluation of small bowel biopsy specimens by electron microscopy may be more sensitive than stool examination for the diagnosis of intestinal microsporidiosis (Figs. 9-26 and 9-27).[214,215] With the development of sensitive diagnostic tests (e.g., ELISA), immunohistochemistry, and PCR,[58] it is likely that low-intensity infections will be more frequently identified, with some probably of little clinical significance.[212]

In all coccidial infections, the small-intestinal mucosa shows nonspecific findings, including normal intestinal mucosa in low-density infections or intraepithelial lymphocytosis, various degrees of villous atrophy, crypt hyperplasia, and mixed inflammation in the lamina propria if the organism burden is high.[216,217] The diagnosis is based on organism morphology by light microscopy and/or ultrastructural examination of biopsy specimens. Microsporidia are difficult to detect in H&E-stained sections, but special stains such as GMS, PAS, modified acid-fast, modified trichrome, auramine, Warthin-Starry, and Brown-Brenn stains can aid greatly in the diagnosis (see Table 9-6).

Helminths

The conventional method used to diagnose gastrointestinal helminth infections is examination of stool for ova and parasites, but pathologists may at times encounter these organisms in endoscopic biopsies or in resection specimens. In this section, helminths that can affect the small intestine are briefly described.

Enterobius vermicularis (Pinworm)

Pinworms are one of the most common human parasites and tend to infest young children. They have a worldwide distribution, but they are more commonly seen in cold or temperate climates and in developed countries. The worms live and reproduce in the ileum, cecum, proximal colon, and appendix; however, pathologists are most likely to encounter them in colonic specimens, usually as an incidental finding in the appendix.

Ascaris lumbricoides

The distribution of ascariasis is worldwide, with the greatest frequency being in moist tropical climates. The mode of infection is fecal contamination of toys, soil, and fingers; contaminated raw vegetables; and drinking water. Usually. children are more vulnerable than adults to *Ascaris* infection. Patients may be asymptomatic, or they may complain of vague abdominal pain. However, massive infection with obstruction, perforation with peritonitis, appendicitis, and pancreatobiliary obstruction does occur.[218-220]

Tissue damage may be seen primarily at the sites of attachment, but adult *A. lumbricoides* in the small intestine usually produces no diagnostic lesions.[218-220] This nematode (round worm) is characterized by its large size, even in its larval form. The female worms reach lengths of greater than 30 cm; males

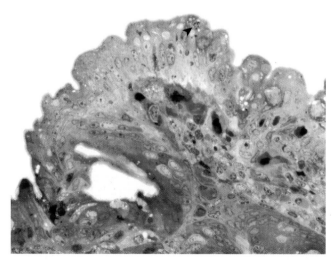

Figure 9-26. *Enterocytozoon bieneusi* infection of duodenum. A mucosal biopsy shows partial villous blunting, with the enterocytes infected with microsporidia spores *(arrowhead)* (toluidine blue stain).

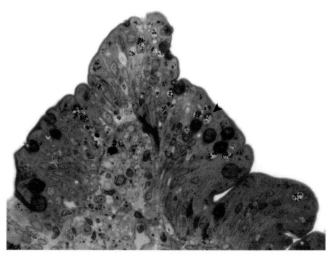

Figure 9-27. *Microspora septata intestinale* infection of duodenum. Spores are grouped in supranuclear vacuoles of enterocytes *(arrowhead)* (toluidine blue stain).

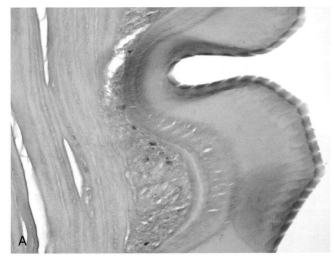 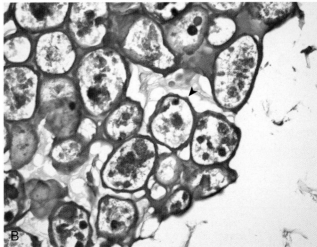

Figure 9-28. A, *Ascaris lumbricoides* with thick annulate cuticle and hypodermis. **B,** The mature ova of *Ascaris* exhibit prominent mamillations *(arrowhead).*

are somewhat smaller. The helminth displays an annulate, multilayered cuticle with prominent hypodermis and conspicuous lateral cords. The female pseudocoelem includes paired genital tubes that contain innumerable ova which, when mature, exhibit prominent mamillations (Fig. 9-28). Even if the organism is no longer viable, it can be readily identified by virtue of its size.

Ancylostomiasis (Hookworm)

The distribution of hookworm (*Necator americanus* and *Ancylostoma duodenale*) is worldwide, with particular prevalence in rural areas of the moist tropics where there is inadequate sanitation and people walk barefoot. The filariform larvae penetrate the skin of the feet or hands, enter venules, and are carried to the capillaries of the lung, where they break through the capillaries into alveolar sacs. They subsequently migrate through proximal airways to the gastrointestinal tract. Adult hookworms are creamy white, cylindrical nematodes with a large buccal capsule that includes teeth or cutting plates.[219,221,222]

The patients are usually asymptomatic, but dyspepsia, nausea, and epigastric discomfort may occur. In addition, because the worms attach to the intestinal mucosa and withdraw blood from villous capillaries, anemia may ensue if the infestation is left untreated.

Mucosal damage is usually minor, but dense eosinophilic infiltrate extending into the submucosa or villous blunting may be seen. Biopsy specimens may occasionally reveal intestinal mucosa in the buccal cavity of the worm.[219,221,222]

Strongyloides stercoralis

The distribution of *S. stercoralis* is worldwide, with the greatest prevalence in warm and wet regions. Adults, especially old, hospitalized, institutionalized, or immunocompromised individuals, are more prone than others to be infected by *Strongyloides.*

Filariform larvae penetrate the skin, enter the venous system, travel to the lung, and migrate up the proximal airways and down into the esophagus, eventually reaching the small intestine. Adult female worms parasitizing human small intestine lay eggs in the intestinal mucosa that hatch into rhabditiform larvae, which are shed in the stool. In an unfavorable environment, rhabditiform larvae transform into filariform larvae (parasitic phase). In the autoinfection cycle, rhabditiform larvae change into infective filiform larvae in the intestine or on the perianal skin and directly invade the host. This autoinfective capability leads to prolonged illness. Disseminated infection (i.e., migration of larvae to organs beyond the range of the autoinfective cycle) can occur in immunocompromised hosts and results in severe, life-threatening illness.[218,219,223-230] Systemic parasitic infection predisposes to gram-negative sepsis.

Adult female worms are 2 to 3 mm in length, with 1- to 2-μm thick cuticles and fine transverse striations. Eggs are 50 to 60 μm, oval, thin shelled, and embryonated when they exit the female. Rhabditiform larvae are 200 to 300 μm, and filariform larvae are 300 to 600 μm.[218,219,223-230]

Many patients are asymptomatic carriers, but abdominal pain, diarrhea, nausea, vomiting, anorexia, weight loss, and gastrointestinal bleeding, in any order or combination, have been reported. Ileus, small-bowel obstruction, and malnutrition also occur. Computed tomography scans occasionally reveal intraabdominal lymphadenopathy. Gastrointestinal manifestations can be accompanied by pruritus, rash, eosinophilia, and pulmonary symptoms.[218,219,223-230]

Mucosal lesions may lead to esophagitis and gastritis in addition to duodenitis, jejunitis, ileitis, and colitis with pseudomembranous colitis. Mucosal ulceration is the most common finding in the small intestine, but it can occur at any level of the gastrointestinal tract. Histologically, the crypts are often distended by numerous larvae and adult worms (Fig. 9-29), but the organisms may be difficult to detect due to their patchy distribution. Other histologic features include villous blunting, ulcers and necrosis, edema, and a dense eosinophilic infiltrate of the lamina propria. Granulomas may also be seen.[218,219,223-230]

Capillaria philippinensis (Intestinal Capillariasis)

Although endemic in the Philippines and Thailand, cases of *C. philippinensis* have been reported in nonendemic areas.

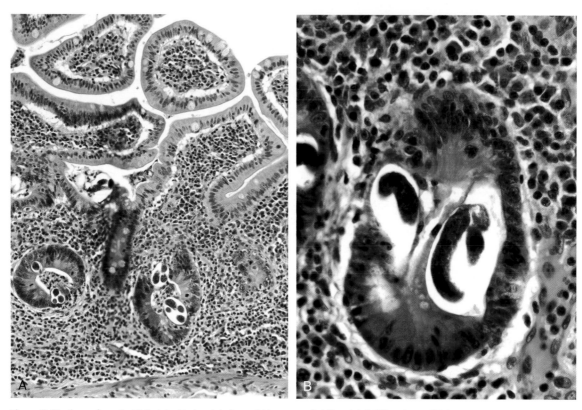

Figure 9-29. Ileum of a patient infected with the adult *Strongyloides stercoralis* **(A)** and rhabditiform larvae **(B)** in crypts.

Transmission to humans is through ingestion of freshwater fish infected by larvae. The worms inhabit both the small and large intestine. At autopsy, as many as 200,000 worms can be recovered from a liter of intestinal contents. Autoinfection is attributed to the huge numbers of the organisms.[219,221,231,232]

The female worms range in size from 2.5 to 4.3 mm, and the male worms are slightly smaller. *C. philippinensis* eggs, 36 to 45 μm long, are barrel shaped with flattened bipolar plugs. *C. philippinensis* resembles *Trichuris* and *Trichinella* species but is distinguished from them by its characteristic ova. The symptoms of infection are nonspecific and include dull gastric pain or generalized abdominal pain, as well as watery and voluminous diarrhea with an increased amount of fat. Intractable diarrhea can lead to ascites and weight loss, followed by cachexia and death. The natural course of the disease is relatively rapid, and the period between onset of symptoms and death is as short as 2 to 3 months.[219,221,231,232]

Grossly, the small intestine is thickened, congested, and distended with fluid. An extremely large number of adult worms, larvae, and ova may be seen within the jejunum, the proximal portion of the ileum, and occasionally the duodenum. Worms are most commonly found in the crypts of the small intestine, but they may also invade the lamina propria. The intestinal villi tend to exhibit secondary changes such as villous atrophy and epithelial sloughing (Fig. 9-30).[219,221,231,232]

Trematodes

Schistosomiasis is the most common disease caused by trematodes worldwide. All *Schistosoma* species cause disease, and any level of

the gastrointestinal tract may be affected. However, pathologists are most likely to encounter the organisms in colonic specimens.

Fasciolopsis buski (Intestinal Fluke)

Fasciolopsis buski infection is prevalent in countries of eastern Asia and the southwest Pacific, and the highest incidence is reported in eastern China. Transmission of the fluke to humans is via ingestion of aquatic plants, such as water chestnuts, containing infective metacercariae. These encyst in the duodenum, attach to the mucosa, and mature into adult worms in about 3 months.[218,233-237]

The adult is a flat, fleshy, ovate trematode that is 2 to 7.5 cm in length (Fig. 9-31). Eggs measure 130 to 140 μm in length and are ellipsoid, with a small operculum at one end.[218,233-237] The majority of infections remain asymptomatic; however, in cases of heavy infection, patients may develop diarrhea, often alternating with constipation, epigastric pain, nausea and vomiting, and hemorrhage, secondary to intestinal obstruction and mucosal injury. Also, the absorption of parasitic metabolites can cause generalized edema, which is most striking in the face. The duodenum and jejunum are most severely affected, with the large adult worms attaching to the mucosa and inducing an intense inflammation with possible ulceration and abscess formation. Leukocytosis and peripheral eosinophilia are also frequently associated with fasciolopsiasis.[218,233-237]

Cestodes

Adult *Taenia saginata* (beef tapeworm), *Taenia solium* (pork tapeworm), and *Diphyllobothrium latum* (fish tapeworm) are

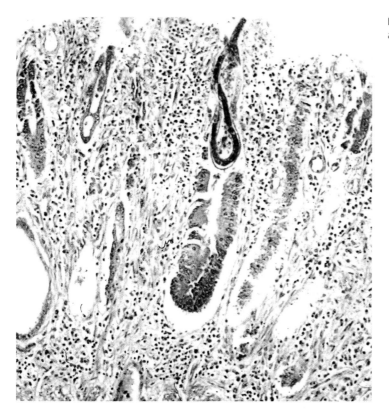

Figure 9-30. *Capillaria philippinensis.* The involved ileum exhibits villous atrophy, epithelial sloughing, and a helminth in a crypt.

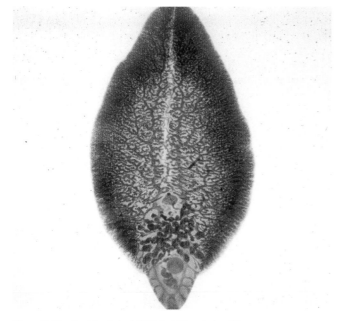

Figure 9-31. *Fasciolopsis buski* (130 to 140 μm in length).

among the largest parasites that infect humans, and they occasionally cause gastrointestinal disease. About 40% of patients with *Hymenolepis nana* (dwarf tapeworm) infection have low vitamin B_{12} levels, because the tapeworm competes with the host for the vitamin.[218,238,239]

Infectious Colitis

Although there is worldwide variation in the most common intestinal infectious agents, diseases that were once considered "tropical" are no longer diagnosed only in distant exotic places but may be encountered anywhere, as a result of international travel and migratory populations. In the West, breakdown in sanitary handling of food and contamination of poultry flocks, as well as the use of raw or partially cooked foods, have led to epidemics of infectious colitis.[240]

Infectious colitis manifests as an acute diarrheal disease frequently associated with hematochezia or microscopic evidence of blood loss. In North America, the diarrheas, commonly of bacterial etiology, are usually self-limited and are commonly referred to as "acute self-limited colitis." However, in immunodeficient patients, presentations may be severe and a benign clinical outcome less certain.

Bacteria

Common Histologic Features of Bacterial (Invasive) Colitis

In response to infection, the colonic mucosa shows remarkable histologic variability. In practice, the dilemma is to distinguish between infectious colitis and the early manifestations of chronic inflammatory bowel disease. Early in the course of infectious colitis, edema of the lamina propria with clusters of neutrophils and ectatic capillaries are the dominant findings. Established crypt abscesses are rare. Commonly, the changes are patchy, and the overall mucosal architecture is preserved. Minimal degenerative changes, limited to the upper half of the mucosa, can be seen. These include mucin depletion and epithelial damage with flattened cytoplasm associated with cryptic dilatation. Concurrently, the inflammatory infiltrate of the lamina propria is mixed, characteristically with more neutrophils than lymphocytes and plasma cells. Microthrombi can plug dilated capillaries and can account for the focal hemorrhage of the lamina propria.

Later in the course of the infection, biopsies may show scattered neutrophils, inflammation with slightly decreased goblet cells, mucin depletion, and cellular degeneration, sometimes with vacuolization. Commonly, a mild increase in plasma cells is noted in the lamina propria, sometimes in association with lymphoid aggregates. However, a well-established dense basal lymphoplasmacytic infiltrate is uncommon. These changes habitually resolve in 2 to 3 weeks, or certainly within a trimester.[241-243]

Histologic Features Associated with Bacterial Infection

Escherichia coli

E. coli is the most prevalent aerobic bacterium of the gut. Five variants are responsible for most common diarrheal illnesses (ETEC, EPEC, EIEC, EHEC, and EAEC species).[244] The ETEC species include O157:H7, which produces a verotoxin and results in a hemorrhagic colitis with features similar to those of ischemic colitis. The diarrheogenic E. coli (ETEC, EAggEC, and EIEC E. coli) account for more than 50% of traveler's diarrhea.[245]

In North America, E. coli O157:H7 is the strain most commonly associated with the hemolytic and uremic syndrome. Its pathogenicity is attributable to two Shiga-like toxins (I and II). These toxins interact with a mucosal receptor in Peyer patches. Eventually, the absorbed toxins cause epithelial and endothelial damage of not only the colon but also the kidneys.[246-248] Incubation takes about 4 days, and the illness lasts about 1 week. In many cases, the disease is self-limited, with minimal or even no diarrhea.

Those who develop a colitis may show various endoscopic appearances, ranging from normal mucosa to edema, erosion, and pseudomembranes. The histologic findings include overlapping features of both ischemic colitis and infectious colitis. Submucosal edema, hemorrhage, pseudomembranes, and withering crypts are seen, along with marked inflammatory infiltrate and cryptitis (Fig. 9-32).[249,250]

Aeromonas

Members of the bacterial genus Aeromonas produce a wide area of virulence factors and have been associated with cases of gastroenteritis, particularly in young children. Chronic symptoms also have been reported.[251]

Campylobacter

Campylobacter bacteria rank among the most common causes of infectious diarrhea. Most infections are self-limited cases of simple diarrhea, occasionally associated with systemic symptoms, but severe infections can occur. Domestic animals, particularly poultry, are reservoirs of infection, and the organism is primarily transmitted by the fecal-oral route. Infections peak in summer and early fall and generally result from ingestion of contaminated food or water.

Campylobacter jejuni, the most important species, produces typical infectious colitis that lasts from 1 to 7 days. The symp-

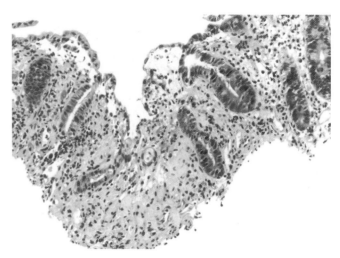

Figure 9-32. Colitis associated with *Escherichia coli* O157:H7 infection. The histology shows evidence of ischemic colitis with hyalinized stroma and withering crypts.

toms usually begin with a prodrome of fever, headache, and myalgias 12 to 24 hours before the onset of gastrointestinal symptoms. Colitis is reported in up to 80% of infections. Colonoscopic findings are nonspecific and range from segmental ulceration to diffuse colitis.[252] Organisms may be seen in the lamina propria by ultrastructural analysis, and granulomatous changes with giant cells may also occur. On biopsy, a focal active colitis is observed.[253] Rare cases produce changes mimicking ulcerative colitis.[252] Complications include toxic megacolon and the development of Guillain-Barré syndrome.[254,255]

Shigella

The enteroinvasive *Shigella* bacteria cause mucosal changes resembling those of chronic inflammatory bowel disease.

Salmonella

Salmonella species are associated with a common form of infectious diarrhea. Classic typhoid fever due to *S. typhi* is primarily an ileal disease (see earlier discussion). However, nontyphoid salmonellosis may involve the colon as well.

At endoscopy, a wide range of nonspecific changes are seen. These include mild edema with petechial hemorrhage and, in severe cases, friability and ulceration. The histologic changes are indistinguishable from other types of bacterial diarrhea and some inflammatory bowel diseases, especially if the specimens were obtained early in the course of inflammatory bowel disease. Complications include the occasional development of toxic megacolon (Fig. 9-33).

Clostridium difficile

C. difficile is a gram-positive bacillus that produces two principal toxins that play a role in pathogenesis of disease. Toxin A is an enterotoxin responsible for food accumulation in the gut and for damage to the enterocolonic mucosa; toxin B is a labile motility-altering cytotoxin that leads to food accumulation.

The spectrum of *C. difficile* colitis ranges from asymptomatic carriage to fulminant colitis. The presence of *C. difficile*

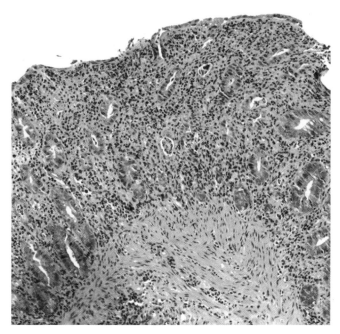

Figure 9-33. Colitis associated with *Salmonella typhi* infection. The lamina propria is moderately expanded by mixed lymphoplasmacytic infiltrate, as well as scattered neutrophils. Cryptitis is present as well. The morphologic features are not specific.

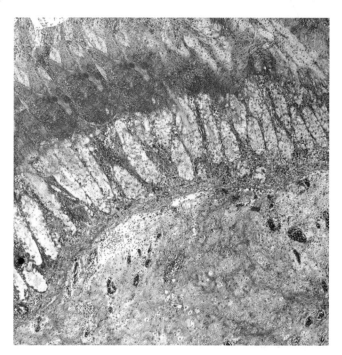

Figure 9-34. Low-power view of specimen from a patient with *Clostridium difficile*–associated pseudomembranous colitis characterized by edema of the submucosa and destructive changes of the mucosa.

infection has been steadily increasing in recent years, particularly among institutionalized patients, and it currently represents a major cause of hospital-acquired diarrhea. *C. difficile* infection is also prevalent in patients with inflammatory bowel disease (particularly ulcerative colitis) who are receiving maintenance immunomodulation therapy, and it is associated with exacerbation of the disease. It appears to play a minor role in sporadic diarrhea. It is well established that *C. difficile* infection follows exposures to antibiotics targeting gut anaerobes, and transmission occurs nosocomially from one host to another.

Toxigenic *C. difficile* is responsible for more than 90% of cases of pseudomembranous colitis and 30% to 40% of cases of antibiotic-associated colitis. The diarrhea usually begins within a few days after antibiotics are started. Some patients develop pseudomembranous colitis, whereas others suffer only mild diarrhea.

Pseudomembranous colitis due to *C. difficile* shows a spectrum of histologic changes, beginning with mild lesions that exhibit a luminal spray of mucus and neutrophils above a background mucosa with minimal inflammation. More advanced disease shows marked inflammatory erosion of the lamina propria covered by a fibrinopurulent cap and cystification of crypts. Finally, mucosal inflammation and erosion extends to form confluent pseudomembranes. In some patients, toxic megacolon ensues.[256] In this setting, the finding of signet-ring cells should not be mistaken as indicating a carcinoma (Figs. 9-34 through 9-36).[257] The standard for diagnosis of *C. difficile* is a toxin test that is positive in more than 90% of patients with classic histologic changes of pseudomembranous colitis.

Yersinia
Y. enterocolitica and *Y. pseudotuberculosis* are gram-negative aerobic coccobacilli. The latter species causes colitis that usually

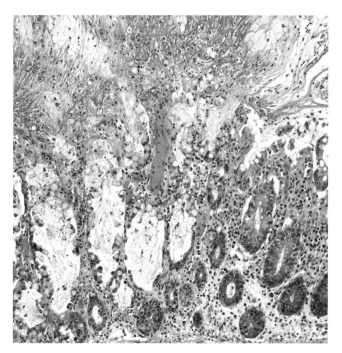

Figure 9-35. At higher power, *Clostridium difficile* pseudomembranous colitis is characterized by sloughing off of superficial epithelial cells. The coating of fibrinopurulent material creates a pseudomembrane.

involves the terminal ileum and mesenteric lymph nodes (see earlier discussion). In *Y. enterocolitica*–associated acute colitis, the mucosa is erythematous and friable, with tiny superficial ulcerations. Granulomas are absent, but aggregates of histiocytes are frequently seen.

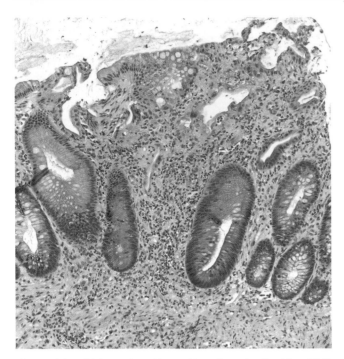

Figure 9-36. Colitis in a patient with a positive toxin test for *Clostridium difficile* colitis but no evidence of pseudomembrane formation. Nonspecific degenerative changes of the surface epithelium, neutrophils, and mild expansion of the lamina propria are present.

Mycobacterium tuberculosis

Tuberculosis of the colon, which is increasing in prevalence due to global travel, is essentially limited to the ileocecal region. Most patients have concomitant pulmonary tuberculosis. The tubercle bacillus can reach the gastrointestinal tract by several routes, including swallowed sputum, infected food, adjacent tissues, lymphatic spread, and via the bloodstream. Colonoscopy can be challenging, given the presence of ulceration and hypertrophic polypoid masses. Ulcerative, hyperplastic, and sclerotic variants may be seen. The differential diagnosis includes ileocecal Crohn disease and carcinoma.[258]

Biopsies reveal mucosal ulceration, granulation tissue, and microabscesses. Characteristic necrotizing granulomas are usually seen in the ulcer bed. The granulomas in tuberculosis are much larger than those seen in Crohn disease. They are confluent, and caseation is a common feature. AFB are demonstrated in 35% to 60% of cases. If *M. tuberculosis* is suspected, acid-fast staining of tissues and cultures is required to establish the diagnosis, and the recent development of PCR technology can increase the diagnostic yield.

Intestinal Spirochetosis

The prevalence of intestinal spirochetosis in rectal biopsies is between 2% and 7% in the West but between 11% and 34% in developing countries. Homosexual men and HIV-infected patients are reported to have the highest prevalence (up to 54%).

Whether the organism is of clinical significance or is a commensal bacterium has been debated. Colonoscopy reveals mucosal erosions and hyperemia. Histologically, the irregular luminal aspect of the surface epithelium seen on H&E-stained

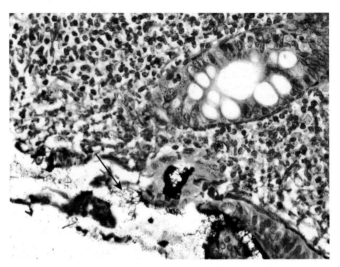

Figure 9-37. Intestinal spirochetosis. With Warthin-Starry stain, numerous tangled spirochetes are seen distributed along the apical surfaces of the mucosa *(arrow)*.

sections is emphasized by PAS or Warthin-Starry stains. Ultrastructural analysis also identifies the spirochetes. The disorder is most frequently seen in the right colon.[259] The spirochetes or brachyspira, *Brachyspira aalborgi* and *Brachyspira pilosicoli*, are found between and parallel to the microvilli and do not penetrate the cytoplasm in most cases (Fig. 9-37). Mild inflammation may be seen in colonic biopsies. Improvement of symptoms and decrease in immunoglobulin E plasma cells within the lamina propria has been observed after treatment with metronidazole. Cases of severe colitis are rare but have been reported.[260,261]

Viruses

Many viruses, including rotavirus, enteric adenovirus, calicivirus, astrovirus, CMV, herpesvirus, and adenovirus can produce colitis. CMV, adenovirus, and HSV are considered here, as the only ones that are likely to be identified on endoscopic biopsies. A wide array of changes, from normal or edematous mucosa to ulcerative colitis, may be seen (Fig. 9-38).

Although CMV infection is usually subclinical, symptoms are common in immunologically suppressed patients, such as patients with AIDS, cancer patients undergoing chemotherapy, transplant recipients, and patients with inflammatory bowel disease.[262,263] CMV colitis can be recognized by the presence of ulceration with or without colitis. The diagnosis of CMV infection depends on the identification of characteristic intranuclear inclusions. Typically, infected cells show endothelial, stromal, or epithelial nuclear and cytoplasmic enlargement with a single, dark red, amphophilic nuclear "bull's-eye" inclusion. However, it is not uncommon for infected cells to show indistinct, smudged, hematophilic nuclei. The cytoplasm of the infected cells can show either granular inclusion or a foamy appearance. The diagnosis can be rendered difficult by granulation tissue arising secondary to the ulceration and the reactive stromal cells. Immunohistochemistry allows a diagnosis to be made in atypical cases.[264]

HSV is a common cause of proctitis in male homosexual patients, in AIDS patients, and in other immunosuppressed indi-

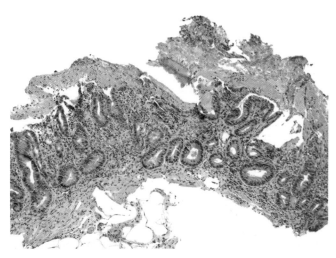

Figure 9-38. Amebiasis of the rectum. The colonic mucosa is moderately inflamed and shows a surface erosion with fibrinopurulent material.

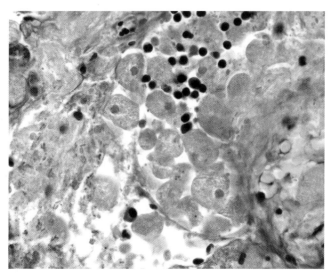

Figure 9-39. Amebiasis of the rectum. Higher magnification shows numerous *Entamoeba histolytica* distributed along the surface epithelium.

viduals. The ulcerations commonly demonstrate peripheral giant cells. Nonspecific cases of severe acute colitis with widespread ulceration have been reported.[265]

Adenovirus is believed to be a common cause of diarrhea in children and patients with HIV infection. Infected vacuolated epithelial cells are found close to the mucosal surface, with amphophilic nuclei that can be either enlarged or crescent-shaped, and the presence of virus can be confirmed by immunocytochemistry. Small intranuclear inclusions are also visible.

Protozoa

The diagnostic identification of protozoa is best done by examination of fresh stool. There is no characteristic histologic pattern on biopsy, and the organisms are usually overlooked on sections unless a careful inspection is made.

Amebiasis

Entamoeba histolytica is found in all climates. Infection is acquired via fecal contamination and ingestion of cysts. In the West, a history of foreign travel to areas of poor sanitation is common, although sexually transmitted cases have been recognized. Infected individuals may present with various symptoms, including toxic megacolon. The range of symptoms is explained in part by the existence of 22 different zymodemes.

Early in infection, edema and nonspecific inflammation with clusters of neutrophils are seen in the lamina propria and surface epithelium. The amebas may be present on the surface, usually in the overlying inflammatory exudate. With time, a large, flask-shaped ulceration may develop. The epithelium shows goblet cell depletion and microulceration with organisms in the exudate overlying the denuded lamina propria (Fig. 9-38). Although there are numerous neutrophils in the lamina propria, crypt abscesses are not conspicuous, and tissue eosinophilia is not a feature.

Deep necrosis with ulceration extending to the submucosa can be seen in severe cases. The mucosa is replaced by a thick,

amorphous inflammatory fibrinoid material with abundant organisms and scattered inflammatory cells. The infective trophozoites are at times substantially larger (10-60 μm) than macrophages, display foamy amphophilic cytoplasm with ingested erythrocytes, and sport a punctate central karyosome (Fig. 9-39). The PAS stain aids in recognition of the amebas but obscures the presence of the diagnostic karyosome and ingested erythrocytes. Of note, antidiarrheal preparations can destroy the protozoa and should be avoided before biopsy. Current diagnostic tools include antigen detection in stool and PCR (Fig. 9-39; see Fig. 9-38).[266]

Coccidia

Coccidia is a collective name for the suborder that includes other human pathogens such as *Isospora*, *Sarcocystis*, and *Toxoplasma*. The diagnosis of these intracellular pathogens is difficult to evaluate on colorectal biopsy. *Cryptosporidium parvum* can be seen in immunocompromised as well as normal subjects, but with a markedly different clinical presentation. The former may present with severe diarrhea, sometimes with toxic megacolon. In the setting of AIDS, several other microorganisms are frequently associated. In immunocompetent individuals, *C. parvum* infection usually manifests as a self-limited, flu-like gastroenteritis; it has also been noted as a cause of traveler's diarrhea.

On biopsy, a nonspecific inflammatory infiltrate and rare ulceration are seen. Cryptosporidia are observed as clusters of tiny hematoxylin dots on the epithelial surface or within the crypt. PAS, silver, or Giemsa stain is also helpful in highlighting the organisms (Fig. 9-40).

Other Protozoan Infections

Giardiasis is more commonly recognized in the small bowel, but rare cases of colonic infection have been documented.

Balantidium coli is a ciliated protozoan. Patients are infected through contact with pigs or rats under conditions of poor personal hygiene. After ingestion of cysts, the trophozoite resides predominantly in the colon. The mucosal lesions are similar to those of amebiasis. Symptoms may include acute diarrhea, fulminant colitis, and perforation. Asymptomatic carriers are recognized.[267]

Helminths

Three classes of helminths can lead to human infection: trematodes (flukes), nematodes (roundworms), and cestodes (tapeworms). Only schistosomiasis leads to colorectal infestation.

Schistosoma mansoni and *Schistosoma japonicum* are the two common trematode worms affecting the colon. The adults reside in the major mesenteric veins, and the disease is caused primarily by an inflammatory reaction to the eggs. The rectal mucosa and submucosa are a good location for identification of *S. mansoni* eggs, whereas those of *S. japonicum* are generally seen in the right colon. The presence of miracidial nuclei indicates that organisms are viable. The ova of *S. mansoni* are characterized by subterminal spines, whereas the eggs of *S. japonicum* have ill-defined subterminal knobs. The eggs are usually surrounded by inflammatory infiltrate in which eosinophils predominate. A granulomatous reaction may develop. In some cases, the eggs are surrounded by an eosinophilic zone of fibrin material, representing an antigen-antibody complex. With time, fibrosis develops around the calcified ova. The lateral spine of *S. mansoni* and the cortical shell stain variably with modified AFB stain; unlike paragonimiasis, the ova are nonrefractile. In countries with endemic infection, the entire colon may become fibrotic, studded with polyps and ulcers. There is an increased incidence of adenocarcinoma in these patients (Figs. 9-41 and 9-42).[268,269]

Strongyloidiasis, trichuriasis, and oxyuriasis are common nematode infestations of the lower gastrointestinal tract. Although *S. stercoralis* is usually restricted to the small intestine, migratory larvae can implant in the colonic mucosa, leading to autoinfection, particularly in the setting of massive infestation. The parasites are found in crypts and superficial mucosae, usually surrounded by transmural eosinophilic inflammation.[270]

Trichuris trichiura (whipworm) preferentially infests the cecum. The body structure of the worm is unique. The anterior three fifths of the worm is threadlike and embeds into the mucosa, whereas the remainder of the organism floats within the lumen. The esophagus shows a characteristic stichosome, and the anterior wall shows characteristic bacillary bands. The posterior part of the worm exhibits the reproductive organs (Fig. 9-43). *Trichuris* causes chronic dysentery. On biopsy, the worm is usually surrounded by an intense focal eosinophilic infiltrate.

Oxyuriasis, or *Enterobius vermicularis*, is the most prevalent parasitic helminth recognized in the West. The adult pinworm attaches to the cecal mucosa, and the worm is commonly

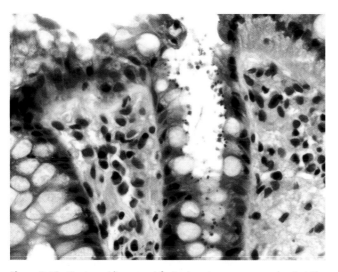

Figure 9-40. *Cryptosporidia parvum* infection in an immunosuppressed patient. The organisms coat the surface epithelium and should not be mistaken for extruded mucin globules.

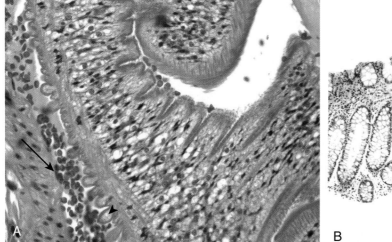

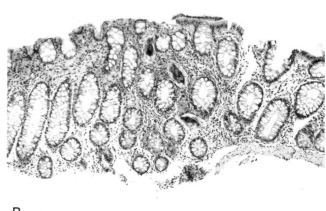

Figure 9-41. A, The tuberculated tegument *(arrowhead)* of an adult male *Schistosoma mansoni* lodged within a mesenteric vein *(arrow).* **B,** Low-power magnification demonstrates degenerating ova within the rectal mucosa.

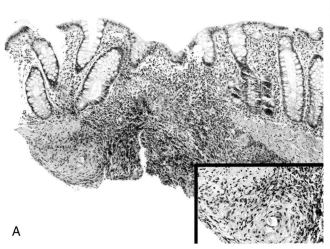

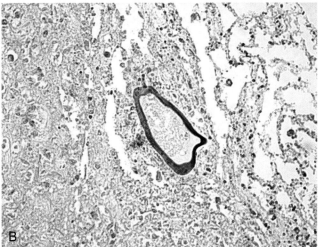

Figure 9-42. A, Colonic schistosomiasis characterized by an ill-formed submucosal granuloma. The inset demonstrates the terminal spine with surrounding ill-formed granulomatous reaction. **B,** A Fite stain highlights the cortex and lateral spine of *Schistosoma mansoni.*

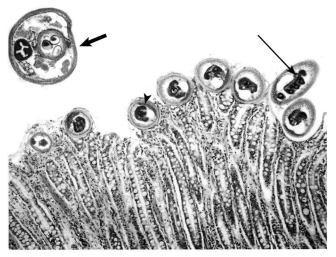

Figure 9-43. *Trichuris trichiura.* The anterior portion of the nematode with stichosome *(arrow)* and bacillary band *(arrowhead)* is embedded in the superficial mucosa, while the posterior two thirds of the helminth containing the sexual organs projects into the bowel lumen *(broad arrow).*

observed in the lumen of the appendix. Symptoms result from the nocturnal migration of the adult female; she lays eggs on the perianal skin, causing intense pruritus. Diagnosis is classically established by adhering the deposited ova to cellophane tape and examining them under the microscope. Refractile ova are characteristically flattened on one side. The helminth is small, shows a muscular wall, and exhibits prominent lateral alae projecting from the cuticle throughout its length. The central oviducts contain the characteristic flattened eggs. The surrounding mucosa is generally inflamed, and tissue eosinophilia may be present (Fig. 9-44). Inflammatory reaction may produce a presenting polyp or even a mass, sometimes mistaken for a carcinoma.[271] Aberrant migration can lead to similar lesions in the vagina and bladder.

Fungi

Fungal infections of the large bowel are rare. They are commonly opportunistic infections of immunocompromised hosts, although in some regions, histoplasmosis, coccidioidomycosis, and paracoccidioidomycosis are endemic. *Histoplasma* is the organism most likely to involve the gut, and the diagnosis depends on identification of the fungus on biopsy. This is best achieved with silver stains. The dimorphic fungus is most often represented in its yeast form, but mycelial growth may be present. The mass mimics carcinoma, from which it must be distinguished.

Sexually Transmitted Diseases

Proctitis is common in homosexual men and is frequently related to infection by *Neisseria gonorrhoeae, Treponema pallidum,* chlamydia, or HSV.[272] The symptoms of gonorrhea, caused by the gram-negative diplococcus *N. gonorrhoeae,* vary from pruritus to severe proctitis and diarrhea. Biopsies frequently are not diagnostic and show either normal mucosa or nonspecific inflammatory change. Fewer than 5% of patients show infectious proctitis.[273]

Secondary syphilis can manifest as proctitis. The changes include marked inflammation, in which small granulomas with giant cells are usually prominent.[272] *Chlamydia trachomatis* is an obligate intracellular bacterium that ranks among the most common causes of sexually transmitted clinical proctitis.[272]

Lymphogranuloma Venereum

In acute cases of lymphogranuloma venereum, the mucosa shows a mixed inflammatory infiltrate. Giant cell granuloma can be seen in association with disrupted crypts. A common differential diagnosis is ulcerative colitis, and the diagnosis is confirmed by immunofluorescent methods. The inflammatory infiltrate may be transmural or may give a pattern of follicular proctitis. Strictures and adenocarcinoma have been reported in chronic infection.

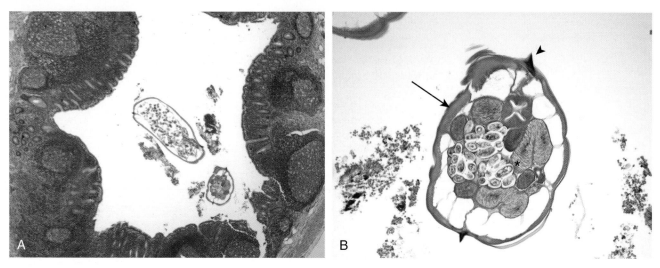

Figure 9-44. A, *Enterobius vermicularis* within the appendiceal lumen. **B,** The helminth shows prominent lateral alae *(arrowhead)*, platymyarian muscle *(arrow)*, and flattened refractile ova *(asterisk)*.

REFERENCES

1. McDonald GB, Sharma P, Hackman RC, et al: Esophageal infections in immunosuppressed patients after marrow transplantation. Gastroenterology 1985;88(5 Pt 1):1111-1117.

2. Walsh TJ, Belitsos NJ, Hamilton SR: Bacterial esophagitis in immunocompromised patients. Arch Intern Med 1986;146:1345-1348.

3. Baehr PH, McDonald GB: Esophageal infections: Risk factors, presentation, diagnosis, and treatment. Gastroenterology 1994;106:509-532.

4. Ezzell JH Jr, Bremer J, Adamec TA: Bacterial esophagitis: An often forgotten cause of odynophagia. Am J Gastroenterol 1990;85:296-298.

5. Fenoglio-Preiser CM: Advances in Pathology, vol 2. St. Louis, Mosby, 1989.

6. Gupta NM, Goenka MK, Vaiphei K, et al: Isolated esophageal tuberculosis. Indian J Gastroenterol 1995;14:25-26.

7. Lockard LB: Esophageal tuberculosis: A critical review. Laryngoscope 1913;23:561-584.

8. Wort SJ, Puleston JM, Hill PD, Holdstock GE: Primary tuberculosis of the oesophagus. Lancet 1997;349(9058):1072.

9. Mokoena T, Shama DM, Ngakane H, Bryer JV: Oesophageal tuberculosis: A review of eleven cases. Postgrad Med J 1992;68(796):110-115.

10. Nagi B, Lal A, Kochhar R, et al: Imaging of esophageal tuberculosis: A review of 23 cases. Acta Radiol 2003;44:329-333.

11. Williford ME, Thompson WM, Hamilton JD, Postlethwait RW: Esophageal tuberculosis: Findings on barium swallow and computed tomography. Gastrointest Radiol 1983;8:119-122.

12. Iwamoto I, Tomita Y, Takasaki M, et al: Esophagoaortic fistula caused by esophageal tuberculosis: Report of a case. Surg Today 1995;25:381-384.

13. Newman RM, Fleshner PR, Lajam FE, Kim U: Esophageal tuberculosis: A rare presentation with hematemesis. Am J Gastroenterol 1991;86:751-755.

14. Gupta SP, Arora A, Bhargava DK: An unusual presentation of oesophageal tuberculosis. Tuber Lung Dis 1992;73:174-176.

15. Prakash K, Kuruvilla K, Lekha V, et al: Primary tuberculous stricture of the oesophagus mimicking carcinoma. Trop Gastroenterol 2001;22:143-144.

16. Sinha SN, Tesar P, Seta W, Sengupta SK: Primary oesophageal tuberculosis. Br J Clin Pract 1988;42:391-394.

17. Damtew B, Frengley D, Wolinsky E, Spagnuolo PJ: Esophageal tuberculosis: Mimicry of gastrointestinal malignancy. Rev Infect Dis 1987;9:140-146.

18. Clouse RE, Abramson BK, Todorczuk JR: Achalasia in the elderly: Effects of aging on clinical presentation and outcome. Dig Dis Sci 1991;36:225-228.

19. De Wit D, Steyn L, Shoemaker S, Sogin M: Direct detection of *Mycobacterium tuberculosis* in clinical specimens by DNA amplification. J Clin Microbiol 1990;28:2437-2441.

20. Eisenach KD, Sifford MD, Cave MD, et al: Detection of *Mycobacterium tuberculosis* in sputum samples using a polymerase chain reaction. Am Rev Respir Dis 1991;144:1160-1163.

21. Kim KM, Lee A, Choi KY, et al: Intestinal tuberculosis: Clinicopathologic analysis and diagnosis by endoscopic biopsy. Am J Gastroenterol 1998;93:606-609.

22. Perosio PM, Frank TS: Detection and species identification of mycobacteria in paraffin sections of lung biopsy specimens by the polymerase chain reaction. Am J Clin Pathol 1993;100:643-647.

23. Centers for Disease Control and Prevention: Revision of the case definition of acquired immunodeficiency syndrome for national reporting—United States. Ann Intern Med 1985;103:402-403.

24. Thom K, Forrest G: Gastrointestinal infections in immunocompromised hosts. Curr Opin Gastroenterol 2006;22:18-23.

25. Walsh TJ, Merz WG: Pathologic features in the human alimentary tract associated with invasiveness of *Candida tropicalis*. Am J Clin Pathol 1986;85:498-502.

26. Geagea A, Cellier C: Scope of drug-induced, infectious and allergic esophageal injury. Curr Opin Gastroenterol 2008;24:496-501.

27. Kirkpatrick CH: Chronic mucocutaneous candidiasis. J Am Acad Dermatol 1994;31(3 Pt 2):S14-S17.

28. Abildgaard N, Haugaard L, Bendix K: Nonfatal total expulsion of the distal oesophagus due to invasive candida oesophagitis. Scand J Infect Dis 1993;25:153-156.

29. Jacobs DH, Macher AM, Handler R, et al: Esophageal cryptococcosis in a patient with the hyperimmunoglobulin E-recurrent infection (Job's) syndrome. Gastroenterology 1984;87:201-203.

30. Jenkins DW, Fisk DE, Byrd RB: Mediastinal histoplasmosis with esophageal abscess: Two case reports. Gastroenterology 1976;70:109-111.

31. Miller DP, Everett ED: Gastrointestinal histoplasmosis. J Clin Gastroenterol 1979;1:233-236.

32. Mineur P, Ferrant A, Wallon J, et al: Bronchoesophageal fistula caused by pulmonary aspergillosis. Eur J Respir Dis 1985;66:360-366.

33. Bibbo M: Comprehensive Cytopathology. Philadelphia, WB Saunders, 1997.

34. Dail DH, Hammer SP: Pulmonary Pathology. New York, Springer-Verlag, 1994.

35. DeMay RM: The Art and Science of Cytopathology. Chicago, ASCP Press, 1996.

36. Tucker LE, Aquino T, Sasser W: Mid-esophageal traction diverticulum: Rare cause of massive upper gastrointestinal bleeding. Mo Med 1994;91:140-142.

37. Nash G, Ross JS: Herpetic esophagitis: A common cause of esophageal ulceration. Hum Pathol 1974;5:339-345.

38. Wandl-Hainberger I, Pichler W, Lechner G, et al: [Ulcerative herpes simplex virus II esophagitis]. Rofo 1988;148:215-216.

39. Whitley RJ: Neonatal herpes simplex virus infections. J Med Virol 1993;(Suppl 1):13-21.

40. Rattner HM, Cooper DJ, Zaman MB: Severe bleeding from herpes esophagitis. Am J Gastroenterol 1985;80:523-525.

41. Byard RW, Champion MC, Orizaga M: Variability in the clinical presentation and endoscopic findings of herpetic esophagitis. Endoscopy 1987;19:153-155.

42. Jenkins D, Wicks AC: Herpes simplex esophagitis in a renal transplant patient: The need for antiviral therapy. Am J Gastroenterol 1988;83:331-332.

43. Shortsleeve MJ, Levine MS: Herpes esophagitis in otherwise healthy patients: Clinical and radiographic findings. Radiology 1992;182:859-861.

44. Watts SJ, Alexander LC, Fawcett K, et al: Herpes simplex esophagitis in a renal transplant patient treated with cyclosporine A: A case report. Am J Gastroenterol 1986;81:185-188.

45. Greenson JK, Beschorner WE, Boitnott JK, Yardley JH: Prominent mononuclear cell infiltrate is characteristic of herpes esophagitis. Hum Pathol 1991;22:541-549.

46. Cardillo MR, Forte F: Brush cytology in the diagnosis of herpetic esophagitis: A case report. Endoscopy 1988;20:156-157.

47. McBane RD, Gross JB Jr: Herpes esophagitis: Clinical syndrome, endoscopic appearance, and diagnosis in 23 patients. Gastrointest Endosc 1991;37:600-603.

48. Singh SP, Odze RD: Multinucleated epithelial giant cell changes in esophagitis: A clinicopathologic study of 14 cases. Am J Surg Pathol 1998;22:93-99.

49. Reed EC, Wolford JL, Kopecky KJ, et al: Ganciclovir for the treatment of cytomegalovirus gastroenteritis in bone marrow transplant patients: A randomized, placebo-controlled trial. Ann Intern Med 1990;112:505-510.

50. Weber JN, Thom S, Barrison I, et al: Cytomegalovirus colitis and oesophageal ulceration in the context of AIDS: Clinical manifestations and preliminary report of treatment with Foscarnet (phosphonoformate). Gut 1987;28:482-487.

51. Levine MS, Loercher G, Katzka DA, et al: Giant, human immunodeficiency virus-related ulcers in the esophagus. Radiology 1991;180:323-326.

52. Connolly GM, Hawkins D, Harcourt-Webster JN, et al: Oesophageal symptoms, their causes, treatment, and prognosis in patients with the acquired immunodeficiency syndrome. Gut 1989;30:1033-1039.

53. Hirsch MS: Herpes group virus infections in the compromised host. In Rubun RH, Young LS (eds): Clinical Approach to Infection in the Compromised Host. New York, Plenum, 1988, pp 347-366.

54. Meigh RE, Getty B, Bone JM, Hart CA: Varicella in an immunocompromised patient: An electron microscopic study. NIPH Ann 1989;12:3-12.

55. Gelb JD: Varicella-zoster virus. In Field BN, Knipe DM (eds): Virology, 2nd ed. New York, Raven Press, 1990, pp 2011-2054.

56. Hording M, Hording U, Daugaard S, et al: Human papilloma virus type 11 in a fatal case of esophageal and bronchial papillomatosis. Scand J Infect Dis 1989;21:229-231.

57. Janson JA, Baillie J, Pollock M: Endoscopic removal of esophageal condylomata acuminatum containing human papilloma virus. Gastrointest Endosc 1991;37:367-370.

58. Schechter M, Pannain VL, de Oliveira AV: Papovavirus-associated esophageal ulceration in a patient with AIDS. AIDS 1991;5:238.

59. Winkler B, Capo V, Reumann W, et al: Human papillomavirus infection of the esophagus: A clinicopathologic study with demonstration of papillomavirus antigen by the immunoperoxidase technique. Cancer 1985;55:149-155.

60. Silverstein FE, Tytgat GNJ: Atlas of Gastrointestinal Endoscopy, 2nd ed. New York, Gower, 1991.

61. Tilbe KS, Lloyd DA: A case of viral esophagitis. J Clin Gastroenterol 1986;8:494-495.

62. Greenspan JS, Greenspan D, Lennette ET, et al: Replication of Epstein-Barr virus within the epithelial cells of oral "hairy" leukoplakia, an AIDS-associated lesion. N Engl J Med 1985;313:1564-1571.

63. Kitchen VS, Helbert M, Francis ND, et al: Epstein-Barr virus associated oesophageal ulcers in AIDS. Gut 1990;31:1223-1225.

64. Wilcox CM, Schwartz DA, Clark WS: Esophageal ulceration in human immunodeficiency virus infection: Causes, response to therapy, and long-term outcome. Ann Intern Med 1995;123:143-149.

65. Akhtar M, Ali MA, Sackey K, et al: Fine-needle aspiration biopsy diagnosis of endodermal sinus tumor: Histologic and ultrastructural correlations. Diagn Cytopathol 1990;6:184-192.

66. Rabeneck L, Popovic M, Gartner S, et al: Acute HIV infection presenting with painful swallowing and esophageal ulcers. JAMA 1990;263:2318-2322.

67. Bonacini M, Young T, Laine L: Histopathology of human immunodeficiency virus-associated esophageal disease. Am J Gastroenterol 1993;88:549-551.

68. Ehrenpreis ED, Bober DI: Idiopathic ulcerations of the oesophagus in HIV-infected patients: A review. Int J STD AIDS 1996;7:77-81.

69. Kotler DP, Wilson CS, Haroutiounian G, Fox CH: Detection of human immunodeficiency virus-1 by 35S-RNA in situ hybridization in solitary esophageal ulcers in two patients with the acquired immune deficiency syndrome. Am J Gastroenterol 1989;84:313-317.

70. Jalfon IM, Sitton JE, Hammer RA, et al: HIV-1 gp41 antigen demonstration in esophageal ulcers with acquired immunodeficiency syndrome. J Clin Gastroenterol 1991;13:644-648.

71. Kotler DP, Reka S, Orenstein JM, Fox CH: Chronic idiopathic esophageal ulceration in the acquired immunodeficiency syndrome: Characterization and treatment with corticosteroids. J Clin Gastroenterol 1992;15:284-290.

72. Gill MJ, Sutherland LR, Church DL: Gastrointestinal tissue cultures for HIV in HIV-infected/AIDS patients. The University of Calgary Gastrointestinal/HIV Study Group. AIDS 1992;6:553-556.

73. Bach MC, Valenti AJ, Howell DA, Smith TJ: Odynophagia from aphthous ulcers of the pharynx and esophagus in the acquired immunodeficiency syndrome (AIDS). Ann Intern Med 1988;109:338-339.

74. Wilcox CM, Schwartz DA:. A pilot study of oral corticosteroid therapy for idiopathic esophageal ulcerations associated with human immunodeficiency virus infection. Am J Med 1992;93:131-134.

75. Bonnet F, Neau D, Viallard JF, et al: Clinical and laboratory findings of cytomegalovirus infection in 115 hospitalized non-immunocompromised adults. Ann Med Intern 2001;152:227-235.

76. Hinnant KL, Rotterdam HZ, Bell ET, Tapper ML: Cytomegalovirus infection of the alimentary tract: A clinicopathological correlation. Am J Gastroenterol 1986;81:944-950.

77. Emory TS, Carpenter HA, Gostout CJ, Sobin LH: Atlas of Gastrointestinal Endoscopy and Endoscopic Biopsies. Washington, DC, Armed Forces Institute of Pathology, 2000.

78. Xiao SY, Hart J: Marked gastric foveolar hyperplasia associated with active cytomegalovirus infection. Am J Gastroenterol 2001;96:223-226.

79. Andrade JS, Bambirra EA, Lima GF, et al: Gastric cytomegalic inclusion bodies diagnosed by histologic examination of endoscopic biopsies in patients with gastric ulcer. Am J Clin Pathol 1983;79:493-496.

80. Goldman H, Hayek J, Federman M: Gastrointestinal Mucosal Biopsy, 1st ed. New York, Churchill Livingstone, 1996.

81. Rivera-Vaquerizo PA, Gomez-Garrido J, Vicente-Gutierrez M, et al: Varicella zoster gastritis 3 years after bone marrow transplantation for treatment of acute leukemia. Gastrointest Endosc 2001;53:809-810.

82. Vieth M, Dirshmid K, Oehler U, et al: Acute measles gastric infection. Am J Surg Pathol 2001;25:259-262.

83. O'Toole PA, Morris JA: Acute phlegmonous gastritis. Postgrad Med J 1988;64:315-316.

84. Bron BA, Deyhle P, Pelloni S, et al: Phlegmonous gastritis diagnosed by endoscopic snare biopsy. Am J Dig Dis 1977;22:729-733.

85. Mittleman RE, Suarez RV: Phlegmonous gastritis associated with the acquired immunodeficiency syndrome/pre-acquired immunodeficiency syndrome. Arch Pathol Lab Med 1985;109:765-767.

86. Staroverov VV, Kisel AT, Sumarokov UA, Kachanova TN: A case of phlegmonous gastritis diagnosed by echography. Eur J Ultrasound 2001;13:197-200.

87. Binmoeller KF, Benner KG: Emphysematous gastritis secondary to gastric infarction. Am J Gastroenterol 1992;87:526-529.

88. Marshall JB: Tuberculosis of the gastrointestinal tract and peritoneum. Am J Gastroenterol 1993;88:989-999.

89. Benson CA: Disease due to the *Mycobacterium avium* complex in patients with AIDS: Epidemiology and clinical syndrome. Clin Infect Dis 1994;18(Suppl 3):S218-S222.

90. Berardi RS: Abdominal actinomycosis. Surg Gynecol Obstet 1979;149:257-266.

91. Chen CY, Chi KH, George RW, et al: Diagnosis of gastric syphilis by direct immunofluorescence staining and real-time PCR testing. J Clin Microbiol 2006;44:3452-3456.

92. Loffeld RJ, Loffeld BC, Arends JW, et al: Fungal colonization of gastric ulcers. Am J Gastroenterol 1988;83:730-733.

93. Jayalakshmi P, Goh KL, Soo-Hoo TS, Daud A: Disseminated histoplasmosis presenting as penile ulcer. Austral N Z J Med 1990;20:175-176.

94. Cherney CL, Chutuape A, Fikrig MK: Fatal invasive gastric mucormycosis occurring with emphysematous gastritis: Case report and literature review. Am J Gastroenterol 1999;94:252-256.

95. Forester G, Sidhom O, Nahass R, Andavolu R: AIDS-associated cryptosporidiosis with gastric stricture and a therapeutic response to paromomycin. Am J Gastroenterol 1994;89:1096-1098.

96. Garone MA, Winston BJ, Lewis JH: Cryptosporidiosis of the stomach. Am J Gastroenterol 1986;81:465-470.

97. Wurtz R, Mirot M, Fronda G, et al: Short report: Gastric infection by *Strongyloides stercoralis*. Am J Trop Med Hygiene 1994;51:339-340.

98. Kim J, Joo HS, Kim DH, et al: A case of gastric strongyloidiasis in a Korean patient. Korean J Parasitol 2003;41:63-67.

99. Choudhuri G, Saha SS, Tandon RK: Gastric ascariasis. Am J Gastroenterol 1986;81:788-790.

100. Warren JR, Marshall B: Unidentified curved bacilli on gastric epithelium in active chronic gastritis. Lancet 1983;321:1273-1275.

101. Kilbridge PM, Dahms BB, Czinn SJ: *Campylobacter pylori*–associated gastritis and peptic ulcer disease in children. Am J Dis Child 1988;142:1149-1152.

102. Malaty HM, Evans DG, Evans DJ Jr, Graham DY: *Helicobacter pylori* in Hispanics: Comparison with blacks and whites of similar age and socioeconomic class. Gastroenterology 1992;103:813-816.

103. Genta RM, Hamner HW: The significance of lymphoid follicles in the interpretation of gastric biopsy specimens. Arch Pathol Lab Med 1994;118:740-743.

104. Collins JS, Hamilton PW, Watt PC, et al: Superficial gastritis and *Campylobacter pylori* in dyspeptic patients: A quantitative study using computer-linked image analysis. J Pathol 1989;158:303-310.

105. Amieva MR, El-Omar EM: Host-bacterial interactions in *Helicobacter pylori* infection. Gastroenterology 2008;134:306-323.

106. Niemela S, Karttunen T, Kerola T: *Helicobacter pylori*-associated gastritis: Evolution of histologic changes over 10 years. Scand J Gastroenterol 1995;30:542-549.

107. Tham TCK, Collins JSA, Sloan JM: Long-term effects of *Helicobacter pylori* on gastric mucosa: An 8 year follow-up. Am J Gastroenterol 1994;89:1355.

108. Villako K, Kekki M, Maaroos HI, et al: A 12-year follow-up study of chronic gastritis and *Helicobacter pylori* in a population-based random sample. Scand J Gastroenterol 1995;30:964-967.

109. Heilmann KL, Borchard F: Gastritis due to spiral shaped bacteria other than *Helicobacter pylori*: Clinical, histological, and ultrastructural findings. Gut 1991;32:137-140.

110. Hilzenrat N, Lamoureux E, Weintrub I, et al: *Helicobacter heilmannii*-like spiral bacteria in gastric mucosal biopsies: Prevalence and clinical significance. Arch Pathol Lab Med 1995;119:1149-1153.

111. Morgner A, Lehn N, Andersen LP, et al: *Helicobacter heilmannii*-associated primary gastric low-grade MALT lymphoma: Complete remission after curing the infection. Gastroenterology 2000;118:821-828.

112. Bentley R, Meganathan R: Biosynthesis of vitamin K (menaquinone) in bacteria. Microbiol Rev 1982;46:241-280.

113. Hudault S, Guignot J, Servin AL: *Escherichia coli* strains colonising the gastrointestinal tract protect germfree mice against *Salmonella typhimurium* infection. Gut 2001;49:47-55.

114. Reid G, Howard J, Gan BS: Can bacterial interference prevent infection? Trends Microbiol 2001;9:424-428.

115. Levine MM: *Escherichia coli* that cause diarrhea: Enterotoxigenic, enteropathogenic, enteroinvasive, enterohemorrhagic, and enteroadherent. J Infect Dis 1987;155:377-389.

116. Rothbaum R, McAdams AJ, Giannella R, Partin JC: A clinicopathologic study of enterocyte-adherent *Escherichia coli*: A cause of protracted diarrhea in infants. Gastroenterology 1982;83:441-454.

117. Chuttani HK, Jain K, Misra RC: Small bowel in typhoid fever. Gut 1971;12:709-712.

118. Kraus MD, Amatya B, Kimula Y: Histopathology of typhoid enteritis: Morphologic and immunophenotypic findings. Mod Pathol 1999;12:949-955.

119. Braunstein H, Tucker EB, Gibson BC: Mesenteric lymphadenitis due to *Yersinia enterocolitica*: Report of a case. Am J Clin Pathol 1971;55:506-510.

120. El-Maraghi NR, Mair NS: The histopathology of enteric infection with *Yersinia pseudotuberculosis*. Am J Clin Pathol 1979;71:631-639.

121. Gleason TH, Patterson SD: The pathology of *Yersinia enterocolitica* ileocolitis. Am J Surg Pathol 1982;6:347-355.

122. Bode RB, Brayton PR, Colwell RR, et al: A new *Vibrio* species, *Vibrio cincinnatiensis*, causing meningitis: Successful treatment in an adult. Ann Intern Med 1986;104:55-56.

123. Brenner DJ, Hickman-Brenner FW, Lee JV, et al: *Vibrio furnissii* (formerly aerogenic biogroup of *Vibrio fluvialis*), a new species

isolated from human feces and the environment. J Clin Microbiol 1983;18:816-824.

124. Davis BR, Fanning GR, Madden JM, et al: Characterization of biochemically atypical *Vibrio cholerae* strains and designation of a new pathogenic species, *Vibrio mimicus.* J Clin Microbiol 1981;14:631-639.

125. Hickman FW, Farmer JJ 3rd, Hollis DG, et al: Identification of *Vibrio hollisae* sp. nov. from patients with diarrhea. J Clin Microbiol 1982;15:395-401.

126. Lee JV, Shread P, Furniss AL, Bryant TN: Taxonomy and description of *Vibrio fluvialis* sp. nov. (synonym group F vibrios, group EF6). J Appl Bacteriol 1981;50:73-94.

127. Love M, Teebken-Fisher D, Hose JE, et al: *Vibrio damsela*, a marine bacterium, causes skin ulcers on the damselfish *Chromis punctipinnis.* Science 1981;214:1139-1140.

128. Mathan MM, Chandy G, Mathan VI: Ultrastructural changes in the upper small intestinal mucosa in patients with cholera. Gastroenterology 1995;109:422-430.

129. Gui L, Subramony C, Fratkin J, Hughson MD: Fatal enteritis necroticans (pigbel) in a diabetic adult. Mod Pathol 2002;15:66-70.

130. Matsuda T, Okada Y, Inagi E, et al: Enteritis necroticans 'pigbel' in a Japanese diabetic adult. Pathol Int 2007;57:622-626.

131. Meinzer U, Esmiol-Welterlin S, Barreau F, et al: Nod2 mediates susceptibility to *Yersinia pseudotuberculosis* in mice. PLoS ONE 2008;3:e2769.

132. Reed RP, Robins-Browne RM, Williams ML: *Yersinia enterocolitica* peritonitis. Clin Infect Dis 1997;25:1468-1469.

133. de Cuenca-Moron B, Solis-Herruzo JA, Moreno D, et al: Spontaneous bacterial peritonitis due to *Yersinia enterocolitica* in secondary alcoholic hemochromatosis. J Clin Gastroenterol 1989;11:675-678.

134. Capron JP, Capron-Chivrac D, Tossou H, et al: Spontaneous *Yersinia enterocolitica* peritonitis in idiopathic hemochromatosis. Gastroenterology 1984;87:1372-1375.

135. Cianciulli P, Trua G, Papa G, et al: *Yersinia enterocolitica* mesenteric adenitis in a thalassaemic adolescent: Conservative management. Eur J Pediatr 1992;151:145-146.

136. Gallant T, Freedman MH, Vellend H, Francombe WH: *Yersinia* sepsis in patients with iron overload treated with deferoxamine. N Engl J Med 1986;314:1643.

137. Green NS: *Yersinia* infections in patients with homozygous beta-thalassemia associated with iron overload and its treatment. Pediatr Hematol Oncol 1992;9:247-254.

138. Cohen JI, Rodday P: *Yersinia enterocolitica* bacteremia in a patient with the acquired immunodeficiency syndrome. Am J Med 1989;86:254-255.

139. Boemi G, Chiesa C, Di Lorenzo M, et al: *Yersinia enterocolitica* peritonitis. Gastroenterology 1985;89:927-928.

140. Brubaker RR: Factors promoting acute and chronic diseases caused by yersiniae. Clin Microbiol Rev 1991;4:309-324.

141. Autenrieth IB, Firsching R: Penetration of M cells and destruction of Peyer's patches by *Yersinia enterocolitica*: An ultrastructural and histological study. J Med Microbiol 1996;44:285-294.

142. Clark MA, Hirst BH, Jepson MA: M-cell surface beta1 integrin expression and invasin-mediated targeting of *Yersinia pseudotuberculosis* to mouse Peyer's patch M cells. Infect Immun 1998;66:1237-1243.

143. Handley SA, Dube PH, Revell PA, Miller VL: Characterization of oral *Yersinia enterocolitica* infection in three different strains of inbred mice. Infect Immun 2004;72:1645-1656.

144. Tuohy AM, O'Gorman M, Byington C, et al: *Yersinia enterocolitis* mimicking Crohn's disease in a toddler. Pediatrics 1999;104:e36.

145. Gold BD, Westra SJ, Graeme-Cook FM: Case records of the Massachusetts General Hospital: Weekly clinicopathological exercises. Case 40-2003: A 14-month-old boy with recurrent abdominal distention and diarrhea. N Engl J Med 2003;349:2541-2549.

146. Anand SS: Hypertrophic ileo-caecal tuberculosis in India with a record of fifty hemicolectomies. Ann R Coll Surg Engl 1956;19:205-222.

147. Hsieh SM, Hung CC, Chen MY, et al: Clinical features and outcome in disseminated mycobacterial diseases in AIDS patients in Taiwan. AIDS 1998;12:1301-1307.

148. Chaisson RE, Gallant JE, Keruly JC, Moore RD: Impact of opportunistic disease on survival in patients with HIV infection. AIDS 1998;12:29-33.

149. Palella FJ Jr, Delaney KM, Moorman AC, et al: Declining morbidity and mortality among patients with advanced human immunodeficiency virus infection. HIV Outpatient Study Investigators. N Engl J Med 1998;338:853-860.

150. Horsburgh CR Jr: The pathophysiology of disseminated *Mycobacterium avium* complex disease in AIDS. J Infect Dis 1999;179(Suppl 3):S461-S465.

151. Horsburgh C: Mycobacterial disease of the gastrointestinal tract. In Blaser M, Amith P, Ravdin JI, et al. (eds): Infections of the Gastrointestinal Tract. New York, Raven Press, 1995, pp 937-955.

152. Sun HY, Chen MY, Wu MS, et al: Endoscopic appearance of GI mycobacteriosis caused by the *Mycobacterium avium* complex in a patient with AIDS: Case report and review. Gastrointest Endosc 2005;61:775-779.

153. Rotterdam H, Tsang P: Gastrointestinal disease in the immunocompromised patient. Hum Pathol 1994;25:1123-1140.

154. Fenollar F, Puechal X, Raoult D: Whipple's disease. N Engl J Med 2007;356:55-66.

155. Fenollar F, Lepidi H, Gerolami R, et al: Whipple disease associated with giardiasis. J Infect Dis 2003;188:828-834.

156. Marth T, Strober W: Whipple's disease. Semin Gastrointest Dis 1996;7:41-48.

157. Marth T, Neurath M, Cuccherini BA, Strober W: Defects of monocyte interleukin 12 production and humoral immunity in Whipple's disease. Gastroenterology 1997;113:442-448.

158. Elssner A, Doseff AI, Duncan M, et al: IL-16 is constitutively present in peripheral blood monocytes and spontaneously released during apoptosis. J Immunol 2004;172:7721-7725.

159. Puechal X: Whipple disease and arthritis. Curr Opin Rheumatol 2001;13:74-79.

160. Gerard A, Sarrot-Reynauld F, Liozon E, et al: Neurologic presentation of Whipple disease: Report of 12 cases and review of the literature. Medicine (Baltimore) 2002;81:443-457.

161. Mahnel R, Kalt A, Ring S, et al: Immunosuppressive therapy in Whipple's disease patients is associated with the appearance of gastrointestinal manifestations. Am J Gastroenterol 2005;100:1167-1173.

162. Dobbins WI: Whipple's Disease. Springfield, Ill., Charles C Thomas, 1987.

163. Marth T, Raoult D: Whipple's disease. Lancet 2003;361:239-246.

164. von Herbay A, Maiwald M, Ditton HJ, Otto HF: Histology of intestinal Whipple's disease revisited: A study of 48 patients. Virchows Arch 1996;429:335-343.

165. Fenollar F, Raoult D: Whipple's disease. Clin Diagn Lab Immunol 2001;8:1-8.

166. Dutly F, Altwegg M: Whipple's disease and *"Tropheryma whippelii."* Clin Microbiol Rev 2001;14:561-583.

167. Owens SR, Greenson JK: The pathology of malabsorption: Current concepts. Histopathology 2007;50:64-82.

168. Peetermans WE, Vonck A: Tropical sprue after travel to Tanzania. J Travel Med 2000;7:33-34.

169. Guerra R, Wheby MS, Bayless TM: Long-term antibiotic therapy in tropical sprue. Ann Intern Med 1965;63:619-634.

170. Ghoshal UC, Ghoshal U, Ayyagari A, et al: Tropical sprue is associated with contamination of small bowel with aerobic bacteria and

reversible prolongation of orocecal transit time. J Gastroenterol Hepatol 2003;18:540-547.

171. Day D, Jass J, Price AB, et al: Morson and Dawson's Gastrointesitnal Pathology. Malden, Mass., Blackwell, 2003.

172. Robert M: Inflammatory disorders of the small intestine. In Odze R, Goldblum J, Crawford J (eds): Surgical Pathology of the Gastrointestinal Tract, Liver, Biliary Tract, and Pancreas. Philadelphia, Saunders, 2004, pp 117-212.

173. Schenk EA, Samloff IM, Klipstein FA: Morphologic characteristics of jejunal biopsy in celiac disease and tropical sprue. Am J Pathol 1965;47:765-781.

174. Swanson VL, Thomassen RW: Pathology of the jejunal mucosa in tropical sprue. Am J Pathol 1965;46:511-551.

175. Wheby MS, Swanson VL, Bayless TM: Comparison of ileal and jejunal biopsies in tropical sprue. Am J Clin Nutr 1971;24:117-123.

176. Prescott RJ, Harris M, Banerjee SS: Fungal infections of the small and large intestine. J Clin Pathol 1992;45:806-811.

177. Cappell MS, Mandell W, Grimes MM, Neu HC: Gastrointestinal histoplasmosis. Dig Dis Sci 1988;33:353-360.

178. Bodily K, Perfect JR, Procop G, et al: Small intestinal histoplasmosis: Successful treatment with itraconazole in an immunocompetent host. Gastrointest Endosc 1996;43:518-521.

179. Halline AG, Maldonado-Lutomirsky M, Ryoo JW, et al: Colonic histoplasmosis in AIDS: Unusual endoscopic findings in two cases. Gastrointest Endosc 1997;45:199-204.

180. Eras P, Goldstein MJ, Sherlock P: Candida infection of the gastrointestinal tract. Medicine (Baltimore) 1972;51:367-379.

181. Leung WK, To KF, Chan PK, et al: Enteric involvement of severe acute respiratory syndrome-associated coronavirus infection. Gastroenterology 2003;125:1011-1017.

182. Walter JE, Mitchell DK: Astrovirus infection in children. Curr Opin Infect Dis 2003;16:247-253.

183. Vernacchio L, Vezina RM, Mitchell AA, et al: Diarrhea in American infants and young children in the community setting: Incidence, clinical presentation and microbiology. Pediatr Infect Dis J 2006; 25:2-7.

184. Chamberlain RS, Atkins S, Saini N, White JC: Ileal perforation caused by cytomegalovirus infection in a critically ill adult. J Clin Gastroenterol 2000;30:432-435.

185. Abu-Elmagd KM, Tzakis A, Todo S, et al: Monitoring and treatment of intestinal allograft rejection in humans. Transplant Proc 1993;25(1 Pt 2):1202-1203.

186. Manez R, Kusne S, Abu-Elmagd K, et al: Factors associated with recurrent cytomegalovirus disease after small bowel transplantation. Transplant Proc 1994;26:1422-1423.

187. Kusne S, Manez R, Frye BL, et al: Use of DNA amplification for diagnosis of cytomegalovirus enteritis after intestinal transplantation. Gastroenterology 1997;112:1121-1128.

188. Keates J, Lagahee S, Crilley P, et al: CMV enteritis causing segmental ischemia and massive intestinal hemorrhage. Gastrointest Endosc 2001;53:355-359.

189. Peterson PK, Balfour HH Jr, Marker SC, et al: Cytomegalovirus disease in renal allograft recipients: A prospective study of the clinical features, risk factors and impact on renal transplantation. Medicine (Baltimore) 1980;59:283-300.

190. Page MJ, Dreese JC, Poritz LS, Koltun WA: Cytomegalovirus enteritis: A highly lethal condition requiring early detection and intervention. Dis Colon Rectum 1998;41:619-623.

191. Teixidor HS, Honig CL, Norsoph E, et al: Cytomegalovirus infection of the alimentary canal: Radiologic findings with pathologic correlation. Radiology 1987;163:317-323.

192. Kotler DP, Shimada T, Snow G, et al: Effect of combination antiretroviral therapy upon rectal mucosal HIV RNA burden and mononuclear cell apoptosis. AIDS 1998;12: 97-604.

193. Clayton F, Kotler DP, Kuwada SK, et al: Gp120-induced Bob/GPR15 activation: A possible cause of human immunodeficiency virus enteropathy. Am J Pathol 2001;159: 1933-1939.

194. Dayanithi G, Yahi N, Baghdiguian S, Fantini J: Intracellular calcium release induced by human immunodeficiency virus type 1 (HIV-1) surface envelope glycoprotein in human intestinal epithelial cells: A putative mechanism for HIV-1 enteropathy. Cell Calcium 1995;18:9-18.

195. Maresca M, Mahfoud R, Garmy N, et al: The virotoxin model of HIV-1 enteropathy: Involvement of GPR15/Bob and galactosylceramide in the cytopathic effects induced by HIV-1 gp120 in the HT-29-D4 intestinal cell line. J Biomed Sci 2003;10:156-166.

196. Schmitz H, Rokos K, Florian P, et al: Supernatants of HIV-infected immune cells affect the barrier function of human HT-29/B6 intestinal epithelial cells. AIDS 2002;16:983-991.

197. Stockmann M, Fromm M, Schmitz H, et al: Duodenal biopsies of HIV-infected patients with diarrhoea exhibit epithelial barrier defects but no active secretion. AIDS 1998;12:43-51.

198. Chui DW, Owen RL: AIDS and the gut. J Gastroenterol Hepatol 1994;9:291-303.

199. Delezay O, Yahi N, Tamalet C, et al: Direct effect of type 1 human immunodeficiency virus (HIV-1) on intestinal epithelial cell differentiation: Relationship to HIV-1 enteropathy. Virology 1997; 238:231-242.

200. Greenson JK, Belitsos PC, Yardley JH, Bartlett JG: AIDS enteropathy: Occult enteric infections and duodenal mucosal alterations in chronic diarrhea. Ann Intern Med 1991;114:366-372.

201. Clayton F, Clayton CH: Gastrointestinal pathology in HIV-infected patients. Gastroenterol Clin North Am 1997;26:191-240.

202. Farthing MJ, Kelly MP, Veitch AM: Recently recognised microbial enteropathies and HIV infection. J Antimicrob Chemother 1996;37(Suppl B):61-70.

203. Farthing MJ: The molecular pathogenesis of giardiasis. J Pediatr Gastroenterol Nutr 1997;24:79-88.

204. Hill DR: Giardiasis. Issues in diagnosis and management. Infect Dis Clin North Am 1993;7:503-525.

205. Feely DE, Gardner MD, Hardin EL: Excystation of *Giardia muris* induced by a phosphate-bicarbonate medium: Localization of acid phosphatase. J Parasitol 1991;77:441-448.

206. Erlandsen SL, Chase DG: Morphological alterations in the microvillous border of villous epithelial cells produced by intestinal microorganisms. Am J Clin Nutr 1974;27:1277-1286.

207. Oberhuber G, Stolte M: Giardiasis: Analysis of histological changes in biopsy specimens of 80 patients. J Clin Pathol 1990;43:641-643.

208. Oberhuber G, Kastner N, Stolte M: Giardiasis: A histologic analysis of 567 cases. Scand J Gastroenterol 1997;32:48-51.

209. Wright SG, Tomkins AM: Quantification of the lymphocytic infiltrate in jejunal epithelium in giardiasis. Clin Exp Immunol 1977;29:408-412.

210. Rosekrans PC, Lindeman J, Meijer CJ: Quantitative histological and immunohistochemical findings in jejunal biopsy specimens in giardiasis. Virchows Arch A Pathol Anat Histol 1981;393:145-151.

211. Huang DB, Chappell C, Okhuysen PC: Cryptosporidiosis in children. Semin Pediatr Infect Dis 2004;15:253-259.

212. Goodgame RW: Understanding intestinal spore-forming protozoa: Cryptosporidia, microsporidia, isospora, and cyclospora. Ann Intern Med 1996;124:429-441.

213. Lewthwaite P, Gill GV, Hart CA, Beeching NJ: Gastrointestinal parasites in the immunocompromised. Curr Opin Infect Dis 2005;18:427-435.

214. Rabeneck L, Gyorkey F, Genta RM, et al: The role of microsporidia in the pathogenesis of HIV-related chronic diarrhea. Ann Intern Med 1993;119:895-899.

215. Beauvais B, Sarfati C, Molina JM, et al: Comparative evaluation of five diagnostic methods for demonstrating microsporidia in stool and intestinal biopsy specimens. Ann Trop Med Parasitol 1993; 87:99-102.

216. Curry A, Smith HV: Emerging pathogens: *Isospora, Cyclospora* and microsporidia. Parasitology 1998;117(Suppl):S143-S159.

217. Connor BA, Reidy J, Soave R: Cyclosporiasis: Clinical and histopathologic correlates. Clin Infect Dis 1999;28:1216-1222.

218. Cook GC: The clinical significance of gastrointestinal helminths: A review. Trans R Soc Trop Med Hyg 1986;80:675-685.

219. Neafie RC, Conner DH, Cross HH, Meyers WH: Diseases caused by other nematodes. In Binford CH, Connor DH (eds): Pathology of Tropical and Extraordinary Disease, vol. 2. Washington, DC, The Armed Forces Institute of Pathology, 1976, pp 397-481.

220. Bundy DA, Cooper ES, Thompson DE, et al: Epidemiology and population dynamics of *Ascaris lumbricoides* and *Trichuris trichiura* infection in the same community. Trans R Soc Trop Med Hyg 1987;81:987-993.

221. Cooper ES, Whyte-Alleng CA, Finzi-Smith JS, MacDonald TT: Intestinal nematode infections in children: The pathophysiological price paid. Parasitology 1992;104(Suppl):S91-S103.

222. Croese J, Loukas A, Opdebeeck J, et al: Human enteric infection with canine hookworms. Ann Intern Med 1994;120:369-374.

223. Milder JE, Walzer PD, Kilgore G, et al: Clinical features of *Strongyloides stercoralis* infection in an endemic area of the United States. Gastroenterology 1981;80:1481-1488.

224. Concha R, Harrington W Jr, Rogers AI: Intestinal strongyloidiasis: Recognition, management, and determinants of outcome. J Clin Gastroenterol 2005;39:203-211.

225. Keiser PB, Nutman TB: *Strongyloides stercoralis* in the immunocompromised population. Clin Microbiol Rev 2004;17:208-217.

226. Ramdial PK, Hlatshwayo NH, Singh B: Strongyloides stercoralis mesenteric lymphadenopathy: Clue to the etiopathogenesis of intestinal pseudo-obstruction in HIV-infected patients. Ann Diagn Pathol 2006;10:209-214.

227. Longworth DL, Weller PF: Hyperinfection syndrome in strongyloidiasis. In Remington JS, Swartz MN (eds): Current Clinical Topics in Infectious Diseases. New York, McGraw-Hill, 1986, pp 1-7.

228. Scaglia M, Brustia R, Gatti S, et al: Autochthonous strongyloidiasis in Italy: An epidemiological and clinical review of 150 cases. Bull Soc Pathol Exot Filiales 1984;77:328-332.

229. Genta RM, Weesner R, Douce RW, et al: Strongyloidiasis in US veterans of the Vietnam and other wars. JAMA 1987;258:49-52.

230. Rivasi F, Pampiglione S, Boldorini R, Cardinale L: Histopathology of gastric and duodenal *Strongyloides stercoralis* locations in fifteen immunocompromised subjects. Arch Pathol Lab Med 2006;130:1792-1798.

231. Dronda F, Chaves F, Sanz A, Lopez-Velez R: Human intestinal capillariasis in an area of nonendemicity: Case report and review. Clin Infect Dis 1993;17:909-912.

232. Cross JH: Intestinal capillariasis. Clin Microbiol Rev 1992;5:120-129.

233. Neafie RC, Connor DH: Fasciolopsiasis. In Binford CH, Connor DH (eds): Pathology of Tropical and Extraordinary Diseases, Vol. 2. Washington, DC, The Armed Forces Institute of Pathology, 1976, pp 528-529.

234. Liu LX, Harinasuta KT: Liver and intestinal flukes. Gastroenterol Clin North Am 1996;25: 627-636.

235. Chai JY, Darwin Murrell K, Lymbery AJ: Fish-borne parasitic zoonoses: Status and issues. Int J Parasitol 2005;35:1233-1254.

236. Fried B, Graczyk TK, Tamang L: Food-borne intestinal trematodiases in humans. Parasitol Res 2004;93:159-170.

237. Park CI, Kim H, Ro JY, Gutierrez Y: Human ectopic fascioliasis in the cecum. Am J Surg Pathol 1984;8:73-77.

238. Despommier DD: Tapeworm infection: The long and the short of it. N Engl J Med 1992;327:727-728.

239. Bruckner DA: Helminthic food-borne infections. Clin Lab Med 1999;19:639-660.

240. Levine MM, Levine OS: Changes in human ecology and behavior in relation to the emergence of diarrheal diseases, including cholera. Proc Natl Acad Sci U S A 1994;91:2390-2394.

241. Nostrant TT, Kumar NB, Appelman HD: Histopathology differentiates acute self-limited colitis from ulcerative colitis. Gastroenterology 1987;92:318-328.

242. Surawicz CM: The role of rectal biopsy in infectious colitis. Am J Surg Pathol 1988;12(Suppl 1):82-88.

243. Surawicz CM, Belic L: Rectal biopsy helps to distinguish acute self-limited colitis from idiopathic inflammatory bowel disease. Gastroenterology 1984;86:104-113.

244. Echeverria P, Savarino SJ, Yamamoto T: *Escherichia coli* diarrhoea. Bailliere Clin Gastroenterol 1993;7:243-262.

245. Adachi JA, Jiang ZD, Mathewson JJ, et al: Enteroaggregative *Escherichia coli* as a major etiologic agent in traveler's diarrhea in 3 regions of the world. Clin Infect Dis 2001;32:1706-1709.

246. Edelman R, Karmali MA, Fleming PA: From the National Institutes of Health. Summary of the International Symposium and Workshop on Infections due to Verocytotoxin (Shiga-like toxin)-producing *Escherichia coli*. J Infect Dis 1988;157:1102-1104.

247. Phillips AD, Navabpour S, Hicks S, et al: Enterohaemorrhagic *Escherichia coli* O157:H7 target Peyer's patches in humans and cause attaching/effacing lesions in both human and bovine intestine. Gut 2000;47:377-381.

248. Tarr PI, Neill MA, Clausen CR, et al: Genotypic variation in pathogenic *Escherichia coli* O157:H7 isolated from patients in Washington, 1984-1987. J Infect Dis 1989;159:344-347.

249. Griffin PM, Olmstead LC, Petras RE: *Escherichia coli* O157:H7-associated colitis: A clinical and histological study of 11 cases. Gastroenterology 1990;99:142-149.

250. Hunt CM, Harvey JA, Youngs ER, et al: Clinical and pathological variability of infection by enterohaemorrhagic (Vero cytotoxin producing) *Escherichia coli*. J Clin Pathol 1989;42:847-852.

251. Lee SD, Surawicz CM: Infectious causes of chronic diarrhea. Gastroenterol Clin North Am 2001;30:679-692, viii.

252. Siegal D, Syed F, Hamid N, Cunha BA: *Campylobacter jejuni* pancolitis mimicking idiopathic ulcerative colitis. Heart Lung 2005;34:288-290.

253. Schneider EN, Havens JM, Scott MA, et al. Molecular diagnosis of *Campylobacter jejuni* infection in cases of focal active colitis. Am J Surg Pathol 2006;30:782-785.

254. Anderson JB, Tanner AH, Brodribb AJ: Toxic megacolon due to *Campylobacter colitis*. Int J Colorectal Dis 1986;1:58-59.

255. Butzler JP: Campylobacter, from obscurity to celebrity. Clin Microbiol Infect 2004;10:868-876.

256. Price AB, Davies DR: Pseudomembranous colitis. J Clin Pathol 1977;30:1-12.

257. Schiffman R: Signet-ring cells associated with pseudomembranous colitis. Am J Surg Pathol 1996;20:599-602.

258. Chatzicostas C, Koutroubakis IE, Tzardi M, et al: Colonic tuberculosis mimicking Crohn's disease: Case report. BMC Gastroenterol 2002;2:10.

259. Calderaro A, Bommezzadri S, Gorrini C, et al: Infective colitis associated with human intestinal spirochetosis. J Gastroenterol Hepatol 2007;22:1772-1779.

260. Christie JD: Intestinal spirochetes: Organisms in search of a disease? Am J Clin Pathol 2003;120:820-821.

261. van Mook WN, Koek GH, van der Ven AJ, et al: Human intestinal spirochaetosis: Any clinical significance? Eur J Gastroenterol Hepatol 2004;16:83-87.

262. Ho M: Epidemiology of cytomegalovirus infections. Rev Infect Dis 1990;12(Suppl 7): S701-S710.

263. Kyriazis AP, Mitra SK: Multiple cytomegalovirus-related intestinal perforations in patients with acquired immunodeficiency syndrome: Report of two cases and review of the literature. Arch Pathol Lab Med 1992;116:495-499.

264. Kambham N, Vij R, Cartwright CA, Longacre T: Cytomegalovirus infection in steroid-refractory ulcerative colitis: A case-control study. Am J Surg Pathol 2004;28:365-373.

265. Surawicz CM, Goodell SE, Quinn TC, et al: Spectrum of rectal biopsy abnormalities in homosexual men with intestinal symptoms. Gastroenterology 1986;91:651-659.

266. Haque R, Huston CD, Hughes M, et al: Amebiasis. N Engl J Med 2003;348:1565-1573.

267. Castro J, Vazquez-Iglesias JL, Arnal-Monreal F: Dysentery caused by *Balantidium coli*: Report of two cases. Endoscopy 1983;15:272-274.

268. Matsumoto T, Iida M, Kimura Y, et al: Anisakiasis of the colon: Radiologic and endoscopic features in six patients. Radiology 1992;183:97-99.

269. Nash TE, Cheever AW, Ottesen EA, Cook JA: Schistosome infections in humans: Perspectives and recent findings. NIH conference. Ann Intern Med 1982;97:740-754.

270. Lemos LB, Qu Z, Laucirica R, Fred HL: Hyperinfection syndrome in strongyloidiasis: Report of two cases. Ann Diagn Pathol 2003;7:87-94.

271. Lee SC, Hwang KP, Tsai WS, et al: Detection of *Enterobius vermicularis* eggs in the submucosa of the transverse colon of a man presenting with colon carcinoma. Am J Trop Med Hygiene 2002;67:546-548.

272. Klausner JD, Kohn R, Kent C: Etiology of clinical proctitis among men who have sex with men. Clin Infect Dis 2004;38:300-302.

273. McMillan A, Gilmour HM, Slatford K, McNeillage GJ: Proctitis in homosexual men: A diagnostic problem. Br J Vener Dis 1983;59:260-264.

10

Liver and Bile Duct Infections

Joseph Misdraji

The liver is the target of many infectious agents, most notably hepatotropic viruses such as hepatitis B virus (HBV) and hepatitis C virus (HCV). Additionally, many infectious organisms can involve the liver in the setting of disseminated infection, in immune-suppressed patients, or as a medical curiosity. The major challenge facing the pathologist in diagnosing these conditions is that many of these diseases have overlapping histopathologic characteristics. Hepatitis, necrosis, or granulomas are characteristic of many liver infections, and distinguishing the exact cause often requires a meticulous search for organisms, attention to subtle morphologic clues, or, not uncommonly, clinical, epidemiologic, or serologic data. Although some organisms can be readily detected in tissue, many are not, even with the use of ancillary techniques. Furthermore, many of the ancillary techniques used to detect organisms in tissue are not widely available. Therefore, although the pattern of injury can provide a differential diagnosis, in some cases, the final diagnosis relies on culture or serologic studies.

Viruses

Hepatitis A

Hepatitis A virus (HAV) is an RNA virus in the Picornaviridae family. Although the incidence of HAV infection has fallen dramatically since the introduction of vaccines, it still causes approximately 60,000 infections per year and occasionally causes dramatic outbreaks with fulminant hepatitis and death.[1] Fecal-oral transmission is facilitated by extensive viral shedding in feces during the 3- to 6-week incubation period, which reaches a maximum just before the onset of hepatocellular injury.[1] An increasing incidence has been noted among urban homosexual men. An effective vaccine has been developed.

The signs and symptoms of hepatitis A are related to patient age. In children younger than 3 years of age, more than 80% of infections are clinically silent, whereas in adolescents and adults, more than 75% of cases are symptomatic.[2] Symptoms include fever, malaise, abdominal pain, and jaundice. Marked transami-

nase elevations are characteristic. About 100 cases of HAV-related fulminant liver failure are reported each year, predominantly in adults.[2] Chronic infection does not occur. However, HAV infection can precipitate autoimmune hepatitis, which can progress to chronic hepatitis with fibrosis or cirrhosis.[3-6]

Liver injury in HAV infection is the result of an immunopathologic response to infected hepatocytes rather than a direct cytopathic effect of the virus.[1] The adaptive immune response is highly effective in eliminating the virus. The earliest antibody response is largely that of immunoglobulin M (IgM), with IgG production beginning shortly thereafter; therefore, the diagnosis is established by the detection of anti-HAV IgM (with or without IgG). Anti-HAV IgG persists for life and confers protection against reinfection.[1]

Acute HAV infection may be indistinguishable from other acute viral hepatitides (see discussion of hepatitis B). However, portal plasma cell infiltrates and periportal necrosis may be prominent, causing confusion with autoimmune hepatitis (Fig. 10-1).[7] In rare cases, perivenular cholestasis with relatively little inflammation mimics cholestatic drug reactions. Fibrin ring granulomas have been reported.[8,9]

Hepatitis B

Chronic hepatitis B affects an estimated 400 million persons worldwide, of whom 1 million die annually.[10,11] Three quarters of patients with chronic hepatitis B in the world are Chinese, and sub-Saharan Africa also has high prevalence.[11] In the United States, the incidence of newly acquired HBV infection has been declining due to screening of pregnant women, vaccination, and safer injection practices.[10]

Virology

HBV is a DNA-containing virus with four overlapping open reading frames.[12] Its four genes are core, surface, X, and polymerase genes. The core gene encodes the core nucleocapsid protein, which is important in viral packaging, and hepatitis B

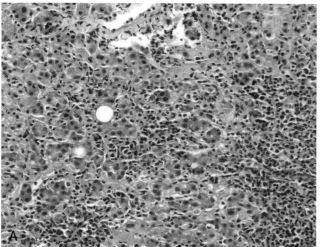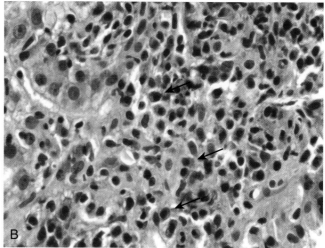

Figure 10-1. Liver biopsy in hepatitis A. **A,** Panlobular inflammation and lobular disarray. **B,** High power shows many plasma cells within the infiltrate *(arrows).*

early antigen (HBeAg). The surface gene encodes pre-S1, pre-S2, and S protein, which are large, middle, and small surface proteins, respectively. The X gene encodes the X protein, which may be important in carcinogenesis. The polymerase gene encodes a large protein that has a role in packaging and DNA replication.[12]

There are eight major HBV genotypes: A is pandemic; B and C are found in Asia, D in southern Europe, E in Africa, F in the United States and South America, G in the United States and France, and H in South America.[11] To some extent, genotype influences the severity of hepatitis and its outcome. The severity of chronic hepatitis is greater with genotype C than with B, and there is a higher frequency of cirrhosis and hepatocellular carcinoma (HCC) in patients infected with HBV genotype C. A higher rate of virologic response is achieved among patients infected with genotype B, compared with genotype C.[13]

Pathophysiology

Hepatitis B is not directly cytotoxic to hepatocytes. Instead, the pathogenesis of HBV infection is related to the host immune response to viral infection. More rigorous immune responses cause more severe liver injury. Patients with a vigorous immune response may suffer fulminant infection with severe liver injury followed by rapid viral clearance, whereas hosts with less vigorous immune responses may become asymptomatic carriers.[10]

Natural History

Transmission of HBV is parenteral. In developed countries, sexual contact, intravenous drug use, acupuncture, and transfusion constitute the most common modes of transmission. In developing countries, vertical transmission is more significant.

Acute hepatitis B manifests as an icteric illness after an incubation period of 6 weeks to 6 months in up to 50% of infected persons.[10] A subset of patients experience a prodromal phase characterized by arthralgias and urticarial skin rash.[14] Acute infection is diagnosed by the detection of hepatitis B surface antigen (HBsAg), IgM antibodies to hepatitis B core antigen (anti-HBcAg), and HBeAg. The outcome of acute hepatitis depends on the immune status and age of the host. Chronic HBV infection develops in as many as 90% of neonates and infants but in only 1% to 5% of immunocompetent adults.[10,11] Patients with chronic HBV infection rarely have extrahepatic manifestations, such as polyarteritis nodosa or glomerulonephritis.[14] Many remain asymptomatic until they present with cirrhosis, HCC, or both.

The presence of HBsAg in serum for 6 months or longer is indicative of chronic HBV infection. Chronic HBV infection manifests in one of several well-defined stages. The immune tolerance phase is seen largely in patients who acquire infection at birth or in early childhood. These patients have high levels of HBV replication but little to no liver inflammation and normal serum aminotransferase levels. Serum HBeAg is detectable, and HBV DNA is markedly elevated.[10,11,15] As the host immune system matures, the patient enters the immune clearance phase, which is characterized by immune mediated liver injury. Patients who acquire infection as children come to clinical attention in this stage, and those who acquire infection as adolescents or adults have a very short or no immune tolerance phase and rapidly move into this second phase of the infection. Viral levels

decrease, but HBV DNA is still elevated, and HBeAg is detectable. Serum aminotransferases increase, and liver histology shows active chronic hepatitis with evolving fibrosis.[10] Although most patients remain asymptomatic, some present with flares that mimic acute hepatitis, and this may precede the development of antibodies to HBeAg and remission of hepatitis activity.[10] Spontaneous seroconversion to HBeAb-positive status occurs in up to 90% of white adults with chronic hepatitis B within 10 years of follow-up, and it is more likely in those with high transaminase levels, which indicate a vigorous immune response to HBV.[10,15]

Seroconversion is followed by the low or nonreplicative HBsAg carrier stage, characterized by normalization of aminotransferases and low or undetectable HBV DNA levels.[10,15] Histologically, minimal to mild hepatitis with variable fibrosis is seen.[10] Most patients remain in this stage, particularly if they acquired the infection as adults; viral clearance may occur, but in patients with established cirrhosis, monitoring for HCC must continue.[10,16] Up to 20% of patients serorevert to HBeAg-positive status, with a flare of activity.[10,16] In up to one third of patients, chronic hepatitis recurs without seroreversion; this is known as HBeAg-negative chronic hepatitis, due to mutations in the precore or core-promoter regions of the HBV genome.[10,16] In this phase, despite the presence of anti-HBeAg antibody (HBeAb) and the absence of HBeAg, HBV DNA is detectable, serum aminotransferases rise, and histologic examination of the liver shows chronic hepatitis.[10] Patients with HBeAg-negative chronic hepatitis tend to be older and to have more advanced liver fibrosis.[10]

Cirrhosis develops at an annual incidence of 8% to 10% in patients with HBeAg-negative chronic hepatitis and 2% to 5% in patients with HBeAg-positive chronic hepatitis.[10] Cirrhosis is the major risk factor for the development of HCC; the annual incidence of HCC is 1% for HBV carriers without cirrhosis and 2% to 3% for those with cirrhosis.[10] The risk factors for cirrhosis and HCC are similar and include high HBV DNA levels, HBeAg positivity, older age, and male gender.[10,15] Additional risk factors for HCC include abnormal alanine aminotransferase levels, long duration of infection, coinfection with HCV or hepatitis D (HDV), a family history of HCC, excessive alcohol intake, cigarette smoking, HBV genotype C, and core-promoter mutations.[10]

Histopathology

Acute HBV infection is indistinguishable from other forms of acute viral hepatitis. Portal tracts exhibit a moderate to marked lymphocytic infiltrate. Lobular mononuclear inflammation is associated with widespread lobular injury in the form of hepatocyte ballooning, although in the early stages the injury may be confined to centrilobular regions. Numerous acidophil bodies, canalicular cholestasis, and Kupffer cell hyperplasia may be seen. In more severe cases, bridging necrosis may span between portal tracts and central veins. Panacinar necrosis or multiacinar necrosis may also be a feature. Fulminant cases are characterized by submassive or massive necrosis with marked ductular reaction. Numerous macrophages laden with lipofuscin and hemosiderin may be seen in necrotic areas. Hepatic lobular regeneration may also be evident, with mitotic figures and lobular disarray. The latter can be highlighted by reticulin stains, which serve to delineate the loss of normal hepatic plate architecture.

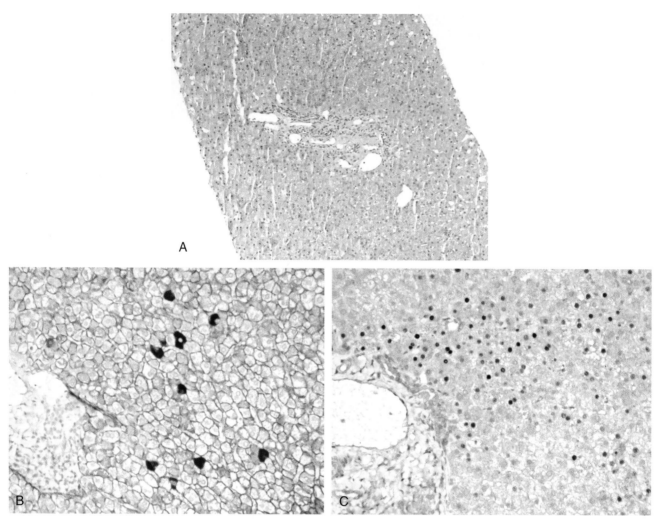

Figure 10-2. Liver biopsy in the immune tolerance phase of hepatitis B. **A,** Portal tract without inflammation or fibrosis. **B,** Immunohistochemical staining for hepatitis B surface antigen (HBsAg) shows strong membranous staining of hepatocytes as well as individual hepatocytes with strong cytoplasmic staining, consistent with high viremia. **C,** Immunohistochemical stain for the core antigen (HBcAg) shows nuclear staining of many hepatocytes, consistent with high viral replication.

The histology of chronic hepatitis B varies according to the phase of the disease and host immunity. The immune tolerance phase may show no or minimal portal and lobular inflammation and no fibrosis, despite rapid viral replication (Fig. 10-2). In the immune clearance phase, chronic hepatitis B shows portal mononuclear infiltrates with interface hepatitis and variable fibrosis (Fig. 10-3). Varying degrees of lobular necroinflammatory activity are present, but typically not to the extent seen in acute viral hepatitis. Hepatocyte anisonucleosis may be conspicuous. A characteristic feature of chronic HBV is the presence of ground glass hepatocytes (Fig. 10-4), which contain HBsAg. These hepatocytes show a finely granular cytoplasmic inclusion that displaces the nucleus and is surrounded by a pale halo. Ground glass hepatocytes can be demonstrated by various histochemical stains such as Victoria blue, orcein, or aldehyde fuchsin[17] and by immunohistochemical stains for HBsAg. In some cases, the hepatocyte nuclei have a "sanded" appearance due to the accumulation of HBcAg, although these are difficult to recognize and also are seen in delta hepatitis.[17]

Immunohistochemistry

Immunohistochemistry for HBV antigens can be used to evaluate the pattern of antigen expression, which correlates with viral replication and disease activity (Table 10-1). Strong cytoplasmic expression of HBsAg in scattered individual hepatocytes, associated with membranous staining of many hepatocytes, indicates high viremia and is seen in the immune tolerance phase.[18,19] In contrast, cytoplasmic expression of HBsAg in clusters of hepatocytes is more often seen in patients with low or absent viremia and without active viral replication; these cells contain integrated HBV DNA, and clonal expansion of such cells may explain their clustering.[18,19]

Expression of HBcAg can be cytoplasmic or nuclear. Nuclear expression correlates with the degree of viral replication; therefore, biopsy specimens from patients in the immune tolerance phase or from immunosuppressed patients often show widespread nuclear staining, whereas those from patients with chronic hepatitis and low-replicative states have rare positive nuclei. Cytoplasmic HBcAg expression is associated with active liver

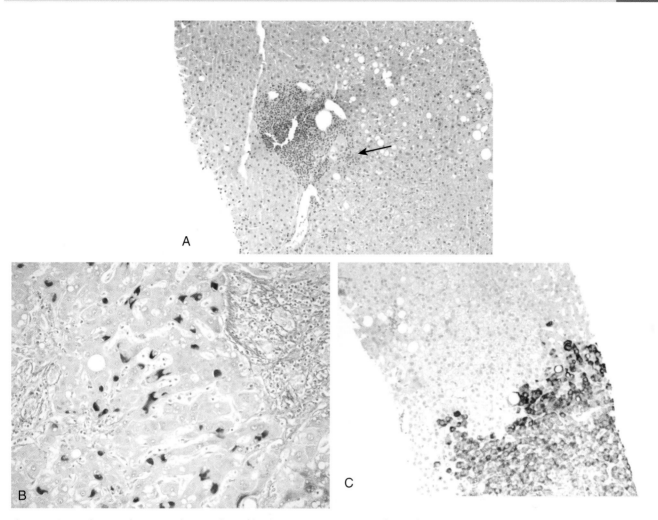

Figure 10-3. Liver biopsy in the immune clearance phase of hepatitis B. **A,** Low-power view of a portal tract with a dense mononuclear infiltrate and focal interface hepatitis *(arrow)*. **B,** Aldehyde fuchsin stain confirms the accumulation of hepatitis B surface antigen (HBsAg) within hepatocytes. **C,** Immunohistochemical stain for HBsAg shows cytoplasmic staining of clusters of hepatocytes, indicative of low viremia.

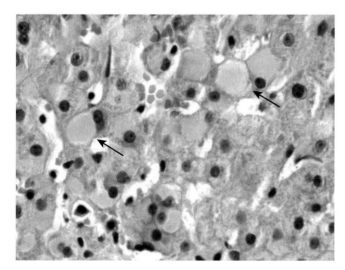

Figure 10-4. Ground glass hepatocytes in chronic hepatitis B *(arrows)*. Ground glass hepatocytes show finely granular cytoplasmic inclusions that displace the nucleus to the edge of the cell and are surrounded by a clear halo.

damage and suggests that HBcAg is the likely target for immune-mediated cytolysis.[18] Coinfection with delta virus can suppress HBcAg production and is one possible cause of a negative HBcAg stain in the setting of active hepatitis.

In general, immunohistochemistry findings for HBV antigens are negative in acute or fulminant hepatitis. Presumably, the inability to detect HBV antigen expression is a result of the short time interval of infection and insufficient accumulation of the proteins in hepatocytes to permit detection by immunohistochemistry.

Management

The management of chronic HBV infection has improved significantly in the last decade with the introduction of nucleoside and nucleotide analogues. These agents are orally administered, safe, well tolerated, and very effective at suppressing HBV DNA replication. However, sustained virologic suppression is not maintained after withdrawal of the agents, and long-term, indefinite therapy is often required. Long-term use of these agents is

Table 10-1 Immunohistochemistry for Hepatitis B

	HBsAg		HBcAg	
	Membranous	**Cytoplasmic**	**Nuclear**	**Cytoplasmic**
Immune tolerance phase	++	++ (individual cells)	++	
Immune clearance phase	–/+	+ (individual cells)	+ (few cells)	+/–
Low-replication states (chronic carriers)	–	++ (clustered cells)	–/+ (rare cells)	–
HDV/HCV coinfection	+	+/–	–	
HBV in immune-deficiency states	++	+/–	++	+

–, absent; +, present; HBcAg, hepatitis B core antigen; HBsAg, hepatitis B surface antigen; HBV, hepatitis B virus; HCV, hepatitis C virus; HDV, hepatitis D virus.

also associated with the development of resistance, loss of clinical response, hepatitis flares, and even death.

Viral Mutants

Precore and Core Gene Mutations

Precore and core gene mutations are associated with decreased production of HBeAg despite continued production of infectious virions. The most common mutation results in a stop codon that prematurely terminates the synthesis of HBeAg.[15] Other mutations in the basic core promoter downregulate HBeAg synthesis at the transcriptional level.[15] Patients infected with these mutants exhibit absent HBeAg but positive HBsAg, elevated serum HBV DNA, and elevated transaminases.

Surface Gene Mutations

Surface gene mutations are responsible for vaccine escape. Although patients infected with these mutants are infectious, HBsAg is not detectable.[12]

Polymerase Gene Mutations

Mutations in the YMDD catalytic site of the polymerase significantly reduce the effectiveness of lamivudine and famciclovir.[12,20] Despite developing this mutation, patients continue to receive some benefit from lamivudine therapy, because the YMDD variant HBV exhibits reduced replication competence and reduced virulence.[12] Discontinuation of lamivudine may cause mutant virus to revert to wild-type, with renewed efficacy of lamivudine.[20]

Post-transplantation Hepatitis B

HBV frequently infects liver allografts after transplantation for HBV and may lead to deterioration of graft function, although some patients enjoy excellent graft function for many years despite active viral replication.[21] The risk of reinfection is greater after transplantation for chronic HBV infection with cirrhosis, compared to acute HBV.[22] The pattern of hepatitis in this setting ranges from purely immunohistochemical evidence of viral antigen expression without histologic features of HBV infection, to acute hepatitis, and to chronic hepatitis with cirrhosis.[21] Acute HBV hepatitis after transplantation may show marked ballooning and degenerative changes in the hepatocytes, scattered acidophil bodies, and extensive immunohistochemical evidence of viral antigen expression, but with remarkably scant inflammation.[21,22]

A distinctive pattern of hepatitis in the transplantation population is known as fibrosing cholestatic hepatitis, initially described by Davies and colleagues in 1991.[21-24] This pattern is characterized by canalicular and cellular cholestasis, ballooning of hepatocytes, and scattered acidophil bodies with relatively scant parenchymal inflammation. Portal tracts are mildly to moderately inflamed and show periportal fibrosis, with immature fibrous tissue extending as thin perisinusoidal strands into the acinus. At the interface, a proliferation of ductal-type cells lends a hypercellularity to the portal areas. Immunohistochemical stains show extensive cytoplasmic and membranous expression with HBsAg and extensive nuclear and cytoplasmic HBcAg.[21,23,24] The combination of high HBV antigen expression, marked hepatocyte injury, and relatively little inflammation suggests that the virus itself may be cytopathic in this setting.[21,22,24] Fibrosing cholestatic hepatitis is associated with a high rate of viral replication, with high serum HBV DNA, high serum HBsAg titers, and rapid deterioration.[22-24] It has also been described in HBV infection in other settings involving immunosuppression, including human immunodeficiency virus (HIV) infection[25] and bone marrow transplantation.[26]

Coinfection with Hepatitis B Virus and Human Immunodeficiency Virus

Approximately 90% of HIV-infected persons show evidence of prior HBV infection, and 5% to 15% have chronic HBV infection.[27] In patients coinfected with HIV and HBV, the rate of clearance of HBsAg and HBeAg is reduced, compared with non–HIV-infected individuals.[28] This reduced clearance rate is most likely due to a weakened immune system. However, the reduced immune reaction is potentially responsible for the relatively reduced inflammation in these patients despite their higher HBV viral replication rates.[28] Even though there is reduced inflammation, HBV infection is more progressive in HIV-positive patients, including development of cirrhosis and its complications.[28] A pattern of hepatitis similar to fibrosing cholestatic hepatitis has been described in HIV patients with concurrent HBV infection.[25] The HBV-related mortality in HIV patients has increased since the introduction of highly active antiretroviral therapy (HAART), possibly because of increased immunologic injury to the liver with immune reconstitution, toxicity of the antiviral drugs, or longer life spans in HIV patients.[28] Conversely, the use of antiretroviral agents that also have activity against HBV may slow the progression of chronic HBV and even result in seroconversion, whereas their discontinuation can cause significant liver disease due to re-emergence of HBV replication.[27]

Hepatitis C

Hepatitis C affects between 123 and 170 million people worldwide.[29]

Virology

HCV is an RNA flavivirus that was characterized in the late 1980s.[29] Its genome is a positive, single-stranded RNA with a large open reading frame that encodes a 3010- to 3030-amino-acid polyprotein.[30] This polyprotein is processed into an array of structural and nonstructural proteins. The structural proteins include the core protein and two envelope proteins, E1 and E2.[30] The nonstructural proteins are NS2, -3, -4A, -4B, -5A, and -5B (RNA polymerase).[30]

There are 6 major genotypes and more than 50 subtypes. However, the genome of HCV is highly mutagenic, and a given host carries a mixture of viral particles with closely related sequences known as quasispecies.[30,31] The high mutation rate may allow the virus to escape the immune system; patients with chronic infection harbor highly diverse quasispecies, whereas those who clear the infection have low virus diversity and patients with fulminant hepatitis have the lowest level of viral diversity.[31] Genotypes 1, 2, and 3 have worldwide distribution, but their relative prevalence varies geographically.[32] Genotype 1a is the predominant genotype in North America (70%).[33] In Japan, subtype 1b is responsible for up to 73% of infections. Subtypes 2a and 2b are common in North America, Europe, and Japan, whereas subtype 2c is common in northern Italy. Genotype 3 is endemic in Southeast Asia, and it is also prevalent among intravenous drug users in Europe and the United States.[33] Genotype 4 is prevalent in North Africa and the Middle East; genotype 5 is largely confined to South Africa; and genotype 6 is found in Hong Kong, Macao, and Vietnam.[32,33]

The genotype affects the rate of evolution to chronic hepatitis, the severity of liver disease, and the response to interferon (IFN) therapy.[32] For example, genotype 1 is associated with a poor response to IFN therapy, whereas genotypes 2 and 3 respond more favorably.[33] An association between genotype 1b and an increased risk of developing severe liver disease and HCC has been reported.[33,34]

Natural History

HCV is primarily transmitted parenterally, such as by recreational drug use, injection with contaminated syringes or needles, or blood transfusion.[29,35] Although sexual and vertical transmission occur, they are less important with HCV than with HBV. The incidence of HCV in the United States has fallen since the introduction of widespread blood donor screening and needle-exchange programs.[31]

Acute infection can be diagnosed in a variety of ways, including documentation of anti-HCV seroconversion and detection of HCV RNA in the absence of HCV antibodies.[36-38] The mean incubation time for HCV is 6 to 8 weeks.[29] Although the majority (60% to 75%) of affected patients do not experience symptoms when acutely infected,[29] acute HCV still accounts for approximately 20% of cases of acute hepatitis.[35,39] The symptoms of acute HCV are malaise, fatigue, lethargy, anorexia, abdominal pain, jaundice, mild hepatosplenomegaly, maculopapular rash, and arthralgia.[29] Fulminant hepatitis is rare.

A minority of patients (approximately 15% to 50%) clear the infection, but most develop chronic viral hepatitis. Symptomatic onset of disease and female gender are associated with a higher chance of viral clearance after acute infection.[39] The serologic diagnosis of chronic HCV infection is made by detection of HCV antibodies, usually by enzyme immunoassay.[29] These assays have a 95% to 99% sensitivity and can detect antibodies 6 to 8 weeks after exposure. Polymerase chain reaction (PCR)–based methods can detect HCV RNA 1 to 3 weeks after exposure.[29] Patients with chronic HCV infection may present with normal transaminases. These patients are often identified during blood donation or screening. The rate of progression to fibrosis or cirrhosis is very low in this group.[35] Patients with elevated transaminases may suffer from fatigue or from nonspecific symptoms.[35]

Extrahepatic manifestations may include mixed essential cryoglobulinemia, membranous or membranoproliferative glomerulonephritis, non-Hodgkin lymphoma, Sjögren syndrome, lichen planus, autoimmune thyroid disease, and porphyria cutanea tarda.[29,35,40] A subset of patients with HCV demonstrate autoantibodies similar to those seen in autoimmune hepatitis, namely antinuclear antibodies (ANA), smooth muscle antibody (SMA), perinuclear antineutrophilic cytoplasmic antibody (p-ANCA), and anti-asialoglycoprotein receptor, although often at lower titer than is typically seen in autoimmune hepatitis.[40] Less often, liver-kidney microsomal (LKM1) autoantibodies are detected, although the epitopes recognized by these antibodies in HCV differ from those in autoimmune hepatitis type 2.[40] Patients with autoantibodies tend to be females and to have higher transaminase levels.[41] Some of these patients experience exacerbation during IFN-α therapy that may respond to steroid therapy, suggesting either preexisting autoimmune hepatitis or induction of autoimmune hepatitis in these patients.

The rate at which chronic hepatitis C progresses to cirrhosis depends on several factors. Factors that increase the rate of progression include male gender, older age at infection acquisition, longer duration of infection, immune suppression (e.g., HIV coinfection), HBV coinfection, alcohol use, and obesity.[29] The risk of developing cirrhosis is approximately 20% to 30% after 10 to 20 years of infection.[35] Once cirrhosis has developed, the risk of liver disease–related mortality is 2% to 5% per year and the risk of developing HCC is 3% to 5% each year.[35]

Histopathology

Acute hepatitis C is characterized by panlobular inflammation, numerous acidophil bodies, and lobular disarray similar to that seen in other acute hepatitides. A sinusoidal pattern of inflammation can mimic EBV hepatitis. More severe patterns of acute hepatitis, such as bridging necrosis or panacinar necrosis, are typically absent. Portal tracts harbor dense mononuclear infiltrates, resembling chronic HCV infection (Fig. 10-5). Bile duct injury may be present. Cholestatic forms of acute HCV

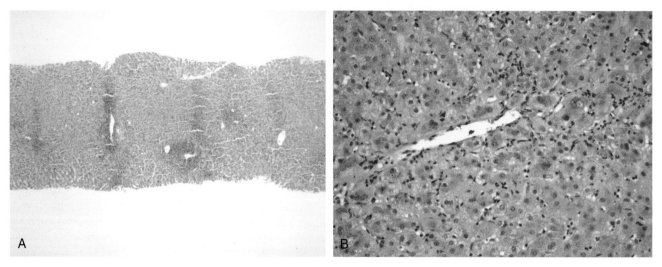

Figure 10-5. Liver biopsy in acute hepatitis C. **A,** Low-power view shows mononuclear cell infiltrates within portal tracts, similar in appearance to chronic hepatitis C virus infection. **B,** High-power view of the centrilobular region shows sinusoidal lymphocytic infiltrates surrounding a central vein.

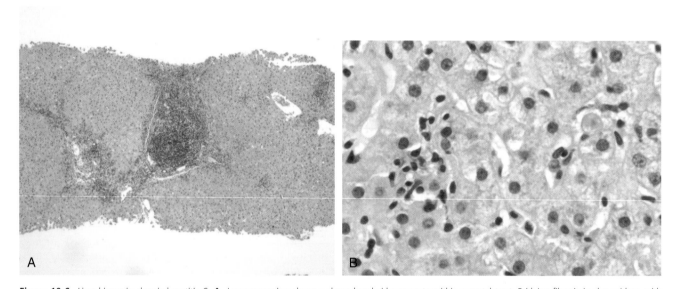

Figure 10-6. Liver biopsy in chronic hepatitis C. **A,** Low-power view shows a dense lymphoid aggregate within a portal tract. Bridging fibrosis is also evident, with mononuclear infiltrates in the septum. **B,** Lobular inflammation shows lytic necrosis on the left with a cluster of mononuclear cells indicating a focus of hepatocyte necrosis and a Councilman body (apoptotic hepatocyte) on the right; the latter is characteristic of hepatitis C virus infection.

infection occur rarely, predominantly in the immunosuppressed population.

Chronic HCV infection is characterized by dense mononuclear cell aggregates or follicles in portal tracts, with mild to moderate interface hepatitis.[42] Bile duct injury may be prominent, although typically it is mild. The lobules show scattered acidophil bodies (Councilman bodies) or foci of lytic necrosis marked by a small cluster of mononuclear cells (Fig. 10-6).[42] Kupffer cell prominence and lymphocytic infiltration of sinusoids may be seen.[17,42] Variable fibrosis is present, and its extent often drives the decision of whether to treat the infection.

Mild to moderate steatosis is characteristic of chronic HCV infection.[42] Steatosis may be related to direct viral cytopathic effects in patients with genotype 3 but to underlying metabolic status in patients with other genotypes.[43,44] HCV core protein

expression produces steatosis in mice through mitochondrial toxicity and production of reactive oxygen species.[43] The severity of steatosis correlates with fibrosis.

Sarcoid-like granulomas are occasionally seen in liver biopsy specimens from patients with HCV. In one series, 9.5% of hepatic granulomas were attributed to HCV.[45] In another series, 5 (10%) of 52 liver explants for HCV-related cirrhosis had granulomas for which no other cause could be identified.[46] In a biopsy series, 14 of 155 biopsies for HCV had granulomas, but half of them could be ascribed to another cause (sarcoidosis, schistosomiasis, primary biliary cirrhosis, or mycobacterial infection).[47] In a large series of 542 biopsies for HCV, only 2% had granulomas. In that series, the presence of granulomas predicted a better response to IFN-α therapy.[48] Others have described granulomas in HCV after treatment with IFN-α in patients who did not respond well to IFN-α.[49-51] In short, when a granulomatous process is encountered in a patient with HCV, other causes of granulomas in the liver must be rigorously excluded before they can be attributed to HCV. A history of IFN-α therapy should be sought.

The granulomas in HCV may occur in portal tracts or in the lobules. It is well known that HCV can be associated with mild bile duct injury. If the granulomas are in the portal area, their presence in conjunction with injured bile ducts may mimic primary biliary cirrhosis. Other clinical information (e.g., AMA, alkaline phosphatase level) may be needed to distinguish the two.

Management

Acute HCV infection is typically observed for 3 months after the onset of symptoms; antiviral therapy is offered to patients who have persistent viremia after that period.[36-38] The management of chronic HCV depends to some extent on viral genotype. Genotype 1 is associated with reduced likelihood of treatment success compared to genotypes 2 and 3. The mainstay of treatment is combination IFN and ribavirin. Treatment success has been improved with the introduction of pegylated IFN, which consists of a polyethylene glycol (PEG) polymer attached to the IFN molecule, which results in reduced drug clearance rates and allows once-weekly dosing.[29] Therapy may need to be continued for up to 24 weeks for genotypes 2 or 3 and up to 48 weeks for genotype 1.[29]

Post-transplantation Hepatitis C

After transplantation for chronic HCV, reinfection of the graft is almost universal. Although most patients do well in the long term, recurrent HCV can be progressive and can lead to graft dysfunction. The histologic features of recurrent HCV hepatitis progress from acute lobular hepatitis with scattered acidophil bodies and sinusoidal lymphocytic infiltration in the early stage to portal-based hepatitis with portal lymphoid aggregates typical of HCV infection in the chronic phase.[52] Progressive fibrosis and cirrhosis of the graft may result. A rapidly progressive cholestatic form of HCV infection has been described in the transplantation population, similar to the fibrosing cholestatic hepatitis described with HBV.[53] Fibrosing cholestatic hepatitis secondary to HCV has also been described in other immunosuppressed patient populations, such as in HIV patients[54] and after heart or kidney transplantation.[55-57]

Coinfection with Hepatitis C Virus and Human Immunodeficiency Virus

In the United States and Europe, 33% of HIV-infected persons are coinfected with HCV.[27] The clearance rate of HCV after acute infection is reduced in HIV-infected patients.[27] In chronic infection, HCV RNA levels are higher in HIV-coinfected patients, the efficacy of anti-HCV therapy is reduced, and the incidence of cirrhosis and HCC is higher.[20,27,28] In hemophiliac patients infected with HCV, coinfection with HIV has been associated with increased severity of hepatitis and increased risk of developing cirrhosis and liver failure.[58,59] Fibrosing cholestatic hepatitis related to HCV has been described in patients with HIV coinfection.[54] With the introduction of HAART, HCV-related liver disease has become an important factor in hospitalizations

and mortality of HIV patients.[28] Patients with HCV are more likely to suffer from hepatotoxicity related to HAART and to have impaired immune reconstitution.[27]

Hepatitis D

HDV (delta virus) is a defective, single-stranded, circular RNA virus that requires the lipoprotein coat of HBV for its replication; therefore, infection from HDV alone does not occur. There are two modes of infection: coinfection with HBV and superinfection of prior HBV infection. Coinfection results in severe acute hepatitis with high mortality, but resolution produces immunity to both viruses. Superinfection is associated with a high likelihood of chronic infection by both viruses and a propensity for more severe inflammation than with HBV alone. HDV infection inhibits HBV replication, resulting in decreased expression of HBcAg, although expression of HBsAg continues.[7] Treatment with IFN-α inhibits HDV replication, but relapse is common.

HDV infection may be associated with autoimmune manifestations in a subset of patients. LKM3 autoantibodies are detected in 13% of patients with HDV.[40] However, one study found liver-specific autoantibodies (anti-asialoglycoprotein receptor) and non–organ-specific autoantibodies (e.g., ANA, anti-SMA) in 60.3% and 22.1% of HBV patients, respectively, regardless of whether HDV was present.[60] The pathology of HBV and delta virus is indistinguishable from that of HBV alone, except that the degree of inflammation and hepatocyte necrosis is often more prominent than with HBV alone.

Hepatitis E

Hepatitis E virus (HEV) is a nonenveloped, positive-sense, single-stranded RNA virus of the calicivirus family. Along with HAV, HEV accounts for the majority of cases of enterically transmitted viral hepatitis worldwide. However, unlike HAV, HEV is not easily transmitted from person to person, so familial clusters are unusual.[61] The virus is spread through fecally contaminated water or food, and epidemics have occurred in central and Southeast Asia, the Middle East, and North Africa.[61,62] Clinically, hepatitis E is indistinguishable from hepatitis A, and serology for anti-HEV IgM or PCR is required to make the diagnosis. Both are acute infections without progression to chronic hepatitis, and both can range from asymptomatic infection to fulminant hepatitis. The mortality rate is 1% to 4% overall, but it is approximately 20% among pregnant women.[61,62]

Although HEV is spread by the fecal-oral route, similar to HAV, there are some curious differences between the two viruses. In some countries where both viruses are endemic, such as India, children are universally infected with HAV by age 5 years, whereas HEV infects young adults and many adults are seronegative. In other countries, such as Egypt, seroconversion to anti-HEV occurs in a greater percentage of the population and at an earlier age. In the United States, anti-HEV is actually more common than anti-HAV, although HAV is more often diagnosed.[61] In developed countries, HEV infection is still only rarely diagnosed, although its incidence is increasing. Some evidence suggests that HEV may be a zoonotic infection: swine have been shown to be frequently infected, and cases of zoonotic transmission to humans via ingestion of undercooked pork or deer meat have been reported.[61]

The histopathology of HEV is similar to HAV in that it can produce a classic acute hepatitis or cholestatic hepatitis with lobular canalicular cholestasis and relatively little inflammation. In some cases, cholangiolar proliferation with bile plugs in dilated cholangioles can be seen.

Epstein-Barr Virus

The liver is involved in more than 90% of cases of infectious mononucleosis, which is caused by Epstein-Barr virus (EBV) infection; hepatomegaly is present in 10% to 15% of cases, splenomegaly in 50%, and jaundice occurs in only 5%. Most often, the hepatic manifestations of EBV infection consist of self-limited elevations of hepatic transaminases. Rarely, EBV hepatitis has more serious consequences, such as the induction of autoimmune hepatitis,[63] severe hepatitis with prolonged jaundice,[64] or liver failure.[65-67]

Liver biopsy shows portal and periportal infiltrates of small and large lymphocytes, with occasional larger immunoblastic cells resembling the Reed-Sternberg cells of Hodgkin disease. A characteristic feature is sinusoidal infiltration by these same lymphocytes, which creates a beaded appearance (Fig. 10-7).[68] Liver cell ballooning is not prominent, although hepatocyte regeneration, canalicular cholestasis, and Kupffer cell hyperplasia are variably seen. Areas of necrosis may be infiltrated by collections of mononuclear cells, creating a granulomatous appearance. Although these histiocytes usually do not form true epithelioid granulomas, well-developed non-necrotizing granulomas[69] and fibrin ring granulomas have been reported in patients with EBV hepatitis.[70] In fatal cases, submassive lobular necrosis has been seen.[65]

Detection of EBV is done by in situ hybridization for EBV-encoded RNA (EBER) (Fig. 10-8) or by PCR for EBV DNA.[71] Immunohistochemistry for EBV latent membrane protein has not proved to be a reliable method for detecting EBV in EBV hepatitis.

Cytomegalovirus

Cytomegalovirus (CMV) infection is clinically mild and self-limited; CMV accounts for 8% of cases of infectious mononucleosis–like syndrome with hepatic involvement. Rare cases of massive hepatic necrosis have been reported, usually in immunocompromised hosts. In immunocompetent hosts, CMV infection can result in a histologic picture virtually identical to that of EBV hepatitis, with sinusoidal beading, atypical lymphocytes within sinusoids, lymphocytic infiltrates in portal tracts, and areas of necrosis with aggregates of Kupffer cells resulting in a granulomatous appearance.[72,73] CMV infection is rarely associated with well-formed non-necrotizing granulomas[74] or fibrin ring granulomas.[75] In immunocompromised patients, viral inclusions may be found in hepatocytes, endothelial cells, Kupffer cells, and duct epithelium (Fig. 10-9). Virally infected cells show a large amphophilic nuclear inclusion surrounded by a halo, known as an "owl's-eye" nuclear inclusion, and coarsely granular cytoplasmic inclusions. The inclusions may be isolated, or they may elicit an inflammatory reaction that can be granulomatous or neutrophilic, the latter being especially common in transplantation patients.[72] In HIV-positive patients, bile duct involvement may result in sclerosing cholangitis (HIV-associated cholangiopathy). Immunohistochemical stains for CMV can highlight cells with inclusions, including atypical inclusions.

Herpes Simplex Virus

Herpes simplex virus (HSV) viremia can result in visceral involvement, affecting mainly the esophagus, lungs, and liver. Liver involvement occurs primarily in neonates, pregnant patients, and immunocompromised patients, although immunocompetent adults are rarely affected as well.[76] HSV hepatitis is rapidly lethal

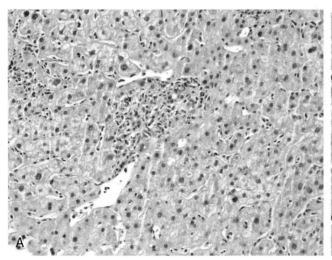
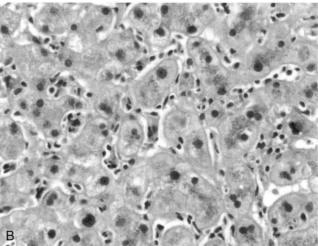

Figure 10-7. Liver biopsy in Epstein-Barr virus infection. **A,** A portal tract shows a mild mononuclear infiltrate, and the lobules show infiltration of sinusoids by mononuclear cells. **B,** High magnification shows prominent sinusoidal lymphocytic infiltration without hepatocyte necrosis.

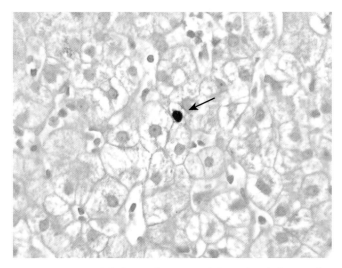

Figure 10-8. In situ hybridization for EBV-encoded RNA (EBER) shows nuclear staining of a single infected lymphocyte *(arrow).*

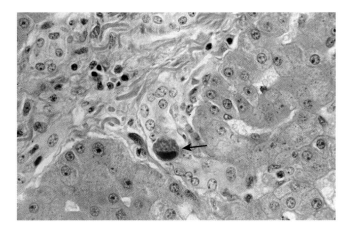

Figure 10-9. Cytomegalovirus (CMV) infection, demonstrating a CMV inclusion in bile duct epithelium *(arrow).* (Courtesy of Dr. Laura Lamps.)

and requires early recognition and institution of antiviral therapy to improve outcome.

HSV hepatitis is characterized by patchy, nonzonal coagulative necrosis with minimal to absent inflammatory response (Fig. 10-10). Intranuclear inclusions of two types can be found in hepatocytes at the edge of the necrotic foci, and virally infected cells are often multinucleated.[76] Cowdry type A inclusions are large, eosinophilic intranuclear inclusions surrounded by a halo, whereas type B inclusions replace the entire nucleus with a basophilic ground glass appearance. Immunohistochemistry for herpes type I and type II antigens highlights the nuclear inclusions, and overlap between the two antibodies is frequent.[76]

Treatment with antiviral drugs before the biopsy is obtained may result in a biopsy specimen with extensive necrosis but without diagnostic inclusions.[76] The main differential is varicella-zoster virus (VZV) infection and adenovirus infection, both of which have a similar histologic appearance; immunohistochemical staining or PCR may be necessary to distinguish these infections. HSV serologic studies are not helpful in establishing the diagnosis.

Varicella-Zoster Virus

Rarely, the rash of VZV can be accompanied by potentially life-threatening noncutaneous manifestations, including encephalitis, pneumonitis, myocarditis, and hepatitis, especially in immuno-compromised patients. In children, the convalescent phase can be associated with Reye's syndrome (microvesicular steatosis, hyperammonemia, coagulopathy, and cerebral edema), particularly if aspirin has been administered. Primary infection in immunocompetent adults can cause severe acute hepatitis and, rarely, fulminant hepatic failure. Transplantation patients and immunocompromised patients are at higher risk for a fatal fulminant hepatitis.

Serology is of little use, especially in the immunocompromised patient. The appearance on liver biopsy resembles HSV. Immunohistochemistry can confirm the presence of a herpes

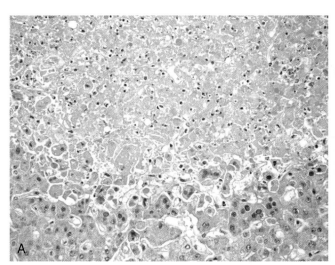

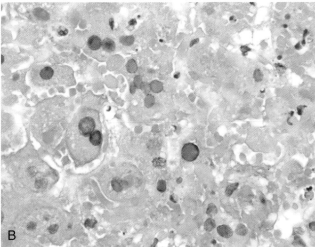

Figure 10-10. Herpes simplex virus (HSV) infection. **A,** The liver shows necrotic regions without an inflammatory response. **B,** Hepatocytes at the edge of the necrotic regions show glassy nuclear inclusions and multinucleation, consistent with HSV infection.

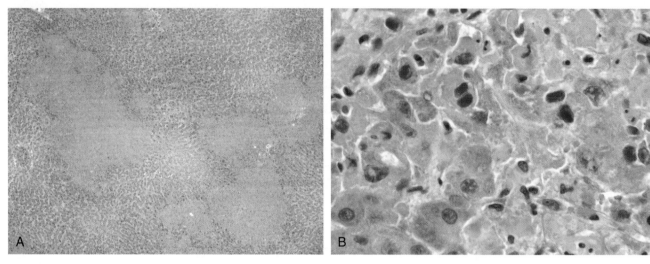

Figure 10-11. Adenovirus hepatitis. **A,** Low-power view shows several regions of necrosis without an inflammatory reaction. **B,** High-power view shows hepatocytes with smudgy nuclear inclusions similar to the Cowdry type A inclusions of herpes simplex virus.

virus, but, depending on the antibody, may not distinguish which one. PCR may be necessary to distinguish HSV from VZV infection.

Adenovirus

Although infection by adenoviruses is generally restricted to the upper respiratory tract and conjunctivae in the normal host, disseminated infection can occur in immunodeficient patients. Postmortem livers in patients with adenovirus hepatitis have shown widespread necrosis with little inflammation, mild steatosis, and viral inclusions similar to the Cowdry type A inclusions of HSV infection (Fig. 10-11).[77,78] Immunohistochemistry, electron microscopy, and viral culture are helpful in making the diagnosis.[78]

Parvovirus B19

Parvovirus B19 produces several clinical manifestations, including erythema infectiosum (fifth disease) in children; hydrops fetalis; arthritis associated with acute infection in adults; various hematologic disorders (e.g., leukopenia, thrombocytopenia, transient aplastic crisis); and, rarely, involvement of other organs, including neurologic, cardiac, hepatic, and vascular disease.

The role of parvovirus B19 infection in acute or fulminant hepatitis is controversial. Parvovirus B19 DNA has been found in the liver of patients with fulminant hepatic failure and in the serum of patients with acute or fulminant hepatitis, suggesting a role for this virus in cases of unexplained acute hepatitis or acute liver failure.[79-81] In one study,[80] parvovirus B19 DNA was found in liver tissue in four of six patients with fulminant hepatic failure associated with aplastic anemia and in two of four patients with cryptogenic acute liver failure (without aplastic anemia), but not in six patients with known causes of acute liver failure. Histology studies in DNA-positive cases showed massive hepatic necrosis and collapse without inflammatory infiltrates or

viral inclusions. In contrast, other investigators found no parvovirus B19 DNA by PCR in 33 cases of cryptogenic acute liver failure but detected parvovirus B19 DNA in several patients with known causes of acute liver failure.[82] In that study, several patients had low-titer IgM positivity without confirmatory PCR positivity. In another study, parvovirus B19 DNA was found with similar frequency in patients with fulminant hepatitis and with hepatitis B or C. Furthermore, RNA transcripts could not be detected in any of the liver tissue samples, arguing against active viral replication.[83] These studies suggest that low levels of PCR positivity may reflect remote infection, and they raise questions about the role of parvovirus B19 in hepatitis and acute liver failure.

Rubella (German Measles)

Acute hepatitis has been reported in adults who acquire rubella. The morphology shows ballooning degeneration of hepatocytes, focal hepatocyte necrosis, and infiltrating mononuclear cells, similar to classic acute hepatitis.[84,85]

Rubeola (Measles)

Measles is a contagious, acute, febrile illness that predominantly affects children and causes a maculopapular rash, Koplik spots, cough, conjunctivitis, fever, and lymphadenopathy. The virus enters the body through the lungs or conjunctivae, replicates at these sites, and then is transported to the reticuloendothelial system, where further replication and lymphoid proliferation occur. Transient transaminase elevation is not uncommon in measles.[86] In one reported case, liver biopsy demonstrated acute cholangitis, periportal inflammation with lymphocytes, eosinophils and neutrophils, periportal hepatocyte necrosis, ballooning degeneration and cholestasis, and multinucleated giant cells (Fig. 10-12). At autopsy, viral inclusions were noted in hepatocytes.[87]

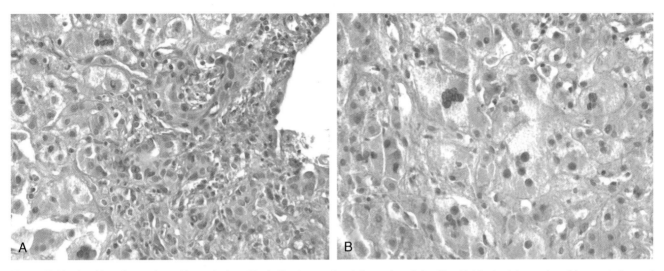

Figure 10-12. Liver biopsy in a patient with measles hepatitis. **A,** Portal tracts show inflammation, cholangitis with bile duct injury, periportal hepatocyte loss, and ballooning degeneration. **B,** The lobules show widespread hepatocyte ballooning degeneration, cholestasis, and multinucleated hepatocytes.

Severe Acute Respiratory Syndrome Coronavirus

In 2003, a novel coronavirus was found to be the causative agent of severe acute respiratory syndrome (SARS), an atypical pneumonia that can progress rapidly to acute respiratory distress syndrome. Hepatic impairment is common in these patients, with elevated transaminases seen in approximately 60% of cases. Liver histology shows lobular hepatitis with occasional acidophil bodies, prominent Kupffer cells, increased numbers of hepatocyte mitoses, focal mild ballooning degeneration, and mild portal tract inflammation.[88]

Human Immunodeficiency Virus

HIV is associated with liver disease in several ways. During seroconversion, a small proportion of patients may experience hepatitis with transaminase elevations, although the histology of this hepatitis has not been described.[89,90] Opportunistic infections such as CMV, *Histoplasma capsulatum*, *Mycobacterium avium-intracellulare* complex (MAC), and *Pneumocystis jiroveci* can infect the liver. HIV can also increase the risk of progression of nonopportunistic pathogens, such as *Mycobacterium tuberculosis*, HBV, or HCV (see earlier discussions). Patients with the acquired immunodeficiency syndrome (AIDS) may develop unusual reactions to certain pathogens, such as bacillary epithelioid angiomatosis secondary to *Bartonella henselae* or *Bartonella quintana* infection (discussed later).[91,92]

Granulomas are a common finding in liver biopsy of patients with HIV infection. The more common causes are *M. tuberculosis*, MAC, *Histoplasma*, *Candida*, CMV, and *Cryptococcus*.[93] In some of these patients, the granulomatous response is poorly developed and composed of loose aggregates of histiocytes, but silver or acid-fast stains show numerous organisms. Therefore, acid-fast and silver stains should be done routinely on biopsy specimens from patients with HIV/AIDS.

AIDS-related cholangiopathy is a syndrome that manifests with right upper quadrant abdominal pain, fever, and marked elevations of serum alkaline phosphatase. On cholangiography, the bile duct shows strictures and irregularities indistinguishable from those of primary sclerosing cholangitis. Several opportunistic pathogens have been implicated in this disorder, including *Cryptosporidium*, CMV, and microsporidia (*Enterocytozoon bieneusi*).[94-99] In a significant minority of cases, there is no identifiable pathogen; it is unclear whether these cases are due to unknown pathogens, occult infection, altered immunity, direct infiltration of the bile duct mucosa by HIV, or primary sclerosing cholangitis coincidentally occurring in patients with AIDS.[98,99]

The liver can be involved by HIV-associated neoplasms such as lymphoma or Kaposi sarcoma.[100] The latter is caused by another virus, Kaposi sarcoma–associated herpesvirus (KSHV), also known as *Human herpesvirus 8* (HHV-8). Finally, immune reconstitution with HAART can precipitate autoimmune hepatitis.[101]

Yellow Fever

Yellow fever is a viral hemorrhagic fever that can vary from subclinical to rapidly fatal. It is transmitted by the *Aedes* mosquito. Classic symptoms include sudden onset of fever, rigors, and headache. Jaundice and hemorrhagic manifestations portend a poor prognosis. The pattern of injury is frequently described as midzonal and sometimes centrilobular.[102-105] Others describe panlobular injury with only a collar (one or two cells thick) of preserved hepatocytes around central veins and portal tracts.[106] The key findings are necrosis with numerous apoptotic hepatocytes (Councilman bodies), microvesicular steatosis, and absence of inflammation (Fig. 10-13).[102-106] Eosinophilic intranuclear inclusions, Torres bodies, are rarely seen in humans.[106] Immunoperoxidase assays are not widely available, but the diagnosis

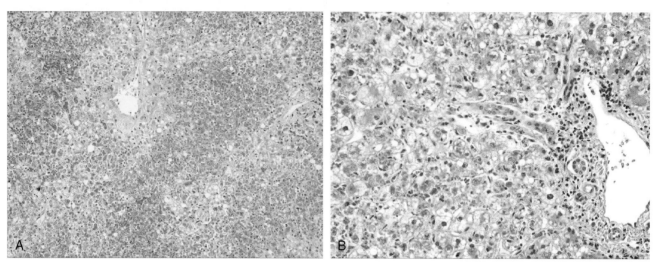

Figure 10-13. Yellow fever. **A,** Low-power view shows panlobular necrosis with numerous necrotic hepatocytes primarily in zones 2 and 3. **B,** High-power view shows relative preservation of periportal hepatocytes with steatosis, ballooning degeneration, and scattered necrotic hepatocytes. (Courtesy of Dr. Shu-Yuan Xiao.)

can be confirmed serologically. The differential diagnosis includes other viral hemorrhagic fevers such as dengue and Rift Valley fever.

Dengue

The dengue virus, a member of the Flaviviridae family, is also transmitted by the *Aedes* mosquito. Dengue virus infection is one of the most important mosquito-borne diseases in the world, and the resurgence of this disease in the last 2 decades may be related to human population growth, inadequate wastewater management, lack of effective mosquito eradication programs, and emergence of more virulent strains.[107] The clinical manifestations include dengue fever, dengue hemorrhagic fever, or dengue shock syndrome. Dengue fever manifests as high fever, severe headache, arthralgias, myalgias, and sometimes a rash. Patients with dengue hemorrhagic fever suffer from bleeding phenomena and circulatory failure. Dengue shock is caused by severe plasma leakage and manifests as cyanosis, hypotension, and encephalopathy.[107] There are four serotypes of dengue virus, and infection with one serotype confers future protective immunity against that serotype only. Infection with a second serotype may result in antibody-dependent enhancement of the illness with immune complex formation.[107]

The severity of hepatic involvement parallels the severity of the dengue infection. Serotypes 3 and 4 are associated with more severe liver disease.[107] The histology is characterized by necrosis, with Councilman bodies involving the centrilobular region or, as in yellow fever, zone 2, although in most cases the degree of necrosis is not as severe as in yellow fever (Fig. 10-14).[105,106] The contributions of virus or shock to the centrilobular necrosis remain uncertain.[106] Microvesicular steatosis is frequent, although relatively mild. As with other arboviruses, little inflammation is present.[108,109] The distinction from yellow fever may require geographic data, clinical features, and virologic studies. Immunohistochemical demonstration of the virus within hepatocytes has been described.[108,109]

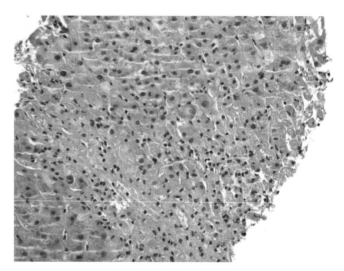

Figure 10-14. Liver biopsy specimen from a patient who died of dengue shock demonstrates centrilobular necrosis with numerous acidophil bodies *(right)* and no inflammatory reaction.

Rift Valley Fever

Rift Valley Fever primarily affects sheep and cattle in Africa, although humans who have direct contact with animals or carcasses may become infected. Fever, severe headache, and myalgia may be followed by facial inflammation, encephalitis, and macular degeneration.[102] Hemorrhage and jaundice are poor prognostic features. Autopsies of cases with hemorrhage show hepatic necrosis, either widespread or predominantly in the periportal and midzonal areas; numerous acidophil bodies; and hemorrhage.[102,106]

Lassa Virus

Lassa virus is associated with severe febrile illness among missionaries and travelers returning from West Africa. Symptoms include chills, malaise, headache, and myalgia. Petechiae, ulcerative tonsillitis, and lymphadenopathy are common.[102] The liver shows haphazardly distributed areas of hepatocyte necrosis, both as foci of contiguous cells and as individual cells, either acidophilic or coagulative in type.[106,110] There is little inflammatory reaction apart from histiocytes phagocytosing necrotic debris.[110] The nonzonal distribution of the necrosis distinguishes this disease from yellow fever.[102,110]

Ebola Virus

Ebola virus causes a severe and frequently fatal viral hemorrhagic fever; outbreaks in Sudan and Zaire have caused international concern. The disease is similar to Marburg virus infection, with disseminated intravascular coagulopathy and bleeding occurring in the majority of patients.[102] The histology is characterized by foci of hepatocellular necrosis randomly distributed throughout the parenchyma and eosinophilic inclusions within hepatocytes.[102,106] Mild to moderate steatosis, mild mononuclear infiltrates in the periportal area, and Kupffer cell activation are additional findings.[106]

Marburg Virus

Marburg virus has been associated with African green monkeys. Fever, malaise, headache, and myalgia may be accompanied by a maculopapular rash and conjunctivitis.[102] The histology is similar to that of Ebola virus infection. On electron microscopy, many hepatocytes contain inclusions composed of uniformly packed filaments arranged in parallel arrays.[102]

Mycobacteria

Tuberculosis

Worldwide, *M. tuberculosis* is one of the most common causes of hepatic granulomas. The organisms may reach the liver hematogenously from the lungs, through the portal circulation in the setting of gastrointestinal tuberculosis, or via lymphatics.[111] Tuberculosis (TB) can affect the liver in several forms. Most often, the liver is affected in the setting of generalized miliary TB.[112] Less often, hepatitic TB manifests as a localized mass lesion that mimics a neoplasm, causes obstructive jaundice from extrinsic compression of the hepatic duct, or causes portal hypertension from compression of the portal vein.[111,113] Localized hepatic involvement can occur in primary infection, in which case there is no evidence of antecedent infection, or as reactivation TB.[114] Tuberculous cholangitis, in which the bacillus primarily infects the biliary tree, is extremely rare.[115]

The most common presentation of hepatic TB is abdominal pain, hepatomegaly, jaundice, fever, and chills. Alkaline phosphatase elevations and hyponatremia usually are prominent features.[114,116,117] In 65% to 78% of patients with hepatic TB, respiratory symptoms or chest radiographs suggest pulmonary TB as well.[111,114,116,117] Abdominal imaging shows liver calcifications in approximately half of patients.[111,112,118] Caseating granulomas are a hallmark of hepatic TB, particularly miliary TB in the setting of primary infection; in reactivation TB, noncaseating granulomas may be present instead (Fig. 10-15). The granulomas may reside in the lobules or in portal tracts. Acid-fast stains or cultures are positive in 0% to 59% of cases, but organisms are more likely to be found with caseating necrosis.[114-116] PCR for *M. tuberculosis* DNA has a 53% to 88% sensitivity and a 96% to 100% specificity for detecting hepatic TB.[111,119,120] Immunocompromised patients may present with a wasting syndrome in which multiple organs, including the liver, contain necrotic miliary nodules surrounded by histiocytes that do not aggregate into well-formed granulomas. Acid-fast stain shows numerous organisms in these lesions.[121]

Localized hepatic TB includes tuberculoma and tuberculous abscess. Radiologically, it mimics tumors except that calcification may be prominent and may assume a bull's-eye configuration.[113] Grossly, localized hepatic TB appears as cheesy or chalky white, irregular nodules. Histologically, tuberculomas are composed of confluent granulomas, contain few organisms, and are encountered in immune-competent patients, whereas tuberculous abscesses are centrally suppurative, contain numerous organisms, and are encountered mainly in immunodeficient patients.

Biliary involvement manifests as obstructive jaundice which might have as its cause compression of the bile duct by a hepatic tuberculoma, small duct involvement by granulomas, or isolated biliary tree involvement.[112] The latter may result in bile duct strictures that can be mistaken for cholangiocarcinoma or primary sclerosing cholangitis.[112,122]

Mycobacterium avium-intracellulare Complex

Of the atypical mycobacteria, *Mycobacterium avium* and *Mycobacterium intracellulare* are significant hepatic pathogens. MAC is commonly encountered in immunocompromised patients, particularly those with AIDS. These organisms cause disseminated infection that commonly affects lung, liver, spleen, lymph nodes, and bone marrow. Patients with hepatic involvement present with fever, elevated alkaline phosphatase, and hepatomegaly.[123] The histopathologic findings range from numerous well-formed, nonnecrotizing granulomas with rare acid-fast organisms on Ziehl-Neelsen stain to less well-formed granulomas with large numbers of acid-fast organisms spilling out of the loose granulomas into nearby Kupffer cells (Fig. 10-16).[121,124] Although the latter pattern differs from the usual case of hepatic TB, the degree of immune compromise, rather than the species of mycobacteria, may be the more important factor in determining the number of organisms and type of granulomas seen, because T-cell function is required for the formation of well-formed granulomas, and hepatic TB in patients with AIDS also may show large numbers of organisms and few well-formed granulomas.[121,123]

Leprosy

Infection by *Mycobacterium leprae* commonly involves the liver, although clinical manifestations are often mild or absent. Hepatic granulomas are found in 90% of patients with lepromatous leprosy but in fewer than 20% of patients with tuberculoid leprosy.[125] The appearance of the granulomas depends on the type of leprosy. In lepromatous leprosy, collections of foam cells within the lobules

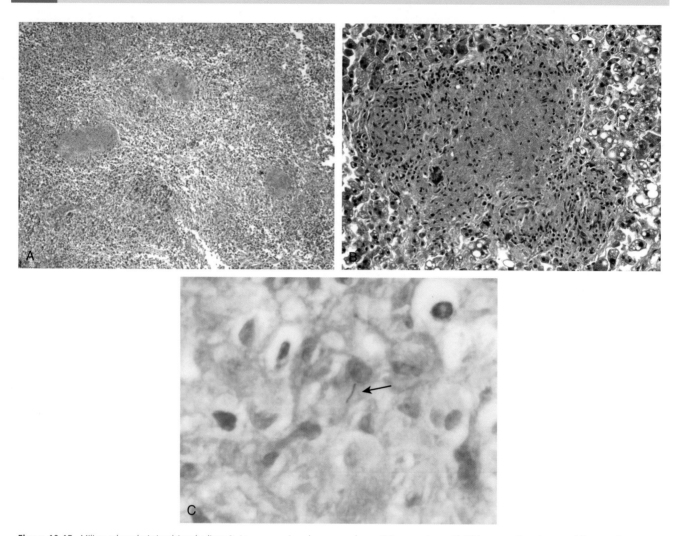

Figure 10-15. Miliary tuberculosis involving the liver. **A,** Low-power view shows several necrotizing granulomas. **B,** High-power view of a necrotizing granuloma. Note the central region of necrosis surrounded by histiocytes and a giant cell. **C,** An acid-fast stain highlights a single bacillus *(arrow)* within the granuloma.

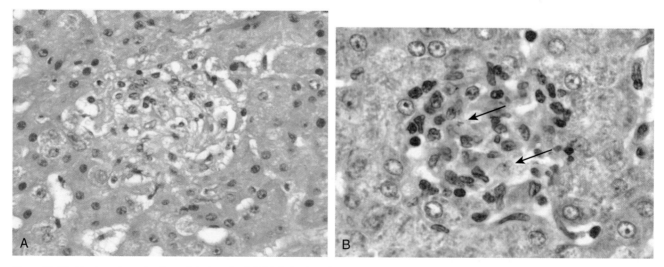

Figure 10-16. *Mycobacterium avium-intracellulare* complex (MAC) infection in an immunocompromised patient. **A,** The liver shows loose collections of histiocytes, suggestive of poorly formed granulomas. **B,** On acid-fast staining, several bacilli are present *(arrows)*.

or portal tracts contain numerous acid-fast bacilli.[125,126] In tuberculoid leprosy, epithelioid granulomas with rare or no acid-fast organisms are seen (Fig. 10-17).[125] An individual patient may have both lepromatous and tuberculoid granulomas.

Bacillus Calmette-Guérin

Bacillus Calmette-Guérin (BCG) is an attenuated form of *Mycobacterium bovis*, immunologically related to *M. tuberculosis*, that has been used as a vaccine against TB, as intralesional treatment of dermal malignancies, and as intravesical therapy for superficial bladder cancer. Hepatic granulomas have been described in patients after intradermal injections of BCG.[127,128] Pneumonitis or granulomatous hepatitis, or both, affect 0.7% of patients who receive multiple intravesical instillations of BCG and are more likely after traumatic catheterization, extensive tumor resection, or bladder perforation.[129] The liver shows noncaseating epithelioid granulomas, mild steatosis, and hepatocyte necrosis. Often, acid-fast bacilli are not identified, and cultures are negative. This

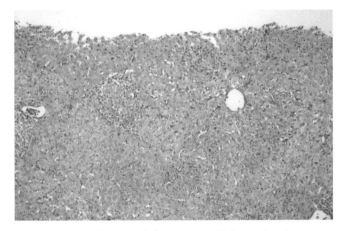

Figure 10-17. Liver biopsy sample from a patient with leprosy. Several noncaseating granulomas are present.

has led to the suggestion that the granulomatous hepatitis represents a hypersensitivity reaction to antigens present in the BCG preparation,[127] particularly because some cases show additional features of extrahepatic granulomas, leukocytoclastic vasculitis, or bile duct injury and eosinophils (Fig. 10-18).[130,131] However, in some reported cases, acid-fast bacilli have been identified in the granulomas, blood cultures have been positive for *M. bovis*, or PCR for mycobacterial DNA has been positive, indicating disseminated BCG infection.[131-133] Some have suggested that two types of adverse reactions may occur, one a disseminated infection that responds to anti-TB therapy and the other a sterile hypersensitivity reaction that is delayed in appearance and responds to steroids.[131]

Nonmycobacterial Bacteria

Bacterial infections of the liver can produce a wide range of pathology, including hepatitis, parenchymal necrosis, microabscesses, pyogenic liver abscess, and granulomatous hepatitis. Mixed patterns are frequent, and many organisms can produce several patterns. Microabscesses or pyogenic liver abscesses can be caused by a multitude of aerobic and anaerobic organisms, fungi, and parasites. Granulomatous hepatitis with or without a necrotizing component can be seen in a number of infections (Table 10-2).[134-136] However, in some entities, the granulomas are not true epithelioid granulomas, but rather aggregates of histiocytes in foci of parenchymal necrosis. Because these "microgranulomas" do not generate the same differential diagnosis as true epithelioid granulomas, the diagnosis of "granulomatous hepatitis" in these cases is best avoided. Biliary involvement can produce acute cholangitis or cholecystitis.

Pyogenic Liver Abscess

Historically, pyogenic liver abscess was associated with acute appendicitis or intra-abdominal infection, and in those settings

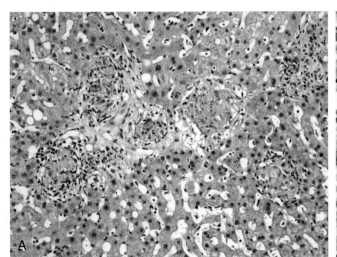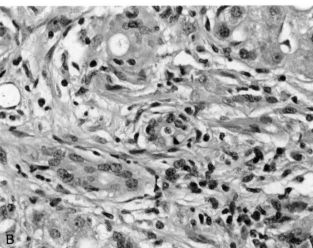

Figure 10-18. Liver biopsy in a patient with bacillus Calmette-Guérin infection. **A,** Several small granulomas are present in this view. **B,** In some portal tracts, bile duct injury and scattered eosinophils are present, suggesting a hypersensitivity reaction.

Table 10-2 Infections Associated with Granulomatous Inflammation in the Liver

Viral

Hepatitis C virus
Cytomegalovirus
Epstein-Barr virus

Mycobacterial

Tuberculosis
Leprosy
Atypical tuberculosis

Bacterial

Brucellosis
Cat-scratch disease
Enteric fever; typhoid fever
Listeriosis
Melioidosis
Tularemia
Whipple disease[134]
Pasteurella multocida[135]
Yersinia enterocolitica[136]
Actinomycosis
Nocardiosis

Rickettsial

Q fever

Chlamydial

Lymphogranuloma venereum
Psittacosis

Spirochetal

Syphilis
Lyme disease

Fungal

Aspergillosis
Blastomycosis
Candidiasis
Coccidioidomycosis
Cryptococcosis
Histoplasmosis
Mucormycosis
Paracoccidioidomycosis
Pneumocystis

Helminthic

Ascariasis
Capillariasis
Fascioliasis
Opisthorchiasis
Schistosomiasis
Strongyloidiasis
Visceral larva migrans

Protozoal

Leishmaniasis
Toxoplasmosis

it was seen more often in children.[137] More recently, biliary disease has emerged as a common etiology, and with that shift, the age of the patients has also increased, to 55 to 60 years of age.[138-140] Diabetes mellitus is a strong risk factor for the development of pyogenic liver abscess.[140,141] Other frequent comorbidities are malignancy, alcohol abuse, cirrhosis, hypertension, recent surgery, and immunosuppression.[138,139,142] A significant minority of cases remain cryptogenic. Although the disease carries a high mortality, improved diagnosis, abscess drainage, and antibiotic therapy have reduced the mortality rate to 5% to 31%.[138,142] Patients typically present with fever, chills, right upper quadrant pain, and elevated alkaline phosphatase.[138,139] Men are affected more often than women in most series.[138-140] Most abscesses are solitary; multiple abscesses occur in 25% to 45% of cases.[138-140,142] Most abscesses are right sided (55% to 70%), with left-sided and bilateral disease occurring less often.[137,138,140]

Culture of aspirated purulent material from the abscess or of blood may yield the offending organisms, although both of these are occasionally negative. Sometimes blood culture results do not correlate with pus culture results; therefore, blood culture alone is not sufficient to determine the etiology.[138] Depending on the organism, serology may be useful. The most commonly isolated organisms are *Escherichia coli, Klebsiella pneumoniae, Enterococcus, Streptococcus,* and *Pseudomonas* species.[138,139,142] A third of infections are polymicrobial (Fig. 10-19). Organisms that produce formic hydrogenlyase, such as *Klebsiella* spp. and *E. coli,* can convert acids that accumulate within the abscess to carbon dioxide and hydrogen gas; infection with these organisms can result in gas-forming pyogenic abscess, which carries a higher risk of septic shock, bacteremia, and mortality.[143] Abscesses secondary to *Yersinia enterocolitica* or *Yersinia pseudotuberculosis* are often associated with underlying hemochromatosis.[144-147] Anaerobes are isolated in up to 25% of cases, sometimes together with aerobes.[139,148,149] Microaerophilic streptococci, *Bacteroides fragilis, Fusobacterium necrophorum,* and *Clostridium* spp. are the most commonly implicated anaerobes. *Actinomyces* spp. are infrequently found by either anaerobic culture of aspirated pus or identification of filamentous bacteria and sulfur granules on histologic examination of resection material (Fig. 10-20); these organisms may be associated with the formation of sinus tracts.[150-153] Rarely, *Francisella tularensis,*[154] *Burkholderia pseudomallei* (the agent of melioidosis),[155,156] or *Listeria monocytogenes*[157] causes liver abscesses. Fungi, such as *Candida* and *Aspergillus,* are found in about 15% of cases.[148,158]

Complications of pyogenic liver abscess include metastatic infections such as endophthalmitis, meningitis, osteomyelitis, pyelonephritis, and pneumonia. The two main risk factors for metastatic infection are infection with *K. pneumoniae* and underlying diabetes mellitus.[142,159,160] Although surgical management was once the mainstay of therapy, percutaneous drainage and antibiotics have become the first-line approach.[138]

Acute Cholangitis

The term *acute cholangitis* refers to an infection of the bile ducts characterized by jaundice, abdominal pain, and sepsis, in combination with biliary obstruction. Bacterial colonization of the biliary tree in the absence of obstruction produces no symptoms; conversely, sterile obstruction of the bile duct produces a picture

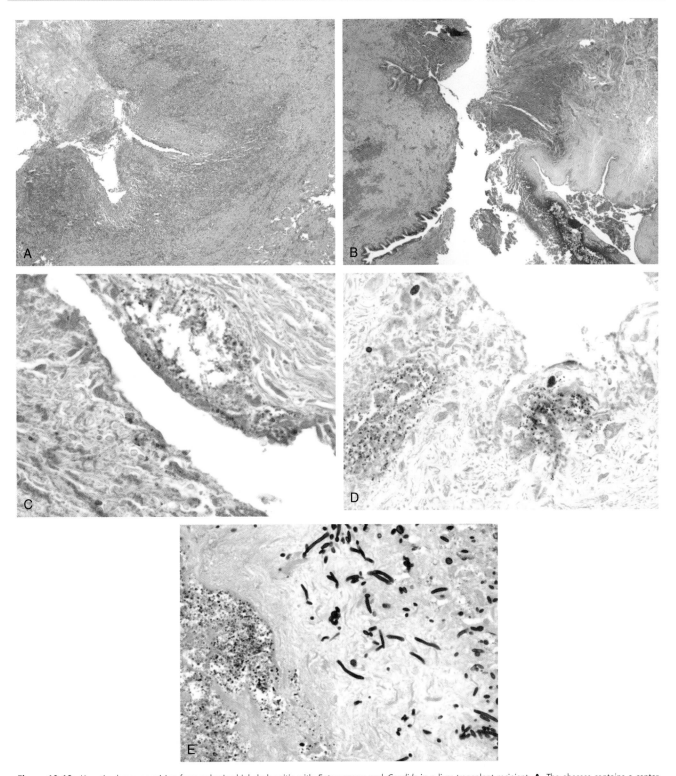

Figure 10-19. Hepatic abscesses arising from polymicrobial cholangitis with *Enterococcus* and *Candida* in a liver transplant recipient. **A,** The abscess contains a center of necrotic debris, fibrin, and neutrophils surrounded by granulation tissue and inflammation, with a fibrotic rim. **B,** In some areas, residual bile duct epithelium at the abscess edge betrays origin from cholangitis. **C,** Yeast forms *(lower left)* are present adjacent to bacterial cocci *(upper right)* in the bile duct lumen. **D,** Gram-positive cocci are revealed by Brown-Hopps stain. **E,** Yeast forms and pseudohyphae consistent with *Candida (upper right)* and bacterial cocci *(lower left)* are present (GMS stain).

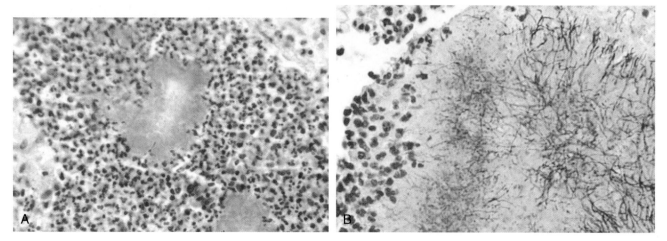

Figure 10-20. *Actinomyces.* **A,** Sulfur granule with aggregate of filamentous bacteria and neutrophils. **B,** Brown-Hopps stain shows gram-positive filamentous bacteria in the sulfur granule. (Courtesy of Dr. Laura Lamps.)

of aseptic obstructive jaundice.[161] The route by which bacteria colonize the bile ducts is uncertain. Possible sources include reflux of intestinal contents through the choledochal sphincter; passage from an infected gallbladder; and lymphatic, hepatic arterial, or portal venous bacteremia.[161] Obstruction is most often due to gallstones. Other causes include strictures, malignancy, and congenital anomalies of the ampulla of Vater. How bactibilia and obstruction leads to biliary septicemia is uncertain. Cholangiovenous reflux with increased intrabiliary pressure can be demonstrated using contrast, and higher biliary pressures are associated with an increased incidence of purulent bile, sepsis, and bacteremia.[161]

Manifestations of acute cholangitis range from mild, recurrent illness to overwhelming sepsis. Most patients are middle aged, and men and women are affected equally. Fever and jaundice are the most common symptoms. In 1877, Charcot proposed a clinical triad: right upper quadrant abdominal pain, fever, and jaundice.[162] About 70% of patients present with the full triad. Reynolds arrived at a pentad in 1959 by adding hypotension and delirium.[163] Although rare, the pentad describes patients with high mortality risk.[164] Alkaline phosphatase and bilirubin are elevated in most patients, but blood cultures are positive in fewer than half of patients.

The bacteria that infect the biliary tree usually derive from the gut. The bacteria most commonly isolated from bile are *E. coli, Enterococcus, Klebsiella, Proteus, Pseudomonas,* and *Enterobacter.*[161,165] Improved culture techniques have shown a significant incidence of infection by anaerobes, such as *B. fragilis* and clostridial species, frequently in association with previous biliary-intestinal anastomosis, an elderly patient, and more severe illness.[161,166] Overall, 56% of cases are polymicrobial. Mycotic infection of the bile duct, principally by *Candida albicans,* is rare and affects older patients, patients with malignancy, immunosuppressed patients, and diabetics.[161]

The histology of acute cholangitis is similar to that of large duct obstruction, with portal edema, neutrophilic portal and periductal inflammation, and neutrophils within duct epithelium.[167,168] In some cases, neutrophils accumulate within the duct lumina; although this is suggestive of infection, the association is not sufficiently reliable to be predictive.[167,168] Microabscesses and

macroscopic abscesses may be seen. Thrombophlebitis may result in portal vein thrombi.[168] Patients suffering from shock may show necrosis of the liver.[168] Chronic changes include strictures, dilatations, portal fibrosis, and. potentially. ductopenia. Histologic findings frequently do not correlate with clinical status, in that most cases of acute cholangitis show relatively minor histologic changes, and patients with mild symptoms can have frank abscesses.[168] Histology is also not predictive of survival.[164] Therefore, clinical and microbiologic correlation is frequently required to make the diagnosis of acute bacterial cholangitis.

Most patients respond well to antibiotics. The efficacy of a specific antibiotic depends on its biliary secretion, which is affected by the size of the compound. The inflammatory process also can cause impairment of secretion. Treatment of the obstruction is necessary to prevent recurrence. Some patients require emergent biliary drainage in addition to antibiotics, and there may be a survival advantage to surgical management of the obstruction.[164] Complications of acute cholangitis include renal failure and the development of hepatic abscesses.[161]

Recurrent Pyogenic Cholangitis (Oriental Cholangiohepatitis)

Recurrent pyogenic cholangitis is a disease that historically was seen largely in the Far East but is reported in increasing numbers in the West, largely among Asian immigrants. The disease is characterized by abdominal pain, fever, chills, and jaundice resulting from recurrent attacks of suppurative cholangitis associated with intrahepatic biliary stones.[169] The cause is not fully known, but bacterial infection of the biliary tree is perhaps the inciting event. Enteric organisms, particularly *E. coli,* are cultured from bile in most cases.[169] Bacteria deconjugate bilirubin glucuronide, which then precipitates with calcium in the bile as soft, brown, friable calcium bilirubinate stones.[169,170] Exactly what predisposes patients to biliary tract infection is unknown, but the geographic distribution of this disease mirrors that of *Clonorchis sinensis* and *Ascaris lumbricoides,* and biliary parasites are detected in a significant minority of patients.[169] Dead flukes and ova within the bile ducts, accompanied by bile stasis, may lead to bacterial infection. However, large numbers of people in endemic areas are infested with liver flukes without recurrent pyogenic cholangitis. In any case, the recurrent cholangitis results in intense periductal inflammation and fibrosis, strictures, and dilated ducts filled with sludge.[170] Morphologically, large ducts show chronic and acute cholangitis, fibrosis, and peribiliary gland hyperplasia. Pigmented stones and pus are seen in ducts; liver abscesses may be present.[169] Bile ductular proliferation with cholangiolitis and periductal fibrosis develops. Cholangiocarcinoma is a complication.

Brucellosis

Brucellosis largely affects handlers of livestock, particularly those in the meatpacking industry. Most patients present with an acute illness characterized by malaise, fever, chills, sweats, weight loss, and headache, but some patients become symptomatic after many years of dormancy or are episodically symptomatic.[171] Viral illness or trauma may precipitate relapse of chronic brucellosis.[171] The most common histopathologic pattern is granulomatous hepatitis.[172,173] In a series of 14 patients with brucellosis, all had hepatic granulomas in both portal tracts and lobules.[174] These granulomas may be indistinguishable from TB or sarcoidosis, and brucellosis should be considered in any patient with hepatic granulomas.[173] The presence of granulomas does not reliably distinguish among the various species of *Brucella*,[175-178] despite a report that *Brucella melitensis* is not associated with granulomas.[179] Other findings may include nonspecific acute hepatitis with hepatocyte necrosis, inflammation, and Kupffer cell hyperplasia.[171,174,178]

Rarely, patients present with a mass mimicking a tumor in the liver or spleen, known as a brucelloma.[171,180] In one series of 15 patients with brucelloma in the liver or spleen, half had suffered from brucellosis many years before, suggesting reactivation of latent disease.[181] Radiologically, brucellomas have central calcification with peripheral necrotic areas.[171,180,181] Histologically, a brucelloma shows necrotic areas surrounded by a palisaded granulomatous reaction.[180,181]

Hepatic pyogenic abscess due to *Brucella* is rare and may be associated with *Brucella suis*.[171] The diagnosis is established by *Brucella* agglutination titer or culture, although the latter is difficult.

Bartonella (Cat-Scratch Disease)

Cat-scratch disease is a self-limited infection caused by infection with *Bartonella* spp. after inoculation by a cat, which usually manifests as a local skin reaction and lymphadenopathy. Most cases are attributed to *B. henselae*, but *B. quintana* has been implicated in some.[182] Approximately 1% to 2% of patients with *Bartonella* infection develop severe systemic disease with involvement of the liver, spleen, bone, central nervous system, or lung.[183] Most patients with hepatosplenic presentation are children 5 to 10 years of age.[182,184,185] Patients often have nonspecific symptoms, including fever, abdominal pain, chills, headache, malaise, and weight loss. About 25% of patients have lymphadenopathy, but often the classic skin papule of cat-scratch disease is absent.[182-184] Hepatic lesions are typically multiple and associated with abdominal lymphadenopathy and, in some cases, splenic lesions; many patients come to biopsy to exclude neoplasia.[183,185,186] On laparotomy, the liver may be found to be studded with hard nodules of varying sizes.[186]

The hallmark lesion in hepatic cat-scratch disease is an irregular, stellate microabscess surrounded by a layer of palisading histiocytes, lymphocytes, and a rim of fibrous tissue (Fig. 10-21).[183,186] Younger lesions may show more necrosis with less organization of the inflammatory granulomatous response, whereas older lesions may show confluent granulomas with scarring and scant residual necrosis.[183] These hepatic lesions are similar to the ones seen in lymph nodes in patients with cat-scratch disease, but they have also been noted in infections with *Y. enterocolitica*, *F. tularensis*, lymphogranuloma venereum, mycobacterial species, *Candida*, and *Actinomyces*.[183] Other lesions may appear as small. rounded granulomas with giant cells and small foci of central necrosis, similar to caseating granulomas in mycobacterial or fungal infections. The background liver parenchyma shows sinusoidal dilatation, portal mixed but predominantly lymphocytic inflammatory infiltrates, portal fibrosis,

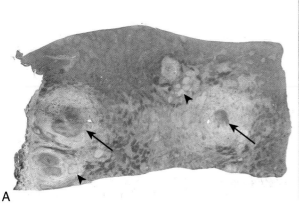
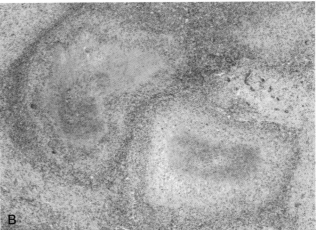

Figure 10-21. Cat-scratch disease involving the liver. **A,** Low-power view of a section of liver shows multiple stellate abscesses *(arrows)* and several older, hyalinized scars *(arrowheads)*. **B,** Medium-power view of stellate abscesses shows central necrosis surrounded by palisaded histiocytes, chronic inflammation, and fibrotic tissue.

periductal concentric fibrosis, and focal bile ductular proliferation.[183] These changes are attributed to mass effect and are also seen in other infections that result in space-occupying lesions, such as pyogenic abscesses.[183]

Warthin-Starry stains identify bacilli in some cases, and the organisms often cluster around vessels or along collagen fibers; the stain is not specific for the organism.[184] Culture is difficult. The diagnosis can be confirmed by PCR and Southern blot for *Bartonella* DNA on tissue, skin testing, or serology.[182,183,187] The disease is self-limited without long-term hepatic dysfunction. The infection responds dramatically to rifampin, erythromycin, or doxycycline, but antibiotics are unnecessary in most cases.

Bartonella also may cause vascular proliferative lesions in the liver. Bacillary epithelioid angiomatosis is a vasoproliferative tissue reaction to *B. henselae* or *B. quintana* that usually occurs in immunocompromised hosts. Hepatic involvement shows sharply demarcated periportal areas in which the normal parenchyma is replaced by vascular tissue with extravasated erythrocytes, delicate spindle cells, neutrophils, and karyorrhexic debris, mimicking Kaposi sarcoma.[91] Similar lesions have been designated as bacillary peliosis hepatis; these are characterized by the presence of multiple blood-filled cystic spaces, foci of necrosis, fibromyxoid stroma, and clumps of granular purple material that correspond to organisms on Warthin-Starry stain and electron microscopy.[92] The latter lesions can be mistaken for nonbacillary peliosis hepatis. Although these infections can be progressive and fatal, they respond to antibiotics.

Enteric Fever (Typhoid and Paratyphoid Fever)

Enteric fever (the inclusive term for typhoid and paratyphoid fever) is caused by infection with *Salmonella enterica* serotype Typhi (*S. typhi*) or serotype Paratyphi (*S. paratyphi*). The disease is transmitted via the fecal-oral route from food or water contaminated by an acutely ill person or a chronic carrier.[188] Human beings are the only known reservoir. Most infections today occur in countries where sanitary conditions are poor; the Indian subcontinent has a particularly high incidence.[188] Travelers to these areas can also be affected. Although *S. typhi* causes 80% of infections, *S. paratyphi* may be more important among travelers, possibly due to a vaccine effect that only protects against *S. typhi*.[188] In indigenous populations, enteric fever is a disease of young children and adolescents, whereas among travelers, the age of the patients reflects the age of travelers.[188]

Ingestion of the organism is followed by an asymptomatic period of about 7 days, during which the organism multiplies within mononuclear phagocytic cells in Peyer patches, mesenteric lymph nodes, liver, and spleen.[189] This is followed by a bacteremic phase, with fever, chills, headache, and rose spots. During this phase, invasion of the gallbladder occurs, either directly or from infected bile. Chronic biliary carriage occurs in 2% to 5% of cases, even after treatment, particularly among women, the elderly, and patients with cholelithiasis.[188,189] In these cases, shedding of virus continues for more than a year and is a public health risk. The majority of patients experience minor degrees of hepatomegaly and elevated transaminases. However, the presentation can resemble acute viral hepatitis, with very high transaminases or even fulminant hepatic failure, although coinfection with HAV or HEV may be responsible for some of these

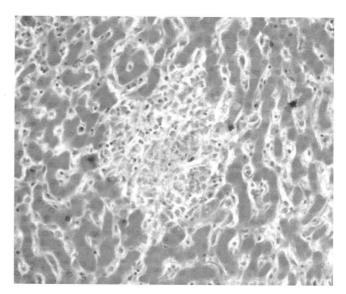

Figure 10-22. Typhoid nodule in typhoid fever. An aggregate of mononuclear cells, including histiocytes and lymphocytes, is present in the lobule. The surrounding liver shows prominent Kupffer cells in the sinusoids.

cases.[188] Intestinal perforation, hemorrhage, and encephalopathy are the most important complications. The diagnosis is made by blood culture or Widal serology assay.

In the liver, hyperplasia of the reticuloendothelial system results in prominence of mononuclear cells in the sinusoids and typhoid nodules (Fig. 10-22).[190,191] Typhoid nodules are lobular collections of macrophages that ingest bacteria, erythrocytes, and degenerated lymphocytes.[191] These nodules may resemble granulomas but are not true epithelioid granulomas, although granulomatous hepatitis has been described as well.[192] Abscesses are rare.

Tularemia

Tularemia is caused by the coccobacillus *Francisella tularensis*. The disease is most often transmitted to humans by ticks or by animal contact, especially with rabbits. Inhalation outbreaks have been associated with lawn mowing and brush cutting in contaminated areas.[154] Most patients have pulmonary involvement. Other features include fever, cutaneous ulcers, lymphadenopathy, headache, and malaise. Hepatic involvement occurs in up to 75% of patients and includes hepatosplenomegaly and mild to moderate elevations of transaminases.[193] Severe cases may show jaundice. Liver histology shows suppurative microabscesses and areas of necrosis (Fig. 10-23). As the lesions age, they become more granulomatous.[194] The diagnosis is often established serologically, because the organism is difficult to culture and is rarely seen on tissue Gram stain. PCR assays for *F. tularensis* in fresh tissue and on formalin-fixed tissue have been described.[154]

Melioidosis

Melioidosis is a glanders-like disease caused by *B. pseudomallei*, a gram-negative aerobic bacillus that survives within phagocytic

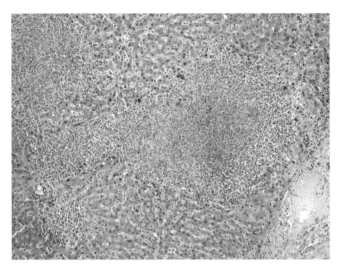

Figure 10-23. Tularemia involving the liver. Several small abscesses are present throughout the lobules.

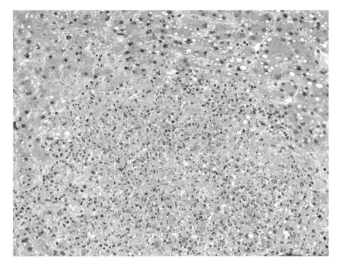

Figure 10-24. Liver from a patient who died of systemic listeriosis, showing microabscess and steatosis in the surrounding hepatocytes.

cells. The organism is a soil saprophyte that prefers wet soils and is an important community-acquired pathogen in Southeast Asia and northern Australia, particularly during rainy seasons.[156] Percutaneous inoculation and inhalation are modes of transmission. Travelers can be exposed when they come in contact with wet soil, such as during adventure tours.[195] Occasionally, patients have chronic disease or reactivation of a latent focus years after leaving an endemic area, a possibility that caused concern for veterans returning from Vietnam.[195] Predisposing factors include diabetes mellitus, renal disease, alcoholism, cirrhosis, and immunosuppression.[155,156] The acute form of the disease is characterized by abscess formation, predominantly in the lung, but seeding and abscess formation also occur in the liver, spleen, skeletal muscle, and lymph nodes; often, multiple sites are involved.[155,156,196] Chronic melioidosis shows granulomatous inflammation with central irregular abscesses, indistinguishable from the stellate abscesses of cat-scratch disease, tularemia, or lymphogranuloma venereum.[196] The granulomas may show caseous-type necrosis, mimicking TB.[196] The lesions in chronic melioidosis are usually confined to a single organ. Serology is not completely reliable, but *B. pseudomallei* can be readily cultured from abscess material.[155]

Listeriosis

Listeria monocytogenes is a gram-positive, facultative intracellular bacillus that is an occasional contaminant of food, even despite proper refrigeration. Infection is associated with pregnancy, extremes of age, diabetes mellitus, and immunosuppression. Transplacental transmission causes granulomatosis infantisepticum, which is characterized by abscesses and granulomas in various fetal organs.[197] After ingestion, the organisms invade the Peyer patches and are transported to the liver, where they are cleared from the bloodstream by Kupffer cells. Some organisms escape from Kupffer cells and invade hepatocytes, where, protected from the host immune response, they replicate. Neutrophils are recruited to the area, forming abscesses, and after a few days, granulomas form in an attempt to impede further spread. Once the organisms escape the granulomas and are released into

the blood, they have a predilection for the central nervous system and placenta.[197]

Hepatic involvement can manifest as solitary liver abscess, multiple liver abscesses, or hepatitis (Fig. 10-24).[157,197] Solitary liver abscess is associated with diabetes mellitus, absence of bacteremia or extrahepatic manifestations, and a relatively good prognosis.[157,197] Multiple liver abscesses are more often associated with bacteremia, extrahepatic sites of involvement, and meningitis and carry a worse prognosis.[157,197] Diffuse hepatitis is associated with underlying conditions such as viral hepatitis, pregnancy, or alcohol abuse.[197,198] Bacteremia is highly likely in cases with diffuse hepatitis. The histology is that of chronic active hepatitis with extensive necroinflammatory activity and occasionally granulomas.[198] The diagnosis is made by culture of the organism from blood or abscess material.

Spirochetes

Syphilis

Treponema pallidum infection can affect the liver in secondary syphilis, in tertiary syphilis, or congenitally. Involvement by the liver in secondary syphilis has been reported in men and women. Several cases have been reported among homosexual men,[199-203] possibly from portal transport of the organism after anal intercourse.[203] A characteristic clinical picture is cholestatic jaundice, hepatomegaly, and a disproportionately elevated alkaline phosphatase level.[199,201,202,204-206] The trademark palmar rash of syphilis may be the key to diagnosis.[204,205] Histologic examination of liver may show a variety of pathologic patterns. In most cases, portal inflammation with mononuclear cells or neutrophils surrounding damaged bile ducts (pericholangitis) is the main finding.[200,201,206,207] Scattered foci of necrosis may be present in the lobules, sometimes accompanied by inflammation around the central veins and Glisson's capsule.[201,203,207,208] Granulomatous hepatitis is described in some cases (Fig. 10-25).[208,209] Spirochetes are only rarely identified in histologic sections with silver stains such as Warthin-Starry or Steiner.[199,204,207]

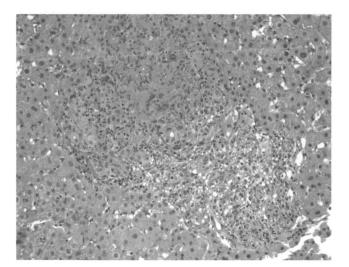

Figure 10-25. Secondary syphilis in the liver. Granulomatous inflammation is seen adjacent to an inflamed portal tract.

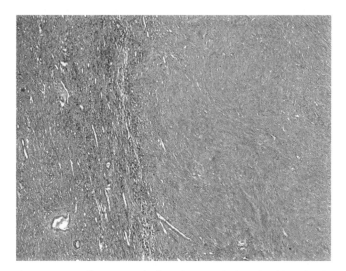

Figure 10-26. Old gumma in the liver, showing a hyalinized nodule with mild chronic inflammation at the periphery. (Courtesy of Dr. Laura Lamps.)

In tertiary syphilis, multiple gummas in the liver may mimic metastatic carcinoma.[210] Histologically, gummas resemble TB, in that they are composed of masses of granulomas with caseating necrosis, surrounding fibrosis, chronic inflammation, and histiocytic inflammation.[210] Healed gummas may be replaced by fibrous scars (Fig. 10-26). Retraction of these scars can distort the liver by producing pseudolobules or so-called hepar lobatum.[210] Scars near the hilum may result in portal hypertension.

Congenital syphilis is frequently fatal, but surviving infants may have hepatomegaly and jaundice, with diffuse fibrosis. Spirochetes can be seen within connective tissue septa, parenchymal cells, and the walls of small vessels.[211]

Leptospirosis

Leptospirosis is an acute febrile illness caused by *Leptospira interrogans* that affects humans and animals in all parts of the world.[212]

The disease is biphasic, with a septicemic phase followed by an immune phase with antibody production and urinary excretion of the organism.[212] Most patients experience a mild anicteric illness, with fever, headaches, and myalgias. Severe cases, characterized by hepatic, renal, and pulmonary involvement, are known as Weil syndrome.[212] Liver pathology is predominantly a cholestatic hepatitis with reactive hepatocellular changes and Kupffer cell hyperplasia.[191,212,213] Scattered Councilman bodies, bile within canaliculi, and mild portal inflammation may be seen.[191,214] Very rarely, spirochetes can be demonstrated on silver stain. The diagnosis is based on serologic assays.

Lyme Disease

Lyme disease is caused by *Borrelia burgdorferi* and is transmitted by *Ixodid* ticks, usually during the months of May through October. Hepatomegaly and symptoms of hepatitis are uncommon. Elevated transaminases indicate mild hepatocellular injury, although a nonhepatic source is possible in the case of Lyme disease–associated myositis.[193] In the liver, mononuclear cells, plasma cells, and granulocytes are seen in sinusoids. Kupffer cell hyperplasia, steatosis, and hepatocyte ballooning are also described.[193,215] Granulomatous hepatitis is uncommon; necrotizing granulomas have been reported.[216] Organisms are only rarely seen in hepatic sinusoids and parenchyma with silver stain such as Dieterle.[215]

Rickettsia

Q fever (*Coxiella burnetii*)

Q fever is a zoonotic rickettsial disease that is caused by the aerosol spread of *Coxiella burnetii* from infected sheep and cattle. The disease is endemic in the southwestern United States and in southwestern Ontario. Most patients suffer an acute, self-limited infection that typically manifests as pneumonitis, although chronic infection with endocarditis is well known. Unlike other rickettsial diseases, Q fever does not produce a rash.[217] Hepatic involvement is common, and the disease may even manifest as hepatic disease without pulmonary symptoms.[218] The diagnosis is established by complement-fixing antibodies to phase II *C. burnetii* antigen in serum.

The classic lesion of Q fever is the fibrin ring granuloma, which can be found in liver or bone marrow (Fig. 10-27).[217-222] Also known as donut or ring granulomas, these lesions contain a central fat vacuole that can lead to their being mistaken for lipogranulomas, but on closer inspection a ring of fibrin surrounds the fat vacuole. The fibrin ring is highlighted on trichrome stain. Q fever is the most commonly reported etiology, but fibrin ring granulomas have also been reported in other infectious and in noninfectious conditions, including hepatitis A,[8,9] *Staphylococcus epidermidis* infection,[223] allopurinol hypersensitivity,[224-227] visceral leishmaniasis,[226,227] giant cell arteritis,[228] CMV,[75] EBV,[70,229] Hodgkin disease,[227,230] toxoplasmosis,[226] and Boutonneuse fever.[226]

In addition to fibrin ring granulomas, epithelioid granulomas with or without central necrosis may be seen and can be mistaken for TB.[217,221,226,231] Other findings in Q fever hepatitis

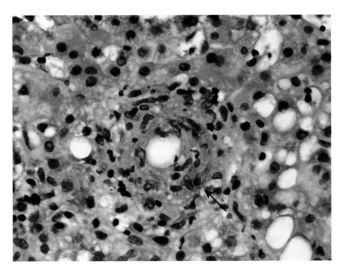

Figure 10-27. Fibrin ring granuloma. A collection of histiocytes contains a central fat droplet surrounded by a rim of histiocytes, a ring of fibrin *(arrow)*, and another rim of histiocytes.

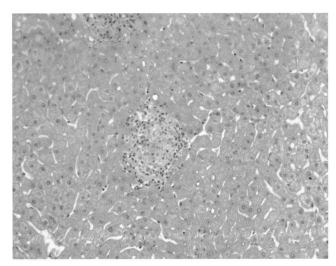

Figure 10-28. Liver biopsy sample in an immune-competent patient with hepatic and splenic histoplasmosis. A solitary, well-formed granuloma is present in the liver.

include moderate steatosis, focal liver cell necrosis, Kupffer cell hyperplasia, hemosiderin deposits, and, rarely, microabscesses.[221]

Ehrlichiosis

Ehrlichiosis is caused by gram-negative obligate intracellular organisms that are transmitted by a tick vector, predominantly in the southeastern United States. Human monocytic ehrlichiosis is caused by *Ehrlichia chaffeensis* and *Ehrlichia canis,* whereas human granulocytic ehrlichiosis is caused by *Ehrlichia phagocytophila* and *Ehrlichia equi.*[193] Symptoms include fever, headache, anorexia, and myalgia. The relatively low incidence of rash (20%) contrasts with the frequent presence of a rash in Lyme disease and Rocky Mountain spotted fever.[232,233] Transaminases are often mildly elevated, although they may be in the range of viral hepatitis. Alkaline phosphatase and bilirubin are less likely to be elevated, but may be so with severe cholestasis.[232,233] Liver biopsy may show lobular lymphohistiocytic aggregates and sinusoidal infiltration by lymphohistiocytic cells associated with erythroleukophagocytosis.[234] In cholestatic cases, bile stasis, duct epithelial injury, and neutrophilic infiltration of medium-sized ducts may suggest extrahepatic obstruction.[232,234] Other reported findings include focal hepatic necrosis, steatosis, granulomas, and foamy Kupffer cells with scattered apoptotic bodies.[233,234]

Rocky Mountain Spotted Fever

Rickettsia rickettsii is transmitted by the wood tick, *Dermacentor andersoni,* in the Rocky Mountain region and by the dog tick, *Dermacentor variabilis,* in the eastern United States. Mild to moderate transaminase elevations and occasionally jaundice may be seen. The main pathologic lesion is vasculitis, and rickettsiae are capable of infecting the endothelial lining cells or portal blood vessels, especially arteries and arterioles, and sinusoidal lining cells.[193,235] Reports of autopsy livers describe portal inflammation, portal vasculitis with subendothelial and intramural mononuclear leukocytes, portal vascular thrombi, portal tract hemorrhage, sinusoidal leukocytosis, and erythrophagocytosis by Kupffer cells.[235,236] Immunofluorescence techniques can be used to identify the organisms in tissue.

Boutonneuse Fever

Boutonneuse fever is caused by *Rickettsia conorii* and is transmitted by the dog tick. The disease is found in Mediterranean countries between the months of June and September. Hepatic involvement shows Kupffer cell swelling and increased sinusoidal cellularity. Small foci of hepatocyte necrosis are seen, associated with collections of histiocytes, a few neutrophils, and lymphocytes.[237,238] The mononuclear cell aggregates in the areas of necrosis may resemble poorly formed granulomas, but they are not true epithelioid granulomas.

Fungi

Histoplasma

Histoplasma is considered to be the most common fungal cause of hepatic granulomas, and it is a common cause of granulomatous hepatitis in areas where *H. capsulatum* is endemic, such as in the Ohio River valley.[239] In one series from that region, 15 (65%) of 23 children with hepatic granulomas had histoplasmosis demonstrated by PCR.[240] In another series, 50% of liver biopsy specimens with granulomas cultured positively for *Histoplasma.* Although histoplasmosis is usually self-limited in infants or immunocompromised patients, it can manifest with progressive disseminated disease requiring treatment.[240] Progressive disseminated histoplasmosis often involves the liver, with hepatomegaly in 62% of patients and abnormal liver function studies in 84%.[241]

Histologically, the appearance is identical to sarcoidosis, with numerous well-formed epithelioid granulomas (Fig. 10-28).[115]

In immunocompromised hosts, loose collections of histiocytes with numerous intracellular organisms can mimic leishmaniasis (Fig. 10-29). The absence of a kinetoplast on Giemsa stain helps distinguish *Histoplasma* from *Leishmania*.[242] The diagnosis can be established with methenamine silver staining of involved tissue, fungal culture, or complement fixation tests.[241]

Candida

Candidiasis is especially problematic in immunocompromised patients, particularly those with leukemia or cytotoxic chemotherapy-related neutropenia.[243] *Candida* accounts for 62% to 91% of fungal infections in the liver transplantation population, affecting 5% to 42% of all liver transplant recipients.[72] Patients present with fever, abdominal pain, and elevated alkaline phosphatase; blood cultures are negative in at least half of the cases.[244]

Usually, patients are in the recovery phase from the neutropenic episode, suggesting a role for the host inflammatory response in defining the lesions.[243] The diagnosis is often not made until postmortem examination.

Radiologically, the lesions appear targetoid and, in the case of older lesions, calcified.[243,244] Grossly, the liver and spleen are studded with white to yellow nodules. In the early stages, the nodule consists of a necrotic center and surrounding neutrophilic infiltrate. Periodic acid–Schiff (PAS) or Gomori methenamine silver (GMS) stains demonstrate yeast or pseudohyphae in the center of the abscess. As the lesion matures, a palisaded histiocytic reaction may develop at the periphery of the lesion, surrounded by a fibrous wall (Fig. 10-30).[244] Eventually, well-defined granulomas with giant cells may be seen.[243] As the lesions progress with increasing fibrosis, organisms become more difficult to detect, so their absence does not exclude the diagnosis. The adjacent liver parenchyma frequently shows sinusoidal dilatation,

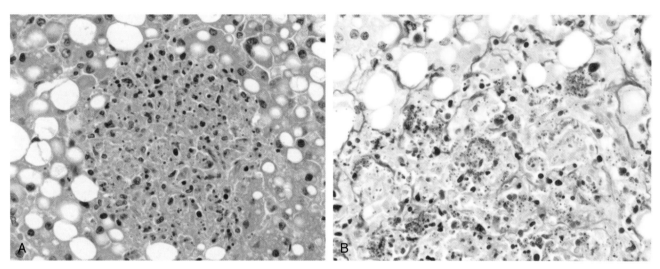

Figure 10-29. Histoplasmosis in an AIDS patient. **A,** Necrotic lesions are composed of histiocytes and debris. **B,** GMS stain shows yeast in macrophages in the necrotic lesion.

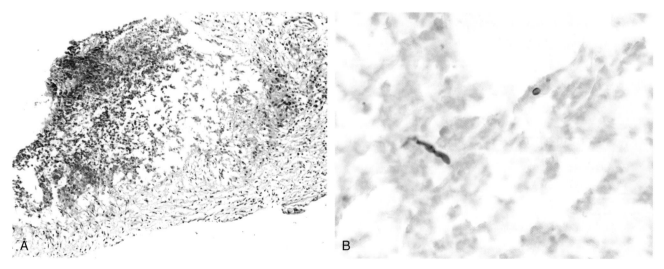

Figure 10-30. Candidal abscess in a patient with leukemia. **A,** Abscess with necrosis and neutrophils *(upper left)* surrounded by a palisaded histiocytic reaction. **B,** Rare yeast and pseudohyphae on GMS staining.

portal edema, neutrophilic infiltrate, and ductular reaction, presumably due to mass effect.[244] Candidal infection of the biliary tree and gallbladder occurs in disseminated candidiasis, with bacterial cholangitis, or as isolated candidal cholangitis or cholecystitis.[245,246]

Pneumocystis jiroveci

Pneumocystis jiroveci (formerly *Pneumocystis carinii*) is a fungal organism that typically causes lung infections in immunocompromised patients. Extrapulmonary infection is rare but has been associated with the use of prophylactic aerosolized pentamidine, which suppresses pulmonary disease but might allow for dissemination of the organism.[247,248] Grossly, the liver is studded with yellow-white nodules. The pathology ranges from caseating granulomas to massive infiltration of sinusoids and vessels by the organism with little inflammatory reaction (Fig. 10-31).[247,248] The organism appears as indented, helmet-shaped "cysts" on silver stains.

Aspergillus

Aspergillus fumigatus involving the liver is seen in cases of disseminated aspergillosis and in immunosuppressed patients. Liver abscess and cholangitis secondary to *Aspergillus* infection have been described.[158,249] The organism is easily demonstrated on methenamine silver or PAS stains and shows characteristic septate hyphae with acute-angle branching.

Zygomycetes

Fungi of the class Zygomycetes are ubiquitous in nature, occurring in decaying material and soil. The members of this class most often implicated in human disease are *Rhizopus, Rhizomucor, Mucor,* and *Absidia*.[250] Hepatic zygomycosis has been reported in immuno-compromised patients, in patients receiving chemo-

therapy, in stem cell transplant recipients, and in solid organ transplant recipients.[250-254] Hepatic infection in the absence of pulmonary disease may be caused by spread from a gastrointestinal source.[250] These fungi have broad (10 to 20 μm), aseptate or hyposeptate, ribbon-like hyphae with right-angle branching, and they have a propensity to invade blood vessels, leading to extensive necrosis, infarctions, and dissemination.[250-253] Diagnosis requires identification of the fungus in tissue or culture. However, tissue culture sensitivity is poor, possibly because the grinding of tissue in preparation for plating destroys the delicate hyphae, and this technique is no longer recommended.[250] Blood cultures are always negative. In tissue identification, erroneous classification as *Aspergillus* may occur if the hyphae are hyposeptate.[250]

Penicilliosis

Penicilliosis is an infection caused by the dimorphic fungus, *Penicillium marneffei*, which is endemic in Southeast Asia.[255] This pathogen has emerged as the third most common opportunistic infection among AIDS patients in Southeast Asia and southern China, although it affects people with apparently normal immunity as well.[256] Pathologic findings include granulomatous inflammation with relatively few organisms, suppurative abscesses, and necrotic lesions consisting of histiocytes filled with organisms, the latter being typical in immuno-compromised patients.[255,256] The organisms appear as small spherules, 2 to 4 μm in diameter, along with some elongated and septate forms; they are highlighted with methenamine silver stain or by PAS stain with diastase digestion (Fig. 10-32).[255,256] The main differential diagnosis is *H. capsulatum*.

Cryptococcosis

Cryptococcosis is caused by the encapsulated yeast, *Cryptococcus neoformans,* and hepatic infection has been reported in both immunocompromised and immune-competent patients.[257,258] In the immune-competent cases, granulomas are seen, whereas in

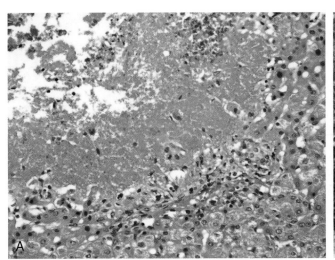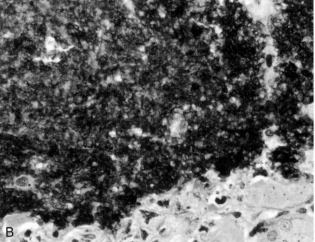

Figure 10-31. *Pneumocystis jiroveci* in the liver. **A,** Necrotic lesion composed of granular eosinophilic material with mild histiocytic reaction at the periphery. **B,** GMS stain demonstrates that the granular material is composed of masses of *Pneumocystis* organisms.

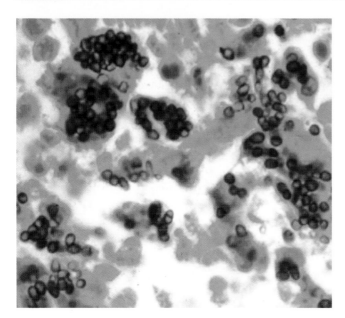

Figure 10-32. Penicilliosis. A GMS stain shows numerous yeast forms in macrophages. The organisms are round to oval, with a few slightly elongate and septate forms. (Courtesy of Drs. David Walker and Laura Lamps.)

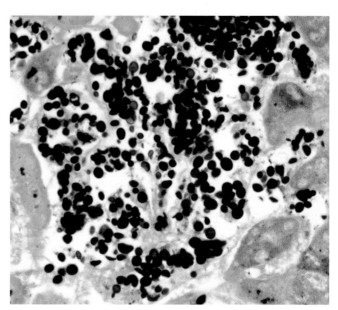

Figure 10-33. Capsule-deficient *Cryptococcus.* A GMS stain shows yeast cells of varying sizes within a collection of histiocytes in the liver. (Courtesy of Dr. Laura Lamps.)

AIDS patients, an inflammatory reaction is poorly developed. Autopsies in cases of disseminated infection have shown areas of necrosis with innumerable yeast cells, yeast cells diffusely within tissue admixed with cellular debris and inflammation, or yeast cells within Kupffer cells (Fig. 10-33).[259] Infection of the bile duct can mimic sclerosing cholangitis.[260] The organism can be demonstrated on silver stains, and mucicarmine stain can be used to highlight the capsule. The capsule is a virulence factor and is helpful in the diagnosis, but in rare instances, capsule-deficient strains can cause infection, particularly in immunocompromised patients (see Fig. 10-33). Capsule-deficient forms can be confused with other yeasts.

Coccidioidomycosis

Coccidioides immitis is endemic to the southwestern United States and northern Mexico. Disseminated infection can show granulomatous hepatitis or microabscesses containing the thick-walled spherules of *C. immitis,* which can be highlighted with PAS and methenamine silver stains.[261-263] The spherules may or may not contain endospores; immature spherules without endospores can be mistaken for *Blastomyces dermatitidis* or *C. neoformans.*[263] Serology and culture results can be used to establish the diagnosis.

Blastomycosis

Blastomyces dermatitidis is a dimorphic fungus that usually involves skin and lungs. The fungus is endemic to the southeastern and south central United States, the areas bordering the Great Lakes, and the Ohio and Mississippi River basins. Hepatic granulomas and cholangitis have been described.[264] Thick-walled yeast forms with broad-based budding are seen on PAS or silver stains (Fig. 10-34).

Paracoccidioidomycosis (South American Blastomycosis)

Paracoccidioides brasiliensis causes a chronic granulomatous disease known as South American blastomycosis. The disease is endemic in rural South America and affects males more often than females. Although pulmonary lesions are typical, extrapulmonary disease can occur. In the liver, the fungus usually causes a granulomatous reaction. Less often, it causes focal necrosis with neutrophilic exudates containing numerous organisms.[265]

Microsporidiosis

Microsporidia are obligate intracellular organisms that were originally believed to be primitive eukaryotes but have recently been reclassified as fungi based on DNA sequence data. Several species have been implicated in human disease. Infection of bile duct epithelium has been described as a cause of AIDS-related cholangitis.[95,97] A case of hepatitis has also been reported, with sinusoidal congestion and microgranulomas on light microscopy.[94] Electron microscopy is necessary to identify the organisms in most cases, but often the organism has already been identified in intestinal biopsy specimens by the time cholangitis develops.

Helminths

Schistosomiasis

Schistosomiasis is the second most common parasitic infection of humans after malaria. Several species of schistosomes affect humans: *Schistosoma japonicum* is associated with hepatic pathology more often than *Schistosoma mansoni.* The intermediate host is a population of snails that is not found in North America

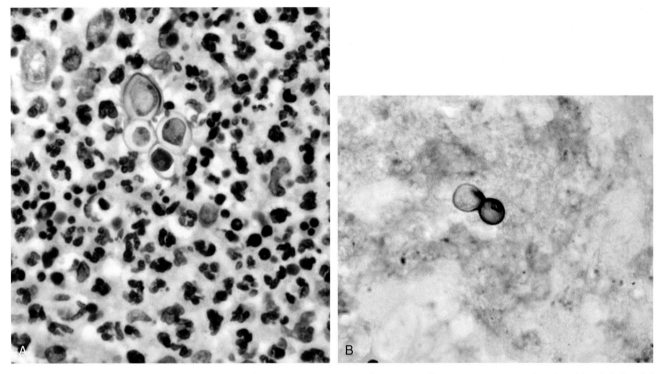

Figure 10-34. Blastomycosis. **A,** Broad-based, budding yeast forms are present in an area of suppurative inflammation. **B,** GMS stain shows broad-based, thick-walled yeast cells. (Courtesy of Dr. Laura Lamps.)

or Europe.[266] Infection occurs when the cercariae exit the snail and penetrate the skin of a vertebrate host. In the human host, the cercariae migrate to the lungs, where they mature, reach the left side of the heart, and then are carried to the portal hepatic circulation. In the mesenteric venous plexus, the male occupies the gynecophoric canal of the female, and the worms remain in a state of continuous copulation for their life span of 3 to 5 years.[266] Eggs released in the mesenteric venous plexus can migrate to the intestine (intestinal form) or into the liver (hepatosplenic form), where they lodge in the small portal vein tributaries. Granuloma formation around the eggs leads to pyelophlebitis and periportal fibrosis.

Histology shows portal fibrosis with partial or complete destruction of the main branches of the portal vein but sparing of arteries and ducts.[266] Adult worms metabolize large amounts of hemoglobin and regurgitate hemozoin pigment, which is engulfed by macrophages in the sinusoids and portal tracts and can be accentuated by Prussian blue stain. Despite the scarring, lobular architecture is maintained, so the fibrosis does not represent true cirrhosis. This pattern of fibrosis is known as Symmers pipe-stem fibrosis because of the clay pipe-stem appearance on gross pathology (Fig. 10-35).[266]

Eventually, portal hypertension supervenes with splenomegaly and esophagogastric varices. However, compensatory increase in hepatic arterial blood flow maintains hepatic perfusion and hepatic function.[266] Often, patients lack other stigmata of chronic liver disease. The diagnosis is based on the demonstration of ova in stool specimens. Serology to detect anti-schistosomal antibodies does not distinguish active from resolved infection. Enzyme-linked immunosorbent assays (ELISA) have been developed that detect schistosomal antigens in the serum and urine of actively infected patients. Antigen levels correlate with worm burden.[266]

Strongyloides

Strongyloides stercoralis exist as rhabditiform larvae in soil and as filariform larvae in humans. The organisms reside in the intestine, where they produce eggs that develop into rhabditiform larvae, which are shed in feces. In certain settings, rhabditiform larvae may develop into the infectious filariform larvae within the intestine; this form is capable of invading the intestinal mucosa and traveling throughout the body, typically the central nervous system, liver, and lungs. This unique cycle of autoinfection is accelerated in immunosuppressed patients. In the liver, the larvae can cause granulomatous hepatitis with or without larval remnants. The larvae measure between 6 and 13 μm, and they may be seen in sinusoids, portal tract lymphatics, or branches of the portal vein (Fig. 10-36).[267] Occasionally, the larvae do not provoke an inflammatory reaction.[267] Steatosis and cholestasis are additional features.

Enterobiasis (Pinworm)

Rarely, *Enterobius vermicularis* travels from the anus to unusual locations, such as the urethra or vagina. Rupture of the appendix or other intestinal disease may also provide the nematode with a mode of reaching the liver.[268] Subcapsular nodules in the liver may be found at the time of surgery; on histologic examination, they prove to be hyalinizing or calcifying granulomas

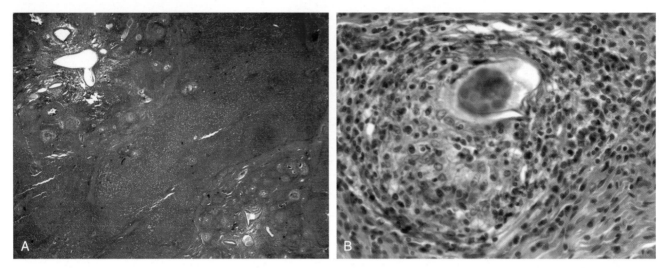

Figure 10-35. Schistosomiasis. **A,** The liver shows marked expansion of two portal areas with fibrosis and numerous granulomas, consistent with Symmers pipe-stem fibrosis. Note the absence of cirrhosis in the background liver. **B,** A high-power view of a granuloma surrounding a schistosome ovum with the characteristic lateral spine.

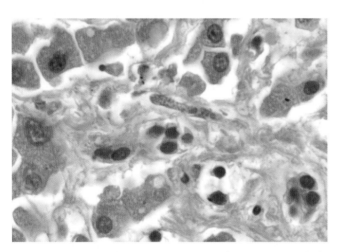

Figure 10-36. *Strongyloides* in an AIDS patient with disseminated *Strongyloides* infestation. A larval form is present in a small portal lymphatic channel.

containing remnants of pinworms with characteristic lateral alae and possibly ova.[268,269]

Echinococcosis

Echinococcosis or hydatid cyst disease is caused by species of the tapeworm, *Echinococcus. Echinococcus granulosus* is endemic in Mediterranean countries, Iran, India, China, Chile, and Argentina, whereas *Echinococcus multilocularis* is endemic in central Europe, the Near East, Russia, China, northern Japan, and Alaska.[270,271] The adult tapeworms live in the jejunum of dogs and other carnivores, the final hosts; the larvae infect herbivores, the intermediate hosts, when they ingest the eggs. Humans are incidental intermediate hosts, because further development of the cestode requires ingestion of the larvae by a carnivore.

Once ingested, the egg develops into a larval oncosphere, which penetrates the intestinal mucosa, enters the portal circula-

tion, and, on reaching the target organ (usually liver or lung), forms a rounded, multinucleated mass that becomes cystic and progressively enlarges.[271] The hydatid cyst consists of an external, acellular, laminated cuticle and an inner germinal membrane that gives rise to brood capsules containing new larvae called protoscolices (Fig. 10-37).[271,272] Hydatid cysts form daughter cysts, either from the germinal membrane or from the protoscolices or brood capsules. In the case of *E. granulosus*, the cysts are slowly enlarging masses that remain asymptomatic for a long period. Eventually, they may cause dull abdominal pain and a palpable mass.[246] About 40% of cases are associated with complications, including erosion into bile ducts, through the hepatic capsule into the peritoneal cavity, into adherent organs, or through the diaphragm.[246] In alveolar hydatid disease due to *E. multilocularis*, the hepatic parenchyma is invaded and replaced by fibrous tissue with numerous embedded vesicles that mimics carcinoma.[270] Dense granulomatous inflammation, microcalcifications, and necrotic cavitation may be present.[272]

Alveolar hydatid disease carries a high mortality without surgery, due to liver failure, invasion of contiguous structures, or, less often, metastases to the brain.[270,272] Transplantation has been attempted, but there is a high risk of recurrence in the donor liver.[272] The diagnosis can be made radiologically and confirmed serologically, although some patients do not develop an immune response.[270,272]

Toxocara

Toxocariasis refers to infection by larvae of the dog ascarid, *Toxocara canis,* or, less commonly, the cat ascarid, *Toxocara cati.* In humans, these larvae do not develop into adult worms but travel throughout host tissue, primarily liver and lungs; therefore, the disease is known as visceral larva migrans.[273] Humans acquire the infection by ingesting the eggs from contaminated soil or by eating raw animal tissue (e.g., cow liver), that is infected by the encapsulated larvae. The larvae are released in the intestines, burrow through the intestinal wall, and reach the liver via the

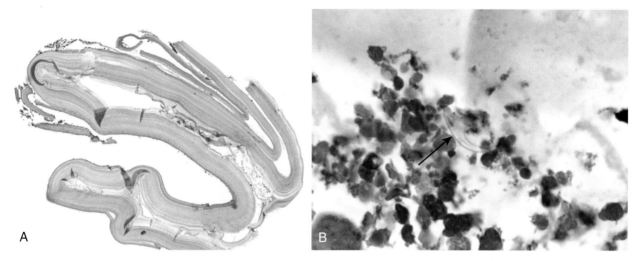

Figure 10-37. Echinococcal cyst. **A,** Collapsed cyst wall is composed of an acellular laminated cuticle. **B,** High-power view of a refractile hooklet *(arrow)* within cyst debris.

portal vein. From there, they travel to various other organs, causing eosinophilic inflammation, granulomas, and abscesses.[273] Most patients are asymptomatic but demonstrate peripheral eosinophilia. Vague abdominal pain, fever, cough, and dyspnea are occasional complaints.[273] Radiologic studies show multiple, ill-defined, oval or angular lesions that improve or resolve spontaneously, similar to *F. hepatica.* Serology is used to detect IgG to *Toxocara* antigens.

In liver biopsy specimens, multiple granulomas and confluent granulomas may be the main finding.[274,275] Grossly, the liver may show 0.3- to 1-cm, white-gray lesions, primarily in the subcapsular region of the right lobe.[276,277] These granulomatous lesions show central necrosis surrounded by a mixed inflammatory infiltrate that includes numerous eosinophils and palisaded granulomas. The central necrotic zone shows granular debris or eosinophilic material. Charcot-Leyden crystals may be seen in the areas of necrosis. Remnants of parasites are found in a minority of cases and measure 15 to 21 μm in diameter.[276] The differential diagnosis includes other causes of visceral larva migrans, including *Capillaria hepatica* and *Ascaris.*

Capillariasis

Capillaria hepatica mainly affects rodents but is also found in carnivores. The organism requires only a single host, with the liver containing both the adult parasite and its ova.[278] Eggs are deposited in soil, where, under favorable conditions, they embryonate. Ingestion of the unembryonated eggs does not result in hepatic disease but only in abdominal discomfort; in these spurious cases, eggs are passed in the stool. Ingestion of embryonated eggs results in hepatic disease and is not associated with passage of eggs in the stool.[278] Infection of humans is rare; children are more commonly affected, probably because of frequent soil-to-mouth contact.[278] Patients present with chronic fever, hepatomegaly, and peripheral eosinophilia. Liver biopsy specimens may show granulomas and eosinophils. Granulomatous lesions with central eosinophilic necrosis rimmed by palisaded histiocytes and

numerous eosinophils similar to toxocariasis may be seen.[276] Remnants of the parasite and its eggs may be identified.[278] The parasite measures 50 μm or larger in diameter.[276] The elliptical eggs are 54 to 64 μm by 29 to 33 μm and have bipolar plugs.[278]

Fascioliasis

Fasciola hepatica and *Fasciola gigantica* are trematode bile duct flukes found primarily in sheep and cattle.[270,279] The leaf-shaped worms reach a size of about 2 cm and may remain viable in the bile ducts for more than a decade. The eggs pass in feces, hatch in water, and infect lymnaeid snails.[270] Snails release a cercarial stage of the parasite that contaminates aquatic plants that are ingested by sheep, cattle, or humans. Watercress is often associated with human infection.[280] Once ingested, metacercariae penetrate the intestine, traverse the peritoneal cavity, and penetrate the liver capsule.[281] They burrow through the liver parenchyma for 1 to 3 months, while maturing, and finally enter the bile ducts to complete the life cycle.

Acute (invasive) fascioliasis manifests with fever, right upper quadrant discomfort, hepatomegaly, and eosinophilia.[279] Infrequently, patients experience respiratory, cardiac, or neurologic symptoms that are believed to be immune-allergic in origin, because the organism only rarely appears at these sites.[279] As the flukes course through the liver, they create tracks of necrosis infiltrated by eosinophils, sometimes surrounded by a reaction of palisaded histiocytes (Fig. 10-38).[280,281] These tracks appear as yellow-white subcapsular nodules or cords at laparoscopy.[280,281] As the lesions age, they become cavities bound by granulation tissue, fibrous tissue, and calcifications.[281] Immature flukes that fail to reach the liver may produce ectopic abscesses, most often in the skin.[279]

Once the flukes penetrate ducts, egg production initiates chronic (obstructive) fascioliasis, characterized by local inflammation, fibrous thickening of the duct wall, ascending cholangitis, episodic biliary pain, and obstructive jaundice.[279] Peripheral eosinophilia is mild or absent in this stage. The flukes attach to the bile duct epithelium using suckers and cause ductal epithelial proliferation, possibly due to their production of proline.[281] Large necrotic granulomas can develop around entrapped eggs, and tissue eosinophilia is typical in these lesions. Adult flukes can be found in the bile ducts or gallbladder, along with stones, hypertrophied muscle coat, and mucosal hyperplasia. Cholangiocarcinoma is not associated with fascioliasis. Diagnosis is made with serologic and antigen-identification tests or stool examination for ova, although the latter is useful only in chronic disease and may be negative if ova production is intermittent.[279]

Clonorchiasis

Clonorchis sinensis, Opisthorchis viverrini, and *Opisthorchis felineus* are similar and are usually considered together. *C. sinensis* infects persons in China and east Asia and is common among immigrants to New York City. *O. viverrini* is limited to Thailand,

Laos, Vietnam, and Cambodia, and *O. felineus* infects cats and humans in parts of Russia and eastern Europe.[282,283] These bile duct flukes are acquired through ingestion of raw fish containing the metacercariae.[282,283]

The flukes migrate into the ducts via the ampulla of Vater, where they mature in about 25 days.[282,283] The adults reside in medium-sized and small intrahepatic ducts, and occasionally in the extrahepatic ducts, gallbladder, or pancreatic duct, where they can live for a decade or longer.[282] Human hosts excrete eggs that hatch in water, pass through snails and fish, and infect other humans or animals. Patients are usually asymptomatic but may present with abdominal pain, hepatomegaly, and eosinophilia or with the syndrome of recurrent pyogenic cholangitis.

Grossly, focal dilatation of segments of smaller ducts may be seen, with thickened walls and possibly worms in the lumen. The left lobe is affected more often, because the left intrahepatic bile duct is straighter and wider, allowing easier access for the worms. Bile ducts that harbor these flukes show dilatation, irregular thickening, adenomatous epithelial hyperplasia, and variable eosinophilia (Fig. 10-39).[282] Eggs are not usually seen in tissues. Ascending cholangitis, usually from *E. coli*, can lead to purulent exudates in dilated ducts. Bile duct obstruction can result from the worms, strictures, or calculus formation.[282] Stones often have dead worms as their nidus. Diagnosis is made by identifying the ova in stool or by ultrasonography. Patients are at risk for cholangiocarcinoma, which is often intrahepatic, multicentric, and mucin-secreting. Serology does not distinguish between present and past infection. Therefore, the diagnosis of active infection may require the detection of ova in stool.[282]

Ascariasis

Ascaris lumbricoides rarely causes biliary ascariasis when the roundworms ascend the bile duct; this occurs usually in patients who live in endemic areas, have biliary abnormalities, or have undergone sphincterotomy. Although children are infected with *Ascaris* commonly, biliary involvement is rare in children, probably because of the narrow ampulla of Vater and bile duct

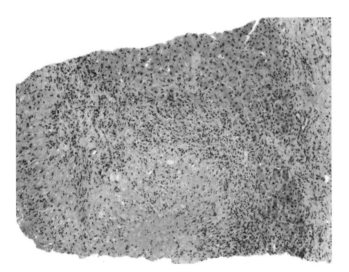

Figure 10-38. Fascioliasis. Necrotic tract is surrounded by a palisaded histiocytic reaction in a patient with *Fasciola* infestation.

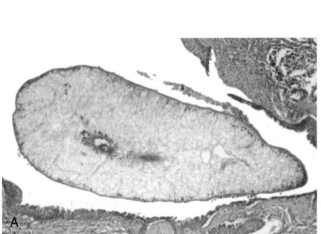

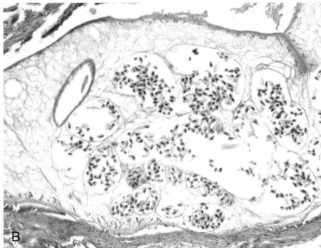

Figure 10-39. *Clonorchis* infestation. **A,** A fluke is present within a large duct that shows squamous metaplasia and periductal chronic inflammation. **B,** Higher magnification shows cross-sections of the uterus filled with ova.

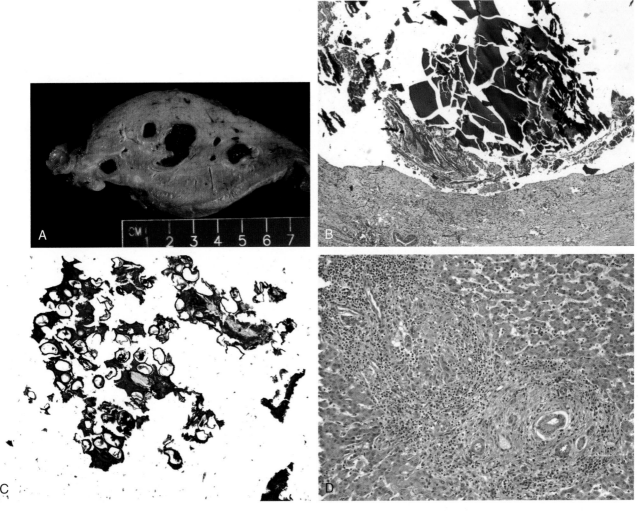

Figure 10-40. *Ascaris* infection in a patient with the clinical diagnosis of recurrent pyogenic cholangitis. **A,** Gross photograph of a section of liver shows dilated bile ducts inspissated with darkly stained sludge. **B,** On microscopic examination, the inspissated sludge is found to contain laminated, bile-stained structures suggestive of dead *Ascaris*. **C,** Focally, a collection of *Ascaris* ova is present in the sludge. **D,** Elsewhere in the liver, granulomatous inflammation was seen in the lobules adjacent to portal tracts.

lumen.[284] Bile duct infestation manifests as biliary colic, obstructive jaundice, or pancreatitis. Dying worms, in conjunction with *E. coli* and other bacteria that they transport into the liver, can cause suppurative cholangitis, liver abscesses, or the syndrome of recurrent pyogenic cholangitis (Fig. 10-40).[167] The worms can also penetrate liver tissue (visceral larva migrans), perforate Glisson's capsule, and exit into the subdiaphragmatic space.[167] The ova can cause granulomas and pseudotumors.[285] Ultrasonography can identify worms within the gallbladder or extrahepatic ducts or the presence of a dilated common bile duct.[284] Ova or adult worms can be found in stool in 91% of patients.[284] In some patients, the worms exit the ducts spontaneously; in others, anti-helminthic therapy or surgery is required.[284]

Protozoans

Amebiasis

Liver abscess is the most common extraintestinal manifestation of amebiasis. Amebic liver abscesses most likely arise from hema-

togenous spread of the trophozoites, probably via the portal circulation.[286] Often, patients with liver abscess have no bowel symptoms, and stool microscopy is negative for *Entamoeba histolytica* trophozoites and cysts.[286] Patients may present years after travel to an endemic area with fever, right upper quadrant pain, and hepatic tenderness.

The histopathologic findings in hepatic amebiasis consists of well-circumscribed regions of dead hepatocytes, liquefied cells, and cellular debris. A rim of connective tissue with few inflammatory cells and amebic trophozoites surrounds the necrotic lesion (Fig. 10-41). The adjacent hepatic parenchyma is often completely unaffected.[286] The number of trophozoites may be surprisingly small relative to the size of the abscess. The diagnosis is often made by identification of a lesion in the liver in the setting of positive amebic serology.

Malaria

The *Plasmodium* parasite has a life cycle that involves both mosquitoes and humans. When the parasite is first transmitted to a

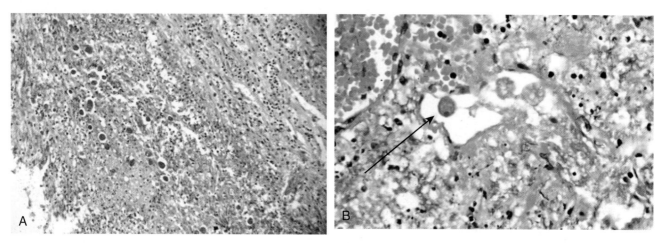

Figure 10-41. Amebic abscess in the liver. **A,** Low-power view shows the edge of an abscess cavity with inflammation and debris. **B,** High-power view of an amebic trophozoite *(arrow)* within the necrotic debris. (Courtesy of Drs. David Walker and Laura Lamps.)

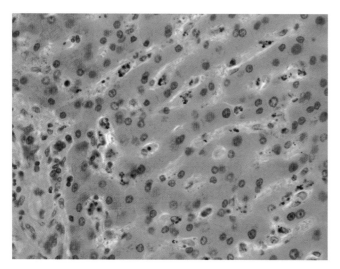

Figure 10-42. Malarial pigment within Kupffer cells.

human host, it is incapable of infecting red blood cells and must first pass through the liver. The parasite grows rapidly within hepatocytes, producing merozoites that can infect red blood cells. Through unknown mechanisms, the parasites render hepatocytes resistant to apoptotic signals.[287]

Hepatic dysfunction is well described in malaria, particularly with infection by *Plasmodium falciparum* or mixed infection with both *P. falciparum* and *Plasmodium vivax,* and usually involves mild abnormalities of liver function studies or jaundice.[288] Hepatic encephalopathy is rare. Hepatic dysfunction and jaundice may be multifactorial in etiology, including hemolysis, sequestration of infected red blood cells in sinusoids, or coexistent viral hepatitis.[288]

The histologic hallmarks of malarial hepatitis are varying degrees of hepatocyte injury and deposition of malarial pigment or hemozoin (Fig. 10-42). Inflammation is generally mild. Sinusoidal congestion and centrilobular necrosis may be caused by adherence of red blood cells in sinusoids, resulting in ischemia. Kupffer cell activation, fatty change, and cholestasis

are other common findings.[288] Exoerythrocytic forms of the parasite in liver biopsy material can be demonstrated by immunofluorescence.[289]

Leishmania

Visceral leishmaniasis, or kala-azar, is caused by an obligate intracellular protozoan, *Leishmania donovani,* that is transmitted to humans by the sandfly, *Phlebotomus argentipes.* Worldwide, India has the highest incidence of kala-azar. Children comprise the majority of patients. In southwest Europe, visceral leishmaniasis affects adults, many of whom are coinfected with HIV.[290] In this population, the majority of patients are intravenous drug users, and the organism is transmitted by the sharing of syringes.[290] Also, reactivation of latent disease may occur in immunocompromised patients years after travel to endemic areas, making the infection difficult to suspect.[291] The organisms exist as flagellated promastigotes in the gut of female sandflies and as amastigotes in animal or human hosts. In visceral leishmaniasis, an incubation period of 10 days to 1 year is followed by low-grade recurrent fevers, malaise, wasting, anemia, and hepatosplenomegaly.[292] Death follows in 2 to 3 years, commonly from secondary infections.

The accumulation of mononuclear phagocytic cells in infected tissues leads to reticuloendothelial hyperplasia affecting the liver, spleen, intestinal mucosa, bone marrow, and lymph nodes.[292] In the liver, the typical pattern consists of marked hyperplasia of Kupffer cells, many of them parasitized by numerous amastigotes (Fig. 10-43).[293] Well-formed granulomas may be seen alongside Kupffer cells with intracellular amastigotes.[292,294] Other patterns include a nodular pattern, with collections of macrophages, lymphocytes, and plasma cells within the lobules and portal tracts harboring few parasites, and a fibrogenic pattern, with perisinusoidal fibrosis that isolates small groups of liver cells with regenerative changes.[293] The differential diagnosis includes *H. capsulatum, P. marneffei,* and *Toxoplasma gondii.*[291] Fibrin ring granulomas have been reported.[227] The diagnosis depends on demonstration of the organism in tissue, typically bone marrow smears or spleen aspirates.[292] In liver tissue, demonstra-

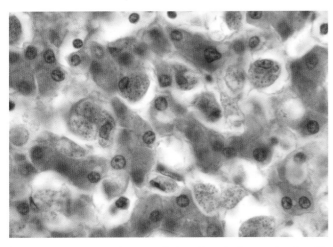

Figure 10-43. Visceral leishmaniasis (kala-azar) in the liver. In the sinusoids, Kupffer cells are filled with amastigotes.

tion of the parasites is best done with Giemsa staining, preferably of touch preparations on glass slides.[289] The presence of a kineto-plast on Giemsa stain is characteristic of *Leishmania* and distinguishes this parasite from *Histoplasma*.[289] Serologic assays are available.

Toxoplasmosis

Toxoplasma gondii is an obligate intracellular parasite usually acquired from ingestion of undercooked pork or lamb, or transplacentally. Cats are a major reservoir. Disseminated infection occurs in bone marrow and solid organ transplant recipients and in AIDS patients. Hepatitis has been reported in apparently healthy persons during acute infection; these patients present with jaundice, rash, and elevated levels of transaminases and alkaline phosphatase.[295,296]

Histologically, *Toxoplasma* hepatitis is characterized as a diffuse hepatitis with infiltration of portal tracts and sinusoids by mononuclear cells associated with focal hepatic necrosis, similar to EBV or CMV hepatitis.[295] Granulomatous hepatitis has also been described.[296] In some cases, *Toxoplasma* cysts have been identified in histiocytes and granulomas.[297] Free tachyzoites have been described within degenerating or necrotic hepatocytes, although they can be difficult to distinguish from detritus.[296] Giemsa stain or immunofluorescent stains may assist in the detection of organisms in tissue. Serologic assay for IgM antibodies to *T. gondii* can be used to establish the diagnosis.

Cryptosporidiosis

Cryptosporidium is a protozoan that causes an opportunistic infection of the gastrointestinal tract resulting in diarrhea. In patients with AIDS, the organism has been known to infect the biliary tree, producing a syndrome similar to primary sclerosing cholangitis.[96] Signs and symptoms include right upper quadrant abdominal pain, nausea, vomiting, fever, and biochemical evidence of anicteric cholestasis.[96] Dilatation of the common bile duct is often seen on ultrasonography or computed tomography

scanning, and cholangiography reveals attenuation and pruning of duct branches, stricturing and beading of the proximal intrahepatic bile ducts, and dilatation or stricturing of the extrahepatic duct.[96] The histologic picture reflects the intense periductal inflammatory response elicited by the organism, with portal edema, inflammation, and hyperplastic periductal glands. The biliary epithelium may be reactive or frankly necrotic. Organisms can be detected on the luminal surface of the epithelial lining of small biliary radicles, peribiliary glands, the pancreatic duct, and the gallbladder.[96] Concomitant CMV infection may be found.

REFERENCES

1. Martin A, Lemon SM: Hepatitis A virus: From discovery to vaccines. Hepatology 2006;43:S164-S172.
2. Leach CT: Hepatitis A in the United States. Pediatr Infect Dis J 2004;23:551-552.
3. Skoog SM, Rivard RE, Batts KP, et al: Autoimmune hepatitis preceded by acute hepatitis A infection. Am J Gastroenterol 2002;97:1568-1569.
4. Huppertz HI, Treichel U, Gassel AM, et al: Autoimmune hepatitis following hepatitis A virus infection. J Hepatol 1995;23:204-208.
5. Hilzenrat N, Zilberman D, Klein T, et al: Autoimmune hepatitis in a genetically susceptible patient: Is it triggered by acute viral hepatitis A? Dig Dis Sci 1999;44:1950-1952.
6. Vento S, Garofano T, Di Perri G, et al: Identification of hepatitis A virus as a trigger for autoimmune chronic hepatitis type 1 in susceptible individuals. Lancet 1991;337:1183-1187.
7. Goldin RD: Viral hepatitis. Curr Diagn Pathol 1994;1:70-76.
8. Ruel M, Sevestre H, Henry-Biabaud E, et al: Fibrin ring granulomas in hepatitis A. Dig Dis Sci 1992;37:1915-1917.
9. Ponz E, Garcia-Pagan JC, Bruguera M, et al: Hepatic fibrin-ring granulomas in a patient with hepatitis A. Gastroenterology 1991;100:268-270.
10. Pungpapong S, Kim WR, Poterucha JJ: Natural history of hepatitis B virus infection: An update for clinicians. Mayo Clin Proc 2007;82:967-975.
11. Lai CL, Ratziu V, Yuen MF, et al: Viral hepatitis B. Lancet 2003;362:2089-2094.
12. Hunt CM, McGill JM, Allen MI, et al: Clinical relevance of hepatitis B viral mutations. Hepatology 2000;31:1037-1044.
13. Akuta N, Kumada H: Influence of hepatitis B virus genotypes on the response to antiviral therapies. J Antimicrob Chemother 2005;55:139-142.
14. Trepo C, Guillevin L: Polyarteritis nodosa and extrahepatic manifestations of HBV infection: The case against autoimmune intervention in pathogenesis. J Autoimmun 2001;16:269-274.
15. Fattovich G, Bortolotti F, Donato F: Natural history of chronic hepatitis B: Special emphasis on disease progression and prognostic factors. J Hepatol 2008;48:335-352.
16. Hsu YS, Chien RN, Yeh CT, et al: Long-term outcome after spontaneous HBeAg seroconversion in patients with chronic hepatitis B. Hepatology 2002;35:1522-1527.
17. Ishak KG: Chronic hepatitis: Morphology and nomenclature. Mod Pathol 1994;7:690-713.
18. Naoumov NV, Portmann BC, Tedder RS, et al: Detection of hepatitis B virus antigens in liver tissue: A relation to viral replication and histology in chronic hepatitis B infection. Gastroenterology 1990;99:1248-1253.
19. Hsu HC, Lai MY, Su IJ, et al: Correlation of hepatocyte HBsAg expression with virus replication and liver pathology. Hepatology 1988;8:749-754.
20. Thomson EC, Main J: Advances in hepatitis B and C. Curr Opin Infect Dis 2004;17:449-459.

21. Walker N, Apel R, Kerlin P, et al: Hepatitis B virus infection in liver allografts. Am J Surg Pathol 1993;17:666-677.

22. Harrison RF, Davies MH, Goldin RD, et al: Recurrent hepatitis B in liver allografts: A distinctive form of rapidly developing cirrhosis. Histopathology 1993;23:21-28.

23. Davies SE, Portmann BC, O'Grady JG, et al: Hepatic histological findings after transplantation for chronic hepatitis B virus infection, including a unique pattern of fibrosing cholestatic hepatitis. Hepatology 1991;13:150-157.

24. Benner KG, Lee RG, Keeffe EB, et al: Fibrosing cytolytic liver failure secondary to recurrent hepatitis B after liver transplantation. Gastroenterology 1992;103:1307-1312.

25. Fang JW, Wright TL, Lau JY: Fibrosing cholestatic hepatitis in patient with HIV and hepatitis B. Lancet 1993;342:1175.

26. McIvor C, Morton J, Bryant A, et al: Fatal reactivation of precore mutant hepatitis B virus associated with fibrosing cholestatic hepatitis after bone marrow transplantation. Ann Intern Med 1994;121:274-275.

27. Sulkowski MS: Viral hepatitis and HIV coinfection. J Hepatol 2008;48:353-367.

28. Thimme R, Spangenberg HC, Blum HE: Hepatitis B or hepatitis C and human immunodeficiency virus infection. J Hepatol 2005;42(Suppl):S37-S44.

29. Wong T, Lee SS: Hepatitis C: A review for primary care physicians. CMAJ Can Med Assoc J 2006;174:649-659.

30. Giannini C, Brechot C: Hepatitis C virus biology. Cell Death Differ 2003;10(Suppl 1):S27-S38.

31. Orland JR, Wright TL, Cooper S: Acute hepatitis C. Hepatology 2001;33:321-327.

32. Zein NN: Clinical significance of hepatitis C virus genotypes. Clin Microbiol Rev 2000;13:223-235.

33. Mondelli MU, Silini E: Clinical significance of hepatitis C virus genotypes. J Hepatol 1999;31(Suppl 1):65-70.

34. Hatzakis A, Katsoulidou A, Kaklamani E, et al: Hepatitis C virus 1b is the dominant genotype in HCV-related carcinogenesis: A case-control study. Int J Cancer 1996;68:51-53.

35. Marcellin P: Hepatitis C: The clinical spectrum of the disease. J Hepatol 1999;31(Suppl 1):9-16.

36. Mondelli MU, Cerino A, Cividini A: Acute hepatitis C: Diagnosis and management. J Hepatol 2005;42(Suppl):S108-S114.

37. Chung RT: Acute hepatitis C virus infection. Clin Infect Dis 2005;41(Suppl 1):S14-S17.

38. Caruntu FA, Benea L: Acute hepatitis C virus infection: Diagnosis, pathogenesis, treatment. J Gastrointestin Liver Dis 2006;15:249-256.

39. Gerlach JT, Diepolder HM, Zachoval R, et al: Acute hepatitis C: High rate of both spontaneous and treatment-induced viral clearance. Gastroenterology 2003;125:80-88.

40. Obermayer-Straub P, Manns MP: Hepatitis C and D, retroviruses and autoimmune manifestations. J Autoimmun 2001;16:275-285.

41. Cassani F, Cataleta M, Valentini P, et al: Serum autoantibodies in chronic hepatitis C: Comparison with autoimmune hepatitis and impact on the disease profile. Hepatology 1997;26:561-566.

42. Scheuer PJ, Ashrafzadeh P, Sherlock S, et al: The pathology of hepatitis C. Hepatology 1992;15:567-571.

43. Negro F: Hepatitis C virus and liver steatosis: When fat is not beautiful. J Hepatol 2004;40:533-535.

44. Castera L, Chouteau P, Hezode C, et al: Hepatitis C virus-induced hepatocellular steatosis. Am J Gastroenterol 2005;100:711-715.

45. Gaya DR, Thorburn D, Oien KA, et al: Hepatic granulomas: A 10 year single centre experience. J Clin Pathol 2003;56:850-853.

46. Emile JF, Sebagh M, Feray C, et al: The presence of epithelioid granulomas in hepatitis C virus-related cirrhosis. Hum Pathol 1993;24:1095-1097.

47. Goldin RD, Levine TS, Foster GR, et al: Granulomas and hepatitis C. Histopathology 1996;28:265-257.

48. Harada K, Minato H, Hiramatsu K, et al: Epithelioid cell granulomas in chronic hepatitis C: Immunohistochemical character and histological marker of favourable response to interferon-alpha therapy. Histopathology 1998;33:216-221.

49. Veerabagu MP, Finkelstein SD, Rabinovitz M: Granulomatous hepatitis in a patient with chronic hepatitis C treated with interferon-alpha. Dig Dis Sci 1997;42:1445-1448.

50. Propst A, Propst T, Dietze O, et al: Development of granulomatous hepatitis during treatment with interferon-alpha 2b. Dig Dis Sci 1995;40:2117-2118.

51. Mert A, Tabak F, Ozaras R, et al: Hepatic granulomas in chronic hepatitis C. J Clin Gastroenterol 2001;33:342-343.

52. Greenson JK, Svoboda-Newman SM, Merion RM, et al: Histologic progression of recurrent hepatitis C in liver transplant allografts. Am J Surg Pathol 1996;20:731-738.

53. Schluger LK, Sheiner PA, Thung SN, et al: Severe recurrent cholestatic hepatitis C following orthotopic liver transplantation. Hepatology 1996;23:971-976.

54. Rosenberg PM, Farrell JJ, Abraczinskas DR, et al: Rapidly progressive fibrosing cholestatic hepatitis: Hepatitis C virus in HIV coinfection. Am J Gastroenterol 2002;97:478-483.

55. Lim HL, Lau GK, Davis GL, et al: Cholestatic hepatitis leading to hepatic failure in a patient with organ-transmitted hepatitis C virus infection. Gastroenterology 1994;106:248-251.

56. Zylberberg H, Carnot F, Mamzer MF, et al: Hepatitis C virus-related fibrosing cholestatic hepatitis after renal transplantation. Transplantation 1997;63:158-160.

57. Toth CM, Pascual M, Chung RT, et al: Hepatitis C virus-associated fibrosing cholestatic hepatitis after renal transplantation: Response to interferon-alpha therapy. Transplantation 1998;66:1254-1258.

58. Makris M, Preston FE, Rosendaal FR, et al: The natural history of chronic hepatitis C in haemophiliacs. Br J Haematol 1996;94:746-752.

59. Hanley JP, Jarvis LM, Andrews J, et al: Investigation of chronic hepatitis C infection in individuals with haemophilia: Assessment of invasive and non-invasive methods. Br J Haematol 1996;94:159-165.

60. McFarlane BM, Bridger CB, Smith HM, et al: Autoimmune mechanisms in chronic hepatitis B and delta virus infections. Eur J Gastroenterol Hepatol 1995;7:615-621.

61. Emerson SU, Purcell RH: Hepatitis E. Pediatr Infect Dis J 2007;26:1147-1148.

62. Wang L, Zhuang H: Hepatitis E: An overview and recent advances in vaccine research. World J Gastroenterol 2004;10:2157-2162.

63. Vento S, Guella L, Mirandola F, et al: Epstein-Barr virus as a trigger for autoimmune hepatitis in susceptible individuals. Lancet 1995;346:608-609.

64. Kimura H, Nagasaka T, Hoshino Y, et al: Severe hepatitis caused by Epstein-Barr virus without infection of hepatocytes. Hum Pathol 2001;32:757-762.

65. Sanchez F, Gimeno-Bayon JL, Esgueva R, et al: Fatal liver failure: Molecular evidence for chronic active Epstein-Barr virus infection. Ann Diagn Pathol 2008;12:368-371.

66. White NJ, Juel-Jensen BE: Infectious mononucleosis hepatitis. Semin Liver Dis 1984;4:301-306.

67. Feranchak AP, Tyson RW, Narkewicz MR, et al: Fulminant Epstein-Barr viral hepatitis: Orthotopic liver transplantation and review of the literature. Liver Transpl Surg 1998;4:469-476.

68. Alshak NS, Jiminez AM, Gedebou M, et al: Epstein-Barr virus infection in liver transplantation patients: Correlation of histopathology and semiquantitative Epstein-Barr virus-DNA recovery using polymerase chain reaction. Hum Pathol 1993;24:1306-1312.

69. Biest S, Schubert TT: Chronic Epstein-Barr virus infection: A cause of granulomatous hepatitis? J Clin Gastroenterol 1989;11:343-346.

70. Nenert M, Mavier P, Dubuc N, et al: Epstein-Barr virus infection and hepatic fibrin-ring granulomas. Hum Pathol 1988;19:608-610.

71. Suh N, Liapis H, Misdraji J, et al: Epstein-Barr virus hepatitis: Diagnostic value of in situ hybridization, polymerase chain reaction, and immunohistochemistry on liver biopsy from immunocompetent patients. Am J Surg Pathol 2007;31:1403-1409.

72. Washington K: Update on post-liver transplantation infections, malignancies, and surgical complications. Adv Anat Pathol 2005;12:221-226.

73. Bonkowsky HL, Lee RV, Klatskin G: Acute granulomatous hepatitis: Occurrence in cytomegalovirus mononucleosis. JAMA 1975;233:1284-1288.

74. Clarke J, Craig RM, Saffro R, et al: Cytomegalovirus granulomatous hepatitis. Am J Med 1979;66:264-269.

75. Lobdell DH: "Ring" granulomas in cytomegalovirus hepatitis. Arch Pathol Lab Med 1987;111:881-882.

76. Goodman ZD, Ishak KG, Sesterhenn IA: Herpes simplex hepatitis in apparently immunocompetent adults. Am J Clin Pathol 1986;85:694-699.

77. Krilov LR, Rubin LG, Frogel M, et al: Disseminated adenovirus infection with hepatic necrosis in patients with human immunodeficiency virus infection and other immunodeficiency states. Rev Infect Dis 1990;12:303-307.

78. Janner D, Petru AM, Belchis D, et al: Fatal adenovirus infection in a child with acquired immunodeficiency syndrome. Pediatr Infect Dis J 1990;9:434-436.

79. Sokal EM, Melchior M, Cornu C, et al: Acute parvovirus B19 infection associated with fulminant hepatitis of favourable prognosis in young children. Lancet 1998;352:1739-1741.

80. Langnas AN, Markin RS, Cattral MS, et al: Parvovirus B19 as a possible causative agent of fulminant liver failure and associated aplastic anemia. Hepatology 1995;22:1661-1665.

81. Yoto Y, Kudoh T, Haseyama K, et al: Human parvovirus B19 infection associated with acute hepatitis. Lancet 1996;347:868-869.

82. Lee WM, Brown KE, Young NS, et al: Brief report: No evidence for parvovirus B19 or hepatitis E virus as a cause of acute liver failure. Dig Dis Sci 2006;51:1712-1715.

83. Wong S, Young NS, Brown KE: Prevalence of parvovirus B19 in liver tissue: No association with fulminant hepatitis or hepatitis-associated aplastic anemia. J Infect Dis 2003;187:1581-1586.

84. Tameda Y, Kosaka Y, Shiraki K, et al: Hepatitis in an adult with rubella. Intern Med 1993;32:580-583.

85. Onji M, Kumon I, Kanaoka M, et al: Intrahepatic lymphocyte subpopulations in acute hepatitis in an adult with rubella. Am J Gastroenterol 1988;83:320-322.

86. McLellan RK, Gleiner JA: Acute hepatitis in an adult with rubeola. JAMA 1982;247:2000-2001.

87. Cheeseman SH, Cleveland RH, Mark EJ: Case records of the Massachusetts General Hospital: Weekly clinicopathological exercises. Case 34-1988: Progressive pulmonary consolidations in a 10-year-old boy with Evans' syndrome. N Engl J Med 1988;319:495-509.

88. Chau TN, Lee KC, Yao H, et al: SARS-associated viral hepatitis caused by a novel coronavirus: Report of three cases. Hepatology 2004;39:302-310.

89. Boag FC, Dean R, Hawkins DA, et al: Abnormalities of liver function during HIV seroconversion illness. Int J STD AIDS 1992;3:46-48.

90. Molina JM, Welker Y, Ferchal F, et al: Hepatitis associated with primary HIV infection. Gastroenterology 1992;102:739.

91. Steeper TA, Rosenstein H, Weiser J, et al: Bacillary epithelioid angiomatosis involving the liver, spleen, and skin in an AIDS patient with concurrent Kaposi's sarcoma. Am J Clin Pathol 1992;97:713-718.

92. Perkocha LA, Geaghan SM, Yen TS, et al: Clinical and pathological features of bacillary peliosis hepatis in association with human immunodeficiency virus infection. N Engl J Med 1990;323:1581-1586.

93. Jagadha V, Andavolu RH, Huang CT: Granulomatous inflammation in the acquired immune deficiency syndrome. Am J Clin Pathol 1985;84:598-602.

94. Terada S, Reddy KR, Jeffers LJ, et al: Microsporidan hepatitis in the acquired immunodeficiency syndrome. Ann Intern Med 1987;107:61-62.

95. Beaugerie L, Teilhac MF, Deluol AM, et al: Cholangiopathy associated with Microsporidia infection of the common bile duct mucosa in a patient with HIV infection. Ann Intern Med 1992;117:401-402.

96. Teixidor HS, Godwin TA, Ramirez EA: Cryptosporidiosis of the biliary tract in AIDS. Radiology 1991;180:51-56.

97. Pol S, Romana CA, Richard S, et al: Microsporidia infection in patients with the human immunodeficiency virus and unexplained cholangitis. N Engl J Med 1993;328:95-99.

98. Cello JP: Acquired immunodeficiency syndrome cholangiopathy: Spectrum of disease. Am J Med 1989;86:539-546.

99. Forbes A, Blanshard C, Gazzard B: Natural history of AIDS related sclerosing cholangitis: A study of 20 cases. Gut 1993;34:116-121.

100. Hasan FA, Jeffers LJ, Welsh SW, et al: Hepatic involvement as the primary manifestation of Kaposi's sarcoma in the acquired immune deficiency syndrome, Am J Gastroenterol 1989;84:1449-1451.

101. O'Leary JG, Zachary K, Misdraji J, et al: De novo autoimmune hepatitis during immune reconstitution in an HIV-infected patient receiving highly active antiretroviral therapy. Clin Infect Dis 2008;46:e12-e14.

102. Howard CR, Ellis DS, Simpson DI: Exotic viruses and the liver. Semin Liver Dis 1984;4:361-374.

103. Quaresma JA, Duarte MI, Vasconcelos PF: Midzonal lesions in yellow fever: A specific pattern of liver injury caused by direct virus action and in situ inflammatory response. Med Hypotheses 2006;67:618-621.

104. Francis TI, Moore DL, Edington GM, et al: A clinicopathological study of human yellow fever. Bull World Health Organ 1972;46:659-667.

105. Monath TP, Barrett AD: Pathogenesis and pathophysiology of yellow fever. Adv Virus Res 2003;60:343-395.

106. Ishak KG, Walker DH, Coetzer JA, et al: Viral hemorrhagic fevers with hepatic involvement: Pathologic aspects with clinical correlations. Prog Liver Dis 1982;7:495-515.

107. Malavige GN, Fernando S, Fernando DJ, et al: Dengue viral infections. Postgrad Med J 2004;80:588-601.

108. de Macedo FC, Nicol AF, Cooper LD, et al: Histologic, viral, and molecular correlates of dengue fever infection of the liver using highly sensitive immunohistochemistry. Diagn Mol Pathol 2006;15:223-228.

109. Huerre MR, Lan NT, Marianneau P, et al: Liver histopathology and biological correlates in five cases of fatal dengue fever in Vietnamese children. Virchows Archiv 2001;438:107-115.

110. Walker DH, McCormick JB, Johnson KM, et al: Pathologic and virologic study of fatal Lassa fever in man. Am J Pathol 1982;107:349-356.

111. Alvarez SZ: Hepatobiliary tuberculosis. J Gastroenterol Hepatol 1998;13:833-839.

112. Chong VH: Hepatobiliary tuberculosis: A review of presentations and outcomes. South Med J 2008;101:356-361.

113. Huang WT, Wang CC, Chen WJ, et al: The nodular form of hepatic tuberculosis: A review with five additional new cases. J Clin Pathol 2003;56:835-839.

114. Essop AR, Posen JA, Hodkinson JH, et al: Tuberculosis hepatitis: A clinical review of 96 cases. Q J Med 1984;53:465-477.

115. Harrington PT, Gutierrez JJ, Ramirez-Ronda CH, et al: Granulomatous hepatitis. Rev Infect Dis 1982;4:638-655.

116. Maharaj B, Leary WP, Pudifin DJ: A prospective study of hepatic tuberculosis in 41 black patients. Q J Med 1987;63:517-522.

117. Wang JY, Hsueh PR, Wang SK, et al: Disseminated tuberculosis: A 10-year experience in a medical center. Medicine (Baltimore) 2007;86:39-46.

118. Maglinte DD, Alvarez SZ, Ng AC, et al: Patterns of calcifications and cholangiographic findings in hepatobiliary tuberculosis. Gastrointest Radiol 1988;13:331-335.

119. Alcantara-Payawal DE, Matsumura M, Shiratori Y, et al: Direct detection of *Mycobacterium tuberculosis* using polymerase chain reaction assay among patients with hepatic granuloma. J Hepatol 1997;27:620-627.

120. Diaz ML, Herrera T, Lopez-Vidal Y, et al: Polymerase chain reaction for the detection of *Mycobacterium tuberculosis* DNA in tissue and assessment of its utility in the diagnosis of hepatic granulomas. J Lab Clin Med 1996;127:359-363.

121. Orenstein MS, Tavitian A, Yonk B, et al: Granulomatous involvement of the liver in patients with AIDS. Gut 1985;26:1220-1225.

122. Hickey N, McNulty JG, Osborne H, et al: Acute hepatobiliary tuberculosis: A report of two cases and a review of the literature. Eur Radiol 1999;9:886-889.

123. Kahn SA, Saltzman BR, Klein RS, et al: Hepatic disorders in the acquired immune deficiency syndrome: A clinical and pathological study. Am J Gastroenterol 1986;81:1145-1148.

124. Farhi DC, Mason UG 3rd, Horsburgh CR Jr: Pathologic findings in disseminated *Mycobacterium avium-intracellulare* infection: A report of 11 cases. Am J Clin Pathol 1986;85:67-72.

125. Chen TS, Drutz DJ, Whelan GE: Hepatic granulomas in leprosy: Their relation to bacteremia. Arch Pathol Lab Med 1976;100:182-185.

126. Ferrari TC, Araujo MG, Ribeiro MM: Hepatic involvement in lepromatous leprosy. Lepr Rev 2002;73:72-75.

127. Bodurtha A, Kim YH, Laucius JF, et al: Hepatic granulomas and other hepatic lesions associated with BCG immunotherapy for cancer. Am J Clin Pathol 1974;61:747-752.

128. Hunt JS, Silverstein MJ, Sparks FC, et al: Granulomatous hepatitis: A complication of B.C.G. immunotherapy. Lancet 1973;2:820-821.

129. Lamm DL, van der Meijden PM, Morales A, et al: Incidence and treatment of complications of bacillus Calmette-Guerin intravesical therapy in superficial bladder cancer. J Urol 1992;147:596-600.

130. Barza MJ, Blum JH, Graeme-Cook FM: Case records of the Massachusetts General Hospital: Weekly clinicopathological exercises. Case 29-1998: A 57-year-old man with fever and jaundice after intravesical instillation of bacille Calmette-Guerin for bladder cancer. N Engl J Med 1998;339:831-837.

131. Schattner A, Gilad A, Cohen J: Systemic granulomatosis and hypercalcaemia following intravesical bacillus Calmette-Guerin immunotherapy. J Intern Med 2002;251:272-277.

132. Proctor DD, Chopra S, Rubenstein SC, et al: Mycobacteremia and granulomatous hepatitis following initial intravesical bacillus Calmette-Guerin instillation for bladder carcinoma. Am J Gastroenterol 1993;88:1112-1115.

133. Leebeek FW, Ouwendijk RJ, Kolk AH, et al: Granulomatous hepatitis caused by bacillus Calmette-Guerin (BCG) infection after BCG bladder instillation. Gut 1996;38:616-618.

134. Saint-Marc Girardin MF, Zafrani ES, Chaumette MT, et al: Hepatic granulomas in Whipple's disease. Gastroenterology 1984;86:753-756.

135. Chateil JF, Brun M, Perel Y, et al: Granulomatous hepatitis in *Pasteurella multocida* infection. Eur Radiol 1998;8:588-591.

136. Stjernberg U, Silseth C, Ritland S: Granulomatous hepatitis in *Yersinia enterocolitica* infection. Hepatogastroenterology 1987;34:56-57.

137. Muorah M, Hinds R, Verma A, et al: Liver abscesses in children: A single center experience in the developed world. J Pediatr Gastroenterol Nutr 2006;42:201-206.

138. Rahimian J, Wilson T, Oram V, et al: Pyogenic liver abscess: Recent trends in etiology and mortality. Clin Infect Dis 2004;39:1654-1659.

139. Ruiz-Hernandez JJ, Leon-Mazorra M, Conde-Martel A, et al: Pyogenic liver abscesses: Mortality-related factors. Eur J Gastroenterol Hepatol 2007;19:853-858.

140. Chan KS, Yu WL, Tsai CL, et al: Pyogenic liver abscess caused by *Klebsiella pneumoniae*: Analysis of the clinical characteristics and outcomes of 84 patients. Chin Med J (Engl) 2007;120:136-139.

141. Thomsen RW, Jepsen P, Sorensen HT: Diabetes mellitus and pyogenic liver abscess: Risk and prognosis. Clin Infect Dis 2007;44:1194-1201.

142. Chen W, Chen CH, Chiu KL, et al: Clinical outcome and prognostic factors of patients with pyogenic liver abscess requiring intensive care. Crit Care Med 2008;36:1184-1188.

143. Chong VH, Yong AM, Wahab AY: Gas-forming pyogenic liver abscess. Singapore Med J 2008;49:e123-e125.

144. Vadillo M, Corbella X, Pac V, et al: Multiple liver abscesses due to *Yersinia enterocolitica* discloses primary hemochromatosis: Three cases reports and review. Clin Infect Dis 1994;18:938-941.

145. Farrer W, Kloser P, Ketyer S: *Yersinia pseudotuberculosis* sepsis presenting as multiple liver abscesses. Am J Med Sci 1988;295:129-132.

146. Santoro MJ, Chen YK, Seid NS, et al: *Yersinia enterocolitica* liver abscesses unmasking idiopathic hemochromatosis. J Clin Gastroenterol 1994;18:253-254.

147. Bergmann TK, Vinding K, Hey H: Multiple hepatic abscesses due to *Yersinia enterocolitica* infection secondary to primary haemochromatosis. Scand J Gastroenterol 2001;36:891-895.

148. Sabbaj J: Anaerobes in liver abscess. Rev Infect Dis 1984;6(Suppl 1):S152-S156.

149. Brook I, Fraizer EH: Role of anaerobic bacteria in liver abscesses in children. Pediatr Infect Dis J 1993;12:743-747.

150. Kazmi KA, Rab SM: Primary hepatic actinomycosis: A diagnostic problem. Am J Trop Med Hygiene 1980;40:310-311.

151. Christodoulou N, Papadakis I, Velegrakis M: Actinomycotic liver abscess: Case report and review of the literature. Chir Ital 2004;56:141-146.

152. Hilfiker ML: Disseminated actinomycosis presenting as a renal tumor with metastases. J Pediatr Surg 2001;36:1577-1578.

153. Sharma M, Briski LE, Khatib R: Hepatic actinomycosis: An overview of salient features and outcome of therapy. Scand J Infect Dis 2002;34:386-391.

154. Lamps LW, Havens JM, Sjostedt A, et al: Histologic and molecular diagnosis of tularemia: A potential bioterrorism agent endemic to North America. Mod Pathol 2004;17:489-495.

155. Apisarnthanarak A, Apisarnthanarak P, Mundy LM: Computed tomography characteristics of *Burkholderia pseudomallei* liver abscess. Clin Infect Dis 2006;42:989-993.

156. White NJ: Melioidosis. Lancet 2003;361:1715-1722.

157. Braun TI, Travis D, Dee RR, et al: Liver abscess due to *Listeria monocytogenes*: Case report and review. Clin Infect Dis 1993;17:267-269.

158. Rieder J, Lechner M, Lass-Floerl C, et al: Successful management of *Aspergillus* liver abscess in a patient with necrotizing fasciitis. Dig Dis Sci 2007;52:1548-1553.

159. Fang CT, Lai SY, Yi WC, et al: *Klebsiella pneumoniae* genotype K1: An emerging pathogen that causes septic ocular or central nervous system complications from pyogenic liver abscess. Clin Infect Dis 2007;45:284-292007.

160. Tan YM, Chee SP, Soo KC, et al: Ocular manifestations and complications of pyogenic liver abscess. World J Surg 2004;28:38-42.

161. Sinanan MN: Acute cholangitis. Infect Dis Clin North Am 1992;6:571-599.

162. Charcot JM: Leçons Sur Les Maladies du Foi des Voies Fliares et des Rins. Paris, Faculté de Médicine de Paris, 1877.

163. Reynolds BM, Dargan EL: Acute obstructive cholangitis: A distinct clinical syndrome. Ann Surg 1959;150:299-303.

164. O'Connor MJ, Schwartz ML, McQuarrie DG, et al: Acute bacterial cholangitis: An analysis of clinical manifestation. Arch Surg 1982;117:437-441.

165. Mukaiya M, Hirata K, Katsuramaki T, et al: Isolated bacteria and susceptibilities to antimicrobial agents in biliary infections. Hepatogastroenterology 2005;52:686-690.

166. Qureshi WA: Approach to the patient who has suspected acute bacterial cholangitis. Gastroenterol Clin North Am 2006;35:409-423.

167. Carpenter HA: Bacterial and parasitic cholangitis. Mayo Clin Proc 1998;73:473-478.

168. Shimada H, Nihmoto S, Matsuba A, et al: Acute cholangitis: A histopathologic study. J Clin Gastroenterol 1988;10:197-200.

169. Lim JH: Oriental cholangiohepatitis: Pathologic, clinical, and radiologic features. AJR Am J Roentgenol 1991;157:1-8.

170. Chung RT, Varghese JC, Sheffer EC: Case records of the Massachusetts General Hospital: Weekly clinicopathological exercises. Case 28-2001: A 44-year-old woman with chills, fever, jaundice, and hepatic abscesses. N Engl J Med 2001;345:817-823.

171. Williams RK, Crossley K: Acute and chronic hepatic involvement of brucellosis. Gastroenterology 1982;83:455-458.

172. Hunt AC, Bothwell PW: Histological findings in human brucellosis. J Clin Pathol 1967;20:267-272.

173. Spink WW, Hoffbauer FW: Histopathology of the liver in human brucellosis. J Lab Clin Med 1949;34:40-58.

174. Akritidis N, Tzivras M, Delladetsima I, et al: The liver in brucellosis. Clinical Gastroenterol Hepatol 2007;5:1109-1112.

175. Jordans HG, DeBruin KD: Granulomas in *Brucella melitensis* infection. Ann Intern Med 1980;92:264-265.

176. Ledro D, Llamas R, Herrerias JM, et al: The presence of granulomas due to *Brucella melitensis* in hepatitis. J Infect Dis 1983;147:606-607.

177. Bruguera M, Cervantes F: Hepatic granulomas in brucellosis. Ann Intern Med 1980;92:571-572.

178. Fernandez Guerrero ML, Diaz Curiel M, Cortes Cansino JM: Hepatic granulomas in brucellosis. Ann Intern Med 1980;92:572.

179. Young EJ: *Brucella melitensis* hepatitis: The absence of granulomas. Ann Intern Med 1979;91:414-415.

180. Villar JM, Garrote D, Villegas MT, et al: Hepatic brucelloma. J Am Coll Surg 2002;194:86.

181. Ariza J, Pigrau C, Canas C, et al: Current understanding and management of chronic hepatosplenic suppurative brucellosis. Clin Infect Dis 2001;32:1024-1033.

182. Arisoy ES, Correa AG, Wagner ML, et al: Hepatosplenic cat-scratch disease in children: Selected clinical features and treatment. Clin Infect Dis 1999;28:778-784.

183. Lamps LW, Gray GF, Scott MA: The histologic spectrum of hepatic cat scratch disease: A series of six cases with confirmed *Bartonella henselae* infection. Am J Surg Pathol 1996;20:1253-1259.

184. Lenoir AA, Storch GA, DeSchryver-Kecskemeti K, et al: Granulomatous hepatitis associated with cat scratch disease. Lancet 1988;1:1132-1136.

185. Ventura A, Massei F, Not T, et al: Systemic *Bartonella henselae* infection with hepatosplenic involvement. J Pediatric Gastroenterol Nutr 1999;29:52-56.

186. Malatack JJ, Jaffe R: Granulomatous hepatitis in three children due to cat-scratch disease without peripheral adenopathy: An unrecognized cause of fever of unknown origin. Am J Dis Child 1993;147:949-953.

187. Liston TE, Koehler JE: Granulomatous hepatitis and necrotizing splenitis due to *Bartonella henselae* in a patient with cancer: Case report and review of hepatosplenic manifestations of bartonella infection. Clin Infect Dis 1996;22:951-957.

188. Connor BA, Schwartz E: Typhoid and paratyphoid fever in travellers. Lancet Infect Dis 2005;5:623-628.

189. Parry CM, Hien TT, Dougan G, et al: Typhoid fever. N Engl J Med 2002;347:1770-1782.

190. Rubin EJ, Graeme-Cook FM: Case records of the Massachusetts General Hospital: Weekly clinicopathological exercises. Case 22-2001: A 25-year-old woman with fever and abnormal liver function. N Engl J Med 2001;345:201-205.

191. Sorabjee JS: The liver in enteric fever and leptospirosis. Indian J Gastroenterol 2001;20(Suppl 1):C44-C46.

192. Pais P: A hepatitis like picture in typhoid fever. Br Med J Clin Res Ed 1984;289:225-226.

193. Zaidi SA, Singer C: Gastrointestinal and hepatic manifestations of tickborne diseases in the United States. Clin Infect Dis 2002;34:1206-1212.

194. Lamps LW: Hepatic granulomas, with an emphasis on infectious causes. Adv Anat Pathol 2008;15:309-318.

195. Currie BJ: Melioidosis: An important cause of pneumonia in residents of and travellers returned from endemic regions. Eur Respir J 2003;22:542-550.

196. Piggott JA, Hochholzer L: Human melioidosis: A histopathologic study of acute and chronic melioidosis. Arch Pathol Lab Med 1970;90:101-111.

197. Scholing M, Schneeberger PM, van den Dries P, et al: Clinical features of liver involvement in adult patients with listeriosis: Review of the literature. Infection 2007;35:212-218.

198. De Vega T, Echevarria S, Crespo J, et al: Acute hepatitis by *Listeria monocytogenes* in an HIV patient with chronic HBV hepatitis. J Clin Gastroenterol 1992;15:251-255.

199. Keisler DS Jr, Starke W, Looney DJ, et al: Early syphilis with liver involvement. JAMA 1982;247:1999-2000.

200. Campisi D, Whitcomb C: Liver disease in early syphilis. Arch Intern Med 1979;139:365-366.

201. Baker AL, Kaplan MM, Wolfe HJ, et al: Liver disease associated with early syphilis. N Engl J Med 1971;284:1422-1423.

202. Ridruejo E, Mordoh A, Herrera F, et al: Severe cholestatic hepatitis as the first symptom of secondary syphilis. Dig Dis Sci 2004;49:1401-1404.

203. Ozaki T, Takemoto K, Hosono H, et al: Secondary syphilitic hepatitis in a fourteen-year-old male youth. Pediatr Infect Dis J 2002;21:439-441.

204. Mullick CJ, Liappis AP, Benator DA, et al: Syphilitic hepatitis in HIV-infected patients: A report of 7 cases and review of the literature. Clin Infect Dis 2004;39:e100-e105.

205. Greenstone CL, Saint S, Moseley RH: Clinical problem solving: A hand-carried diagnosis. N Engl J Med 2007;356:2407-2411.

206. Pareek SS: Liver involvement in secondary syphilis. Dig Dis Sci 1979;24:41-43.

207. Sobel HJ, Wolf EH: Liver involvement in early syphilis. Arch Pathol Lab Med 1972;93:565-568.

208. Longstreth P, Hoke AW, Elroy C: Hepatitis and bone destruction as uncommon manifestations of early syphilis: Report of a case. Arch Dermatol 1976;112:1451-1454.

209. Koff RS, Gang DL: Case records of the Massachusetts General Hospital: Weekly clinicopathological exercises. Case 27-1983: A 25 year old man with liver disease. N Engl J Med 1983;309:1127-1128.

210. Maincent G, Labadie H, Fabre M, et al: Tertiary hepatic syphilis: A treatable cause of multinodular liver. Dig Dis Sci 1997;42:447-450.

211. Vainrub B: Bacterial infections of the liver and biliary tract: Laboratory studies to determine etiology. Lab Res Methods Biol Med 1983;7:119-128.

212. de Brito T, Menezes LF, Lima DM, et al: Immunohistochemical and in situ hybridization studies of the liver and kidney in human leptospirosis. Virchows Archiv 2006;448:576-583.

213. de Brito T, Penna DO, Hoshino S, et al: Cholestasis in human leptospirosis: A clinical, histochemical, biochemical and electron microscopy study based on liver biopsies. Beitr Pathol Anat 1970;140:345-361.

214. de Brito T, Machado MM, Montans SD, et al: Liver biopsy in human leptospirosis: A light and electron microscopy study. Virchows Arch Pathol Anat Physiol Klin Med 1967;342:61-69.

215. Goellner MH, Agger WA, Burgess JH, et al: Hepatitis due to recurrent Lyme disease. Ann Intern Med 1988;108:707-708.

216. Zanchi AC, Gingold AR, Theise ND, et al: Necrotizing granulomatous hepatitis as an unusual manifestation of Lyme disease. Dig Dis Sci 2007;52:2629-2632.

217. Srigley JR, Vellend H, Palmer N, et al: Q-fever: The liver and bone marrow pathology. Am J Surg Pathol 1985;9:752-758.

218. Hofmann CE, Heaton JW, Jr.: Q fever hepatitis: Clinical manifestations and pathological findings. Gastroenterology 1982;83:474-479.

219. Modol JM, Llamazares JF, Mate JL, et al: Acute abdominal pain and Q fever. Eur J Clin Microbiol Infect Dis 1999;18:158-160.

220. Travis LB, Travis WD, Li CY, et al: Q fever: A clinicopathologic study of five cases. Arch Pathol Lab Med 1986;110:1017-1020.

221. Qizilbash AH: The pathology of Q fever as seen on liver biopsy. Arch Pathol Lab Med 1983;107:364-367.

222. Silver SS, McLeish WA: "Doughnut" granulomas in Q fever. Can Med Assoc J 1984;130:102-104.

223. Font J, Bruguera M, Perez-Villa F, et al: Hepatic fibrin-ring granulomas caused by *Staphylococcus epidermidis* generalized infection. Gastroenterology 1987;93:1449-1451.

224. Stricker BH, Blok AP, Babany G, et al: Fibrin ring granulomas and allopurinol. Gastroenterology 1989;96:1199-1203.

225. Vanderstigel M, Zafrani ES, Lejonc JL, et al: Allopurinol hypersensitivity syndrome as a cause of hepatic fibrin-ring granulomas. Gastroenterology 1986;90:188-190.

226. Marazuela M, Moreno A, Yebra M, et al: Hepatic fibrin-ring granulomas: A clinicopathologic study of 23 patients. Hum Pathol 1991;22:607-613.

227. Moreno A, Marazuela M, Yebra M, et al: Hepatic fibrin-ring granulomas in visceral leishmaniasis. Gastroenterology 1988;95:1123-1126.

228. de Bayser L, Roblot P, Ramassamy A, et al: Hepatic fibrin-ring granulomas in giant cell arteritis. Gastroenterology 1993;105:272-273.

229. Voigt JJ, Delsol G, Fabre J: Liver and bone marrow granulomas in Q fever. Gastroenterology 1983;84:887-888.

230. Delsol G, Pellegrin M, Voigt JJ, et al: Diagnostic value of granuloma with fibrinoid ring. Am J Clin Pathol 1980;73:289.

231. Pellegrin M, Delsol G, Auvergnat JC, et al: Granulomatous hepatitis in Q fever. Hum Pathol 1980;11:51-57.

232. Moskovitz M, Fadden R, Min T: Human ehrlichiosis: A rickettsial disease associated with severe cholestasis and multisystemic disease. J Clin Gastroenterol 1991;13:86-90.

233. Nutt AK, Raufman J: Gastrointestinal and hepatic manifestations of human ehrlichiosis: 8 Cases and a review of the literature. Dig Dis 1999;17:37-43.

234. Sehdev AE, Dumler JS: Hepatic pathology in human monocytic ehrlichiosis: *Ehrlichia chaffeensis* infection. Am J Clin Pathol 2003;119:859-865.

235. Jackson MD, Kirkman C, Bradford WD, et al: Rocky mountain spotted fever: Hepatic lesions in childhood cases. Pediatr Pathol 1986;5:379-388.

236. Adams JS, Walker DH: The liver in Rocky Mountain spotted fever. Am J Clin Pathol 1981;75:156-161.

237. Walker DH, Staiti A, Mansueto S, et al: Frequent occurrence of hepatic lesions in boutonneuse fever. Acta Trop 1986;43:175-181.

238. Guardia J, Martinez-Vazquez JM, Moragas A, et al: The liver in boutonneuse fever. Gut 1974;15:549-551.

239. Mir-Madjlessi SH, Farmer RG, Hawk WA: Granulomatous hepatitis: A review of 50 cases. Am J Gastroenterol 1973;60:122-134.

240. Collins MH, Jiang B, Croffie JM, et al: Hepatic granulomas in children: A clinicopathologic analysis of 23 cases including polymerase chain reaction for histoplasma. Am J Surg Pathol 1996;20:332-338.

241. Smith JW, Utz JP: Progressive disseminated histoplasmosis: A prospective study of 26 patients. Ann Intern Med 1972;76:557-565.

242. Maekelt GA: Diagnostic procedures in the evaluation of hepatic diseases: Studies to determine mycotic etiology. Lab Res Methods Biol Med 1983;7:141-144.

243. Thaler M, Pastakia B, Shawker TH, et al: Hepatic candidiasis in cancer patients: The evolving picture of the syndrome. Ann Intern Med 1988;108:88-100.

244. Johnson TL, Barnett JL, Appelman HD, et al: Candida hepatitis: Histopathologic diagnosis. Am J Surg Pathol 1988;12:716-720.

245. Diebel LN, Raafat AM, Dulchavsky SA, et al: Gallbladder and biliary tract candidiasis. Surgery 1996;120:760-764, discussion 4-5.

246. Uflacker R, Wholey MH, Amaral NM, et al: Parasitic and mycotic causes of biliary obstruction. Gastrointest Radiol 1982;7:173-179.

247. Kates DM, Sparling TG, Jetha N, et al: Alteration of the natural history of *Pneumocystis carinii* infection in patients with acquired immunodeficiency syndrome receiving aerosolized pentamidine. West J Med 1991;154:721-723.

248. Boldorini R, Guzzetti S, Meroni L, et al: Acute hepatic and renal failure caused by *Pneumocystis carinii* in patients with AIDS. J Clin Pathol 1995;48:975-978.

249. Erdman SH, Barber BJ, Barton LL: Aspergillus cholangitis: A late complication after Kasai portoenterostomy. J Pediatr Surg 2002;37:923-925.

250. Padmanabhan S, Battiwalla M, Hahn T, et al: Two cases of hepatic zygomycosis in allogeneic stem cell transplant recipients and review of literature. Transplant Infect Dis 2007;9:148-152.

251. Marco del Pont J, De Cicco L, Gallo G, et al: Hepatic arterial thrombosis due to *Mucor* species in a child following orthotopic liver transplantation. Transplant Infect Dis 2000;2:33-35.

252. Mekeel KL, Hemming AW, Reed AI, et al: Hepatic mucormycosis in a renal transplant recipient. Transplantation 2005;79:1636.

253. Suh IW, Park CS, Lee MS, et al: Hepatic and small bowel mucormycosis after chemotherapy in a patient with acute lymphocytic leukemia. J Korean Med Sci 2000;15:351-354.

254. Oliver MR, Van Voorhis WC, Boeckh M, et al: Hepatic mucormycosis in a bone marrow transplant recipient who ingested naturopathic medicine. Clin Infect Dis 1996;22:521-524.

255. Tsui WM, Ma KF, Tsang DN: Disseminated *Penicillium marneffei* infection in HIV-infected subject. Histopathology 1992;20:287-293.

256. Duong TA: Infection due to *Penicillium marneffei*, an emerging pathogen: Review of 155 reported cases. Clin Infect Dis 1996;23:125-130.

257. Bonacini M, Nussbaum J, Ahluwalia C: Gastrointestinal, hepatic, and pancreatic involvement with *Cryptococcus neoformans* in AIDS. J Clin Gastroenterol 1990;12:295-297.

258. Das BC, Haynes I, Weaver RM, et al: Primary hepatic cryptococcosis. Br Med J Clin Res Ed 1983;287:464.

259. Sabesin SM, Fallon HJ, Andriole VT: Hepatic failure as a manifestation of cryptococcosis. Arch Intern Med 1963;111:661-669.

260. Bucuvalas JC, Bove KE, Kaufman RA, et al: Cholangitis associated with *Cryptococcus neoformans*. Gastroenterology 1985;88:1055-1059.

261. Knapp WA, Seeley TT, Ruebner BH: Fatal coccidioidomycosis: Report of two cases. Calif Med 1972;116:86-90.

262. Zangerl B, Edel G, von Manitius J, et al: Kokzidioidomykose als Ursache einer granulomatosen Hepatitis. Med Klin 1998;93:170-173.

263. Howard PF, Smith JW: Diagnosis of disseminated coccidioidomy-cosis by liver biopsy. Arch Intern Med 1983;143:1335-1338.

264. Ryan ME, Kirchner JP, Sell T, et al: Cholangitis due to *Blastomyces dermatitidis*. Gastroenterology 1989;96:1346-1349.

265. Teixeira F, Gayotto LC, De Brito T: Morphological patterns of the liver in South American blastomycosis. Histopathology 1978;2:231-237.

266. Bica I, Hamer DH, Stadecker MJ: Hepatic schistosomiasis. Infect Dis Clin North Am 2000;14:583-604.

267. Poltera AA, Katsimbura N: Granulomatous hepatitis due to *Strongyloides stercoralis*. J Pathology 1974;113:241-246.

268. Mondou EN, Gnepp DR: Hepatic granuloma resulting from *Enterobius vermicularis*. Am J Clin Pathol 1989;91:97-100.

269. Daly JJ, Baker GF: Pinworm granuloma of the liver. Am J Trop Med Hygiene 1984;33:62-64.

270. Garcia HH, Moro PL, Schantz PM: Zoonotic helminth infections of humans: Echinococcosis, cysticercosis and fascioliasis. Curr Opin Infect Dis 2007;20:489-494.

271. Filippou D, Tselepis D, Filippou G, et al: Advances in liver echinococcosis: Diagnosis and treatment. Clin Gastroenterol Hepatol 2007;5:152-159.

272. Craig P: *Echinococcus multilocularis*. Curr Opin Infect Dis 2003;16:437-444.

273. Lim JH: Toxocariasis of the liver: Visceral larva migrans. Abdom Imaging 2008;33:151-156.

274. Hartleb M, Januszewski K: Severe hepatic involvement in visceral larva migrans. Eur J Gastroenterol Hepatol 2001;13:1245-1249.

275. Kaushik SP, Hurwitz M, McDonald C, et al: *Toxocara canis* infection and granulomatous hepatitis. Am J Gastroenterol 1997;92:1223-1225.

276. Kaplan KJ, Goodman ZD, Ishak KG: Eosinophilic granuloma of the liver: A characteristic lesion with relationship to visceral larva migrans. Am J Surg Pathol 2001;25:1316-1321.

277. Inan M, Sakru N, Vatansever U, et al: Visceral larva migrans presenting as acute abdomen in a child. J Pediatr Surg 2006;41:e7-e9.

278. Berger T, Degremont A, Gebbers JO, et al: Hepatic capillariasis in a 1-year-old child. Eur J Pediatr 1990;149:333-336.

279. Arjona R, Riancho JA, Aguado JM, et al: Fascioliasis in developed countries: A review of classic and aberrant forms of the disease. Medicine (Baltimore) 1995;74:13-23.

280. MacLean JD, Graeme-Cook FM: Case records of the Massachusetts General Hospital: Weekly clinicopathological exercises. Case 12-2002: A 50-year-old man with eosinophilia and fluctuating hepatic lesions. N Engl J Med 2002;346:1232-1239.

281. Acosta-Ferreira W, Vercelli-Retta J, Falconi LM: *Fasciola hepatica* human infection: Histopathological study of sixteen cases. Virchows Archiv A Pathol Anat Histol 1979;383:319-327.

282. Marcos LA, Terashima A, Gotuzzo E: Update on hepatobiliary flukes: Fascioliasis, opisthorchiasis and clonorchiasis. Curr Opin Infect Dis 2008;21:523-530.

283. Lim JH, Kim SY, Park CM: Parasitic diseases of the biliary tract. AJR Am J Roentgenol 2007;188:1596-1603.

284. Al Absi M, Qais AM, Al Katta M, et al: Biliary ascariasis: The value of ultrasound in the diagnosis and management. Ann Saudi Med 2007;27:161-165.

285. Fogaca HS, Oliveira CS, Barbosa HT, et al: Liver pseudotumor: A rare manifestation of hepatic granulomata caused by *Ascaris lumbricoides* ova. Am J Gastroenterol 2000;95:2099-2101.

286. Stanley SL Jr: Amoebiasis. Lancet 2003;361:1025-1034.

287. Mikolajczak SA, Kappe SH: A clash to conquer: The malaria parasite liver infection. Mol Microbiol 2006;62:1499-1506.

288. Bhalla A, Suri V, Singh V: Malarial hepatopathy. J Postgrad Med 2006;52:315-320.

289. Maekelt GA: Diagnostic procedures in the evaluation of hepatic diseases: Studies to determine parasitologic etiology. Lab Res Methods Biol Med 1983;7:129-139.

290. Cruz I, Nieto J, Moreno J, et al: Leishmania/HIV co-infections in the second decade. Indian J Med Res 2006;123:357-388.

291. Albrecht H, Sobottka I, Emminger C, et al: Visceral leishmaniasis emerging as an important opportunistic infection in HIV-infected persons living in areas nonendemic for *Leishmania donovani*. Arch Pathol Lab Med 1996;120:189-198.

292. Malla N, Mahajan RC: Pathophysiology of visceral leishmaniasis: Some recent concepts. Indian J Med Res 2006;123:267-274.

293. Duarte MI, Corbett CE: Histopathological patterns of the liver involvement in visceral leishmaniasis. Rev Inst Med Trop Sao Paulo 1987;29:131-136.

294. Koshy A, Al-Azmi WM, Narayanan S, et al: Leishmaniasis diagnosed by liver biopsy: Management of two atypical cases. J Clin Gastroenterol 2001;32:266-267.

295. Tiwari I, Rolland CF, Popple AW: Cholestatic jaundice due to toxoplasma hepatitis. Postgrad Med J 1982;58:299-300.

296. Weitberg AB, Alper JC, Diamond I, et al: Acute granulomatous hepatitis in the course of acquired toxoplasmosis. N Engl J Med 1979;300:1093-1096.

297. Bonacini M, Kanel G, Alamy M: Duodenal and hepatic toxoplasmosis in a patient with HIV infection: Review of the literature. Am J Gastroenterol 1996;91:1838-1840.

Infectious Lymphadenitis

Judith A. Ferry

Lymph nodes play an important role in the reaction to infectious processes. In many cases, the histologic changes are nonspecific and a particular etiology cannot be assigned; in other cases, the findings are characteristic of specific entities. This chapter focuses on histologically distinctive types of infectious lymphadenitides and on their differential diagnosis.

Lymphadenitis of Viral or Possible Viral Etiology

Infectious Mononucleosis

Infectious mononucleosis is defined as symptomatic primary infection by Epstein-Barr virus (EBV). Infectious mononucleosis was first described as a distinct entity in 1920, when six college students with pharyngitis, fever, and lymphadenopathy (a syndrome then referred to as glandular fever) were all found to have an absolute lymphocytosis in the peripheral blood, with mononuclear cells with unusually abundant cytoplasm. Subsequently, Paul and Bunnell found that the serum of patients with infectious mononucleosis caused sheep red blood cells to agglutinate due to the presence of what they called a heterophile antibody, and this provided a laboratory test for the diagnosis of infectious mononucleosis. The definition of infectious mononucleosis was further refined when a laboratory worker exposed to EBV, which had only recently been discovered and identified as being associated with endemic Burkitt's lymphoma,[1] developed heterophile-positive infectious mononucleosis, establishing EBV as the causative agent.[2]

Currently, the diagnosis of infectious mononucleosis is usually established clinically, but if enlarged lymph nodes or tonsils are biopsied, problems in differential diagnosis may arise.

Clinical Features

Infectious mononucleosis is a fairly common disease of adolescents and young adults. Cases of infectious mononucleosis in young children have been reported, although EBV infection in this age group is usually subclinical. Rare cases are also described in older adults. Males and females are affected equally. Infectious mononucleosis is more commonly encountered among individuals in higher socioeconomic groups, who are less likely to be exposed to EBV during early childhood. Transmission is through close contact with another individual who is EBV infected.

The classic findings at presentation are fever, pharyngitis, and cervical lymphadenopathy accompanied by an atypical peripheral blood lymphocytosis and a positive heterophile antibody (Monospot) test. Lymphadenopathy is usually symmetric and tender.[2] Splenomegaly is also common. A maculopapular or urticarial rash may develop, mainly among patients who are treated with a β-lactam antibiotic.[2]

Supportive therapy is usually sufficient, and spontaneous recovery is the rule in almost all cases, except for those with serious complications. In more severe cases, generalized lymphadenopathy, hepatomegaly with hepatic dysfunction, splenic rupture, peripheral cytopenias, and development of a hemophagocytic syndrome may occur. In most cases, the illness is self-limited, but rarely, intercurrent infection, Guillain-Barré syndrome, or splenic rupture with hemorrhage results in death.

Problems in establishing a diagnosis on clinical and laboratory grounds sometimes arise because the heterophile antibody test may not be positive, especially early in the illness and among children; repeated Monospot testing is sometimes required. In some individuals, particularly those at the extremes of age, the heterophile antibody is never detected.[2] In such cases, serologic studies for EBV-associated antigens help establish a diagnosis. Another scenario creating diagnostic difficulties is the patient who has clinical features diverging from the classic presenting symptoms, such as a presentation with diffuse lymphadenopathy without prominent pharyngitis. Patients with unusual clinical or laboratory features are more likely than those with classic infectious mononucleosis to undergo lymph node excision to establish a diagnosis.

Pathologic Features

The lymph nodal architecture is typically distorted but not effaced by an expanded paracortex containing a polymorphous population of lymphoid cells, including small lymphocytes, intermediate-sized lymphoid cells, immunoblasts, tingible body macrophages, and mature and immature plasma cells. The immunoblasts may be atypical, with pleomorphic or lobated nuclei. Binucleated cells resembling Reed-Sternberg cells may be identified. Mitotic figures may be numerous. Apoptosis is common, and zonal necrosis may be present. Primary follicles or reactive follicles are often present at the periphery of the lymph node, but follicular hyperplasia is not usually a prominent feature. Sinuses are patent in at least some areas, and frequently they are dilated. Sinuses contain histiocytes and a polymorphous population of lymphoid cells similar to that found in the paracortex, including immunoblasts. Lymphoid cells sometimes infiltrate the capsule and extend into perinodal fat. Similar histologic features are found in the tonsils of patients with infectious mononucleosis (Fig. 11-1). In tonsils, crypts are usually present, although the epithelium lining them may be necrotic.[3-7]

The small and intermediate-sized cells in the paracortex are predominantly T cells, including many that are activated in response to the presence of the virus. The CD4/CD8 ratio is decreased. The paracortical immunoblasts are CD20+ B cells. They typically coexpress MUM1/IRF4 but not bcl6 or CD10; some are bcl2+. Therefore, the EBV+ immunoblasts have a post–germinal center immunophenotype.[8] With the use of immunostains or in situ hybridization for κ and λ immunoglobulin light chains, the plasma cells are demonstrated to be polytypic. Polytypic light chain expression can often be demonstrated in the immunoblasts as well.[8] The blasts typically show focal staining for the activation antigen CD30; they are CD15–.[3,4,9-11] With in situ hybridization, EBV-encoded RNA (EBER) can be detected in the paracortical immunoblasts.[9] Rarely, patients with acute infectious mononucleosis or a recent history of infectious mononucleosis have florid follicular hyperplasia with large follicles,

rather than the more common paracortical immunoblastic reaction. EBER+ cells may be found in follicles and in the interfollicular areas in such cases.[12]

Differential Diagnosis

The differential diagnosis of infectious mononucleosis is broad. A variety of infectious processes can be associated with an infectious mononucleosis–like illness, including cytomegalovirus (CMV), Human herpesvirus 6 (HHV-6), herpes simplex virus type 1 (HSV-1), human immunodeficiency virus (HIV), group A β-hemolytic *Streptococcus pyogenes* (strep throat), *Toxoplasma gondii,* and others.[2] Careful clinical evaluation, augmented by laboratory studies, is required to establish a diagnosis.

The differential diagnosis based on pathologic features includes a variety of reactive and neoplastic conditions. If immunoblasts are numerous, the possibility of diffuse large B-cell lymphoma is often a consideration. In favor of infectious mononucleosis are lack of architectural effacement, presence of areas readily recognizable as reactive hyperplasia, a polymorphous background of lymphoid cells, patent sinuses containing lymphoid cells including immunoblasts, and lack of monotypic immunoglobulin expression on immunophenotyping.[4,7] The typical immunophenotype of the immunoblasts (CD10–, bcl6–, bcl2+/–, MUM1+) may also be helpful, because the majority of diffuse large B-cell lymphomas express bcl6. Diffuse large B-cell lymphomas are usually EBV– unless the patient is immunocompromised, so the presence of EBV should raise the possibility of infectious mononucleosis.

Classic Hodgkin lymphoma is often included in the differential diagnosis, because Reed-Sternberg–like cells are often seen in infectious mononucleosis (see Fig. 11-1C); however, most large cells in infectious mononucleosis have the appearance of immunoblasts rather than Reed-Sternberg cells or variants. Hodgkin lymphoma is more often associated with obliteration of the lymph nodal architecture. The polymorphous background of lymphoid cells ranging from small to intermediate and large in the paracortex and sinuses in infectious mononucleosis is very helpful in excluding Hodgkin lymphoma, in which background lymphocytes are all typically small. Granulocytes, especially eosinophils, and a background of fibrosis are more common in Hodgkin lymphoma. Immunoblasts in infectious mononucleosis are CD20+, CD15–, in contrast to the CD20–, CD15+ status typically found with Reed-Sternberg cells. The CD4/CD8 ratio is usually normal or elevated in Hodgkin lymphoma, in contrast to the CD8 predominance typically seen in infectious mononucleosis. Reed-Sternberg cells in approximately 50% of cases of classic Hodgkin lymphoma are EBV+, so the presence of EBV does not exclude Hodgkin lymphoma. Obtaining adequate clinical information is important to make the correct diagnosis. If the patient is known to have clinical or laboratory evidence of infectious mononucleosis, a diagnosis of Hodgkin disease or non-Hodgkin lymphoma should be made with caution.

Other viral infections, vaccination, certain drugs, and acute reaction to severe necrotizing processes can produce lymphadenopathy with histologic features similar to or indistinguishable from those of infectious mononucleosis. Clinical information can be helpful in investigating the cause of the lymphadenopathy. In addition, in infectious mononucleosis, EBV+ immunoblasts are typically present in large numbers, whereas in other conditions,

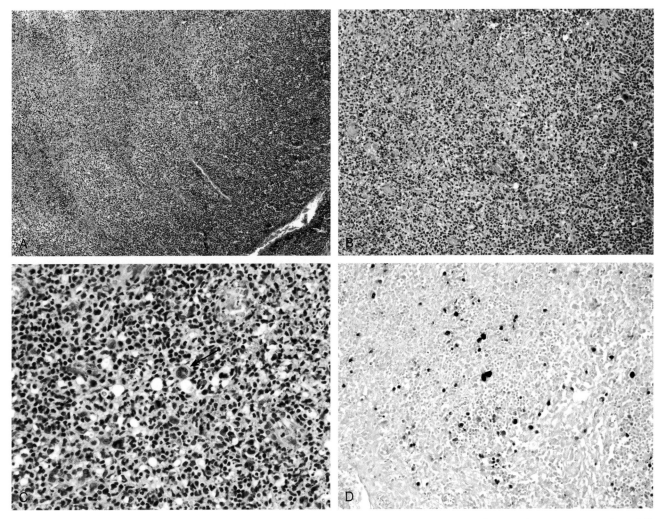

Figure 11-1. Infectious mononucleosis in the tonsil. **A,** Low-power view shows a dense, polymorphous lymphoid proliferation with extensive necrosis *(upper left).* **B,** Higher power shows numerous small to medium-sized cells and scattered large cells, as well as numerous apoptotic cells *(upper left).* **C,** High power shows a Reed-Sternberg–like trinucleate cell *(arrow)* with prominent nucleoli in a background of lymphoid cells of various sizes. **D,** Scattered small and large cells are positive for Epstein-Barr virus (in situ hybridization using Epstein-Barr virus–encoded RNA [EBER] probe).

EBV+ cells are usually absent.[9,13-16] The Monospot test and serologic testing for EBV-specific antibodies can be helpful in establishing a diagnosis.

Cytomegaloviral Lymphadenitis

Clinical Features

CMV is an uncommon cause of lymph nodal enlargement; lymphadenopathy may be localized or generalized.[17,18] CMV lymphadenitis may occur in the setting of an infectious mononucleosis–like illness in which patients have sore throat, fatigue, and malaise; it may also be found in patients who are otherwise asymptomatic.[2,19-21]

CMV lymphadenitis can occur in individuals of any age; males and females are equally affected. The risk of CMV lymphadenitis is increased in the setting of congenital or acquired immunodeficiency, and CMV infection is described in patients who have, or have had, Hodgkin lymphoma or non-Hodgkin

lymphoma.[22] However, CMV lymphadenitis also occurs in immunologically normal individuals. CMV infection is common in patients with common variable immunodeficiency.[17,22,23] Most patients have a self-limited illness and require no specific therapy. Patients with associated lymphoproliferative disorder or immunodeficiency may have a more severe course.

Pathologic Findings

On microscopic examination, involved lymph nodes most often show follicular hyperplasia and monocytoid B-cell hyperplasia; this may be sufficiently florid to distort the nodal architecture. Paracortical hyperplasia may also be prominent. Infected cells contain a large eosinophilic intranuclear inclusion (mean size, 9 μm) and often also contain multiple tiny eosinophilic to amphophilic cytoplasmic inclusions.[22] Cells with inclusions are usually present focally in relatively small numbers, but occasionally they are numerous.[18,22] Neutrophils and histiocytes are often scattered around the infected cells. Inclusions are typically found among monocytoid B cells, but the infected cells are most likely histiocytes rather than lymphocytes; inclusions in the paracortex have also been described. Occasionally, endothelial cells are infected.[17,22,24]

Immunoperoxidase stains for CMV-associated antigens can be used to confirm the diagnosis when inclusions are found on routine sections and can help identify CMV-infected cells when inclusions are difficult to find.[18,22] Cells containing inclusions express CD15, usually with a Golgi-region or diffuse cytoplasmic pattern of staining, but membrane staining is less common.[22]

Differential Diagnosis

The differential diagnosis of CMV lymphadenitis includes reactive hyperplasia due to causes other than CMV and lymphoma, including both Hodgkin and non-Hodgkin lymphoma. If the viral inclusions are overlooked, the changes may be interpreted as nonspecific reactive lymphoid hyperplasia. The histologic features of CMV lymphadenitis overlap with those of *Toxoplasma* lymphadenitis and early cat-scratch disease, in that all three are characterized by follicular and monocytoid B-cell hyperplasia. *Toxoplasma* lymphadenitis is characterized in addition by clusters of epithelioid histiocytes, and cat-scratch disease, even at an early stage, typically also shows small foci of necrosis with fibrin and neutrophils.

Cells with nuclear viral inclusions may resemble Reed-Sternberg cells and variants on routinely stained sections, raising the possibility of classic Hodgkin lymphoma. CD15 expression by the virally infected cells enhances the resemblance to Hodgkin lymphoma. However, CMV lymphadenitis is much less likely to cause obliteration of the nodal architecture, and Hodgkin lymphoma is unlikely to be found in a lymph node occupied by florid follicular hyperplasia. Cells harboring virus may contain numerous granular cytoplasmic inclusions, in contrast to the agranular cytoplasm of Reed-Sternberg cells. Membrane staining by CD15 is more common in Reed-Sternberg cells than in CMV-infected cells.[22]

Occasionally, the follicular and monocytoid B-cell hyperplasia can be so florid as to distort the nodal architecture, potentially suggesting follicular lymphoma or nodal marginal zone lymphoma. Identification of CMV-infected cells, confirmed by immunostaining for CMV in a background of a follicular and monocytoid B-cell proliferation, establishes a diagnosis of CMV lymphadenitis.

Herpes Simplex Viral Lymphadenitis

Clinical Features

HSV-1 or HSV-2 infection is rarely associated with lymphadenitis. In some cases, primary infection with HSV-1 occurs in the setting of an infectious mononucleosis–like syndrome, with pharyngitis, fever, and cervical lymphadenopathy.[2] This type of lymphadenitis has been described in individuals over a wide age range. Males and females are equally affected. The risk of HSV lymphadenitis appears to be increased among the immunodeficient; some patients have also had a hematologic malignancy. The most common associated disorder is chronic lymphocytic leukemia, but other B-cell lymphomas and myeloid leukemias

are also occasionally associated with HSV lymphadenitis. HSV can cause localized or generalized lymphadenitis, or it can involve lymph nodes in the setting of widespread visceral infection. When localized, the lymphadenopathy most often affects inguinal nodes, with cervical nodes next most often affected. The enlarged lymph nodes are characteristically tender or even painful. The presence of concurrent ulcerated cutaneous or mucosal lesions provides a clue to the diagnosis, but such lesions are not always present and, if present, may be inconspicuous and overlooked. Rarely, HSV-1 is responsible for Parinaud's oculoglandular syndrome; manifestations include conjunctivitis, periorbital swelling and tenderness, and enlarged, painful preauricular lymph nodes.[25]

Some patients have had no specific therapy, and some have received acyclovir. In those with an associated hematologic disorder, therapy may be directed at that condition rather than directly at the HSV infection. The prognosis depends on the extent of infection and on the prognosis of any underlying hematologic disorder or immunodeficiency. Disseminated HSV infection has a poor prognosis, but isolated HSV lymphadenitis is self-limited in most cases.[26-35]

Pathologic Features

HSV infection results in a necrotizing lymphadenitis. Viable areas show prominent paracortical hyperplasia, often with numerous immunoblasts. Necrosis appears to begin in the paracortex and often shows prominent extension into perinodal soft tissue. The necrotic areas contain neutrophils, karyorrhectic or amorphous eosinophilic debris, and a variable number of viral inclusions, ranging from rare to abundant. Most infected cells are uninucleated, although a few multinucleated cells are seen (Fig. 11-2). This is in contrast to HSV infection of squamous epithelial cells, in which multinucleated cells with nuclear molding are characteristic. Intact neutrophils are most abundant in early lesions and may be absent in long-standing lymphadenitis. Histiocytes often surround the necrotic areas, but granulomas are not found.[26-28,30-33] Similar changes are seen in the tonsils in herpetic tonsillitis.[34] Varicella-zoster virus rarely causes lymphadenitis; the histologic features are similar to those of HSV lymphadenitis.[36,37]

The diagnosis can be confirmed readily with the use of immunohistochemical stains for antigens associated with HSV-1 and HSV-2; polymerase chain reaction (PCR), in situ hybridization, electron microscopy, or viral culture can also be used.

Differential Diagnosis

The differential diagnosis includes other types of necrotizing lymphadenitis as well as lymphoma. The lack of granulomatous inflammation with epithelioid or palisading histiocytes provides evidence against infections caused by mycobacteria, fungi, *Yersinia*, cat-scratch bacilli, and lymphogranuloma venereum.[31] Infectious mononucleosis typically shows paracortical expansion with immunoblasts and some necrosis, but EBV does not produce viral inclusions. In those cases with marked paracortical expansion with numerous immunoblasts, a high-grade lymphoma with necrosis may enter the differential diagnosis. In HSV lymphadenitis, the nodal architecture may be distorted, although it is not obliterated, in contrast to most nodes involved by

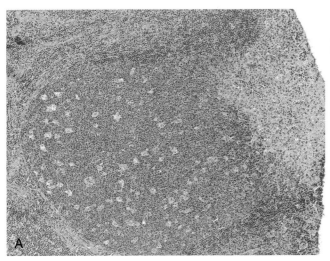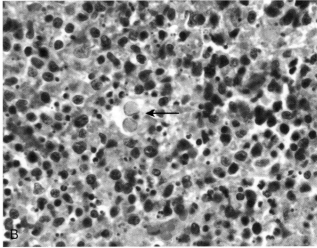

Figure 11-2. Herpes simplex lymphadenitis. **A,** A discrete focus of necrosis lies adjacent to a floridly hyperplastic lymphoid follicle. **B,** Within the necrotic focus, there are small and large lymphoid cells, necrotic debris, and rare cells with nuclei replaced by homogeneous, glassy viral inclusions *(arrow)*.

lymphoma. Viral inclusions are absent in lymphoma, except in cases in which HSV and lymphoma concurrently involve the same lymph node.[27,29,35]

Human Immunodeficiency Virus–Associated Lymphadenopathy

Reactive changes in lymph nodes directly related to HIV infection are discussed here. Lymphadenitis and lymphadenopathy in HIV+ patients related to infectious agents other than HIV are discussed separately in those sections.

Clinical Features

Most patients are young to middle-aged adult males, but women and children of either sex may occasionally be affected. There are a number of different clinical settings in which HIV-associated lymphoid hyperplasia can be found:

- Lymphadenopathy, occurring in the setting of an infectious mononucleosis–like illness, in association with primary infection by HIV
- Persistent generalized or isolated lymphadenopathy, which may be accompanied by constitutional symptoms
- Cystic lymphoid hyperplasia, involving periparotid lymph nodes and causing multicystic, often bilateral, masses in the area of the parotid glands
- Hyperplasia of extranodal lymphoid tissue, with symptoms related to mass effect

On acute infection by HIV, some patients develop an infectious mononucleosis–like illness with fever, pharyngitis, and cervical lymphadenopathy.[38] This has been referred to as the acute retroviral syndrome.[2] Persistent generalized lymphadenopathy, defined as extrainguinal lymphadenopathy persisting for at least 3 months, involving at least two noncontiguous node groups, is common among HIV+ patients. Persistent generalized lymphadenopathy mainly affects adult men and is often accompanied

by fever, weight loss, headaches, and malaise. If the periparotid nodes are affected, the hyperplastic lymphoid tissue can obstruct intranodal ductal structures, resulting in the formation of cysts within the nodes. This produces multicystic, often bilateral lesions in the area of the parotid. The process has been called cystic lymphoid hyperplasia or lymphoepithelial cysts.[39,40] If the lymphoid tissue of Waldeyer's ring is affected, patients may present with a large, obstructive nasopharyngeal mass, nasal stuffiness, or nasal bleeding. The hyperplastic lymphoid tissue may obstruct the eustachian tubes and cause hearing loss.[41]

Therapy is directed against the HIV infection itself. Outcome is related to the underlying HIV infection, but with the availability of highly active antiretroviral therapy (HAART) in recent years, the prognosis has significantly improved.

Pathologic Features

A range of changes is found in lymphadenopathy associated with HIV infection. Similar changes may be found in organized extranodal lymphoid tissue. In early stages of HIV infection, lymph nodes show florid follicular hyperplasia. Follicle centers are often large and irregularly shaped and have an expanded dark zone with numerous blast cells, numerous mitoses, many tingible body macrophages, and attenuated or absent follicle mantles. Follicle lysis, in which the follicle center appears disrupted and fragmented by irregularly infiltrating small lymphocytes, sometimes accompanied by tiny foci of hemorrhage, is common. The interfollicular region contains a mixture of immunoblasts, plasma cells, lymphocytes, and histiocytes. Monocytoid B cells are often prominent. Sinuses are patent and may show sinus histiocytosis, sometimes with erythrophagocytosis. Scattered epithelioid histiocytes and polykaryocytes or Warthin-Finkeldey–type giant cells may be seen.

In advanced stages of immunodeficiency, there is lymphoid depletion. Follicles are decreased in number. The follicles that are present are small and may be ill-defined and difficult to identify. Follicle centers are "burnt out" or regressively transformed and contain a decreased number of B cells. The paracortex appears hypocellular. It is occupied by scattered lymphocytes and immunoblasts, often with prominent vascularity. As in early stages of infection, plasma cells are often abundant. Amorphous eosinophilic interstitial material may be present, or there may be fibrosis, and the node may have a pale, depleted appearance. In some cases, lymph nodes show changes intermediate between florid follicular hyperplasia and lymphoid depletion.[42-45]

Cutaneous rashes are common among HIV+ patients; these individuals often have a component of dermatopathic lymphadenopathy.

In both early and late stages, B cells in follicles are polytypic. T cells show a decreased, usually reversed CD4/CD8 ratio.[44,46] Follicles with follicle lysis show a fragmented follicular dendritic cell network; this may be seen with antibodies to CD21 or CD23. Few to many scattered cells infected by EBV may be found with the use of in situ hybridization for EBER, reflecting poor immunologic control of EBV+ B cells.

The pathologic changes are not completely specific, but if a patient has lymphadenopathy with the features described here and is not known to be HIV+, a test for HIV is warranted. HIV+ patients, particularly those with histologic changes consistent with advanced immunodeficiency, are at increased risk for opportunistic infections, Kaposi sarcoma, or malignant lymphoma, and lymph nodes should be examined carefully to be certain one of these serious complications of HIV infection is not present. If follicles show changes of the type that may be seen in Castleman disease, a stain for HHV-8 (also called Kaposi sarcoma–associated virus, or KSHV) should be performed, to investigate the possibility of HHV-8–associated multicentric Castleman disease (see later discussion).

Most patients who have been treated with HAART show improvement in lymphoid architecture as well as an increase in CD4+ T cells and a decrease in CD8+ T cells within lymphoid tissue. However, HIV often is detectable in follicular dendritic cells in lymphoid tissue, even after a prolonged course of HAART, and even in the absence of detectable virus in the peripheral blood.[47]

Measles Lymphadenitis

Measles is an infectious disease caused by a paramyxovirus of the genus *Morbillivirus*. Measles is uncommon in the United States because of widespread inoculation of children. Lymphadenitis in the setting of measles therefore occurs only rarely. Lymph nodes show follicular hyperplasia; the most distinctive feature is the presence of Warthin-Finkeldey giant cells within reactive germinal centers. Warthin-Finkeldey giant cells are found in the prodromal stage of infection and usually disappear as a rash develops.

Human Herpesvirus 6–Associated Lymphadenitis

HHV-6 is the etiologic agent of a common febrile illness among young children that is known as exanthem subitum, roseola infantum, or sixth disease. Adults infected by HHV-6 may develop a heterophile-negative mononucleosis-like illness with cervical lymphadenopathy.[2] Rare cases of lymphadenitis in the setting of a severe acute febrile illness due to HHV-6 in adults

have been described.[48] Lymph nodes in these systemically ill patients showed marked paracortical expansion by a polymorphous population of cells of varying size, including many atypical-appearing cells containing large eosinophilic nuclear and/or cytoplasmic viral inclusions. Virally infected cells appeared to be CD4+ T cells. The differential diagnosis in such cases may include CMV lymphadenitis, because the inclusions bear some resemblance to those of CMV. The paracortical expansion, in conjunction with many immunoblasts or virally infected cells resembling immunoblasts, could raise the possibility of lymphoma.[48] A small proportion of cases of lymphadenitis with the morphology of Kikuchi disease (discussed later) may be caused by HHV-6 infection. Immunostains for HHV-6–associated antigens, electron microscopy, PCR for HHV-6, and serologic studies may help establish the diagnosis.[2]

Kawasaki Disease

Kawasaki disease, also known as mucocutaneous lymph node syndrome or infantile polyarteritis, is a systemic vasculitis of uncertain etiology. It is included in this chapter because evidence strongly suggests that an infection, most likely viral, underlies the development of Kawasaki disease.

Clinical Features

Kawasaki disease is an acute febrile disease of young children, with 85% of patients younger than 5 years of age. Boys are more often affected than girls, with a male-to-female ratio of approximately 2 : 1. In the United States, the annual incidence is approximately 17 cases per 100,000 children younger than 5 years of age. The prevalence is higher in Asia than in the United States. There is also a higher risk among family members of patients with Kawasaki disease.

The Centers for Disease Control and Prevention has published requirements for the diagnosis of Kawasaki disease that include fever of 5 or more days, no response to antibiotics, and at least four of the following:

1. Bilateral conjunctival congestion
2. Abnormalities of the lips and oral cavity, including diffuse erythema, dry fissured lips, and prominent lingual papillae (strawberry tongue)
3. Abnormalities of the skin of the distal extremities, including erythema of palms and soles with edema early on and desquamation of fingertips later in the course of the disease
4. Polymorphous, nonvesicular, primarily truncal, rash
5. Acute, nonsuppurative cervical lymphadenopathy not due to any other identifiable cause

In addition to the diagnostic criteria noted, patients may have cardiac abnormalities (electrocardiographic changes, cardiomegaly, murmurs), diarrhea, arthritis or arthralgia, peripheral blood abnormalities (neutrophilic leukocytosis with a leftward shift, anemia, thrombocytosis), elevated erythrocyte sedimentation rate, aseptic meningitis, mild jaundice, proteinuria, sterile pyuria, elevated transaminases, or a combination of these conditions. Most patients recover after an illness of 3 to 4 weeks' duration, but without therapy 20% to 25% develop complications of coronary arteritis (aneurysm, thrombosis), which may be fatal, sometimes years later. A subset of patients present initially with fever and cervical lymphadenopathy alone; these patients are slightly older on average than those with a more classic presentation of Kawasaki disease. They may be thought to have some form of infectious lymphadenitis, potentially leading to a delay in diagnosis and delay in instituting appropriate therapy.[49]

Kawasaki disease can often be treated successfully with intravenous immunoglobulin (IVIG) and aspirin; steroids and other anti-inflammatory agents may be used if symptoms persist. Prompt administration of IVIG reduces the risk of coronary arterial changes and resulting serious or fatal complications of this disease.

Pathologic Features

Only a limited amount of information is available on histologic findings in lymph nodes of patients with Kawasaki disease. Lymph nodes are reported to show paracortical expansion by lymphocytes and a variable number of immunoblasts, plasma cells, and histiocytes, as well as small to large areas of necrosis containing karyorrhectic debris, sometimes with admixed neutrophils. Increased numbers of blood vessels lined by swollen endothelial cells and containing fibrin thrombi may surround the necrotic areas. Activation of the immune response is believed to underlie the pathogenesis of the disease; important components are proposed to be immunoglobulin A, cytotoxic T cells, and monocyte-macrophages.[50-54]

Kikuchi Disease

Kikuchi disease, also known as histiocytic necrotizing lymphadenitis, subacute necrotizing lymphadenitis, Kikuchi lymphadenitis, or Kikuchi-Fujimoto disease, is an uncommon cause of lymphadenopathy. This disease is of unknown etiology, but an infectious cause, with various viruses most often implicated, is a strong possibility for at least a subset of cases of Kikuchi disease.

Clinical Features

Almost all patients with Kikuchi disease are between adolescence and middle age, but it is mainly a disease of young adults, with the mean and median age in the third decade. There is a female preponderance that ranges from modest to pronounced in different series. Kikuchi disease appears to be more prevalent among Asians than in Western populations.[55-62] Most patients present with unilateral, often painful, cervical lymphadenopathy. Other lymph nodes are affected much less often.[61] Infrequently, there is generalized lymphadenopathy.[56] Approximately one half of patients have fever at presentation. Some patients have anemia or neutropenia; one quarter have an atypical lymphocytosis. Leukocytosis is uncommon. Occasionally, patients have a rash.

Kikuchi disease is typically self-limited, and most patients recover without therapy. A small number develop recurrent lymphadenopathy. Rarely, Kikuchi disease occurring in immunocompromised patients results in a severe illness. A few patients thought to have Kikuchi disease later develop systemic lupus erythematosus; this may be coincidental, or the patient may have had systemic lupus erythematosus mimicking Kikuchi disease from the outset.[55,57-59,61,62]

A variety of viral and other types of infectious etiologies have been suggested as potential causes of Kikuchi disease, including EBV, parvovirus B19,[63] human T-cell lymphotropic virus 1 (HTLV-1),[64] HHV-6,[61] HIV,[65] and others. We have seen two cases of lymphadenitis with pathologic features typical of Kikuchi disease in which one patient had clinically typical infectious mononucleosis and one patient had HIV infection (unpublished results). However, no single infectious agent stands out as the principal cause of Kikuchi disease, and when large series of Kikuchi disease are studied, the majority of cases have no associated specific, identifiable infectious agent.[56,61] The apparent evolution to systemic lupus erythematosus in a small number of cases raises the question of whether Kikuchi disease is an autoimmune disease that is self-limited in the vast majority of cases. Some patients have developed lymphadenitis with features of Kikuchi disease as a reaction to foreign material or other type of noninfectious conditions. Kikuchi disease appears to be more common among individuals with certain human leukocyte antigen (HLA) class II genes.[55-58,66] It is possible that the histologic and immunohistologic features of Kikuchi disease can be produced by a variety of stimuli depending on the susceptibility of the individual affected.

Pathologic Features

Lymph nodes show prominent paracortical hyperplasia with one or more round or irregular, discrete or confluent eosinophilic areas in the cortex or paracortex containing histiocytes, lymphocytes, immunoblasts, plasmacytoid dendritic cells, and karyorrhectic and eosinophilic granular debris. The necrotic debris is most abundant in the centers of these areas, whereas immunoblasts are most numerous at the periphery. The cytologically bland histiocytes have oval, indented, or twisted nuclei and typically include a mixture of phagocytic and nonphagocytic forms. Vacuolated or xanthomatous histiocytes may be present. Histiocytes with eccentric sickle-shaped nuclei have been called crescentic histiocytes. Plasmacytoid dendritic cells are medium-sized cells with round nuclei, dispersed chromatin, small nucleoli, and a moderate amount of faintly amphophilic cytoplasm. In Kikuchi lymphadenitis, aggregates of plasmacytoid dendritic cells are frequently seen in viable areas; necrosis appears to begin within clusters of plasmacytoid dendritic cells. The necrosis is predominantly apoptotic. Thrombosed vessels may be seen around necrotic foci. Epithelioid histiocytes, plasma cells, eosinophils, and neutrophils are virtually absent (Fig. 11-3). The characteristic foci may be relatively small and confined to the paracortex or may occupy the majority of the lymph node. The infiltrate may extend beyond the capsule into perinodal soft tissue. Reactive lymphoid follicles may be present, but they are not important as a diagnostic feature of Kikuchi disease.[55-59,61,62]

Kikuchi disease can be classified into three histologic types: proliferative, necrotizing, and xanthomatous. The proliferative and necrotizing patterns are more common than the xanthomatous pattern.[61] These may represent different stages in the evolution of the disease. In the proliferative type, microscopic examination reveals the mixture of cells described earlier, with apoptosis but without coagulative necrosis. In the necrotizing type, lymph nodes show large areas of necrosis in addition to the changes characteristic of the proliferative type. In the

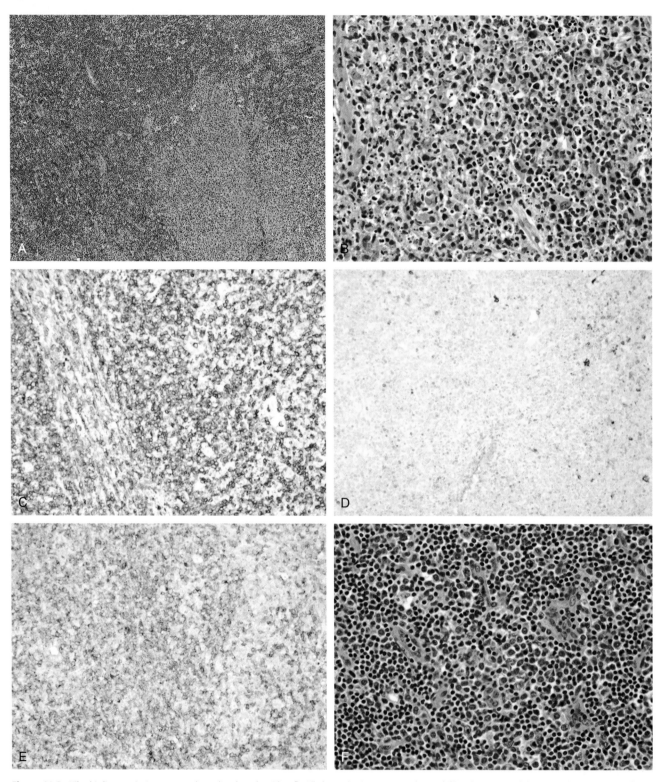

Figure 11-3. Kikuchi disease. **A,** Low power shows lymph node with a floridly hyperplastic paracortex *(upper left)* and an eosinophilic zone rich in histiocytes *(lower right)*. **B,** Higher-power view of the eosinophilic zone shows histiocytes, necrotic debris, lymphocytes, and occasional immunoblasts. The histiocyte-rich zone contains numerous CD3+ T cells **(C)** and rare to absent (CD20+) B cells **(D)**. **E,** Almost all T cells are CD8+. **F,** Plasmacytoid dendritic cells with nuclei slightly larger and paler than in small lymphocytes, and with slightly more cytoplasm, form a loose cluster in the center of the field.

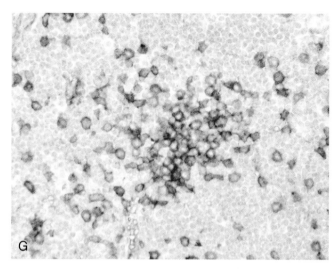

Figure 11-3, cont'd. G, An immunostain for CD123 highlights the plasmacytoid dendritic cells. (**C, D, E,** and **G,** immunoperoxidase technique on paraffin sections.)

xanthomatous type, there is a predominance of foamy histiocytes, and necrosis can be present or absent.[55,59,62]

Immunohistochemical analysis confirms the presence of a mixture of lymphoid cells, histiocytes, and plasmacytoid monocytes. The lymphoid cells in the necrotic areas, including the immunoblasts, are almost all T cells. In most cases, the majority of T cells are CD8+ (see Fig. 11-3C, E), often with coexpression of cytotoxic granule proteins, such as TIA-1, granzyme B, and perforin. The histiocytes are lysozyme+ and CD68+; surprisingly, they are reported to coexpress myeloperoxidase.[55,59,66,67] The plasmacytoid dendritic cells express CD123 (see Fig. 11-3G) and CD68. They also express CD2, CD4, and CD43, markers that may be expressed by both T cells and monocytes, and lack T cell–specific antigens such as CD3.[67-69] Although B cells are found if reactive follicles are present, B cells are sparse to absent in the areas of the lymph node with histiocytes and cellular debris (see Fig. 11-3D).

Differential Diagnosis

A variety of reactive and neoplastic disorders can enter the differential diagnosis of Kikuchi disease. The most important entity in the differential diagnosis is non-Hodgkin lymphoma. The distinction may be difficult if immunoblasts are abundant. Familiarity with the spectrum of changes found in Kikuchi disease and identification of areas with the characteristic polymorphous infiltrate are essential to rendering the correct diagnosis. In addition, Kikuchi disease shows partial nodal involvement more often than lymphoma does. The vast majority of lymphomas in Western countries are B-cell lymphomas. Only a minority of lymphomas in the United States are T-cell lymphomas, and most lymph node–based T-cell lymphomas are CD4+. The predominance of T cells in Kikuchi disease, usually with a predominance of CD8+ T cells, is an important clue in avoiding a misdiagnosis of lymphoma.

Because necrosis is such a prominent component of Kikuchi disease, infectious lymphadenitis is often a consideration. However, neutrophils, suppurative necrosis, and granulomas—

features characteristic of many types of infectious lymphadenitis—are not found in Kikuchi disease. HSV lymphadenitis can resemble Kikuchi disease, particularly in older lesions with few intact neutrophils. Although histiocytes may be prominent in herpetic lymphadenitis, the histiocytic infiltrate is usually even more pronounced in Kikuchi disease, and viral inclusions are absent.

If crescentic histiocytes are prominent, metastatic carcinoma of the signet ring cell type may enter the differential diagnosis. However, histiocytes in Kikuchi disease are cytologically typical, may contain cellular debris but do not contain mucin, and express histiocyte-related antigens rather than cytokeratin.[62] In addition, the classic clinical setting for Kikuchi disease—a young woman with isolated cervical lymphadenopathy—differs greatly from the usual clinical setting expected in a patient with signet ring cell carcinoma.

Lymphadenitis in patients with systemic lupus erythematosus can closely resemble Kikuchi disease.[59] The finding of hematoxylin bodies, plasma cells, or deposition of nuclear material on the basement membranes of blood vessels (Azzopardi phenomenon) supports a diagnosis of lupus lymphadenitis over Kikuchi disease, but these features may not be evident in every case of lupus lymphadenitis. Clinical features are sometimes helpful in making a definitive distinction. Because of the difficulty of excluding lupus on microscopic examination, and because a minority of patients diagnosed with Kikuchi disease have developed lupus later, clinicians may consider performing a workup for autoimmune disease in cases showing histologic features of Kikuchi disease.[55]

Bacterial Lymphadenitis

Pyogenic Bacterial Lymphadenitis

Lymphadenitis due to pyogenic bacteria, such as *Streptococcus* or *Staphylococcus*, although not often biopsied, may be the most common cause of acute cervical lymphadenopathy in children in the United States. Microscopic examination usually shows follicular hyperplasia and a variably prominent paracortical infiltrate of neutrophils.[70,71]

Cat-Scratch Disease

Clinical Features

Cat-scratch disease is among the most common causes of subacute or chronic, benign lymphadenopathy in the United States, with about 24,000 cases occurring per year.[72] For reasons that may be related to the breeding patterns of cats, it is more common between July and December than between January and June.[73-76] *Bartonella henselae* is the cause of almost all cases of cat-scratch disease. It is possible that a small subset of cases are due to infection by *Afipia felis*.[73,75-78] A few cases are due to *Bartonella quintana*, the louse-borne agent of the infamous trench fever of World War I.[79] Although cat-scratch disease can affect patients of any age, at least half are younger than 18 years old.[74,80,81] A history of exposure to a cat can be found in almost every case.[74,81] *B. henselae* bacteremia is common among cats, but it is not associated with a serious illness. Kittens are more likely to be bacteremic than adult cats and could be more likely to transmit the disease. The infectious agent has been identified within the gastrointestinal tract of fleas; flea feces contaminating a cat scratch or bite could possibly initiate cat-scratch disease.[82] Three to 10 days after exposure, a red papule or papules develop in the skin at the inoculation site (usually the site of a cat scratch); the papules typically become vesiculated and then crusted over during the next several days. Regional lymphadenopathy is usually found 1 to 2 weeks after the papule appears.[74,77]

The frequently tender lymphadenopathy usually involves only one node or one group of nodes.[74,81] Surrounding soft tissue may be edematous or inflamed.[83] Noncontiguous lymphadenopathy is occasionally found, probably because there is more than one inoculation site or because the inoculation site is midline, allowing organisms to drain to lymph nodes bilaterally. The axilla is the most common site for lymphadenopathy. Also commonly involved are cervical, supraclavicular, and epitrochlear lymph nodes. Femoral or inguinal nodes may be involved.[74,80,83] In approximately 5% of cases, the inoculation site is the eye, and patients may develop the oculoglandular syndrome of Parinaud (granulomatous conjunctivitis and preauricular or submandibular lymphadenopathy). Cat-scratch disease is the most common cause of this syndrome.[25] Rarely *B. quintana* rather than *B. henselae* is the cause of oculoglandular syndrome of Parinaud.[79] Up to half of patients have fever, which is usually low grade.[74,81] Patients may also experience malaise, anorexia, or, rarely, nausea or abdominal pain. The disease is usually mild and self-limited and may have resolved by the time a diagnosis is established. Some patients receive antibiotics,[83] although it is not clear that antibiotics shorten the course of the illness or are required if the patient is immunocompetent and without severe manifestations of the *B. henselae* infection.[82]

Severe complications, occurring in up to 2% of cases, include involvement of the nervous system, skeleton, lung, liver, spleen, or heart. Neurologic manifestations include seizures, encephalitis, meningitis, and involvement of cranial or peripheral nerves. Ocular disease can result in retinitis or uveitis. Splenic or hepatic abscesses may develop. The skeleton is rarely involved by a necrotizing granulomatous osteomyelitis, sometimes in the vicinity of an affected lymph node. Pulmonary involvement may take the form of pneumonia or pleural effusions.[72,77,81,83,84] Rarely, patients have died of complications of their infection.[80] In some patients with severe manifestations of cat-scratch disease, there is an underlying immunodeficiency.[83] Older patients (>60 years) are infrequently affected by cat-scratch disease, but when it does occur, they are slightly less likely than younger patients to have lymphadenopathy and more likely to have malaise, endocarditis, encephalitis, and fever of unknown origin. The uncommon occurrence of cat-scratch disease in older patients and its atypical clinical presentation may lead to a delay in diagnosis.[80]

Pathologic Features

The appearance of the infected lymph nodes changes over time. The earliest changes are follicular hyperplasia with a prominent proliferation of monocytoid B cells. Foci of necrosis with a few neutrophils, scant fibrin, and cellular debris appear within aggregates of monocytoid B cells. Necrotic foci are adjacent to, or encroach upon, follicle centers, or are adjacent to the subcapsu-

lar sinus (Fig. 11-4). *B. henselae* is an intracellular organism with tropism for endothelial cells, and for this reason, these foci may be found in the vicinity of small blood vessels. Sinuses may contain a mixture of immunoblasts, neutrophils, and histiocytes. Over time, necrotic foci enlarge, extending deeper into the node. They contain pus, fibrin, and debris and acquire a rim of histiocytes. The foci continue to enlarge and coalesce and are surrounded by palisading histiocytes, replacing the node with the classic stellate microabscesses or granulomas.

The cat-scratch bacillus is a tiny, slender, pleomorphic, weakly gram-negative rod up to 3 μm long. Its very small size makes it difficult to see, but when a silver stain such as a Warthin-Starry stain or a Steiner stain is used, the bacilli are coated with the black reaction product, making them appear larger and more readily visualized (see Fig. 11-4D). Bacilli are present singly, in chains or large clumps, along the walls of blood vessels, in macrophages in necrotic areas, or admixed with necrotic debris. Bacilli are most numerous in the early stages of inflammation within clusters of monocytoid B cells. By the time well-developed stellate abscesses have formed, the organisms can be difficult to detect (Fig. 11-5).[77,78,83,85]

The tiny cat-scratch bacilli may be difficult to recognize in histologic sections and are difficult to culture. For these reasons, serologic studies and PCR for *Bartonella* can help establish a diagnosis.[77,83,86,87] Immunohistochemistry using antibodies specific for *B. henselae* is also reported to be helpful in identifying the microorganisms.[86]

B. henselae infection in immunocompromised patients is not likely to produce a localized granulomatous lymphadenitis. Disseminated cat-scratch disease with granulomatous inflammation, bacillary angiomatosis, bacillary peliosis, or bacteremia may occur instead.[77] Bacillary angiomatosis is the term used to describe a vasoproliferative disorder in skin, lymph nodes, and other sites caused by *Bartonella* species. When lymph nodes are involved by bacillary angiomatosis, *B. henselae* is almost always responsible, whereas *B. quintana* may cause bacillary angiomatosis in sites such as subcutaneous tissue and bone.[88] Bacillary peliosis is the term used to describe this disorder in the liver and spleen. Bacillary angiomatosis occurs mainly in HIV+ patients. It has also been described in transplant recipients.[88] Bacillary angiomatosis in lymph nodes shows a proliferation of variably sized vascular structures lined by plump endothelial cells, sometimes without a recognizable lumen. Many neutrophils, extravasated red cells, and cellular debris may be present. Microorganisms in these cases may be numerous. Prompt antibacterial infection therapy is required.

The florid vascular proliferation in an immunocompromised host may suggest Kaposi sarcoma, but Kaposi sarcoma typically lacks neutrophils and debris, tumor cells are positive for HHV-8, and bacteria should be absent unless there is some form of superimposed infection.

Differential Diagnosis

A variety of microorganisms cause necrotizing lymphadenitis that can mimic the lymphadenitis of cat-scratch disease. Clinical features, including age, possible exposure to various infectious agents, anatomic distribution of lymphadenopathy, and severity of symptoms, as well as special stains on tissue sections, serologic studies, and culture are helpful in establishing a definite diagno-

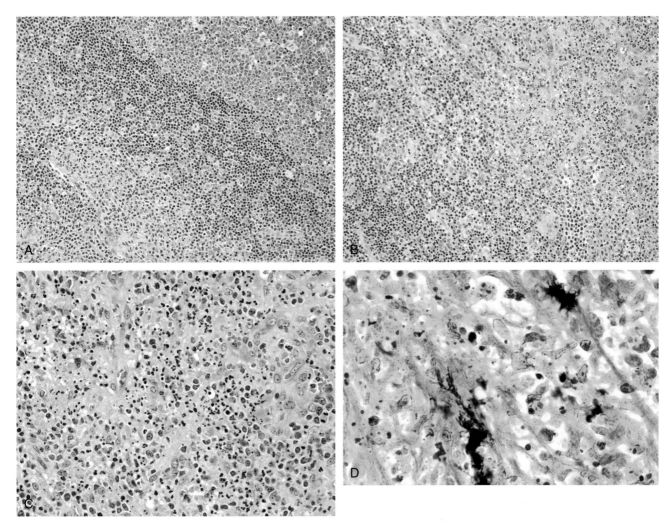

Figure 11-4. Cat-scratch disease, early stage. **A,** A hyperplastic follicle is present adjacent to a band of pale monocytoid B cells with a small amount of interstitial fibrin and scant apoptotic debris, consistent with very early involvement by cat-scratch disease. **B,** Inflammation is more advanced in this focus, which is from the same lymph node as in **A. C,** Higher power shows an aggregate of monocytoid B cells that has been mostly replaced by neutrophils, fibrin, cellular debris, and blood vessels lined by endothelial cells with plump nuclei. **D,** A Warthin-Starry stain shows bacteria consistent with *Bartonella* in clumps.

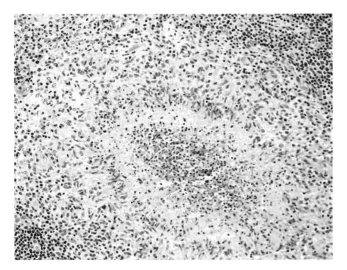

Figure 11-5. Cat-scratch disease, late stage. This lymph node was almost entirely replaced by small and large granulomas with suppurative necrosis. Palisading histiocytes surround the central area of necrosis.

sis. Infection by bacteria such as *Chlamydia trachomatis* (lymphogranuloma venereum), *Francisella tularensis* (tularemia), *Hemophilus ducreyi* (chancroid), *Yersinia enterocolitica* (pseudotuberculous mesenteric lymphadenitis), *Listeria monocytogenes* (listeriosis), *Pseudomonas mallei* (glanders), and *Pseudomonas pseudomallei* (melioidosis) can be associated with a necrotizing lymphadenitis with histologic features that may be indistinguishable from that of cat-scratch disease. These infections are all likely to be associated with significantly greater morbidity than cat-scratch disease. The florid follicular hyperplasia and monocytoid B-cell hyperplasia of early cat-scratch disease may suggest CMV or *Toxoplasma* lymphadenitis.

As noted previously, infection by pyogenic cocci may be associated with an acute suppurative lymphadenitis with follicular hyperplasia that could suggest cat-scratch disease, except that the pyogenic cocci typically do not elicit a rim of palisading histiocytes around areas of suppurative necrosis. One exception is in cases of chronic granulomatous disease (CGD) of childhood (discussed later), in which palisading granulomas with suppurative necrosis may be found in association with infection due to a variety of bacteria and fungi. The appearance may resemble that of cat-scratch disease.[71,87,89]

The necrotizing granulomas of mycobacterial and fungal lymphadenitis may resemble those of cat-scratch disease. As in cat-scratch disease, atypical mycobacterial infection usually affects the cervical lymph nodes of children. In the late stages of cat-scratch disease, the necrotic material may acquire an amorphous quality that resembles the caseation necrosis of tuberculosis. Special stains for microorganisms may be helpful in establishing a diagnosis.

Syphilitic Lymphadenitis

Syphilis, an infectious disease caused by *Treponema pallidum*, is much less prevalent in the population now than in the past, because it responds to readily available antibiotics; syphilitic lymphadenitis is only rarely encountered. In primary and secondary syphilis, lymph nodes show marked follicular hyperplasia and a prominent plasmacytosis. They may also contain non-necrotizing or suppurative granulomas and show capsular and perinodal fibrosis, endarteritis, and phlebitis. Blood vessels, germinal centers, and granulomas may harbor spirochetes. The changes characteristic of syphilis are best seen in lymph nodes that drain the site of the primary infection, usually the inguinal lymph nodes (Fig. 11-6).[90,91] In the infrequent instance in which the primary site is the oropharynx (e.g., the tonsil), cervical lymph nodes may show well-developed changes of syphilitic lymphadenitis.[92] The tonsils may show histologic changes similar to those typical of lymphadenitis; an ulcerated tonsillar chancre containing spirochetes may be present.[92]

Recently, some cases of nodal inflammatory pseudotumor have been found to be related to infection by *T. pallidum*. A clue to the diagnosis of syphilis in such cases is prominent follicular hyperplasia, in addition to the usual spindle-cell proliferation and polymorphous inflammatory cell infiltrate of inflammatory pseudotumors.[93]

Spirochetes may be detected with silver stains such as Warthin-Starry or Steiner stains. Immunohistochemistry using antibody to *T. pallidum* is reported to be a sensitive technique

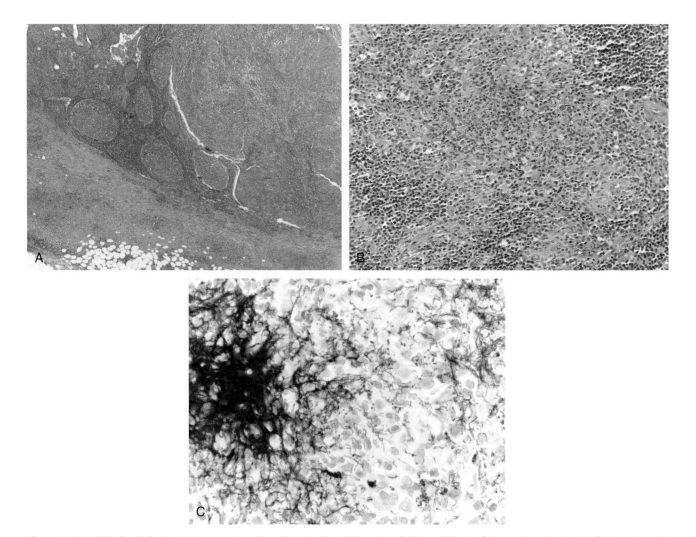

Figure 11-6. Syphilitic lymphadenitis. **A,** Low-power view shows a lymph node with hyperplastic follicles and fibrosis of the capsule and perinodal soft tissue. A vaguely nodular expansion of the paracortex is seen at the right of the image. **B,** Higher-power view of the nodular area shows increased numbers of blood vessels and focal suppurative necrosis. **C,** A Steiner stain highlights numerous spirochetes.

for detecting microorganisms.[93] Although secondary syphilis may be associated with diffuse lymphadenopathy, nodes away from the inguinal region may show only nonspecific follicular hyperplasia.[90,91]

Brucellosis

Clinical Features

Brucellosis, also known as undulant fever, is an acute, intermittent or chronic febrile illness caused by infection with *Brucella* species. The incidence is highly variable. Up to 3.5 cases per 100,000 persons occur annually in endemic areas, but brucellosis is rare in the United States. Both children and adults and both males and females are affected, depending on their exposure, which includes close animal contact, particularly among individuals such as shepherds or goatherds; ingestion of unpasteurized milk; and consumption of uncooked meat. *Brucella melitensis* is the most common cause of brucellosis in humans and is especially prevalent in developing countries.

The constellation of symptoms and their severity are highly variable from one case to another. However, fever is almost always present, and almost all patients complain of malaise and night sweats. Other common complaints include arthralgia, myalgia, back pain, headache, abdominal pain, and gastrointestinal symptoms such as diarrhea, nausea, and vomiting. Splenomegaly is common. Hepatomegaly and lymphadenopathy are slightly less common. Lymphadenopathy appears to be more common in children than in adults and it seems to be more conspicuous early in the course of the disease. Some patients have evidence of cardiac and even central nervous system involvement. Laboratory abnormalities that may be found include anemia, leukopenia, monocytosis, and eosinophilia. The presence of splenomegaly tends to correlate with the finding of leukopenia and with fever lasting longer than 1 week.

Pathologic Features

Involved tissues show non-necrotizing, sarcoidal granulomas and necrotizing granulomas, sometimes with suppurative necrotic abscesses or diffuse infiltrates of mononuclear cells. The microorganisms are gram-negative, intracellular coccobacilli.

Diagnosis can be established with blood culture; biopsy of involved lymph nodes (or other tissue) with microscopic examination and culture; serologic studies; the standard tube agglutination test; or the Rose-Bengal slide agglutination test.

Brucellosis responds well to treatment with appropriate antibiotics, which should be given for a sufficiently long course to help prevent relapse. Proactive animal testing and treatment could decrease the incidence of disease in humans.[94-96]

Mycobacterial Lymphadenitis

Mycobacterial lymphadenitis may be found in conjunction with pulmonary tuberculosis or disseminated infection, or it may occur in isolation. The clinical picture varies widely with the type of mycobacteria and the age and immune status of the affected patient.

Tuberculous Lymphadenitis

Tuberculous lymphadenitis is the result of lymph nodal infection by tuberculous mycobacteria, such as *Mycobacterium tuberculosis* or *Mycobacterium bovis*. *M. tuberculosis* is a serious global health problem, with approximately one third of the world's population infected by this microorganism. In Central Africa, for example, the most common finding among patients who undergo a superficial lymph node biopsy, almost all of whom are HIV+, is tuberculous lymphadenitis.[97] *M. tuberculosis* was also the most common specific cause of cervical lymphadenopathy in children in a study from South Africa.[98] Although tuberculosis is much less common among residents of the United States compared to those in other parts of the world, the number of cases in this country has recently increased due to homelessness and poor living conditions. Incomplete courses of antibiotic treatment resulting from poor patient compliance has led to the emergence of increased numbers of drug-resistant strains.[99]

Patients with lymphadenitis due to *M. tuberculosis* are usually adults who present with constitutional symptoms (fever, fatigue, and weight loss) and have associated pulmonary tuberculosis. When peripheral lymph nodes are involved, they tend to be in the supraclavicular fossa or posterior cervical triangle. Frequently, multiple lymph nodes are involved bilaterally, and there are draining sinuses. The purified protein derivative (PPD) test is usually strongly positive.

Lymph nodes in immunocompetent patients show well-formed granulomas composed of epithelioid histiocytes and Langhans-type giant cells. Granulomas may be non-necrotizing or necrotizing. Necrosis is typically caseation necrosis. A Ziehl-Neelsen stain is used to identify acid-fast bacilli; they are usually few in number in immunocompetent patients. PCR or culture is needed to diagnose cases in which organisms cannot be identified in tissue sections and to distinguish definitively between infections by *M. tuberculosis* and those caused by atypical mycobacteria.[99]

Atypical Mycobacterial Lymphadenitis

Non-tuberculous mycobacterial lymphadenitis is due to infection by the atypical mycobacteria, most often *Mycobacterium avium-intracellulare*. Among immunocompetent individuals with atypical mycobacterial lymphadenitis, the majority are children younger than 5 years of age. Some studies report boys and girls to be affected equally; others report a higher proportion of female patients. Atypical mycobacterial infection is the most common cause of chronic lymphadenitis among previously healthy children; in some developing countries, however, tuberculous lymphadenitis is more prevalent than atypical mycobacterial lymphadenitis. The annual incidence is estimated to be 1.2 to 2.1 cases per 100,000 persons, although the incidence appears to have increased in recent years.[98,100-102]

Patients present with firm, nontender cervical lymphadenopathy that is typically unilateral. In general, constitutional symptoms are absent. Lymph nodes other than those from the cervical area are rarely affected. The mycobacteria are believed to gain access to the patient via the oropharynx, skin, or conjunctiva; involved lymph nodes correspond to those with lymphatic drainage from these sites. Over time, necrosis develops within the infected nodes, and the lymph nodes become fluctuant. Discoloration of the overlying skin and sinus tracts may

Table 11-1 Tuberculous Lymphadenitis versus Atypical Mycobacterial Lymphadenitis in Immunocompetent Patients

	Tuberculous Mycobacterial Lymphadenitis	Atypical Mycobacterial Lymphadenitis
Definition	Lymphadenitis due to tuberculous mycobacteria (e.g., *M. tuberculosis, M. bovis*)	Lymphadenitis due to atypical mycobacteria (e.g., *M. avium-intracellulare*)
Risk factors	Poor living conditions	None known
Age	Any age	Mostly young children
Sex	Males = Females	Boys and girls affected
Constitutional symptoms	Often present	Uncommon; mild if present
Sites	Cervical nodes, mediastinal nodes, lungs	Cervical nodes; unilateral; most often submandibular, jugulodigastric, or preauricular lymph nodes
Chest radiograph	Frequently abnormal	Almost always negative
Communicable	Yes	No
PPD	Positive	Negative or weakly positive
Preferred treatment	Full course of appropriate antibiotics	Complete excision

M., genus *Mycobacterium*; PPD, purified protein derivative test.

develop. The PPD test is typically negative or only weakly positive, and the chest radiograph is typically normal.

Patients have enlarged, sometimes matted lymph nodes with necrotizing and non-necrotizing granulomas, often with Langhans-type giant cells. The necrosis may be caseous or noncaseous. Necrotic areas may contain neutrophils and nuclear debris focally or diffusely. Diagnosis can be established by complete excision of affected lymph nodes, with special stains for microorganisms and culture. Complete excision is usually also effective treatment. Biopsy or aspiration of a lymph node may be performed but can be complicated by draining sinuses and scarring. Ziehl-Neelsen stain typically reveals small numbers of acid-fast bacilli, particularly at the periphery of the necrotic area, but these may be very infrequent and very difficult to identify. The organisms are slow-growing, so diagnosis by culture can require a protracted period of time. In selected instances, such as for infection for *M. tuberculosis*, PCR may be used to subclassify the organisms (Table 11-1).

Antibiotics do not typically influence the course of the disease. Surgical excision of the abnormal lymph nodes is effective therapy and is associated with a very low rate of recurrence. If incomplete removal of the lymph nodes is undertaken by incision and drainage or by curettage, the infection often persists. It may result in sinus tract formation, and additional surgery may be required. A delay in therapy increases the chance for development of sinus tracts and scarring, leading to a permanent cosmetic defect.

Mycobacterial Lymphadenitis in Immunocompromised Patients

Disseminated atypical mycobacterial infection can develop in HIV+ patients. Lymph nodes are often involved in this setting. The immune system in these patients sometimes proves unable to produce well-formed granulomas, and involved tissues may contain only loose aggregates of histiocytes containing numerous microorganisms. We have seen a remarkable case of an HIV+ patient with splenomegaly due to concurrent infection by both atypical mycobacteria (Fig. 11-7) and pneumocystis (see Fig.

11-11); a case of lymphadenitis with dual infection by *M. avium-intracellulare* and *Pneumocystis* in an HIV+ patient has been described.[103]

HIV+ patients with subclinical *M. avium-intracellulare* infection who initiate HAART may develop so-called immune restoration disease in the form of symptomatic *M. avium-intracellulare* infection including lymphadenitis. Other types of opportunistic infections may also produce a similar phenomenon.[104]

Differential Diagnosis

The differential diagnosis of mycobacterial lymphadenitis is broad; it includes a variety of infectious disorders and some neoplastic processes. A wide variety of microorganisms, including fungi, *Bartonella* species, *Brucella* species, syphilis, and *Leishmania*,[105] can be associated with granulomatous lymphadenitis. Caseation necrosis is more common in mycobacterial infections, although necrosis resembling caseation may be seen in fungal infections and in late stages of suppurative granulomatous infections, such as cat-scratch disease. In syphilitic lymphadenitis, there may be non-necrotizing or suppurative granulomas, but they are found in the setting of marked follicular hyperplasia and plasmacytosis. Uncommon entities that may enter the differential diagnosis include CGD of childhood and leprosy, particularly the tuberculoid form.

Noninfectious granulomatous diseases may be considered in the differential diagnosis of mycobacterial lymphadenitis. Cases with little or no necrosis may mimic sarcoidosis. A Ziehl-Neelsen stain and culture are helpful in establishing a diagnosis; however, this stain is often negative in mycobacterial infections lacking necrosis. Wegener granulomatosis can infrequently cause necrotizing lymphadenitis with granulomatous vasculitis and could potentially enter the differential of mycobacterial lymphadenitis.[106,107] Results of stains for microorganisms, culture, and clinical information can be helpful in such cases.

Classic Hodgkin lymphoma is often associated with necrosis and granulomatous inflammation. Identification of Reed-Sternberg cells and variants, typically found in greatest numbers

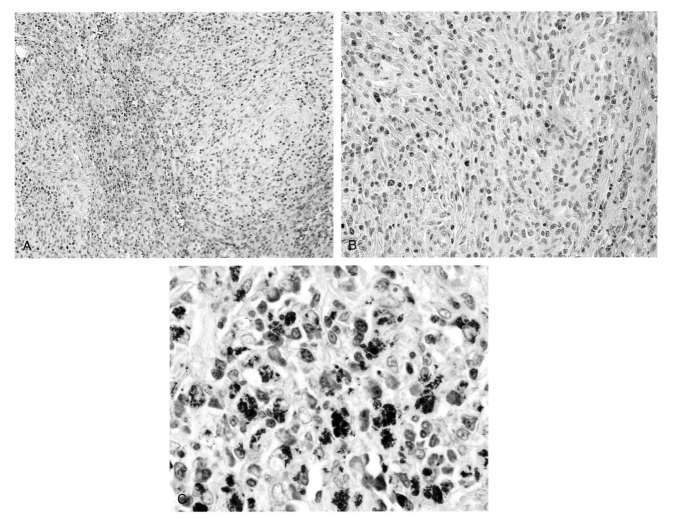

Figure 11-7. *Mycobacterium avium-intracellulare* infection in the spleen of an HIV-positive patient. This patient had concurrent splenic involvement by *Pneumocystis jiroveci* (see Fig. 11-11). **A,** The markedly enlarged spleen contained multiple loose aggregates of histiocytes, consistent with poorly formed granulomas. **B,** Plasma cells are scattered among the histiocytes. **C,** A stain for acid-fast bacilli shows histiocytes containing numerous microorganisms.

at the periphery of necrotic areas, confirms the diagnosis of Hodgkin lymphoma. The presence of a polymorphous inflammatory cell infiltrate, with eosinophils and plasma cells, is more common in Hodgkin lymphoma than in mycobacterial infection. Non-Hodgkin lymphomas are also occasionally associated with granulomas, but this is less common.

Metastatic carcinoma is rarely associated with granuloma formation in lymph nodes. The granulomas may draw the pathologist's attention away from a neoplastic infiltrate if it is subtle, and the carcinoma may potentially be overlooked.

Bacille Calmette-Guérin Lymphadenitis

Clinical Features
Bacille Calmette-Guérin (BCG) vaccine is administered in some developing countries to decrease the risk of tuberculosis. BCG lymphadenitis is defined as ipsilateral regional lymphadenopathy occurring after BCG vaccination; it develops in approximately 1% of vaccinated patients. Other infrequent complications of BCG vaccination include inoculation site abscesses and inflam-

mation involving bones, joints, and other sites. Immunocompetent individuals who develop lymphadenopathy usually do so within 6 months after vaccination. Lymphadenopathy is usually nontender. Immunodeficient individuals with disorders such as severe combined immunodeficiency, CGD, or HIV infection may develop severe disease, manifested by generalized lymphadenopathy and disseminated BCG infection.

The nonsuppurative form usually resolves spontaneously. The suppurative form is accompanied by erythema and edema of overlying skin and sometimes by ulceration and sinus tract formation. Incision and drainage of suppurative lymphadenitis can expedite healing and help prevent development of sinus tracts. Immunodeficient individuals urgently require prompt diagnosis and treatment. For such patients, this serious complication of vaccination can be fatal and requires anti-tuberculosis therapy as well as treatment of the immunodeficiency.

Pathologic Features
Lymphadenitis comes in suppurative and nonsuppurative forms. Microscopic examination reveals epithelioid granulomas with

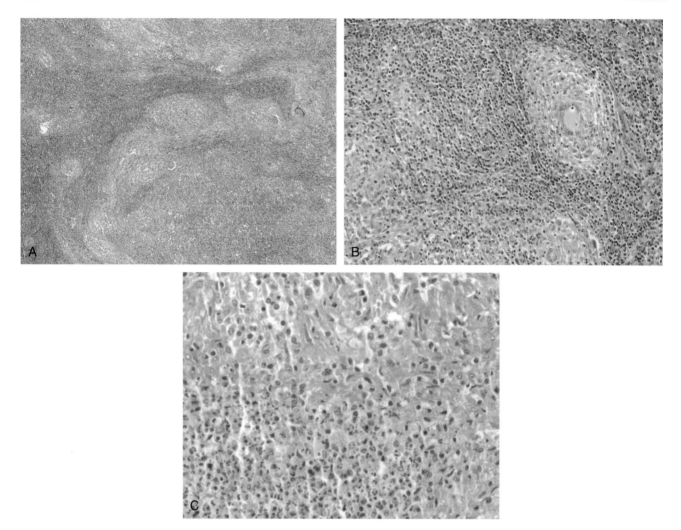

Figure 11-8. Bacille Calmette-Guérin lymphadenitis in a 3-year-old child. **A,** Large and small granulomas replace most of the lymph node. **B,** Higher power shows well-formed granulomas with occasional Langhans-type giant cells. **C,** Some granulomas show suppurative necrosis.

or without necrosis. If necrosis is present, it is usually suppurative rather than caseous (Fig. 11-8). Acid-fast bacilli are usually present in small numbers. Among immunodeficient patients, depending on the severity of the immunodeficiency, there may be epithelioid granulomas with few acid-fast bacilli or diffuse infiltrates of histiocytes laden with numerous acid-fast bacilli.[70,108-113]

Whipple Disease

Clinical Features

Understanding of Whipple disease took a major step forward when the causative infectious agent, the actinobacterium *Tropheryma whippelii*, was identified.[114] In the older literature, the disease was known as intestinal lipodystrophy.[115] It is a rare disorder, with an estimated annual incidence of less than 1 per 1 million persons. Whipple disease predominantly affects white men, with a male-to-female ratio ranging from 5 : 1 to 8 : 1. Patients can be affected from childhood to old age, but most are in the fourth to sixth decade of life, and the mean age at diag-

nosis is approximately 50 years. Transmission from one person to another has not been described.

The constellation of symptoms and signs related to Whipple disease varies with the patient. The classic findings are diarrhea, weight loss, abdominal pain, and arthralgia, but anemia, cutaneous hyperpigmentation, and fever all occur in 50% or more of patients. Some patients have intermittent low-grade fever. Lymphadenopathy is found in about half of the cases. Peripheral lymphadenopathy is common; intra-abdominal and mediastinal nodes may also be enlarged. The disease can affect the heart and lungs, with inflammation or fibrosis of endocardium, myocardium, or pericardium; thickened, distorted cardiac valves; chronic cough; pleuritic pain; or some combination of these. Whipple disease can produce a wide variety of manifestations, with central nervous system involvement including cognitive changes, motor and sensory deficits, altered consciousness, and hypothalamic dysfunction. Ocular involvement, which is almost always found in patients who have central nervous system disease, can result in retinitis or uveitis and loss of vision. Central nervous system involvement is identified in up to 50% of patients. Although symptoms related to gastrointestinal involvement are generally the most prominent, some patients have presented with lymphadenopathy without diarrhea or malabsorption; in some of these unusual cases, the diagnosis was delayed by years or was made only at autopsy.[116]

Whipple disease is a chronic, slowly progressive disease; if left untreated, it can be fatal. Whipple disease usually responds to antibiotics, but the duration of therapy must be long (approximately 12 months) to avoid relapse. The antibiotic should cross the blood-brain barrier to treat any central nervous system disease and to prevent relapse in the central nervous system, which is associated with a high mortality rate.

Pathologic Features

Diagnosis is most readily established on biopsy of the small intestine, but, occasionally, the first tissue submitted for pathologic examination is a lymph node. In lymph nodes, the distinctive finding is the presence of dilated sinuses distended by cystic-appearing, lipid-filled spaces surrounded by foreign-body giant cells and lipogranulomas, with clusters of foamy and epithelioid histiocytes. The histiocytes have granular, PAS+, diastase-resistant cytoplasm. However, in some cases, especially in the peripheral lymph nodes, non-necrotizing granulomas, similar to those seen in sarcoidosis, are identified. In such cases, the PAS stain may be negative or only focally positive, and bacilli may be rare or absent.[115,117] The high lipid content of the lymph nodes makes them somewhat distinctive radiographically.[117]

Electron microscopy reveals that the PAS+ histiocytes are filled with intact and degenerated bacilli. The Whipple bacilli are bacteria with an unusual trilaminar membrane and a cell wall similar to that seen in gram-positive bacteria.

PCR has been used on fluids, such as cerebrospinal fluid and blood, and on biopsy specimens to detect the presence of Whipple bacilli. However, *T. whippelii* DNA has reportedly been found by PCR in healthy individuals, so PCR should not be used in isolation to establish a diagnosis of Whipple disease. PCR is useful to confirm a diagnosis in patients with clinical or pathologic features suspicious for Whipple disease. PCR may also play a role in monitoring the efficacy of therapy.

Differential Diagnosis

Based on pathologic features, Whipple disease has a broad differential diagnosis. When lymph nodes have sinus histiocytosis lipogranulomas, the appearance closely resembles the effect of a diagnostic lymphangiogram; a PAS stain can exclude this possibility. Lymphangiograms are now done much less often than they were in the past, so this error is less likely.

Sarcoidosis, Crohn disease, and mycobacterial infections are included in the differential diagnosis when non-necrotizing granulomas are found. Special stains for acid-fast bacilli and culture are useful in excluding a mycobacterial infection. Intestinal biopsies are helpful in distinguishing Crohn disease from Whipple disease. A PAS stain and electron microscopy may be helpful in differentiating between Whipple disease and sarcoidosis, but in some lymph node biopsies in Whipple disease, particularly in samples from peripheral lymph nodes, the appearance may be similar to that of sarcoidosis. *M. avium-intracellulare* infection in immunodeficient patients and lepromatous leprosy can both be associated with prominent infiltrates of histiocytes with finely granular or vacuolated cytoplasm containing numerous microorganisms and can enter the differential diagnosis of Whipple

disease. Special stains for microorganisms and correlation with clinical features establish the diagnosis.

If the clinical features suggest the possibility of Whipple disease, biopsy of the proximal small bowel should be considered to establish a diagnosis.[114,115,118-123]

Chronic Granulomatous Disease

Clinical Features

CGD is a genetically determined, heterogeneous disorder characterized by leukocytes with impaired intracellular killing of microorganisms after phagocytosis, leading to recurrent, severe infections by bacteria and, less often, by fungi. Phagocytes are able to ingest microbes normally, but microbicidal activity is diminished because of abnormal nicotinamide adenine dinucleotide phosphate oxidase (NADPH oxidase), an enzyme complex found in granulocytes, monocytes, and macrophages that normally generates the superoxide ions and hydrogen peroxide that are toxic to microbes. NADPH oxidase has membrane-bound components (gp91-phox, p22-phox, and rap1a, which together make cytochrome b_{558}) and also cytosolic components (p47-phox, p40-phox, p67-phox, Rac2). Defects in the gp91-phox of cytochrome b_{558} account for most cases; these cases have X-linked inheritance. A defect with autosomal recessive inheritance accounts for the remaining cases. Among autosomal recessive defects, an abnormal p47-phox is most common; abnormal p67-phox and abnormal p22-phox each account for a small proportion of cases. CGD is usually inherited but may occur as the result of a germline mutation. More than 400 mutations giving rise to CGD have been described. Approximately 95% result in complete or partial loss of protein, and 5% are associated with normal levels of abnormal protein.[124]

The severity of the disease is dependent on the underlying genetic defect: X-linked inheritance with absence of cytochrome b_{558} expression is associated with more severe disease, compared with other defects. CGD accounts for fewer than 10% of primary immunodeficiencies, but it is the most common inherited disorder of phagocytic dysfunction. Its prevalence is approximately 1 in 1.2 million individuals, with an incidence of approximately 1 in 250,000 live births. The age at onset of symptoms is usually less than 1 year. Boys are more often affected than girls, because the most common form of CGD has X-linked transmission. There is a male-to-female ratio of 2:1 to 4:1. Consanguinity is a risk factor for developing this inherited disease.

CGD leads to recurrent suppurative infections, with lymphadenitis, pulmonary infection, upper respiratory infection, cutaneous abscesses, gastrointestinal infections, hepatic abscesses, sepsis, osteomyelitis, or some combination of these. The offending organisms are *Staphylococcus aureus*, *Klebsiella*, *Salmonella*, *Burkholderia*, *M. tuberculosis*, *Nocardia*, *Aspergillus*, or *Candida*.

Patients also have certain noninfectious manifestations, such as poor wound healing, overly exuberant inflammatory reactions, and autoimmune-type phenomena, including symptoms resembling those of inflammatory bowel disease symptoms or lupus. Prophylactic use of antibiotics can forestall a significant proportion of bacterial infections; prophylactic antifungal agents and interferon-γ are administered to some patients. Bone marrow transplantation and gene therapy may eventually have a role in the treatment of this disorder. The most common cause of death is infection by *Aspergillus*. The mortality rate is an estimated 2% to 5% per year.

Pathologic Features

Lymphadenopathy is common in CGD. Microscopic examination of enlarged lymph nodes reveals non-necrotizing or necrotizing granulomas with suppurative necrosis and occasional acute lymphadenitis.[124] Diagnosis can be established by the nitroblue tetrazolium reduction test or with chemiluminescent or fluorescent assays of oxidase activity or assays that detect peroxide. If the specific genetic defect is known, prenatal diagnosis can be performed.

Differential Diagnosis

Based on morphologic findings in an involved lymph node, the differential diagnosis includes a variety of other types of necrotizing lymphadenitis, including *Bartonella* infection, atypical mycobacterial lymphadenitis, brucellosis, and others. The lack of specificity of the pathologic findings and the rarity of the disease often result in delay, sometimes for years, in establishing a diagnosis. CGD is distinctive in that there are recurrent, often severe, pyogenic infections, usually beginning in the first year of life and almost always present by the age of 2 years.[124-129]

Fungal Lymphadenitis

Fungal lymphadenitis is uncommon. Patients with fungal lymphadenitis are often immunosuppressed because of HIV infection, malignancy (most often, hematolymphoid neoplasia), or iatrogenic immunosuppression. Immunologically normal individuals are occasionally affected. *Histoplasma capsulatum* and *Cryptococcus neoformans* are the most common fungi to cause lymphadenitis. Symptomatic fungal lymphadenitis is usually not an isolated finding; patients often also have pulmonary involvement or disseminated disease. Immunocompetent patients who develop fungal pulmonary infection may also have hilar lymph node involvement. Lymphadenitis in this setting can be asymptomatic, although histoplasmosis involving mediastinal nodes may be associated with inflammation and severe scarring of the surrounding tissue, producing sclerosing mediastinitis. During institution of HAART in HIV+ patients harboring fungi, symptomatic fungal lymphadenitis may emerge as the patient becomes capable of mounting an immune response to the fungi.[130]

Infection is typically associated with necrotizing or nonnecrotizing granulomatous inflammation (Fig. 11-9). Granulomas may be poorly formed or absent in immunosuppressed patients. Fibrosis and even calcification may develop in old lesions, especially in cases of histoplasmosis. The differential diagnosis is similar to that of *M. tuberculosis* and atypical mycobacteria.[43,131-134]

Protozoal Lymphadenitis

Toxoplasmosis

Clinical Features

Although lymphadenitis due to other types of protozoal infection has been reported,[105] infection by *T. gondii* is the only one encountered with any frequency in the United States. Toxoplasmosis is a relatively common infectious disease.[135] Transmission occurs via contact with cat feces containing *Toxoplasma* oocysts or by ingestion of undercooked meat containing *Toxoplasma* cysts.[2] Most patients are children or young adults; *Toxoplasma* lymphadenitis is more common among females than males.

Toxoplasmosis may cause encephalitis, chorioretinitis, disseminated disease, and congenital infection, as well as lymphadenitis.[136] Immunodeficient patients are at risk for the more severe manifestations of toxoplasmosis. Among the various clinical manifestations, *Toxoplasma* lymphadenitis is the most common. Patients with *Toxoplasma* lymphadenitis typically have unilateral or bilateral cervical lymphadenopathy, especially in the posterior cervical area. They may have malaise or be asymptomatic.[137] Some patients have an atypical lymphocytosis. This type of lymphadenopathy was first described by Piringer-Kuchinka in 1952,[136] and it is sometimes called Piringer-Kuchinka lymphadenitis.

Patients with *Toxoplasma* lymphadenitis typically have a self-limited illness and need no specific therapy. Immunodeficient patients may develop lymphadenopathy but are at high risk for severe manifestations, especially encephalitis. Infection during pregnancy may be associated with fetal morbidity or mortality. Rarely, immunocompetent patients develop serious complications, such as myocarditis or encephalitis, which can be fatal.

Adults with more severe manifestations may respond to drug therapy. Congenital infection may cause irreversible damage.

Pathologic Features

Lymph nodes are slightly to moderately enlarged. The triad of histologic features classically associated with *Toxoplasma* lymphadenitis includes florid follicular hyperplasia; prominent bands of parasinusoidal and parafollicular monocytoid B cells; and many small, irregular paracortical clusters of histiocytes, some of which encroach on germinal centers (Fig. 11-10). Large granulomas and granulomas with necrosis are not features of *Toxoplasma* lymphadenitis. The monocytoid B cells are CD20+, CD5−, CD10−, bcl2−, bcl6−, and CD23−. Analysis of the immunoglobulin heavy chain genes of the monocytoid B cells of *Toxoplasma* lymphadenitis has shown that they are clonally related, with intraclonal variation. Preferential usage of certain V_H gene segments is also reported; it is suggested that this may be due to stimulation of the monocytoid B cells by a superantigen expressed by *T. gondii*.[138]

The microorganisms are identified in lymph nodes only rarely,[24] although *Toxoplasma* DNA has reportedly been identified by PCR.[139] The diagnosis can be confirmed by serologic studies; in 95% of cases with the classic triad of histologic findings, results of serology document infection by *T. gondii*.[135]

Differential Diagnosis

Other causes of reactive lymphoid hyperplasia with follicular hyperplasia and histiocytes form the differential diagnosis of *Toxoplasma* lymphadenitis. Early or partial nodal involvement by cat-scratch disease, sarcoidosis or mycobacterial infection, or primary or secondary syphilis, can result in an appearance that resembles *Toxoplasma* lymphadenitis, except that in none of

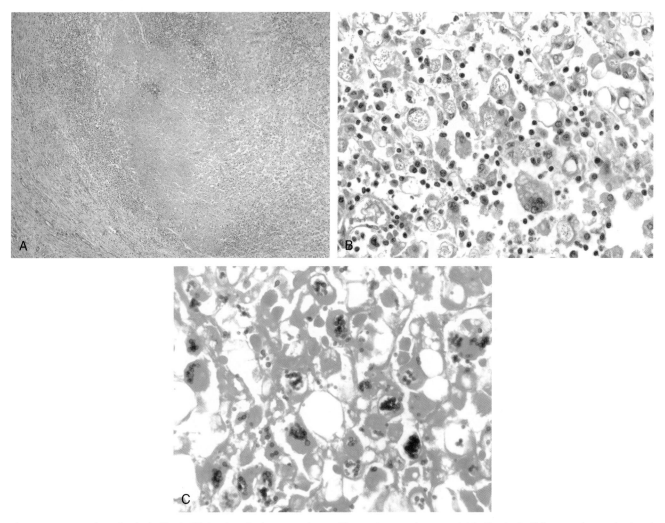

Figure 11-9. *Histoplasma* lymphadenitis. **A,** This lymph node shows granulomas with extensive necrosis, surrounded by fibrosis. **B,** High power shows uninucleated and multinucleated histiocytes, many containing numerous microorganisms with a dot-like appearance on this hematoxylin and eosin–stained section. **C,** The Grocott methenamine silver stain shows numerous intracellular yeast forms.

these disorders is there a tendency for epithelioid histiocytes to encroach on lymphoid follicles. Granulomas, necrosis, and necrotizing granulomas are unusual in toxoplasmosis. Leishmania can produce a lymphadenitis closely resembling that of *Toxoplasma*; it can also be associated with a necrotizing or non-necrotizing granulomatous lymphadenitis.[105] With *Leishmania* infection, however, microorganisms are usually identifiable in epithelioid histiocytes. Unlike *Toxoplasma*, *Leishmania* have kinetoplasts (see later discussion).[140]

Leishmanial Lymphadenitis

Clinical Features

Leishmaniasis is an infectious disease caused by *Leishmania* species and transmitted by sandflies (*Phlebotomus* species). Leishmaniasis occurs in the Middle East; in parts of Africa, South America, and Asia; and in Central America. Information about the patient's origin or travel history may provide a clue to the diagnosis. *Leishmania* can infect lymph nodes in two settings:

localized lymphadenopathy, often draining a focus of cutaneous infection, and widespread lymphadenopathy in the setting of visceral leishmaniasis (kala-azar).

Pathologic Features

The localized lymphadenitis associated with cutaneous leishmaniasis can show follicular and paracortical hyperplasia with necrotizing or non-necrotizing granulomatous inflammation, sometimes with numerous plasma cells. Plasma cells may contain crystalline inclusions of various shapes. The necrosis may be suppurative or caseating. The granulomas may resemble those seen in tuberculosis or mimic the granulomas of cat-scratch disease.[105,141] Identification of Leishman-Donovan bodies establishes a diagnosis.[140] In some cases, diagnosis can be established by cytologic examination of a fine-needle aspiration specimen.[140]

In visceral leishmaniasis, organisms reside in mononuclear phagocytes, but follicular hyperplasia and paracortical hyperplasia may not be prominent, and discrete granulomas are typically

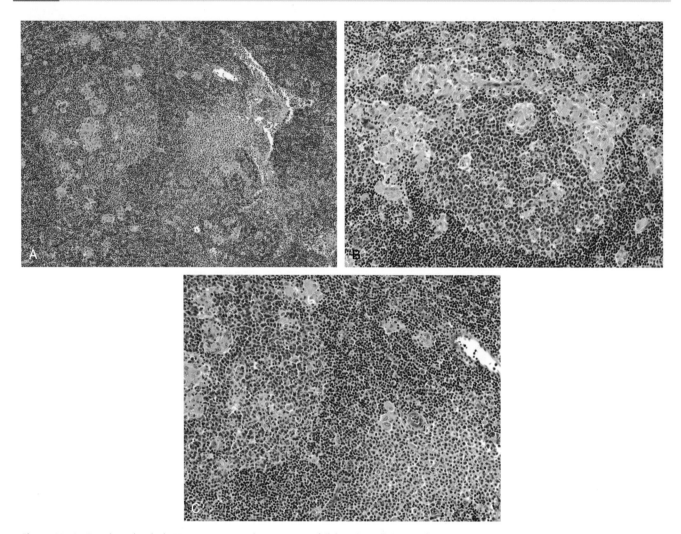

Figure 11-10. *Toxoplasma* lymphadenitis. **A,** Low power shows a reactive follicle with small clusters of epithelioid histiocytes outside and within follicle centers. An aggregate of monocytoid B cells with pale cytoplasm is present to the right of the follicle. **B,** A reactive follicle center is surrounded by clusters of epithelioid histiocytes; histiocytes also infiltrate the follicle center. **C,** A follicle containing clusters of epithelioid histiocytes *(left)* is seen adjacent to an aggregate of monocytoid B cells *(lower right)*.

absent.[141-143] The organisms can be seen on routinely stained sections, on Giemsa stains, and on reticulum stains, although they are sometimes present in small numbers.[142,143]

Pneumocystis jiroveci Lymphadenitis

Clinical Features

Pneumocystis jiroveci (formerly *Pneumocystis carinii*) lymphadenitis is a very rare disorder. Fewer than 1% of all cases of pneumocystosis affect extrapulmonary sites. Among extrapulmonary sites, however, lymph nodes are the site most commonly affected,[144,145] followed by liver and spleen (Fig. 11-11).[145] Patients are HIV+ individuals, children with congenital immunodeficiency, organ transplant recipients, and patients with malignancies. The HIV+ patients typically have an advanced stage of immunodeficiency and already carry a diagnosis of AIDS at the time of development of *P. jiroveci* lymphadenitis. Treatment with aerosolized pentamidine, which prevents *P. jiroveci*

pneumonia but not extrapulmonary infections, may lead to increased risk of *P. jiroveci* infection in extrapulmonary sites. Patients are typically febrile and quite ill. *P. jiroveci* lymphadenitis usually occurs in association with or after *P. jiroveci* pneumonia, or it occurs in the setting of widespread extrapulmonary infection. Infection may involve multiple lymph nodes. Specific symptoms vary depending on the site of disease. Treatment consists of prompt administration of the appropriate antibiotics. Without therapy, mortality is high.[103,144]

Pathologic Features

Diagnosis can be established with microscopic examination of a biopsy specimen of affected tissue, although, in many cases, the diagnosis is made only at autopsy. Involved tissues show frothy material with scattered helmet-shaped organisms that can be detected with a Grocott methenamine silver stain.[144] Lymphadenitis with concurrent infection by *P. jiroveci* and *M. tuberculosis* has been described.[103]

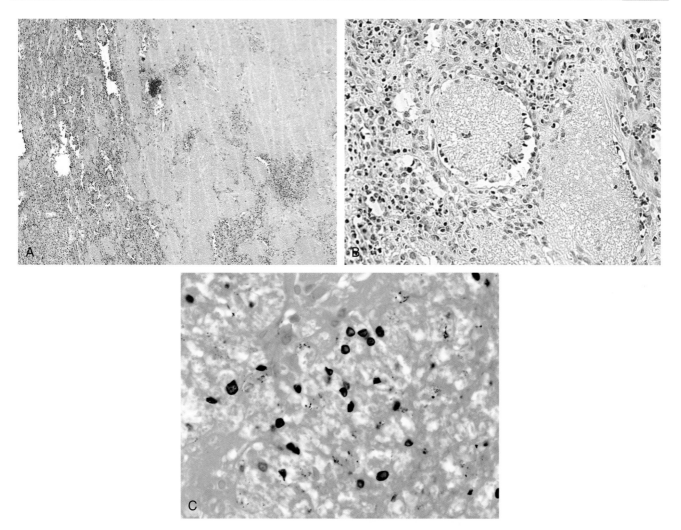

Figure 11-11. *Pneumocystis jiroveci* infection of the spleen in an HIV-positive patient (same case as in Fig. 11-7). **A,** Low-power view shows pale pink material replacing large zones of splenic parenchyma. **B,** High power shows frothy and granular pink material. **C,** Grocott methenamine silver stain shows occasional *Pneumocystis* organisms.

Filarial Infections

Clinical Features

Among helminthic infections, only filariasis is likely to be encountered in lymph nodes. Lymphatic filariasis affects an estimated 120 million persons worldwide. Among some, the disease is mild or asymptomatic, whereas others have a severe, disabling illness related to lymphatic obstruction. Manifestations include lymphedema, lymphadenopathy, elephantiasis of the extremities, and hydrocele.[146] Most cases are due to infection by *Wuchereria bancrofti*, which affects patients in equatorial Africa, India, the Mediterranean coast, the Caribbean, the eastern and northern coastal areas of South America, and some parts of Central America.[147,148] *Brugia malayi*, another type of lymphatic filaria, affects patients in coastal areas of Southeast Asia and India.[147,148] Another source of infection, particularly for individuals living in the United States who have not traveled to an endemic area, is one of the various zoonotic *Brugia* species. Typically, in zoonotic infections, only a single adult worm is present, and excision of the involved lymph node is curative.[147] Patients with *W. bancrofti* or *B. malayi* infection require additional anthelminthic therapy.

Pathologic Features

Histologic examination reveals adult worms in lymphatics and in lymph nodes. Within lymph nodes, the worms may be found within sinuses. Lymph nodes typically show prominent hyperplastic changes, which may include follicular hyperplasia, monocytoid B-cell hyperplasia, and a mixed infiltrate of lymphocytes, plasma cells, eosinophils, and neutrophils. When the worms present are degenerated or dead, there may be a particularly striking infiltrate of eosinophils, sometimes with formation of eosinophilic microabscesses, as well as granuloma formation. Dead worms may undergo dystrophic calcification.[147] Capsular and intranodal fibrosis may be prominent. *Brugia* species have smaller maximum midbody diameters (approximately 160 μm for females and 90 μm for males), compared with *Wuchereria* species (females, 250 μm; males, 150 μm).[147,148] Serial sections may be required to identify the worm (Fig. 11-12).[147]

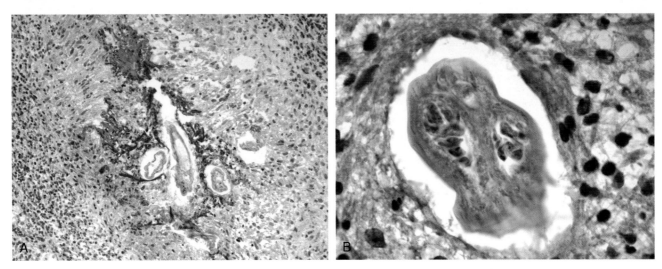

Figure 11-12. Filarial lymphadenitis. **A,** Low-power view shows an adult worm surrounded by palisading granulomatous inflammation. **B,** High power shows a cross-section of the worm distinct cuticle and oviducts.

Castleman Disease

The term *Castleman disease* encompasses a heterogeneous group of disorders with some overlapping histologic features but with differing etiologies and widely differing clinical features. Castleman disease occurs in two clinical forms: localized and multicentric. Almost all HIV+ patients and about half of HIV− patients with multicentric Castleman disease have evidence of HHV-8 infection, and HHV-8 is believed to underlie the development of Castleman disease in these cases.[149,150] The discussion here focuses on multicentric Castleman disease related to HHV-8 infection, an uncommon cause of lymphadenopathy that straddles the border between an infectious disease and a lymphoproliferative disorder.

Multicentric Castleman Disease

Multicentric Castleman disease is a systemic disease with a poor prognosis. Most patients are middle-aged to older adults; HIV+ patients are overall younger than HIV− patients and show a striking male preponderance.[151-153] Patients present with multifocal peripheral and/or internal lymphadenopathy, often accompanied by hepatomegaly, splenomegaly and peripheral edema. Patients almost always have some systemic symptoms, including fever, fatigue, weight loss, or night sweats. Common laboratory abnormalities include anemia, polyclonal hypergammaglobulinemia, elevated C-reactive protein, and elevated erythrocyte sedimentation rate.[151,152,154,155] A few patients have a serum M component.[151] Infrequently, HHV-8+ multicentric Castleman disease without concomitant HIV infection is associated with the POEMS syndrome (polyneuropathy, organomegaly, endocrinopathy, M component, and skin changes).[150]

A majority of HIV+ patients and a minority of HIV− patients have cutaneous Kaposi sarcoma.[150,151,154] The etiology may be related to elevated levels of human or viral interleukin 6 (IL-6), possibly produced in the affected tissues in follicular dendritic cells.[156] IL-6 is believed to be responsible for the plasmacytosis seen in multicentric Castleman disease.[154] Serum levels of IL-6

and also of IL-10 appear to correlate with disease activity.[151,156,157] Some patients respond to treatment with chemotherapy, steroids, irradiation, antiviral agents, or anti-IL-6 antibodies.[152,155,158] Promising results have been described with the use of rituximab in HIV-associated multicentric Castleman disease.[151] However, the best therapy for this disorder has not been established.[155,158] It is suggested that radiographic studies including positron-emission tomographic scanning and determination of plasma HHV-8 levels can be helpful in monitoring disease activity and response to treatment.[151,152]

Patients with multicentric Castleman disease are at increased risk for severe infections and also have an increased incidence of lymphoma, in particular HHV-8+ primary effusion lymphoma and HHV-8+ plasmablastic lymphoma[149,159]; the latter is also known as large B-cell lymphoma arising in HHV-8–associated multicentric Castleman disease.[160] The prognosis of patients with multicentric Castleman disease has traditionally been considered poor, but some of the morbidity and mortality associated with this disorder, particularly among HIV+ patients, stems from the development of lymphoma and opportunistic infections and the development or progression of Kaposi sarcoma. Immune reconstitution with HAART may therefore improve the outlook for patients with multicentric Castleman disease.[154,161]

Cases of multicentric Castleman disease may have the histologic features of plasma cell Castleman disease, hyaline-vascular Castleman disease, or mixed-type Castleman disease.[150] Some cases, almost all in HIV+ patients, have pathologic features of so-called plasmablastic Castleman disease (discussed separately).

The familiar hyaline-vascular variant of Castleman disease is characterized by lymphoid follicles with small, hyalinized germinal centers and broad mantle zones. Each follicle may contain one or more germinal centers; some follicles contain no recognizable germinal center. The germinal centers contain an increased proportion of follicular dendritic cells and endothelial cells. Mantle-zone lymphocytes are arranged in concentric rings (onion-skin pattern) around the germinal center. Follicles are often radially penetrated by a blood vessel (lollipop follicle). The interfollicular region shows increased numbers of high endothelial venules and of small vessels with flat endothelium and hyalinized walls. Lymphocytes are fewer in number than in a normal lymph node, and there may be an admixture of scattered plasma cells, few immunoblasts, few eosinophils, and clusters of plasmacytoid monocytes. Sheets of plasma cells are absent. Epithelioid histiocytes and granulomas are inconspicuous or absent. In some cases, patent sinuses may be found in residual normal lymphoid tissue at the periphery of the lesion, but in general, they are absent within the lesion. Fibrosis is common peripherally and also in bands running through the lesion. There may be prominent perivascular fibrosis.[156,162-164]

The plasma cell variant of Castleman disease is characterized by enlarged lymph nodes with sheets of mature plasma cells in the interfollicular area, sometimes with Russell bodies; occasional immunoblasts may be seen. The follicles may be hyperplastic follicles of the usual type or hyaline-vascular follicles or a mixture of the two types of follicles. Blood vessels are less conspicuous than in hyaline-vascular Castleman disease. Sinuses are usually obliterated but may be patent focally.

The mixed or transitional type of Castleman disease has features intermediate between those of hyaline-vascular Castleman disease and the plasma cell variant of Castleman disease.

Plasmablastic Castleman Disease

Subsequent to the finding of HHV-8 in many cases of multicentric Castleman disease,[149,150] cases of multicentric Castleman disease in HIV+ patients were described in which immunoblasts or plasmablasts in expanded follicle mantles were HHV-8+ and expressed monotypic immunoglobulin M λ chain. Interfollicular plasma cells were polytypic. This entity was named plasmablastic Castleman disease. Additional studies showed that the plasmablasts could also cluster and replace part of the follicle (microlymphoma) or proliferate to form sheets of plasmablasts (frank lymphoma), referred to in the classification of the World Health Organization as large B-cell lymphoma arising in HHV-8–associated multicentric Castleman disease.[160] The monotypic plasmablasts in plasmablastic Castleman disease and in microlymphomas are usually polyclonal by molecular techniques, although frank lymphomas are usually clonal.[165,166] This raises the question of whether HHV-8 preferentially infects λ+ lymphoid cells.

The plasmablasts are characteristically negative for EBV, although we have seen a case of multicentric Castleman disease in an HIV+ man complicated by the development of EBV+ plasmablastic microlymphoma and then frank lymphoma.[153] In our case, a hemophagocytic syndrome developed.[153] Hemophagocytic syndromes are typically precipitated by infections, often by EBV, and may be seen in association with EBV+ malignancies of natural killer (NK) cell lineage, including extranodal NK/T-cell lymphoma, nasal type, and aggressive NK-cell leukemia.[153,167,168] Rare cases of hemophagocytic syndrome have also been described in association with HHV-8 infection.[169] In one recent case report, an HIV– man developed an HHV-8+, EBV– plasmablastic microlymphoma associated with a hemophagocytic syndrome, with a rapidly fatal disease course.[170]

Careful examination of lymph nodes with multicentric Castleman disease often reveals concurrent involvement by Kaposi sarcoma; foci of Kaposi sarcoma are often small and tend to involve the nodal capsule, trabeculae, or hilum.[171]

Differential Diagnosis

In cases of HHV-8+ multicentric Castleman disease in HIV+ patients, the histologic features may not be as distinctive as in classic hyaline-vascular Castleman disease or in the plasma cell variant of Castleman disease in immunocompetent hosts. The lymph nodes may have a depleted appearance, and in some cases only careful examination reveals a few follicles with features suggesting Castleman disease. Performing a stain for HHV-8 on lymph nodes with changes that are suggestive of Castleman disease helps avoid overlooking the diagnosis.

REFERENCES

1. Burkitt D: The discovery of Burkitt's lymphoma. Cancer 1983; 51:1777-1786.
2. Hurt C, Tammaro D: Diagnostic evaluation of mononucleosis-like illnesses. Am J Med 2007;120:911.e1-911.e8.
3. Abbondanzo SL, Sato N, Straus SE, et al: Acute infectious mononucleosis: CD30 (Ki-1) antigen expression and histologic correlations (see comments). Am J Clin Pathol 1990;93:698-702.
4. Childs CC, Parham DM, Berard CW: Infectious mononucleosis: The spectrum of morphologic changes simulating lymphoma in lymph nodes and tonsils. Am J Surg Pathol 1987;11:122-132.
5. Custer RP, Smith EB: The pathology of infectious mononucleosis. Blood 1948;3:830-857.
6. Mroczek EC, Weisenburger DD, Grierson HL, et al: Fatal infectious mononucleosis and virus-associated hemophagocytic syndrome. Arch Pathol Lab Med 1987;111:530-535.
7. Salvador AH, Harrison EGJ, Kyle RA: Lymphadenopathy due to infectious mononucleosis: Its confusion with malignant lymphoma. Cancer 1971;27:1029-1040.
8. Louissaint A, Soupir C, Ganguly A, et al: Infectious mononucleosis: Morphology and immunophenotype in cervical lymph nodes and Waldeyer's ring. Mod Pathol 2008;21(Suppl 1):263A.
9. Niedobitek G, Herbst H, Young LS, et al: Patterns of Epstein-Barr virus infection in non-neoplastic lymphoid tissue. Blood 1992;790:2520-2526.
10. Segal GH, Kjeldsberg CR, Smith GP, et al: CD30 antigen expression in florid immunoblastic proliferations: A clinicopathologic study of 14 cases. Am J Clin Pathol 1994;102:292-298.
11. Shin SS, Berry GJ, Weiss LM: Infectious mononucleosis: Diagnosis by in situ hybridization in two cases with atypical features. Am J Surg Pathol 1991;15:625-631.
12. Kojima M, Nakamura S, Shimizu K, et al: Reactive lymphoid hyperplasia of the lymph nodes with giant follicles: A clinicopathologic study of 14 Japanese cases, with special reference to Epstein-Barr virus infection. Int J Surg Pathol 2005;13:267-272.
13. Abbondanzo SL, Irey NS, Frizzera G: Dilantin-associated lymphadenopathy: Spectrum of histopathologic patterns. Am J Surg Pathol 1995;19:675-686.
14. Hartsock RJ: Postvaccinial lymphadenitis: Hyperplasia of lymphoid tissue that simulates malignant lymphomas. Cancer 1968;21:632-649.
15. Hartsock RJ, Bellanti JA: Postvaccinial lymphadenitis. GP 1969;39:99-105.
16. Segal GH, Clough JD, Tubbs RR: Autoimmune and iatrogenic causes of lymphadenopathy. (Review). Semin Oncol 1993;20:611-626.
17. Abramowitz A, Livni N, Morag A, et al: An immunoperoxidase study of cytomegalovirus mononucleosis. Arch Pathol Lab Med 1982;106:115-118.
18. Younes M, Podesta A, Helie M, et al: Infection of T but not B lymphocytes by cytomegalovirus in lymph node: An immunophenotypic study. Am J Surg Pathol 1991;15:75-80.

19. Abgueguen P, Delbos V, Chennebault JM, et al: Vascular thrombosis and acute cytomegalovirus infection in immunocompetent patients: Report of 2 cases and literature review. Clin Infect Dis 2003;36:E134-E139.

20. Sinha AK, Lovett M, Pillay G: Cytomegalovirus infection with lymphadenopathy. BMJ 1970;3:163.

21. Weller TH: The cytomegaloviruses: Ubiquitous agents with protean clinical manifestations: 1. (Review). N Engl J Med 1971;285:203-214.

22. Rushin JM, Riordan GP, Heaton RB, et al. Cytomegalovirus-infected cells express Leu-M1 antigen: A potential source of diagnostic error. Am J Pathol 1990;136:989-995.

23. Case records of the Massachusetts General Hospital: Case 7-1995. N Engl J Med 1995;332:663-671.

24. Ferry J, Harris N: Atlas of Lymphoid Hyperplasia and Lymphoma, 1st ed. Bordin G (ed): Atlases in Diagnostic Surgical Pathology. Philadelphia: WB Saunders, 1997, p 271.

25. Parentin F, Molin GD, D'Agaro P, et al: Parinaud's oculoglandular syndrome due to herpes simplex virus type 1. Ocul Immunol Inflamm 2007;15:139-141.

26. Audouin J, Le Tourneau A, Aubert JP, et al: Herpes simplex virus lymphadenitis mimicking tumoral relapse in a patient with Hodgkin's disease in remission. Virch Archiv A Pathol Anat Histopathol 1985;408:313-321.

27. Epstein JI, Ambinder RF, Kuhajda FP, et al: Localized herpes simplex lymphadenitis. Am J Clin Pathol 1986;86:444-448.

28. Gaffey MJ, Ben-Ezra JM, Weiss LM: Herpes simplex lymphadenitis. Am J Clin Pathol 1991;95:709-714.

29. Higgins J, Warnke R: Herpes lymphadenitis in association with chronic lymphocytic leukemia. Cancer 1999;86:1210-1215.

30. Howat AJ, Campbell AR, Stewart DJ: Generalized lymphadenopathy due to herpes simplex virus type 1. Histopathology 1991;19:563-564.

31. Miliauskas JR, Leong AS: Localized herpes simplex lymphadenitis: Report of three cases and review of the literature. (Review). Histopathology 1991;19:355-360.

32. Tamaru J, Mikata A, Horie H, et al: Herpes simplex lymphadenitis: Report of two cases with review of the literature. (Review). Am J Surg Pathol 1990;14:571-577.

33. Taxy JB, Tillawi I, Goldman PM: Herpes simplex lymphadenitis: An unusual presentation with necrosis and viral particles. Arch Pathol Lab Med 1985;109:1043-1044.

34. Wat PJ, Strickler JG, Myers JL, et al: Herpes simplex infection causing acute necrotizing tonsillitis. Mayo Clinic Proc 1994;69:269-271.

35. Witt M, Torno M, Sun N, et al: Herpes simplex virus lymphadenitis: Case report and review of the literature. Clin Infect Dis 2002;34:1-6.

36. Miliauskas JR, Webber BL: Disseminated varicella at autopsy in children with cancer. Cancer 1984;53:1518-1525.

37. Patterson SD, Larson EB, Corey L: Atypical generalized zoster with lymphadenitis mimicking lymphoma. N Engl J Med 1980;302:848-851.

38. Vanhems P, Allard R, Cooper D, et al: Acute human immunodeficiency virus type 1 disease as a mononucleosis-like illness: Is the diagnosis too restrictive? Clin Infect Dis 1997;24:965-970.

39. Dave SP, Pernas FG, Roy S: The benign lymphoepithelial cyst and a classification system for lymphocytic parotid gland enlargement in the pediatric HIV population. Laryngoscope 2007;117:106-113.

40. Harris N: Lymphoid proliferations of the salivary glands. Am J Clin Pathol Pathol Patterns 1999;111(Suppl 1):S94-S103.

41. Shahab I, Osborne B, Butler J: Nasopharyngeal lymphoid tissue masses in patients with human immunodeficiency virus-1: Histologic findings and clinical correlation. Cancer 1994;74:3083-3088.

42. Ioachim HL, Gonin W, Roy M, et al: Persistent lymphadenopathies in people at high risk for HIV infection: Clinicopathologic correlations and long-term follow-up in 79 cases. Am J Clin Pathol 1990;93:208-218.

43. Quijano G, Siminovich M, Drut R: Histopathologic findings in the lymphoid and reticuloendothelial system in pediatric HIV infection: A postmortem study. Pediatr Pathol Lab Med 1997;17:845-856.

44. Said JW: AIDS-related lymphadenopathies. Semin Diagn Pathol 1988;5:365-375.

45. Wenig BM, Thompson LDR, Frankel SS, et al: Lymphoid changes of the nasopharyngeal and palatine tonsils that are indicative of human immunodeficiency virus infection: A clinicopathologic study of 12 cases. Am J Surg Pathol 1996;20:572-587.

46. Burns BF, Wood GS, Dorfman RF: The varied histopathology of lymphadenopathy in the homosexual male. Am J Surg Pathol 1985;9:287-297.

47. Alos L, Navarrete P, Morente V, et al: Immunoarchitecture of lymphoid tissue in HIV-infection during antiretroviral therapy correlates with viral persistence. Mod Pathol 2005;18:127-136.

48. Maric I, Bryant R, Abu-Asab M, et al: Human herpesvirus-6-associated acute lymphadenitis in immunocompetent adults. Mod Pathol 2004;17:1427-1433.

49. Yanagi S, Nomura Y, Masuda K, et al: Early diagnosis of Kawasaki disease in patients with cervical lymphadenopathy. Pediatr Int 2008;50:179-183.

50. Burns J, Glode M: Kawasaki syndrome. Lancet 2004;364:533-544.

51. Du Z, Zhang T, Liang L, et al: Epidemiologic picture of Kawasaki disease in Beijing from 1995 through 1999. Pediatr Infect Dis J 2002;21:103-107.

52. Kao CH, Hwang B, Jan SL, et al: Kawasaki disease presenting as cervical lymphadenitis or deep neck infection. J Nucl Cardiol 2002;9:41-46.

53. Muzaffer MA, Al-Mayouf SM: Pattern of clinical features of Kawasaki disease. Saudi Med J 2002;23:409-412.

54. Shulman S, Rowley A: Advances in Kawasaki disease. Eur J Pediatr 2004;163:285-291.

55. Bosch X, Guilabert A, Miquel R, et al: Enigmatic Kikuchi-Fujimoto disease: A comprehensive review. Am J Clin Pathol 2004;122:141-152.

56. Cho MS, Choi HJ, Park HK, et al: Questionable role of human herpesviruses in the pathogenesis of Kikuchi disease. Arch Pathol Lab Med 2007;131:604-609.

57. Dorfman R, Berry G: Kikuchi's histiocytic necrotizing lymphadenitis: An analysis of 108 cases with emphasis on differential diagnosis. Semin Diagn Pathol 1988;5:329-345.

58. Kikuchi M, Takeshita M, Eimoto T, et al: Histiocytic necrotizing lymphadenitis: Clinicopathologic, immunologic and HLA typing study. In Hanaoka M, Kadin ME, Mikata A (eds): Lymphoid Malignancy: Immunocytology and Cytogenetics. New York, Fields and Wood, 1990, pp 251-257.

59. Kuo T: Kikuchi's disease (histiocytic necrotizing lymphadenitis): A clinicopathologic study of 79 cases with an analysis of histologic subtypes, immunohistology and DNA ploidy. Am J Surg Pathol 1995;19:798-809.

60. Lin H, Su C, Huang C, et al: Kikuchi's disease: A review and analysis of 61 cases. Otolaryngol Head Neck Surg 2003;128:650-653.

61. Maeda N, Yamashita Y, Kimura H, et al: Quantitative analysis of herpesvirus load in the lymph nodes of patients with histiocytic necrotizing lymphadenitis using a real-time PCR assay. Diagn Mol Pathol 2006;15:49-55.

62. Tsang WYW, Chan JKC, Ng CS: Kikuchi's lymphadenitis: A morphologic analysis of 75 cases with special reference to unusual features. Am J Surg Pathol 1994;18:219-231.

63. Yufu Y, Matsumoto M, Miyamura T, et al: Parvovirus B19-associated haemophagocytic syndrome with lymphadenopathy resembling histiocytic necrotizing lymphadenitis (Kikuchi's disease). Br J Haematol 1997;96:868-871.

64. Bataille V, Harland CC, Behrens J, et al: Kikuchi disease (histiocytic necrotizing lymphadenitis) in association with HTLV1. Br J Dermatol 1997;136:610-612.

65. Pasquinucci S, Donisi PM, Cavinato F, et al: Kikuchi's disease in a patient infected with AIDS. AIDS 1991;5:235.

66. Sumiyoshi Y, Kikuchi M, Takeshita M, et al: Alpha-interferon in Kikuchi's disease. Virchows Arch B Cell Pathol 1991;61:201-207.

67. Sumiyoshi Y, Kikuchi M, Takeshita M, et al: Immunohistologic studies of Kikuchi's disease. Hum Pathol 1993;24:1114-1119.

68. Facchetti F, deWolf-Peters C, Mason D, et al: Plasmacytoid T cells: Immunohistochemical evidence for their monocyte/macrophage origin. Am J Pathol 1988;133:15-21.

69. Hansmann ML, Kikuchi M, Wacker HH, et al: Immunohistochemical monitoring of plasmacytoid cells in lymph node sections of Kikuchi-Fujimoto disease by a new pan-macrophage antibody Ki-M1P. Hum Pathol 1992;23:676-680.

70. Beiler H, Eckstein T, Roth H, Daum R: Specific and nonspecific lymphadenitis in childhood: etiology, diagnosis, and therapy. Pediatr Surg Intern 1997;12:108-112.

71. Segal GH, Perkins SL, Kjeldsberg CR: Benign lymphadenopathies in children and adolescents. Semin Diagn Pathol 1995;12:288-302.

72. Adal KA, Cockerell CJ, Petri WA: Cat scratch disease, bacillary angiomatosis and other infections due to *Rochalimaea*. N Engl J Med 1994;330:1509-1515.

73. Bergmans AM, Groothedde JW, Schellekens JF, et al: Etiology of cat scratch disease: Comparison of polymerase chain reaction detection of *Bartonella* (formerly *Rochalimaea*) and *Afipia felis* DNA with serology and skin tests. J Infect Dis 1995;171:916-923.

74. Carithers HA: Cat-scratch disease: An overview based on a study of 1,200 patients. Am J Dis Child 1985;139:1124-1133.

75. Grossniklaus HE: The cat scratch disease-bacillary angiomatosis puzzle. (Editorial). Am J Ophthalmol 1994;118:246-248.

76. Min KW, Reed JA, Welch DF, et al: Morphologically variable bacilli of cat scratch disease are identified by immunocytochemical labeling with antibodies to *Rochalimaea henselae*. Am J Clin Pathol 1994;101:607-610.

77. Lamps LW, Scott MA: Cat-scratch disease: Historic, clinical, and pathologic perspectives. Am J Clin Pathol 2004;121(Suppl):S71-S80.

78. Wear D, Margileth A, Hadfield T, et al: Cat-scratch disease: A bacterial infection. Science 1983;221:1403-1404.

79. Borboli S, Afshari NA, Watkins L, et al: Presumed oculoglandular syndrome from *Bartonella quintana*. Ocul Immunol Inflamm 2007;15:41-43.

80. Ben-Ami R, Ephros M, Avidor B, et al: Cat-scratch disease in elderly patients. Clin Infect Dis 2005;41:969-974.

81. Massei F, Messina F, Talini I, et al: Widening of the clinical spectrum of *Bartonella henselae* infection as recognized through serodiagnostics. Eur J Pediatr 2000;159:416-419.

82. Koehler JE, Duncan LM: Case records of the Massachusetts General Hospital. Case 30-2005: A 56-year-old man with fever and axillary lymphadenopathy. N Engl J Med 2005;353:1387-1394.

83. Ridder-Schroter R, Marx A, Beer M, et al: Abscess-forming lymphadenopathy and osteomyelitis in children with *Bartonella henselae* infection. J Med Microbiol 2008;57(Pt 4):519-524.

84. Case records of the Massachusetts General Hospital. Case 22-1992: A 6 1/2-year-old girl with status epilepticus, cervical lymphadenopathy, pleural effusions, and respiratory distress (see comments). N Engl J Med 1992;326:1480-1489.

85. Miller-Catchpole R, Variakojis D, Vardiman JW, et al: Cat scratch disease: Identification of bacteria in seven cases of lymphadenitis. Am J Surg Pathol 1986;10:276-281.

86. Lin YY, Hsiao CH, Hsu YH, et al: Immunohistochemical study of lymph nodes in patients with cat scratch disease. J Formos Med Assoc 2006;105:911-917.

87. Ridder G, Boedeker C, Technau-Ihling K, et al: Role of cat-scratch disease in lymphadenopathy in the head and neck. Clin Infect Dis 2002;35:643-649.

88. Juskevicius R, Vnencak-Jones C: Pathologic quiz case: A 17-year-old renal transplant patient with persistent fever, pancytopenia, and axillary lymphadenopathy: Bacillary angiomatosis of the lymph node in the renal transplant recipient. Arch Pathol Lab Med 2004;128:e12-e14.

89. Case records of the Massachusetts General Hospital: Case 19-1993. N Engl J Med 1993;328:1406-1414.

90. Hartsock RJ, Halling LW, King FM: Luetic lymphadenitis: A clinical and histologic study of 20 cases. Am J Clin Pathol 1970;53:304-314.

91. Turner DR, Wright DJM: Lymphadenopathy in early syphilis. J Pathol 1973;110:305-308.

92. Oddo D, Carrasco G, Capdeville F, et al: Syphilitic tonsillitis presenting as an ulcerated tonsillar tumor with ipsilateral lymphadenopathy. Ann Diagn Pathol 2007;11:353-357.

93. Facchetti F, Incardona P, Lonardi S, et al: Nodal inflammatory pseudotumor caused by luetic infection. Am J Surg Pathol 2009;33:447-453.

94. Al-Shamahy HA, Wright SG: A study of 235 cases of human brucellosis in Sana'a, Republic of Yemen. East Mediterr Health J 2001;7:238-246.

95. Galanakis E, Bourantas K, Leveidiotou S, et al: Childhood brucellosis in north-western Greece: A retrospective analysis. Eur J Pediatr 1996;155:1-6.

96. Malik G: A clinical study of brucellosis in adults in the Asir region of southern Saudi Arabia. Am J Trop Med Hyg 1997;56:375-377.

97. Bem C, Patil P, Bharucha H: Importance of human immunodeficiency virus-associated lymphadenopathy and tuberculous lymphadenitis in patients undergoing lymph node biopsy in Zambia. Br J Surg 1996;83:75-78.

98. Moore DF Jr, Garrett C, Goyle V, et al: Diagnostic aspects of cervical lymphadenopathy in children in the developing world: A study of 1,877 surgical specimens. Am J Clin Oncol 2003;26:473-476.

99. Simon HB: Infections due to mycobacteria. Infect Dis 1995;7:1-25.

100. Chesney P: Nontuberculous mycobacteria. Pediatr Rev 2002;23:300-309.

101. O'Brien DP, Currie BJ, Krause VL: Nontuberculous mycobacterial disease in northern Australia: A case series and review of the literature. Clin Infect Dis 2000;31:958-967.

102. Panesar J, Higgins K, Daya H, et al: Nontuberculous mycobacterial cervical adenitis: A ten-year retrospective review. Laryngoscope 2003;113:149-154.

103. Khawcharoenporn T, Apisarnthanarak A, Sakonlaya D, et al: Dual infection with *Mycobacterium tuberculosis* and *Pneumocystis jiroveci* lymphadenitis in a patient with HIV infection: Case report and review of the literature. AIDS Patient Care STDS 2006;20:1-5.

104. Shelburne SA 3rd, Hamill RJ: The immune reconstitution inflammatory syndrome. AIDS Rev 2003;5:67-79.

105. Azadeh B, Sells PG, Ejeckam GC, et al: Localized leishmania lymphadenitis: Immunohistochemical studies. Am J Clin Pathol 1994;102:11-15.

106. Banerjee AK, Tungekar MF, Derias N, et al: Lymph node cytology in Wegener's granulomatosis. Diagn Cytopathol 2001;25:112-114.

107. Hashizume T, Yamaguchi T, Matsushita K: Supraclavicular and axillary lymphadenopathy as the initial manifestation in Wegener's granulomatosis. Clin Rheumatol 2002;21:525-527.

108. Ahmad Al-Bhlal L: Pathologic findings for bacille Calmette-Guerin infections in immunocompetent and immunocompromised patients. Am J Clin Pathol 2000;113:703-708.

109. Evans M, Smith N, Thornton C, et al: Atypical mycobacterial lymphadenitis in childhood: A clinicopathological study of 17 cases. J Clin Pathol 1998;51:925-927.

110. Goraya JS, Virdi VS: Bacille Calmette-Guerin lymphadenitis. Postgrad Med J 2002;78:327-329.

111. Kanlikama M, Gokalp A: Management of mycobacterial cervical lymphadenitis. World J Surg 1997;21:516-519.

112. Suskind D, Handler S, Tom L, et al: Nontuberculous mycobacterial cervical adenitis. Clin Pediatr (Phila) 1997;36:403-409.

113. Turnbull F, McIntyre P, Achat H, et al: National study of adverse reactions after vaccination with bacille Calmette-Guerin. Clin Infect Dis 2002;34:447-453.

114. Relman DA, Schmidt TM, McDermott RP, et al: Identification of the uncultured bacillus of Whipple's disease. N Engl J Med 1992;327:293-301.

115. Black-Schaffer B: The tinctorial demonstration of a glycoprotein in Whipple's disease. Proc Soc Exp Biol Med 1949;72:225-227.

116. Southern JF, Moscicki RA, Magro C, et al: Lymphedema, lymphocytic myocarditis, and sarcoidlike granulomatosis: Manifestations of Whipple's disease. JAMA 1989;261:1467-1470.

117. Craven DE, Tronic BS, Scholz FJ, et al: A man with chronic leg edema, purpuric skin lesions, and abdominal lymphadenopathy. Clin Infect Dis 2005;41:519-520, 557-559.

118. Alkan S, Beals T, Schnitzer B: Primary diagnosis of Whipple disease manifesting as lymphadenopathy: Use of polymerase chain reaction for detection of Tropheryma whippelii. Am J Clin Pathol 2001; 116:898-904.

119. Caples S, Petrovic L, Ryu J: Successful treatment of Whipple disease diagnosed 36 years after symptom onset. Mayo Clin Proc 2001;76:1063-1066.

120. Durand D, Lecomte C, Cathebras P, et al: Whipple disease: Clinical review of 52 cases. Medicine (Baltimore) 1997;76:170-184.

121. Dutly F, Altwegg M: Whipple's disease and "Tropheryma whippelii." Clin Microbiol Rev 2001;14:561-583.

122. Ereno C, Lopez JI, Elizalde JM, et al: A case of Whipple's disease presenting as supraclavicular lymphadenopathy: A case report. APMIS 1993;101:865-868.

123. Magira EE, Gounaris T, Sioula E: Whipple's disease: Multiple hospital admissions of a man with diarrhoea, fever and arthralgia. J Infect 2005;51:E35-E37.

124. Levine S, Smith VV, Malone M, et al: Histopathological features of chronic granulomatous disease (CGD) in childhood. Histopathology 2005;47:508-516.

125. Case records of the Massachusetts General Hospital: Case 35-1993. N Engl J Med 1993;329:714-721.

126. Liese J, Kloos S, Jendrossek V, et al: Long-term follow-up and outcome of 39 patients with chronic granulomatous disease. J Pediatr 2000;137:687-693.

127. Movahedi M, Aghamohammadi A, Rezaei N, et al: Chronic granulomatous disease: A clinical survey of 41 patients from the Iranian primary immunodeficiency registry. Int Arch Allergy Immunol 2004;134:253-259.

128. Segal BH, Leto TL, Gallin JI, et al: Genetic, biochemical, and clinical features of chronic granulomatous disease. Medicine (Baltimore). 2000;79:170-200.

129. Winkelstein JA, Marino MC, Johnston RB Jr, et al: Chronic granulomatous disease: Report on a national registry of 368 patients. Medicine (Baltimore). 2000;79:155-169.

130. Trevenzoli M, Cattelan A, Rea F, et al: Mediastinitis due to cryptococcal infection: A new clinical entity in the HAART era. J Infect 2002;45:173-179.

131. Chan YH, Wong KM, Lee KC, et al: Pneumonia and mesenteric lymphadenopathy caused by disseminated Penicillium marneffei infection in a cadaveric renal transplant recipient. Transplant Infect Dis 2004;6:28-32.

132. Neubauer MA, Bodensteiner DC: Disseminated histoplasmosis in patients with AIDS. South Med J 1992;85:1166-1170.

133. Weinberg GA, Kleiman MB, Grosfeld JL, et al: Unusual manifestations of histoplasmosis in childhood. Pediatrics 1983;72:99-105.

134. Witt D, McKay D, Schwam L, et al. Acquired immune deficiency syndrome presenting as bone marrow and mediastinal cryptococcosis. Am J Med 1987;82:149-150.

135. Tuzuner N, Dogusoy G, Demirksen C, et al: Value of lymph node biopsy in the diagnosis of toxoplasmic lymphadenitis. J Laryngol Otol 1996;110:348-352.

136. Rose I: Morphology and diagnostics of human toxoplasmosis. Diagn Pathol 1997;142:257-270.

137. Montoya JG, Remington JS: Studies on the serodiagnosis of toxoplasmic lymphadenitis. Clin Infect Dis 1995;20:781-789.

138. Lazzi S, Bellan C, Tiacci E, et al: IRTA1+ monocytoid B cells in reactive lymphadenitis show a unique topographic distribution and immunophenotype and a peculiar usage and mutational pattern of IgVH genes. J Pathol 2006;209:56-66.

139. Lin M, Kuo T: Specificity of the histopathological triad for the diagnosis of toxoplasmic lymphadenitis: Polymerase chain reaction study. Pathol Int 2001;51:619-623.

140. Daneshbod Y, Daneshbod K, Khademi B, et al: New cytologic clues in localized Leishmania lymphadenitis. Acta Cytol 2007;51:699-710.

141. Gaafar A, Ismail A, El Kadaro A, et al: Necrotizing and suppurative lymphadenitis in Leishmania major infections. Trop Med Int Health 1996;1:243-250.

142. Connor D, Neafie R: Cutaneous leishmaniasis. In Binford C, Connor D (eds): Pathology of Tropical and Extraordinary Diseases. Washington, DC, Armed Forces Institute of Pathology, 1976, pp 258-264.

143. Neafie R, Connor D: Visceral leishmaniasis. In Binford C, Connor D (eds): Pathology of Tropical and Extraordinary Diseases. Washington, DC, Armed Forces Institute of Pathology, 1976, pp 265-272.

144. Raviglione M: Extrapulmonary pneumocystosis. Rev Infect Dis 1990;12:1127-1138.

145. Anuradha SA: Extrapulmonary Pneumocystis carinii infection in an AIDS patient: A case report. Acta Cytol 2007;51:599-601.

146. Fox LM, Furness BW, Haser JK, et al: Ultrasonographic examination of Haitian children with lymphatic filariasis: A longitudinal assessment in the context of antifilarial drug treatment. Am J Trop Med Hyg 2005;72:642-648.

147. Elenitoba-Johnson KS, Eberhard ML, Dauphinais RM, et al: Zoonotic Brugian lymphadenitis: An unusual case with florid monocytoid B-cell proliferation. Am J Clin Pathol 1996;105:384-387.

148. Meyers W, Neafie R, Connor D: Bancroftian and Malayan filariasis. In Binford C, Connor D (eds): Pathology of Tropical and Extraordinary Diseases. Washington, DC, Armed Forces Institute of Pathology, 1976, pp 340-355.

149. Cesarman E, Knowles D: Kaposi's sarcoma-associated herpesvirus: A lymphotropic human herpesvirus associated with Kaposi's sarcoma, primary effusion lymphoma and multicentric Castleman's disease. Sem Diagn Pathol 1997;14:54-66.

150. Soulier J, Grollet L, Oksenhendler E, et al: Kaposi's sarcoma-associated herpesvirus-like DNA sequences in multicentric Castleman's disease. Blood 1995;84:1276-1280.

151. Bower M, Powles T, Williams S, et al: Brief communication: Rituximab in HIV-associated multicentric Castleman disease. Ann Intern Med 2007;147:836-839.

152. Dieval C, Bonnet F, Mauclere S, et al: Multicentric Castleman disease: Use of HHV8 viral load monitoring and positron emission tomography during follow-up. Leuk Lymphoma 2007;48:1881-1883.

153. Seliem RM, Griffith RC, Harris NL, et al: HHV-8+, EBV+ multicentric plasmablastic microlymphoma in an HIV+ man: The spec-

trum of HHV-8+ lymphoproliferative disorders expands. Am J Surg Pathol 2007;31:1439-1445.

154. Collins LS, Fowler A, Tong CY, et al: Multicentric Castleman's disease in HIV infection. Int J STD AIDS 2006;17:19-24; quiz 25.

155. Herrada J, Cabanillas F, Rice L, et al: The clinical behavior of localized and multicentric Castleman disease. Ann Intern Med 1998;128:657-662.

156. Cokelaere K, Debiec-Rychter M, De Wolf-Peeters C, et al: Hyaline-vascular Castleman's disease with HMGIC rearrangement in follicular dendritic cells: Molecular evidence of mesenchymal tumorigenesis. Am J Surg Pathol 2002;26:662-669.

157. Oksenhendler E, Carcelain G, Aoki Y, et al: High levels of human herpesvirus 8 viral load, human interleukin-6, interleukin-10, and C reactive protein correlate with exacerbation of multicentric castleman disease in HIV-infected patients. Blood 2000;96:2069-2073.

158. Dispenzieri A, Kyle R, Lacy M, et al: POEMS syndrome: Definitions and long-term outcome. Blood 2003;101:2496-2506.

159. Oksenhendler E, Boulanger E, Galicier L, et al: High incidence of Kaposi sarcoma-associated herpesvirus-related non-Hodgkin lymphoms in patients with HIV infection and multicentric Castleman's disease. Blood 2002;99:2331-2336.

160. Isaacson P, Campo E, Harris N: Large B-cell lymphoma arising in HHV8-associated multicentric Castleman's disease. In Swerdlow S, Campo E, Harris NL, et al. (eds): WHO Classification of Tumours of Haematopoietic and Lymphoid Tissues. WHO Classification of Tumours, vol 2. Lyon, International Agency for Research on Cancer, 2008, pp 258-259.

161. Aaron L, Lidove O, Yousry C, et al: Human herpesvirus 8-positive Castleman disease in human immunodeficiency virus-infected patients: The impact of highly active antiretroviral therapy. Clin Infect Dis 2002;35:880-882.

162. Castleman B, Iverson L, Menendez VP: Localized mediastinal lymph node hyperplasia resembling thymoma. Cancer 1956;9:822-830.

163. Frizzera G: Castleman's disease and related disorders. (Review). Semin Diagn Pathol 1988;5:346-364.

164. Keller AR, Hochholzer L, Castleman B: Hyaline-vascular and plasma-cell types of giant lymph node hyperplasia of the mediastinum and other locations. Cancer 1972;29:670-683.

165. Du M-Q, Liu H, Diss T, et al: Kaposi sarcoma-associated herpesvirus infects monotypic (IgMlambda) but polyclonal naive B cells in Castleman disease and associated lymphoproliferative disorders. Blood 2001;97:2130-2136.

166. Dupin N, Diss T, Kellam P, et al: HHV-8 is associated with a plasmablastic variant of Castleman disease that is linked to HHV-8-positive plasmablastic lymphoma. Blood 2000;95:1406-1412.

167. Chan J, Quintanilla-Martinez L, Ferry J, et al: Extranodal NK/T-cell lymphoma, nasal type. In Swerdlow S, Campo E, Harris NL, et al. (eds): WHO Classification of Tumours of Haematopoietic and Lymphoid Tissues. WHO Classification of Tumours, vol 2. Lyon, International Agency for Research on Cancer, 2008, pp 285-288.

168. Janka G, Imashuku S, Elinder G, et al: Infection and malignancy-associated hemophagocytic syndromes: Secondary hemophagocytic lymphohistiocytosis. Hematol Oncol Clin North Am 1998;12:435-444.

169. Low P, Neipel F, Rascu A, et al: Suppression of HHV-8 viremia by foscarnet in an HIV-infected patient with Kaposi's sarcoma and HHV-8 associated hemophagocytic syndrome. Eur J Med Res 1998;3:461-464.

170. Li CF, Ye H, Liu H, et al: Fatal HHV-8-associated hemophagocytic syndrome in an HIV-negative immunocompetent patient with plasmablastic variant of multicentric Castleman disease (plasmablastic microlymphoma). Am J Surg Pathol 2006;30:123-127.

171. Naresh KN, Rice AJ, Bower M: Lymph nodes involved by multicentric Castleman disease among HIV-positive individuals are often involved by Kaposi sarcoma. Am J Surg Pathol 2008;32:1006-1012.

Infectious Diseases of the Bone Marrow and Spleen

Robert P. Hasserjian

Introduction

The bone marrow and spleen may be affected by a wide variety of infectious agents. Pathologists must be aware of the clinical concern for infection, in order to initiate appropriate studies to detect microorganisms, and be prepared to recognize features of infection even when it is not clinically suspected. Bone marrow sampling may be performed to evaluate fever of unknown origin (most commonly in immunosuppressed patients, but sometimes in immunocompetent patients) or to evaluate for systemic infec-tion in a patient known or suspected to harbor a particular infec-tious agent. Anemia and other peripheral cytopenias are the most frequent indications for bone marrow sampling and may be the presenting signs of a clinically unsuspected infection identifiable within the bone marrow.

Bone marrow morphologic changes related to infections are most often nonspecific, and confirmation of a specific infectious agent may require special stains, immunohistochemistry, micro-biologic cultures, serologic studies, and molecular studies. However, it is important to understand the spectrum of mor-phologic changes elicited by specific infectious agents and to recognize how comparable changes can at times be caused by noninfective or neoplastic processes. The first part of this chapter discusses the various patterns of bone marrow changes that can be associated with infections; although most are nonspecific, in some instances they suggest a particular causative agent and can elicit appropriate ancillary studies. In the second part of the chapter, the pathologies of specific infectious agents involving the bone marrow are described. Infections involving the spleen are discussed at the end of the chapter.

Patterns of Bone Marrow Response to Infections

Hyperplasia

Bone marrow cellularity (i.e., the percentage of cellular marrow elements occupying the hemopoietic marrow space of the bone marrow biopsy specimen) is frequently increased in infection. This may reflect either an appropriate reaction against the offend-ing agent or ineffective hemopoiesis due to the effects of the infectious agent on the maturing hemopoietic cells and marrow microenvironment. In the former situation, the peripheral smear shows leukocytosis, often with increased band neutrophils, cir-culating immature myeloid elements, neutrophil toxic granula-tion, or some combination of these characteristics. If ineffective hemopoiesis is present, leukopenia or pancytopenia may be present despite the marrow hypercellularity. The marrow may show hyperplasia of all lineages, or it may show relative myeloid, erythroid, or megakaryocytic hyperplasia. Although the type of hyperplasia is not specific for any particular infectious agent, marked myeloid hyperplasia is often seen in sepsis, and the bone marrow in a region affected by osteomyelitis may show a marked predominance of neutrophils.[1,2] Megakaryocytic hyperplasia is frequently observed in human immunodeficiency virus (HIV) infection (see later discussion).

Hypoplasia

Global marrow hypocellularity may occur in severe, overwhelming infections such as sepsis; in such cases of acute marrow injury, a necrotic background of eosinophilic granular material, reflecting products of massive cell death, may be observed (Fig. 12-1).[1,2] Marked erythroid hypoplasia or pure red cell aplasia (defined as <5% red cell precursors in the bone marrow) can be produced by a variety of infectious agents but is commonly associated with parvovirus B19 infection. Dengue hemorrhagic fever, caused by a single-stranded RNA flavivirus that can infect hemopoietic cells, is associated with cytopenias and marked bone hypocellularity, often with a maturation arrest in erythroid and myeloid lineages.[3,4] Aplastic anemia may occur after acute hepatitis (including hepatitis A, B, and C viruses); the mechanism of marrow failure and definite implication of a viral etiology are uncertain in these cases.[5]

Serous Atrophy (Gelatinous Transformation)

Serous atrophy of the bone marrow represents an alteration of the bone marrow stroma whereby the adipocytes and hemopoietic cells are replaced by pale pink, amorphous, extracellular ground substance. The adipocytes are often smaller in size than normal marrow adipocytes.[6] Serous atrophy is usually observed in late stages of HIV infection; in that context, it is always associated with anemia (usually severe, with a median hemoglobin concentration of 7.9 g/dL) or, less often, with other cytopenias.[7] The bone marrow aspirates are typically difficult to obtain and may result in a dry tap. If an aspirate is obtained, gelatinous pink material may be present in the background of the Wright-Giemsa–stained smears.[7] In the trephine biopsy on hematoxylin and eosin (H&E) stain, the material appears amphophilic or eosinophilic and homogeneous, although a fibrillar or granular appearance may be observed on high power (Fig. 12-2). This contrasts to the eosinophilic background material of acute marrow injury (such as that observed after cytotoxic chemotherapy), which is granular at low power and appears to be more eosinophilic than serous atrophy material. The material in serous atrophy stains with periodic acid–Schiff (PAS) stain and is also positive for Alcian blue at acidic pH (2.5 and 1.0). Because predigestion with hyaluronidase abrogates the Alcian blue staining, serous atrophy material appears to comprise the extracellular ground substances hyaluronic acid and sulfated glycosaminoglycans.[8,9] Disruption of the normal extracellular matrix marrow microenvironment likely explains the ineffective erythropoiesis and marked anemia typically associated with serous atrophy. The marrow is hypocellular in about half of the cases and may

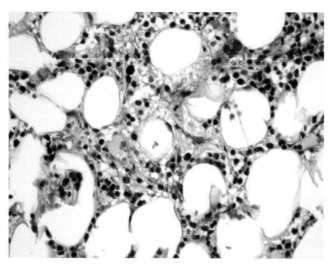

Figure 12-1. Acute marrow injury due to sepsis. The marrow is hypocellular, with interstitial eosinophilic fibrillar material representing products of intramedullary cell death. The marrow in sepsis may be either hypercellular or hypocellular (H&E stain).

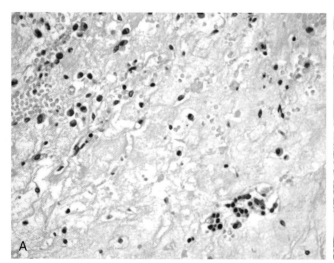
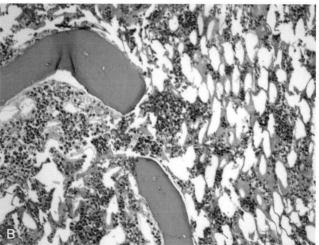

Figure 12-2. Serous atrophy (gelatinous transformation). **A,** The marrow is usually hypocellular, with background amorphous pale eosinophilic material; hemopoiesis is confined to islands within the background material (H&E stain). **B,** Serous atrophy may be focal, and in this photomicrograph from the bone marrow biopsy of a patient with widespread carcinoma it is present on the right-hand side. The fat cells within the area of serous atrophy are smaller than normal and have clearly demarcated cell borders (H&E stain).

occasionally be hypercellular. Serous atrophy may be either focal or diffuse (see Fig. 12-2B). When associated with HIV infection, megakaryocytes are usually increased and show the typical abnormal features observed in HIV-infected patients (see later discussion).

Serous atrophy may also occur in HIV-negative patients. In fact, some reports have suggested that, since the advent of highly effective antiretroviral therapy (HAART), HIV infection has become a relatively uncommon cause of serous atrophy[10]; cachexia due to tumors or malnutrition was a more common cause in one recent series. Other infections associated with serous atrophy include bacterial endocarditis, pneumonia, and tuberculosis.[10] In such cases, the histologic features are similar to those of HIV-associated serous atrophy, but serous atrophy in HIV− patients usually does not exhibit reticulin fibrosis and may be associated with less marked anemia.[7]

Morphologic Dysplasia

Myelodysplastic syndromes (MDSs) characteristically exhibit morphologic abnormalities of the erythroid, myeloid, and megakaryocytic lineages, reflecting abnormal maturation of the clonal, defective hematopoiesis. These changes include nuclear irregularities, nuclear fragmentation, binucleation, megaloblastoid change, and cytoplasmic vacuolation of erythroid elements; hypogranularity, vacuolization, and abnormal nuclear lobation of myeloid cells; and small size and nuclear hypolobulation of megakaryocytes. Reactive conditions that disrupt the marrow microenvironment, including many inflammatory and infectious processes, may produce morphologic changes resembling those of MDS. In particular, the erythroid cells of HIV+ patients often exhibit nuclear irregularities, megaloblastic change, vacuolation, and, occasionally, ring sideroblasts on iron stain (Fig. 12-3A).

The megakaryocytes in HIV+ patients are frequently small and increased in number. However, in contrast to many cases of MDS, the myeloid lineage is usually spared; the megakaryocytes have very sparse cytoplasm (so-called naked or bare megakaryocyte nuclei) but do not have the small, hypolobated nuclei of MDS (see Fig. 12-3B).[11] Hemopoietic elements show a lower rate of proliferation and apoptosis in HIV infection than in MDS.[12] These morphologic changes are reversible after treatment of HIV infection, because they reflect a disrupted bone marrow microenvironment rather than an intrinsic, clonal hemopoietic stem cell abnormality as seen in MDS. Nevertheless, HIV infection should be considered in the differential diagnosis of bone marrow samples showing dysplastic changes, particularly if the dysplasia is most prominent in the erythroid lineage, if it is accompanied by numerous bare megakaryocyte nuclei and increased plasma cells, and if it occurs in young patients, in whom MDS is uncommon.

Similar to HIV infection, a reactive morphologic dysplasia of erythroid elements may be observed in other infections involving the bone marrow, such as leishmania.[13] The morphologic dysplasia in HIV and other infections is most likely due to effects of the infection on histiocytes, macrophages, and marrow stromal cells; these cells provide important microenvironmental structural and cytokine factors required for normal maturation of hemopoietic elements.[14]

Lymphoid Aggregates

Aggregates of small, mature lymphocytes (that may or may not contain germinal centers) are nonspecific and can occur in normal individuals as well as in a variety of neoplastic and nonneoplastic conditions. Lymphoid aggregates in the setting of HIV infection are often large, are admixed with histiocytes and plasma cells, and have ill-defined borders; they may occasionally be paratrabecular, thus mimicking lymphomatous aggregates in some cases.[15,16] Flow cytometry and/or immunohistochemistry on bone marrow can be helpful in such cases to exclude the possibility of lymphomatous involvement of the bone marrow.

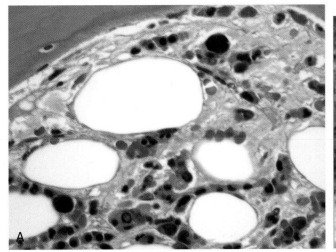
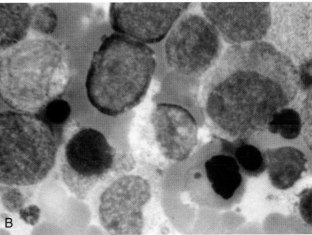

Figure 12-3. Reactive morphologic dysplasia in the bone marrow of HIV-infected patients. **A,** The megakaryocytes in HIV-infected patients are often small, with irregular nuclei and very scant cytoplasm (naked megakaryocyte nuclei) (H&E stain). **B,** Erythroid elements, in particular, often show morphologic dysplasia such as cytoplasmic vacuolization and nuclear irregularities, features that may lead to an erroneous diagnosis of a myelodysplastic syndrome (H&E stain).

Granulomas

Granulomas are identified in approximately 1% of bone marrow samples and in about 20% of studies performed to evaluate a fever of unknown origin.[17] Granulomas are readily identified in trephine biopsy sections. Granulomas are usually not well represented in the aspirate smear due to associated reticulin fibrosis that limits aspiration of the tell-tale histiocytic and giant cell aggregates.[18] An associated infection is diagnosed in only about 30% of bone marrow granuloma cases. In many cases, bone marrow granulomas are the result of noninfectious processes, including sarcoidosis, drug reactions, and paraneoplastic phenomena caused by hematologic or nonhematologic malignancies. In up to 5% of cases, bone marrow granulomas are idiopathic with no known cause identified.[17]

The pattern of granulomas, including the ratio of histiocytes to lymphocytes and the presence or absence of multinucleated giant cells, eosinophils, and plasmacytosis, does not appear to be predictive of an infectious versus a noninfectious etiology.[17] However, granuloma localization within the marrow can be helpful, because the granulomas in *Mycobacterium tuberculosis* infections are often paratrabecular.[2] Granulomas are most commonly associated with mycobacterial and fungal infections but can also occur with other infections, including Epstein-Barr virus (EBV),[19] leishmaniasis and toxoplasmosis,[20] brucellosis, and Q fever.

Diffuse histiocytosis in the absence of granulomas may occur in immunosuppressed patients with mycobacterial infections. Acid-fast bacilli (AFB) stain should be performed on samples from any immunosuppressed patient with increased bone marrow histiocytes or unexplained lymphohistiocytic aggregates. Whipple disease can rarely involve the bone marrow as histiocytosis containing PAS+ inclusions and occasionally PAS+ *Tropheryma whippelii* organisms.[21] Although the presence of PAS+ inclusions in bone marrow macrophages is nonspecific, it may raise the differential diagnosis of Whipple disease, which can be confirmed by PCR or additional clinical investigations.[21]

Bone marrow fibrin ring granulomas (also called doughnut granulomas) represent a distinctive type of granuloma associated with cytomegalovirus (CMV), EBV, and Q fever (caused by the rickettsial organism, *Coxiella burnetii*).[22,23] Fibrin ring granulomas represent annular granulomas composed of concentric rings of neutrophils and epithelioid histiocytes surrounding a central empty space (Fig. 12-4). The granulomas are often encircled by a lamellated ring of fibrin (highlighted by Masson trichrome or fibrin stains).[24] The nature of the central clear space is uncertain; in the bone marrow and the liver, the fibrin ring granulomas are typically located adjacent to blood vessels or sinusoids and have been termed a perivasculitis. The central material appears to be lipid rather than a vascular lumen, however, because vascular components have not been identified within ring granulomas.[25] Of note, fibrin ring granulomas are not specific for an infectious process, because they also may occur as a paraneoplastic phenomenon in lymphomas.[22,26]

Plasmacytosis

Bone marrow plasma cells (normally comprising <2% of all marrow cells) may increase, often to prominent levels, in a wide

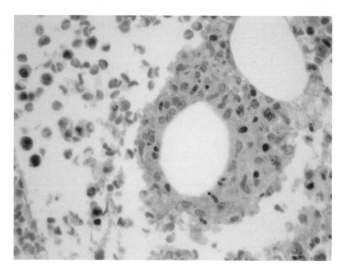

Figure 12-4. A fibrin ring granuloma is characterized by a central empty space surrounded by histiocytes and neutrophils that may or may not be encircled by a concentric ring of fibrin (Giemsa stain).

variety of infections and inflammatory conditions. In such cases, the plasma cells are usually perivascular and can be demonstrated to be polyclonal by immunoglobulin light chain immunohistochemistry or in situ hybridization; this is particularly important to avoid a misdiagnosis of plasma cell myeloma in HIV+ patients, who may have serum paraproteins. Sheets of mature, polyclonal plasma cells replacing the marrow space may be seen in chronic osteomyelitis.

Hemophagocytosis

Hemophagocytosis represents the presence of intact hemopoietic cells (erythrocytes, leukocytes, or both) within the cytoplasm of phagocytic histiocytes in any tissue; hemophagocytic histiocytes can be readily identified in both bone marrow biopsy sections and aspirate smears (Fig. 12-5). Note that the phagocytic histiocytes that are commonly present in high-turnover tissues such as germinal centers and that contain pyknotic cellular debris are not equivalent to hemophagocytic histiocytes. Hemophagocytic lymphohistiocytosis (HLH), also known as hemophagocytic syndrome, is an inherited or acquired histiocyte activation syndrome that is potentially fatal. The identification of hemophagocytic histiocytes in bone marrow (or, less commonly, in spleen or lymph node tissue) represents a key diagnostic feature of HLH. However, hemophagocytosis is nonspecific and in isolation cannot confirm a diagnosis of HLH; conversely, a diagnosis of HLH can be made even if hemophagocytosis is not present in biopsied tissues.[27] The diagnostic criteria of HLH were revised in 2004 and are shown in Table 12-1.

Bone marrow sampling is often performed to evaluate for clinically suspected HLH. These cases require careful review, because hemophagocytic cells may be rare: the median number in confirmed cases of HLH is only 1 in 500 cells in bone marrow aspirates. As mentioned earlier, the lack of hemophagocytosis does not exclude a diagnosis of HLH, and this diagnosis can be made based on clinical and molecular features in such cases. Although the sensitivity of the first bone marrow sample to

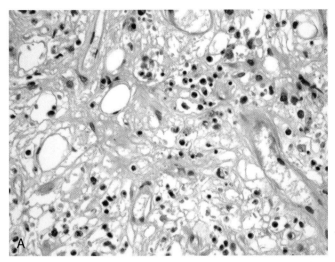
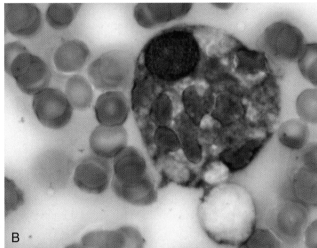

Figure 12-5. Bone marrow findings in hemophagocytic lymphohistiocytosis. **A,** The bone marrow biopsy specimen may show hypocellularity or, as in this case, marked hypocellularity (H&E stain). **B,** Phagocytic histiocytes contain intact red blood cells (or other hemopoietic elements) within the cytoplasm (bone marrow aspirate; Wright-Giemsa stain).

Table 12-1 Diagnostic Criteria for Hemophagocytic Lymphohistiocytosis

The diagnosis of hemophagocytic lymphohistiocytosis (HLH) can be established if either criterion A or criterion B is fulfilled.

Criterion A. A molecular diagnosis consistent with HLH (primary HLH)

Criterion B. At least five of the following eight diagnostic criteria for HLH fulfilled

1. Fever
2. Splenomegaly
3. Cytopenias (affecting at least two of three lineages in the peripheral blood)
   a. Hemoglobin <90 g/L (in infants <4 wk of age, hemoglobin <100 g/L)
   b. Platelets <100 × 10⁹/L
   c. Neutrophils <1.0 × 10⁹/L
4. Hypertriglyceridemia and/or hypofibrogenemia
   a. Fasting triglycerides ≥3.0 mmol/L (i.e., ≥265 mg/dL)
   b. Fibrinogen ≤1.5 g/L
5. Hemophagocytosis in bone marrow or spleen or lymph nodes
6. Low or absent NK-cell activity (according to local laboratory reference)
7. Serum ferritin ≥500 µg/L
8. Soluble CD25 (i.e., soluble IL-2 receptor) ≥2400 U/mL

IL-2, interleukin 2; NK, natural killer.
Adapted from Henter JI, Horne A, Arico M, et al: HLH-2004: Diagnostic and therapeutic guidelines for hemophagocytic lymphohistiocytosis. Pediatr Blood Cancer 2007;48:124-131.

Table 12-2 Secondary Causes of Hemophagocytic Lymphohistiocytosis (HLH)

I. Infections
   A. Viruses
      1. Herpesviruses (HSV, VZV, CMV, EBV, HHV-6, HHV-8)
      2. HIV
      3. Other viruses: adenovirus, hepatitis viruses, parvovirus, influenza
   B. Other infections
      1. Bacteria including mycobacteria and spirochetes
      2. Parasites
      3. Fungi
II. Malignancy (most commonly lymphomas)
III. Macrophage activation syndrome (associated with autoimmune disease)

CMV, cytomegalovirus; EBV, Epstein-Barr virus; HHV, human herpesvirus; HSV, herpes simplex virus; VZV, varicella-zoster virus.
Adapted from Rouphael NG, Talati NJ, Vaughan C, et al: Infections associated with haemophagocytic syndrome. Lancet Infect Dis 2007;7:814-822, 898; and Verbsky JW, Grossman WJ: Hemophagocytic lymphohistiocytosis: Diagnosis, pathophysiology, treatment, and future perspectives. Ann Med 2006;38:20-31.

document HLH is only about 60%, serial bone marrow samples in suspected disease yield a higher sensitivity[27]; therefore, repeat bone marrow sampling is indicated if HLH is suspected but cannot be diagnosed on the initial sample nor confirmed on clinical and molecular criteria alone. Aside from the presence of hemophagocytic histiocytes, the bone marrow appearance of HLH is variable. The marrow can be hypocellular or hypercellular, and the myeloid-to-erythroid ratio is variable. Because HLH commonly occurs secondary to infection or a neoplastic process, the bone marrow may be concurrently involved by the inciting process, such as a lymphoma (Table 12-2). Other abnormal clinical and laboratory findings that can be clues to the diagnosis of HLH but do not represent diagnostic criteria are cerebromeningeal symptoms, lymphadenopathy, jaundice, edema, skin rash, hepatic enzyme abnormalities, hypoproteinemia, and hyponatremia.[27]

Primary (familial) HLH is a rare, autosomal recessive disease that usually manifests in infancy or early childhood.[28] The main gene defect in familial HLH (25% to 50% of cases) is a mutation in the perforin gene.[29] Defects in other genes, including *UNC13D* and *syntaxin11*,[30] have been shown to cause HLH in smaller subsets of patients. These mutations result in impaired cytotoxic T-cell and NK-cell function that leads to inappropriate activation of macrophages; uncontrolled macrophage phagocytosis of hemopoietic elements, erythrocytes, and platelets ensues, with resulting severe and often life-threatening pancytopenia. Primary HLH may also occur during the course of inherited immunodeficiency syndromes such as Chediak-Higashi and X-linked lymphoproliferative syndrome.[31]

Secondary HLH is an acquired disorder characterized by a similar histiocyte activation induced by an infection, neoplasm, or chronic inflammatory condition. Causes of secondary HLH are shown in Table 12-2.[32] It is important to note that infections, especially EBV, can precipitate the first episode of hemophagocytosis in patients with familial HLH.[33] Therefore, the presence of an infection concurrent with HLH does not exclude a genetic or familial etiology, because these forms may not manifest until adolescence or even adulthood.[34] The identification of unexplained hemophagocytosis in a bone marrow sample in which some clinical features of HLH are present should precipitate a search for possible infectious, neoplastic, or inflammatory causes as well as consideration that this may be a manifestation of familial HLH. Infection-associated HLH can occur in either immunocompetent or immunodeficient patients. However, in cases associated with EBV infection, viral titers are usually very high compared with uncomplicated infectious mononucleosis, suggesting an underlying immune abnormality even in patients lacking a known immunodeficiency syndrome.[35]

Hemophagocytosis is not specific for HLH and can be identified in up to 50% of patients who undergo bone marrow examination as part of a workup for fever and also in bone marrow after blood transfusions.[36-38] Hemophagocytic histiocytes are less frequent in these nonspecific settings than in most cases fulfilling diagnostic criteria for HLH.

Bone Marrow Features of Specific Infections

Parvovirus B19 Infection

Parvovirus B19 is a small, unenveloped DNA virus that causes erythema infectiosum, a childhood infection characterized by rash and sometimes arthralgias, hydrops fetalis and intrauterine fetal death in pregnancy, and anemia. The virus is highly transmissible through respiratory secretions. Parvovirus B19 infects erythroid precursors and arrests red blood cell production.[39] In immunocompetent patients, this arrest is transient except in patients with markedly decreased red blood cell survival, in which case severe anemia (so-called transient aplastic crisis) may result. Transient aplastic crisis is most commonly associated with sickle cell disease but has also been reported with hereditary spherocytosis, thalassemia, pyruvate kinase deficiency, and autoimmune hemolytic anemia.[40,41] Unlike the severe but short-term anemia of infected immunocompetent individuals with hemolytic anemia, parvovirus-infected immunodeficient patients may develop chronic anemia in spite of normal red cell survival due to a prolonged, chronic infection. These patients may remain transfusion-dependent for up to 12 months.[42,43] Parvovirus-related anemia has been described in patients with AIDS, congenital immunodeficiencies, or chronic lymphatic leukemia and in patients undergoing chemotherapy; in such immunocompromised patients, the myeloid-to-erythroid ratio may be preserved or even increased.[39,42]

The bone marrow in transient aplastic crisis typically shows marked erythroid hypoplasia or aplasia with preserved megakaryopoiesis and granulopoiesis. The few erythroid forms that are present are large, early precursors termed giant pronormoblasts; they may be identified in the bone marrow aspirate or biopsy specimen (Fig. 12-6). Viral inclusions usually are not identifiable by routine microscopy in the bone marrow of immunocompetent individuals with transient aplastic crisis.[44] Transient aplastic crisis typically lasts only 7 to 10 days, but the anemia may be severe enough to require transfusions and can be fatal if not treated.[45] Parvovirus infection in patients with known underlying hemolytic anemia is in the differential diagnosis of acute-onset severe anemia in such patients and can be confirmed by PCR identification of virus in peripheral blood or serologic tests. In such a setting, bone marrow sampling is now rarely performed. The pathologist is more likely to encounter a bone marrow sample from an immunosuppressed patient with chronic anemia, in whom parvovirus infection may not be suspected.

In immunocompromised patients, the bone marrow in parvovirus infection is usually hypercellular and commonly shows preserved erythropoiesis. Although giant pronormoblasts are infrequent, maturing erythroid forms contain prominent intranuclear eosinophilic inclusions with peripheral condensation of the nuclear chromatin.[42] These inclusions are better demonstrated in the bone marrow biopsy sample than in the aspirate. Fixation artifact may sometimes produce nuclear changes resembling parvovirus inclusions; however, in such cases, the nuclear abnormalities are present in all hemopoietic lineages, rather than being limited to the erythroid series.[42] Parvovirus infection can be confirmed by demonstration of viral protein on immunohistochemistry, or of RNA sequences on in situ hybridization, or by PCR identification of parvovirus DNA in peripheral blood (see Fig. 12-6D).[46] These confirmatory studies may be necessary, because serologic studies (anti-parvoviral IgM and IgG) may be negative due to immunosuppression or early-stage infection.[42] Transmission electron microscopy also demonstrates electron-dense amorphous intranuclear material representing viral particles, but this technique is rarely required for diagnosis.[42]

Human Immunodeficiency Virus Infection

Bone marrow biopsies are performed in HIV+ patients to evaluate cytopenias that may occur during the course of disease, to stage lymphomas and other neoplasms that develop, or to assess for the presence of suspected systemic infections (often evidenced by unexplained fevers). HIV infection causes changes in the bone marrow that appear to be independent of concurrent infections or the effects of antiretroviral or other drugs.[47] These changes most likely relate to both disruption of the bone marrow microenvironment and HIV infection of hemopoietic elements. Normal maturation of hemopoietic elements depends on cytokines secreted by local T cells and macrophages, both of which are affected by HIV.[48] HIV also has been shown to infect

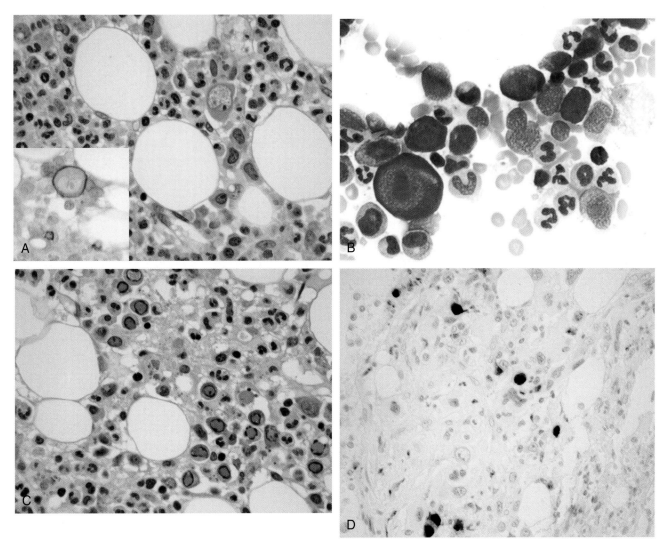

Figure 12-6. Bone marrow findings in parvovirus infection. **A,** The bone marrow biopsy specimen shows a marked paucity of maturing erythroids; the rare erythroid forms present are giant pronormoblasts (H&E stain); they are positive for the erythroid markers glycophorin by immunohistochemistry *(inset)*. **B,** Giant pronormoblasts can also be identified in the bone marrow aspirate and exhibit prominent nucleoli (Wright-Giemsa stain) (courtesy of Dr. Tracy George, Stanford University). **C,** In immunosuppressed patients, eosinophilic inclusions may be seen on routine histology within early erythroid forms (H&E stain). **D,** An immunostain for parvovirus highlights the inclusions and aids in confirming the diagnosis.

hemopoietic precursors, megakaryocytes, and macrophage-myeloid progenitors, potentially with direct effects on their maturation.[49,50] The retention of iron within histiocytes and the paucity of sideroblastic iron (so-called reticuloendothelial iron blockade) resembles that of anemia of chronic disease and may represent another mechanism of HIV-associated anemia. The changes observed in the bone marrow of HIV+ patients are summarized in Table 12-3, and examples are shown in Fig. 12-7.

The morphologic changes in the maturing hemopoietic cells were termed "dysplastic" in older literature. Although these morphologic abnormalities overlap with some findings in MDS, they are reactive in nature and, unlike MDS, are not associated with increased risk of developing acute myeloid leukemia. In particular, there is no increase in myeloblasts, and dysplasia of the myeloid lineage (hypogranulation and pseudo–Pelger-Huet neutrophils) is uncommon in HIV infection.[11] Moreover, the megakaryocytic abnormalities differ from those of MDS: the

megakaryocytes in HIV infection typically have hyperchromatic nuclei lacking discernable cytoplasm (bare or naked megakaryocyte nuclei), as opposed to the small megakaryocytes with round nuclei or with separated nuclear lobes that typify MDS (see Fig. 12-3A).[12,15,51] The morphologic "dysplasia" observed in HIV infection is associated with ineffective hemopoiesis and, analogous to the ineffective hemopoiesis of MDS, leads to cytopenias. Anemia is the most common manifestation; unlike most MDS cases which are macrocytic, HIV-associated anemias are usually normocytic.

Although HIV patients often receive drugs that can affect the bone marrow and cause cytopenias, the characteristic changes described here are observed independent of drug therapy, concurrent infection, or concurrent neoplasm and therefore are attributable to infection by HIV itself.[11,52] Moreover, abnormal maturation of erythroid and granulocytic elements is associated with anemia and leukopenia, respectively, as well as with more

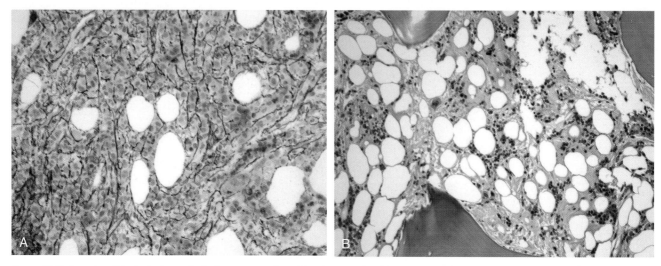

Figure 12-7. Examples of histologic changes in the bone marrow of HIV-infected patients (in addition to morphologic dysplasia and abnormal megakaryocytes, shown in Figure 12-3). **A,** Increased reticulin fibrosis (reticulin silver stain). **B,** Serous atrophy (H&E stain).

Table 12-3 Changes Commonly Described in the Bone Marrow of HIV-Infected Patients That Are Directly Attributed to the Viral Infection[7,51,52]

1. Hypercellularity (majority of cases)
2. Hypocellularity (5%-15% of cases)
3. Serous atrophy* (10%-30% of cases)
4. Megakaryocyte abnormalities (clustering, bare nuclei, small size)
5. Erythroid lineage abnormalities* (left shift, megaloblastic changes, morphologic dysplasia); the erythroid lineage is the lineage that most often shows dysplastic changes
6. Myeloid lineage abnormalities* (left shift, nuclear hypolobation or hyperlobation, giant metamyelocytes)
7. Increased plasma cells
8. Lymphoid aggregates (often with admixed plasma cells and histiocytes)
9. Increased reticulin fibrosis*
10. Increased iron stores within bone marrow histiocytes*
11. Ring sideroblasts (rarely)
12. Granulomas (10% to 15% of cases, not necessarily associated with identifiable opportunistic infections)

*Features that are associated with advanced acquired immunodeficiency syndrome (Centers for Disease Control and Prevention class IV-C).

advanced AIDS. In contrast, megakaryocyte abnormalities are not associated with the occurrence of thrombocytopenia in HIV+ patients.[11,52] Peripheral platelet destruction mediated by antiplatelet antibodies (idiopathic thrombocytopenic purpura) represents a common mechanism of thrombocytopenia in HIV+ patients,[53] and antibodies to granulocytes also occur.[54] In the thrombocytopenic HIV+ patient, the main role of bone marrow biopsy is to exclude an infectious or infiltrative process as a cause for the thrombocytopenia. When confronted with a bone marrow specimen from a cytopenic HIV+ patient, provided that infections or neoplasms are excluded, the presence of the morpho-

logic abnormalities described here implicates HIV infection (with or without the effects of any concomitant drugs) as the cause for the cytopenias.

Unexplained fever is a common clinical scenario in which a bone marrow biopsy is performed in HIV+ patients; in such cases, a combination of bone marrow biopsy and aspirate morphology with bone marrow culture yields a specific infectious agent in 30% to 40% of cases.[55,56] Lymphoid aggregates and increased interstitial T cells represent a nonspecific finding in HIV+ patients and do not correlate with the stage of disease or the presence of opportunistic infections involving the marrow. The lymphocytes are predominantly T cells with varied CD4/CD8 ratios. In contrast, granulomas in the bone marrow usually correlate with opportunistic infections; even in the setting of low CD4+ counts, infectious agents can incite granuloma formation in the bone marrow of HIV+ patients. However, in some cases, granuloma formation may be impaired. In these cases, organisms may be present in large numbers within the marrow, often within the cytoplasm of histiocytes. In particular, abundant intrahistiocytic mycobacteria can give the impression of pseudo-Gaucher cells due to the cytoplasmic striations (Fig. 12-8). The specific organisms commonly identified in infection of the bone marrow of HIV+ patients and the associated morphologic patterns of marrow reaction are shown in Table 12-4.[57]

Mycobacterial cultures of blood and bone marrow are more sensitive at detecting systemic mycobacterial infections in HIV+ patients than AFB stain of bone marrow, and AFB stain is positive in only about half of culture-positive cases.[58-60] For these reasons, some investigators have questioned the utility of special stains or even histologic examination of the bone marrow in the workup of AIDS patients with suspected infections.[61] However, AFB staining (as well as PAS or Grocott methenamine silver [GMS] staining for suspected fungi) of a bone marrow biopsy sample allows a more rapid diagnosis of infection and prompt institution of therapy.[58,62,63] Acid-fast organisms may be detected in rare cases in which granulomas are lacking, so the absence of granuloma formation does not exclude mycobacterial infection in HIV+ patients.[62] Conversely, granulomas or lymphohistiocytic

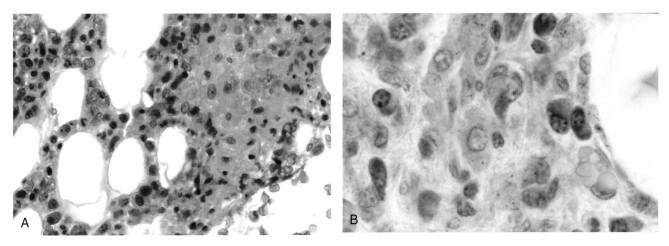

Figure 12-8. *Mycobacterium avium-intracellulare* infection involving the bone marrow of an HIV-positive patient. **A,** Discrete granulomas often are not present, but histiocytes are increased and form some vague clusters (H&E stain). **B,** Acid-fast bacilli are identified in the cytoplasm of histiocytes (AFB stain).

Table 12-4 Pathologic Patterns of Bone Marrow Opportunistic Infections in HIV-Positive Patients[57,60,78,84]

Infectious Agent	Pattern	Special Stain
Mycobacteria (*M. tuberculosis* or *M. avium-intracellulare*)	Granulomas Diffuse histiocytic proliferation with intracellular organisms	AFB
Histoplasma capsulatum	Diffuse histiocytic proliferation with intracellular organisms Occasionally granulomas	GMS or PAS
Cryptococcus neoformans	Granulomas	GMS or PAS
Leishmania	Diffuse histiocytic proliferation with intracellular organisms	Giemsa Direct examination of Wright-Giemsa–stained bone marrow aspirate
Pneumocystis jiroveci	Diffuse reticulin fibrosis Granulomas	GMS Immunohistochemistry
Cytomegalovirus	Viral inclusions	Immunohistochemistry

AFB, acid-fast bacilli stain; GMS, Gomori methenamine silver stain; *M., Mycobacterium* genus; PAS, periodic acid–Schiff stain.

aggregates may be present in the absence of any demonstrable infection or neoplasm.[60] Both fungal cultures and PAS or GMS stains are generally effective at detecting fungal infections, although fungal cultures are more sensitive.[58,60]

Aside from HIV-related bone marrow abnormalities and opportunistic infections, HIV patients undergoing bone marrow biopsy for fever or other nonspecific systemic symptoms may have a neoplasm. The most common neoplasms involving the bone marrow in HIV+ patients are Burkitt lymphoma, diffuse large B-cell lymphoma, classic Hodgkin lymphoma, and Kaposi sarcoma. Lymphomas in HIV+ patients are more likely to involve the marrow than lymphomas in immunocompetent patients, and they more commonly manifest with cytopenias and bone marrow infiltration lacking identifiable lymphadenopathy. For example, the bone marrow may be the initial site of presentation of HIV+ patients with Hodgkin lymphoma.[64] The neoplastic cells in HIV-associated bone marrow lymphomas usually exhibit infection of the neoplastic cells by EBV (but not HIV).

Epstein-Barr Virus Infection

Bone marrow sampling is only rarely performed in infectious mononucleosis, particularly in the pediatric and young adult age group most commonly infected. However, given the rarity of infectious mononucleosis in adults (<3% of patients are >40 years old),[65] bone marrow sampling may be performed in older individuals with fever, constitutional symptoms, or atypical lymphocytosis, for which infectious mononucleosis is not seriously considered. Patients with infectious mononucleosis may also develop hemolytic anemia, neutropenia, or pancytopenia, prompting a bone marrow biopsy.[39] The bone marrow biopsy in infectious mononucleosis is typically normocellular or mildly hypocellular and frequently contains small lymphoid aggregates and small, non-necrotizing granulomas.[66] It is unknown whether in situ hybridization for EBV-encoded RNAs (EBER) is positive in the bone marrow of infectious mononucleosis affecting immunocompetent patients.

Hemophagocytic syndrome (HLH) is a potentially fatal complication of EBV infection and is present in most cases of fatal infectious mononucleosis.[67] Fatal cases usually occur in patients with inherited or iatrogenic immunodeficiency but can occasionally occur in immunocompetent individuals. Patients usually develop pancytopenia, and the bone marrow often exhibits massive marrow necrosis and diffuse marrow histiocytic infiltrates in addition to hemophagocytosis.[67,68]

Cytomegalovirus Infection

CMV may produce an infectious mononucleosis–like picture similar to that of EBV infection in immunocompetent individuals, and in such cases the bone marrow findings are similar to those of infectious mononucleosis (discussed earlier). Viral inclusions are often not detected. In immunosuppressed patients, the viral inclusions may be readily detected in the bone marrow endothelial cells and may precede positive antibody titers.[69] Viral inclusions can also be identified within the cytoplasm of endothelial cells in the blood of infected immunosuppressed patients.[70] Small, non-necrotizing granulomas and fibrin ring granulomas in the bone marrow have been associated with CMV infection in immunosuppressed patients.[23]

Brucellosis

Adults and children with brucellosis may present with pancytopenia eliciting bone marrow examination; fever and hepatosplenomegaly are commonly present concurrently.[71] The bone marrow in patients with brucellosis is usually hypercellular (but can rarely be hypocellular) and shows non-necrotizing granulomas or aggregates of histiocytes lacking giant cells; hemophagocytosis may be present.[72,73]

Rickettsial Infections

In Q fever, the bone marrow characteristically shows nodular areas of fibrinoid necrosis, small epithelioid granulomas, and characteristic fibrin ring granulomas (see earlier discussion and Fig. 12-4). The organism typically cannot be demonstrated on microbacterial stains, and the diagnosis requires confirmation by serologic studies.[24,25]

Leishmaniasis

Visceral leishmaniasis is a parasitic disease endemic to the Mediterranean basin, but since the advent of AIDS it has been seen more frequently in other geographic regions. *Leishmania* usually affects HIV+ patients with advanced disease and is most common in AIDS patients in southern Europe, where it affects about 1% of AIDS patients over the course of their disease.[74] Visceral leishmaniasis also can affect immunocompetent infants and children.[74] Visceral leishmaniasis affects the liver, spleen, and bone marrow and is most commonly diagnosed by splenic aspiration and bone marrow sampling.[75]

In biopsy sections, the *Leishmania* amastigotes are present as extracellular organisms, occasionally associated with granulomas.[76] Direct examination of the bone marrow aspirate and Giemsa-stained bone marrow biopsy specimens for *Leishmania* amastigotes is an effective method of diagnosing visceral leishmaniasis, with a sensitivity of 90% (Fig. 12-9).[77] Bone marrow culture and serologic studies are somewhat less sensitive but do improve the diagnostic yield of morphologic examination.[74] Recently, PCR of peripheral blood or bone marrow has been shown to rapidly detect species-specific *Leishmania* in both HIV+ and immunocompetent patients, with excellent specificity and sensitivity superior to bone marrow morphologic examination.[77]

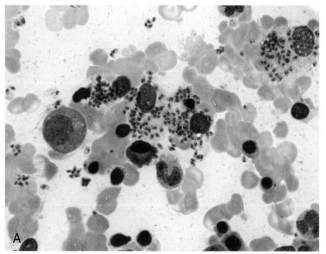
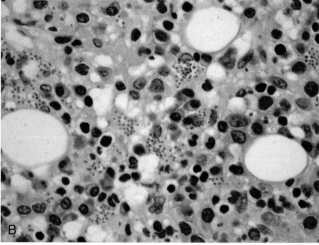

Figure 12-9. Bone marrow leishmaniasis. **A,** The *Leishmania* amastigotes in this aspirate smear are both extracellular and within histiocytes (Wright-Giemsa stain) (courtesy of Dr. Laurence de Leval, Liege, Belgium). **B,** Intrahistiocytic amastigotes can also be visualized on a thin trephine biopsy section (H&E stain).

Pneumocystis

Pneumocystis jiroveci (formerly *Pneumocystis carinii*) only rarely involves the bone marrow, but marrow involvement has been reported in AIDS patients and in patients with immunosuppression due to chemotherapy.[78,79] The bone marrow may appear fibrotic or hypocellular, and interstitial amorphous, frothy eosinophilic material similar to that seen in the lung may be present.[78] The organism can be visualized by GMS stain of the bone marrow specimen, which reveals the characteristic cyst wall. Immunohistochemistry using a monoclonal antibody to *Pneumocystis* appears to be more sensitive than GMS stain in detecting extrapulmonary disease, and it stains the *Pneumocystis* trophozoites as well as cyst walls.[80,81]

Fungal Infections

Cryptococcus neoformans involves the bone marrow mainly in the setting of HIV infection[82] and may be the presenting manifestation of AIDS.[83] Patients usually present with concurrent cryptococcal meningitis and cytopenias.[84] The bone marrow almost always contains granulomas, but these may be poorly formed, and the bone marrow may also exhibit loosely cohesive histiocytic aggregates or gelatinous change (Fig. 12-10).[84] The cryptococcal organisms can be seen in biopsy sections on routine H&E staining; the capsule can be visualized by mucicarmine or PAS staining. Intrahistiocytic organisms can also be identified on Wright-Giemsa–stained aspirate smears. *Histoplasma capsulatum* also usually involves the marrow only in immunosuppressed patients, but it may rarely be present in the marrow of immunocompetent individuals. In rare cases, fungal forms of *Cryptococcus* or *Histoplasma* may be identified within megakaryocytes.[85]

Infections Involving the Spleen

The spleen has two major anatomic compartments, the red pulp and the white pulp. The red pulp comprises a network of vascular sinuses, blood vessels, and associated accessory cells such as histiocytes and serves largely as a filter and reservoir of blood cells. The white pulp consists of specialized lymphoid tissue (B cells and T cells) organized around splenic arterioles. The splenic red pulp often manifests infections that involve the blood and bone marrow, whereas the white pulp typically reflects changes of infections similar to those observed in lymph nodes. Rare infections involving the spleen may form masses detected on radiologic studies.

Diffuse Red Pulp Reactions to Infection

The term *splenitis* refers to massive infiltration of the red pulp sinusoids with neutrophils and is usually associated with typhoid fever; it is only rarely seen in typical bacterial infections occurring in the Western world. The spleen in sepsis is often enlarged, with red pulp hyperplasia caused by increased activated macrophages. Postmortem autolysis of the macrophages can lead to massive lysis of the red pulp, as observed at autopsy in patients dying of

sepsis. However, massive red pulp autolysis at autopsy is not specific to sepsis and can result from splenomegaly of any cause.[86] Splenic red pulp macrophages filter red blood cell debris and remove *Plasmodium* parasites from red cells passing through the sinusoids in malaria patients. The spleen is almost always enlarged in such cases; in a recent series of patients dying of malaria in Vietnam, the median spleen weight was 300 g.[87,88] Spleens affected by malaria show expansion of both red and white pulp, with red pulp congestion and disrupted B- and T-cell architecture in the white pulp (Fig. 12-11A,B).[88] Chronic malaria infection may produce massive splenomegaly, known as the tropical splenomegaly syndrome or hyperreactive malarial splenomegaly. This is an important differential diagnosis of massive splenomegaly in areas endemic for malaria.[89] The median spleen weight in hyperreactive malarial splenomegaly is greater than 3 kg, and patients are cytopenic due to hypersplenism. On histology, the affected spleen shows marked sinusoidal dilatation with foci of extramedullary hemopoiesis.[90]

The spleen in hemophagocytic syndromes is enlarged, with prominent erythrophagocytosis observed in the red pulp; the red pulp histiocytes also contain intracellular neutrophils and lymphocytes. If the hemophagocytic syndrome is secondary to lymphoma, the spleen may be concomitantly involved by lymphomas, particularly peripheral T-cell lymphomas.[91]

The spleen is often enlarged in infectious mononucleosis and may rupture spontaneously or with minimal abdominal trauma, representing a rare but potentially fatal complication of the disease.[92] Although infectious mononucleosis is associated with lymphadenopathy and usually does result in splenic white pulp hyperplasia (see later discussion), the splenic red pulp shows more prominent expansion. The red pulp cords and sinuses contain numerous immunoblasts with prominent nucleoli.[93] Some cells may resemble Reed-Sternberg cells, mimicking Hodgkin lymphoma, and frequent large nucleolated immunoblasts may also mimic a non-Hodgkin lymphoma. EBER staining and a clinical history of infectious mononucleosis are helpful in avoiding misdiagnosis as lymphoma. EBV infection may also be associated with hemophagocytic syndrome in the spleen.

White Pulp Reactions to Infection

Follicular hyperplasia is the most common white pulp reaction that can occur as an incidental finding or as a nonspecific finding secondary to a variety of inflammatory or infectious conditions. Hyperplasia of the white pulp without prominent germinal centers can also occur in infectious mononucleosis and other viral infections, such as herpes simplex and HIV infection.[91,94]

Mass-Forming and Cystic Splenic Infections

Mycobacterial infections in HIV+ patients may produce solid spindle-cell nodules within the spleen. Special stains to demonstrate the mycobacteria within the spindle-shaped histiocytes are helpful in avoiding misdiagnosis as a splenic inflammatory pseudotumor or sarcoma.[95] Infections involving the spleen that manifest with splenic cyst are uncommon. Splenic abscesses are rare in the developed countries and usually occur in the setting of

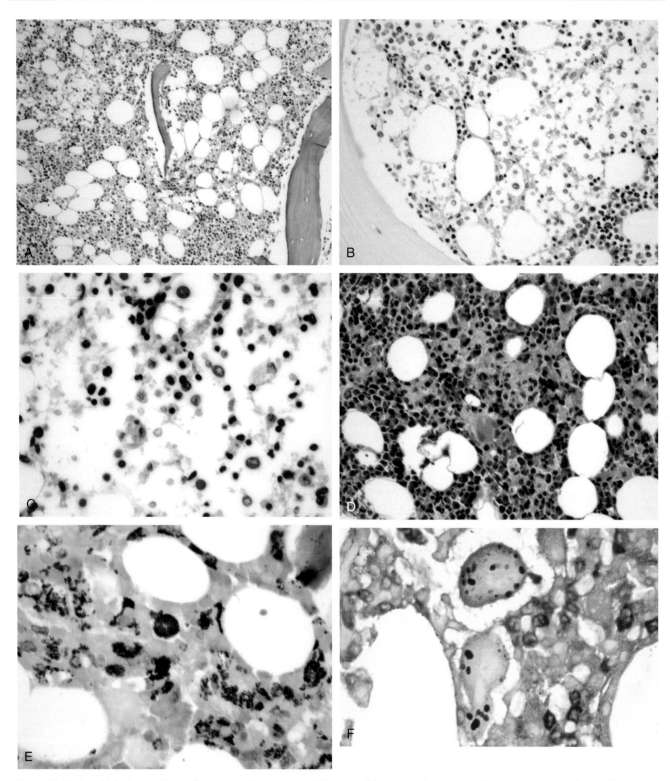

Figure 12-10. Fungal infections involving the bone marrow. **A,** In cryptococcal infection, well-formed granulomas may not be evident, but there is often a diffuse increase in histiocytes (H&E stain). **B,** On special staining of the bone marrow biopsy sample, the yeast forms are visualized (PAS stain). **C,** The yeast forms show characteristic narrow-based budding (PAS stain). **D,** In disseminated histoplasmosis involving the bone marrow, there is usually a diffuse proliferation of histiocytes (H&E stain). **E,** Special stains reveal the numerous intracellular and extracellular organisms; unlike *Leishmania*, the *Histoplasma* yeast forms are Giemsa negative (GMS stain). **F,** Fungal and yeast forms may be demonstrated within megakaryocytes in some cases (GMS stain) (Courtesy of Dr. Judith Ferry, Massachusetts General Hospital).

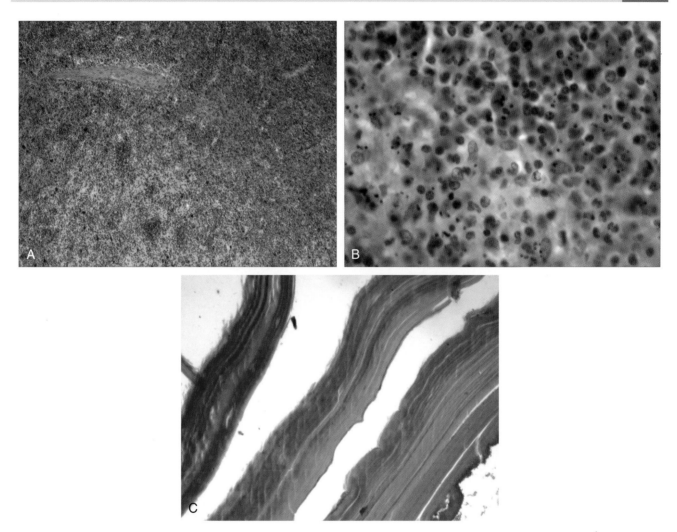

Figure 12-11. Infections involving the spleen. **A,** The spleen in malaria shows disorganization of the white pulp and red pulp congestion (H&E stain). **B,** High-power view of a spleen from a patient with malaria. Malarial pigment (hemozoin) is visible within histiocytes in the red pulp cords (H&E stain). **C,** The wall of an echinococcal (hydatid) cyst is acellular and eosinophilic with a characteristic lamellated appearance (H&E stain).

bacterial endocarditis, immunosuppression, intravenous drug use, or splenic trauma.[96,97] Bacterial agents such as *Staphylococcus* or *Streptococcus* species are the most common pathogens.[98] The diagnosis may be made with splenic aspiration or splenectomy and microbiologic cultures, but splenectomy is recommended for successful therapy.[96]

Hydatid cysts due to *Echinococcus granulosus* infection can rarely occur in the spleen. They manifested as a splenic cyst in only 3% of cases in one large recent series (see Fig. 12-11C).[99]

REFERENCES

1. Wickramasinghe S: Pathology of the marrow. In Wickramasinghe SN Mccullough J, (eds.): Blood and Bone Marrow Pathology. London, Churchill Livingstone, 2003, pp 89-128.
2. Diebold J, Molina T, Camilleri-Broet S, et al: Bone marrow manifestations of infections and systemic diseases observed in bone marrow trephine biopsy review. Histopathology 2000;37:199-211.
3. Bierman HR, Nelson ER: Hematodepressive virus diseases of Thailand. Ann Intern Med 1965;62:867-884.
4. Nakao S, Lai CJ, Young NS: Dengue virus, a flavivirus, propagates in human bone marrow progenitors and hematopoietic cell lines. Blood 1989;74:1235-1240.
5. Kaplan C, Morinet F, Cartron J: Virus-induced autoimmune thrombocytopenia and neutropenia. Semin Hematol 1992;29:34-44.
6. Murugan P, Chandrakumar S, Basu D, Hamide A: Gelatinous transformation of bone marrow in acquired immunodeficiency syndrome. Pathology 2007;39:287-288.
7. Mehta K, Gascon P, Robboy S: The gelatinous bone marrow (serous atrophy) in patients with acquired immunodeficiency syndrome: Evidence of excess sulfated glycosaminoglycan. Arch Pathol Lab Med 1992;116:504-508.
8. Cornbleet PJ, Moir RC, Wolf PL: A histochemical study of bone marrow hypoplasia in anorexia nervosa. Virch Arch A Pathol Anat Histol 1977;374:239-247.
9. Seaman JP, Kjeldsberg CR, Linker A: Gelatinous transformation of the bone marrow. Hum Pathol 1978;9:685-692.
10. Bohm J: Gelatinous transformation of the bone marrow: The spectrum of underlying diseases. Am J Surg Pathol 2000;24:56-65.
11. Kaloutsi V, Kohlmeyer U, Maschek H, et al: Comparison of bone marrow and hematologic findings in patients with human immuno-

deficiency virus infection and those with myelodysplastic syndromes and infectious diseases. Am J Clin Pathol 1994;101:123-129.

12. Thiele J, Zirbes TK, Bertsch HP, et al: AIDS-related bone marrow lesions: Myelodysplastic features or predominant inflammatory-reactive changes (HIV-myelopathy)? A comparative morphometric study by immunohistochemistry with special emphasis on apoptosis and PCNA-labeling. Anal Cell Pathol 1996;11:141-157.

13. Wickramasinghe SN, Abdalla SH, Kasili EG: Ultrastructure of bone marrow in patients with visceral leishmaniasis. J Clin Pathol 1987;40:267-275.

14. Moses A, Nelson J, Bagby GC Jr: The influence of human immunodeficiency virus-1 on hematopoiesis. Blood 1998;91:1479-1495.

15. Harbol AW, Liesveld JL, Simpson-Haidaris PJ, Abboud CN: Mechanisms of cytopenia in human immunodeficiency virus infection. Blood Rev 1994;8:241-251.

16. McClain K, Gehrz R, Grierson H, et al: Virus-associated histiocytic proliferations in children: Frequent association with Epstein-Barr virus and congenital or acquired immunodeficiencies. Am J Pediatr Hematol Oncol 1988;10:196-205.

17. Bhargava V, Farhi DC: Bone marrow granulomas: Clinicopathologic findings in 72 cases and review of the literature. Hematol Pathol 1988;2:43-50.

18. Bain BJ: Bone marrow trephine biopsy. J Clin Pathol 2001;54:737-742.

19. Fiala M, Colodro I, Talbert W, et al: Bone marrow granulomas in mononucleosis. Postgrad Med J 1987;63:277-279.

20. Brouland JP, Audouin J, Hofman P, et al: Bone marrow involvement by disseminated toxoplasmosis in acquired immunodeficiency syndrome: The value of bone marrow trephine biopsy and immunohistochemistry for the diagnosis. Hum Pathol 1996;27:302-306.

21. Walter R, Bachmann SP, Schaffner A, et al: Bone marrow involvement in Whipple's disease: Rarely reported, but really rare? Br J Haematol 2001;112:677-679.

22. Chung HJ, Chi HS, Cho YU, et al: [Bone marrow fibrin-ring granuloma: review of 24 cases]. Korean J Lab Med 2007;27:182-187.

23. Young JF, Goulian M: Bone marrow fibrin ring granulomas and cytomegalovirus infection. Am J Clin Pathol 1993;99:65-68.

24. Delsol G, Pellegrin M, Familiades J, Auvergnat JC: Bone marrow lesions in Q fever. Blood 1978;52:637-638.

25. Okun DB, Sun NC, Tanaka KR: Bone marrow granulomas in Q fever. Am J Clin Pathol 1979;71:117-121.

26. Delsol G, Pellegrin M, Voigt JJ, Fabre J: Diagnostic value of granuloma with fibrinoid ring. Am J Clin Pathol 1980;73:289.

27. Henter JI, Horne A, Arico M, et al: HLH-2004: Diagnostic and therapeutic guidelines for hemophagocytic lymphohistiocytosis. Pediatr Blood Cancer 2007;48:124-131.

28. Janka GE: Familial hemophagocytic lymphohistiocytosis. Eur J Pediatr 1983;140:221-230.

29. Stepp SE, Dufourcq-Lagelouse R, Le Deist F, et al: Perforin gene defects in familial hemophagocytic lymphohistiocytosis. Science 1999;286:1957-1959.

30. Zur Stadt U, Beutel K, Kolberg S, et al: Mutation spectrum in children with primary hemophagocytic lymphohistiocytosis: Molecular and functional analyses of PRF1, UNC13D, STX11, and RAB27A. Hum Mutat 2006;27:62-68.

31. Rouphael NG, Talati NJ, Vaughan C, et al: Infections associated with haemophagocytic syndrome. Lancet Infect Dis 2007;7:814-822.

32. Verbsky JW, Grossman WJ: Hemophagocytic lymphohistiocytosis: Diagnosis, pathophysiology, treatment, and future perspectives. Ann Med 2006;38:20-31.

33. Henter JI, Ehrnst A, Andersson J, Elinder G: Familial hemophagocytic lymphohistiocytosis and viral infections. Acta Paediatr 1993;82:369-372.

34. Clementi R, Emmi L, Maccario R, et al: Adult onset and atypical presentation of hemophagocytic lymphohistiocytosis in siblings carrying PRF1 mutations. Blood 2002;100:2266-2267.

35. Yamashita N, Kimura H, Morishima T: Virological aspects of Epstein-Barr virus infections. Acta Med Okayama 2005;59:239-246.

36. Risdall RJ, McKenna RW, Nesbit ME, et al: Virus-associated hemophagocytic syndrome: A benign histiocytic proliferation distinct from malignant histiocytosis. Cancer 1979;44:993-1002.

37. Favara BE: Hemophagocytic lymphohistiocytosis: A hemophagocytic syndrome. Semin Diagn Pathol 1992;9:63-74.

38. Suster S, Hilsenbeck S, Rywlin AM: Reactive histiocytic hyperplasia with hemophagocytosis in hematopoietic organs: A reevaluation of the benign hemophagocytic proliferations. Hum Pathol 1988;19:705-712.

39. Rosenfeld SJ, Young NS: Viruses and bone marrow failure. Blood Rev 1991;5:71-77.

40. Young N: Hematologic and hematopoietic consequences of B19 parvovirus infection. Semin Hematol 1988;25:159-172.

41. Brown KE: Haematological consequences of parvovirus B19 infection. Baillieres Best Pract Res Clin Haematol 2000;13:245-259.

42. Crook TW, Rogers BB, McFarland RD, et al: Unusual bone marrow manifestations of parvovirus B19 infection in immunocompromised patients. Hum Pathol 2000;31:161-168.

43. Kurtzman GJ, Ozawa K, Cohen B, et al: Chronic bone marrow failure due to persistent B19 parvovirus infection. N Engl J Med 1987;317:287-294.

44. Krause JR, Penchansky L, Knisely AS: Morphological diagnosis of parvovirus B19 infection: A cytopathic effect easily recognized in air-dried, formalin-fixed bone marrow smears stained with hematoxylin-eosin or Wright-Giemsa. Arch Pathol Lab Med 1992;116:178-180.

45. Leads from the MMWR: Risks associated with human parvovirus B19 infection. JAMA 1989;261:1406-1408.

46. Vadlamudi G, Rezuke WN, Ross JW, et al: The use of monoclonal antibody R92F6 and polymerase chain reaction to confirm the presence of parvovirus B19 in bone marrow specimens of patients with acquired immunodeficiency syndrome. Arch Pathol Lab Med 1999;123:768-773.

47. Zon LI, Arkin C, Groopman JE: Haematologic manifestations of the human immune deficiency virus (HIV). Br J Haematol 1987;66:251-256.

48. Fauci AS: Multifactorial nature of human immunodeficiency virus disease: Implications for therapy. Science 1993;262:1011-1018.

49. Kowalska MA, Ratajczak J, Hoxie J, et al: Megakaryocyte precursors, megakaryocytes and platelets express the HIV co-receptor CXCR4 on their surface: Determination of response to stromal-derived factor-1 by megakaryocytes and platelets. Br J Haematol 1999;104:220-229.

50. Lee B, Ratajczak J, Doms RW, et al: Coreceptor/chemokine receptor expression on human hematopoietic cells: Biological implications for human immunodeficiency virus-type 1 infection. Blood 1999;93:1145-1156.

51. Gordon S, Lee S: Naked megakaryocyte nuclei in bone marrows of patients with acquired immunodeficiency syndrome: A somewhat specific finding. Mod Pathol 1994;7:166-168.

52. Karcher DS, Frost AR: The bone marrow in human immunodeficiency virus (HIV)-related disease: Morphology and clinical correlation. Am J Clin Pathol 1991;95:63-71.

53. Karpatkin S: HIV-1-related thrombocytopenia. Hematol Oncol Clin North Am 1990;4:193-218.

54. Murphy MF, Metcalfe P, Waters AH, et al: Incidence and mechanism of neutropenia and thrombocytopenia in patients with human immunodeficiency virus infection. Br J Haematol 1987;66:337-340.

55. Benito N, Nunez A, de Gorgolas M, et al: Bone marrow biopsy in the diagnosis of fever of unknown origin in patients with acquired

immunodeficiency syndrome. Arch Intern Med 1997;157:1577-1580.

56. Engels E, Marks PW, Kazanjian P: Usefulness of bone marrow examination in the evaluation of unexplained fevers in patients infected with human immunodeficiency virus. Clin Infect Dis 1995;21:427-428.

57. Kurtin PJ, McKinsey DS, Gupta MR, Driks M: Histoplasmosis in patients with acquired immunodeficiency syndrome: Hematologic and bone marrow manifestations. Am J Clin Pathol 1990;93:367-372.

58. Kilby JM, Marques MB, Jaye DL, et al: The yield of bone marrow biopsy and culture compared with blood culture in the evaluation of HIV-infected patients for mycobacterial and fungal infections. Am J Med 1998;104:123-128.

59. Volk EE, Miller ML, Kirkley BA, Washington JA: The diagnostic usefulness of bone marrow cultures in patients with fever of unknown origin. Am J Clin Pathol 1998;110:150-153.

60. Luther JM, Lakey DL, Larson RS, et al: Utility of bone marrow biopsy for rapid diagnosis of febrile illnesses in patients with human immunodeficiency virus infection. South Med J 2000;93:692-697.

61. Marques MB, Waites KB, Jaye DL, et al: Histologic examination of bone marrow core biopsy specimens has limited value in the diagnosis of mycobacterial and fungal infections in patients with the acquired immunodeficiency syndrome. Ann Diagn Pathol 2000;4:1-6.

62. Hussong J, Peterson LR, Warren JR, Peterson LC: Detecting disseminated *Mycobacterium avium* complex infections in HIV-positive patients: The usefulness of bone marrow trephine biopsy specimens, aspirate cultures, and blood cultures. Am J Clin Pathol 1998;110:806-809.

63. Akpek G, Lee SM, Gagnon DR, et al: Bone marrow aspiration, biopsy, and culture in the evaluation of HIV-infected patients for invasive mycobacteria and histoplasma infections. Am J Hematol 2001;67:100-106.

64. Karcher DS: Clinically unsuspected Hodgkin disease presenting initially in the bone marrow of patients infected with the human immunodeficiency virus. Cancer 1993;71:1235-1238.

65. Horwitz CA, Henle W, Henle G, et al: Heterophil-negative infectious mononucleosis and mononucleosis-like illnesses: Laboratory confirmation of 43 cases. Am J Med 1977;63:947-957.

66. Krause JR, Kaplan SS: Bone marrow findings in infectious mononucleosis and mononucleosis-like diseases in the older adult. Scand J Haematol 1982;28:15-22.

67. Wick MJ, Woronzoff-Dashkoff KP, McGlennen RC: The molecular characterization of fatal infectious mononucleosis. Am J Clin Pathol 2002;117:582-588.

68. Harrington DS, Weisenburger DD, Purtilo DT: Epstein-Barr virus–associated lymphoproliferative lesions. Clin Lab Med 1988;8:97-118.

69. Penchansky L, Krause JR: Identification of cytomegalovirus in bone marrow biopsy. South Med J 1979;72:500-501.

70. Pooley RJ Jr, Peterson L, Finn WG, Kroft SH: Cytomegalovirus-infected cells in routinely prepared peripheral blood films of immunosuppressed patients. Am J Clin Pathol 1999;112:108-112.

71. Karakukcu M, Patiroglu T, Ozdemir MA, et al: Pancytopenia, a rare hematologic manifestation of brucellosis in children. J Pediatr Hematol Oncol 2004;26:803-806.

72. Sari I, Altuntas F, Hacioglu S, et al: A multicenter retrospective study defining the clinical and hematological manifestations of brucellosis and pancytopenia in a large series: Hematological malignancies, the unusual cause of pancytopenia in patients with brucellosis. Am J Hematol 2008;83:334-339.

73. Yildirmak Y, Palanduz A, Telhan L, et al: Bone marrow hypoplasia during *Brucella* infection. J Pediatr Hematol Oncol 2003;25:63-64.

74. Pintado V, Martin-Rabadan P, Rivera ML, et al: Visceral leishmaniasis in human immunodeficiency virus (HIV)-infected and non-HIV-infected patients: A comparative study. Medicine (Baltimore) 2001;80:54-73.

75. Pearson RD, Sousa AQ: Clinical spectrum of leishmaniasis. Clin Infect Dis 1996;22:1-13.

76. Browne PM, Sharma OP, Salkin D: Bone marrow sarcoidosis. JAMA 1978;240:2654-2655.

77. Antinori S, Calattini S, Longhi E, et al: Clinical use of polymerase chain reaction performed on peripheral blood and bone marrow samples for the diagnosis and monitoring of visceral leishmaniasis in HIV-infected and HIV-uninfected patients: A single-center, 8-year experience in Italy and review of the literature. Clin Infect Dis 2007;44:1602-1610.

78. Rossi JF, Eledjam JJ, Delage A, et al: *Pneumocystis carinii* infection of bone marrow in patients with malignant lymphoma and acquired immunodeficiency syndrome: Original report of three cases. Arch Intern Med 1990;150:450-452.

79. Heyman MR, Rasmussen P: *Pneumocystis carinii* involvement of the bone marrow in acquired immunodeficiency syndrome. Am J Clin Pathol 1987;87:780-783.

80. Amin MB, Mezger E, Zarbo RJ: Detection of *Pneumocystis carinii*: Comparative study of monoclonal antibody and silver staining. Am J Clin Pathol 1992;98:13-18.

81. Radio SJ, Hansen S, Goldsmith J, Linder J: Immunohistochemistry of *Pneumocystis carinii* infection. Mod Pathol 1990;3:462-469.

82. Wong KF, Ma SK, Chan JK, Lam KW: Acquired immunodeficiency syndrome presenting as marrow cryptococcosis. Am J Hematol 1993;42:392-394.

83. Witt D, McKay D, Schwam L, et al: Acquired immune deficiency syndrome presenting as bone marrow and mediastinal cryptococcosis. Am J Med 1987;82:149-150.

84. Pantanowitz L, Omar T, Sonnendecker H, Karstaedt AS: Bone marrow cryptococcal infection in the acquired immunodeficiency syndrome. J Infect 2000;41:92-94.

85. Ferry JA, Pettit CK, Rosenberg AE, Harris NL: Fungi in megakaryocytes: An unusual manifestation of fungal infection of the bone marrow. Am J Clin Pathol 1991;96:577-581.

86. Van Krieken JHJM, Te Velde J: Normal histology of the Spleen. In Sternberg S (ed.): Histology for Pathologists. New York, Raven Press, 1992, pp 253-260.

87. Angus BJ, Chotivanich K, Udomsangpetch R, White NJ: In vivo removal of malaria parasites from red blood cells without their destruction in acute falciparum malaria. Blood 1997;90:2037-2040.

88. Urban BC, Hien TT, Day NP, et al: Fatal *Plasmodium falciparum* malaria causes specific patterns of splenic architectural disorganization. Infect Immun 2005;73:1986-1994.

89. Sundaresan JB, Dutta TK, Badrinath S, et al: A hospital-based study of splenomegaly with special reference to the group of indeterminate origin. J Indian Med Assoc 2008;106:150, 152, 154 passim.

90. Pitney WR: The tropical splenomegaly syndrome. Trans R Soc Trop Med Hyg 1968;62:717-728.

91. Neiman RS, Orazi A: Histopathologic manifestations of lymphproliferative and myeloproliferative disorders involving the spleen. In Knowles D (ed.): Neoplastic Hematopathology, 2nd ed. Philadelphia, Lippincott Williams & Wilkins, 2001.

92. Frecentese DF, Cogbill TH: Spontaneous splenic rupture in infectious mononucleosis. Am Surgeon 1987;53:521-523.

93. Burke JS: Surgical pathology of the spleen: An approach to the differential diagnosis of splenic lymphomas and leukemias. Part II: Diseases of the red pulp. Am J Surg Pathol 1981;5:681-694.

94. Klatt EC, Meyer PR: Pathology of the spleen in the acquired immunodeficiency syndrome. Arch Pathol Lab Med 1987;111:1050-1053.

95. Suster S, Moran CA, Blanco M: Mycobacterial spindle-cell pseudo-tumor of the spleen. Am J Clin Pathol 1994;101:539-542.

96. Fotiadis C, Lavranos G, Patapis P, Karatzas G: Abscesses of the spleen: Report of three cases. World J Gastroenterol 2008;14:3088-3091.

97. Chun CH, Raff MJ, Contreras L, et al: Splenic abscess. Medicine (Baltimore) 1980;59:50-65.

98. Chang KC, Chuah SK, Changchien CS, et al: Clinical characteristics and prognostic factors of splenic abscess: A review of 67 cases in a single medical center of Taiwan. World J Gastroenterol 2006;12:460-464.

99. Bal N, Kocer NE, Arpaci R, et al: Uncommon locations of hydatid cyst. Saudi Med J 2008;29:1004-1008.

Bone Infections

Andrew E. Rosenberg, Susan V. Kattapuram, and G. Petur Nielsen

Osteomyelitis is defined literally as inflammation of bone and marrow, although in common use the term almost always implies infection. Infection of the skeleton, the largest organ system of the body, is important, because it is a major site of microbial infestation that is often morbid and sometimes fatal. All types of organisms, including bacteria, mycobacteria, fungi, viruses, and parasites, can cause osteomyelitis, but infections associated with certain pyogenic bacteria and mycobacteria are the most common. The microbes and their interplay with the host produce a wide spectrum of clinical manifestations that are further influenced by the causative event, the bone involved, the specific pathogen and its virulence, the medical condition of the host, the type of therapy, and the clinical course of the disease. Many of the molecular mechanisms underlying these biologic interactions have been elucidated, and this knowledge has facilitated advances in the stalwarts of therapy—surgery and antibiotics. However, the complexities and problems in diagnosing and treating osteomyelitis have become ever more challenging because of the increase in the elderly population, the widespread prevalence of diabetes, the high frequency of antibiotic-resistant pathogens, and the expanding population of immunocompromised patients and their exotic opportunistic infections.

Pathophysiology

The fundamental biologic processes active in bone infection are independent of pathogen type. Entry of the organism into bone is the first step in osteomyelitis and occurs by three main mechanisms: hematogenous seeding, extension from a contiguous site, and direct implantation (Table 13-1).

Hematogenous Spread

Hematogenous osteomyelitis is usually caused by bacteria and most commonly affects rapidly growing long bones. It frequently manifests as a primary, solitary focus of disease but, importantly, may occur as a complication of any localized or systemic infection. Within a long bone, the site first infected depends on whether the patient is an infant, child, or adult, and the relationship between age and localization is based on the vascular anatomy of the bone. Briefly, the nutrient artery supplies the majority of blood flow to bone; during growth and development after the first year of life, its terminal branches end as capillaries at the base of the growth plate (Fig. 13-1). As the capillaries approach the epiphyseal plate, they reverse direction by forming

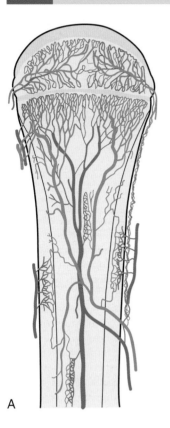
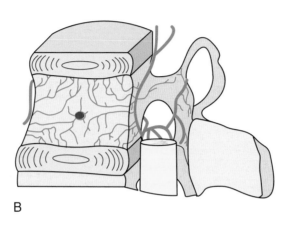

A

B

Figure 13-1. A, Vascular supply to a long bone in a child. The nutrient artery arborizes to small capillary loops at the base of the growth plate. **B,** Vascular supply to the vertebral body. The subchondral region has the richest capillary network.

Table 13-1 Routes of Entry of Infection into Bone
Hematogenous spread
Contiguous extension
Direct implantation

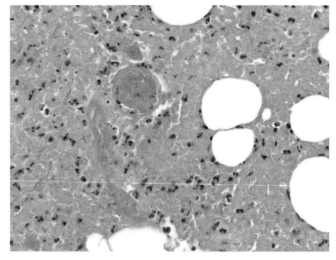

Figure 13-2. Early stage of acute osteomyelitis with thrombosis, neutrophils, fibrin, platelets, hemorrhage, and necrosis.

a loop and then merge into a network of sinusoidal venous blood lakes, which in turn empty into the venous drainage system of the medullary cavity. The blood flow in the capillary-sinusoid loop region is sluggish and turbulent, and phagocyte function is suboptimal; together, these features facilitate deposition of the organism into the metaphyseal tissue.[1,2] In infants younger than 1 year old, some of the terminal branches of the nutrient artery penetrate the growth plate; as they end near the base of the articular cartilage, their diameter expands, forming large venous lakes resembling metaphyseal sinusoids.[1,2] Therefore, in neonates, microbes may settle in the epiphysis or quickly spread into this region from a metaphyseal focus of disease.[3] In adults, after closure of the growth plate, the metaphyseal and epiphyseal vessels establish reconnections, and bacteria entering the nutrient artery are directed to the vascular loops beneath the articular cartilage. Accordingly, acute hematogenous osteomyelitis in infants and adults often affects the epiphysis, whereas in children, the growth plate acts as an effective barrier and the infection is usually limited to the metaphysis.

Once microbes seed the tissue, they adhere to the organic matrix or invade into cells, where they reproduce, forming growing colonies. The enlarging morass of organisms can obstruct blood flow, causing thrombosis and infarction, which creates an environment conducive to further propagation. Structural elements of the microbes or their secreted byproducts that are detected by the host trigger the innate and adaptive immune responses, which may vary according to the type of microbe. Once initiated, the immunologic reaction causes the contaminated area to become inundated with fluid, fibrin, degranulated platelets, extravasated red blood cells, and inflammatory cells (Fig. 13-2).[4] This phlegmon and developing abscess increases intraosseous pressure, which forces the inflammatory reaction

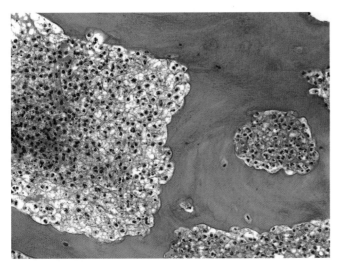

Figure 13-3. Sheets of neutrophils filling haversian systems. The bone is viable but shows scalloping of the surfaces, indicative of previous osteoclastic activity.

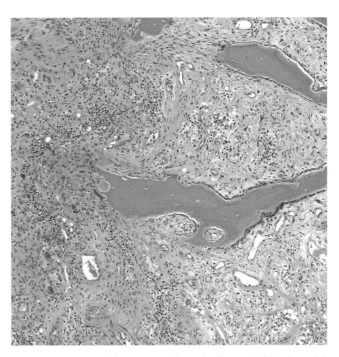

Figure 13-4. Acute and chronic osteomyelitis with inflammation filling the medullary cavity. Osteoclasts are resorbing the preexisting trabecular bone.

Table 13-2 Cytokines and Molecules Implicated in Stimulating Bone Cells in the Immune Response to Infection

Receptor activator of nuclear factor-κB ligand (RANKL)

Receptor activator of nuclear factor-κB (RANK)

Osteoprotegerin (OPG)

Macrophage colony-stimulating factor

Tumor necrosis factor

Interleukin 1

Interleukin 6

Interleukin 7

Interleukin 8

Interleukin 10

Interleukin 12

Interleukin 15

Interleukin 17

Interleukin 18

Interleukin 23

Interferon

through the medullary cavity and into haversian systems and Volkmann canals, causing necrosis of sometimes a sizable segment of bone. The devitalized bone is known as a sequestrum (Fig. 13-3). In infants and young children, the periosteum is not tightly bound to the cortex, so it may be mechanically lifted off the bone surface over large distances, disrupting periosteal feeding vessels and significantly enlarging the region of bone necrosis. The pus also may perforate the periosteum and extend into neighboring soft tissues, forming an abscess that can burrow to the skin surface, creating one or more sinus tracts that drain discolored exudates and necrotic tissue. The pus may extend into the epiphysis, where it can penetrate the articular surface or spread along capsular and tendoligamentous insertions into the joint. Consequently, septic or suppurative arthritis develops and can be associated with severe destruction of the articular cartilage and eventual permanent disability. This complication most frequently affects articulations whose joint capsules insert into cortices beyond the confines of the epiphysis.

As the acute phase intensifies over a period of several days to weeks, the inflammatory cells and their released enzymes and cytokines (Table 13-2) form a biologic broth that has powerful effects on the resident cells and biomaterials that comprise the bone tissue. Accordingly, osteoclasts are generated. and in this setting their numbers and activity are more extreme than in any other disease process. The osteoclasts target and resorb necrotic bone, thereby creating space for the expanding inflamed granulation tissue (Fig. 13-4). The evolving response leads to the arrival of lymphocytes, plasma cells, macrophages, collagen-producing fibroblasts, and newly formed blood vessels, which herald the so-called chronic phase of osteomyelitis. Mesenchymal stem cells located in the medullary cavity, cortex, and periosteum are stimulated simultaneously to produce osteoblasts that manufacture and secrete newly formed viable bone, usually woven in architecture. The living bone forms a subperiosteal shell, known as the involucrum, that envelops the necrotic cortical sequestrum, as well as a zone of sclerosis around the intramedullary extent of infection (Fig. 13-5). Over time, bone remodeling continues, and the nidus of infection may become walled off by the host reaction, forming an intraosseous abscess, also known

as a Brodie abscess (Fig. 13-6).[5] Some infections, especially those in the jaw bones, are associated with extensive new bone formation that obscures much of the underlying osseous structure; this form of disease is known as sclerosing osteomyelitis of Garré.

Hematogenous osteomyelitis also affects other portions of the skeleton. The more common locations include metaphyseal equivalent sites in long bones (e.g., adjacent to the femoral trochanters and tibial tuberosity) and flat and irregular bones (e.g., ilium adjacent to the triradiate cartilage, ilium adjacent to

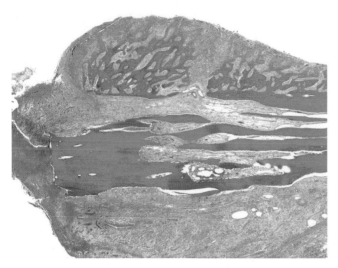

Figure 13-5. Medullary cavity filled with inflammation extending through the necrotic cortex (sequestrum) and associated with abundant viable subperiosteal reactive bone (involucrum).

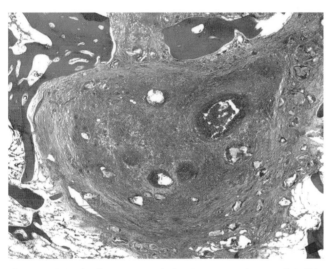

Figure 13-6. Brodie abscess composed of an intraosseous abscess walled off by reactive bone.

the acetabular roof, ilium adjacent to the anterior inferior spine, ilium adjacent to the sacroiliac joint, ilium adjacent to the crest).[6] The organisms preferentially seed these regions, leading to an inflammatory reaction and bone destruction.

In the spine, bloodborne pathogens usually localize to the subchondral regions of the vertebral body. These areas have the richest vascular supply; they are fed by branches of the spinal artery and drained by a venous plexus.[7] The proliferating organisms and inflammatory reaction digest and transgress the hyaline cartilage end plate and extend into and destroy the intervertebral disc. Spread to adjacent vertebral bodies is common. If the inflammatory process violates the periosteum, inflammation can accumulate in the surrounding soft tissue, such as in the epidural space or along or in the iliopsoas and paravertebral muscles.

Contiguous Spread

Osteomyelitis resulting from contiguous spread occurs after organisms from a neighboring anatomic site gain direct access to the bone. This can affect any bone adjacent to a soft tissue abscess, and it is most commonly seen in the setting of periodontal and sinus disease, cellulitis of diabetic feet, epidural abscess, decubitus ulcer, or septic arthritis. In these situations, the inflammatory process must first destroy the periosteum or articular surface before it accesses the bone. Unlike hematogenous osteomyelitis, the cortex instead of the medullary cavity is initially infected, and the site at which this occurs influences the rapidity of spread and extent of disease.

Direct Implantation

Direct implantation of pathogens into bone takes place in a variety of circumstances. Common scenarios are contamination of an open fracture, penetration of fomites such as shrapnel or orthopaedic hardware into bone, and exposure of bone during an operation. In these situations, the causative event and the extent of associated hemorrhage, tissue fragmentation, and necrosis influences important aspects of the infection.[8]

The balance between the biologic characteristics of the pathogen and the host determines the extent of the osseous manifestations of the infection and the ability of the host to confine and eradicate the organism. All too frequently, the pathogens remain viable and continue to proliferate in an environment of necrotic tissue inaccessible to the immune response and therapeutic antibiotics. In this fashion, a smoldering chronic infection is generated that maintains the potential to cause future havoc when conditions permit.

Bacterial Osteomyelitis

Bacterial infection of the skeleton accounts for the vast majority of microbial diseases of bone. It causes a variety of different clinicopathologic conditions which are related to the mode of infection, anatomic site, type of organism, and condition of the host. Approximately 20% of cases of bacterial osteomyelitis are hematogenous in origin, with the remainder secondary to contiguous spread and direct inoculation.

Bacterial Osteomyelitis from Hematogenous Spread

Bacterial hematogenous osteomyelitis is typically acute and most often develops in children. Half of the patients are younger than 5 years of age, and more than 85% of them are 16 years or younger. The annual incidence has remained relatively constant over the past several decades and is estimated to be 1 in every 5000 to 10,000 children annually.[9] Males are affected almost twice as frequently as females. Predisposing factors include indwelling catheters; infections of the skin, throat, ears, lung, heart, and genitourinary tract; nonpenetrating trauma; and underlying diseases or conditions such as diabetes, renal failure, hemoglobinopathies, and immunosuppression. More often than not, the host is healthy and the source of the bacteria is obscure, with the initiating bacteremia possibly complicating trivial occurrences, such as occult injury to the intestinal mucosa during defecation, vigorous chewing of hard foods, or minor infections of the skin.

The bones most commonly affected in children are the long tubular bones of the extremities, especially the femur (36%), tibia (33%), and humerus (10%).[9] In most instances, the infection involves a single osseous site, but in 5% to 20% of cases, it is multifocal in distribution.[10] In adults, the spine is most commonly involved, accounting for 2% to 4% of all bone infections. Most cases originate in the lumbar vertebrae (58%), followed by the thoracic (30%) and cervical vertebrae (11%).[11,12] The spine is also the most frequent site of infection in intravenous drug abusers. In patients with sickle cell disease, osteomyelitis usually occurs in the long bones, followed by the vertebrae.[13]

Clinically, hematogenous osteomyelitis may manifest as an acute systemic illness with malaise, fever, chills, leukocytosis, elevated erythrocyte sedimentation rate (ESR), and elevated C-reactive protein (CRP) level, as well as edema, swelling, warmth and marked-to-intense throbbing pain over the affected region. The presentation may be more subtle, with only unexplained fever, particularly in infants, or with only localized pain in the absence of fever in the adult.

Imaging studies reveal changes that vary with the stage of infection. The technetium bone scan becomes positive within 24 to 48 hours after the development of symptoms. Radiographs may reveal deep soft tissue swelling after several days, but it takes 10 to 21 days for changes to manifest in bone, because 30% to 50% of the osseous tissue must be resorbed before the infection becomes apparent on plain films.[14] The focus of infection first appears as a poorly defined area of radiolucency in the metaphysis that increases in breadth over time; in children, it may extend to the growth plate by an irregular channel (Figs. 13-7 through 13-9). Subsequently, reactive new bone is deposited, both beneath the raised periosteum and within the medullary canal at the boundary of disease. Extraosseous spread may be associated with a cortical cloaca and a contiguous abscess (Fig. 13-10). Computed tomography (CT) more precisely delineates the presence of gas, the extent of bone destruction, the formation of sequestra and involucra, and soft tissue involvement (see Figs. 13-9B and 13-10B).[14] Magnetic resonance imaging (MRI) detects edema and the inflammatory changes 3 to 5 days after the beginning of infection. It does not demonstrate the bony changes as well as CT but is better at revealing the extent of disease, the presence of intraosseous and soft tissue abscesses, the zone of surrounding edema, and joint effusions and joint involvement (see Figs. 13-7B, 13-8B, 13-10C).[14] If the changes are confined over time, an intraosseous abscess (Brodie abscess) may develop and can mimic a neoplasm (Fig. 13-11).

Vertebral infection usually localizes to the anterior subchondral portion of the vertebral body, in close proximity to the intervertebral disc. Within several weeks, the disc becomes involved, and this is associated with loss of height and blurring of the normal contour of the subchondral bone plate. Progressive destruction of the bone and disc ensues, and the neighboring vertebrae and soft tissue may become involved (Figs. 13-12 through 13-14).

Pathologically, bacterial infection usually elicits a suppurative inflammatory response with edema, fibrin, hemorrhage, and necrosis. Necrosis of bone manifests as osseous tissue with empty lacunae, and, in the setting of infection, many of its surfaces are either covered by osteoclasts or pockmarked by Howship lacunae (Fig. 13-15). Colonies of bacteria may be found in the inflammatory infiltrate and necrotic tissue (Fig. 13-16). After several weeks, the marrow becomes replaced by reactive fibrovascular tissue, and the inflammatory infiltrate becomes enriched with lymphocytes, plasma cells, and macrophages (Fig. 13-17). In some cases, the plasma cells are so numerous (plasma cell osteo-

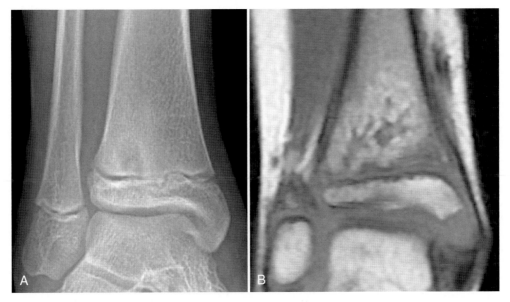

Figure 13-7. Acute osteomyelitis of distal tibia. **A,** Anteroposterior radiograph shows poorly defined area of osteolysis with minimal surrounding sclerosis in the distal tibial metaphysis. **B,** Coronal T1-weighted magnetic resonance image demonstrates an irregular dark area composed of inflammatory tissue surrounded by a dark zone of edema adjacent to the plate medially.

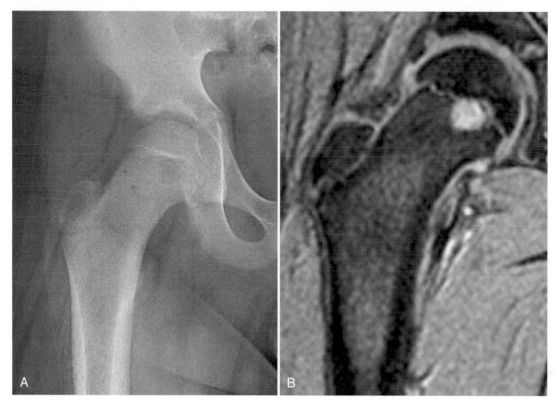

Figure 13-8. Acute osteomyelitis of proximal femur. **A,** Anteroposterior radiograph showing central area of bone lucency adjacent to the growth plate. **B,** The area is very bright on the coronal T2-weighted magnetic resonance image.

myelitis) they can cause confusion with plasma cell neoplasms (Fig. 13-18).[15] Intraosseous abscesses consist of granulation tissue admixed with inflammatory cells. The reactive bone that forms is frequently woven and is deposited beneath the periosteum and within the medullary cavity de novo or on the surfaces of preexisting living or necrotic trabecular bone (see Fig. 13-5).

Importantly, some bacteria are associated with granulomatous inflammation, including multinucleated Langhans-type giant cells. This type of inflammatory response can be associated with infections by *Salmonella, Brucella, Bartonella, Coxiella burnetii* (Q fever), and *Burkholderia pseudomallei* (melioidosis).[16-21]

Most specimens from bacterial hematogenous osteomyelitis are derived from curettage specimens, so the gross findings may be difficult to appreciate; however, they may contain green-tan discolored pus that can be putrid. Resection specimens are typically derived from patients with long-standing chronic disease. In these instances, the necrotic tissue is discolored green-tan-brown and the fibrotic marrow is white-gray. The cancellous bone in the center of the infection is largely destroyed by the fibrous tissue, and the surrounding bone is sclerotic, having been rebuttressed. The cortex is frequently thickened in an irregular fashion by subperiosteal reactive bone, and a cloaca appears as a round or oval hole in the cortex that is in continuity with soft tissue involvement (Fig. 13-19).

Staphylococcus aureus is responsible for 80% to 90% of the cases of bacterial hematogenous osteomyelitis in which an organism is recovered.[22] Group A and B streptococci and gram-negative organisms are important etiologic agents in neonates. *Haemophilus influenzae* has become less important since the introduction of the vaccine against this organism. *Salmonella* complicates sickle cell disease, and *Escherichia coli, Pseudomonas,* and *Klebsiella* are more frequently isolated from patients who have genitourinary tract infections or who are intravenous drug abusers.

The diagnosis can be strongly suggested by the characteristic findings on clinical and imaging studies. However, in some cases, especially in children, the destructive process may mimic a primary malignancy such as Ewing sarcoma or osteosarcoma. In many untreated cases, blood cultures are positive, but biopsy and bone cultures are required to identify the pathogen in most instances. The combination of antibiotics and surgical drainage is usually curative, but in 5% to 25% of cases, acute osteomyelitis fails to resolve and persists as chronic infection. Chronicity may develop if there is delay in diagnosis, extensive bone necrosis, abbreviated antibiotic therapy, inadequate surgical débridement, or weakened host defenses. Acute flare-ups may mark the clinical course of chronic infection; they are usually spontaneous, have no obvious cause, and may occur after years of dormancy.[23] Other complications of chronic osteomyelitis include pathologic fracture, secondary amyloidosis, endocarditis, sepsis, development of squamous cell carcinoma in the sinus tract, and, rarely, sarcoma in the infected bone.

Bacterial Osteomyelitis from Contiguous Spread

Bacterial infection can spread from a poorly controlled neighboring juxtaosseous infection to involve bone. In this situation, the

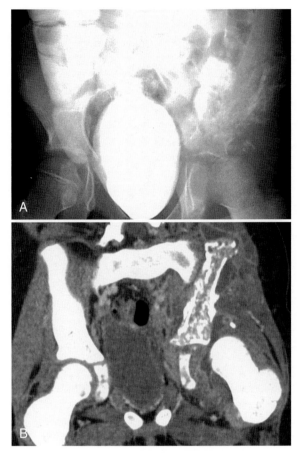

Figure 13-9. Acute and chronic osteomyelitis of the pelvis. **A,** Anteroposterior radiograph of the left pelvis in a child shows marked destruction of bone with irregular periosteal reactive bone. **B,** Coronal computed tomogram shows extensive bone lysis and new bone formation with multiple low-density areas (abscesses) in the gluteal and iliopsoas muscles. There is a joint effusion.

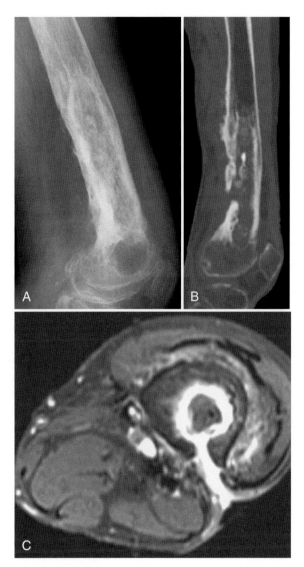

Figure 13-10. Acute and chronic osteomyelitis with soft tissue abscess and sinus tract. **A,** Lateral radiograph of the distal femur shows a large area of lysis and sclerosis. Irregular subperiosteal new bone deposition is present. **B,** Sagittal reformatted image from computed tomography scan demonstrates marked bone destruction and sclerosis. Cortical cloaca is present, adjacent to the soft tissue abscess sinus tract. **C,** Axial T2-weighted magnetic resonance image illustrates the intraosseous inflammation which extends into the soft tissues through the sinus tract and exits through the skin.

proliferating bacteria devitalize the periosteum or digest the articular cartilage and thereby gain entry to the cortex or medullary cavity. Patients with common conditions such as periodontal disease, caries, sinusitis, cellulitis of the feet and toes (in patients with severe peripheral vascular disease, especially diabetics), or immobility with decubitus ulcers are prone to this type of infection.

Osteomyelitis of the jaw frequently occurs as a result of periodontal disease and caries (Fig. 13-20). Many patients also have a history of irradiation, which compromises the gingiva and induces necrosis of the underlying bone. The exposed bone acts as a good medium for bacterial pathogens, which frequently becomes infected by multiple organisms, including *S. aureus, Streptococcus* species, and *Actinomyces.*[24]

Actinomycosis most commonly occurs in the jaws and is often associated with chronic infection, including draining sinuses.[25] It is often seen in the setting of osteoradionecrosis and in patients who have been treated with bisphosphonates.

Bisphosphonate-induced osteonecrosis has recently been the focus of attention because of the widespread use of bisphosphonates and the controversy regarding the pathogenesis of this disease.[26,27] The first large series of patients with bisphosphonate-induced osteonecrosis was described in 2003 and involved

patients who had a malignancy, frequently myeloma, and were receiving intravenous bisphosphonates.[28] Typically, patients have a history of a recent dental procedure and present with exposed bone that is necrotic but also infected with actinomycetes (Fig. 13-21). It is unclear whether the infection is the primary causative event or is secondary, nor whether it begins in the gingiva or in the bone. Pathologic examination of surgical specimens shows gingival inflammation and ulceration and necrotic bone infiltrated by actinomycetes and neutrophils (Fig. 13-22). The organisms are pleomorphic branching, filamentous, gram-positive bacteria that frequently aggregate into sulfur granules and exhibit the Splendore-Hoeppli phenomenon. The disease can be

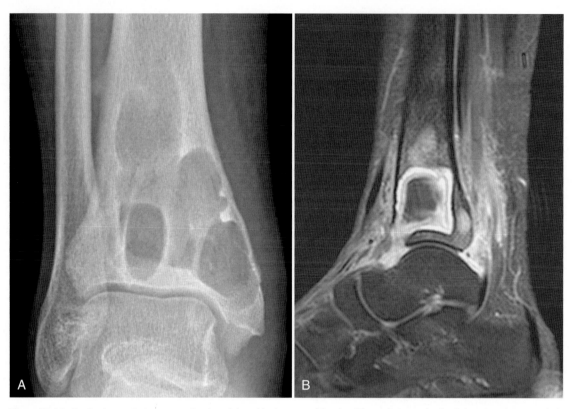

Figure 13-11. Brodie abscess. **A,** Anteroposterior view of the ankle shows a multiloculated, lucent lesion in the distal tibia. The margins are fairly well defined. No internal matrix is visible. **B,** Sagittal, contrast-enhanced T1-weighted sequence shows a characteristic appearance, with a nonenhancing, low-signal-intensity central area (abscess) surrounding hyperintense granulation tissue. There is also enhancement of the surrounding marrow and the synovium.

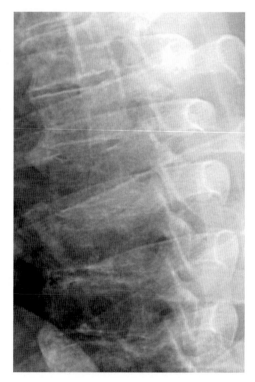

Figure 13-12. Osteomyelitis of spine. Lateral radiograph shows loss of subchondral bone plate and adjacent bone lysis.

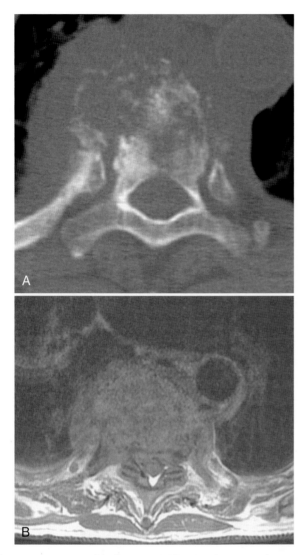

Figure 13-13. Osteomyelitis of spine. **A,** Axial computed tomogram demonstrates irregular destruction of bone with extension into the anterior soft tissues. **B,** T1-weighted magnetic resonance image shows extensive marrow involvement and extensions into the soft tissues.

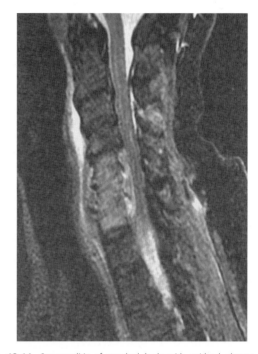

Figure 13-14. Osteomyelitis of vertebral body with epidural abscess. Sagittal T2-weighted magnetic resonance image shows involvement of several cervical vertebral bodies with an epidural abscess and involvement of anterior soft tissues.

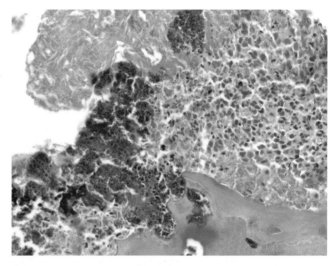

Figure 13-16. Acute osteomyelitis involving primary spongiosa adjacent to the growth plate. Dark purple aggregates of bacteria are adjacent to dying inflammatory cells.

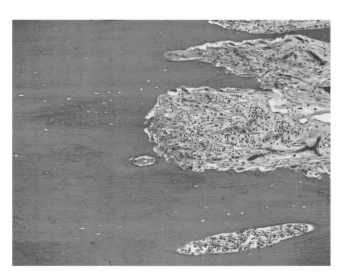

Figure 13-15. Necrotic cortical bone being resorbed by osteoclasts in expanded haversian canal.

chronic and recurrent, and treatment commonly includes surgical débridement and antibiotics.[28,29]

The development of osteomyelitis as a complication of bacterial sinusitis is uncommon. Patients range from adolescents to the elderly and present with headache, swelling, fever, and discharge. The most common site of involvement is the frontal sinus.[30] In this region, osteomyelitis may produce a subperiosteal abscess that may manifest as a soft tissue mass of the forehead known as Pott's puffy tumor.[31] The more common pathogens include *S. aureus,* nonenterococcal streptococci, and oral anaerobes.[30]

Osteomyelitis of the feet in patients with vascular insufficiency, particularly in diabetics, is a serious problem. The ulcers develop because of a combination of neuropathic, ischemic, and local biomechanical changes that subject the skin and soft tissues to excessive pressure, friction, breakdown, and necrosis while eliciting sometimes only minimal local symptoms (Fig. 13-23). The development of osteomyelitis in these patients is usually

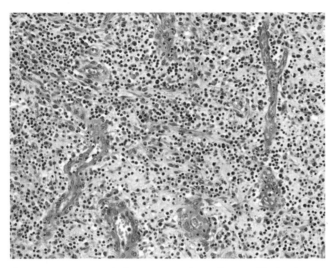

Figure 13-17. Acute and chronic osteomyelitis with neutrophils, lymphocytes, plasma cells, macrophages, and capillaries.

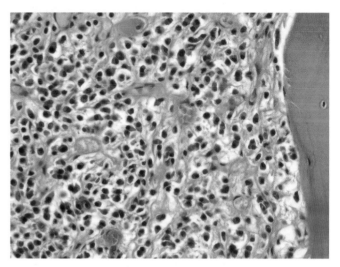

Figure 13-18. Chronic osteomyelitis with numerous plasma cells. Sometimes this can be confused with myeloma.

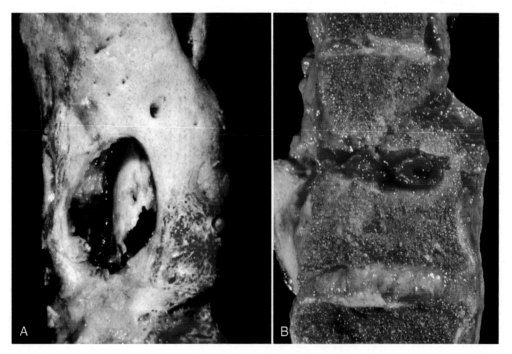

Figure 13-19. Gross specimens of osteomyelitis. **A,** Chronic osteomyelitis of long bone with cortical sequestrum and its cloaca, and with a well-formed involucrum which also has a cloaca. **B,** Vertebral bodies removed at autopsy. The disk space is replaced by hemorrhagic inflammatory tissue, and the adjacent vertebral bodies show replacement of the marrow by tan tissue with focal disruption of the bone.

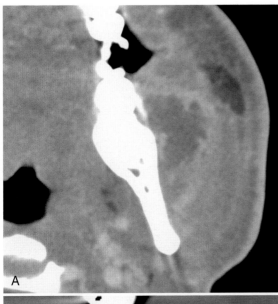

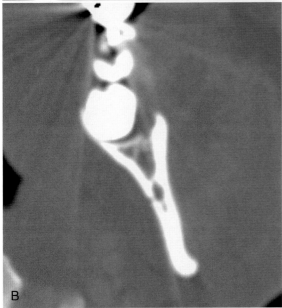

Figure 13-20. Periodontal abscess of mandible. **A,** Axial computed tomogram of mandible with soft tissue windows showing low-density abscess in the soft tissues. **B,** Bone window shows a small focus of cortical disruption with a lytic focus within the bone.

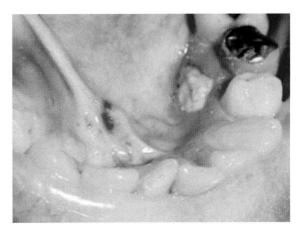

Figure 13-21. This patient was treated with intravenous bisphosphonate; after an extraction, the patient developed exposed bone infected with actinomycosis which was also necrotic.

a complication of a nonhealing ulcer that gradually involves the deeper soft tissues until the periosteum is breached. Once the bone is exposed, the cortex may undergo necrosis, with the infection spreading along its length and into the medullary cavity via the haversian systems. Joint involvement is relatively common in severe disease (Fig. 13-24). As the bone is resorbed, it may undergo secondary fracture with callus formation. Bone cultures frequently isolate *S. aureus*, which may be methicillin resistant, followed by *Staphylococcus epidermidis*. *E. coli, Klebsiella pneumoniae,* and *Proteus* spp., with *Pseudomonas aeruginosa* the most common pathogen among Enterobacteriaceae.[32]

Infection of bone beneath a decubitus ulcer typically develops when a pressure sore fails to resolve and the bacteria and inflammation extend into the underlying osseous tissue. This complication develops in 17% to 32% of infected decubiti.[33] The patients usually lack sensation in the affected region and are immobile and poorly nourished. Common sites for this problem are the sacrum, posterior calcaneus, ischial tuberosities, greater trochanters, elbows, scapulae, and lateral malleoli.[33] The infection is polymicrobial and includes aerobes (*Proteus mirabilis, E. coli,* enterococci, staphylococci, and *Pseudomonas* spp.) and anaerobes (*Peptostreptococcus* spp., *Bacteroides fragilis,* and *Clostridium perfringens*).[34] The infection may involve only the superficial portion of the bone, or it may be more extensive.[35] The histologic findings frequently show the features of chronic osteomyelitis.[35]

Bacterial Osteomyelitis from Direct Inoculation

Bone infection caused by direct implantation of bacteria into bone has diverse etiologies. The common thread to all is that the bone is either exposed or violated, giving bacteria direct access to osseous tissue. Degloving injuries or open fractures in which the fractured ends of the bone pierce the skin and become contaminated are serious injuries. The extent of the trauma, the amount of tissue necrosis, the degree of contamination, the amount of available soft tissue coverage, the rapidity and skill of surgical intervention, and the state of the host influence wound healing.[36] Between 3% and 30% of open fractures eventually become infected with bacteria residing in pieces of necrotic bone. Many patients are young, and the long bones of the lower extremities, especially the tibia and fibula, are frequently affected. A host of different bacteria may behave as pathogens, including those that normally colonize the skin, bacteria from the contaminating soil, and nosocomial organisms acquired during hospitalization and restorative surgical procedures. The most frequent offenders are staphylococci and aerobic gram-negative bacilli; however, enterococci are also infrequently implicated. The osteomyelitis often manifests as a non-union with local and systemic symptoms such as swelling, fever, and pain. Crucial to preventing this complication are successful débridement and wash-out of the wound, fixation of the bone, and closure of the

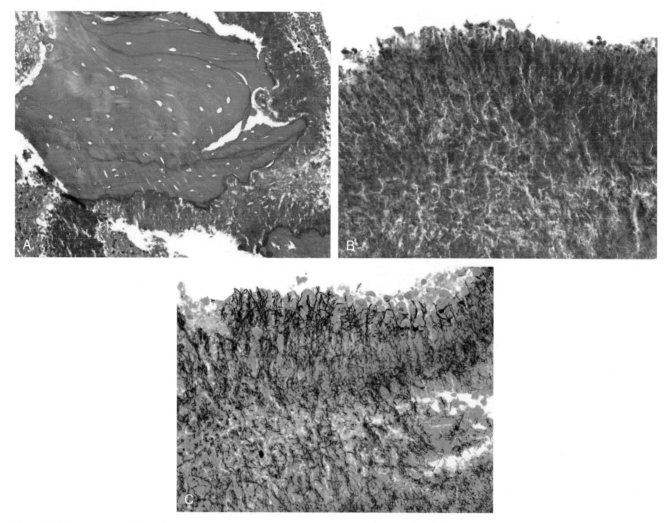

Figure 13-22. Actinomycosis of mandible. **A,** Necrotic bone infiltrated by colonies of actinomycetes. **B,** High-power view of actinomycetes in tissue exhibits the Splendore-Hoeppli phenomenon. **C,** Actinomycetes stained with Grocott methenamine silver (GMS) stain highlighting the filamentous nature of the bacteria.

surrounding soft tissue envelope. Ideally, this should be accomplished within 6 hours after the injury.[37,38]

Orthopedic implants, including prosthetic joints and internal fixation devices, are being used at a steadily increasing rate. More than 1 million reconstructive prosthetic joint arthroplasties and significantly more trauma-related implant surgeries are performed annually in the United States. The impetus for this rise in orthopedic implant surgery is the longer lifespan of the population, which is associated with a higher prevalence of significant osteoarthritis (joint replacement) and osteoporosis (pathologic fracture); active lifestyles; improved prosthetic materials and hardware; and more refined and safer surgical techniques, especially for the elderly. Orthopedic implants have high success rates, but they may fail because of metal fatigue with fracture, corrosion, generation of wear debris, and infection. Although there have been great strides in preventing and treating implant-associated infections, the total number is increasing because the devices have a lifelong risk of becoming seeded by bacteria. The risk of developing infection within 2 years after primary joint replacement is less than 1% for hip and shoulder prostheses, less than 2% for knee prostheses, and less than 9% for artificial

elbows.[39-42] The rate increases to 5% to 40% with revision joint arthroplasties.[40] Approximately 5% of internal fixation devices become infected; the infection rate after closed fractures is 0.5% to 2%, and that after reconstruction of open fractures is 30%.[40]

Orthopedic implant–associated infections can be divided into those that are perioperative or early (<3 months after surgery), delayed (3 to 24 months after implantation), and late (>24 months after surgery).[42] The early and delayed infections are believed to result from contamination occurring at the time of implantation surgery, whereas the late infections are hematogenous in origin.[42]

Infections developing soon after implantation are usually acute in onset and manifest with warmth, swelling, and pain at the operative site and the systemic findings of fever, leukocytosis, elevated ESR and CRP. The organisms usually responsible are virulent and include *S. aureus* and gram-negative bacilli. Delayed infections are more subtle clinically, and the patients may present with loosening of the implant and pain (Fig. 13-25). The presentation may be very similar to loosening caused by prosthetic particulate wear debris. The cause of the loosening is stimulation of osteoclastic resorption of bone adjacent to the implant by cytokines released by the inflammatory reaction to the pathogen. The normally thin layer of reactive fibrous tissue between the host and the implant or its anchoring cement, which is frequently designated the membrane by orthopedic surgeons, becomes thickened by inflammatory cells, collagen, and blood vessels. In severe cases, pus develops. The organisms are usually not very virulent and include coagulase-negative staphylococci and *Propionibacterium acnes*. Although these pathogens are acquired at the time of implantation, they attach to the devices by proteinaceous cell wall and capsular polysaccharide–associated adhesins and remain protected from antibiotics and the host immune response by secreted biofilms.

The distinction between delayed infection and failure related to prosthetic wear debris can be very difficult. In many instances, it requires correlation of the clinical findings, imaging studies, and laboratory tests such as the ESR and CRP. All too frequently,

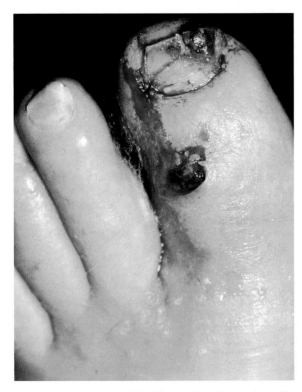

Figure 13-23. Great toe of elderly diabetic patient. The toe is swollen and erythematous with several ischemic ulcers.

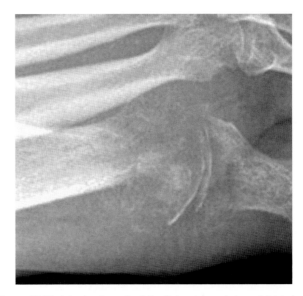

Figure 13-24. Lateral radiograph of the first metatarsophalangeal joint shows osteopenia, loss of joint space, and destruction of the adjacent bones, especially the metatarsal head.

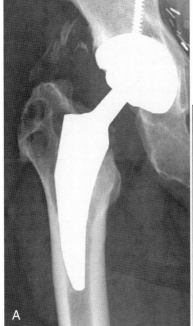
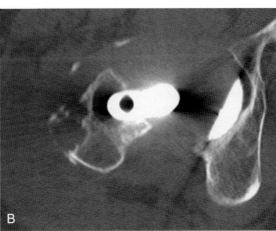

Figure 13-25. Hip prosthesis with heterotopic bone in soft tissues and infection of the femoral component. **A,** Plain radiograph shows large radiolucencies in the greater trochanter. **B,** Axial computed tomogram shows destruction of bone around the implant involving the greater trochanter.

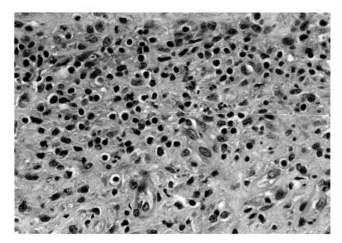

Figure 13-26. Synovial-like tissue removed from the region around the femoral component. The neutrophils are indicative of infection.

Table 13-3 Histologic Criteria for Diagnosis of Osteomyelitis Complicating Prosthesis Placement

Five or more neutrophils in each of five consecutive high-power fields

Neutrophils enmeshed in fibrin

Exclude surface exudates

these data are nonconclusive, and the next step is frozen-section histologic examination of the tissue adjacent to the implant at the time of joint replacement.[43] Studies have shown that the identification of five neutrophils in five consecutive separate high-power fields, excluding surface exudates and neutrophils enmeshed within fibrin aggregates, correlates with culture-proven infection (Fig. 13-26, Table 13-3). This technique has relatively low sensitivity (29%) but high specificity (95%).[43] Practical suggestions for performing this technique include the following: (1) prepare a minimum of three cassettes per specimen, and (2) identify the surface of the tissue that abutted the prosthesis (it is shiny and frequently smooth), and section it in a perpendicular plane—if neutrophils are present, they will be most numerous in the superficial portion of the tissue.

The treatment of an infected prosthesis frequently involves surgical and medical therapy. The surgical procedures range from reimplantation, either at the time of resection (one-stage replacement) or in a second surgery (two-stage replacement); excision of diseased tissue with preservation of the prosthesis; complete resection with or without arthrodesis; and amputation. The type of pathogen, the amount and condition of the residual bone and soft tissues, the antimicrobial susceptibility of the infecting microorganism, and the patient's medical condition are factors that influence the surgical treatment strategy. The two-stage reconstruction is optimal. After removal of the implant, the structural integrity of the site can be temporarily maintained by an antibiotic-impregnated spacer or cement. The patient is also treated with parenteral antibiotics, and 4 to 6 weeks after the site is sterilized, a new prosthesis is implanted. The cost for the treatment of this complication is more than $50,000.

Mycobacterial Osteomyelitis

Mycobacteria are aerobic and usually nonmotile bacteria that are acid-alcohol fast and have thick cell walls that are hydrophobic and rich in mycolic acids. Currently, within the genus *Mycobacterium*, more than 120 different species are recognized.[44] The majority are not pathogenic and are ubiquitous in the environment, with their natural reservoirs being water, soil, aerosols, dust, animals, and foods. The major human pathogenic mycobacterium is *Mycobacterium tuberculosis*, but *Mycobacterium leprae* and *Mycobacterium ulcerans* are also responsible for significant human disease. The major differences between *M. tuberculosis* and the non-tuberculous mycobacteria are the virulence of the organisms and the potential for human-to-human transmission. Non-tuberculous mycobacteria are generally of low virulence and are not associated with human-to-human spread. The successful pathogens have the capability to reside and proliferate within host macrophages, despite the bactericidal properties of these cells. The macrophages are a component of the complex immune response involving both innate and adaptive systems that sequesters the microorganisms within granulomas. Overall, mycobacterial infection of the skeletal system is much less frequent than bacterial osteomyelitis.

Tuberculous Osteomyelitis

Tuberculosis is defined as an infectious disease caused by *M. tuberculosis*. It kills 1.8 million people annually and is the leading cause of death associated with an infectious disease. It is responsible for the death of approximately 3 million people annually.

Tuberculous osteomyelitis has plagued mankind for millennia. Evidence of bone disease has been found in Egyptian mummies and in skeletal remains dating from the Iron Age. A resurgence of tuberculous osteomyelitis has occurred in industrialized nations that has been attributed to the influx of immigrants from underdeveloped countries and to greater numbers of immunosuppressed people. In developing countries, the affected individuals are usually adolescents or young adults, whereas in the indigenous population of the United States, the victims tend to be older, except for those who are immunosuppressed. Currently, in the United States, the incidence of tuberculosis is on the decline, but it remains an important health problem. Approximately 1% to 3% of patients with pulmonary tuberculosis also have osseous disease, and 10% of all cases of extrapulmonary tuberculosis are caused by bone infection.

Mycobacteremia is the mechanism that underlies most cases of bone disease. The organisms originate from foci of active visceral disease that are in the initial stages of primary infection. Direct extension (e.g., from a pulmonary focus into a rib, from tracheobronchial nodes into adjacent vertebrae) or spread via draining lymphatics or Batson's venous plexus from the lung to the spine may also occur. The bone infection is usually solitary and in some cases may be the only clinical manifestation of the disease. Infection in the bone can fester for years before being recognized. Patients with acquired immunodeficiency syndrome (AIDS) frequently have multifocal bone involvement resulting from widespread hematogenous dissemination.

The spine is affected in 40% to 50% of cases of tuberculous osteomyelitis, followed in frequency by the hips in 25% and the knees in 20% of cases. Spinal infection occurs 2 to 10 times more frequently in patients infected with the human immunodeficiency virus (HIV). In the spine, 98% of infections are centered in the anterior column, and the involved level is usually located in the region of T6 through L3.[45,46] Thoracic disease is more frequent in children; in adults, the lumbar area is more often involved.

Patients present with insidious symptoms that develop over a period of months to 1 year or longer. Common manifestations are low-grade fevers, weight loss, pain that is regional and ranges from mild to severe, swelling, local warmth without erythema, muscle spasms and atrophy, limitation of range of motion, limping, gibbus formation, and soft tissue masses (typically a manifestation of a cold abscess).

Radiographically, nuclear magnetic resonance is the modality of choice for assessing spinal tuberculosis, because plain films and CT are not very sensitive and do not adequately demonstrate marrow involvement. The disease first begins in the anterior subchondral region of the vertebral body (Fig. 13-27). Initially it may appear as a localized area of osteoporosis with loss of the subchondral bone plate. On MRI, the inflammatory bone marrow changes manifest as patchy high signal intensities on T2-weighted images and low signal intensity on T1-weighted images.[47] Continued expansion of the infection produces disruption of the cortex and spread into the neighboring disc. In comparison to purulent bacterial discitis, the disc space in tuber-

culosis may show only limited narrowing on imaging studies, despite the presence of extensive bone destruction, and this is an important diagnostic feature of tuberculous spondylitis. Progressive disease causes erosion of the anterior and lateral cortices, leading to angular collapse with posterior projection and deformity (Pott's disease). The angle of the projection is most severe when only one or two vertebral bodies have collapsed (Fig. 13-28). If the bony collapse involves one side of the vertebral body more than the other, lateral angulation may also occur.

Within the bone, bright signal intensity on T2-weighted images surrounding a central region of low signal intensity on T1-weighted images reflects the presence of an intraosseous abscess. The rim of the abscess shows intense enhancement after the administration of contrast agents such as gadolinium. Craniocaudal spread beneath the anterior longitudinal ligament produces involvement of multiple vertebral bodies, and sometimes this is associated with the sparing of one or more intervening vertebrae (skip lesions).[47] Extensive disease may be associated with involvement of the posterior elements and epidural space and with large paravertebral abscesses (Fig. 13-29). In exceptional cases, the abscesses may dissect along tissue planes and produce large distant masses that can compress organs, erode bones, and manifest as soft tissue masses. Those growing along the psoas fascia can extend beneath the inguinal ligament and manifest as a thigh mass (Fig. 13-30). The wall of abscess may calcify in long-standing disease, and the abscess can continue to burrow and form fistulas and draining sinuses.

Tuberculous osteomyelitis of the appendicular skeleton usually begins in the metaphysis and extends into the epiphysis; joint involvement is commonplace. As a result, subchondral bone

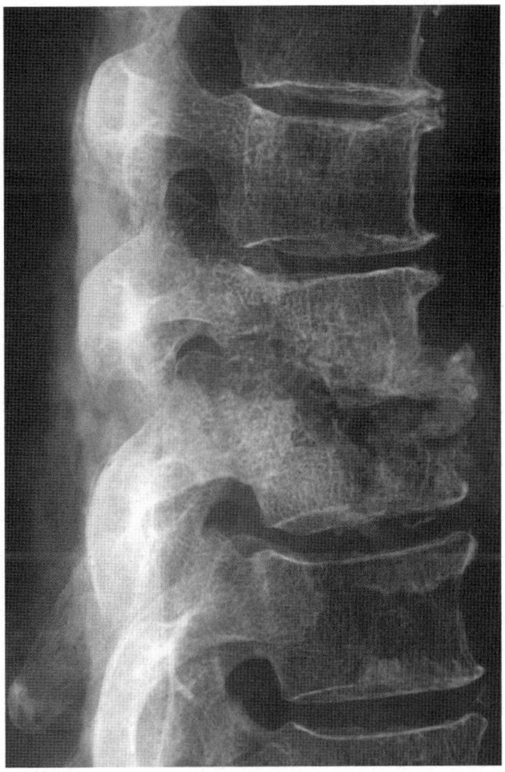

Figure 13-27. Tuberculosis of thoracic spine with destruction of adjacent vertebral bodies and the intervening disc. The anterior portions of the bodies are most severely affected.

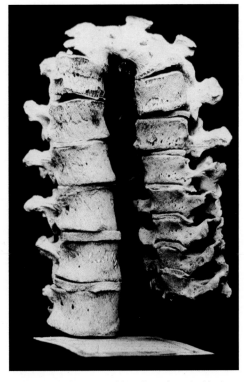

Figure 13-28. Severe kyphosis caused by collapsed vertebral body as a result of tuberculosis. (Courtesy of Dr. W. Putschar.)

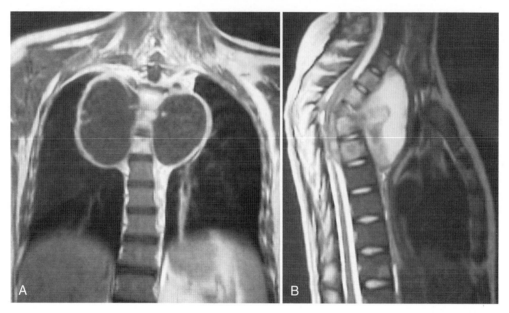

Figure 13-29. Magnetic resonance images of tuberculosis of vertebrae with abscess extending bilaterally. **A,** Coronal T1-weighted image shows a large hypointense mass on both sides of the upper thoracic spine. **B,** Sagittal T2-weighted sequence without fat saturation shows significant anterior wedging of the sixth thoracic vertebral body, leading to the gibbus deformity. Also note the large anterior hyperintense collection and the epidural mass causing pressure effect on the spinal cord. The hypointense foci within the anterior mass represent debris.

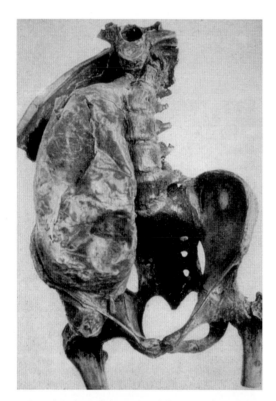

Figure 13-30. Tuberculosis of the spine with formation of a large abscess that dissected along the psoas. The wall of the abscess is calcified. (Courtesy of Dr. W. Putschar.)

destruction and periarticular erosions occur on both sides of the joint and are characteristic of the disease (Fig. 13-31). Large regions of bone may be destroyed and exhibit poorly defined margins, sequestrate, and periosteal reaction.[48] Accompanying spread into the soft tissue and abscess formation may develop.

Grossly, infected bone is discolored pale tan-yellow-white-gray; the involved area is poorly defined and may extend through the cortex into the soft tissues. In miliary disease, the individual granulomas appear as pinpoint round, white-gray nodules. In regions of bone destruction, firm fibroinflammatory tissue replaces the bone, except in areas of abscess formation. Abscess cavities are filled with liquid of variable viscosity and range in color from light green-yellow to brown. They sometimes contain pieces of bone which may be finely granular (so-called bone sand).

Histologically, the sine qua non of tuberculous osteomyelitis is necrotizing granulomatous inflammation (Fig. 13-32). The granulomas or tubercles are round to oval and are composed of aggregates of polyhedral macrophages that have oval or kidney bean–shaped vesicular nuclei and abundant eosinophilic cytoplasm. Admixed are multinucleated giant cells, including Langhans-type giant cells. Scattered around the granulomas are small, mature-appearing lymphocytes, all of which are enmeshed in fibrovascular connective tissue. Areas of necrosis vary in size from microscopic, occurring in the centers of the granulomas, to large, grossly visible regions. The necrosis is caseous in nature, being an admixture of coagulative and liquefactive devitalization. Histologically, the necrotic tissue is amorphous and eosinophilic; it contains scattered neutrophils, nuclear debris, and coagulated fibrin and is bordered by histiocytes. The surrounding tissue consists of granulation tissue with variable numbers of granulomas. The involved bone is necrotic and shows evidence of previous osteoclastic resorption. The neighboring uninvolved bone is

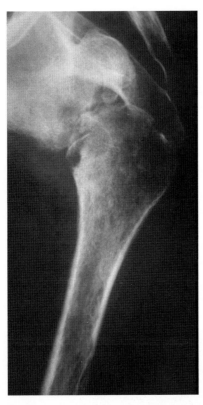

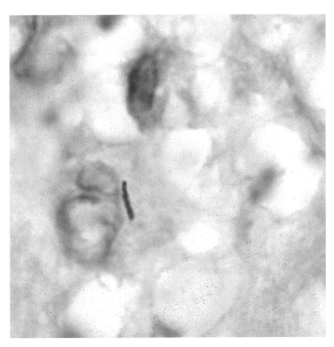

Figure 13-33. Acid-fast stain shows beaded rod shape of *Mycobacterium tuberculosis* in the cytoplasm of a histiocyte.

Figure 13-31. Tuberculosis of the shoulder. Axillary view of the shoulder shows subchondral and marginal erosions of the glenoid and the adjacent humeral head. Note the osteopenia.

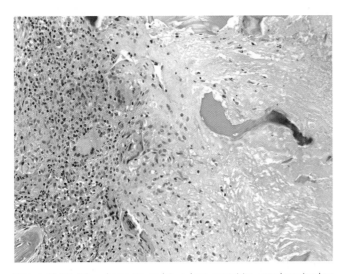

Figure 13-32. Tuberculous osteomyelitis. A large necrotizing granuloma involves the medullary cavity. The dead trabecula is surrounded by caseous debris. Scattered Langhans-type giant cells, lymphocytes, and plasma cells are present in the viable portion of the granuloma.

sclerotic with reactive new bone formation, and loose granulation tissue fills the intertrabecular spaces.

The microorganisms are usually most numerous in the areas of necrosis, but they can also be found in the cytoplasm of macrophages. *M. tuberculosis* are gram positive. With acid-fast

histochemical stains such as the Ziehl-Neelsen stain, they appear as red, rod-shaped structures 2 to 4 μm in length and 0.2 to 0.5 μm in diameter (Fig. 13-33).

Spinal tuberculosis causes significant bone destruction, which can result in permanent severe scoliotic or kyphotic deformities with subluxations, contractures, and neurologic deficits, including paralysis secondary to spinal cord and nerve compression. Tuberculous osteomyelitis tends to be more destructive and resistant to control than pyogenic osteomyelitis. Treatment is usually a combination of multi-drug therapy and surgery and is not always successful.

Non-Tuberculous Mycobacterial Osteomyelitis

Non-tuberculous mycobacteria are relatively nonvirulent and are present throughout the environment. Although infection in humans has been well established since the 1930s, the introduction of immunosuppressive therapy and the HIV epidemic have created the conditions for a significant increase in the frequency of this type of disease. Approximately 60 species of non-tuberculous mycobacteria have been documented to cause human illness, and new species are still being reported.[49,50] Nevertheless, relatively few species are responsible for the majority of infections, with *Mycobacterium avium-intracellulare* causing 61% of cases, followed by *Mycobacterium fortuitum* (19%) and *Mycobacterium kansasii* (10%).[49,50] Currently, non-tuberculous mycobacterial infection accounts for 0.5% to 30% of all mycobacterial diseases, and this percentage is on the rise.[51] A strong relationship exists between the type of infecting mycobacterial species and the geographic area of the population. The gamut of clinical infections caused by these organisms is broad, and they can be classified into chronic pulmonary infection, lymphadenitis, soft tissue and osteoarticular infection, disseminated disease, and iatrogenic illnesses.[49]

Approximately 5% to 10% of patients with non-tuberculous mycobacterial disease have involvement of the musculoskeletal system.[52] The predisposing factors of bone infection are trauma, surgery, and immunocompromise. The patients tend to be young and are infected by inoculation of the organism into the soft tissues, with secondary spread into the adjacent bone or directly into osseous structures, as a result of penetrating trauma, contamination of open wounds, or introduction into the body via medical devices such as catheters, shunts, injections, and surgical procedures. The organisms responsible for this type of infection are usually *Mycobacterium abscessus*, *M. fortuitum*, *Mycobacterium chelonae*, *Mycobacterium haemophilum*, *Mycobacterium marinum*, *M. avium-intracellulare*, *M. kansasii*, and *Mycobacterium terrae*. Patients who are immunosuppressed often have disseminated disease, and the mycobacteria spread to the skeleton hematogenously, causing multiple lesions that tend to affect the metaphyseal and diaphyseal regions of the long bones. Patients with osteomyelitis caused by *M. chelonae* or *M. haemophilum* are usually immunosuppressed.

Several clinical associations are well known. First, *M. marinum* produces a condition known as swimming pool granuloma or fish tank granuloma in people exposed to a marine environment. Local trauma, especially in the extremities, provides a pathway of access for the organism into the tissues. Second, *M. ulcerans* produces chronic necrotizing skin lesions of the distal extremities, known as Buruli ulcer.[53] It is associated with secondary bone involvement in approximately 15% of cases and is most prevalent in West Africa and Australia.

Patients with non-tuberculous mycobacterial osteomyelitis frequently present with localized pain, swelling, erythema, and induration of the involved site. They may also exhibit low-grade fever, sweats, chills, anorexia, malaise, and weight loss. In Buruli ulcer, the lesion is nonpainful and is associated with deep ulcers that undermine the skin edges.

The radiographic findings of non-tuberculous mycobacterial infection are similar to those caused by acute pyogenic bacterial osteomyelitis, but the rate of progression is slower; in the spine, the changes resemble tuberculous spondylitis.[52] The infection results in bone resorption, sequestrum formation, deposition of reactive new bone (involucrum), and the development of sinus tracts. In some cases, the plain films show a honeycomb pattern of bone dissolution or lytic cystic-appearing areas of bone destruction with limited surrounding sclerosis. In immunosuppressed patients, the lesions are usually multifocal and lytic.

The histologic reaction to the mycobacteria is variable and depends to some degree on the immune status of the host. The infection may elicit caseating and non-necrotizing granulomas, nonspecific chronic inflammation with lymphocytes, plasma cells and macrophages, and areas of tissue necrosis with little inflammation (Fig. 13-34). Immunosuppressed patients frequently have no granulomatous inflammation, and innumerable organisms may be present in histiocytes. The mycobacteria stain with Ziehl-Neelsen and Fite special stains.

The treatment of non-tuberculous mycobacterial osteomyelitis is usually a combination of surgery and multidrug antimycobacterial chemotherapy. Excision of infected tissue should be performed if feasible, and contaminated prostheses or hardware should be removed.

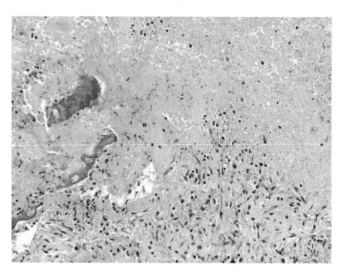

Figure 13-34. Necrotizing granulomas with pieces of dead bone in *Mycobacterium avium-intracellulare* osteomyelitis of the tibia.

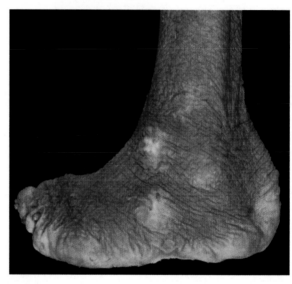

Figure 13-35. Leprosy of the foot. The toes have been largely resorbed. The skin shows areas of depigmentation. (Courtesy of Dr. W. Putschar.)

Lepromatous Osteomyelitis

The bone changes associated with leprosy may result from direct infection of the organism or from complications of the disease, including deep ulceration and superimposed infection and neuropathic changes. It is estimated that 3% to 5% of hospitalized leprosy patients have bone involvement.[54] The bones most commonly affected are the small bones of the face, especially the nose, and the hands and feet. The slowly progressive and relentless infection spreads from the skin, mucosa, and soft tissues into the underlying bone, producing lytic lesions and gradual resorption of the involved bone (Figs. 13-35 through 13-38).[54] The pathology reveals bone necrosis and resorption, marrow fibrosis and histiocytes sometimes forming granulomas, and occasional Langhans giant cells (Fig. 13-39). Bone involvement is usually

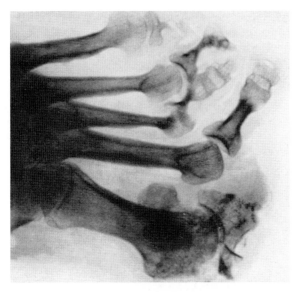

Figure 13-36. Leprosy. Lateral radiograph of the foot shows resorption (mutilans) of the phalanges and distal metatarsals and the soft tissues. There is atrophy of the remaining soft tissues. (Courtesy of Dr. W. Putschar.)

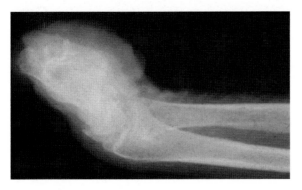

Figure 13-37. Oblique lateral radiograph of the wrist and hand in leprosy shows resorption of the phalanges and distal metacarpals and the soft tissues. There is atrophy of the remaining soft tissues. No significant demineralization is evident. (Courtesy of Dr. W. Putschar.)

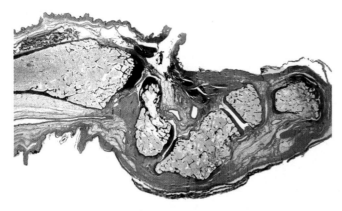

Figure 13-38. Whole-mount section of the hand in severe leprosy. The bones of the fingers have been resorbed, with only carpal bones remaining. (Courtesy of Dr. W. Putschar.)

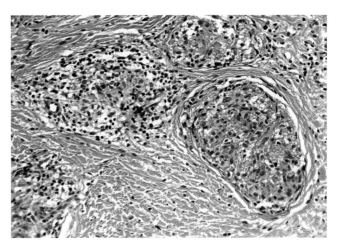

Figure 13-39. Tuberculoid leprosy with well-formed granulomas.

indicative of chronic disease and is treated with antibiotics and surgery.

Treponemal Osteomyelitis

Treponema are anaerobic host-associated spirochetes that represent one of six genera of the family Spirochaetaceae. Spirochetes are long, thin, gram-negative bacteria that are helical or spiral shaped. They can be visualized in tissue with silver stains, such as the Warthin-Starry stain, immunofluorescence, immunohisto-chemistry, and DNA analysis. The treponemes produce venereal and endemic (nonvenereal) disease, and those that most commonly cause bone infection are venereal syphilis (*Treponema pallidum* subspecies *pallidum*) and yaws (*Treponema pallidum* subspecies *pertenue*).

Skeletal Syphilis

The incidence of syphilis has waxed and waned over the past several decades, and this fluctuation has correlated with changes in behavior associated with drug abuse and homosexuality, as well as the reaction of the medical community to these behaviors. Currently, syphilis is experiencing a resurgence as a result of homosexual physical contact.[55] Despite this, bone involvement remains infrequent, because the disease is readily diagnosed and treated before this complication develops.

Syphilis can be acquired by physical contact, transmission through the placenta, blood transfusion, and accidental inoculation. Most cases result from direct contact with active lesions during sexual intimacy. Hematogenous dissemination leads to skeletal involvement, and the manifestations of bone disease vary according to whether the infection is congenital or acquired.

Congenital syphilis or infection of the fetus in utero may complicate the pregnancy of any untreated or inadequately treated woman and usually occurs during the early stages of the disease. The osseous lesions characteristic of congenital syphilis are osteochondritis, diaphyseal osteomyelitis, and periostitis. The lesions do not appear before the fifth month of gestation and are often fully developed at birth. They tend to be distributed in a bilateral and symmetric fashion but with variable severity from one bone to another. The spirochetes localize to areas of greatest growth; namely, regions of active enchondral ossification (osteochondritis) and the cellular layer of the periosteum (periostitis). The sites commonly involved are the metaphyseal regions of long tubular bones and costochondral junctions. In syphilitic osteochondritis, the zone of mineralization and the region of primary spongiosa are first affected.

The organisms infect osteoblasts, causing a significant decrease in their number and in the amount of new bone formed. As a consequence, the struts and latticework of partially resorbed mineralized cartilage elongate and occupy a greater amount of the metaphysis. Grossly, this appears as an irregular, jagged white line at the junction of the metaphysis and the base of the growth plate cartilage; in severe cases, this is discolored yellow, is 1 to 2 mm thick, and becomes visible on radiographs (Fig. 13-40). Filling the spaces between the bars of cartilage and bony trabeculae is granulation tissue with perivascular lymphocytes, plasma cells, macrophages, and neutrophils. The granulation tissue progressively occupies a greater amount of the metaphysis, with small groups of preserved chondrocytes remaining as isolated islands in the juxtaepiphyseal portion of the metaphysis. With more severe involvement, much of the metaphysis is replaced by the inflamed granulation tissue. This zone of connective tissue produces the lytic regions seen on radiographs at the ends of the long bones and can cause separation of the epiphysis and pathologic fracture, with displacement and impaction of the terminal fragment and attached epiphysis into the shaft (Fig. 13-41A). All of these changes are manifestations of

chronic infection and are part of the generalized proliferation of connective tissue that is responsible for the characteristic lesions of syphilis wherever they occur in the body; they are not pathognomonic and may occur in the setting of other chronic infections. After treatment, the lesions may heal completely.

During the first months of infancy, distinctive foci of osteomyelitis may involve the diaphysis. The granulation tissue and inflammation may originate from the metaphysis or develop de novo through seeding of the organism. Pathologically, necrosis,

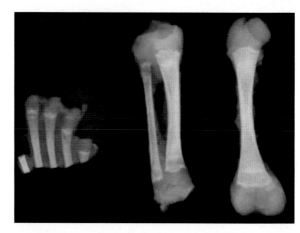

Figure 13-40. Congenital syphilis radiographs of the costochondral region, femur, tibia, and fibula. The metaphyseal-epiphyseal junctions are mildly widened, serrated, and radiopaque.

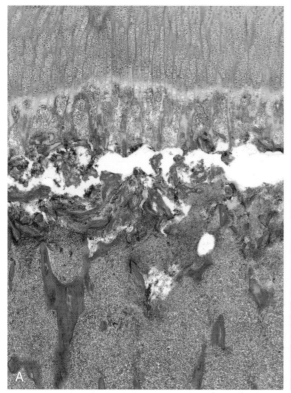

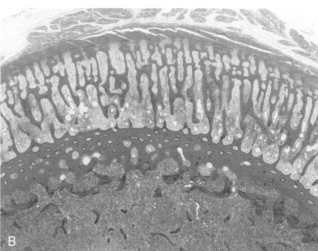

Figure 13-41. Congenital syphilis. **A,** Osteochondritis showing metaphysis with fracture and separation of the epiphysis. **B,** Marked periostitis with parallel struts of subperiosteal new bone deposited on the surface of the cortex.

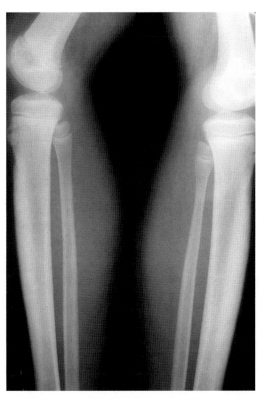

Figure 13-42. Radiograph of tibia in an 8-year-old child shows saber-shin deformity with abundant periosteal bone deposited along the anterior surface of the tibia. (Courtesy of Dr. W. Putschar.)

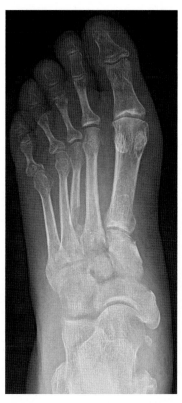

Figure 13-43. Syphilis of the foot. Anteroposterior view of the foot shows destruction of the adjacent bones along the navicular cuneiform and the second and third tarsometatarsal joints. Small erosions are noted along the medial cuneiform and the adjacent base of the first metatarsal. A large lytic focus is seen along the base of the third metatarsal.

granulation tissue, and acute and chronic inflammatory cells are present, with osteoclastic resorption of the adjacent bone.

Periostitis also develops in infants who survive intrauterine infection. In this situation, the infected periosteum deposits layers of reactive new bone that completely or partially encircle the shafts of the long bones (see Fig. 13-41B). This produces the so-called saber shin of the tibia (Fig. 13-42). The flat bones, such as the ilium and scapula, may also be affected. The thickness of the reactive bone is maximum in the midportion of the bone and gradually tapers down toward each end. The reactive bone is initially woven and then becomes remodeled into lamellar bone and disappears soon after effective treatment is initiated. The underlying cortex may remain intact, or it may become osteoporotic with dilated haversian systems. During active disease, the organism can be found in the cambium layer of the periosteum, as well as within the bone.

In acquired disease, bone involvement may begin early in the tertiary stage, which is usually 2 to 5 years after the initial infection, or, less frequently, in the secondary stage (Figs. 13-43 and 13-44). The bones most frequently involved are those that are superficial, such as the nose (saddle deformity), palate, skull, clavicle, and long bones of the extremities, especially the tibia. The lesions can vary drastically in size and are associated with a prominent inflammatory periostitis that causes the saber shin of adults. Involvement of the underlying medullary cavity often occurs and manifests as lytic destructive areas surrounded by regions of sclerosis. The lesion causing the destruction is known as the gumma. Grossly, the gumma, named after its resemblance to Arabic gum, is yellow and has a dry, crumbly consistency.

Histologically, it consists of eosinophilic necrotic inflammatory cells and connective tissue surrounded by granulation tissue containing lymphocytes, numerous plasma cells, macrophages (which may be epithelioid), and occasional Langhans giant cells. The gumma forms as the organism proliferates in the walls of small vessels and causes an obliterative endotheliitis and thrombosis. Consequently, the tissue undergoes necrosis and in the early stages contains many neutrophils surrounded by numerous lymphocytes, plasma cells, and epithelioid histiocytes; it can resemble the granulomas seen in tuberculosis. As the lesion enlarges, the neutrophils undergo apoptosis, and viable mononuclear cells surround the periphery of the large areas of necrosis (Fig. 13-45). Organisms may be difficult to identify in this stage of infection.

The treatment of syphilitic bone disease is antibiotic therapy, which usually is effective in curing congenital disease. The large, destructive lesions of tertiary disease can be irreversible, and surgical intervention may be required.

Yaws Bone Infection

Yaws is an endemic form of treponemal infection caused by *T. pallidum* subsp. *pertenue*. The name of the disease may come from the Carib word *yaya*, which means "sore." Yaws is a contagious, chronic, relapsing disease that is found in remote, humid tropical, rural settings in South America, Asia, Africa, and Oceania. Most patients are young and range in age from 2 to 15 years old. The disease is contracted through direct, nonsexual skin contact with infected material. In most instances, a child with a scratch or cut comes in contact with the exudate or serum of an infected ulcerated lesion from another person.[56] After gaining entry into tissue, the organism disseminates hematogenously throughout the body.

Bone infection as a component of yaws is seen in untreated patients in the secondary and uncommon tertiary stages of the disease. It usually manifests as prominent periostitis and osteomyelitis and often affects the long bones of the extremities, including those of the hands and feet, forearm, leg, pelvis, skull and face; it is also the cause of tibial saber shin (Fig. 13-46).[57] The bone disease may be associated with gummas that can be large and destructive, arthritis mutilans with marked resorption of bones similar to what may occur in leprosy, and severe contractures with pathologic fractures (Fig. 13-47). Histologically, the inflammatory reaction is similar to that of venereal syphilis. Microscopically, the organism is identical in appearance to *T. pallidum* subsp. *pallidum*.

Fungal Osteomyelitis

Fungi occur worldwide, reside within the soil and dead tissue, and have a symbiotic relationship with plants, animals, and other fungi. Certain species are restricted to specific geographic conditions and locations, and this fact has implications for human disease.

Fungi cause a variety of different human afflictions, which range from insignificant to life-threatening infections. Fungal osteomyelitis is a serious illness and is most virulent in individuals with depressed immune systems. Fungus causes bone infection by hematogenous dissemination, direct inoculation, and spread from a neighboring site of disease. Fungal osteomyelitis may occur as a component of a multisystem infection or as an isolated condition.[58] *Candida* spp., *Blastomyces dermatitidis, Coccidioides immitis, Histoplasma capsulatum,* and *Cryptococcus neoformans* commonly spread to bone via the vascular system as a complication of pulmonary or other type of deep internal

Figure 13-44. Macerated femur from a migrant 55-year-old man with tertiary syphilis. **A,** The entire shaft of the bone is distorted by a prominent periostitis. **B,** The reactive new bone produces an irregular surface. (Courtesy of Dr. W. Putschar.)

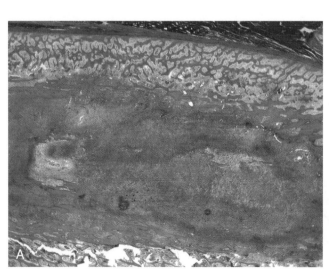

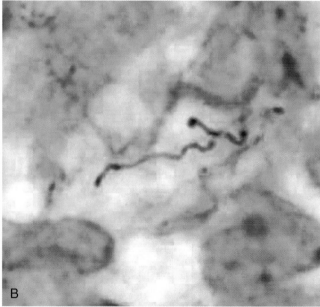

Figure 13-45. Gumma of tertiary syphilis. **A,** The inflammatory focus has destroyed the preexisting trabecular bone and is surrounded by reactive new bone. **B,** Steiner stain shows coiled *Treponema pallidum.*

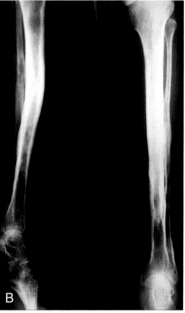

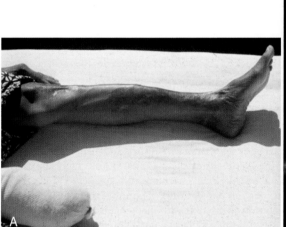

Figure 13-46. Tertiary yaws in an adult. **A,** Clinical photograph showing tibial saber shin. **B,** Anteroposterior and lateral radiographs of the lower leg demonstrate anterior bowing, marked periostitis, medullary sclerosis, and cortical thickening of the tibia. Similar changes are also noted in the fibula. (Courtesy of Dr. W. Putschar.)

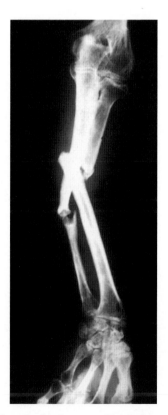

Figure 13-47. Radiograph of tertiary yaws with lytic destruction and pathologic fracture through diaphyses of ulna and radius. (Courtesy of Dr. W. Putschar.)

infection. *Histoplasma, Blastomyces,* and *Coccidioides* bone infections are usually endemic and occur secondary to hematogenous dissemination in immunocompetent people. Opportunistic mycotic osteomyelitis is usually caused by *Candida, Aspergillus,* and cryptococcal organisms. *Aspergillus* species, *Sporothrix schenckii,* and the fungi that cause mycetomas usually access bone by first forming a soft tissue infection and then spreading via direct extension into the adjacent bone.

The diagnosis of fungal osteomyelitis can be difficult, because the disease may evolve slowly and may mimic other conditions such as tuberculosis, myeloma, and metastatic disease. The clinical presentation and outcome vary according to the specific pathogen, the location of the infection, and host factors. Invariably, the infection causes pain, localized swelling, bone destruction with reactive changes, and a prominent inflammatory reaction. Definitive diagnosis usually requires identification of the organism in tissue specimens or cultures. Treatment consists of a combination of antibiotics and surgical débridement.

Candida Osteomyelitis

The genus *Candida* includes almost 200 species, of which about 20 cause disease in humans and animals. In humans, *Candida albicans* is the major pathogenic species. Over the past decade, however, there has been an increase in infection by non-*albicans* species, including the *Candida* species *glabrata, guilliermondii, lambica, krusei, parapsilosis, tropicalis, stellatoidea,* and *zeylanoides.* Traditionally considered to be commensal organisms and part of the normal flora of humans, *Candida* species can cause significant disease in the situation of impaired host immunity or repeated intravascular cannulation. *Candida* is the fourth leading organism causing bloodstream infections in the United States and accounts for 5% to 10% of such infections.[59] In 1% to 2% of these cases, osteomyelitis becomes a clinical complication. Accordingly, *Candida* osteomyelitis is often seen in the background of invasive candidiasis, and the patients are frequently immunosuppressed, debilitated, or critically ill. Other risk factors include exposure to broad-spectrum antibiotics, indwelling catheters, diabetes, malnutrition, cirrhosis, or parenteral drug abuse. The skeletal disease may not manifest until several months or years after the candidemia has been treated. Occasionally, *Candida* osteomyelitis results from contamination during a surgical procedure such as a coronary bypass or spine surgery. If it occurs in a patient with no known predisposing factors, then conditions associated with polymorphonuclear leukocyte dysfunction should be suspected.

Most patients are adults and range in age from 40 to 80 years; younger patients often have a history of intravenous drug abuse. Pain localized to the site of disease is a common complaint, but constitutional findings may be minimal or absent, because fewer than half of affected patients have fever or elevated ESR.[58] Disease progression is usually insidious and slow. Common sites of involvement are the spine, especially the lumbar vertebrae (two adjacent vertebral bodies), a long bone such as the femur, and the sternum. Most cases are solitary, but in approximately 10% of cases, two or more sites are involved.[60] Drug addicts have an increased incidence of costochondral involvement.

Radiographic studies show destruction of bone with surrounding sclerosis. Vertebral infection is frequently accompanied by discitis; at other sites, such as the sternum, sinus tracts may form. Histologically, the oval budding yeast, which are 5 to 12 μm in diameter, and hyphal forms elicit a dense acute and chronic inflammatory infiltrate and abundant granulation tissue. Treatment is with antibiotic therapy, and surgical débridement is frequently required. The prognosis is good, with the infection usually curable, but some patients who are severely ill die from the fungemia.

Aspergillus Osteomyelitis

Aspergillus species normally reside in soil and are ubiquitous in the environment. There are more than 250 different species, but only a few act as pathogens in humans. These include *Aspergillus fumigatus*, *Aspergillus flavus*, *Aspergillus niger*, and *Aspergillus terreus*. Aspergillosis is the most common invasive fungal infection, although bone involvement is very uncommon.

The most important route of infection in aspergillosis is inhalation of the spores, which eventually settle in the pulmonary alveoli and on the surface of the sinus mucosa.[61] Additional factors leading to infection are trauma (e.g., severe burns), indwelling catheters, and intravenous drug use. Many patients have predisposing conditions associated with immune system dysfunction, including chronic granulomatous disease in children and immunosuppressive drug therapy in adults.

Affected individuals are usually adults who present with pain and symptoms related to the site of involvement. Imaging studies show that the infection destroys bone and induces surrounding reactive changes. Sometimes, an associated soft tissue mass is present. In children, the thoracic vertebrae are the most common locus of disease, because the infection spreads from a contiguous focus in the lung. The vertebral column, especially the lumbar vertebrae, is the most frequent site of osteomyelitis in adults, and most cases are hematogenous in origin or result from direct inoculation during previous spine surgery (Fig. 13-48).[62] Spine infection is often associated with discitis and involvement of both neighboring vertebral bodies. Other bones reported to be affected include the skull, sternum, ribs, tibia, and ilium.[58] The tissue response to the growing dimorphic septate organism is usually a purulent reaction with many neutrophils, plasma cells, lymphocytes, and macrophages. Granulomatous inflammation is uncommon but may be seen in patients with chronic granulomatous disease. The treatment of *Aspergillus* osteomyelitis is antibiotics and surgical débridement.

Cryptococcal Osteomyelitis

Cryptococcus is a genus of fungi that includes almost 20 different species. The encapsulated organism is found worldwide in the soil, in trees, and in pigeon dung. The most common species that is pathogenic to humans is *C. neoformans*. Although most patients infected with *Cryptococcus* are adults and immunosuppressed, approximately 20% to 34% are otherwise normal hosts.[63,64] Common underlying conditions include AIDS, treatment with steroids, organ transplantation, cancer, diabetes, and sarcoidosis.

The organism usually gains access to the body via the respiratory system, with direct inoculation occurring in a small

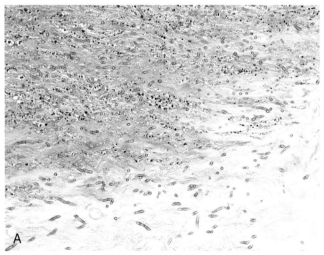
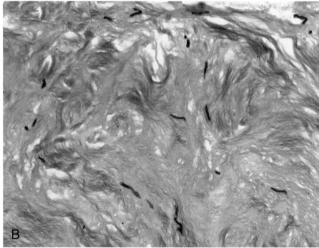

Figure 13-48. *Aspergillus* discitis. **A,** Necrotic annulus fibrosus of intervertebral disc with neutrophils, inflammatory debris, and infiltrating organisms. **B,** Grocott methenamine silver stain demonstrates septate hyphae growing between collagen fibers of the annulus fibrosus.

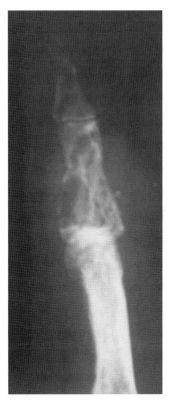

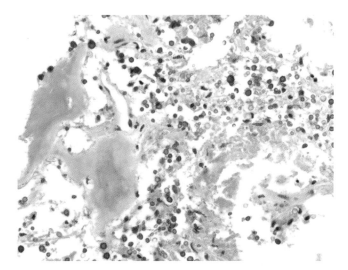

Figure 13-50. Mucicarmine stain shows cryptococcal budding yeast forms surrounded by inflammatory cells and trabeculae of woven bone.

Figure 13-49. Cryptococcosis involving the finger. Anteroposterior view demonstrates lytic lesions involving the middle phalanx. Note the osteopenia in the distal phalanx. (Courtesy of Dr. W. Putschar.)

number of cases. Cryptococcal osteomyelitis is frequently hematogenous in origin and develops in approximately 10% of patients with disseminated disease.[58] Patients commonly present with localized pain and swelling, and the bones involved include the vertebrae, femur, tibia, rib, humerus, clavicle, and scapula.[63,64] In approximately 75% of cases, only one bone is involved; in the remainder, multiple sites are involved. Radiographically, the infection manifests with bone destruction and sometimes an accompanying soft tissue abscess (Fig. 13-49). The histologic findings show round, yeast-like cells that are 3 to 6 μm in diameter. The tissue reaction varies with the immune status of the host and ranges from a very limited inflammatory response to numerous granulomas with caseous necrosis (Fig. 13-50). Treatment requires antibiotics and surgical débridement.

Sporotrichosis Osteomyelitis

Sporothrix schenckii, the pathogen that causes sporotrichosis, is the only active member of the genus *Sporothrix*. The thermally dimorphic fungus is found worldwide in tropical zones and inhabits soil and plant material. *S. schenckii* infection varies in frequency with regard to geographic location and tends to be related to occupation, because it most often develops in farmers, gardeners, fruit and vegetable pickers and packers, and workers in other related industries.[65] Classically, the infection is acquired by minor penetrating trauma, such as a prick by a rose thorn, and manifests as skin and subcutaneous disease with spread to

regional lymphatics. Osteoarticular infection is the most common form of extracutaneous disease and may result from direct spread from an abscess in the soft tissue, from septic arthritis, or through the vascular system. Uncommonly, the infection originates in the lungs or gastrointestinal tract and disseminates from there throughout the body, causing severe, life-threatening disease especially in persons who are immunosuppressed.

S. schenckii osteomyelitis can take several forms. It can manifest as eccentric erosions from a subcutaneous or synovial focus of disease, or it can appear as solitary or multiple lytic lesions secondary to hematogenous spread. The bones frequently affected include the tibia, fibula, femur, humerus, and short tubular bones of the hands and feet.[65] The patients are adults and present with pain and swelling. Radiographically, the lesions are destructive and lytic, with periarticular erosions and osteoporosis. Histologically, the branching hyphae induce a granulomatous reaction with necrosis and multinucleated giant cells. The treatment is antibiotics and surgical débridement.

Coccidioidomycosis Osteomyelitis

Coccidioides is a genus of fungi that is endemic to the arid southwestern United States and portions of Mexico and South America that have high summer temperatures, low rainfall, and low altitude.[66] The only species, *C. immitis*, lives in alkaline soil and accesses the human body via inhalation of arthroconidia. Most afflicted individuals are immunocompetent and are employed in jobs that involve working in or with the soil. Immunosuppressed individuals who develop infection are at risk for severe disseminated disease.

The vast majority of *C. immitis* infections are pulmonary in nature. Fewer than 5% of infections are extrapulmonary, and many of these occur in immunocompromised patients. Between 20% and 50% of extrapulmonary infections involve the skeletal system.[67] It is believed that most cases of coccidioidomycosis of the skeleton follow hematogenous dissemination from a primary focus of disease in the lung, even if it has completely resolved by the time the bone infection is diagnosed.

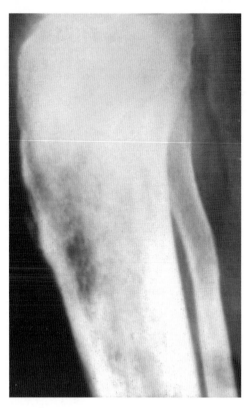

Figure 13-51. Radiograph of proximal tibia in patient with coccidioidomycosis. In the proximal tibia, there is a permeative lytic lesion with surrounding sclerosis. (Courtesy of Dr. W. Putschar.)

The patient presents with pain, swelling, limitation of function, and, sometimes, sinus tracts. The bone involvement is solitary in approximately 60% of cases and multifocal in the remainder. Any bone can be infected, but most cases involve the spine, skull, sternum, ribs, or pelvis. The metaphyses of long bones and carpal and tarsal bones are affected less commonly. In the spine, the disease is frequently multifocal, with extension into the soft tissues and development of a paraspinal abscess and relative sparing of intervening discs. In the ribs, the lesions are often marginal in location and associated with subpleural abscesses. Infection of the tubular bones frequently involves bony prominences, where the disease often extends into neighboring joints. On radiography, the infected site ranges from well-demarcated to poorly defined lytic foci with limited surrounding reactive bone formation (Fig. 13-51).[67] Histologically, the thick-walled spherules of organisms elicit a granulomatous reaction that may be associated with neutrophils. Grocott methenamine silver (GMS) and periodic acid–Schiff (PAS) stains highlight the fungus, which can also be seen with H&E (Fig. 13-52).

The infection is chronic, progressive, and destructive. Treatment consists of antibiotics and surgery, which results in a high rate of disease control and cure.

Paracoccidioidomycosis Osteomyelitis

Paracoccidioidomycosis is a systemic fungal disease caused by *Paracoccidioides brasiliensis*, which is the only member of its

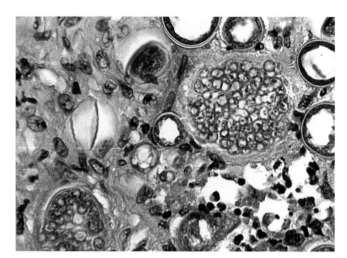

Figure 13-52. *Coccidioides* with numerous spherules containing endospores (hematoxylin and eosin stain).

genus and is endemic to Central and South America. *P. brasiliensis* is a saprophyte and a natural inhabitant of the protein-rich soil native to this hot and humid geographic region. In this environment, the fungus grows in the mycelial phase, producing airborne conidia, which, if inhaled, result in inoculation. Consequently, pulmonary disease is the most common manifestation of paracoccidioidomycosis and is most often observed in male agricultural workers in rural communities.[68] The disease has its highest incidence in Brazil.

Paracoccidioidomycosis produces a variety of clinical manifestations, which can be classified into acute and chronic forms. Chronic paracoccidioidomycosis is the most common type (>90% of cases) and is usually diagnosed in adults. The disease typically begins in the pulmonary parenchyma, where the fungus propagates and enters draining lymphatics, resulting in regional lymphadenitis. Depending on the host immune response, the infection may then be cleared, remain dormant, or become active. In chronic cases, the disease progresses slowly, and in many instances the burden of infection is confined to the lungs, where it may produce varying degrees of parenchymal damage or become quiescent. In some individuals, however, the organism spreads through bronchogenic, lymphatic, or hematogenous routes, producing symptomatic involvement of one or more organs (chronic multifocal form). The pathophysiology underlying most cases of bone involvement in paracoccidioidomycosis is believed to be hematogenous spread of the organism from a primary site of infection in the lung.[68] Less frequently, but more commonly in the jaw area, the bone becomes involved by contiguous spread from a neighboring site of infection, such as the gingiva. Most cases of joint involvement are believed to represent direct extension from a focus of adjacent osteomyelitis.

Bone and joint involvement in paracoccidioidomycosis is relatively uncommon and, based on radiographic studies, ranges from 5.9% to 27% of cases. Most patients are adult men who have the chronic form of the disease. In children, the acute type of disease is more frequent, and there is a higher incidence of skeletal involvement. The bones commonly affected are the scapula including the acromion, clavicle, rib, humerus, radius, and phalanges. Infection centered in the long bones is usually

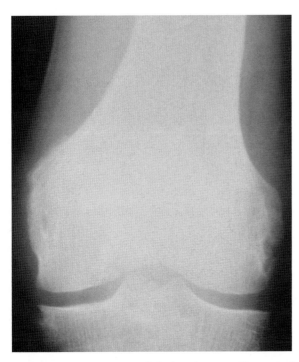

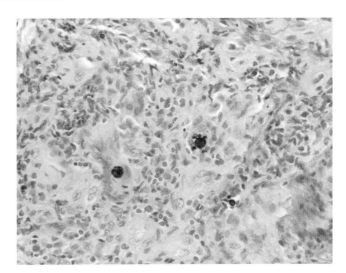

Figure 13-54. *Paracoccidioides* with budding yeast produces a ship's-wheel configuration seen on silver stain.

Figure 13-53. Anteroposterior view of the knee in paracoccidiomycosis shows poorly defined area of lysis in the femoral condyles. An erosion is also seen in the medial proximal tibia.

located in the diaphyseal or metaphyseal-epiphyseal regions. Radiographically, *Paracoccidioides* infection of bone produces lytic destruction that may have well-circumscribed or permeative margins with usually limited surrounding sclerosis and periostitis (Fig. 13-53). Joint involvement should be suspected if periarticular erosions are present.

Histologically, the fungus elicits an inflammatory response containing loose and compact granulomas with scattered multinucleated giant cells, acute and chronic inflammatory cells, and foci of caseous-type necrosis. The organisms are round, are 5 to 30 μm in greatest dimension, have refractile double walls, and exhibit multiple budding daughter cells that protrude from and surround the mother cell, forming a ship's-wheel configuration. They are most numerous in the loosely formed granulomas and are easily identified on PAS or GMS histochemical stains (Fig. 13-54).

The treatment of paracoccidioidomycosis bone disease includes antibiotics and surgery when necessary. The outcome is generally good, but relapses occur and can be problematic.[69]

Histoplasmosis Osteomyelitis

The genus *Histoplasma* contains one species, *H. capsulatum*, which comprises two varieties: *Histoplasma capsulatum* var. *capsulatum* and *Histoplasma capsulatum* var. *duboisii*. The organisms live in soil with high nitrogen content that is contaminated by bird droppings or bat guano. *Histoplasma* is endemic to the midwestern and south central United States and portions of western, central, and southern Africa. Histoplasmosis is usually initiated by inhalation of conidia from contaminated soil, fol-

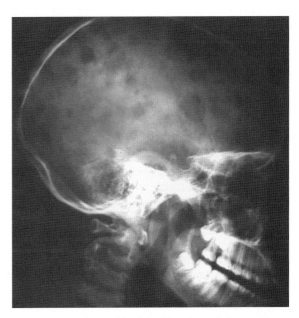

Figure 13-55. *Histoplasma duboisii* involving the skull in an African man. Lateral view of the skull shows multiple lytic foci of varying size. (Courtesy of Dr. W. Putschar.)

lowed by pulmonary infection. Hematogenous dissemination results in bone infection in a very small percentage of cases and is most common with the *duboisii* variant. Adult men are most frequently affected. Bone involvement can be multifocal and often affects the pelvis, skull, ribs, and the short tubular bones (Fig. 13-55).[70] Histologically, the infection induces a granulomatous reaction, with budding yeast surrounded by the inflammatory infiltrate.

Blastomycosis Osteomyelitis

Blastomyces dermatitidis is the only species included in the genus *Blastomyces*. *B. dermatitidis* includes two distinct serotypes that

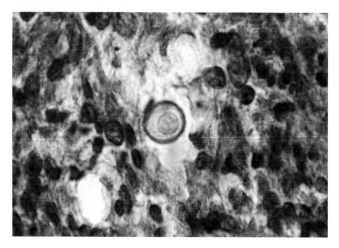

Figure 13-56. Thick refractile wall of blastomycetes seen in PAS stain.

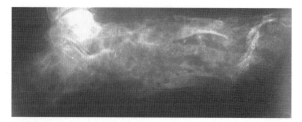

Figure 13-57. Madura foot. Lateral radiograph of the foot shows osteopenia with lytic foci within the tarsals, metatarsals, and phalanges. There is atrophy of the soft tissues. (Courtesy of Dr. W. Putschar.)

are endemic to the Mississippi, Ohio, and St. Lawrence River valleys. Cases have been reported from around the world, including Africa, South America, and Asia. Blastomycosis is a chronic infection with protean clinical manifestations; it is initiated by inhalation of airborne conidia and the subsequent development of pulmonary disease. The fungus then disseminates through the vascular system and frequently involves the cutaneous and skeletal systems. In 10% of patients, the primary presenting symptoms are related to bone manifestations.

Approximately one third of patients with disseminated disease develop bone lesions. Affected patients are usually middle-aged men. The anatomic regions most commonly affected include the axial skeleton and lower extremities; however, any bone may be targeted, including the vertebrae, ribs, facial bones, skull, metaphyses of long bones, small bones, pelvis, and scapula.[71] In most cases, only one bone is involved, but almost 20% of patients have disease affecting two or more osseous sites. Patients with multifocal disease frequently have accompanying septic arthritis. The osteomyelitis causes pain, swelling, and, in many cases, adjacent soft tissue abscesses and draining sinuses. Radiographically, the lesions produce either well-circumscribed areas of bone destruction with sclerotic margins or a more diffuse pattern of bone resorption with moth-eaten margins.[71] In the spine, the changes may mimic tuberculosis, with extensive involvement of the vertebral body, loss of disc space, and paraspinal soft tissue abscess formation. Histologically, the fungus is frequently associated with neutrophilic microabscesses and granulomatous inflammation with numerous lymphocytes and plasma cells. The organism is optimally visualized with PAS and GMS stains and appears as multinucleated yeast forms 8 to 15 μm in diameter with a thick, refractile wall (Fig. 13-56).[72] Budding occurs singly, and the bud is attached by a broad base.

The treatment of skeletal blastomycosis is usually antibiotics and surgical débridement. Outcome is generally good.

Mycetoma

Mycetoma is a chronic, frequently subcutaneous, granulomatous infection that commonly affects the feet, where it is also known as Madura foot.[73] The infecting organism is either actinomycetes

bacteria (*Nocardia brasiliensis*, *Nocardia asteroides*, *Streptomyces somaliensis*, *Actinomadura madurae*, or *Actinomadura pelletieri*) or Eumycetes fungi (>20 different species, including *Madurella mycetomatis*, *Madurella grisea*, *Fusarium* spp., and *Acremonium* spp.).[73] The disease usually occurs in tropical and subtropical areas and is endemic to Latin America, India, and Africa. It develops when organisms that are usually saprophytes in the soil are traumatically inoculated into tissue. This may occur on the plantar aspect of the feet of persons who are frequently barefoot or on the extremities or backs of workers carrying contaminated vegetation or other objects. Patients are typically poverty-stricken, young or middle-aged adult men who present with tumefactive indurated areas of infection of the subcutis with draining sinuses. Exiting from the sinuses are pus-containing grains (their color depending on the infectious agent) which are composed of aggregates of organisms. Long-term infection is associated with spread to the neighboring bones and resultant osteomyelitis. The osteomyelitis often manifests as multifocal lytic bone destruction with minimal reactive new bone formation (Fig. 13-57).[74] Histologically, the organisms elicit a purulent and granulomatous reaction with fibrosis and granulation tissue (Fig. 13-58). The disease can be progressive and very destructive, and it can spread through draining lymphatics.

Treatment consists of identifying the pathogen and then administering the appropriate antibiotics and surgical débridement as required. In some cases, amputation is necessary. Superinfection with other types of bacteria can result in sepsis and death.

Helminthic Osteomyelitis

Helminthic infection of humans occurs worldwide and causes significant disease-related morbidity. The organisms can infect many different organ systems, but involvement of the skeleton is extremely uncommon. The worm that has the greatest propensity to infect bone is *Echinococcus*.

Echinococcal Osteomyelitis

Echinococcus, a parasitic tapeworm, includes 12 different species; however, *Echinococcus granulosa* is the most important human pathogen and the only one that causes significant bone disease.[75] Human echinococcal infections occur across the globe and result from the ingestion of contaminated water and food, handling of live animals that act as definitive hosts (e.g., dogs), or working

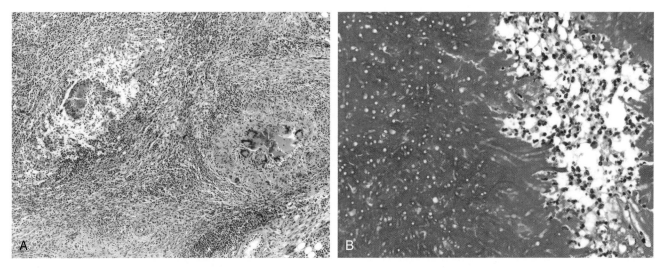

Figure 13-58. Madura foot. **A,** Numerous granulomas with giant cells surrounding organisms of pigmented fungi. **B,** PAS stain demonstrates branching septate fungi.

with their pelts. The swallowed eggs hatch in the small intestine and release minute hooked embryos, which burrow through the bowel wall and are then transported by the bloodstream to various sites such as the lung, liver, brain, skeletal muscle, and eyes. Involvement of the skeletal system is rare and occurs in 0.2% to 4% of cases. Once organisms reach their final destination, they produce hydatid larval cysts. These unilocular cysts are filled with fluid and lined by an inner germinal membrane that produces brood capsules. The inner wall of the brood capsules facilitates an asexual budding process that generates thousands of new larval tapeworms (protoscolices) in daughter cysts. The hydatid cysts can achieve large size (2 to 30 cm), have a thick wall, and contain clear, pale-yellow fluid that has a neutral pH and contains sodium chloride, proteins, glucose, ions, lipids, and polysaccharides. The fluid is antigenic.

The sites of bone disease commonly include the spine, pelvis, and long bones. Once lodged within bone, the hydatid cyst fills the spaces between the bony trabeculae; this eventually results in resorption of the trabeculae and the neighboring cortex, so that the cyst extends into the adjacent soft tissues. These changes cause the patient to complain of pain, swelling, and sometimes pathologic fracture, with other symptoms specific to the anatomic site of involvement.[76] Radiographically, the cyst appears as an expanded portion of bone with irregular areas of bone destruction that may have sclerotic, well-defined or moth-eaten margins (Fig. 13-59). By MRI, the mass is bright on T2-weighted sequences because of the prominent water content of the cyst.

Grossly, *Echinococcus* infection of bone is centered in the medullary cavity and frequently distorts the bone by expansion and destruction. On cross-section, the bone contains many small, thin-walled cysts that range from 1 millimeter to several centimeters or larger in greatest dimension; a mother cyst is not present. The cysts percolate between the trabeculae, eventually resulting in their resorption by osteoclasts and the production of reactive fibrous tissue infiltrated by a dense population of lymphocytes, eosinophils, plasma cells, and scattered granulomas with multinucleated histiocytes, all of which surround the cysts (Fig. 13-60).[76] The nucleated germinal cyst wall is thin and

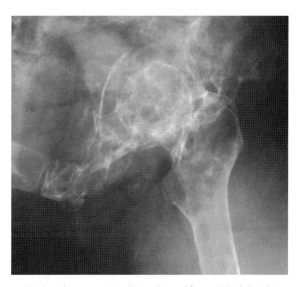

Figure 13-59. Echinococcosis involving pelvis and femur. Multiple lytic lesions are seen within the proximal femur and acetabulum. There is protrusio acetabuli with a pathologic fracture through the iliopectineal line.

eosinophilic; rarely, protoscolices are attached to its inner surface (Fig. 13-61).

The treatment of hydatid disease of bone is anthelminthic chemotherapy and surgery—either curettage and packing with cement or en bloc excision. Because the disease evolves slowly, many patients have extensive osseous changes by the time they are diagnosed. This complicates adequate therapy and results in a high rate of local recurrence.[75]

Viral Osteomyelitis

Viral osteomyelitis is an uncommon clinical problem, with arthritis being one of its more common complications. The infections that most commonly cause bone changes include smallpox, vaccinia, and intrauterine rubella and cytomegalic inclusion disease.

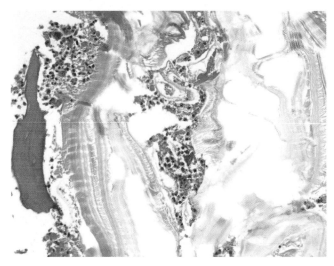

Figure 13-60. Echinococcal cyst walls infiltrating the medullary cavity and surrounded by inflammatory cells and necrotic bone.

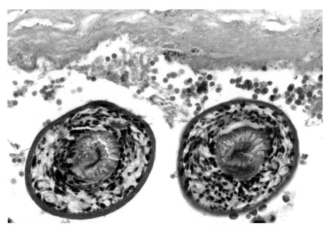

Figure 13-61. Echinococcal cyst wall with protoscolices.

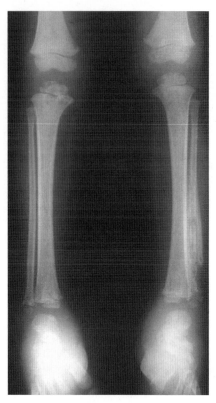

Figure 13-62. A 3-year-old child with smallpox. Radiograph of the legs shows metaphyseal lysis and sclerosis of proximal and distal tibia and prominent periostitis of fibula. (Courtesy of Dr. W. Putschar.)

Variola Osteomyelitis

The variola virus, one of the most virulent pathogens of humans, is the cause of smallpox, a disease that is now considered extinct. Smallpox osteomyelitis is a well-recognized phenomenon that complicates 2% to 5% of childhood cases and has been termed osteomyelitis variolosa. There is no relationship between the severity of the initial smallpox infection and the occurrence or degree of severity of bone involvement.[77] The patients usually complain of pain and swelling one to several weeks after the smallpox becomes clinically evident. Musculoskeletal involvement can affect the joints and the bones, frequently simultaneously, and in a symmetric fashion. Tubular bones, especially those about the elbow and those of the hands and feet, are commonly affected. The spine and pelvis may also be targeted. The radiographic findings include juxtametaphyseal lysis and destruction with extension into the epiphysis, which sometimes separates from the bone, and prominent periosteal reactive new bone formation (Fig. 13-62).[78] Histologically, the bone undergoes

necrosis with medullary fibrosis and osteoclastic activity. In severe cases, draining sinuses, pathologic fractures, contractures, growth deformities, and secondary bacterial infection may develop. Treatment is supportive, unless there is secondary infection, and uncomplicated cases usually heal and resolve over time.

Rubella Osteomyelitis

Rubella (German measles) infrequently involves the skeleton, and when it does, it is in the setting of intrauterine infection. Radiographically, the findings are most notable along the distal femoral and proximal tibial metaphyses, where radiolucent horizontal bands may be present. Additionally, linear "celery stalk" type radiolucencies are sometimes evident. They begin adjacent to an irregular zone of calcification of the growth plate and extend into the diaphysis, are delineated by a thin zone of radiodensity and are oriented parallel to the long axis of the bone.[78] Periostitis is absent. Histologically, there is reduced bone formation, with marrow fibrosis and increased numbers of plasma cells in the marrow and periosteum.[79] The changes usually resolve spontaneously, but, infrequently, they may persist or progress.

Other Types of Viral Bone Infection

Infrequently, other types of viral infection can involve the skeleton. Intrauterine cytomegalic inclusion disease can produce changes similar to those of rubella. Rarely, vaccinia or varicella can induce alterations in bone.

Differential Diagnosis of Osteomyelitis

The differential diagnosis of osteomyelitis includes other conditions in which an inflammatory infiltrate is present in bone. Based on histologic findings alone, it can be difficult or impossible to determine whether inflammation is a manifestation of infection or of some other process. Features that support the possibility of infection include the density of inflammation and its distribution. Situations prone to potential misinterpretation include subchondral acute inflammation in severe arthritis, acute inflammation associated with acute fracture, autoinflammatory diseases (chronic recurrent multifocal osteomyelitis), sarcoidosis, hematopoietic malignancies, and histiocytic proliferations (Table 13-4).

Subchondral acute inflammation in severe arthritis may occur secondary to disruption of the articular surface. This gives rise to acute inflammation of the subchondral tissues and a neutrophilic exudate in the synovial fluid (Fig. 13-63).[80] This process is usually identified as an incidental finding in large-joint arthroplasty specimens. Patients frequently have a history of rheumatoid arthritis, osteonecrosis, or osteoarthritis. Two distinct patterns of subchondral inflammation may be present. In specimens demonstrating osteonecrosis, the suppurative inflammation diffusely

Table 13-4 Radiographic and Histologic Mimics of Osteomyelitis
Subchondral acute inflammation
Acute fracture
Autoinflammatory diseases (chronic recurrent multifocal osteomyelitis), sarcoidosis
Hematopoietic malignancies
Histiocytic proliferations

fills the marrow space in necrotic cancellous bone. Because the trabecular bone is necrotic, the histologic resemblance to acute bacterial osteomyelitis can be striking. The inflammation does not extend beyond the confines of the necrotic tissue and is sharply demarcated from the surrounding viable bone.

The second and more frequent type of inflammation is centered on subchondral cysts (geodes). In these examples, the center of the cyst is distended by sheets of neutrophils associated with a fibrinous exudate. The suppurative exudate is admixed with granular eosinophilic to basophilic debris resembling bone dust. The fibrous lining of the "cyst" is edematous and contains a mild chronic inflammatory infiltrate, scattered foamy or vacuolated histiocytes, and occasional multinucleated giant cells within its walls. The nodular nature of the acute inflammatory process, in addition to the frequent presence of histiocytes within the wall, can create a distinctly granulomatous appearance. However, the adjacent sclerotic subchondral bone is viable, and the surrounding marrow spaces may show mild fibrosis that extends for only a short distance from the edge of the inflammatory infiltrate. In contrast, untreated osteomyelitis is frequently associated with a dense inflammatory infiltrate that involves a large area of bone and has a poorly defined margin with abundant reactive fibrosis at the periphery.

In the acute stages of fracture, abundant neutrophils may be present at the traumatized site, and the involved bone may be necrotic if enough time has passed to permit breakdown of osteoblast and osteocyte nuclei (Fig. 13-64). This combination of features can resemble osteomyelitis. An important distinguishing feature is extensive hemorrhage, which is present in fracture but usually not nearly as prominent in infection.

Autoinflammatory conditions of bone, especially chronic recurrent multifocal osteomyelitis (CRMO), can be confused with infectious bone disease based on clinical, radiographic, and histologic features.[81] Diagnostic criteria for CRMO include (1) multiple bone lesions; (2) extended clinical course spanning years, with remissions and exacerbations; (3) no response to antibiotics; and (4) appearance on radiographs as foci of lysis surrounded by sclerosis.[81] The cause is unknown but is unlikely

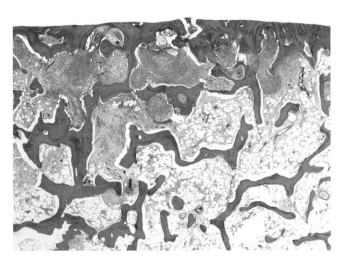

Figure 13-63. Femoral head with severe osteoarthritis. Neutrophils fill subchondral cysts. The adjacent marrow is relatively unremarkable.

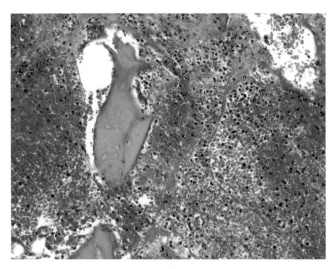

Figure 13-64. Recent fracture with abundant hemorrhage containing many neutrophils and pieces of focally necrotic bone.

to be infectious in nature. Recent studies have suggested that genetic abnormalities may be important in its genesis. CRMO usually manifests in children (median age, 10 years), who complain of pain and tenderness; fever and swelling, although common, are sometimes absent. Some patients have been reported to have other conditions, such as palmar-plantar pustulosis, psoriasis vulgaris, generalized pustulosis, severe acne, Sweet syndrome, and inflammatory bowel disease. It is also a component of SAPHO syndrome (synovitis, acne, pustulosis, hyperostosis, and osteitis). Frequent laboratory abnormalities include an elevated ESR, increased concentration of tumor necrosis factor-α, and, sometimes, a high white blood cell count. Patients have one or more sites of active bone disease; this most often is localized to the metaphyseal region of long bones, followed by the clavicle, but may involve essentially any bone, including the pelvis, spine, and craniofacial skeleton.[82] The lesions are hot on bone scan, and on radiography are irregular, radiolucent, and surrounded by a zone of sclerosis. Tissue from biopsy specimens resembles that from patients with bacterial infection with regard to the inflammatory infiltrate and bone changes. In the early stage of the disease, neutrophils predominate; over time, these are replaced by lymphocytes, plasma cells, and scattered macrophages. The bone shows areas of necrosis, osteoclastic activity, and reactive bone formation. Cultures of the tissue and blood are negative. The clinical course is characterized by cycles of waxing and waning, with new lesions developing. Treatment usually consists of nonsteroidal anti-inflammatory drugs, because antibiotics are ineffective.

Hematopoietic malignancies containing large numbers of mature-appearing inflammatory cells can cause confusion with osteomyelitis. This is especially relevant when the population of inflammatory cells consists of small lymphocytes, plasma cells, or the mixed inflammatory infiltrate that characterizes some forms of Hodgkin disease. The monomorphous nature of the cells in the setting of lymphoma or plasma-cell malignancies is a key finding that helps separate them from infection. If doubt persists, immunohistochemistry can be helpful in demonstrating clonality of the infiltrating cells. Regarding Hodgkin disease, the identification of Reed-Sternberg cells and their variants is crucial for accurate diagnosis. Some cases of Hodgkin disease exhibit so many neutrophils and eosinophils that the distinction from infection is challenging and requires immunohistochemistry (Fig. 13-65).

Sarcoidosis is a granulomatous systemic disease of uncertain etiology. It most frequently involves the pulmonary parenchyma and mediastinal lymph nodes, but any organ system can be affected. Skeletal disease is present in 1% to 13% of cases and is frequently accompanied by pulmonary and skin lesions. Bone involvement is often bilateral, and bones commonly affected include the middle and distal phalanges (sausage finger), wrist, skull, vertebral column, and long bones (Fig. 13-66). Radiographically. the lesions are lytic or lacelike, frequently involve the cortex, and may have moth-eaten margins. Histologically, sarcoidosis is characterized by compact, round or oval granulomas composed of epithelioid histiocytes that have oval or kidney bean–shaped, pale nuclei (Fig. 13-67). Langerhans and conventional multinucleated giant cells may be present. The granulomas may contain limited amounts of central fibrinoid necrosis, but caseation is absent. Lymphocytes are frequently distributed around the periphery of the histiocytes, and the inflammatory

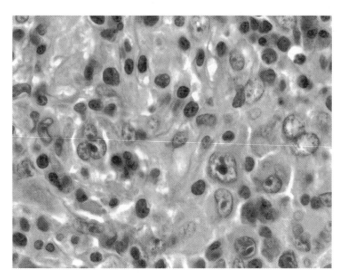

Figure 13-65. Hodgkin disease with Reed-Sternberg cells and scattered inflammatory cells.

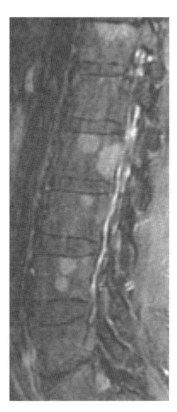

Figure 13-66. Sarcoidosis of the spine. Sagittal T1-weighted post-gadolinium image with fat saturation shows multiple enhancing lesions in several vertebral bodies.

infiltrate is enmeshed in reactive fibrous tissue. Special stains for microorganisms are negative. The differential diagnosis includes granulomatous osteomyelitis caused by mycobacteria, fungi, and bacteria. Helpful distinguishing features are the clinical findings and histologic features such as the cohesive aggregation of the epithelioid histiocytes and the absence of caseous necrosis and demonstrable microorganisms.

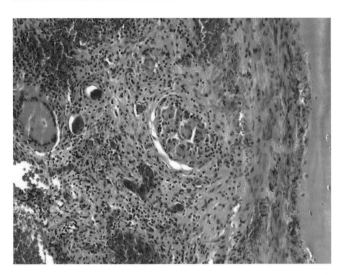

Figure 13-67. Sarcoidosis of bone. Well-formed granuloma with giant cells enmeshed in reactive fibrous tissue with scattered lymphocytes.

Langerhans cell histiocytosis of bone, previously known as histiocytosis X, is defined as an intraosseous mass of proliferating Langerhans cells. Langerhans cell histiocytosis is associated with a variety of clinical syndromes that vary according to the number, site, and size of the tumors. Traditionally, single or multiple lesions restricted to the skeleton have been termed "eosinophilic granuloma." Langerhans cell histiocytosis is usually diagnosed during the first three decades of life, and men are affected approximately twice as frequently as women. The disease usually manifests in the skeleton, and solitary bone lesions are encountered twice as often as multiple bone lesions. The tumors can develop in any bone but most commonly originate in the skull and jaw, followed by vertebral bodies, ribs, pelvis, and long bones. The lesions are well defined and lytic on radiographs, but in a minority of cases, they have ill-defined and permeative margins (Fig. 13-68). Cortical involvement may elicit a periosteal reaction.

Histologically, the proliferating Langerhans cells are ovoid or round, histiocyte-like cells, 10.0 to 15.0 μm in diameter, that are arranged in aggregates, sheets, or individually, within a loose fibrous stroma. The cells have eosinophilic cytoplasm and contain central ovoid coffee-bean–shaped nuclei with pale chromatin and inconspicuous nucleoli. The coffee-bean appearance is produced by deep indentations, clefts, and folds of the nuclear membranes, which form linear grooves that traverse the length of the nuclei (Fig. 13-69). One of the morphologic hallmarks of Langerhans cell histiocytosis is an accompanying infiltrate of eosinophils, which may be so dense that the underlying Langerhans cells are obscured. The eosinophils are distributed evenly or arranged in clusters, producing eosinophilic abscesses. Other types of inflammatory cells, including lymphocytes, plasma cells, macrophages, neutrophils, and osteoclast-type giant cells, are also frequently present. The diagnosis of Langerhans cell histiocytosis is principally based on the light microscopic appearance of the Langerhans cells and the appropriate mixed cellular background; however, adjuvant diagnostic techniques, including electron microscopy and immunohistochemistry, help confirm their presence. Langerhans cells strongly express S-100 protein,

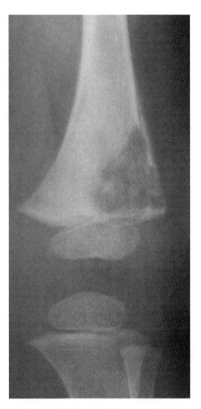

Figure 13-68. Langerhans cell histiocytosis. Radiograph of the distal femur shows an eccentric destructive lesion in the lateral metaphysis with significant reactive sclerosis in the adjacent bone and overlying periosteal new bone formation.

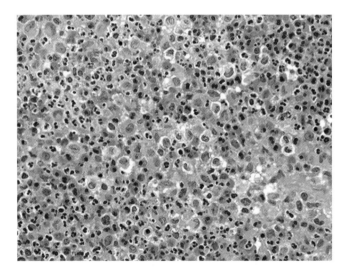

Figure 13-69. Cell-cell histiocytes associated with many eosinophils.

CD1a, and langerin. Langerhans cell histiocytosis can be distinguished from osteomyelitis by virtue of the fact that the Langerhans cells grow in clusters and are not randomly distributed as single cells in the setting of infection. Other helpful features are the predominance of neutrophils in acute osteomyelitis and the relative paucity of eosinophils in most types of bacterial infection.

REFERENCES

1. Trueta J: The three types of acute hematogenous osteomyelitis: A clinical and vascular study. J Bone Joint Surg 1959;41B:671-680.

2. Waldvogel FA, Medoff G, Swartz MN: Osteomyelitis: A review of clinical features, therapeutic considerations and unusual aspects. 3: Osteomyelitis associated with vascular insufficiency. N Engl J Med 1970;282:316-322.

3. Kahn DS, Pritzker KP: The pathophysiology of bone infection. Clin Orthop Relat Res 1973;(96):12-19.

4. Bar-Shavit Z: Taking a toll on the bones: Regulation of bone metabolism by innate immune regulators. Autoimmunity 2008;41:195-203.

5. Kandel SN, Mankin HJ: Pyogenic abscess of the long bones in children. Clin Orthop Relat Res 1973;(96):108-117.

6. Nixon GW: Hematogenous osteomyelitis of metaphyseal-equivalent locations. AJR Am J Roentgenol 1978;130:123-129.

7. Wiley AM, Trueta J: The vascular anatomy of the spine and its relationship to pyogenic vertebral osteomyelitis. J Bone Joint Surg 1959;41B:796-809.

8. Tsukayama D: Pathophysiology of post-traumatic osteomyelitis. Clin Orthop Relat Res 1999;(360):22-29.

9. Weichert S, Sharland M, Clarke NM, et al: Acute haematogenous osteomyelitis in children: Is there any evidence for how long we should treat? Curr Opin Infect Dis 2008;21:258-262.

10. Dahl LB, Hoyland AL, Dramsdahl H, et al: Acute osteomyelitis in children: A population-based retrospective study 1965 to 1994. Scand J Infect Dis 1998;30:573-577.

11. Lew DP, Waldvogel FA: Osteomyelitis. Lancet 2004;364:369-379.

12. Mylona E, Samarkos M, Kakalou E, et al: Pyogenic vertebral osteomyelitis: A systematic review of clinical characteristics. Semin Arthritis Rheum 2008 Jun 10 [Epub ahead of print].

13. Chambers JB, Forsythe DA, Bertrand SL, et al: Retrospective review of osteoarticular infections in a pediatric sickle cell age group. J Pediatr Orthop 2000;20:682-685.

14. Pineda C, Vargas A, Rodriguez AV: Imaging of osteomyelitis: Current concepts. Infect Dis Clin North Am 2006;20:789-825.

15. Gurelik M, Goze F, Karadag O, et al: Vertebral plasma cellular osteomyelitis. Br J Neurosurg 2003;17:357-360.

16. Landais C, Fenollar F, Constantin A, et al: Q fever osteoarticular infection: Four new cases and a review of the literature. Eur J Clin Microbiol Infect Dis 2007;26:341-347.

17. Ma J, Chan JK: Granulomatous osteomyelitis caused by bacteria other than mycobacteria: A report of two cases. Pathology 2002;34:477-479.

18. Maman E, Bickels J, Ephros M, et al: Musculoskeletal manifestations of cat scratch disease. Clin Infect Dis 2007;45:1535-1540.

19. Sirikulchayanonta V, Subhadrabandhu T: Melioidosis: Another etiology of granulomatous osteomyelitis. Report of 2 cases. Clin Orthop Relat Res 1994;(308):183-186.

20. Wu PC, Khin MM, Pang SW: Salmonella osteomyelitis: An important differential diagnosis of granulomatous osteomyelitis. Am J Surg Pathol 1985;9:531-537.

21. Zwass A, Feldman F: Case report 875: Multifocal osteomyelitis—a manifestation of chronic brucellosis. Skeletal Radiol 1994;23:660-663.

22. Gutierrez K: Bone and joint infections in children. Pediatr Clin North Am 2005;52:779-794, i.

23. Ciampolini J, Harding KG: Pathophysiology of chronic bacterial osteomyelitis: Why do antibiotics fail so often? Postgrad Med J 2000;76:479-483.

24. Prasad KC, Prasad SC, Mouli N, et al: Osteomyelitis in the head and neck. Acta Otolaryngol 2007;127:194-205.

25. Sharkawy AA: Cervicofacial actinomycosis and mandibular osteomyelitis. Infect Dis Clin North Am 2007;21:543-556, viii.

26. Dodson TB, Raje NS, Caruso PA, et al: Case records of the Massachusetts General Hospital. Case 9-2008: A 65-year-old woman with a nonhealing ulcer of the jaw. N Engl J Med 2008;358:1283-1291.

27. Reid IR: Osteonecrosis of the jaw: Who gets it, and why? Bone 2009;44:4-10.

28. Silverman SL, Landesberg R: Osteonecrosis of the jaw and the role of bisphosphonates: A critical review. Am J Med 2009;122:S33-S45.

29. Hansen T, Kunkel M, Springer E, et al: Actinomycosis of the jaws: Histopathological study of 45 patients shows significant involvement in bisphosphonate-associated osteonecrosis and infected osteoradionecrosis. Virchows Arch 2007;451:1009-1017.

30. Goldberg AN, Oroszlan G, Anderson TD: Complications of frontal sinusitis and their management. Otolaryngol Clin North Am 2001;34:211-225.

31. Kombogiorgas D, Seth R, Athwal R, et al. Suppurative intracranial complications of sinusitis in adolescence: Single institute experience and review of literature. Br J Neurosurg 2007;21:603-609.

32. Hartemann-Heurtier A, Senneville E: Diabetic foot osteomyelitis. Diabetes Metab 2008;34:87-95.

33. Bluestein D, Javaheri A: Pressure ulcers: Prevention, evaluation, and management. Am Fam Physician 2008;78:1186-1194.

34. Livesley NJ, Chow AW: Infected pressure ulcers in elderly individuals. Clin Infect Dis 2002;35:1390-1396.

35. Turk EE, Tsokos M, Delling G: Autopsy-based assessment of extent and type of osteomyelitis in advanced-grade sacral decubitus ulcers: A histopathologic study. Arch Pathol Lab Med 2003;127:1599-1602.

36. Kadas I, Magyari Z, Vendegh Z, et al: Changing the treatment to reduce complication rate in open tibial fractures. Int Orthop 2008 Oct 29 [Epub ahead of print].

37. Crowley DJ, Kanakaris NK, Giannoudis PV: Debridement and wound closure of open fractures: The impact of the time factor on infection rates. Injury 2007;38:879-889.

38. Murray CK, Hsu JR, Solomkin JS, et al: Prevention and management of infections associated with combat-related extremity injuries. J Trauma 2008;64:S239-S251.

39. Jamsen E, Huhtala H, Puolakka T, et al: Risk factors for infection after knee arthroplasty: A register-based analysis of 43,149 cases. J Bone Joint Surg 2009;91A:38-47.

40. Trampuz A, Widmer AF: Infections associated with orthopedic implants. Curr Opin Infect Dis 2006;19:349-356.

41. Trampuz A, Zimmerli W: Prosthetic joint infections: Update in diagnosis and treatment. Swiss Med Wkly 2005;135:243-251.

42. Zimmerli W, Trampuz A, Ochsner PE: Prosthetic-joint infections. N Engl J Med 2004;351:1645-1654.

43. Kanner WA, Saleh KJ, Frierson HF Jr: Reassessment of the usefulness of frozen section analysis for hip and knee joint revisions. Am J Clin Pathol 2008;130:363-368.

44. Tortoli E: The new mycobacteria: An update. FEMS Immunol Med Microbiol 2006;48:159-178.

45. Gardam M, Lim S: Mycobacterial osteomyelitis and arthritis. Infect Dis Clin North Am 2005;19:819-830.

46. Jain AK, Dhammi IK: Tuberculosis of the spine: A review. Clin Orthop Relat Res 2007;(460):39-49.

47. De Vuyst D, Vanhoenacker F, Gielen J, et al: Imaging features of musculoskeletal tuberculosis. Eur Radiol 2003;13:1809-1819.

48. Teo HE, Peh WC: Skeletal tuberculosis in children. Pediatr Radiol 2004;34:853-860.

49. Jarzembowski JA, Young MB: Nontuberculous mycobacterial infections. Arch Pathol Lab Med 2008;132:1333-1341.

50. Wagner D, Young LS: Nontuberculous mycobacterial infections: A clinical review. Infection 2004;32:257-270.

51. Ding LW, Lai CC, Lee LN, et al: Disease caused by non-tuberculous mycobacteria in a university hospital in Taiwan, 1997-2003. Epidemiol Infect 2006;134:1060-1067.

52. Theodorou DJ, Theodorou SJ, Kakitsubata Y, et al: Imaging characteristics and epidemiologic features of atypical mycobacterial infections involving the musculoskeletal system. AJR Am J Roentgenol 2001;176:341-349.

53. Demangel C, Stinear TP, Cole ST: Buruli ulcer: Reductive evolution enhances pathogenicity of *Mycobacterium ulcerans.* Nat Rev Microbiol 2009;7:50-60.

54. Moonot P, Ashwood N, Lockwood D: Orthopaedic complications of leprosy. J Bone Joint Surg 2005;87B:1328-1332.

55. Kent ME, Romanelli F: Reexamining syphilis: An update on epidemiology, clinical manifestations, and management. Ann Pharmacother 2008;42:226-236.

56. Antal GM, Lukehart SA, Meheus AZ: The endemic treponematoses. Microbes Infect 2002;4:83-94.

57. Sengupta S: Musculoskeletal lesions in yaws. Clin Orthop Relat Res 1985;(192):193-198.

58. Kohli R, Hadley S: Fungal arthritis and osteomyelitis. Infect Dis Clin North Am 2005;19:831-851.

59. Mean M, Marchetti O, Calandra T: Bench-to-bedside review: Candida infections in the intensive care unit. Crit Care 2008;12:204.

60. Gathe JC Jr, Harris RL, Garland B, et al: Candida osteomyelitis: Report of five cases and review of the literature. Am J Med 1987;82:927-937.

61. Tack KJ, Rhame FS, Brown B, et al: *Aspergillus* osteomyelitis: Report of four cases and review of the literature. Am J Med 1982;73:295-300.

62. Vinas FC, King PK, Diaz FG: Spinal aspergillus osteomyelitis. Clin Infect Dis 1999;28:1223-1239.

63. Al-Tawfiq JA, Ghandour J: *Cryptococcus neoformans* abscess and osteomyelitis in an immunocompetent patient with tuberculous lymphadenitis. Infection 2007;35:377-382.

64. Liu PY: Cryptococcal osteomyelitis: Case report and review. Diagn Microbiol Infect Dis 1998;30:33-35.

65. Altner PC, Turner RR: Sporotrichosis of bones and joints: Review of the literature and report of six cases. Clin Orthop Relat Res 1970;(68):138-148.

66. Parish JM, Blair JE: Coccidioidomycosis. Mayo Clin Proc 2008;83:343-348; quiz 348-349.

67. Blair JE: State-of-the-art treatment of coccidioidomycosis skeletal infections. Ann N Y Acad Sci 2007;1111:422-433.

68. Amstalden EM, Xavier R, Kattapuram SV, et al: Paracoccidioidomycosis of bones and joints: A clinical, radiologic, and pathologic study of 9 cases. Medicine (Baltimore) 1996;75:213-225.

69. Travassos LR, Taborda CP, Colombo AL: Treatment options for paracoccidioidomycosis and new strategies investigated. Expert Rev Anti Infect Ther 2008;6:251-262.

70. Cockshott WP, Lucas AO: Histoplasmosis duboisii. Q J Med 1964;33:223-238.

71. Oppenheimer M, Embil JM, Black B, et al: Blastomycosis of bones and joints. South Med J 2007;100:570-578.

72. Taxy JB: Blastomycosis: Contributions of morphology to diagnosis. A surgical pathology, cytopathology, and autopsy pathology study. Am J Surg Pathol 2007;31:615-623.

73. Ameen M, Arenas R: Developments in the management of mycetomas. Clin Exp Dermatol 2009;34:1-7.

74. Putschar W: Osteomyelitis including fungal. In Ackerman LV, Spjut HJ, Abele MR (eds): Bones and Joints. International Academy of Pathology Monographs in Pathology No. 17. Baltimore, Williams & Wilkins, 1976.

75. Song XH, Ding LW, Wen H: Bone hydatid disease. Postgrad Med J 2007;83:536-542.

76. Howorth M: Echinococcosis of bone. J Bone Joint Surg 1945;27A:401-411.

77. Davidson JC, Bulawayo PE: Osteomyelitis variolosa. J Bone Joint Surg 1963;45B:687-693.

78. Silverman FN: Virus diseases of bone: Do they exist? The Neuhauser Lecture. AJR Am J Roentgenol 1976;126:677-703.

79. Reed GB Jr: Rubella bone lesions. J Pediatr 1969;74:208-213.

80. O'Connell JX, Nielsen GP, Rosenberg AE: Subchondral acute inflammation in severe arthritis: A sterile osteomyelitis? Am J Surg Pathol 1999;23:192-197.

81. Ferguson PJ, El-Shanti HI: Autoinflammatory bone disorders. Curr Opin Rheumatol 2007;19:492-498.

82. El-Shanti HI, Ferguson PJ: Chronic recurrent multifocal osteomyelitis: A concise review and genetic update. Clin Orthop Relat Res 2007;(462):11-19.

Infections of Joints, Synovium-Lined Structures, and Soft Tissue

Elizabeth G. Demicco, Susan L. Kattapuram, Richard L. Kradin, and Andrew E. Rosenberg

14

CHAPTER

Involvement of joints and other synovium-lined structures, including tendon sheaths and bursae, by pathogens is a relatively uncommon but important form of infection. Its significance is related to the severe destruction of musculoskeletal structures it can cause, which often results in permanent disability and, in some instances, even death.

Synovial tissue is vital to the normal functioning of the musculoskeletal system. It helps maintain joints, tendons, bursae, and ligaments; is the source of nourishment for articular cartilage; and participates in the immune surveillance and activity of these tissues.[1] The synoviocytes secrete the fluid that provides lubrication, protection, and nourishment to the adjacent structures. Articular cartilage, which lacks its own vascular supply, is wholly dependent on synovial fluid for the provision of oxygen and other essential metabolites. The fluid is also rich in glycoproteins, hyaluronic acid, and lysosomal enzymes that are important in the homeostasis of chondrocytes, fibroblasts, and the structural matrix. Histologically, synoviocytes are cuboidal to elongate and are arranged in a layer, two to four cells thick, which is supported by loose fibrofatty connective tissue containing abundant blood vessels, lymphatics, and nerves. The synovial lining lacks a protective basement membrane, and this, in conjunction with its rich vascular network, makes it a prime target for invasion by a wide variety of microorganisms (Table 14-1).[1]

Mechanistically, the initial entry of an organism into a joint or synovial structure occurs by the same pathways involved in osteomyelitis; namely, hematogenous seeding, extension from a contiguous site, and direct implantation. In many situations, hematogenous seeding is the most common etiology, followed in frequency by spread from a neighboring infection in bone or soft tissue. Trauma with direct implantation is a common cause of tenosynovitis and bursitis, which often affects the digits of the hands and feet and may less frequently involve larger joints. Because tendon sheaths may communicate with bursae,

Table 14-1 Organisms That Cause Septic Arthritis

Gram-Positive Bacteria (60-70%)	
Staphylococcus aureus	44%
Streptococcus pyogenes	7%
Streptococcus pneumoniae	7%
Coagulase-negative staphylococci	4%
Streptococcus agalactiae	3%
Other β-hemolytic streptococci	4%
Gram-Negative Bacteria (20-30%)	
Mycobacterium tuberculosis	4%
Escherichia coli	4%
Haemophilus influenzae	4%
Neisseria gonorrhoeae	3%
Pseudomonas aeruginosa	2%
Neisseria meningitidis	1%
Salmonella species.	1%
Other gram-negatives	5%
Polymicrobial/Anaerobic Bacteria (2-5%)	
Bacteroides	
Fusobacterium	
Peptostreptococcus	
Clostridium	
Fungal (4%)	
Candida species	
Sporothrix schenckii	
Coccidioides immitis	
Blastomyces dermatitidis	
Cryptococcus neoformans	
Histoplasma capsulatum	
Miscellaneous (1%)	

Data from Ross JJ: Septic arthritis. Infect Dis Clin North Am 2005;19:799-817.

infection of these structures can produce complicated patterns of extension.

Once an organism infects the synovium, there is usually an acute inflammatory response with vascular dilatation and increased permeability, resulting in tissue edema and hyperemia. The inflamed synovium undergoes architectural changes to accommodate its increased girth by forming papillary structures lined by hypertrophied and hyperplasic synoviocytes. The synoviocytes increase their secretion of fluid, and this, in conjunction with serum leakage from reactive vessels and fibrin production, results in effusion of the affected joint, bursa, or tendon sheath. Both pathogenic infiltration and the reactive host inflammatory reaction can trigger necrosis of synoviocytes, chondrocytes, and tendinocytes and digestion of crucial structural components, with subsequent destruction of the tissues. The closed physical nature of joints, tendon sheaths, and bursae limits their expansion, so, once they are inundated by the infectious

process, secondary ischemia and its complications (e.g., compartment syndromes) may occur. Over time, chronic inflammatory cells appear and are accompanied by reactive fibrosis and scarring. If located near bone, the infection can initiate osteoclastic activity and erosion of the bone; this frequently manifests as juxta-articular erosions in joint infections. Eventually, there can be severe and permanent destruction of the joint and periarticular structures, resulting in significant dysfunction. In some instances, the infectious agent, because of molecular mimicry between the host and the pathogen, initiates an autoimmune reaction that may be short-lived or chronic and may cause further significant damage and disability.

Bacterial Arthritis

Bacteria are the most common cause of infection of the synovium. Large weight-bearing joints, such as the knee, are particularly prone to hematogenous seeding. Small joints of the hands and feet are more likely to develop septic arthritis secondary to penetrating trauma.[2] Iatrogenic causes of infection include arthroscopy, corticosteroid injection, surgery, and implantation of prosthetic joints.

The primary risk factor for septic arthritis is preexisting joint disease, and up to 47% of patients have prior joint problems or rheumatologic disorders, including rheumatoid arthritis, systemic lupus erythematosus (SLE), osteoarthritis, gout, pseudogout, trauma, or prior joint surgery.[2,3] Rheumatoid arthritis is most frequently associated with septic arthritis and tends to have worse outcomes. Chronic breach in skin integrity (e.g., psoriasis, chronic skin ulcers, intravenous drug use) is also a risk factor. An immunocompromised state (e.g., malignancy, corticosteroid use, chronic disease, acquired immunodeficiency syndrome [AIDS]) is strongly linked to increased risk for infectious arthritis, in particular with atypical microorganisms, such as *Listeria*, *Salmonella*, and *Actinobacillus*, as well as fungal and mycobacterial arthritides.[4]

Most cases of bacterial arthritis are due to occult bacteremia with gram-positive organisms, typically *Staphylococcus aureus*. Gram-negative bacilli account for 10% of community-acquired septic arthritis and are associated with intravenous drug use.[4,5] Gram-positive bacteria are thought to more efficiently bind extracellular matrix proteins, thereby facilitating adhesion to affected tissues. A number of bacterial adhesion genes that may be involved in this process have been identified, including those encoding fibrinogen-binding proteins (fib, cflA, fbpA), fibronectin-binding proteins (fnbA, fnbB), an elastin-binding protein (ebpS), a collagen receptor (cna), and a less specific binding protein (map).[5] Bacterial invasion and proliferation result in direct soft tissue and cartilage damage through the production of bacterial enzymes and toxins (e.g., staphylococcal TSST-1, enterotoxins, α-hemolysin). The host inflammatory response further damages articular cartilage through activation of matrix metalloproteinases (MMPs) and release of reactive oxygen species, lysosomal enzymes, and pro-inflammatory cytokines including interleukin 2 (IL-2), interferon-γ (IFN-γ), and tumor necrosis factor-α (TNF-α).[5] Articular cartilage is also subjected to ischemia as accumulation of pus within the joint space leads to increased joint pressure and tamponade of synovial blood flow.[4-6] If left untreated, infection may spread to adjacent bone and soft tissues, leading to the formation of sinus tracts, osteo-myelitis, and possible destruction of tendons and ligaments.

S. aureus accounts for 40% to 50% of cases of septic arthritis, followed by *Streptococcus pyogenes* (8%), *Streptococcus pneumoniae* (7%), *Haemophilus influenzae* (4-7%), *Escherichia coli* (4%), coagulase-negative staphylococci (4%), *Neisseria gonorrhoeae* (3%), *Streptococcus agalactiae* (3%), *Pseudomonas aeruginosa* (2%), *Neisseria meningitidis* (1%), and *Salmonella* species (1%).[4] Other gram-negative rods and β-hemolytic streptococci are responsible for 5% and 4% of cases, respectively, and 1% to 2% of cases are polymicrobial. *Staphylococcus* and *Streptococcus* are the primary bacterial pathogens in pediatric septic arthritis, whereas vaccination against *H. influenzae* has significantly reduced the incidence of arthritis associated with that organism.[7] *Kingella kingae*, a fastidious gram-negative rod once thought to be a rare cause of disease, is gaining recognition as a growing pathogen in children younger than 2 years of age and has been implicated in septic arthritis, osteomyelitis, and spinal discitis.[8] Anaerobic pathogens are fastidious and difficult to culture and therefore are often overlooked as a cause of septic arthritis.[9] The infections are often polymicrobial, and their true incidence is uncertain. *Bacteroides, Peptostreptococcus, Fusobacterium, Clostridium,* and *Propionibacterium acnes* are the primary culprits, and pigmented *Prevotella, Porphyromonas,* and *Fusobacterium* are all associated with bite infections. *Bacteroides fragilis* has a predilection for hand and foot infections.[9] Risk factors for anaerobic infection include collagen vascular disease, bites, trauma, prosthetic joints, prior surgery, and peripheral neuropathy. Adults are more frequently affected than children.

Bacterial arthritis is usually monoarticular. The knee is the primary site for bacterial arthritis, with 30% to 50% of cases, followed by hip (15-22%), ankle (6-9%), elbow (8-9%), wrist (4-6%) and shoulder (5-12%).[2,3,10] In the pediatric population, the most common sites of septic arthritis are the hip and knee, and 90%

of cases are monoarticular.[11] Polyarticular disease occurs in approximately 15% of cases and is associated with immunocompromise.[3] Gonococcal, pneumococcal, group B streptococcal, and gram-negative infections also may result in polyarthritis.[12] Septic polyarthritis is asymmetric, and 72% of cases involve the knee.[12] The cartilaginous joints of the axial skeleton are relatively resistant to infection, although an association with intravenous drug use has been established.[13]

The classic presentation of septic arthritis is fevers and rigor accompanying a swollen, warm, erythematous, and painful joint. High-grade fever is present only in 58% of cases, whereas low-grade fever is present 90% of the time.[14] Fewer than 60% of patients present with a serum leukocytosis,[3,14] and immunocompromised patients may not report pain. Therefore, a high index of suspicion should be maintained, even in the absence of classic symptoms, and arthrocentesis should be performed. Synovial fluid chemistries, including protein, glucose, and lactate dehydrogenase concentrations, as well as synovial white blood cell (WBC) counts, are relatively nonspecific for infection. Infectious etiologies should be considered in all synovial fluids with a WBC count greater than 50,000 cells/μL; however, a low WBC count does not exclude septic arthritis (Table 14-2). Gram staining and culture should be routinely performed whenever infection is suspected, as well as polymerase chain reaction (PCR) or serologic testing where indicated.

Historically, plain films have been of use only in late-stage disease, demonstrating joint effusions, cartilage loss, or bone destruction (Fig. 14-1).[15] Magnetic resonance imaging (MRI) may be helpful in diagnosing early lesions, including those that involve tendon sheaths, with findings such as effusion, synovial thickening and enhancement, bone marrow edema, and perisynovial edema and enhancement (Fig. 14-2).[16] Reactive bone marrow edema in septic arthritis can be mistaken on imaging for periarticular osteomyelitis. However, in osteomyelitis, the edema

Table 14-2 Synovial Fluid Analysis by Etiology*

Parameter	Normal	Noninflammatory	Inflammatory, Viral, or Reactive	Bacterial	Fungal	Crystal	Trauma
Color	Yellow	Yellow	Yellow	Gray-green	Variable	Yellow-white	Red-brown
Clarity	Clear	Slightly cloudy	Cloudy	Cloudy	Variable	Cloudy	Bloody
Viscosity	High	Reduced	Low	Low	Low	Low	Reduced
Clot	No	Rare	Rare	Frequent	—	Rare	Yes
WBCs/μL	0-200	0-2000	2,000-100,000	20-200,000	10,000-100,000	500-200,000	50-10,000
% Neutrophils	<25	<30	>50	>75	>50	<90	<50
Serum glucose concentration (mg/dL)	0-10	0-10	0-40	20-100	10-20	0-80	0-20
Crystals	No	No	±	±	±	Yes	±
Culture	Negative	Negative	Negative	Most organisms	Some organisms	Negative	Negative
PCR/Serology	Negative	Negative	Positive	Some organisms	Some organisms	Negative	Negative
Stains	Negative	Negative	Negative	Gram stain, AFB, silver stain	Silver stain, PAS, Gram stain	Negative	Negative

*Synovial WBCs, glucose, protein, and lactate dehydrogenase concentrations are relatively nonspecific indicators of infection.
Presence of crystals does not exclude septic arthritis. Gram stain, culture, PCR, or serologic studies remain essential for definitive diagnosis and organism identification.
AFB, acid-fast bacteria stain; PAS, periodic acid–Schiff stain; PCR, polymerase chain reaction; WBCs, white blood cells.

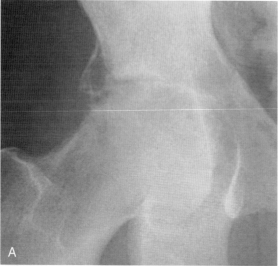

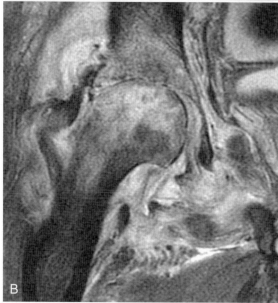

Figure 14-1. Septic arthritis of the hip joint. **A,** Plain radiograph of the hip shows near-complete loss of the joint space, destruction of the superomedial acetabulum and the superolateral femoral head, and acetabulum with bone fragments in the soft tissues. **B,** Coronal T2-weighted magnetic resonance image demonstrates bright signal intensity within the acetabulum and femoral head and in and around the joint, representing inflammation and edema. Note the destruction of the cortical bone along the femoral head and adjacent acetabulum.

demonstrates markedly low signal on T1-weighted images and is more diffuse and robust than that seen in association with septic joints, although these findings are not specific.[15] Ultrasound may also be used to detect early effusion. Echo-free effusions, resulting from clotting hemorrhagic fluid collections, are thought to be characteristic of septic arthritis.[17] Imaging studies can also be used to monitor the response to treatment or to demonstrate underlying conditions such as osteoarthritis.[5]

Histologic examination of infected synovial tissue from native joints is rarely performed, because diagnosis relies on clinical findings, arthrocentesis, and analysis and culture of synovial fluid. Animal models have shown that joint injury is rapid,

with synovial hypertrophy visible within 24 hours after intravascular bacterial injection, whereas bone erosions and pannus formation may develop within 3 days. Early septic arthritis is dominated by dense neutrophilic infiltration of the synovium, which may coat articular cartilage and result in its necrosis and digestion (Fig. 14-3). Eventually, lymphocytes, plasma cells, and histiocytes appear, and an acute and chronic papillary synovitis with fibrin aggregates develops. These changes resemble those seen in noninfectious inflammatory arthritides, such as rheumatoid arthritis.[18] In long-standing disease, the entire articular cartilage may be eroded, resulting in osteomyelitis (Fig. 14-4).

Treatment of septic arthritis should be prompt and involves appropriate antimicrobial therapy. Intra-articular antibacterial therapy is not usually indicated. Drainage should be performed by needle aspiration or open drainage, and may be repeated. Débridement may be required.[5]

Outcomes in septic arthritis may be poor, especially if the infection accompanies systemic sepsis, with an overall mortality rate as high as 11%.[3,14] Morbidity is also high, with secondary osteomyelitis occurring in 8% and poor functional outcome in 24% to 40% of cases.[3,14] Poor outcome is associated with polyarticular arthritis, age greater than 65 years, delay in presentation, existence of medical comorbidities, chronic illness, and rheumatoid arthritis.[3,4]

Gonococcal Arthritis

Neisseria gonorrhoeae, a gram-negative diplococcus, is the most common sexually transmitted bacterium associated with infective arthritis. In the 1970s through the 1980s, it was the most common cause of infective arthritis in the United States.[19] Safer sex practices resulted in a steep decline in disease prevalence through the 1990s. More recently, gonococcal infections have been on the rise, primarily due to high-risk sexual behavior among young gay men. Of further concern is the appearance of antibiotic-resistant strains. These two trends ensure that gonorrhea will continue to be of clinical importance for the foreseeable future.

Patients with gonococcal arthritis are usually young, healthy, and sexually active. Gonococcal arthritis may take one of two forms: a classic suppurative arthritis similar to the septic arthritis seen with other bacterial infections or a syndrome of disseminated gonococcal infection (DGI) including tenosynovitis, skin lesions, and polyarthralgias without true septic arthritis.[19] Some authors have postulated an immunologic basis for DGI. However, the presence of positive blood cultures in up to 50% of cases and an inability to identify circulating immune complexes argue against this theory.[19]

Gonococcal infection begins with localized mucosal disease. In fewer than 3% of cases, the organism rapidly enters the circulation and produces DGI.[20-22] Risk factors associated with DGI include delayed diagnosis, SLE, deficiency of the complement system, menstruation, and pregnancy, as well as socioeconomic factors, promiscuity, urban residence, male homosexuality, and educational status.[5] Bacterial strains also play a role, with higher risk associated with piliated *N. gonorrhoeae* strains that are capable of phase variation. Women have four times the risk of men for development of DGI,[23] most likely because of asymptomatic infection and delayed diagnosis.

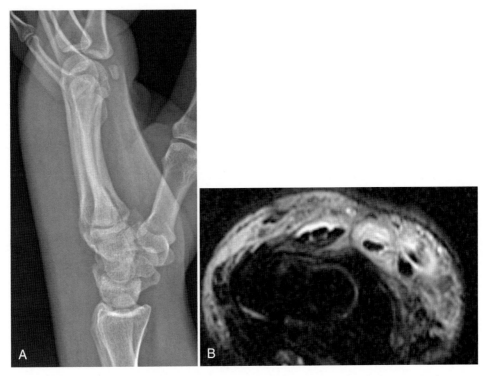

Figure 14-2. Septic tenosynovitis. **A,** Lateral radiograph shows edema of the dorsal soft tissues. **B,** Axial magnetic resonance image demonstrates marked T2-intense edema around the dark tendon.

Patients with DGI present with migratory arthralgias, fever, chills, dermatitis, and tenosynovitis. Most are found to have asymptomatic mucosal gonococcal infection involving the genitals, anus, or pharynx.[20] Skin lesions are classically limited to the extremities and trunk and begin as small, inconspicuous erythematous papules which progress to vesicular or pustular lesions. The papules may overlie affected joints. Tenosynovitis causes pain, swelling, and erythema. Polyarthralgias may involve knees, elbows, and distal joints, whereas arthritis and tenosynovitis are polyarticular and preferentially involve the distal joints, including those of the hands and fingers, wrists, elbows, knees, and ankles.[5,19]

Suppurative gonococcal arthritis is monoarticular or oligoarticular and involves the knees, wrists, ankles, and elbows. Symptoms of bacteremia, skin lesions, or prior polyarthralgias are not present.

The radiographic and histopathologic findings in gonococcal arthritis are similar to those seen in other septic bacterial arthritides. However, imaging studies and synovial biopsy are rarely performed. In rare biopsied cases, the periarticular soft tissues show granulation tissue with mixed polymorphonuclear and mononuclear cell infiltrates (Fig. 14-5).

Synovial fluid analysis and culture are required for diagnosis. Treatment requires appropriate antibacterial therapy in conjunction with aspiration. Surgery is rarely necessary. Patients should be tested for concomitant infection with *Chlamydia trachomatis.* Appropriate treatment is associated with a good outcome.

The differential diagnosis of DGI includes *N. meningitidis* infection, which manifests with similar skin lesions and arthralgias. Other bacterial infections also must be ruled out and can usually be distinguished by their clinical features or by culture.

Meningococcal Arthritis

Infection with *N. meningitidis* is associated with a sterile monoarticular or oligoarticular arthritis that is thought to be secondary to a hypersensitivity reaction with immune complex deposition. Recovery from this form of arthritis is usually complete. Infrequently, meningococcus may lead to a monoarticular septic arthritis.

Lyme Arthritis (Borreliosis)

Lyme borreliosis was first described in 1975 in the United States, after the perplexing outbreak of juvenile rheumatoid arthritis in the vicinity of Lyme, Connecticut.[24] The causative agent, the spirochete *Borrelia burgdorferi,* was not identified until 1982.[25,26] Lyme disease is now recognized as the most common vector-borne disease in North America and Europe, with annual incidence rates as high as 31.6 cases per 100,000 population in endemic areas.[27] In the United States, it is localized to three endemic areas: the East Coast (Maine to Maryland), the Midwest (Minnesota and Wisconsin), and the Northwest (Northern California and Oregon). However, these regions continue to enlarge as the geographic range of the vector ticks infected with *B. burgdorferi* expands.

Three members of the *Borrelia* genus are known to cause Lyme disease in humans: *B. burgdorferi* (endemic to North America), *Borrelia garinii,* and *Borrelia afzelii* (endemic to Europe and Asia). More recently, *Borrelia lonestari* has been implicated in a Lyme disease–like illness in the southern United States. Borreliosis is a vector-borne disease, with pathogens

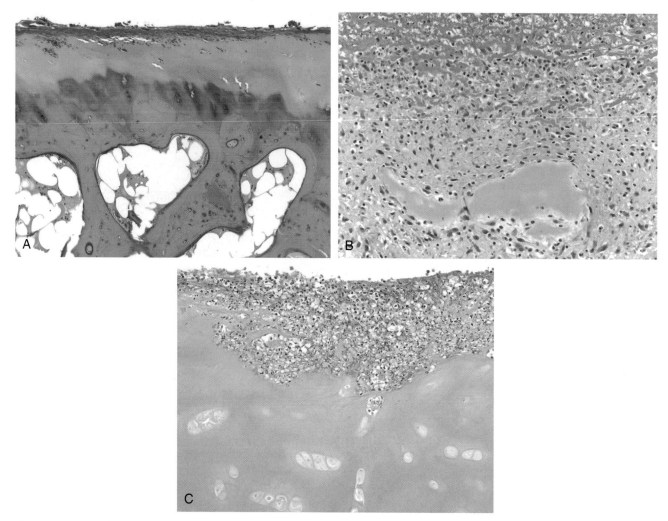

Figure 14-3. Septic arthritis. **A,** Neutrophils coat the articular cartilage surface. **B,** Synovial surface covered by neutrophils and fibrin. Note embedded fragment of articular cartilage. **C,** Chondrocytes digesting necrotic articular hyaline cartilage.

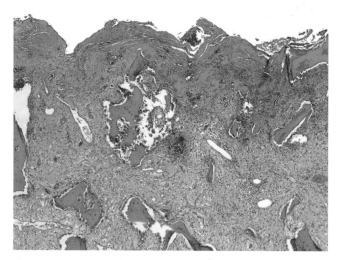

Figure 14-4. Articular surface with destruction of cartilage. The irregular bone surface is covered by a fibrous synovial pannus.

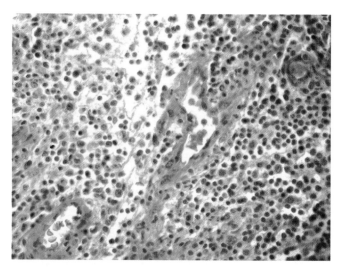

Figure 14-5. Gonococcus causes a periarticular inflammation with granulation tissue, neutrophils, and mononuclear cells.

transmitted by the bite of infected *Ixodes ricinus* ticks. In the larval and nymph stages of the tick life cycle, ticks feed primarily on small rodents—predominantly, the white-footed mouse in the United States and the vole in Europe and Asia. These animals then serve as a disease reservoir for horizontal transmission between nymphs and larval ticks. In contrast, larger mammals such as deer or humans, preferred as a food source for adult ticks, are dead-end hosts for *Borrelia*.[28,29] For *Borrelia* transmission to occur, the tick must be attached to its host for at least 24 hours[30]; this allows the bacteria to migrate from the tick midgut into the salivary gland, a process mediated by cell surface adhesion molecules, including OspA and Ospc.[31]

A number of factors have been implicated in disease transmission. Tick saliva is thought to contain vasodilators, anticoagulants, and immunomodulators, which may facilitate *Borrelia* transmission to the host.[29] Factors on the spirochete membrane function as adhesion molecules, such as p66, which binds to β_3-chain integrins, and BBK32, which binds to fibronectin. *B. burgdorferi* then binds to host plasmin and urokinase, resulting in plasmin-mediated MMP activation and proteolysis of extracellular matrix, which allows dissemination of bacteria throughout the host.[28,29]

The pathognomonic lesion of early acute Lyme disease is the erythema migrans rash, which appears at the site of tick bite within 5 to 14 days, then spontaneously resolves after several days to weeks.[32] The rash is erythematous, often with a central clearing, or bull's eye, and is usually painless and nonpruritic. Erythema migrans has been reported to have an incidence of up to 90% in some studies of Lyme disease patients.[33,34] Within a few weeks of infection, untreated patients develop symptoms of early disseminated disease, including fever, malaise, aseptic meningitis, facial palsy, radiculoneuropathy, or carditis, as well as migratory arthralgias and myalgias. Typically, true arthritis develops weeks or months after the initial infection.

Acute Lyme arthritis occurs in up to 50% to 60% of untreated patients infected with *B. burgdorferi*[35]; the incidence is lower with *B. garinii* or *B. afzelii* infection.[36] Lyme arthritis is usually a monoarticular or oligoarticular arthritis that typically affects the knee or other large joints.[37] Joints of the digits are occasionally involved, and tendonitis and bursitis may also occur. In most patients, arthritis occurs in flares, which resolve over a period of years. In a minority of patients, chronic synovitis may develop despite appropriate antibiotic treatment. Chronic synovitis is accompanied by joint injury and results in permanent joint damage in 2% of patients.[37]

Autoimmunity has been implicated in chronic Lyme disease, because the arthritis persists despite eradication of spirochetes in the affected joint. Mechanistically, this immune response is thought to be caused by focal homology between the *B. burgdorferi* membrane antigen OspA and hLFA-1α, an adhesion molecule expressed by most lymphoid and myeloid cells that is upregulated during an inflammatory response. An association with major histocompatibility complex (MHC) class II human leukocyte antigens HLA-DRB1*0401 and 0101 has also been identified. Therefore, infection by *B. burgdorferi* is thought to lead to antigen presentation of OspA epitopes, resulting in activation and expansion of OspA-specific T cells. These T cells then secrete IFN-γ in the infected joint, leading to inflammation and subsequent upregulation of MHC class II molecules and hLFA-

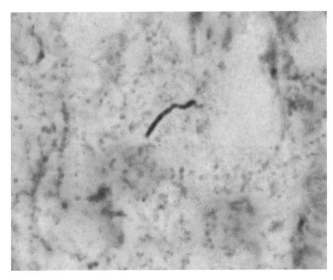

Figure 14-6. Lyme disease with Warthin-Starry stain demonstrating coiled *Borrelia burgdorferi* spirochete.

1α in the microenvironment. After elimination of *B. burgdorferi*, T cells may remain active in the affected joint due to cross-reaction with hLFA-1α, leading to progressive and chronic joint injury.[29,38]

On imaging, acute Lyme arthritis shows effusion of the knee joint. Intra-articular edema can be seen, along with a spectrum of soft tissue changes involving the infrapatellar fat pad, periarticular soft tissues, and entheses. In chronic Lyme arthritis, an inflammatory arthritis is seen, with juxta-articular osteoporosis, loss of cartilage, and bony erosions. Rarely, degenerative changes, such as subarticular sclerosis and osteophyte formation, may be seen.[39]

The histologic features of acute Lyme synovitis are similar to those observed in other septic arthritides, with edema and abundant neutrophilic infiltration of synovium and adjacent soft tissues. Organisms have been demonstrated in synovial tissues in the early stages of infection by Warthin-Starry silver stain (Fig. 14-6), and PCR has been shown to improve detection.[40] Histologic examination of synovial tissue from chronic Lyme arthritis demonstrates nonspecific features of chronic inflammatory or rheumatoid arthritis. Fibrin deposition is seen, along with synovial hypertrophy, neovascularization, and infiltration by histiocytes, plasma cells, and a subsynovial mixed lymphocyte population (Fig. 14-7).[41] In this setting, the morphologic changes overlap with those of other, noninfectious inflammatory arthropathies.

Diagnosis of Lyme arthritis should be considered in patients who have recently been in areas endemic for *B. burgdorferi* and present with acute or subacute monoarthritis. A history of erythema migrans is helpful, but not required, to proceed to serologic or synovial fluid testing. Treatment of acute Lyme arthritis involves oral or intravenous antibiotic therapy. If arthritis does not resolve with two courses of an appropriate antibiotic regimen and PCR testing of synovial fluid is negative for *B. burgdorferi*, chronic Lyme arthritis should be considered, and it should be treated with immunosuppressive therapy.

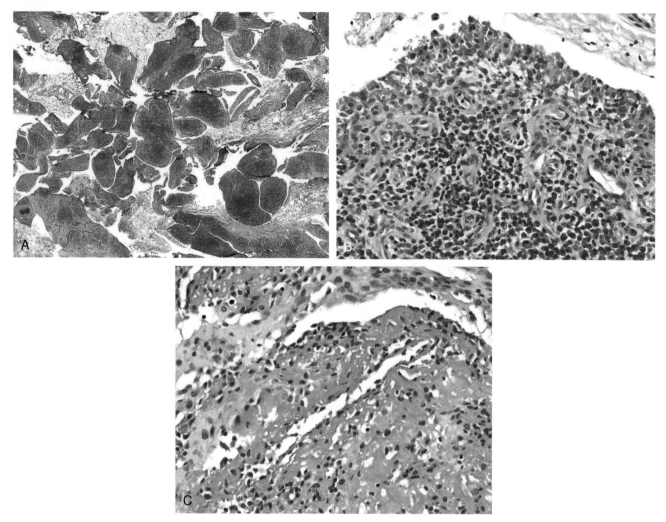

Figure 14-7. Lyme disease. **A,** Low-power view of chronic papillary synovitis. **B,** Hyperplastic synoviocytes overlie a dense infiltrate composed of lymphocytes and plasma cells. **C,** Synoviocytes cover a layer of fibrin.

Tuberculous Mycobacterial Arthritis

Joint involvement follows infection of the spine as the most common manifestation of musculoskeletal tuberculosis. Peripheral large and medium-sized joints, especially the hip and knee, are most frequently affected.[42] Risk factors for development of tuberculous arthritis include female gender and older age; children rarely develop this form of infection.[43,44] Seeding of the joint space is thought to occur as a complication of bone infection or through direct inoculation.[42] Hematogenous spread can also result in multifocal joint involvement, especially in immunocompromised patients.[45]

Pain and local swelling are common presenting complaints. Fever and weight loss are rarely present. Tuberculous arthritis has an indolent course, with the gradual development of a nonspecific synovitis and joint effusion.

Radiographically, Phemister's triad is characteristic. It consists of juxta-articular osteoporosis, osseous erosions, and slight narrowing of the joint space (Fig. 14-8).[46] In contrast, the MRI findings of synovitis with pannus formation, effusions, and peripheral and central erosions are relatively nonspecific.[47] On

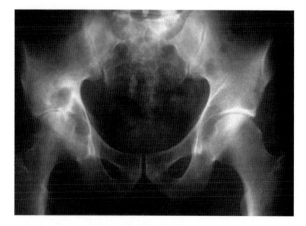

Figure 14-8. Anteroposterior radiograph of the pelvis showing tuberculous arthritis of the right hip. There is mild narrowing of the joint space, and round lucencies are seen in the femoral head and acetabulum. Sclerosis surrounds the lytic foci.

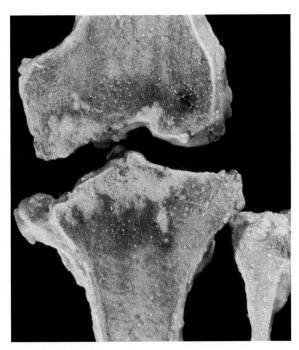

Figure 14-9. Gross specimen of tuberculous arthritis involving the knee. The articular cartilage is eroded, and caseous necrotic tissue has infiltrated into the subchondral bone of the distal femur and the proximal tibia and fibula.

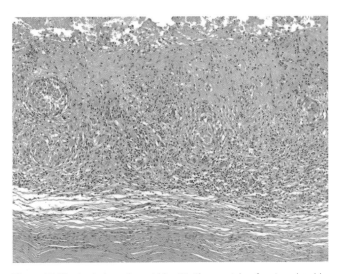

Figure 14-10. Atypical mycobacterial bursitis. The synovial surface is replaced by granulomas with scattered lymphocytes and fibrin deposition on the surface.

T2-weighted images, tuberculous synovitis demonstrates low signal in areas of granuloma formation.[48]

Grossly, the inflamed synovial tissue is tan-yellow, with destruction of the articular cartilage and possible erosion into bone (Fig. 14-9). Histologically, the synovium shows acute and chronic inflammation with necrotizing granulomas. The infection frequently extends into bursae and synovial tendon sheaths. Treatment consists of local débridement with multidrug anti-tuberculosis chemotherapy.

Non-Tuberculous Mycobacterial Arthritis

Non-tuberculous mycobacterial infections rarely affect the joints and are usually associated with underlying immunocompromise or rheumatologic disorders. Occasionally, direct inoculation or trauma is the route of infection.[49,50] Hematogenous spread from a primary pulmonary lesion may also occur. Non-tuberculous mycobacterial arthritis has also been seen in association with foreign bodies, including prosthetic joints.[42] Among the non-tuberculous mycobacteria, *Mycobacterium kansasii* is the most common cause of monoarthritis, whereas *Mycobacterium marinum* and *Mycobacterium avium* complex are the most frequent causes of tenosynovitis. *Mycobacterium chelonae*, *Mycobacterium fortuitum*, *Mycobacterium abscessus*, and *Mycobacterium terrae*, among others, have also been implicated.[50,51]

Patients with non-tuberculous mycobacterial arthritis typically present with an insidious onset of localized swelling and pain over the affected joint. A joint effusion may be present, and erosive changes may be seen on imaging.[49,52,53] Non-tuberculous mycobacterial tenosynovitis and arthritis most frequently involve the hands, although other sites, including the feet, shoulder, and knee, have been reported.[54] Histologically, the findings range from chronic synovitis with scattered macrophages to florid necrotizing granulomas (Fig. 14-10).

The differential diagnosis for non-tuberculous mycobacterial arthritis includes sarcoidosis, especially if the small joints are involved; however, the histopathologic changes, special stains for microorganisms, and culture can establish the correct diagnosis.

Treatment of non-tuberculous mycobacterial arthritis usually involves a prolonged course of multidrug antimycobacterial therapy with or without local débridement.

Fungal Arthritis

Fungal (mycotic) arthritis is a rare disease that arises mainly from hematogenous dissemination, although direct inoculation or extension from an adjacent region of infection may also occur.[55] As with bacterial arthritis, predisposing factors include chronic disease, immunosuppression, and prolonged use of intravenous antibiotics, as well as the presence of indwelling catheters and joint prostheses.[56,57] Since the advent of the human immunodeficiency virus (HIV) epidemic, the incidence of fungal arthritis has markedly increased. Although the true incidence is unknown, candidal infection is thought to account for most cases. However, other species, including *Sporothrix schenckii*, *Coccidioides immitis*, *Blastomyces dermatitidis*, *Cryptococcus neoformans*, and *Histoplasma capsulatum*, are also known to cause articular disease.[56]

Mycotic arthritis tends to manifest indolently, with an extended course between symptom onset and diagnosis. Although any joint may be affected, the knee and other large joints are the most common sites. Clinical symptoms are nonspecific, and common complaints are decreased range of motion, pain, erythema, and joint effusion.[55,57]

Radiographic findings demonstrate soft tissue swelling, periarticular bone erosions, effusions, and narrowing of the joint space.

Synovial fluid analysis may be suggestive of an inflammatory aseptic arthritis, although *Candida* and *Cryptococcus* are associated with purulent synovial fluid. Routine cultures are frequently negative. Histologically, there is an acute and chronic synovitis, and in some cases necrotizing granulomas are present. Special histochemical stains are useful in identifying the offending organism.

Treatment invariably involves intravenous antifungal therapy, and surgical drainage or débridement is often required.

Candidiasis

Nine species of *Candida* are known to be pathogenic in humans. *Candida albicans, Candida parapsilosis, Candida tropicalis, Candida glabrata, Candida guilliermondii, Candida krusei,* and *Candida zeylanoides* have been identified in cases of candidal arthritis.[56,57] Joint infections involving *Candida* species occur in the setting of disseminated disease in most cases. Other factors predisposing to *Candida* infection are indwelling catheters, intravenous drug use, parenteral hyperalimentation, malignancy, multiple surgeries, use of broad-spectrum antibiotics, and prosthetic joints.[56,58] Candidal arthritis may also occur secondary to intra-articular corticosteroid injection.[56]

Candidal arthritis most frequently involves the knee (67% of cases), although hip, shoulder, ankle, and other joints have been reported to be affected.[55,56] Candidal infection from hematogenous spread usually causes a monoarticular or oligoarticular arthritis.[59,60] Patients are febrile and may have leukopenia or leukocytosis. There may be a long latency between fungemia or joint surgery and onset of arthritis, and in rare cases symptoms have been reported for up to 4 years before diagnosis.[56,57,61] Patients may present with a normal WBC count and no fever. Clinical symptoms include pain, inability to bear weight, and restricted range of motion.[62] The affected joints are swollen, painful, and warm.

Radiologic examination reveals nonspecific soft tissue swelling, joint effusion, and destructive joint changes. If a prosthesis is present, there may be evidence of loosening.[56]

Candidal arthritis begins as a synovitis and spreads to adjacent bone. Grossly, the synovium may be thickened and hyperemic, with scarring and erosion of articular cartilage.[63] Histologic examination of infected synovium reveals histiocytic and mononuclear cell infiltration and fibrosis. Granulomas are rarely present.[57,64] Silver stain or tissue Gram stain may demonstrate fungal organisms, but culture of synovial fluid or tissue is more sensitive. Blood cultures are often negative.

Treatment usually involves intravenous antifungal chemotherapy, with or without local débridement and synovectomy. Infected prostheses must be removed. Use of intra-articular antifungal chemotherapy is controversial.[55] The mortality rate in cases involving a systemic fungal infection may be as high as 50%.[56]

Candida is the prototypical fungal pathogen involved in pediatric arthritis. Affected patients are primarily neonates and infants younger than 6 months of age. Typically, joint infections are a result of hematogenous spread in the setting of systemic invasive candidiasis.[55] Risk factors include prematurity, low birth weight, respiratory distress syndrome, aspiration pneumonia, gastrointestinal defects, surgery, malnutrition, and use of broad-spectrum antibiotics.[55] Maternal vaginal candidiasis may also be a factor. Patients present with fever and a swollen, tender joint,

with abnormal positioning of the infected limb. Thirty percent of cases are polyarticular, and the knee is most frequently involved. There may be associated metaphyseal osteomyelitis, either by direct extension from synovium or by concurrent hematogenous spread. Radiographic findings include joint effusion, joint dislocation, or metaphyseal abnormalities.[60] Intravenous antifungal therapy is the treatment of choice.

Cryptococcosis

Cryptococcus neoformans infection primarily involves the lungs and central nervous system. Disseminated disease is thought to occur by hematogenous spread from infected lungs.[65] Cryptococcal joint infection is an extremely rare event that usually occurs by direct spread from adjacent infected bone.[65] Cryptococcal arthritis may affect one or several joints, and the knee is the most common site of involvement.[66] In one case, cryptococcal infection was documented in tendonitis and tenosynovitis of the forearm.[66] Patients are usually immunocompromised as a result of organ transplantation, malignancy, corticosteroid use, or AIDS.[55]

Patients present with warmth, swelling, tenderness, and limited range of motion in the affected joint. Symptoms of systemic disease may also be present. Radiographs show narrowing of the joint space along with bony changes of osteomyelitis. MRI demonstrates synovial thickening and enhancement if tenosynovitis is present.[66]

Histologic examination reveals epithelioid granulomas with multinucleated giant cells, moderate lymphocytic infiltration, and areas of necrosis. Intracytoplasmic and extracytoplasmic spheroidal budding organisms ranging in diameter from 5 to 20 µm can be seen on silver or periodic acid–Schiff (PAS) stains (Fig. 14-11).[65] Organisms may be cultured from synovial tissue or fluid.

Treatment requires débridement and intravenous antifungal chemotherapy. Despite treatment, patients may develop postinfectious degenerative arthritis.[65]

Coccidioidomycosis

Coccidioides immitis infection begins with a pulmonary infection in immunocompetent individuals. In fewer than 1% of cases, infection disseminates, with involvement of meninges, skin and subcutaneous tissues, lymph nodes, and bones and joints.[57,67] Acute polyarticular arthritis with fever, rash, eosinophilia, and bilateral hilar lymphadenopathy may develop as part of a hypersensitivity syndrome in 30% of cases during primary infection.[68] The arthritis is migratory, and joints are tender and painful on motion. Effusions are generally not present. The ankle and knee are the primary joints affected, and the arthritis resolves within 1 month without permanent sequelae. In disseminated disease, arthritis arises from hematogenous seeding or direct extension from areas of osteomyelitis. Symptoms begin as intermittent, painful swelling of one joint and progress to large effusions, swelling, and development of draining sinus tracts.[57] The knee is affected in 50% to 70% of cases, but any joint may be involved. Tenosynovitis may also occur.

Imaging findings include effusion, joint space narrowing, and bone destruction. Histology demonstrates villonodular

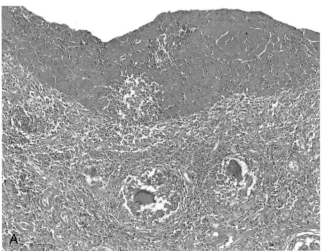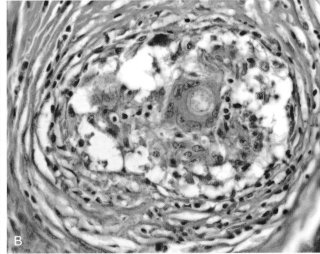

Figure 14-11. Cryptococcal synovitis. **A,** Synovial tissue is covered by a thick layer of fibrin. Well-formed granulomas are surrounded by reactive fibrous tissue. **B,** Granuloma containing organism. Note refractile capsule.

synovitis, or pannus formation with non-necrotizing granulomas, and spherules containing coccidioidal endospores. Treatment is with antifungal chemotherapy. Drainage and débridement may be necessary.

Blastomycosis

Blastomyces dermatitidis arthritis is a monoarticular arthritis that usually affects men from the third to the fifth decade of life. The knee is the main site of involvement, followed by ankle, elbow, wrist, and hand. Joint infection may occur by hematogenous seeding or by spread from a focus of osteomyelitis. If left untreated, infection may spread to additional joints. The clinical onset may be abrupt, and pain and swelling are associated with fever and weight loss. Synovial fluid can be purulent. Diagnosis requires evidence of fungus, in synovial fluid or in any other site, and can be made on wet mount microcopy. Treatment with antifungal agents results in resolution of arthritis. Drainage of infected fluid may be necessary.[55,57]

Histoplasmosis

Joint manifestations of *Histoplasma capsulatum* infection occur as part of a hypersensitivity reaction during primary infection. This self-limited arthritis is migratory and polyarticular and may coexist with other hypersensitivity reactions, such as erythema nodosum, pleuritis, or pericarditis.[69] Disseminated disease rarely results in more serious articular involvement, which is associated with immunocompromise. *Histoplasma* arthritis manifests as a monoarthritis, typically of the knee. Tenosynovitis involving the flexor tendon sheaths of the hand has been reported. Radiologically, destructive joint lesions, erosions, sclerosis, and joint space narrowing may be present. Diagnosis depends on detection of fungal organisms or on serology. Treatment is with antifungals, with or without débridement.[57]

Sporotrichosis

Infection with *S. schenckii* occurs after cutaneous inoculation or, less commonly, after inhalation of spores. Dissemination develops infrequently but may involve any organ system. The arthritis is chronic and can be monoarticular or polyarticular; it primarily involves the knee or, less often, the wrist or joints of the hands and feet.[57] Symptoms are chronic, with an insidious onset. The diagnosis is often delayed, sometimes up to several years from symptom onset, and requires culture of synovial fluid or tissue. Radiographic findings include joint space narrowing, effusions, periarticular erosions, soft tissue swelling, and periarticular osteopenia.[55] Treatment is with intravenous or intra-articular antifungal agents. Synovectomy may also be effective.

Aspergillosis

Aspergillus fumigatus and *Aspergillus flavus* are the most frequently identified *Aspergillus* species in human infection. *Aspergillus* infection in an immunosuppressed host very rarely causes arthritis and is usually associated with adjacent osteomyelitis. *Aspergillus* arthritis manifests with fever, chills, or malaise, as well as pain, swelling, and tenderness of the affected joint. A synovial effusion is present, and there is a restricted range of motion. On imaging, soft tissue swelling and osteomyelitis may be present. Diagnosis requires isolation of fungus from tissue or synovial fluid. Treatment requires both débridement and intravenous antifungal agents.[57]

Mycetoma

Pseudallescheria boydii is a saprophyte found in soil, polluted water, and sewage. Although infection may result in a wide variety of clinical manifestations, mycetoma is by far the most common. The infection typically is seen in men living in rural areas who have a prior history of local trauma. *Ascheria boydii* infection manifests with a monoarticular arthritis, usually involving the knee, with joint pain, swelling, and restricted range of motion. Arthritis develops within days to 1 year after trauma. Imaging findings consist of osteopenia, soft tissue swelling, and lytic lesions of the articular surface. Treatment involves surgery and intra-articular antifungal agents.[57]

Viral Arthritis

A wide range of viral infections can lead to reactive arthritis and subsequent rheumatic syndromes. Acute or chronic persistent viral infection can lead to direct tissue damage as a result of inflammation or the immune response. The immune response to viral infection is complicated by homology between viral and host antigen epitopes, which leads to induction of autoantibodies,[70] many of which have been implicated in rheumatologic disorders. Viral infection may result in the formation of antinuclear antibodies (ANA), rheumatoid factor, antibodies to cardiolipin, double-stranded DNA, SS-A (Ro), SS-B (La), antineutrophil cytoplasmic antibody (ANCA), and cryoglobulin, among others.[71] Viruses may also directly infect synovium and can lead to persistent or recurrent infection.

The radiographic findings of chronic viral arthritis typically resemble those seen in rheumatoid arthritis, with bony erosions and cartilage destruction. Synovitis may be seen on MRI.

Histologically, viral infection causes a nonspecific synovitis or tenosynovitis. Biopsy is rarely performed, because the diagnosis usually can be made on the basis of clinical presentation and serology.

Treatment is usually symptomatic.

Parvovirus B19

Parvovirus B19 is a member of the non-enveloped, single-stranded Parvoviridae family of DNA viruses, which was first identified in 1975 as the cause of erythema infectiosum, or fifth disease, in children. It may also lead to nonspecific fever or, more seriously, arthritis, vasculitis, Still disease, SLE-like disorders, or aplastic crisis. Articular symptoms, usually arthralgias or joint swelling, affect 8% of infected children.[71,72] In adults, rash is rare, and B19 infection manifests with acute onset of symmetric polyarticular arthralgia or arthritis.[72] Joint involvement can mimic rheumatoid arthritis, and patients may suffer from morning stiffness. However, to date, studies have been contradictory as to the role of B19 in the etiology of rheumatoid arthritis.[71] Joints are tender and swollen and may be erythematous.[73] In immunocompetent patients, arthritis resolves with no permanent swelling or functional limitation. Immunocompromised patients may fail to clear an acute infection, and persistent infection may develop. B19 may be associated with presence of rheumatoid factor, ANA, anti-DNA antibodies, anti-lymphocyte antibodies, and antiphospholipid antibodies.[73] Diagnosis is by serology.

B19 may persist in synovium, as well as in other tissues, but persistent B19 infection alone is insufficient to cause arthritis, and the pathophysiology of chronic B19 arthritis is not well understood.

Treatment is usually symptomatic, although intravenous immunoglobulin therapy may be necessary to clear the virus in immunosuppressed patients. Nonsteroidal anti-inflammatory drugs (NSAIDs) and supportive care with appropriate pain control are sufficient for management of chronic B19 arthritis.

Rubella

Rubella virus is a member of the Togaviridae family of enveloped, positive-sense, single-stranded RNA viruses.[74] Rubella typically infects young adults, who present with suboccipital lymphadenopathy and a maculopapular rash that begins on the face and spreads to the torso and extremities. Constitutional symptoms may be present.[72] Rubella may lead to arthritis or arthralgia in 30% of infected adults and is more common in women. Of note, vaccination against rubella has demonstrated an association with acute arthropathy and arthritis similar to that seen in rubella virus infection.[71] Rubella arthritis is symmetric and occurs in a rheumatoid arthritis–like pattern, although it may be migratory. Metacarpophalangeal and proximal interphalangeal joints are frequently affected, as are knees, wrists, ankles, and elbows. Periarthritis, tenosynovitis, and carpal tunnel syndrome may occur.[75] The arthritis usually resolves within 2 weeks, but in some cases it persists for years.[72]

Diagnosis relies on serology for antirubella seroconversion. Treatment is supportive, with NSAIDs. Steroids may also be used for symptom control.

Hepatitis C

Hepatitis C virus (HCV) is an enveloped, single-stranded RNA flavivirus that infects approximately 3% of the world's population.[76] HCV is a leading cause of chronic liver disease and is associated with numerous extrahepatic disorders, including cryoglobulinemia, as well as arthritis in a small percentage of patients. The exact pathophysiology of HCV arthritis is unclear, but several theories have been proposed, including the hypotheses that HCV initiates or exacerbates an inflammatory arthritis and that HCV directly causes a distinct arthritis syndrome of its own.[72] HCV-associated joint disease manifests as a monoarticular or oligoarticular arthritis and tenosynovitis. Radiographically, erosions are absent and the arthritis is nonprogressive.[77] Aggressive antiviral therapy may be attempted, but underlying rheumatologic disorders should also be ruled out or treated appropriately.

Hepatitis B

Hepatitis B (HBV), a member of the Hepadnaviridae family, is an enveloped, partially double-stranded DNA virus that affects approximately 30% of the world's population.[78] Infection is usually self-limited but may become chronic in 5% to 10% of patients. HBV is not associated with chronic arthritis, but acute HBV infection can cause rapid onset of a polyarticular arthritis mimicking rheumatoid arthritis.[72] The arthritis resolves with the onset of jaundice. Only supportive care is indicated.

Human Immunodeficiency Virus

HIV is now a worldwide pandemic, with more than 30 million infected individuals.[79] HIV is a risk factor for the development of septic arthritis and has been associated with articular symptoms including arthralgia, spondyloarthropathy, reactive arthritis, and avascular necrosis. Arthritis may occur at any stage in HIV infection but is more prevalent later in the course of disease. The pathogenesis of HIV-associated arthritis is not well understood, but direct invasion of synovium by the virus, the host immune response, and genetic factors are all thought to play a role. Patients with HIV-associated arthritis are usually adult, although children may also be affected. There is a male predominance.[80,81]

HIV-associated arthritis in children is frequently polyarticular (40%), although spondyloarthropathy-like symptoms and oligoarthritis have been documented in 34% and 26% of cases. Systemic symptoms including fever, lymphadenopathy, hepatomegaly, and rash may be present.[81] In adults, HIV can cause nonspecific intermittent arthralgias or arthritis,[82] which are likely to be oligoarticular (47%) or monoarticular (38%).[83] Reactive arthritis may also occur, typically accompanied by extra-articular features such as urethritis or skin lesions.[82] The knee is most commonly involved, followed by ankles, wrists, and small joints of the hands and feet.[84] Enthesial involvement may occur, usually in the Achilles tendon, plantar fascia, tibial tendons, or extensor tendons.[84] Erosive changes are not seen.

Histologically, there may be nonspecific chronic inflammation of synovium.[81] HIV may be isolated from synovial fluid,[85] and HIV p24 antigen may be detected within synovial cells and in synovial histiocytes.[86] HIV-associated arthritis usually resolves within 1 year. In a minority of cases, it may persist or recur.

Approximately 1% of HIV-infected patients develop septic arthritis, with *S. aureus* as the number one pathogen. Atypical mycobacterial or fungal infections may also occur.

Alphavirus

Alphaviruses belong to the Togaviridae family and include a number of mosquito-borne entities. O'nyong-nyong is a disease that originated in Uganda and is characterized by fever, rash, and arthritis. Ross River virus is a source of epidemic polyarthritis in Australia and the South Pacific. The virus attacks the knees and the small joints of the hands and feet. Systemic systems including fever and rash may be present. Barmah Forest virus is found only in Australia and may cause a polyarthritis similar to that of Ross River virus. Pogosta disease occurs in epidemics every 7 years and causes joint symptoms in 93% of patients, with polyarthritis in 40%. Kokobera virus, Alfuy virus, Edge Hill virus, Kunjin virus, Stratford virus, dengue and Gan Gan virus also may be associated with arthritis.[71,72] Alphaviral arthritis usually resolves within weeks, but severe cases may be symptomatic for month to years. Treatment is supportive with NSAIDs, although aspirin is contraindicated.

Reactive Arthritis

In addition to septic arthritis, bacterial infection may result in a postinfectious reactive arthritis. The prototype for this manifestation of disease is post-streptococcal reactive arthritis, which is part of a spectrum of reactive syndromes that includes acute rheumatic fever. Reactive arthritis occurs as a result of the formation of antibodies against bacterial or viral antigens, which then cross-react with synovial antigens, leading to the deposition of immune complex in the synovium. Immune complex deposition stimulates a local inflammatory reaction that may damage tissue through release of inflammatory cytokines, cytolytic enzymes, and reactive oxygen species. Host genetic factors are important, and reactive arthritis has been linked to MHC class II HLA-DRβ1*16 and β1*01. Bacteria known to be associated with reactive arthritis include *N. meningitidis, Salmonella, Shigella, Yersinia enterocolitica,* and *Campylobacter jejuni.*[87] Rare parasitic infections, such as with the helminth *Strongyloides stercoralis,* may also result in a reactive arthritis syndrome.[88]

Acute Rheumatic Fever

Formerly one of the most common vascular diseases of children, acute rheumatic fever has waned in importance in developed countries over the last 60 years. The disease is exemplified by arthritis, carditis, Sydenham chorea, and skin manifestations such as erythema marginatum and subcutaneous nodules. Acute rheumatic fever arises after an untreated infection with group A streptococci in genetically susceptible individuals; it has been linked to the HLA-DRβ1*16 allele.[89] In this syndrome, arthritis develops approximately 3 weeks after streptococcal infection. Immune response to bacterial antigens is thought to result in formation of cross-reactive antibodies or cell-mediated processes that recognize human antigens within affected tissue, leading to tissue damage. Arthritis may, on occasion, be the single major manifestation of acute rheumatic fever. Large joints are involved by an asymmetric migrating polyarthritis; the axial skeleton is rarely affected. Pain in a joint may resolve within 24 hours, only to be followed by arthritis in a different joint.[87] Some patients experience only mild arthralgias. Articular symptoms typically resolve within a few weeks, without permanent sequelae. Treatment with aspirin leads to complete resolution of joint pain.

Post-Streptococcal Reactive Arthritis

The symptoms of post-streptococcal reactive arthritis occur acutely, within a few days to 2 weeks after streptococcal infection. Fever and rash may be present during the initial infection, but they disappear with the onset of arthritis. In contrast to acute rheumatic fever, post-streptococcal arthritis is nonmigratory, is associated with morning stiffness, and may affect both large and small joints. Knees, ankles, wrists, and interphalangeal joints are frequent sites of involvement. The axial skeleton is affected in up to 20% of cases. The clinical course is chronic, and symptoms may persist for up to 8 months.[89] Post-streptococcal arthritis responds poorly to treatment with NSAIDs.

Soft Tissue Infections

Soft tissue infections are a common problem after local trauma or systemic infection. Superficial infections of the skin, such as impetigo or folliculitis, may develop into cellulitis with local spread or may hematogenously seed distant tissue. More severe infections, including necrotizing fasciitis, gas gangrene, or myositis, may occur in the setting of severe trauma, immunocompromise, vascular insufficiency, or prior infection (Table 14-3). In

Table 14-3 Bacterial Soft Tissue Infections

Infection	Site	Type	Organism	Treatment
Cellulitis	Extremities	Monomicrobial	*Staphylococcus aureus*	Antibiotics
Necrotizing fasciitis	Extremities, abdomen	Polymicrobial	*Streptococcus, Bacteroides,* enteric species	Débridement, antibiotics
Gas gangrene	Extremities	Monomicrobial or polymicrobial	*Clostridium,* anaerobes	Débridement, antibiotics, hyperbaric oxygen
Pyomyositis	Lower extremities	Monomicrobial	*S. aureus*	Drainage, antibiotics
Psoas abscess	Psoas muscle	Monomicrobial or polymicrobial	*S. aureus, Mycobacterium tuberculosus,* enteric species	Drainage, antibiotics
Necrotizing myositis	Extremities	Monomicrobial or polymicrobial	*Streptococcus, Peptostreptococcus*	Débridement, antibiotics

many parts of the world, parasitic soft tissue infections continue to pose a significant health problem, resulting in myositis, lymphadenitis, and lymphedema, among other conditions. Less commonly, fungi may also contribute to soft tissue infections, especially in the setting of immunocompromise (e.g., HIV infection).

Necrotizing Soft Tissue Infections

Necrotizing soft tissue infection (fasciitis) is a serious but uncommon, rapidly progressive bacterial infection involving dermis, subcutaneous tissue, fascia, or muscle. Historically, necrotizing lesions of the soft tissue have been subclassified into entities such as streptococcal gangrene, Fournier gangrene, Meleney bacterial synergistic gangrene, necrotizing fasciitis, and clostridial cellulitis. However, the initial diagnosis and management of each entity is identical, and subclassification is best left until after identification of the causative organism or organisms. Characteristic of this disease is its rapid spread along fascial planes, frequently with only minimal involvement of adjacent tissues such as muscle or subcutaneous fat. Accordingly, necrotizing soft tissue infections cause significant morbidity and are associated with a relatively high mortality rate, ranging between 20% and 28%.[90-92] Speedy diagnosis and treatment are essential to avoid serious complications.

Infection commonly develops from a cutaneous lesion and usually originates in the extremities or perineum (Fournier gangrene), although any site may be affected. The primary risk factors are immunocompromise, smoking, diabetes mellitus, intravenous drug use, and vascular insufficiency, as well as older age and chronic renal insufficiency.[90,93] Trauma, burns, dermal abscess, or recent surgery may be antecedent events.[93,94] Risk factors for death include age older than 60 years, female gender, delay in diagnosis or débridement, extent of tissue involvement, degree of organ system dysfunction, and other medical comorbidities. In addition, infections in the perineum and those associated with burn wounds or perforated bowel are all linked to higher mortality. Myonecrosis is not linked to increased mortality.[90]

Most cases of necrotizing infection are polymicrobial, with as many as six pathogens being present simultaneously. Only 30% are monomicrobial, with group A β-hemolytic streptococci the

Table 14-4 Causative Organisms in Necrotizing Soft Tissue Infections

Pathogen Group	% of Cases
Bacteroides	40-50
Streptococcus	40-50
Enterococcus	30-40
Peptostreptococcus	30-35
Staphylococcus	30-40
Escherichia coli	30-35
Proteus	20-25
Gram-negative rods	40-45
Clostridium	20-25
Other anaerobes	20
Fungal	5

Data from Edlich RF, et al: Modern concepts of the diagnosis and treatment of necrotizing fasciitis. J Emerg Med 2008 Dec 10 (Epub ahead of print).

most common culprit.[93] Most polymicrobial necrotizing infections involve a mixed population of aerobes and anaerobes. Other common organisms involved in monomicrobial and polymicrobial infections are *Bacteroides* species, staphylococci, enterococci, *E. coli*, *Proteus* species, *Peptostreptococcus*, *Clostridium perfringens*, *Fusobacterium*, and *Prevotella* species, as well as fungi and other aerobic and anaerobic organisms (Table 14-4).[90,95] Pure clostridial myonecrosis (gas gangrene) is rare and highly lethal.

Clinically, necrotizing fasciitis is divided into three subtypes based on the microorganisms involved. Type 1 is a polymicrobial infection that usually affects diabetic patients or those with peripheral vascular disease. It occurs after operations for abdominal or perineal infectious disease and is caused by non–group A streptococci in combination with anaerobes or facultative anaerobes. Enterobacteriaceae may also be involved. Type 2 infection usually arises in the extremities and involves group A β-hemolytic streptococci, such as *S. pyogenes*, with or without staphylococcal involvement.[96] Infection with methicillin-resistant *S. aureus* in type 2 necrotizing fasciitis is becoming an increasingly serious problem. Type 3 necrotizing fasciitis is caused by marine *Vibrio* species such as *Vibrio vulnificus* or *Vibrio parahaemolyticus* and often is the result of a puncture injury.[97]

The pathogenesis of necrotizing soft tissue infection is hypothesized to be related to the relative paucity of blood supply to the fascia. Local toxin-induced thrombosis is believed to induce fascial ischemia,[93] while other bacterial toxins, such as hyaluronidase, contribute to tissue breakdown.[98] The host inflammatory response causes extravasation of fluid that becomes entrapped between the layers of infected fascia and adjacent tissues. This undermines the effectiveness of the immune response by impeding phagocytosis. Together, inadequate perfusion and ineffective phagocytic clearance of damaged tissue and microorganisms produce an ideal milieu for pathogen proliferation. The polymicrobial nature of the necrotizing infection is also thought to play an important role, because there is a synergistic interaction among certain bacterial species, such as β-hemolytic streptococci and *S. aureus*.[93]

The clinical manifestations vary with the stage of disease. Initially, patients typically present with high fever, tachycardia, erythema and swelling of involved skin, and pain out of proportion to physical findings. As the infection progresses, skin lesions evolve into a reticulated pattern of purpura, with anesthesia over the affected area. Eventually, blistering, cutaneous hemorrhage with purpuric bullae, or gross necrosis may develop.[94] Crepitus may be apparent on palpation. As the region of local spread expands, bacteria invade the local vasculature, leading to bacteremia. As a result of hematologic spread of infection, there is an accompanying increase in the severity of systemic symptoms, with a markedly elevated WBC count, signs of sepsis, and, eventually, septic shock leading to multiorgan failure.[93] Disease progression can be extremely rapid, with death ensuing mere days after presentation.

MRI findings include irregular, hyperintense fascial signals on T2-weighted scans of affected areas, although there is some debate as to the specificity of this finding (Fig. 14-12).[98] CT, MRI, and ultrasonography are helpful in detecting fluid accumulations along fascial planes and tissue edema in soft tissue around the fascia (Fig. 14-13). However, it is important to note that the presence of edema and fluid are not specific for necrotizing infections.[92,98]

Grossly, incision of the infected area in necrotizing fasciitis yields a murky, "dishwater" exudative fluid. Diseased tissue is discolored gray-white to yellow. Fascia may be easily separated from subcutaneous tissues using only a finger, whereas in healthy tissue, fascia tightly adheres to adjacent tissues.[93,99,100]

In the early stages of necrotizing fasciitis, histopathologic examination of infected tissue demonstrates edema of the subcutaneous soft tissue and superficial fascia, with obliterative vasculitis and thrombosis of the dermal vasculature with scattered neutrophils (Fig. 14-14). The overlying skin may appear uninvolved, although it is invariably affected by progressive necrosis. As the lesions progress, liquefactive necrosis of surrounding fascia and subcutaneous tissue develops, and acute neutrophilic inflammation and hemorrhage extends into the dermis (Fig. 14-15). Accompanying the neutrophils are T lymphocytes, macrophages, and monocytes.[101] Full-thickness necrosis may extend from the skin surface to the superficial fascia. Infection may then rapidly

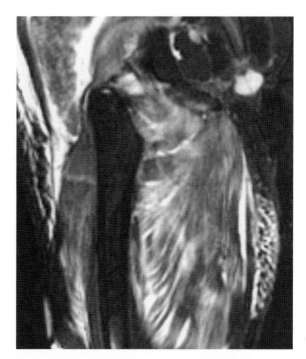

Figure 14-12. Necrotizing fasciitis. Coronal T2-weighted magnetic resonance image of thigh shows diffuse edema within all compartments of the right upper thigh, hyperintense deep fascia, and focal stranding of the subcutaneous fat.

Table 14-5 Histopathologic Findings in Necrotizing Fasciitis

Variegated appearance at low power
Dermal edema and necrosis
Fascial necrosis and interstitial fibrin deposition
Lobular panniculitis
Sparing of deep striated muscle
Neutrophils
Macrophages and lymphocytes
Vascular thrombi

spread along the horizontal plane of the superficial fascia, undermining normal-appearing skin.[98] The thick fascia of the underlying muscle may be spared until late in the course of infection, when a vertical infectious phase may develop (Fig. 14-16).[93]

Necrotizing fasciitis may be diagnosed on frozen section using criteria developed by Stamenkovic and Lew (Table 14-5).[102] According to this diagnostic scheme, infected tissue is characterized by a marked neutrophilic infiltrate of the fascia, with accompanying liquefactive necrosis, and fat necrosis. Thrombosis and obliterative vasculitis with fibrinous necrosis of vessel walls is present. Abundant bacterial forms are seen within the necrotic tissue.[102]

Treatment of all necrotizing soft tissue infections requires early diagnosis, aggressive surgical débridement, and widespectrum antibiotic therapy. Hyperbaric oxygen therapy has also been shown to be beneficial in accelerating wound closure and reducing mortality in some studies,[90] although its use remains

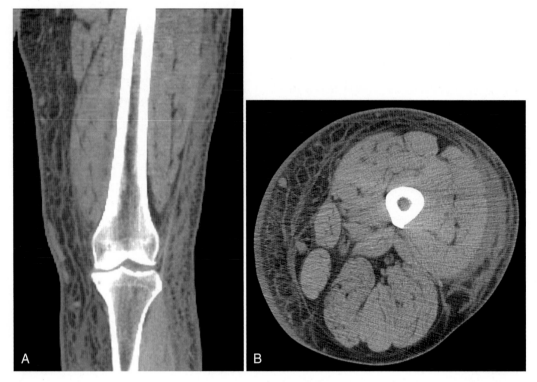

Figure 14-13. Necrotizing fasciitis. **A,** Coronal computed tomogram demonstrates extensive stranding of the subcutaneous tissues of much of the leg. **B,** Axial CT scan shows that the stranding is almost circumferential around the thigh.

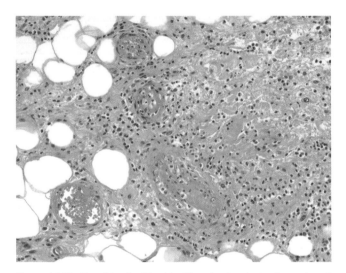

Figure 14-14. Necrotizing fasciitis with obliterative thrombosis of several small vessels. Focal fibrinoid necrosis is present with surrounding neutrophilic infiltrate.

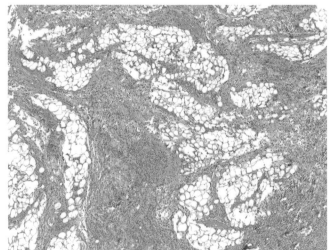

Figure 14-15. Necrotizing fasciitis with extensive necrosis of the subcutaneous adipose tissues, which contain a dense neutrophilic infiltrate dissecting between the septa.

controversial in non-clostridial infections.[103] Repeated débridement or amputation is often necessary to halt disease progression. Patients are frequently in critically unstable condition due to sepsis and must be managed in the intensive care unit with hemodynamic, respiratory, and nutritional support as required. Delay in diagnosis or treatment may result in serious morbidity or death.

Care must be taken to exclude mimickers of necrotizing fasciitis, such as acute necrotizing neutrophilic dermatosis (ANND), a recently described variant of Sweet syndrome arising in conjunction with hematologic malignancy or granulocyte-macrophage colony-stimulating factor (GM-CSF) therapy (Fig. 14-17). This entity should be suspected, in the appropriate clinical setting, if necrotic lesions fail to respond to débridement and antibiotic therapy and no organisms can be isolated from the suspected site of infection. Unlike necrotizing fasciitis, ANND rapidly resolves with corticosteroid therapy, and débridement is not necessary.[104]

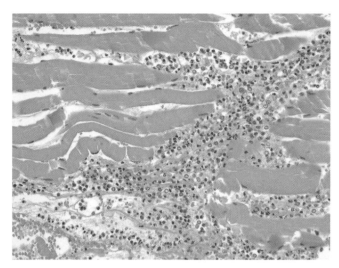

Figure 14-16. Necrotizing fasciitis extending into edematous and viable skeletal muscle. Numerous neutrophils and macrophages infiltrate between individual myofibers.

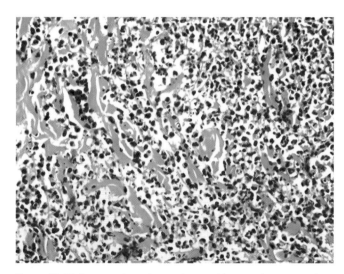

Figure 14-17. Sweet syndrome in a patient receiving granulocyte-macrophage colony-stimulating factor (GM-CSF) therapy. The microscopic appearance suggests an acute pyogenic infection with large numbers of infiltrating neutrophils, but no organisms were isolated, and findings resolved with corticosteroids.

Gas Gangrene

Clostridial myonecrosis (gas gangrene) is a type of rapidly progressive necrotizing soft tissue infection caused by *Clostridium* species; *C. perfringens*, *Clostridium septicum*, *Clostridium histolyticum*, and *Clostridium novyi* have all been identified as causative agents. The primary risk factor is severe penetrating trauma or crush injury with disruption of blood flow, because low oxygen concentration is required for clostridial infection to produce the toxins that lead to tissue damage and systemic symptoms.[94] *C. perfringens* is the most frequent pathogen in this setting. Infections have also been reported at sites of injection in intravenous drug users and secondary to malignancy or colonic perforation.[94] Presence of a foreign body has also been identified as a risk factor.[105]

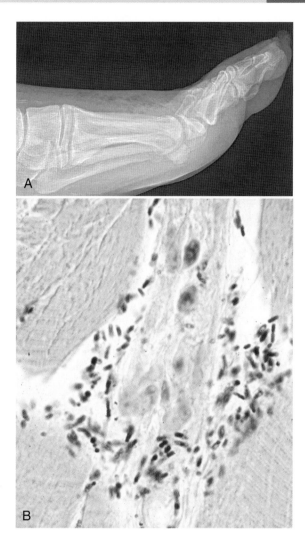

Figure 14-18. A, Subcutaneous gas is present in the dorsal soft tissue on lateral radiograph of the foot in a patient with diabetes. **B,** Tissue Gram stain shows numerous gram-positive bacilli infiltrating muscle, with pauci-inflammatory response. Cultures were positive for *Clostridium* spp.

Gas gangrene not related to trauma is most commonly caused by *C. septicum* and is associated with neutropenia and gastrointestinal malignancy.[94] Infection is usually a result of hematogenous spread, and the lesion may rapidly progress.

Cutaneous findings are the same as in other necrotizing soft tissue infections, with purpuric bullae, skin sloughing, edema, and systemic symptoms of fever, chills, tachycardia, or hypotension. Necrosis of skin, subcutaneous tissue, and muscle is often present. The palpation of gas in the infected tissues is a classic finding on physical examination and imaging studies; however, the diagnosis may be made even in the absence of this finding.[105] Radiographically, gas is seen in the soft tissue, together with edema and fluid collection along fascial planes. On histologic examination, large numbers of bacilli may be seen percolating through the interstices of the skeletal muscle, evoking a pauci-inflammatory response (Fig. 14-18).

Early recognition and extensive débridement and fasciotomy with appropriate wide-spectrum antibiotic therapy are critical. Hyperbaric oxygen therapy may be used as adjunctive treatment. Prognosis is poor, with a mortality rate approaching 25%[106] and significant morbidity in survivors due to extensive tissue destruction.

Non-Necrotizing Cellulitis

The term *non-necrotizing cellulitis* refers to diffuse, spreading skin infections that are not associated with underlying abscess or necrotizing processes such as osteomyelitis or septic arthritis.[94] Classically, non-necrotizing cellulitis has been divided into two overlapping entities: erysipelas and cellulitis. Erysipelas is characterized by lesions that are elevated above the surrounding normal skin and show a clear line of demarcation between involved and uninvolved tissue.[92] In contrast, cellulitis is a deeper infection involving the dermis and subcutaneous tissue. In practice, however, it may be difficult to distinguish between the two, and some clinicians use the term *erysipelas* to refer to both lesions.[94]

Non-necrotizing cellulitis without an associated portal skin lesion is usually caused by group A β-hemolytic streptococci or other streptococcal species,[94] although other causative species, such as *H. influenzae*, pneumococcus, and *S. aureus*, have also been reported. Risk factors are associated with breaches in skin integrity and include ulcers, fungal infections, and inflammatory dermatoses, as well as alterations in vascularity or lymphatic drainage (e.g., prior surgery, lymph node dissection, venous insufficiency). Immunocompromise is another significant risk factor.[92] Erysipelas is more commonly seen in infants, young children, or older adults.[94]

Both erysipelas and cellulitis manifest with rapidly spreading areas of edema, erythema, and heat. Lymphadenitis may be present,[92] and regional lymph nodes may be enlarged. Superficial skin edema may result in a peau d'orange appearance. Vesicles, bullae, and petechiae or ecchymoses may eventually form.[94] Systemic manifestations include fever, tachycardia, hypotension, and leukocytosis. Signs of severe toxicity with widespread cutaneous lesions should raise suspicion for a more severe underlying process, such as necrotizing fasciitis.

Histopathologic changes in cellulitis are notable for edema of subcutaneous fat and a mixed inflammatory infiltrate, including a preponderance of neutrophils. The vasculature within adipose tissue may be dilated and may contain focal thrombi.[100]

Diagnosis is usually based on clinical symptoms; blood cultures are rarely positive. Care must be taken to exclude a necrotizing process or more serious condition. The differential diagnosis includes acute dermatitis, gout, herpes zoster, and acute lipodermatosclerosis.[94] Treatment is antibiotic therapy based on empirical diagnosis. Any underlying disorder or chronic skin condition that may have contributed to infection should also be treated.

Myositis

Bacterial infections of the muscle are uncommon and may result from penetrating trauma, contiguous spread from an adjacent site of infection, vascular insufficiency, or hematogenous spread.[105] The causative organisms are related to the mechanism of infection. Trauma most commonly results in a polymicrobial infection, whereas myositis secondary to hematogenous infection usually is due to *S. aureus*.

Pyomyositis

Pyomyositis, also known as pyogenic myositis, suppurative myositis, tropical myositis, temperate myositis, myositis purulenta tropica, or epidemic abscess, is a rare and frequently misdiagnosed infection of skeletal muscle. It is often mistaken for a variety of other conditions including thrombophlebitis, osteomyelitis, malignancy, hematoma, and muscle strain. Severe complications such as compartment syndrome, osteomyelitis, sepsis, or death may occur if diagnosis and treatment are delayed.[99] The lower limbs and pelvic girdle muscles are most frequently affected, and the quadriceps is the most commonly involved muscle, followed by the gluteal and iliopsoas muscles, although any muscle may be affected.[99] Most cases involve only one site; however, multisite infection is present in 16%.[107]

Pyomyositis most often occurs as a result of hematogenous spread.[105] Although the exact pathophysiology of disease is unknown, infection is thought to develop secondary to skin compromise and the resultant bacteremia in the setting of muscle injury. Risk factors consist of infections, chronic inflammatory skin disease, local injections, and immunocompromised condition (e.g., HIV infection, diabetes).[94,105] In tropical areas, any age group may be affected, although the disease is more prevalent in children and immunocompetent adults. In contrast, in temperate regions, pyomyositis affects younger adults and immunocompromised patients. Men are more frequently affected than women and often have a history of local trauma. *S. aureus* is identified in 90% of cases; streptococci, *H. influenzae, Aeromonas hydrophila, Fusobacterium, Bartonella, Klebsiella pneumoniae*, other gram-negatives, and anaerobes, as well as fungi and mycobacterial species, are reported less frequently.[99,105]

In the initial stages, pyomyositis manifests with fever, anorexia, and nonspecific local symptoms such as muscle cramps and swelling. There may be restricted range of motion and pain on weight bearing. In the second, suppurative phase, patients develop high fever and chills along with muscle swelling, pain, and fluctuance of the affected region due to abscess formation. Erythema may be absent. Without treatment, patients eventually become septic.[99]

Radiographic findings in early stages of pyomyositis are nonspecific. Ultrasonography demonstrates hyperechogenicity caused by muscle swelling and edema, intermixed with areas of hypoechogenicity reflecting muscle necrosis.[108] CT imaging demonstrates muscle swelling and fluid attenuation, with ring enhancement in areas of abscess formation.[109] MRI is the most sensitive imaging modality and is useful for defining the extent of disease and tissue damage.[99]

Diagnosis requires Gram staining and culture of infected tissue or aspirated fluid. Histologically, pyomyositis is defined by the presence of pus within individual muscle groups. Examination of affected tissue reveals muscle edema with separation of myofibers, along with a lymphocytic and plasmacytic inflammatory infiltrate. Muscle necrosis with disintegration of myofibers is present.[94,110]

Treatment requires appropriate antibiotic coverage. If abscess is present, drainage must be performed. The prognosis is generally good, and the mortality rate is usually less than 4%. Most patients experience a complete recovery, although recurrence may occur in immunocompromised patients.[105]

Psoas Abscess

A psoas abscess is an uncommon variant of pyomyositis in which a purulent infection affects the psoas muscle. Infection is normally unilateral and usually arises by hematogenous spread or by contiguous spread from local infection. Primary abscess arising from hematogenous spread is commonly caused by occult *S. aureus* bacteremia and usually is associated with intravenous drug use or immunocompromise. Other pathogens, including *S. pneumoniae, Streptococcus milleri,* group A streptococci, *E. coli, Pseudomonas, Haemophilus, Proteus,* and *Pasteurella* species, have been reported. Historically, secondary psoas abscess was most often due to *Mycobacterium tuberculosis* infection occurring after Pott's disease, with local spread from adjacent involved vertebral bodies, or, less frequently, after bloodborne infection (Fig. 14-19).[105] In recent decades, with the decline in tuberculosis in the developed world, there has been a shift to psoas abscess arising from genitourinary or gastrointestinal infections, especially in immunocompromised patients. Any age group may be affected, and there is no gender bias. Secondary psoas abscesses arising from intra-abdominal infection are more likely to be polymicrobial and to involve enteric species such as *E. coli, Enterobacter, Salmonella,* and *Klebsiella,* as well as anaerobic species. Psoas abscess arising from adjacent osteomyelitis may involve *Salmonella, Brucella, Nocardia,* or fungi such as *B. dermatitidis* or *C. immitis.*[105]

Clinically, patients may present with fever or other systemic symptoms such as malaise, anorexia, or weight loss. Pain and limp are only occasionally present, and the pain may involve the back or flank. A mass or fullness may be apparent in the groin. Immunocompromised patients may be afebrile with minimal symptoms.

Blood cultures may be positive, and cultures of abscess fluid should be performed. Imaging is the gold standard for detection of psoas infection. CT and MRI are the preferred modalities and clearly demonstrate the abscess. Ultrasonography is less effective. Treatment involves drainage and intravenous antibiotics. Adjacent or concomitant infection elsewhere in the body should be identified and treated appropriately with débridement, resection, or antibiotics as indicated. The prognosis is often good, especially in primary or early disease. Secondary psoas abscess has a less favorable outcome depending on the type and extent of adjacent infections.

Bacterial Myositis

Bacterial myositis is a diffuse muscle infection without abscess formation. It occurs less frequently than pyomyositis and tends to be seen more often in adults rather than children. *Streptococcus* is the primary pathogen, although many other organisms have been reported. If *Staphylococcus* is involved, infection may rarely result in diffuse myositis with rhabdomyolysis.[105]

Group A streptococci may cause a spectrum of muscle infection, ranging from pyomyositis to necrotizing myositis, also known as spontaneous streptococcal gangrenous myositis. This disease is rare but very aggressive and often fatal. The portal of disease entry is usually unknown, with no prior trauma or illness. Clinically, streptococcal necrotizing myositis manifests with flu-like symptoms, including rash and myalgia, which progress to severe muscle pain with local swelling and fevers. Overlying skin lesions such as those found in fasciitis are not typically present. Multiple sites may be involved. The course is rapidly progressive and can lead to septic shock within days. Compartment syndrome may occur as a result of rapid muscle swelling.[105]

Histologic examination demonstrates muscle necrosis with abundant streptococcal organisms. Treatment requires repeated débridement and high-dose antibiotics. Fasciotomy may be necessary to prevent compartment syndrome.

Fungal Myositis

Fungal myositis is an uncommon infection predominantly affecting immunocompromised patients. *Candida* species are the most common fungal pathogens reported in myositis, although *C. neoformans, H. capsulatum, Coccidioides, Aspergillus,* and *Pneumocystis jiroveci* have all been reported.[105] Symptoms are similar to those seen in bacterial infection, with fever and muscle tenderness the most frequent presenting symptoms.

Diagnosis is by tissue biopsy and culture. Histologic examination typically reveals diffuse microabscesses or granulomatous inflammation, with rare larger fungal abscesses. Fungal organisms may be identified within tissues (Fig. 14-20). Treatment requires débridement and antifungal therapy. Mortality rates are often high.

Parasitic Soft Tissue Infection

A variety of parasites have been identified in soft tissue infections. Most result in myositis and are only rarely found in subcutaneous

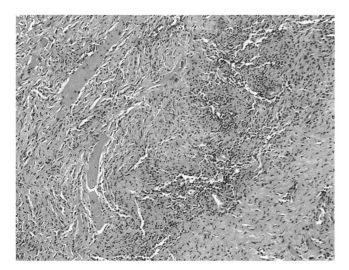

Figure 14-19. Granulomatous inflammation and degenerating skeletal muscle fibers in a patient with soft tissue swelling of the anterior chest wall. Cultures were positive for *Mycobacterium tuberculosis.* No contiguous lesion was present.

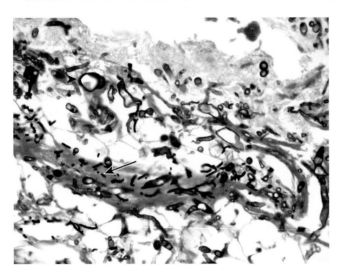

Figure 14-20. Soft tissue infection due to mixed infection by zygomycetes *(arrowhead)* and *Candida* spp. *(arrow)* is demonstrated in a GMS-stained section.

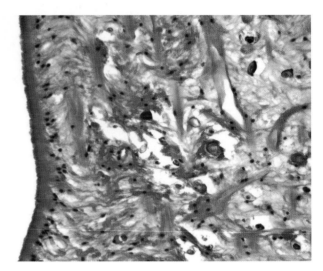

Figure 14-21. This sparganum was removed as a soft tissue tumor in the breast. It shows a tegument with loose internal structure and multiple calcareous bodies that are expressed by cestode larval forms. There is no evidence of a protoscolex.

soft tissues. *Trichinella, Taenia solium* (cysticercosis), and *Toxoplasma gondii* are the most commonly reported causes of parasitic myositis. Many other parasites are less frequently implicated, including *Trypanosoma cruzi, Plasmodium falciparum, Echinococcus, Entamoeba histolytica, Sarcocystis, Microsporidia, Toxocara, Schistosoma,* and *Onchocerca volvulus.*[105] Parasitic soft tissue infections are uncommon in the United States and are usually acquired during travel abroad. Typically, parasitic larvae or ova are ingested, then migrate out of the gastrointestinal tract and into the bloodstream, from whence systemic dissemination occurs. Many parasites display a tropism for certain organs, such as muscle, skin, or the central nervous system. On entry into muscle or soft tissue, organisms usually encyst and remain dormant in preparation for the next stage of their life cycle. Many infections, such as cysticercosis or trichinosis, manifest with subclinical symptoms or as an incidental finding. When present, symptoms usually result from an inflammatory response to waste or shed material from parasites, or to dead and degenerating organisms, and only rarely from direct tissue damage caused by migrating parasites.[105,111]

Patients with symptomatic parasitic infection of muscle present with myalgias, muscle swelling, and weakness.[105] Some parasites, such as *Toxoplasma* or filarial worms, display a tropism for lymphatics and can cause acute or chronic lymphadenitis. Chronic lymphadenitis in filarial infection may result in lymphedema and eventual elephantiasis.

Radiographs may demonstrate calcified, encysted organisms within affected tissue. Cysticerci, for example, are often found incidentally as 5- to 7-μm, spindle-shaped, calcified cysts within infected tissue.[112] Other aberrantly migrating cestode larvae, including spargana and coenuri, also cause disease. The sparganum (Fig. 14-21) is distinguished by the absence of protoscolices, although so-called racemose cysticerci also lack protoscolices. Inflammatory reactions with prominent eosinophils may be present.

Viral Myositis

A number of viruses have been implicated in myalgia, myositis, or viral-associated rhabdomyolysis. In the United States, influenza A and B are most frequently reported; other responsible pathogens include enterovirus, human T-cell lymphoma virus, HBV, and HCV. However, a wide range of other viruses have also been reported as causes of myositis.[105]

Myalgias are a common symptom of influenza infection and may be diffuse and transitory. In contrast, myositis is less common, occurs later in the course of infection, and is characterized by a more focal, sudden onset of severe pain. Myositis in influenza infection tends to affect children but may also be seen in adults. The calf is the most frequent site of involvement. Enterovirus targets costochondral muscles, resulting in severe chest pain. Rhabdomyolysis is a rare complication of infection by influenza viruses, coxsackieviruses, and enteric cytopathologic human orphan (ECHO) viruses, among others.

Muscle biopsy in viral myositis is rarely performed; however, histologic examination of affected muscle demonstrates focal muscle fiber degeneration and necrosis with a mild inflammatory infiltrate. Although viral particles have been isolated from muscle tissue, many studies postulate an immune-mediated etiology for viral myositis. Treatment is symptomatic, and myositis spontaneously resolves within 1 month.

Other Unusual Soft Tissue Infections

Mycetoma

As described in Chapter 13, both bacteria and true fungi can produce localized infections of the soft tissues. The most common soft tissue mycetoma in the United States is caused by *P. boydii,* but a variety of other fungi can yield mycetomas (Fig. 14-22). Tissue Gram and silver stains, such as the Gomori methenamine silver (GMS) stain, are required to identify the cause of the granule, and culture is required for confirmation. These infections are characterized by the presence of exudate granules—proteinaceous structures that can be white, yellow, or black, depending on the nature of the infection. Organisms are present at the core of the "granule," which consists of a cortical

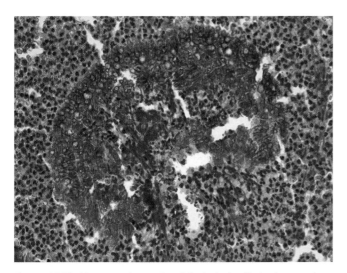

Figure 14-22. Mycetoma due to *Pseudallescheria boydii* showing prominent Splendore-Hoeppli phenomenon. The diagnosis was confirmed by isolation of the fungus in culture.

shell of plasma proteins, the Splendore-Hoeppli phenomenon. Treatment includes surgical excision.

Chromoblastomycosis and Phaeohyphomycosis

Soft tissue infections due to pigmented dematiaceous fungi can be caused by pigmented yeast or hyphal fungi. The subcutaneous infections form fluctuant, painless masses, often in the extremities. The generic diagnosis depends on whether yeast or hyphate fungi are detected. Infection in these cases is often the result of introduction of a foreign body (Fig. 14-23A). In chromoblastomycosis, the pigmented yeast forms show septation (sclerotic bodies or Medlar bodies) (see Fig. 14-23B). The histologic responses are often granulohistiocytic, with microabscess formation. In phaeohyphomycosis, cyst formation is common. Pigmentation of the fungi is generally apparent on hematoxylin and eosin (H&E)–stained sections (see Fig. 14-23C), but a Fontana-Masson stain can be applied if uncertainty persists. Specific identification of the causative fungus requires microbio-

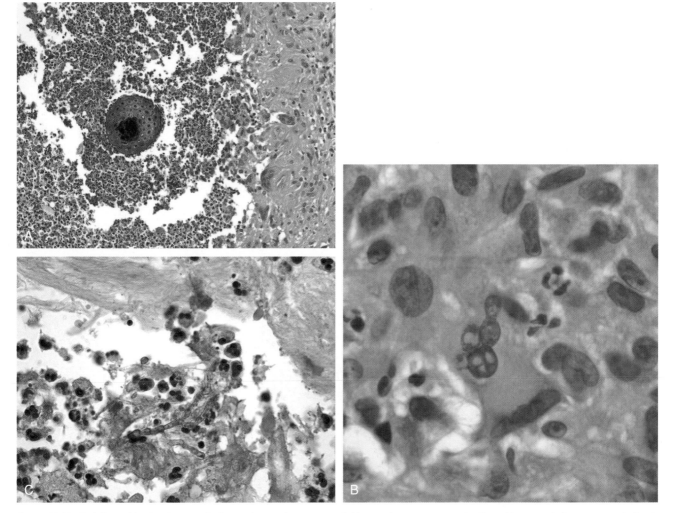

Figure 14-23. A, Splinter with microabscess and adjacent pigmented yeast surrounded by granulomatous response. **B,** Chromoblastomycosis shows a septated sclerotic (Medlar) body. **C,** Phaeohyphomycosis shows pigmented hyphal fungi and microabscess formation. Definitive classification of the offending organisms in these disorders requires fungal culture and isolation.

logic culture, because a large variety of fungi can produce these syndromes.

Protothecosis

This disease is caused by a nonpigmented algae of the genus *Prototheca*. Two members of the species are pathogenic in humans, *Prototheca wickerhamii* (2-12 μm) and *Prototheca zopfii* (10-25 μm). *Prototheca* organisms produce two major syndromes in humans—a cutaneous hyperkeratotic maculopapular eruption and olecranon bursitis—although tenosynovitis at other sites has been reported. The host response to infection includes histiocytic and granulomatous inflammation with fibrinous exudates (Fig. 14-24A). The organisms can be seen in H&E-stained sections and are highlighted to advantage by both PAS and GMS stains (see Fig. 14-24B). The diagnostic morphologic finding is a morula sporangium that includes a central endospore surrounded by multiple encapsulated and molded endospores (see Fig. 14-24C). The diagnostic sporulating forms can be sparse and difficult to identify.

Green algae of the genus *Chlorella* rarely cause soft tissue infections. They are difficult to distinguish from *Prototheca* by light microscopy but characteristically produce green, discolored lesions; contain chloroplasts that can be seen on electron microscopy; and can be specifically identified by immunohistochemical methods.

Surgical Site Infections

Surgical site infections (SSIs) are the most common adverse events occurring after surgical procedures; they account for 38% of nosocomial infections in surgical patients.[113] The frequency of SSI is highly dependent on the type of operation, with high-risk and contaminated surgeries carrying the highest risk. SSIs can be categorized by the depth of involvement.[113]

- Superficial SSIs extend into the subcutaneous space but do not penetrate the underlying muscular fascia. They occur within 1 month after the operation.
- Deep incisional SSI extend into the fascia and muscle and can occur as late as 1 year after the operation. Deep SSI may be associated with prosthetic implants.
- An organ or space SSI may also occur up to 1 year after an operation and involves any organ or space that may have been exposed during surgery.

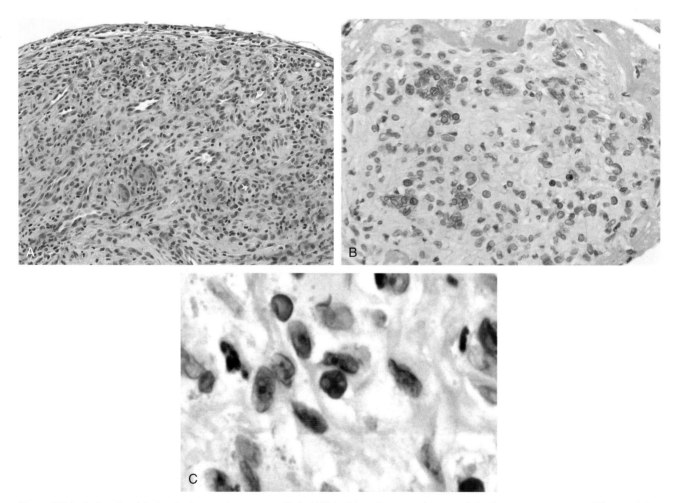

Figure 14-24. A, *Prototheca* infection showing granulomatous synovitis. **B,** Multiple PAS-positive, septated, nonsporulating forms are seen in an area of fibrin exudation. **C,** The diagnostic morula shows a central endospore surrounded by molded and septated spores.

Most SSIs do not develop until at least 5 days after operation, although *S. pyogenes* or clostridial infection may occur within 2 days of surgery. The type of organism found in an incisional SSI tends to depend on the operation: abdominal procedures may lead to SSIs with polymicrobial mixed gram-positive and gram-negative species, whereas extra-abdominal procedures more frequently result in *S. aureus* or streptococcal infection.[94]

Diagnosis of an incisional SSI is usually based on the appearance of the incision. Both superficial and deep SSIs are characterized by purulent incisional drainage, positive culture of wound fluid or tissue, and local pain, tenderness, swelling, and erythema.[94]

Treatment involves opening of the incision, with débridement and drainage of infected material. Antibiotic therapy has not been shown to be of use.[94]

Soft Tissue Infection after Military Trauma

Military trauma resulting from gunshot wounds, shrapnel, burns, blast injuries, or other penetrating or crushing injuries incurs a high risk of infection. Not only are wounds often deeply contaminated with soil and foreign material, but the injury may be extensive and associated with tissue devitalization. This allows microbes to proliferate beyond the bounds of the immune response. The type of organisms responsible for post-traumatic infection largely depends on the site of injury. Abdominal wounds are most frequently infected with enteric gram-negative species, whereas burns and extremity wounds are most likely to be contaminated by *Pseudomonas* or *Klebsiella*.[114] Clostridial infections are now uncommon, primarily because of early surgical débridement and appropriate antibiotic therapy.[114] In many cases, the infections are polymicrobial,[115] and they may include unusual multidrug-resistant organisms such as *Acinetobacter* species.[115-117] *Acinetobacter* infection preferentially affects the extremities and manifests as a well-defined, edematous and erythematous cellulitis arising at the edges of a contaminated wound. As the disease progresses, the skin develops a sandpaper appearance, followed by the development of vesicles that may be hemorrhagic.[117] Bacteremia may ensue, leading to life-threatening sepsis. Treatment requires débridement and intravenous antibiotics. The mortality rate approaches 12%.[117]

REFERENCES

1. O'Connell JX: Pathology of the synovium. Am J Clin Pathol 2000;114:773-784.
2. Kaandorp CJ, et al: Incidence and sources of native and prosthetic joint infection: A community based prospective survey. Ann Rheum Dis 1997;56:470-475.
3. Weston VC, et al: Clinical features and outcome of septic arthritis in a single UK Health District 1982-1991. Ann Rheum Dis 1999;58:214-219.
4. Ross JJ: Septic arthritis. Infect Dis Clin North Am 2005;19:799-817.
5. Shirtliff ME, Mader JT: Acute septic arthritis. Clin Microbiol Rev 2002;15:527-544.
6. Stevens CR, et al: Hypoxia and inflammatory synovitis: Observations and speculation. Ann Rheum Dis 1991;50:124-132.
7. Goergens ED, et al: Acute osteomyelitis and septic arthritis in children. J Paediatr Child Health 2005;41:59-62.
8. Yagupsky P: *Kingella kingae:* From medical rarity to an emerging paediatric pathogen. Lancet Infect Dis 2004;4:358-367.
9. Brook I: Microbiology and management of joint and bone infections due to anaerobic bacteria. J Orthop Sci 2008;13:160-169.
10. Le Dantec L, et al: Peripheral pyogenic arthritis: A study of one hundred seventy-nine cases. Rev Rhum Engl Ed 1996;63:103-110.
11. Marin C, et al: Magnetic resonance imaging of osteoarticular infections in children. Curr Probl Diagn Radiol 2004;33:43-59.
12. Dubost JJ, et al: Polyarticular septic arthritis. Medicine (Baltimore) 1993;72:296-310.
13. Brancos MA, et al: Septic arthritis in heroin addicts. Semin Arthritis Rheum 1991;21:81-87.
14. Goldenberg DL, Cohen AS: Acute infectious arthritis: A review of patients with nongonococcal joint infections (with emphasis on therapy and prognosis). Am J Med 1976;60:369-377.
15. Clement JP 4th, Kassarjian A, Palmer WE: Synovial inflammatory processes in the hand. Eur J Radiol 2005;56:307-318.
16. Karchevsky M, et al: MRI findings of septic arthritis and associated osteomyelitis in adults. AJR Am J Roentgenol 2004;182:119-122.
17. Zieger MM, Dorr U, Schulz RD: Ultrasonography of hip joint effusions. Skeletal Radiol 1987;16:607-611.
18. Bremell T, Abdelnour A, Tarkowski A: Histopathological and serological progression of experimental *Staphylococcus aureus* arthritis. Infect Immun 1992;60:2976-2985.
19. Rice PA: Gonococcal arthritis (disseminated gonococcal infection). Infect Dis Clin North Am 2005;19:853-861.
20. O'Brien JP, Goldenberg DL, Rice PA: Disseminated gonococcal infection: A prospective analysis of 49 patients and a review of pathophysiology and immune mechanisms. Medicine (Baltimore) 1983;62:395-406.
21. Holmes KK, Counts GW, Beaty HN: Disseminated gonococcal infection. Ann Intern Med 1971;74:979-993.
22. Kerle KK, Mascola JR, Miller TA: Disseminated gonococcal infection. Am Fam Physician 1992;45:209-214.
23. Al-Suleiman SA, Grimes EM, Jonas HS: Disseminated gonococcal infections. Obstet Gynecol 1983;61:48-51.
24. Steere AC, et al: Lyme arthritis: An epidemic of oligoarticular arthritis in children and adults in three connecticut communities. Arthritis Rheum 1977;20:7-17.
25. Barbour AG: Isolation and cultivation of Lyme disease spirochetes. Yale J Biol Med 1984;57:521-525.
26. Burgdorfer W, et al: Lyme disease: A tick-borne spirochetosis? Science 1982;216:1317-1319.
27. Centers for Disease Control and Prevention: Lyme disease—United States, 2003-2005. MMWR Morb Mortal Wkly Rep 2007:56:573-576.
28. Hu L: Lyme arthritis. Infect Dis Clin North Am 2005;19:947-961.
29. Guerau-de-Arellano M, Huber BT: Development of autoimmunity in Lyme arthritis. Curr Opin Rheumatol 2002;14:388-393.
30. des Vignes F, et al: Effect of tick removal on transmission of *Borrelia burgdorferi* and *Ehrlichia phagocytophila* by *Ixodes scapularis* nymphs. J Infect Dis 2001;183:773-778.
31. Schwan TG, Piesman J: Temporal changes in outer surface proteins A and C of the Lyme disease-associated spirochete, *Borrelia burgdorferi,* during the chain of infection in ticks and mice. J Clin Microbiol 2000;38:382-388.
32. Nocton JJ, Steere AC: Lyme disease. Adv Intern Med 1995;40:69-117.
33. Krause PJ, et al: Concurrent Lyme disease and babesiosis: Evidence for increased severity and duration of illness. JAMA 1996;275:1657-1660.
34. Gerber MA, et al: Lyme disease in children in southeastern Connecticut. Pediatric Lyme Disease Study Group. N Engl J Med 1996;335:1270-1274.

35. Steere AC, Schoen RT, Taylor E: The clinical evolution of Lyme arthritis. Ann Intern Med 1987;107:725-731.

36. Berglund J, et al: An epidemiologic study of Lyme disease in southern Sweden. N Engl J Med 1995;333:1319-1327.

37. Steere AC, et al: Clinical manifestations of Lyme disease. Zentralbl Bakteriol Mikrobiol Hyg A 1986;263:201-205.

38. Steere AC, et al: Autoimmune mechanisms in antibiotic treatment-resistant lyme arthritis. J Autoimmun 2001;16:263-268.

39. Lawson JP, Steere ac: Lyme arthritis: Radiologic findings. Radiology 1985;154:37-43.

40. El-Gabalawy H: The challenge of early synovitis: Multiple pathways to a common clinical syndrome. Arthritis Res 1999;1:31-36.

41. Steere AC, Duray PH, Butcher EC: Spirochetal antigens and lymphoid cell surface markers in Lyme synovitis: Comparison with rheumatoid synovium and tonsillar lymphoid tissue. Arthritis Rheum 1988;31:487-495.

42. Gardam M, Lim S: Mycobacterial osteomyelitis and arthritis. Infect Dis Clin North Am 2005;19:819-830.

43. Crow HE, et al: A limited clinical, pathologic, and epidemiologic study of patients with pulmonary lesions associated with atypical acid-fast bacilli in the sputum. Am Rev Tuberc 1957;75:199-222.

44. Jutte PC, et al: Increase of bone and joint tuberculosis in The Netherlands. J Bone Joint Surg Br 2004;86:901-904.

45. Nightingale SD, et al: Incidence of *Mycobacterium avium-intracellulare* complex bacteremia in human immunodeficiency virus-positive patients. J Infect Dis 1992;165:1082-1085.

46. Resnick D, Niwayama G: Osteomyelitis, septic arthritis and soft tissue infection: Organisms. In Resnick D (ed): Diagnosis of Bone and Joint Disorders. Philadelphia, Saunders, 1995, pp 2461-2492.

47. Suh JS, et al: MR imaging of tuberculous arthritis: Clinical and experimental studies. J Magn Reson Imaging 1996;6:185-189.

48. Sawlani V, et al: MRI features of tuberculosis of peripheral joints. Clin Radiol 2003;58:755-762.

49. Loddenkemper K, et al: Granulomatous synovialitis with erosions in the shoulder joint: A rare case of polyarthritis caused by *Mycobacterium kansasii*. Ann Rheum Dis 2005;64:1088-1090.

50. Mateo L, et al: *Mycobacterium chelonae* tenosynovitis of the hand. Semin Arthritis Rheum 2004;34:617-622.

51. Wallace RJ Jr, Brown BA, Griffith DE: *Mycobacterium chelonae* vs. abscessus. Pediatr Infect Dis J 1997;16:829.

52. Iwata H, et al: Emergence of erosive polyarthritis coincident with *Mycobacterium kansasii* pulmonary infection in a patient with systemic sclerosis-rheumatoid arthritis overlap syndrome. Clin Exp Rheumatol 1999;17:757-758.

53. Girard DE, Bagby GC Jr, Walsh JR: Destructive polyarthritis secondary to *Mycobacterium kansasii*. Arthritis Rheum 1973;16:665-669.

54. Nakamura T, et al: *Mycobacterium kansasii* arthritis of the foot in a patient with systemic lupus erythematosus. Intern Med 2001;40:1045-1049.

55. Kohli R, Hadley S: Fungal arthritis and osteomyelitis. Infect Dis Clin North Am 2005;19:831-851.

56. Hansen BL, Andersen K: Fungal arthritis: A review. Scand J Rheumatol 1995;24:248-250.

57. Cuellar ML, Silveira LH, Espinoza LR: Fungal arthritis. Ann Rheum Dis 1992;51:690-697.

58. Gathe JC Jr, et al: *Candida* osteomyelitis: Report of five cases and review of the literature. Am J Med 1987;82:927-937.

59. Cuende E, et al: *Candida* arthritis in adult patients who are not intravenous drug addicts: Report of three cases and review of the literature. Semin Arthritis Rheum 1993;22:224-241.

60. Silveira LH, et al: *Candida* arthritis. Rheum Dis Clin North Am 1993;19:427-437.

61. Gumbo T, et al: *Candida glabrata* fungemia: Clinical features of 139 patients. Medicine (Baltimore) 1999;78:220-227.

62. Choi IS, et al: *Candida* polyarthritis in a renal transplant patient: Case report of a patient successfully treated with amphotericin B. Transplant Proc 2000;32:1963-1964.

63. Bayer AS, Guze LB: Fungal arthritis: I. *Candida* arthritis: Diagnostic and prognostic implications and therapeutic considerations. Semin Arthritis Rheum 1978;8:142-150.

64. Kemper CA, Deresinski SC: Fungal diseases of bone and joint. In Kibbler CC, Mackenzie DWR, Odds FC (eds): Principles and Practice of Clinical Mycology. Chichester, GB, John Wiley & Sons, 1996, pp 49-68.

65. Bosch X, et al: Bilateral cryptococcosis of the hip: A case report. J Bone Joint Surg 1994;76A:1234-1238.

66. Bruno KM, et al: Cryptococcal arthritis, tendinitis, tenosynovitis, and carpal tunnel syndrome: Report of a case and review of the literature. Arthritis Rheum 2002;47:104-108.

67. Lantz B, et al: Coccidioidomycosis of the knee with a 26-year follow-up evaluation: A case report. Clin Orthop Relat Res 1988;(234):183-187.

68. Bayer AS, Guze LB: Fungal arthritis: II. Coccidioidal synovitis: Clinical, diagnostic, therapeutic, and prognostic considerations. Semin Arthritis Rheum 1979;8:200-211.

69. Bayer AS, et al: Fungal arthritis: V. Cryptococcal and histoplasmal arthritis. Semin Arthritis Rheum 1980;9:218-227.

70. Hansen KE, Arnason J, Bridges AJ: Autoantibodies and common viral illnesses. Semin Arthritis Rheum 1998;27:263-271.

71. Ytterberg SR: Viral arthritis. Curr Opin Rheumatol 1999;11:275-280.

72. Calabrese LH, Naides SJ: Viral arthritis. Infect Dis Clin North Am 2005;19:963-980, x.

73. Naides SJ, et al: Rheumatologic manifestations of human parvovirus B19 infection in adults: Initial two-year clinical experience. Arthritis Rheum 1990;33:1297-1309.

74. Frey TK: Molecular biology of rubella virus. Adv Virus Res 1994;44:69-160.

75. Smith CA, Petty RE, Tingle AJ: Rubella virus and arthritis. Rheum Dis Clin North Am 1987;13:265-274.

76. World Health Organization: Hepatitis C. Fact sheet 164. Geneva, WHO, 2009.

77. Lovy MR, Starkebaum G, Uberoi S: Hepatitis C infection presenting with rheumatic manifestations: A mimic of rheumatoid arthritis. J Rheumatol 1996;23:979-983.

78. World Health Organization: Hepatitis B. Fact sheet 204. Geneva, WHO, 2009.

79. Joint United Nations Programma on HIV/AIDS: 2008 Report on the global AIDS epidemic. Geneva, UNAIDS, 2008.

80. Berman A, et al: Rheumatic manifestations of human immunodeficiency virus infection. Am J Med 1988;85:59-64.

81. Chinniah K, et al: Arthritis in association with human immunodeficiency virus infection in Black African children: Causal or coincidental? Rheumatology (Oxford) 2005;44:915-920.

82. Vassilopoulos D, Calabrese LH: Virally associated arthritis 2008: Clinical, epidemiologic, and pathophysiologic considerations. Arthritis Res Ther 2008;10:215.

83. Berman A, et al: Human immunodeficiency virus infection associated arthritis: Clinical characteristics. J Rheumatol 1999;26:1158-1162.

84. Calabrese LH, Kirchner E, Shrestha R: Rheumatic complications of human immunodeficiency virus infection in the era of highly active antiretroviral therapy: Emergence of a new syndrome of immune reconstitution and changing patterns of disease. Semin Arthritis Rheum 2005;35:166-174.

85. Withrington RH, et al: Isolation of human immunodeficiency virus from synovial fluid of a patient with reactive arthritis. Br Med J (Clin Res Ed) 1987;294:484.

86. Espinoza LR, et al: HIV associated arthropathy: HIV antigen demonstration in the synovial membrane. J Rheumatol 1990;17:1195-1201.

87. Shulman ST, Ayoub EM: Poststreptococcal reactive arthritis. Curr Opin Rheumatol 2002;14:562-565.

88. Akoglu T, et al: Parasitic arthritis induced by *Strongyloides stercoralis*. Ann Rheum Dis 1984;43:523-525.

89. Ahmed S, et al: Poststreptococcal reactive arthritis: Clinical characteristics and association with HLA-DR alleles. Arthritis Rheum 1998;41:1096-1102.

90. Elliott DC, Kufera JA, Myers RA: Necrotizing soft tissue infections: Risk factors for mortality and strategies for management. Ann Surg 1996;224:672-683.

91. Mok MY, et al: Necrotizing fasciitis in rheumatic diseases. Lupus 2006;15:380-383.

92. May AK: Skin and soft tissue infections. Surg Clin North Am 2009;89:403-420, viii.

93. Childers BJ, et al: Necrotizing fasciitis: A fourteen-year retrospective study of 163 consecutive patients. Am Surg 2002;68:109-116.

94. Stevens DL, et al: Practice guidelines for the diagnosis and management of skin and soft-tissue infections. Clin Infect Dis 2005;41:1373-1406.

95. Brook I, Frazier EH: Clinical and microbiological features of necrotizing fasciitis. J Clin Microbiol 1995;33:2382-2387.

96. Giuliano A, et al: Bacteriology of necrotizing fasciitis. Am J Surg 1977;134:52-57.

97. Green RJ, Dafoe DC, Raffin TA: Necrotizing fasciitis. Chest 1996;110:219-229.

98. Wong CH, Wang YS: The diagnosis of necrotizing fasciitis. Curr Opin Infect Dis 2005;18:101-106.

99. Torralba KD, Quismorio FP Jr: Soft tissue infections. Rheum Dis Clin North Am 2009;35:45-62.

100. Yamashiro E, et al: Necrotizing fasciitis caused by *Streptococcus pneumoniae*. J Dermatol 2009;36:298-305.

101. Saenz AJ, et al: Immune cell subsets in necrotizing fasciitis: An immunohistochemical analysis. Virchows Arch 2009:455:87-92.

102. Stamenkovic I, Lew PD: Early recognition of potentially fatal necrotizing fasciitis: The use of frozen-section biopsy. N Engl J Med 1984;310:1689-1693.

103. Edlich RF, et al: Modern concepts of the diagnosis and treatment of necrotizing fasciitis. J Emerg Med 2008 Dec 10 (Epub ahead of print).

104. Sepehr A, Kroshinsky D: Acute necrotizing neutrophilic dermatosis: A new variant of Sweet's syndrome mimicking necrotizing fasciitis. Poster 178. Presented at the 45th Annual Meeting of the American Society of Dermatopathology, San Francisco, 2008. Available at http://www.asdp.org/meeting/2008_Final-Program/Poster%20 Abstracts.pdf (accessed July 28, 2009).

105. Crum-Cianflone NF: Bacterial, fungal, parasitic, and viral myositis. Clin Microbiol Rev 2008;21:473-494.

106. Hart GB, Lamb RC, Strauss MB: Gas gangrene. J Trauma 1983;23:991-1000.

107. Bickels J, et al: Primary pyomyositis. J Bone Joint Surg 2002;84A:2277-2286.

108. Chau CL, Griffith JF: Musculoskeletal infections: Ultrasound appearances. Clin Radiol 2005;60:149-159.

109. Fayad LM, Carrino JA, Fishman EK: Musculoskeletal infection: Role of CT in the emergency department. Radiographics 2007;27:1723-1736.

110. Small LN, Ross JJ: Tropical and temperate pyomyositis. Infect Dis Clin North Am 2005;19:981-989, x-xi.

111. Fayer R: *Sarcocystis* spp. in human infections. Clin Microbiol Rev 2004;17:894-902.

112. Struk DW, et al: Imaging of soft tissue infections. Radiol Clin North Am 2001;39:277-303.

113. Mangram AJ, et al: Guideline for prevention of surgical site infection, 1999. Centers for Disease Control and Prevention (CDC) Hospital Infection Control Practices Advisory Committee. Am J Infect Control 1999;27:97-132; quiz 133-134; discussion 96.

114. Simchen E, Sacks T: Infection in war wounds: Experience during the 1973 October War in Israel. Ann Surg 1975;182:754-761.

115. Petersen K, et al: Trauma-related infections in battlefield casualties from Iraq. Ann Surg 2007;245:803-811.

116. Hofmeister EP, Mazurek M, Ingari J: Injuries sustained to the upper extremity due to modern warfare and the evolution of care. J Hand Surg Am 2007;32:1141-1147.

117. Sebeny PJ, Riddle MS, Petersen K: *Acinetobacter baumannii* skin and soft-tissue infection associated with war trauma. Clin Infect Dis 2008;47:444-449.

15

Genitourinary Infectious Disease Pathology

Alton B. Farris and G. Petur Nielsen

Infections of the genitourinary tract can be caused by a number of viral, bacterial, fungal, and parasitic organisms (Table 15-1). Although many of these organisms are also seen in other locations, some of them have a predilection for the genitourinary area. Their clinical manifestations, in conjunction with their gross and microscopic appearances, are useful in characterizing these infections, and ancillary tests are often useful in their diagnosis.

Genitourinary Cutaneous Infections

Bacterial Infections

Erythrasma is a chronic bacterial infection of the genitourinary region caused by *Corynebacterium minutissimum*, particularly in humid cutaneous recesses such as the vulva and inguinal folds, and especially on the inner aspect of the thigh just below the crural fold. Diabetics and institutionalized patients are predisposed. Clinically, it is characterized by a sharply demarcated, brown to red, scaly plaque that fluoresces under a Wood's lamp because of the presence of bacterial porphyrins, often giving a coral-red or orange-red color. Corynebacteria are pleomorphic, small, gram-positive rods, also referred to as diphtheroid.[1,2] The diagnosis is often one of exclusion, after fungal infections are ruled out. Fungal organisms may be visualized with the use of potassium hydroxide (KOH) on various microscopic preparations or with periodic acid–Schiff (PAS) and methenamine silver stains.[2-6]

Trichomycosis pubis and axillaris is an asymptomatic colonization of hair follicles by various corynebacteria (particularly *Corynebacterium tenuis*), which can lead to a red, cream, yellow, or, less commonly, black coating around pubic or axillary hairs and produce an offensive odor. Pubic involvement is less common than axillary involvement. Microscopically, large bacterial colonies are present and may invade the superficial hair cortex. *C. tenuis* was once thought to be the primary offending organism, but now multiple species are recognized. The so-called corynebacterial triad is the combination of erythrasma, trichomycosis axillaris, and pitted keratolysis. However, pitted keratolysis usually affects the plantar surface of the feet, leading to multiple asymptomatic pits and superficial erosions; it is less common in the genitourinary region.[2,3,5-8]

Cellulitis of the scrotum and penis can result from bacteria (particularly β-hemolytic streptococci but also *Escherichia coli, Vibrio vulnificus, Vibrio cholerae, Pasteurella multocida,* and others) that gain an entry after a disruption of the epidermal surface, such as after circumcision. Genital skin in this condition is red, hot, and tender, and histologically there is prominent edema with dermal perivascular and interstitial acute inflammation. *P. multocida* cellulitis may occur after animal bites.[2,3,9,10]

Staphylococcus aureus produces primary lesions in the genital tract, including impetigo, bullous impetigo, furuncles, and folliculitis. Impetigo usually occurs on the face or extremities but may also spread to the genital area; although it was previously thought that group A β-hemolytic streptococci most commonly caused impetigo, *S. aureus* is currently the most common cause.

Table 15-1 Summary of Some of the Important Genitourinary Infectious Disorders

Disorder	Microbe
Chancroid	*Haemophilus ducreyi*
Dermatophytosis	*Trichophyton, Epidermophyton,* and *Microsporum* species
Encrusted cystitis	*Corynebacterium urealyticum*
Granuloma inguinale	*Klebsiella granulomatis*
Lymphogranuloma venereum	*Chlamydia trachomatis*
Malakoplakia	*Escherichia coli* (frequently)
Pityriasis versicolor (tinea versicolor)	*Malassezia furfur*
Syphilis	*Treponema pallidum*

Bullous impetigo consists of 0.5- to 3-cm in diameter flaccid bullae, with thin roofs and erythematous rims and erosions; the bullae may coalesce. The roof may rupture, forming a thin crust. A furuncle (boil) is an infection of the pilosebaceous unit that occurs at sites of friction such as the inner aspects of the thighs and the buttocks. Histologically, the furuncle consists of an abscess in the deep dermis centered on a hair follicle. Folliculitis, usually caused by *S. aureus*, has a number of manifestations that clinically consist of small pustules developing around follicular ostia, sometimes pierced by hair. Histologically, folliculitis consists of a subcorneal pustule with abundant neutrophils and some macrophages and lymphocytes overlying the follicular infundibulum. *S. aureus* can also cause secondary infections in atopic dermatitis, psoriatic plaques, and lichen simplex chronicus, as well as superinfections of candidiasis, genital herpes, or syphilitic chancres.[2,3]

Group A or B β-hemolytic streptococci can cause superficial erosive intertrigo.[3] In addition, perianal streptococcal dermatitis can be caused by group A β-hemolytic streptococci. Perianal streptococcal dermatitis occurs most commonly in children and is recognized by a perianal erythema with a well-demarcated border that may desquamate as a scale and subsequently heal.[2]

Hidradenitis Suppurativa

Hidradenitis suppurativa (also known as acne inversa or apocrine acne) is caused by bacterial infection of the apocrine glands, usually in the axilla, but it can also involve apocrine glands in the perineum and vulvar region.[2] Some studies have suggested that coagulase-negative staphylococci are the most common cause,[11] but others have found the microbiologic flora to be variable.[12-14]

Fournier Gangrene

Fournier gangrene is a necrotizing subcutaneous infection of the genital and anorectal regions caused by a mixture of aerobic and anaerobic enteric organisms. Risk factors include genitourinary trauma, periurethritis, diabetes, immunosuppression, poor nutritional status, septic injection into the penile vein, and,

rarely, *trans*-retinoic acid treatment for hematologic malignancies. A rapidly developing cellulitis, fasciitis, myositis, and systemic toxicity may result; however, the external physical findings may not be prominent and may be out of proportion to the severity of the infection. A localized vasculitis results from a Schwartzman-like reaction. The Schwartzman reaction is the inflammatory process brought about by injection of endotoxin, which on first injection results only in mild inflammation but on second injection results in a thrombohemorrhagic lesion, similar to that seen in Fournier gangrene.[15] The mortality rate ranges from 10% to 30%. Treatment is typically with débridement and broad-spectrum antibiotics, as necrotizing fasciitis in other locations.[3,16-20]

Pseudomonal Cellulitis (Ecthyma Gangrenosum)

Pseudomonal sepsis may be complicated by a cellulitis known as ecthyma gangrenosum, which starts with an erythematous or purpuric cutaneous macule that may rapidly develop into a bulla, which sometimes ulcerates. This is caused by a bacterial vasculitis that may eventually result in cutaneous infarction. Penile ecthyma gangrenosum has been reported in patients with a history of drug abuse and neutropenia.[3,21-23]

Mycobacterial Disease

Genital tuberculosis can result from sexual contact with individuals who have active oral or genital tuberculosis. *Mycobacterium tuberculosis* is the most common organism, but infections due to *Mycobacterium celatum* have also been reported.[24] Clinically, subacute or chronic, painful ulcers with or without lymphadenopathy may be present, and the lesions may even mimic tumors grossly, notably in scrotal lesions.[25] Lupus vulgaris, which is the most frequent form of reinfection tuberculosis, can affect the penis. Confluent papules may coalesce into plaques; when viewed by diascopy, these plaques have an "apple-jelly" deposit representing cellular infiltrates. Involvement of the glans may occur. Bacillus Calmette-Guérin (BCG) balanitis after instillation for bladder carcinoma has rarely been reported.[3,25,26]

Syphilis

The spirochetal organism, *Treponema pallidum*, is the causative agent of syphilis. The anogenital area may be affected by primary, secondary, tertiary, or congenital lesions of syphilis. Three weeks after initial exposure, a primary syphilitic chancre occurs at the site of inoculation, usually the inner prepuce, coronal sulcus, penile shaft, vulvovaginal area, or anus.[3,4]

The painless, button-like papule ulcerates centrally, and adjacent "kissing" lesions may also be present. Histologically, there is a prominent lymphoplasmacytic infiltrate in an edematous ulcer bed with prominent capillary proliferation containing swollen endothelial cells. Spirochetes may be identified with the use of Warthin-Starry or Steiner stains or immunohistochemically.[27,28] Smears can be analyzed by darkfield examination or by immunofluorescence with antitreponemal antibodies.[28] Secondary syphilis occurs if the primary lesion is left untreated and the spirochete spreads systemically. It typically forms 3 to 6 weeks after the chancre but may arise up to 6 months after healing of the primary lesion. Clinically large, red to pale, moist, flat-topped or verruciform papules may develop in the anogenital region (condyloma lata). In 80% of patients, there is a diffuse, non-pruritic, papulosquamous eruption. In dark-skinned patients, annular polycyclic lesions may occur. Microscopically, many spirochetes are present, explaining the highly contagious nature of secondary syphilis. Pseudoepitheliomatous hyperplasia may be prominent. The composition of the inflammatory cells is similar to that of the primary lesion; additionally, a neutrophilic infiltrate may be present.[3,4,29]

Tertiary syphilis targets bones, the central nervous system, the cardiovascular system, and skin with ulcerative and nodular lesions. In tertiary syphilis, the classic lesion is a gumma, a type of granuloma with a focus of necrobiosis surrounded by multinucleated giant cells, histiocytes, plasma cells, lymphocytes, and fibroblasts. Obliterative endarteritis may be present. A nodular presentation consists of tuberculoid granulomas with a mixed inflammatory cell reaction including plasma cells. Treponemes cannot usually be detected with silver stains, but polymerase chain reaction (PCR) may be useful.[3,29]

Chancroid

Haemophilus ducreyi is the gram-negative, facultative anaerobic bacterium that causes chancroid. It is uncommon in the United States but is a common cause of genital ulcers in Africa. Chancroid is transmitted by sexual contact during the active phase of lesions, which in untreated patients lasts about 6 weeks. A papule or pustule appears at the exposure site after approximately 1 week. This usually develops into a painful ulcer or ulcers with a gray-yellow exudate and sharp, undermined, ragged erythematous borders. Many lesions can arise in the location of the original lesion through autoinoculation, and lesions may merge with serpiginous borders. After 1 to 2 weeks, adenopathy with suppuration (buboes) occurs in approximately 25% to 50% of untreated patients, sometimes leading to inguinal abscesses and draining sinuses. Microscopically, microvascular and endothelial proliferation with overlying surface ulceration and necrotic debris is typically seen. Vessels may be thrombosed. There is often a dense lymphoplasmacytic infiltrate. Special culture medium is required for isolation.[3,4,30] Chancroid is treated with antibiotics. Large lymph nodes may need to be drained.

Lymphogranuloma Venereum

Chlamydia trachomatis, an obligate intracellular parasite, particularly serovars L1, L2, and L3, cause lymphogranuloma venereum; the organisms spread through sexual transmission, travel through lymphatic channels, and multiply within draining lymph nodes of the genital and anorectal region. Serotypes D to K are associated with sexually transmitted oculogenital disease.[3,4,29]

In the primary stage, eroded papules or groups of small herpetiform ulcers form at the inoculation site (coronal sulcus, frenulum, prepuce, shaft, glans, scrotum, or vulva). Urethritis with a mucopurulent discharge may be present. In the secondary stage, occurring several weeks later, inguinal lymphadenitis and formation of buboes (enlarged lymph nodes, from the Greek *boubón*, "groin") occur, often with concurrent cord-like lymphangitis of the dorsal penis and suppurative inguinal bubo formation. The so-called groove sign may be present, which results from a cleft formed by the inguinal (Poupart) ligament between enlarged involved femoral and inguinal lymph nodes. Proctocolitis may occur.

A third stage comprises various sequelae from inflammation and includes fistula formation, fibrosis, and scarring.[3,4,29,31] This may be complicated by sinuses and tracts between the skin and urethra and deforming scars of the penis. In the anogenital syndrome, proctocolitis and hyperplasia of the perirectal lymph nodes may occur, and fistulas and rectal strictures may form. Obstruction of chronic lymphedema may lead to elephantiasis.[3,4]

Histologically, the ulcers of lymphogranuloma venereum consist of a chronic inflammatory process with scattered giant cells, plasma cells, lymphocytes, necrosis, and granulation tissue. Non-necrotizing granulomas composed of epithelioid histiocytes may be present. Fibrosis and, eventually, prominent scarring occur as the process becomes more chronic. Pseudoepitheliomatous hyperplasia may be present. Lymph nodes show accumulation of neutrophils, often with prominent necrosis, particularly in the early stages of the infection. Plasma cell infiltration and lymphocytic hyperplasia follow. Eventually, what are referred to as stellate abscesses form; these are suppurative foci that have coalesced and are surrounded by epithelioid cells and multinucleated giant cells.[4,29]

Culture of the lesions is the best method to identify the organisms in oculogenital chlamydial infections. The obligate intracellular organisms can typically be identified in vacuoles of vacuolated macrophages.[32] The organisms stain faintly blue with hematoxylin and eosin (H&E), are gram-negative, and can be identified with Warthin-Starry stain. Electron microscopy, immunohistochemistry, and PCR for the 16S ribosomal DNA of the organisms are sometimes needed for a definitive diagnosis. Serology may be useful in confirming the diagnosis.[4,31,29]

Granuloma Inguinale (Donovanosis)

Klebsiella granulomatis (formerly called *Calymmatobacterium granulomatis*), a gram-negative bacillus, leads to donovanosis, a sexually transmitted genital ulcer disease. It is rare in the United States and occurs primarily in the southern states.[33] Clinically, well-defined, single or multiple, painless ulcers with beefy-red granulation tissue at the base and elevated, rolled, serpiginous, or hyperplastic borders form the primary lesion. The ulcer may heal with prominent fibrosis. Lymphedema with eventual elephantiasis of the penis and scrotum can result in chronic disease. Subcutaneous nodules (pseudobuboes) can simulate lymph node involvement. Lesions may be nodular, hypertrophic, cicatricial, and ulcerovegetative. Microscopically, there is prominent granulation-type tissue with an inflammatory infiltrate including plasma cells, neutrophils, and histiocytes that contain 0.6- to 2-μm Donovan bodies, which are encapsulated rods with bipolar granules (Fig. 15-1). Pseudoepitheliomatous hyperplasia may be prominent. The gram-negative coccoid to bacillary bacteria may be difficult to identify, requiring Wright/Giemsa, toluidine blue, or Warthin-Starry stains. Cytologic identification of Donovan bodies in granuloma inguinale (see Fig. 15-1) can be accomplished with Papanicolaou-stained smears. Ultrastructural studies have identified the organism in greater detail, demonstrating it in the phagosomes of macrophages.[3,4,34-38] Squamous cell carcinomas of the vulva secondary to granuloma inguinale have been reported.[4,29,39,40]

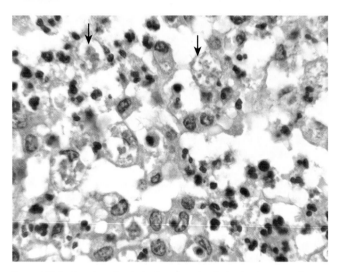

Figure 15-1. Granuloma inguinale. Granuloma inguinale, also known as donovanosis, is characterized histologically by the presence of dense acute inflammation in lesional ulcers, which are usually painless. Donovan bodies *(arrows)*, intracellular inclusions of engulfed bacteria, are present within macrophages.

Fungal Infections

Certain superficial fungal infections, such as dermatophytosis, pityriasis versicolor, and candidiasis, occur in the genitourinary area and are discussed in this section. Deep mycotic infections, including blastomycosis, histoplasmosis, coccidioidomycosis, and paracoccidioidomycosis, also occur in this area. Diagnosis is aided by identification of hyphae in skin scrapings treated with potassium-hydroxide (KOH). Fungal infections are usually superficial, but deep infections may occur, and phycomycosis (an older term for zygomycosis) of the vulva has been reported in diabetic women.[3,4,41,42]

Dermatophytosis

Dermatophytosis (tinea) is a superficial fungal infection of keratinized tissues caused by species such as *Trichophyton*, *Epidermophyton*, and *Microsporum*. Tinea cruris is an infection of the inguinal area. An infection of the genital area can result from a transfer by hand from a dermatophytosis of the feet (tinea pedis).[3,4]

Pityriasis Versicolor (Tinea Versicolor)

Although pityriasis versicolor is usually located on the upper trunk or upper arms, this superficial fungal infection, caused by the lipophilic yeast of the genus *Malassezia*, can cause hypopigmented or hyperpigmented, white to red-brown, macular eruptions in genital areas, notably on the penile shaft.[43,44] Scales show pale yellow fluorescence with a Wood's lamp. Pityriasis versicolor is usually considered to be noncontagious. The organism to which this disorder is usually attributed is *Malassezia globosa*, which was formerly classified as *Malassezia furfur*.[2,3]

Candidiasis

The normal flora of the intertriginous skin, prepuce, and perineal area includes *Candida albicans*. Candidal balanoposthitis is the most common fungal infection of the penis.[45] Obesity and uncontrolled diabetes mellitus are predisposing factors, as are other immunocompromised states. The infection can be sexually transmitted. More than 75% of women experience at least one symptomatic episode of vulvovaginal candidiasis. Small pustules may be present. Microscopically, there is epidermal thickening and spongiosis with dermal chronic inflammation. Yeast and pseudohyphae are present on the surface, together with degenerated squamous cells and neutrophils.[3,4]

Viral Infections

Molluscum Contagiosum

Molluscum contagiosum is caused by a large poxvirus (molluscum contagiosum virus), which is a double-stranded, brick-shaped DNA virus. It manifests as solitary or multiple, 2- to 8-mm, dome-shaped, pearly, centrally umbilicated papules that may cluster, become more keratotic with trauma, and simulate condyloma acuminata. The lesion may express a white caseous material (caseum). Transmission is via fomites or sexual contact. Children often have a primary inoculation in the anogenital region, and autoinoculation may lead to additional lesions. Microscopically (Fig. 15-2), a lobular epidermal acanthosis is present and causes an inverted pattern of epidermal hyperplasia. Intracytoplasmic eosinophilic inclusions, referred to as Henderson-Paterson bodies, can be identified in the stratum spinosum and granulosum. The lesions usually regress spontaneously within 1 year, although scarring may occur. About 60% of individuals with skin lesions have antibodies to the virus, but this fraction is less among patients with the acquired immunodeficiency syndrome (AIDS), who, along with other immunocompromised patients, may have numerous lesions, some of which may manifest as tumor-like lesions. Ultrastructurally, large, brick-shaped viral particles can be seen.[2,3,29,46-51]

Herpetic Infections

Herpes simplex virus type 2 (HSV-2), a double-stranded linear DNA virus, is the most common organism that leads to sexually transmitted genital herpes; however, HSV-1 has been shown to cause almost half of genital herpes cases in developing countries.[52] The incubation period is approximately 5 days, and the virus is harbored for life in sensory ganglia. Vesicles consisting of clear lesions with an erythematous base form the primary lesions, which may rupture and leave behind erosions. The primary lesion may be accompanied by lymphadenopathy, but the lymphadenopathy usually subsides and does not recur. Histologically, the lesions start with epidermal cell peripheral nuclear chromatin clumping, ballooning degeneration, and homogeneous ground glass changes with eosinophilic nuclear inclusions. Cytoplasmic vacuolization may also be present. Eventually, affected cells swell, losing their attachment to and separating from adjacent cells (a process referred to as secondary acantholysis). Cellular cytoplasm becomes homogeneous and intensely eosinophilic, and multinucleated cells (Tzanck cells)

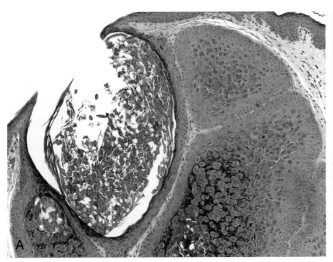
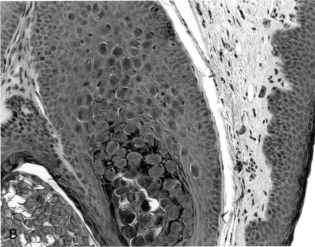

Figure 15-2. Molluscum contagiosum. **A,** Medium-power view shows a crateriform lesion with an inverted pattern of epidermal hyperplasia and epidermal acanthosis. **B,** High-power view shows characteristic viral inclusions, the intracytoplasmic eosinophilic inclusions of which are known as Henderson-Paterson bodies.

may be present. The basal layer of the epidermis may be destroyed, leading to the formation of a subepidermal vesicle. Reticular degeneration, a process whereby the epidermal cells undergo progressive hydropic swelling and cytoplasmic clearing with peripheral cytoplasmic strands remaining, can occur. Eventually, these break, and further vesicle formation occurs. Vesicles may contain neutrophils, and accompanying vasculitis may be present. Late lesions are often ulcerated, with ghosts of acantholytic, multinucleate epithelial cells. Primary infection and viral excretion last approximately 3 weeks. Extragenital lesions occur in about 20% of cases, and aseptic meningitis in about 10%.[2,3,51]

Recurrences are less severe. Burning and tingling may manifest 1 to 2 days before a recurrence. Vesicles are limited in number and heal in about 10 days, and virus is shed for only a few days. The glans, prepuce, and shaft are the primary sites of involvement; however, the scrotum may be involved. Perianal lesions may also be present, particularly in homosexual men.[3] Chronic HSV disease manifests as painful ulcers with rolled borders. Chronic persistent herpes lesions may suggest and help define the presence of AIDS if they last for longer than 1 month, and they may also occur in other immunosuppressed states (e.g., history of transplantation, chemotherapy, hematologic disorders).[3] The herpes varicella-zoster virus (VZV) may infect the anogenital area in a dermatomal distribution through involvement of the third and fourth sacral sensory nerves.[3,51]

Immunohistochemical stains may be useful in distinguishing HSV from VZV in biopsy specimens. Monoclonal antibodies to the VZV envelope protein gp1 are sensitive and specific in distinguishing between HSV and VZV.[53-56] Cultures and molecular probes for viral antigens can also be useful. Viral antigen can be detected in inflamed nerve twigs. Electron microscopy may reveal the 90- to 130-nm viral particles.[2,3]

Human Papillomavirus

Human papillomavirus (HPV) is a member of the Papovaviridae family, which consists of circular, double-stranded DNA viruses.

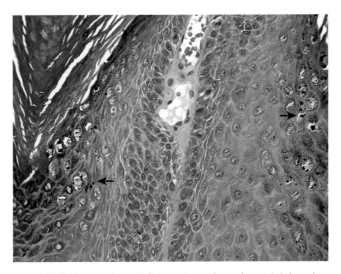

Figure 15-3. Verruca vulgaris. High-power image shows characteristic keratohyaline granules in a lesion associated with human papillomavirus (arrows).

HPV is involved in a number of pathologic lesions, from the benign end of the spectrum, the common wart (verruca vulgaris) (Fig. 15-3), to frankly malignant squamous cell carcinoma. More than 100 genotypes are known.[2,3,51,57] Relationships between different HPV types and particular lesions have been recognized (Table 15-2).

HPV was first recognized to have oncogenic potential in patients with epidermodysplasia verruciformis. This is an autosomal recessive condition, associated with a gene locus on chromosome 17, that leads to decreased defenses against several HPV subtypes (HPV 2, 3, 5, 10, and 8), resulting in exophytic lesions on the trunk and upper extremities which appear in the first decade of life. These lesions may undergo malignant transformation into squamous cell carcinoma during young adulthood. Unlike common warts caused by HPV, epidermodysplasia verruciformis lesions are not transmissible to healthy individuals.

Table 15-2 Human Papillomavirus (HPV) Types and Associated Lesions

HPV Type	Lesion
1	Plantar, common (verruca vulgaris) warts (see Fig. 15-3) and anogenital warts
2	Common warts; also plantar, oral, and anogenital lesions
3	Plane warts (verruca planae) and epidermodysplasia verruciformis
4	Plantar and common warts
5	Epidermodysplasia with subsequent development of carcinoma Psoriatic skin lesions (detected in research setting)
6	Anogenital warts and epidermodysplasia Condyloma acuminatum (other types detected include HPV 2, 6, 11, 16, 18, 31, 33, 35, 39, 41-45, 51, 56, 59, and others) (see Fig. 15-4) Oral and laryngeal squamous papilloma Verrucous carcinoma
7	Warts in meat and fish handlers
8, 9, 10, 12, 14, 17, 19, 22, 24, and others	Epidermodysplasia
10	Plane warts
11	Anogenital lesions (e.g., condyloma acuminatum) Oral and laryngeal squamous papilloma Verrucous carcinoma
16 and 18	Bowenoid papulosis (which sometimes progresses to invasive carcinoma) Anogenital warts Cervical squamous dysplasia and invasive squamous cell carcinoma (types 16, 18, 31, 33, and 35) Cervical adenocarcinoma in situ (AIS) and invasive cervical adenocarcinoma (type 18 > type 16) Squamous cell carcinoma in other nongenital sites Verrucous carcinoma
13 and 32	(Oral) Focal epithelial hyperplasia (Heck disease)
57	Plantar epidermoid cysts and nail dystrophy
60	Plantar warts and epidermal cysts
63, 65, 66	Plantar warts
75, 76, 77	Common warts in immunosuppressed patients

Data from Weedon D, Strutton G: Skin Pathology. 2nd ed. Edinburgh, Churchill Livingstone, 2002; and Mais DD: Quick Compendium of Clinical Pathology, 2nd ed. Chicago, American Society of Clinical Pathology Press, 2008.

Lesions resembling epidermodysplasia verruciformis are sometimes seen in organ transplant recipients.[57]

Condyloma acuminatum is one of the most common sexually transmitted diseases. In males, the frenulum, corona, glans, shaft, and scrotum are affected. Multiple lesions may become confluent, forming a cobblestone appearance. Microscopically, condyloma acuminatum typically has some degree of epidermal hyperplasia or hyperkeratosis, acanthosis, parakeratosis, and numerous koilocytes which cytologically are characterized by perinuclear clearing and wrinkled or crenated ("raisinoid") nuclei[3,51] (Fig. 15-4). Condyloma acuminatum is usually caused by HPV types 6 and 11, and there is little risk of squamous cell carcinoma from infection with these HPV types. HPV types 16 and 18 are the high-risk types, leading to anogenital squamous intraepithelial lesions and squamous cell carcinomas (e.g., penile squamous cell carcinoma, cervical carcinoma; see Fig. 15-23). HPV 16 and 18 account for more than 70% of all malignancies in the anogenital region and are present in more than 98% of cases of high-grade dysplasia and squamous cell carcinoma of the cervix. After treatment, latent HPV in perilesional skin may lead to recurrent lesions.[3,57]

Bowenoid papulosis due to HPV (mostly type 16) manifests on the anogenital skin as multiple small (2-3 mm), pearly papules. Histologically, it resembles squamous cell carcinoma in situ (also known as Bowen disease). Bowenoid papulosis rarely results in invasive carcinoma and often spontaneously regresses. It can usually be distinguished clinically from Bowen disease (also known as erythroplasia of Queyrat).[57]

Verrucous carcinoma (giant condyloma of Buschke and Lowenstein) is sometimes associated with HPV. It is a slow-growing, well-differentiated variant of squamous cell carcinoma with an exophytic papillary appearance, typically 1 to 3 cm in diameter, that arises in the skin (usually the genital skin), oral cavity, larynx, and esophagus. It is defined by a broad base between the tumor and the underlying stroma with minimal atypia and mitoses at the base, although focal stromal invasion may be observed; dense chronic inflammation may also be present at this interface. Microscopically, verrucous carcinoma is hyperkeratotic and acanthotic, with orthokeratosis (the presence of keratohyaline granules), parakeratosis, and papillomatosis. Papillae may have fibrovascular cores, and papillae may also have a central keratin plug with peripherally located tumor cells. Occasional vacuolated (nonkoilocytotic) clear cells may be present. Verrucous carcinoma has been associated with HPV 6, 11, 16, and 18, although koilocytosis is not present. Verrucous carcinoma is sometimes distinguished from giant condyloma by the absence of koilocytic change,[29,57] and it has been suggested that the term "warty (condylomatous) squamous cell carcinoma" should be used for exophytic warty tumors of the penis and similar lesions that occur on the vulva and are related to HPV-16. These warty carcinomas are described as having more prominent, long, condylomatous papillae and fibrovascular cores with rounded, irregular, jagged bases, and more obvious koilocytotic atypia. Penile warty carcinoma appears to have a better prognosis than typical squamous cell carcinoma.[2,58-60]

Both in situ hybridization and immunohistochemistry are available for the detection of HPV in formalin-fixed tissue. In situ hybridization, which is typically considered to be more sensitive, has largely replaced immunohistochemistry for this purpose (except for specific diagnostic purposes in the cervix, discussed

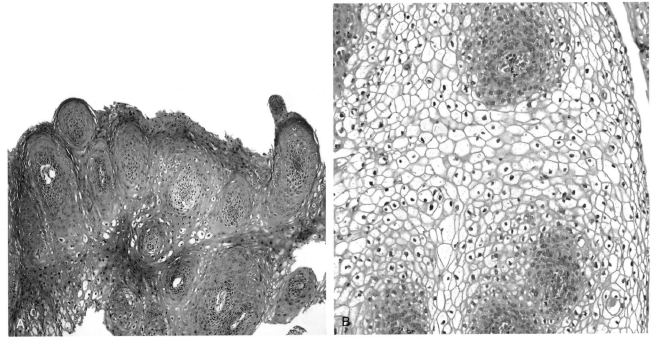

Figure 15-4. Condyloma. **A,** Low-power view shows hyperkeratosis, parakeratosis, acanthosis, and koilocytes with cytoplasmic clearing. **B,** High-power view shows cytoplasmic clearing, primarily in a perinuclear location, which is characteristic of the koilocytes that make up a large proportion of cells in condylomas.

later). Immunohistochemistry detects only productive and not latent infections, and it cannot be used to determine the type of virus present, whereas other molecular techniques are useful for some of these purposes.[56,61-64]

Parasitic Infections

The perineal skin can be affected by *Entamoeba histolytica* when infection extends from the anus in a patient with *E. histolytica* colitis. This can result from spread by anal intercourse and may also involve the penis. Clinically, ulcerated, painful nodules with serpiginous borders result. An amebic ulcer may present as balanoposthitis resistant to antibiotics.[3,65]

Wuchereria bancrofti, Brugia malayi, and *Brugia timori* are filarial worms that can involve lymphatic vessels, resulting in obstruction, chronic lymphedema leading to elephantiasis, and chronic inflammation. Up to 25% of the male population are affected in tropical areas. The scrotum is often swollen, erythematous, and tender. Histologically, there may be thickening of the scrotal skin and verruciform epidermal hyperplasia. Vulvar elephantiasis may also occur from lymphatic obstruction by filariform worms.[3,4,66]

Schistosomiasis

Schistosoma mansoni is a fluke that can colonize pelvic veins. Adult organisms within abdominopelvic veins can involve surrounding visceral or cutaneous tissue with a granulomatous reaction. Eggs are typically conducted to the bladder lumen and are excreted during micturition. Sinuses, fistulas, and masses may be present. Ulcers and papillary nodules may simulate condyloma acuminata.[3,4,67]

Scabies and Lice

Scabies (caused by the mite *Sarcoptes scabiei*) can form tunnels under the stratum corneum of the penis, scrotum, buttock, and waist. Immunocompromised patients may have crusted lesions (known as Norwegian scabies). Lice may also infect the genital region.[3,4,29]

Kidney Infections

Acute Interstitial Nephritis

Acute interstitial nephritis was first thoroughly defined by Councilman in 1898.[68] Before the advent of widespread antibiotic use, acute interstitial nephritis was most commonly caused by bacterial infections such as scarlet fever (scarletina, caused by *Streptococcus* spp.) or diphtheria. Currently, acute interstitial nephritis is most commonly observed in the setting of an allergic reaction (such as to a drug[69]) or acute transplant rejection; however, bacteria and viruses are still important causes of acute interstitial nephritis.[70-74] Councilman was astute in observing that many cases of acute interstitial nephritis do not arise as a direct infection by organisms filling the kidney but rather from an indirect influence in which inflammatory cells are attracted to the kidney by, as he surmised, "soluble substances that may exert a positive chemotaxis for them."[68,74]

Grossly, the kidneys are enlarged, soft, and pale due to edema. Microscopically, edema expands the interstitium, and there is usually a mixed inflammatory cell infiltrate composed primarily of lymphocytes and monocytes with a smaller number of plasma cells and eosinophils. Granulomas may be present in rejection, allergic reactions, or sarcoidosis, in which they are usually noncaseating.[75] Tubulitis, a lymphocytic infiltration of tubular epithelial cells, and vasculitis may be present.[70,73,74]

Bacterial organisms, particularly *Streptococcus*, were formerly the common causes of acute interstitial nephritis. Glomerulonephritis was formerly rare compared to interstitial nephritis in streptococcal infections. However, interstitial nephritis due to *Streptococcus* declined around the beginning of the 20th century. Specific bacteria involving the kidney are discussed in the following paragraphs. In general, acute interstitial nephritis due to bacterial organisms contains a mixed infiltrate of neutrophils, plasma cells, and eosinophils amid interstitial edema and tubular injury.[70-74]

Cytomegalovirus (CMV), adenovirus, and polyomavirus produce characteristic intranuclear viral inclusions in tubular epithelial cells and occasionally in the endothelium and glomerular epithelium.[70,73,74] Adenovirus may produce smudgy intranuclear inclusions that may have a glassy appearance. Intranuclear inclusions may have a distinct halo surrounded by a ring of marginated chromatin (Cowdry A inclusion). Necrotizing tubulointerstitial nephritis due to adenovirus has been reported, notably in patients who are immunosuppressed. Mass-forming lesions and granulomatous inflammation have also been reported. Immunofluorescence or immunohistochemistry for viral antigens may aid the diagnosis.[70,73,76-80]

CMV produces large eosinophilic intranuclear inclusions with halos, most often in proximal tubules but also in the loops of Henle and collecting ducts. Microscopically, interstitial inflammation is typically observed to be composed of lymphocytes, plasma cells, and macrophages. CMV-infected renal tubular cells or stromal cells may show enlargement and a single eosinophilic nuclear inclusion surrounded by a clear halo (Fig. 15-5). CMV acute interstitial nephritis can occur as a congenital infection during the neonatal period. Another setting for CMV acute interstitial nephritis is in renal allografts. CMV may result in impairment of renal graft function and glomerular and interstitial injury. Immunohistochemistry for viral antigens may help solidify the diagnosis.[73,74,81-83]

Epstein-Barr virus (EBV), the cause of infectious mononucleosis, may also produce an acute interstitial nephritis. In EBV acute interstitial nephritis, there is usually a prominent lymphocytic infiltrate with plasma cells and macrophages producing tubular injury and necrosis. Lymphocytes may be atypical and are usually CD8-positive. Granulomas may be present. It has been argued that EBV acute interstitial nephritis is simply an immunologic phenomenon. In situ hybridization for EBV RNA and immunohistochemistry findings may be negative; however, EBV DNA has been identified on PCR studies in biopsy material involved by EBV-associated acute interstitial nephritis.[74,84]

Other infectious agents that may cause acute interstitial nephritis include viruses such as HSV, rubeola virus (measles), and human immunodeficiency virus (HIV); bacteria including *Brucella* species, *Legionella*, *Mycoplasma*, and *Yersinia*; and parasites including *Toxoplasma gondii* and *Leishmania* (acute visceral leishmaniasis or kala-azar). Only rare cases have been reported of HSV and measles leading to acute interstitial nephritis. *Brucella* may produce a caseating granulomatous infiltrate with neutrophils, lymphocytes, and interstitial edema. *Legionella* often has an infiltrate rich in lymphocytes, plasma cells, macrophages, and sometimes even neutrophils. *T. gondii* can lead to an acute interstitial nephritis rich in lymphocytes and neutro-

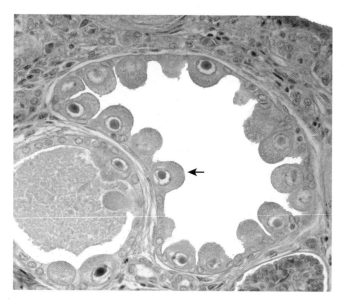

Figure 15-5. Cytomegalovirus acute interstitial nephritis. Characteristic eosinophilic intranuclear inclusions surrounded by a clear halo can be seen in enlarged renal tubular epithelial cells *(arrow)*.

phils. Acute visceral leishmaniasis results in an inflammatory infiltrate of plasma cells and lymphocytes without eosinophils. The renal parenchyma is spared. Patients with HIV infection (AIDS) can have a severe interstitial nephritis composed of an infiltrate rich in lymphocytes and plasma cells. AIDS also predisposes individuals to infectious with a number of organisms such as *Pneumocystis*.[74]

Certain disorders are in the differential diagnosis of granulomatous interstitial nephritis and other granulomatous diseases of the kidney; they include xanthogranulomatous pyelonephritis, malakoplakia, brucellosis, mycobacterial infection, fungal infection, parasitic infection, urate nephropathy, oxalosis, sarcoidosis, vasculitis, drug hypersensitivity, tubulointerstitial nephritis with uveitis syndrome (TINU), granulomatous vasculitis (Wegener granuloma), and cholesterol granulomas. Many infectious agents that may produce a granulomatous interstitial nephritis are listed in Table 15-3. Ultimately, many cases are idiopathic.[85,86]

Immune complex deposits may be seen on immunofluorescence in tubular basement membranes or peritubular capillaries in cases of interstitial nephritis, but this is a nonspecific finding that merely indicates that an immunologic reaction has taken place. Immunoperoxidase stains may be useful to confirm the presence of adenovirus, cytomegalovirus, or BK polyomavirus. However, in many cases of acute interstitial nephritis, a specific etiology cannot be determined.[70,73,74]

Acute Pyelonephritis

Acute pyelonephritis occurs as a result of infection of the kidney, usually from bacteria.[70,73] Most pediatric cases occur in boys, and most adult cases occur in women. Infections can be ascending, from lower urinary tract infection, or hematogenous, from sepsis or endocarditis.[70,73,87,88]

Lower urinary tract infections that can involve the kidney include *E. coli*, followed by *Proteus*, *Klebsiella*, and *Enterobacter*.

Table 15-3 Differential Diagnosis and Pharmacotherapy of Interstitial Nephritis*

Causes	Selected Drugs
Viral Infection	Antibiotics
Cytomegalovirus (CMV)	β-Lactams
Epstein-Barr virus (EBV)	Amoxicillin
Polyomavirus (e.g., BK virus)	Ampicillin
Human immunodeficiency virus (HIV)	Nafcillin
Hantavirus	Oxacillin
Bacterial Infection	Penicillin G
Scarlet fever (*Streptococcus*)	Cephalexin
Diphtheria	Cefotaxime
Typhoid fever	Others
Brucellosis	Chloramphenicol
Leptospira	Ethambutol
Rickettsia	Gentamicin
Fungal Infection	Rifampin
Histoplasma	Sulfonamides
Parasitic Infection	Tetracyclines
Leishmania	Diuretics
Toxoplasma gondii	Non-steroidal
Ascaris	anti-inflammatory
Systemic disorders	drugs (NSAIDs)
Connective tissue disorders	Allopurinol
Systemic lupus erythematosus	Rifampicin
Sjögren's syndrome	Cimetidine
Sarcoidosis	Sulfa drugs
Transplant rejection	Phenytoin
Irradiation	
Ischemia	
Protein accumulation (e.g., amyloid, light chain, myeloma)	
Hereditary (e.g., Alport syndrome, medullary cystic disease, nephrophthisis, familial interstitial nephritis)	
Metals (e.g., cadmium, lithium, gold)	
Metabolic disorders (e.g., oxalosis, hypercalcemia, gout, cystinosis)	
Toxins (e.g., snake bite, CCl_4, mushroom)	
Anti-tubular basement membrane disease	
Tubulointerstitial nephritis-uveitis syndrome (Dobrin syndrome)	
Idiopathic	

*Organisms, agents, and disorders listed include entities that affect the kidney directly (e.g., through direct infection) or indirectly (e.g., through an immunologic reaction or other reactive state).
Data from Colvin RB, Fang LST: Interstitial nephritis. In Tisher CC, Brenner BM (eds): Renal Pathology with Clinical and Functional Correlations, vol 2, 2nd ed. Philadelphia, JB Lippincott, 1994; and Bonsib SM: Non-neoplastic disease of the kidney. In Bostwick DG, Eble JN (eds): Urologic Surgical Pathology. St. Louis, Mosby, 1997.

Vesicoureteral reflux in cases of bacterial cystitis can lead to pyelonephritis. Congenital predisposition toward vesicoureteral reflux leads to more frequent cases of pyelonephritis.[70] Incompetence of the vesicoureteric junction causes congenital (primary) reflux.[73] Some cases of congenital obstruction are familial. Reflux may also result from neurogenic bladder, cystitis, or other causes of distal obstruction. Intrarenal reflux leads to infection of the kidney.[70,73,87,88]

Hematogenous infections involve organisms such as *S. aureus* and are usually composed of numerous small abscesses scattered throughout the parenchyma, particularly the cortex; this is sometimes termed multiple cortical abscesses, diffuse suppurative nephritis, or diffuse bacterial nephritis. This process is sometimes considered distinct from acute pyelonephritis.[73] Prolonged infectious endocarditis or sepsis is a common cause of hematogenous pyelonephritis, and gram-positive bacteria and fungi are the most common culprits in these instances. *Pyonephrosis* is the term used for near-total destruction of an obstructed kidney by acute pyelonephritis. Pyonephrosis or renal abscesses may lead to perinephric abscesses.[70,73,87,88]

Clinically, the patients are often febrile with flank pain and have leukocytosis. Urinalysis usually shows pyuria and white blood cell casts. Treatment is usually medical with antibiotic therapy, although surgical intervention with either débridement or nephrectomy may be required in severe cases.[70,73,87,88]

Grossly, the kidneys are often yellow-white with suppurative foci and sometimes frank abscesses, particularly in ascending acute pyelonephritis. The abscesses may be smaller and scattered, with a concentration in the cortex, in the hematogenous form.[70,73] Microscopically, there are numerous neutrophils in the tubules and interstitium. Neutrophils and bacteria can be seen in the tubules and collecting ducts of the cortex and medulla (Fig. 15-6). Glomeruli are affected only in severe cases in which there is extensive parenchymal destruction with abscess formation. Vascular thromboses, ischemic necrosis, and cyst formation may be seen.[70,73,87,88]

Focal Bacterial Nephritis (Lobar Nephronia)

Acute focal bacterial nephritis (lobar nephronia) is a rare form of renal infection. It typically involves the renal cortex and may manifest as a renal mass and be mistaken for a neoplasm, even after cytologic examination. It is thought to be the early stage of an intrarenal abscess. Clinically, flank pain, fever, leukocytosis, pyuria, and bacteriuria may be present; all of these features may also be present in renal abscesses or acute pyelonephritis. Radiologic studies may detect lobar nephronia as focal imaging abnormalities. Microscopically, microabscesses with foci of hemorrhage and necrosis can be appreciated. *E. coli* is thought to be the most common causative organism, but other organisms have also been implicated, including *S. aureus* and *Klebsiella pneumoniae*. Lobar nephronia has been reported in renal allografts.[89-93]

Emphysematous Pyelonephritis

Emphysematous pyelonephritis is an uncommon, life-threatening condition in which bubble-like collections of gas develop in the renal parenchyma, particularly in areas of coagulative necrosis, and extend into the perinephric space or retroperitoneum or both. The emphysematous foci may be cystic and multiple. Approximately 90% of the patients have diabetes mellitus, and signs of diabetic glomerulosclerosis may be present. Urinary tract obstruction is present in approximately 40% of patients.[70,73,94,95] Cortical and papillary necrosis and vascular thromboses may result.[73] *E. coli* is the most common organism (about 68% of the cases), and *Klebsiella* is present in approximately 9% of patients.

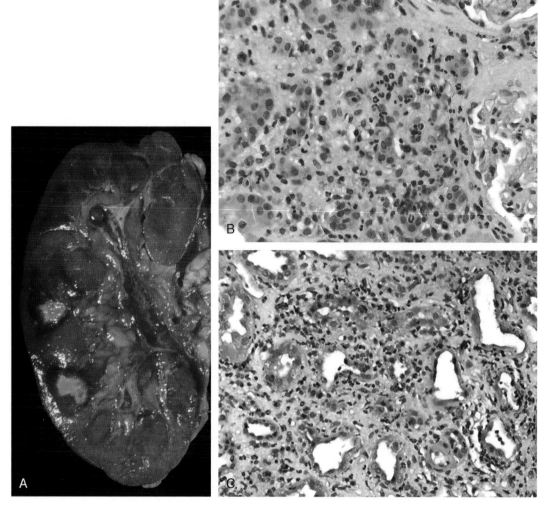

Figure 15-6. Acute pyelonephritis. **A,** Nephrectomy specimen grossly shows acute pyelonephritis with abscess formation. **B,** Acute pyelonephritis with abundant neutrophils invading tubules and filling the interstitium adjacent to a relatively normal-appearing glomerulus. **C,** Acute pyelonephritis with a mixed inflammatory infiltrate in the interstitium composed of lymphocytes, neutrophils, and abundant eosinophils. Tubulitis is multifocal.

Mixed infections are detected in 19% of patients.[70] The infectious route is usually thought to be hematogenous, and gas-forming bacteria, high tissue glucose levels, decreased tissue perfusion, and an inadequate immune response are the four factors that are considered important in the development of emphysematous pyelonephritis.[73,96] Emphysematous pyelonephritis has also been described in the parenchyma of tumors.[97] Surgical intervention is ultimately required, because antibiotics are usually not effective.[70,73]

Chronic Pyelonephritis

Chronic pyelonephritis is a chronic tubulointerstitial disease caused by bacterial infection, vesicoureteral reflux (also termed chronic nonobstructive pyelonephritis), or urinary tract obstruction (also termed obstructive pyelonephritis). It is responsible for 5% to 15% of cases of end-stage renal disease. Other causes of chronic interstitial nephritis include exogenous agents such as

drugs, including analgesics (nonsteroidal anti-inflammatory drugs), chemotherapeutic agents (cis-platinum, methyl CCMU), cyclosporine, and lithium, and heavy metals such as lead and cadmium.[70,73,85,88]

Patients with reflux nephropathy often present with flank pain but may be asymptomatic. Uremia, polyuria, and polydipsia may result.[70,73,88]

Grossly, diffuse scarring may be present in reflux nephropathy. Microscopically, there may be tubular atrophy, interstitial fibrosis, chronic inflammation (Fig. 15-7), and glomerulosclerosis that may manifest in a focal segmental glomerulosclerosis pattern.[70,73,88]

Xanthogranulomatous Pyelonephritis

Xanthogranulomatous pyelonephritis is a chronic inflammatory condition that is caused by pyogenic infection of the kidney, usually secondary to staghorn calculi (70% of cases), most commonly by *Proteus* or *E. coli*.[70] The process usually begins with

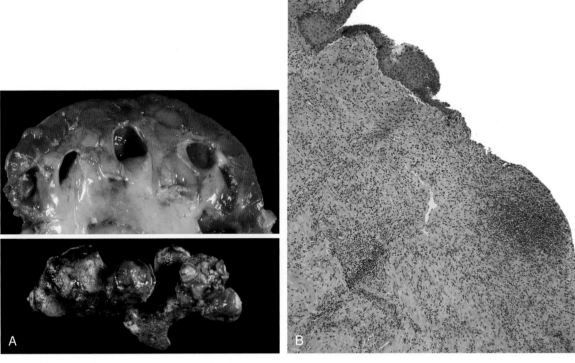

Figure 15-7. Chronic pyelonephritis. **A,** Gross specimen that microscopically exhibited chronic pyelonephritis. The chronic pyelonephritis in this case was caused, at least in part, by a large staghorn calculus, which caused the dilated renal pelvis and calyces. **B,** Chronic pyelonephritis characterized microscopically by numerous mononuclear lymphocytes singly and in aggregates in the interstitium and underneath the urothelium.

suppurative inflammation that may extend into the pelvic mucosa and sinus fat with edema and fat necrosis. Eventually, the cortex, retroperitoneal tissue, and perinephric fat may be involved.[70,73,88]

Approximately 70% of the patients are women who present clinically with fever, flank pain, and pyuria. Imaging studies demonstrate a lipid-rich mass, and calculi may be seen. The affected kidney may be completely destroyed; eventually, a nephrectomy may be required.[70,73,88]

Grossly, the renal pelvis is dilated, with thickened walls containing a staghorn calculus, and there may be a yellow, tumor-like nodular mass replacing the renal pyramids. A diffuse form with widespread involvement of the renal parenchyma is most common; however, a segmental form, often involving a pole of the kidney, may be present, particularly in children. A focal form, also referred to as the tumefactive form, lacks communication with the pelvis and is not associated with pyelitis, calculi, or urinary tract obstruction. Nephrectomy is often required.[70,73,88]

Microscopically, there is a central nidus of necrotic debris and neutrophils surrounded by a zone of foamy macrophages (Fig. 15-8). Peripherally, there is a fibroblastic proliferation. Immunohistochemical stains for CD68 may be used to demonstrate the prominent population of macrophages. The reactive fibrous tissue is vimentin-positive and keratin-negative. This is helpful in ruling out carcinoma, which can mimic xanthogranulomatous pyelonephritis histologically, because the foamy macrophages can look like clear cell renal cell carcinoma. The presence of mitoses and atypia favors a diagnosis of carcinoma. The spindled areas often raise the possibility of a spindle-cell

neoplasm.[70,73,88] Xanthogranulomatous pyelonephritis also needs to be distinguished from inflammatory malignant fibrous histiocytoma that contains numerous acute inflammatory cells in addition to scattered atypical neoplastic cells.

Malakoplakia

Malakoplakia is an inflammatory disorder that occurs in the urinary tract[98-101] and in a number of other organs, including the prostate,[102] testis,[103] vagina, gastrointestinal tract (primarily the large intestine),[104] lung, bone, brain, and skin.[70,73] Early descriptions were by von Hansemann[105] and by Michaelis and Gutman.[106] It is rather uncommon, and the bladder is involved 4 to 10 times more commonly than the upper urinary tract; renal involvement is relatively rare. *E. coli* is the most common agent. It is thought that megalocytic interstitial nephritis (MIN) is a precursor lesion (see later discussion).[70,73,107]

Clinically, patients have fever, flank pain, and renal dysfunction, eventually leading to renal failure in most cases of renal involvement.[70,73,108] Females are affected more commonly than males (4:1 for malakoplakia in general,[109] 3:1 for the renal form[110]). Patients from childhood to older adulthood are affected,[110,111] and involvement is bilateral in up to 50% of patients.[70,73,112]

Macroscopically, the kidneys show dilated pelves and calyces due to the obstructive process. The mucosa of the bladder and, less commonly, the ureter and renal pelvis shows yellow-brown, soft (*malakos*) plaques (*plakos*), often with a central umbilication

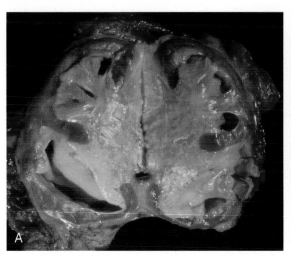

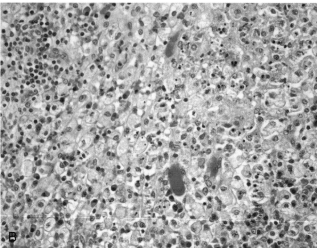

Figure 15-8. Xanthogranulomatous pyelonephritis. **A,** Gross specimen of a kidney with xanthogranulomatous pyelonephritis showing yellow areas in the renal parenchyma. **B,** Microscopic appearance showing abundant foamy macrophages in a case of xanthogranulomatous pyelonephritis.

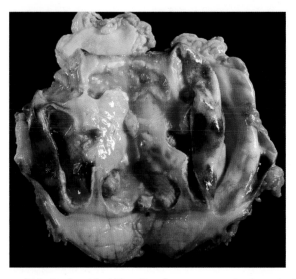

Figure 15-9. Renal malakoplakia with yellow areas appreciated grossly that histologically were malakoplakia.

(Fig. 15-9). Similar nodules may be present in the parenchyma. Microscopically, there are large masses of eosinophilic histiocytes in the interstitium (von Hansemann histiocytes), many of which contain granular eosinophilic cytoplasm and basophilic inclusions (Michaelis-Gutman bodies), which can be highlighted with PAS, iron, or calcium stains. The histologic appearance is similar in the testis (see Fig. 15-26). Renal tubules may be destroyed.[70,73]

Megalocytic Interstitial Nephritis

MIN is similar to malakoplakia characterized by a prominent histiocytic infiltrate, often leading to tumor formation. Unlike malakoplakia, MIN does not contain Michaelis-Gutmann bodies (Fig. 15-10).[70,73]

Grossly, MIN may be solitary, sometimes forming a cortical nodule, and tumor-like. Alternatively, MIN may consist of multiple foci, comprising numerous gray nodules. Microscopically, there are large numbers of polygonal cells with coarse granular eosinophilic cytoplasm containing PAS-positive material. Some contend that MIN is simply malakoplakia that cannot be strictly diagnosed as such, possibly because it is an early stage of malakoplakia.[70,73,113]

Transplant-Related Renal Infections

A number of infections occur in the post-transplantation setting. These include a variety of bacterial, viral, and fungal infections that are typically seen in any postsurgical patient or in immuno-compromised patients. The most characteristic infections are BK virus nephropathy and post-transplantation lymphoproliferative disorder (PTLD) (Table 15-4).[114]

BK Nephropathy

BK polyomavirus, a member of the Papovaviridae family composed of double-stranded circular DNA viruses, causes nucleo-megaly, pale intranuclear inclusions, and karyolysis. It was first observed in 1971, in a Sudanese renal transplant recipient who had ureteral obstruction secondary to a virally induced distal ureteral mass; the name "BK" came from the initials of that first patient.[51,73,115-125]

The virus is small and nonenveloped, with structural similarities to simian virus 40 (SV40). BK virus is a normal inhabitant of urothelium but rarely causes morbidity in immunocompetent individuals. Polyomavirus typically has striking intranuclear viral inclusions in a background of interstitial nephritis and tubular injury (Fig. 15-11). The intranuclear viral inclusions have been classified into four types: type 1 has classic basophilic inclusions; type 2 is eosinophilic and granular with an incomplete halo; type 3 is finely granular without a halo; and type 4 has markedly

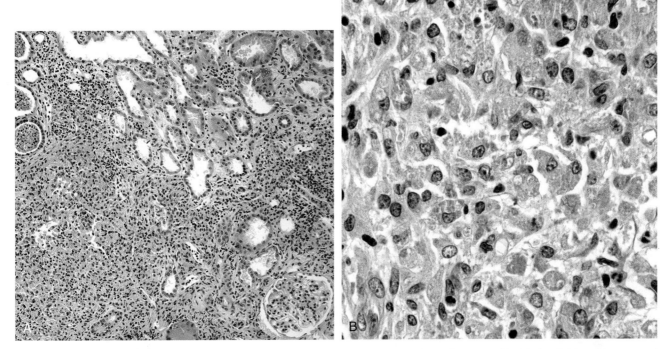

Figure 15-10. Megalocytic interstitial nephritis (MIN). **A,** Low-power view of renal parenchyma shows a dense inflammatory infiltrate in the tubulointerstitium composed of mononuclear cells including lymphocytes and macrophages and abundant eosinophilic cytoplasm with tubular atrophy, necroinflammatory tubular debris, and a relatively preserved glomerulus (H&E stain). **B,** High-power view of a PAS-stained specimen shows abundant polygonal macrophages with PAS-positive cytoplasmic material; some have convoluted nuclei with prominent nucleoli and a few admixed neutrophils. Some consider this entity to be in the spectrum of malakoplakia. In contrast to malakoplakia, MIN does not produce Michaelis-Gutmann bodies.

Table 15-4 Typical Time Course of Selected Common Infections after Transplantation

Interval (mo)	Infection
<1	Bacteria (MRSA, VRE, *Clostridium difficile, Pseudomonas*), fungi (*Candida, Aspergillus*) Wound infections and other common infections Donor-derived infections: HSV, LCMV, rhabdovirus (rabies), WNV, HIV, *Trypanosoma cruzi*
1-6	BK nephropathy, *C. difficile*, HCV, adenovirus, influenza, *Cryptococcus, Mycobacterium tuberculosis*
>6	Community-acquired pneumonia and other bacterial and viral infections, fungi (e.g., *Aspergillus*), CMV, HBV, HCV, BK nephropathy, PTLD

CMV, cytomegalovirus; HBV, hepatitis B virus; HCV, hepatitis C virus; HIV, human immunodeficiency virus; HSV, herpes simplex virus; LCMV, lymphocytic choriomeningitis virus; MRSA, methicillin-resistant *Staphylococcus aureus*; PTLD, post-transplantation lymphoproliferative disorder; VRE, vancomycin-resistant enterococci; WNV, West Nile virus.
Data from Fishman JA: Infection in solid-organ transplant recipients. N Engl J Med 2007;357:2601-2614.

enlarged nuclei with clumped irregular chromatin and prominent nucleoli.

In addition to the viral cytopathic effect, which is most notably observed in renal tubular epithelial cells, there is usually prominent tubulointerstitial nephritis, composed primarily of lymphocytes. Active polyomavirus can be detected in approximately 65% of renal transplant recipients through careful microscopic examination or urinary cytology (which shows the characteristic "decoy cells" that display inclusions and mimic urothelial carcinoma in situ); however, only about 26% of patients show functional renal impairment.[126]

Immunohistochemistry, which typically employs antibodies to the large T antigen of SV40, has proved to be useful in demonstrating virally infected cells, although the SV40 antibody can cross-react with the large T antigen of BK and JC viruses. The virus can also be seen ultrastructurally. Plasma viral loads may be useful in the diagnosis of BK nephropathy.[56,73,114,127-131]

Post-Transplantation Lymphoproliferative Disorder

PTLD is a lymphoproliferative disorder that in many cases manifests as a frank lymphoma; it arises in immunocompromised hosts such as recipients of solid organ or bone marrow allografts. Many cases of PTLD are driven by EBV, and most are of the B-cell type. Some are of the T-cell type. PTLD is estimated to occur in 1% of renal allograft recipients. Among renal allograft patients with PTLD, the allograft kidney is affected in more than 30% of the cases. PTLD restricted to the kidney transplant (approximately 12% of cases) occurs early (about 5

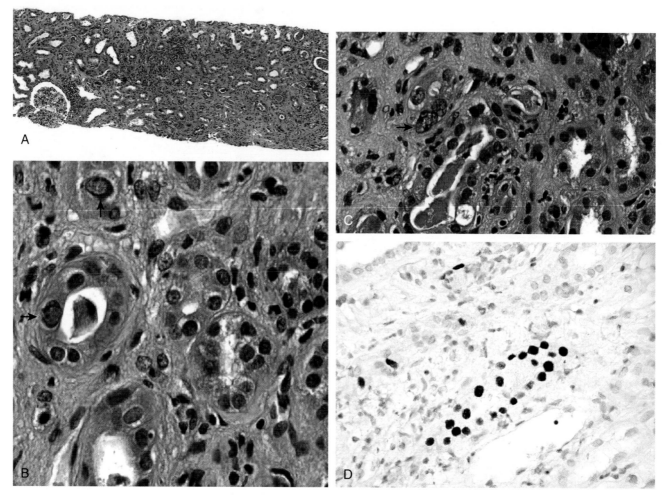

Figure 15-11. BK nephropathy. **A,** Low-power view shows prominent interstitial nephritis. **B** and **C,** High-power views show nuclear viral cytopathic effect. **D,** Immunohistochemistry for the simian virus 40 (SV40) antigen is used to detect the BK virus in BK nephropathy.

months) after surgery. PTLD is most often of donor origin, and the prognosis can be favorable with treatment, which may include reduction in immunosuppression, irradiation, antiviral drugs (acyclovir, ganciclovir, interferon-alfa), or chemotherapy.[132] Chemotherapy regimens using anti-CD20 (rituximab) have been useful.[114,132,133]

Pathologic features of PTLD involving the kidney include swollen kidneys with blurring of the corticomedullary junction and diffuse petechiae. Involvement is usually vaguely nodular and composed of mononuclear cells with enlarged nuclei, prominent nucleoli, and mitoses; the cells of PTLD may be monomorphic or polymorphic (Fig. 15-12). Necrosis, often described as presenting a serpiginous pattern, may be present. Cells may have blast-like features. PTLD may be confused with allograft rejection, because features mimicking rejection, such as tubulitis and endarteritis, may be present. In PTLD, there may be admixed plasma cells, but granulocytes and macrophages are not seen as commonly as they are in rejection.[114,132]

Most PTLD cases (85-90%) express CD20, and in-situ hybridization for EBV-encoded RNA (EBER) usually shows prominent staining in the atypical lymphoid cells. By contrast,

rejection usually shows a predominance of CD3- and CD68-positive cells.[114,132]

Other Infections

Direct infection of the kidney is an important cause of illness, particularly in immunocompromised patients and transplant recipients; however, various renal diseases are observed in different geographic areas around the world as disorders normally considered endemic to those regions.[73]

Mycobacterial Infections

According to studies in the United States and other Western countries, approximately 5% of patients with tuberculosis have renal involvement. However, individuals in areas of the world other than the United States appear to have a higher incidence of renal involvement, and it is possible that renal disease is underestimated as an extrapulmonary manifestation of tuberculosis infection.[73,134] Additionally, mycobacterial organisms other than

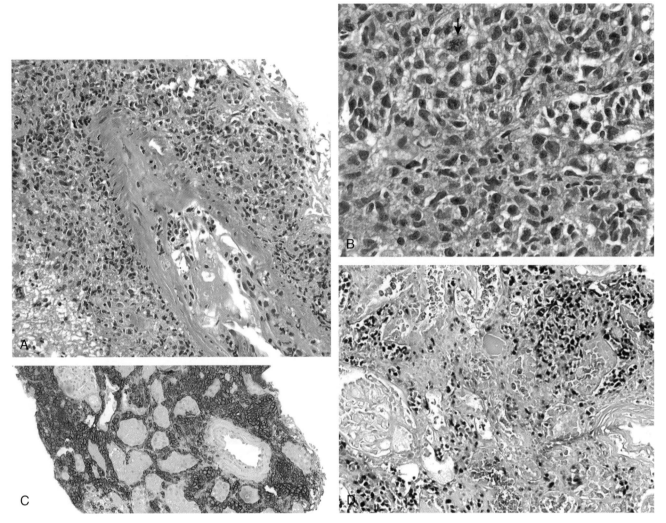

Figure 15-12. Post-transplantation lymphoproliferative disorder (PTLD) involving the kidney. **A,** Prominent lymphoid infiltrate is appreciable at low power. **B,** Prominent lymphoid infiltrate with mitosis. **C,** CD20 immunohistochemical stain is positive, indicating the majority of cells are B cells. **D,** In situ hybridization for Epstein-Barr virus (EBV)–encoded RNA is positive in numerous cells, indicating that the PTLD is EBV-driven.

M. tuberculosis also cause renal disease, including *Mycobacterium avium-intracellulare, Mycobacterium bovis, Mycobacterium kansasii,* and *Mycobacterium leprae.* Risk factors for renal mycobacterial infection include transplantation, HIV, and other causes of immunosuppression. Renal tuberculosis may be cavitary or miliary.[73,134]

Cavitary tuberculosis of the kidney often occurs through an ascending infection from a lower urinary tract infection. The renal medulla is severely affected, with epithelioid caseating granulomas that become confluent and eventually form cavities, often with associated papillary necrosis. Renal involvement is frequently unilateral, and renal function may be largely preserved. Renal failure occurs in approximately 12% of patients.[73,134,135,137]

Grossly, in cavitary tuberculosis, the kidney may be smaller or larger than normal, and there may be irregular surface scarring. The pelves and calyces may be dilated, constricted, or deformed. The parenchyma may show atrophy, calcification, and foci of caseating necrosis (sometimes termed tuberculous pyonephrosis or a "chalk," "cement," or "putty" kidney) (Fig. 15-13).

The appearance may even mimic a neoplasm (i.e., renal cell carcinoma). Microscopically, caseating necrosis with surrounding granulomatous inflammation with plasma cells and calcification (i.e., tubercles) are observed. Langhans-type giant cells may be seen as a component of the granulomatous inflammation. Stains to detect acid-fast bacilli are often useful.[73,134,136]

Miliary tuberculosis of the kidney occurs as a consequence of disseminated infection. Grossly, there are white nodules (tubercles) approximately 1 mm in diameter occurring at a higher density in the cortex than in the medulla. Microscopically, there is granulomatous inflammation with caseating granulomas containing epithelioid histiocytes and a mixed inflammatory infiltrate of neutrophils, lymphocytes, monocytes, and plasma cells.

Tuberculoid forms of leprosy (*M. leprae*) may involve the kidney, affecting about 70% of patients based on autopsy studies. Microscopically, there is diffuse infiltration of macrophages and cells filled with bacilli. Chronic tubulointerstitial nephritis composed of a mononuclear infiltrate with interstitial fibrosis and

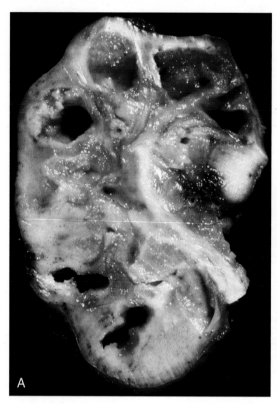

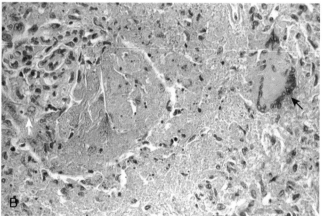

Figure 15-13. Renal tuberculosis. **A,** Gross appearance of renal tuberculosis with extensive parenchymal destruction. **B,** Microscopic appearance of renal tuberculosis showing extensive caseating cortical necrosis (with the amorphous background) and a Langhans giant cell embedded in the necrosis.

tubular atrophy may be present. Coexisting glomerulonephritis and amyloidosis may be present.[73,134,138]

Fungal Infections

The most common fungal organisms affecting the kidney are of the genus *Candida*, including *C. albicans*, *Candida* (formerly *Torulopsis*) *glabrata*, and other *Candida* species. Other organisms implicated include *Aspergillus, Cryptococcus, Coccidioides, Histoplasma, Blastomyces, Paracoccidioides,* and *Mucor* species. Infection of the kidney often results from hematogenous dissemination, particularly in cases of fungal sepsis. Histologically, fungal infections often show a prominent granulomatous inflammation. Because the PAS stain is frequently used as routine stain to evaluate basement membranes in renal biopsy specimens, it is also a good stain to evaluate for fungi.[73,139]

Candida infections, mostly *C. albicans*, spread to the kidney from other locations through hematogenous dissemination, particularly in immunosuppressed, newborn, diabetic, or granulocytopenic patients. Grossly, papillary necrosis may be present. Abscesses with a miliary pattern may be recognized. Fungus balls may be present in the pelves and calices. Microscopically, the inflammatory response may be brisk or practically nonexistent. Cortical abscesses that destroy glomeruli may be seen. Pseudohyphae and budding yeast 2 to 4 μm in diameter can usually be identified and may be recognized with PAS or Grocott methenamine silver (GMS) stains (Fig. 15-14). *C. albicans* infection may also result in emphysematous pyelonephritis. *C. glabrata* produces manifestations similar to those of *C. albicans.* Immu-

nohistochemistry may be useful in the identification of *Candida* species, which may sometimes be difficult to distinguish from *Histoplasma, Cryptococcus,* or *Pneumocystis.*[56,73,140-142]

Aspergillosis is caused by *Aspergillus* species, the most common of which is *Aspergillus fumigatus.* Hematogenous dissemination is the usual route of infection. *Aspergillus* affects a similar patient population as *Candida* and in addition affects patients with invasive bronchial infections or pneumonitis and those receiving corticosteroid therapy. There is usually a mononuclear inflammation with neutrophils, abscesses, and infarcts, and branching septated hyphae 3 to 5 μm in size can be identified with PAS or GMS stains (Fig. 15-15). Immunohistochemistry may be useful in confirming the identity of the organisms.[56,73,140-144]

Cryptococcus neoformans infection usually results from hematogenous dissemination, often from the respiratory tract and classically from avian (e.g., pigeon) exposure. Immunosuppressed and neutropenic patients are particularly susceptible. Parenchymal abscesses, granulomas, and necrosis are identified in the cortex and medulla, sometimes with papillary necrosis, severe tubular injury, and destruction. However, there may be a paucity of inflammation. The organisms are 4 to 20 μm in diameter and are surrounded by a polysaccharide capsule, which stains with mucicarmine, Alcian blue, and PAS. Immunohistochemistry is also available.[56,73,140-142]

Histoplasma capsulatum, the causative agent of histoplasmosis, is endemic in the Mississippi and Ohio River valleys and in South and Central America. It is usually contracted through inhalation of soil that is contaminated with bird or bat droppings

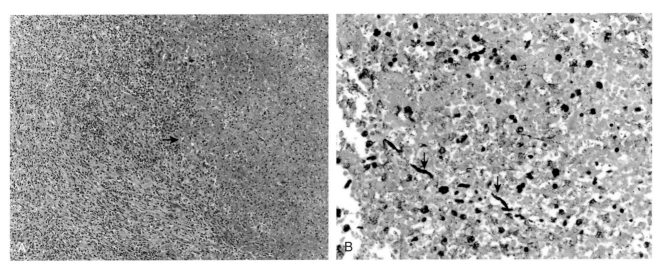

Figure 15-14. *Candida* pyelonephritis. **A,** *Candida* pyelonephritis forming an abscess cavity *(arrow).* **B,** GMS stain reveals several yeast cells (blastoconidia) and pseudohyphae with constrictions or septations between the cells *(arrows).*

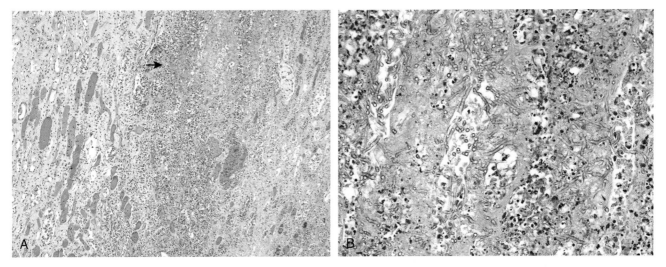

Figure 15-15. *Aspergillus* pyelonephritis. **A,** Low-power appearance of *Aspergillus* causing a pyelonephritis. The infection in this case was caused by a disseminated systemic *Aspergillus* infection. **B,** High-power appearance of *Aspergillus,* showing dichotomously branching hyphae on an H&E-stained section.

containing the fungus. The kidneys are affected in 40% of patients with progressive disseminated histoplasmosis. Histologically, there is typically a significant degree of tubulointerstitial inflammation, which may be granulomatous and caseating. Macrophages show large numbers of nonencapsulated, intracellular, oval or round yeast forms measuring up to 5 μm in diameter, some of which may display budding (Fig. 15-16). GMS stains, immunohistochemistry, and immunofluorescence are useful for their recognition.[56,73,142,145,146]

Coccidioides immitis, the causative agent of coccidioidomycosis, is endemic in the southwestern United States. The infective form consists of arthrospores from arthroconidia. The fungus also exists in nature in a mycelial form. The kidneys are affected in approximately one third of patients who die of disseminated infection. Multiple abscesses and minute granulomas may be present, along with caseous or suppurative necrosis. Thick-walled spherules (Fig. 15-17), approximately 100 μm in diameter, contain endospores 5 to 30 μm in diameter. Special stains, such as GMS and PAS, may be useful in highlighting the organisms. Immunohistochemistry is available but is usually not needed for diagnosis.[73,141,142]

Blastomyces dermatitidis, the causative agent of blastomycosis, is present notably in the southeastern United States and in the Ohio and Mississippi River areas. It affects males approximately four times more frequently than females. Grossly, the renal capsule may have perinephric abscesses and draining sinuses. Microscopically, microabscesses and epithelioid and giant cell granulomas, some of which are caseating, are present. Yeast cells measure 8 to 15 μm and may have a double-contoured appearance with broad-based budding of the daughter cells. GMS stains and immunohistochemistry may be useful in the diagnosis.[73,141,142]

Paracoccidioidomycosis (i.e., South American blastomycosis) is caused by *Paracoccidioides brasiliensis,* which is endemic

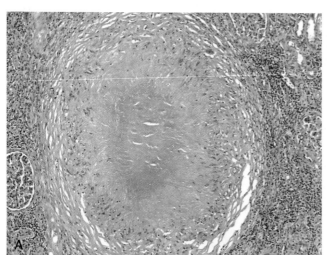

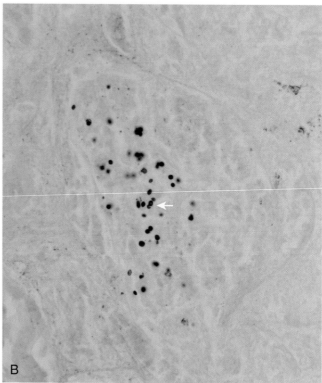

Figure 15-16. Granulomatous pyelonephritis due to histoplasmosis. **A,** Caseating granulomas that were found throughout the kidney. **B,** GMS stain reveals small, black-staining, 2- to 3-μm, budding yeast cells *(arrow).*

to South America, Central America, and Mexico. Infection is by inhalation with pulmonary involvement and secondary spread to other organs, including the kidneys. Microscopically, there is often prominent granulomatous inflammation with giant cells, often with caseating necrosis. Nonbudding forms, approximately 10 μm in diameter, predominate, but multiple buds may radiate from a single cell, resembling the steering wheel of a ship (mariner's wheel). GMS stains and immunohistochemistry may be useful.[73,142]

Mucormycosis infection (i.e., zygomycosis) occurs through hematogenous dissemination, usually from respiratory infections. Immunocompromised patients and diabetics are particularly susceptible to disseminated infection. On microscopic examination, there is suppurative necrotizing inflammation with interlobular and arcuate artery thrombosis. The hyphae are broad and non-septated, with right-angle branching.[73,140,142]

Syphilis

The kidney may be affected in tertiary and congenital syphilis. Primarily glomeruli are affected, leading to membranous nephropathy with granular immune deposits in glomeruli and the tubular basement membrane and the resultant nephrotic syndrome, particularly in congenital syphilis. Microscopically, gumma and tubulointerstitial nephritis composed of mononuclear cells, plasma cells, and interstitial fibrosis may be present. Attachment of *Treponema* organisms to endothelium, as mediated by fibronectin, complement, and humoral- and cell-

mediated immune responses, are thought to be important mechanisms for infection.[73,147]

Filamentous Bacteria: Actinomycosis and Nocardiosis

The filamentous bacteria from the genuses *Actinomyces* (*Actinomyces israelii*) and *Nocardia* (mainly *Nocardia asteroides* but also *Nocardia farcinica*) may involve the kidneys, primarily in immunocompromised individuals. Microscopically, both organisms produce suppurative infections. In *Actinomyces* infections, necrosis may be present. So-called sulfur granules (bacterial macrocolonies) may be present in the urine or sinus tracts and may be appreciated on sections stained with H&E, Gram, or GMS stains or immunofluorescence. In nocardial infections, vascular thromboses may be present with solitary or multiple abscesses, diffuse pyelonephritis, or draining sinus tracts. *Nocardia* can also form granules and large colonies, which can be classified as mycetomas. *Nocardia* can be identified with Gram, PAS, or GMS stains.[73,145] Unlike *Actinomyces*, *Nocardia* also stains with acid-fast stain.[139]

Rickettsia

Rickettsial infections are arthropod-borne zoonoses that are caused by small, gram-negative, rod-shaped bacteria. These include Rocky Mountain spotted fever (caused by *Rickettsia rickettsii*), Mediterranean spotted fever (*Rickettsia conorii*), scrub typhus (*Rickettsia tsutsugamushi*) transmitted by mites, and epi-

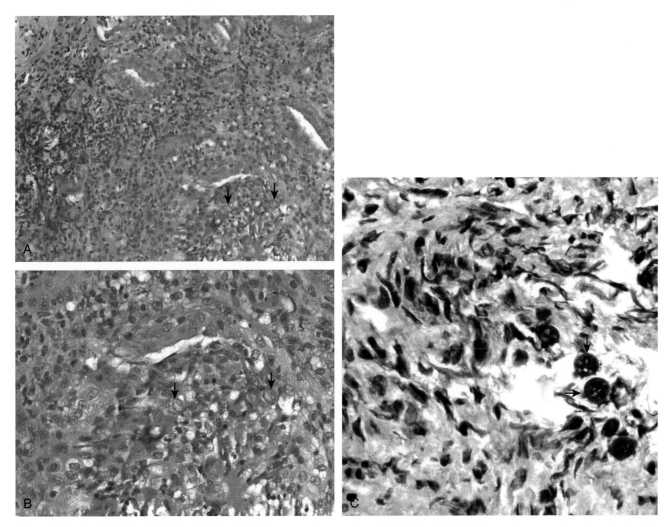

Figure 15-17. *Coccidioides immitis* involving the kidney. **A,** Medium power shows prominent interstitial nephritis. **B,** High power shows several organism spherules with vaguely defined endospores. **C,** High power shows several organism spherules with endospores highlighted with a PAS stain.

demic typhus (*Rickettsia prowazekii*) transmitted by body lice. All cause varying degrees of tubulointerstitial nephritis and tubular injury, and the inflammation is often vasculocentric and composed of an infiltrate of lymphocytes and histiocytes. Rocky Mountain spotted fever and epidemic typhus in particular show vasculitis, sometimes with appreciable rickettsial organisms or antigens in the endothelial cells. Scrub typhus is milder, with less severe vascular changes and only rare thrombosis and necrosis. Acute renal failure may occur.[73,74]

R. rickettsii, the causative agent of Rocky Mountain spotted fever, is transmitted by the bites of ticks. Small mammals are reservoirs. In the early stage of infection, there is often fever and a rash. Histologically, in the kidney, there is often a tubulo-interstitial nephritis composed of a mononuclear infiltrate with mononuclear cells, neutrophils, edema, and tubular cell necrosis. Inflammation is often vasculocentric, and endothelial cell necrosis is a characteristic feature. Death due to renal failure may occur, particularly in the elderly and in those who do not obtain rapid treatment. Immunofluorescence and immunohistochemis-

try can be useful in the diagnosis, because *Rickettsia* antigens may be demonstrated in the capillary endothelium; serologic methods are also helpful to detect antibodies to spotted fever group (SFG) rickettsiae.[56,73,148-151]

Leptospirosis

Leptospira species, including *Leptospira icterohaemorrhagiae*, the causative agent of Weill disease; *Leptospira pomona; Leptospira bataviae; Leptospira canicola; Leptospira shermani;*, and *Leptospira grippotyphosa*, are long, thin aerobic spirochetes that can be responsible for human infection. Patients typically present with jaundice, renal dysfunction, or even acute renal failure. *Leptospira* are typically considered to be enzootic diseases with reservoirs in skunks, foxes, rodents, livestock, and ducks. The organism is present in the urine of these animals, and humans are infected through direct contact or via contaminated water. In Weill disease, the kidneys are enlarged, edematous, and brownish yellow. Histologically, there is prominent acute tubular injury and necrosis with a mixed inflammatory infiltrate of monocytes, plasma cells, and neutrophils with petechial hemorrhages and vasculitis. A special stain that is sometimes used is the Levaditi stain, which is a special silver nitrate stain, although it requires special expertise.[73,74,152]

Parasitic Infections

Parasitic infections can cause renal dysfunction and gross and microscopic abnormalities in the kidney through direct and indirect mechanisms. Some changes result from the direct effects of parasitic infestation or deposition of parasitic eggs in the kidney, but changes may also occur due to inflammatory mediators released by or as a response to the parasites. Parasitic infections that may affect the kidney include malaria, schistosomiasis, filariasis, microsporidiosis, amebiasis, and hydatidosis. Microfilariae incite granulomatous inflammatory responses. Amebic abscesses in the kidneys (primarily caused by *E. histolytica*) may occur. Microsporidia may lead to tubulointerstitial nephritis, and spores may be deposited in the kidney. Other major parasitic infections affecting the kidney are discussed later in this chapter.[73,74]

Malaria
Plasmodium species, transmitted by the bite of the *Anopheles* mosquito, lead to malaria. However, malaria may also be transmitted by blood transfusion or organ transplantation. Glomerular disease may be caused by malaria, leading to proteinuria, hematuria, and nephrotic syndrome. Glomerular disease is particularly a feature of *Plasmodium malariae*. However, *P. malariae* and *Plasmodium falciparum* may also lead to tubulointerstitial injury. Hemoglobinuric acute renal failure may result in the so-called blackwater fever, which occurs in 1% to 4% of patients in endemic areas. Histologically, acute tubular injury and necrosis are seen, along with interstitial nephritis composed primarily of mononuclear cells (lymphocytes) and edema with tubular hemoglobin casts. Parasitized red blood cells become adherent to the endothelium and platelets, leading to occlusion of the microcirculation, which explains many of the pathogenic effects of malaria.[73,153-156]

Schistosomiasis
S. mansoni and *Schistosoma hematobium* are the primary schistosomal organisms that affect the kidney. *S. mansoni* causes glomerulonephritis, leading to nephrotic syndrome. *S. hematobium* causes obstructive uropathy, leading to prominent interstitial inflammation with mononuclear cells and fibrosis. Schistosomal eggs (notably from *S. mansoni*, *S. hematobium*, and *Schistosoma japonicum*) may be localized to the kidney and may incite a granulomatous inflammatory reaction. The eggs of *S. mansoni* (with characteristic large lateral spines) and *S. japonicum* (with small lateral spines) are acid fast, but those of *S. hematobium* (with characteristic terminal spines) are not acid fast.[73,157,158]

Hydatidosis
Larval forms of *Echinococcus granulosus* cause cystic hydatid disease, which is endemic in parts of Latin America, Africa, Turkey, and the Mediterranean region. Cystic hydatid disease is most common in the liver and the lungs, and renal involvement is usually accompanied by hydatid disease in other organs. Isolated disease is rare. Hydatid cysts or grapelike material may be passed in the urine, but only in a minority (5-25%) of cases. Renal cysts may be treated by cystectomy or marsupialization, although nephrectomy may be required.[73,159,160]

Renal Glomerular Disease Caused by Infection

A number of infections can cause renal dysfunction and various renal diseases that affect the glomeruli as a prominent pattern of injury, including bacteria (post-streptococcal and other post-infectious glomerulonephritides), viruses (particularly hepatitis), malaria, schistosomal infection, echinococcal infection (hydatid disease), and filarial infection (Table 15-5).[161,162] Clinically, these disorders often lead to nephrotic syndrome, but disease may range from mild proteinuria or hematuria to the nephrotic syndrome, the nephritic syndrome, renal insufficiency, or rapidly progressive glomerulonephritis. Organisms that produce glomerular disorders may give rise to a number of patterns of glomerular injury (Table 15-6), primarily proliferative disorders such as diffuse proliferative, membranoproliferative, or mesangioproliferative glomerulonephritis. Membranous nephropathy, focal segmental glomerulosclerosis (FSGS) (Fig. 15-18), minimal change disease, and minimal change disease–like lesions may all be the glomerular manifestations of systemic infections.[73,163]

Postinfectious (Post-streptococcal) Glomerulonephritis
One of the classic glomerular diseases associated with infection is post-streptococcal glomerulonephritis (PSGN) and other postinfectious glomerulonephritides. Acute glomerulonephritis has been recognized as a disorder for some time, since before it was recognized histologically. Hippocrates first noticed the association between flank pain and dark urine (hematuria) which eventually leads to oliguria or anuria. The English physician Richard Bright realized the association between scarletina and swelling of the face and lower-extremity edema, and he further described the hematuria and eventual chronic renal failure in some cases of the disorder.[73,163-165]

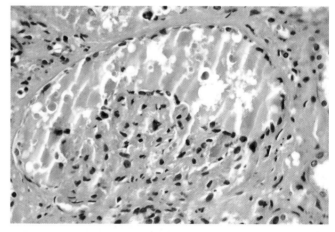

Figure 15-18. Collapsing focal segmental glomerulosclerosis (FSGS) caused by acquired immunodeficiency syndrome (AIDS). The glomerular tuft is collapsed, making Bowman's space appear relatively larger. This is one of many manifestations of viral and other infectious diseases that affect glomeruli. Collapsing FSGS is not observed as commonly as it once was, before the advent of more effective antiviral agents for AIDS.

Table 15-5 Selected Infectious Diseases and Their Renal Glomerular and Other Manifestations

Organism	Pattern of Injury	Presentation and Comments
Bacteria		
Streptococcus	Diffuse proliferative GN	Nephritic syndrome
Treponema pallidum (syphilis)	Membranous GN	
Other	Postinfectious, from organisms other than *Streptococcus* IgA nephropathy IgA-dominant postinfectious GN, often with *Staphylococcus aureus,* MRSA, and *Staphylococcus epidermidis,* particularly in diabetics[161]	IgG and C3 in a "starry sky" pattern[166] Infections of the gastrointestinal and respiratory tracts Predominance of IgA deposits in mesangium and subepithelial "humps"
Viruses		
Hepatitis B	Membranous GP[162] MPGN[167-170]	Proteinuria/nephrotic syndrome
Hepatitis C	Membranous GP MPGN (type I) Cryoglobulinemic GP Glomerular intracapillary proliferation with or without extracapillary proliferation	Proteinuria/nephrotic syndrome Usually has the pattern of MPGN type I "Pseudolinear" deposits of IgG/IgM and C3[166]
HIV	CGP/HIVAN	Resembles a collapsing variant of FSGS but is now thought to be a distinct entity[166]
Parvovirus B19	Non–HIV–associated CGP	
CMV	Non–HIV–associated CGP CMV glomerulitis	Characteristic inclusions seen in tubulointerstitial disease may be present
Parasites		
Plasmodium malariae	Mesangioproliferative GN MPGN Membranous GP FSGS	Proteinuria/nephrotic syndrome Nephrotic syndrome
Plasmodium falciparum	Tubulointerstitial damage Mesangio-MPGN	Acute renal failure Proteinuria/nephrotic syndrome
Schistosoma hematobium	Hydronephrosis and pyelonephritis	Chronic renal failure
Schistosoma mansoni	Mesangio-MPGN FSGS Membranous GP Amyloidosis (rare) Crescentic GN	Proteinuria Nephrotic syndrome Acute renal failure
Leishmania donovani (kala-azar)	Mesangioproliferative GN MPGN, amyloidosis	Proteinuria Nephrotic syndrome
Trypanosoma brucei subsp. *rhodesiense* and *T. brucei* subsp. *gambiense*	Mesangioproliferative GN (rare)	Proteinuria
Toxoplasma gondii	MPGN FSGS (rare) Tubulointerstitial nephritis	Proteinuria/nephrotic syndrome Nephrotic syndrome (especially congenital toxoplasmosis) Acute renal failure
Trichinella spiralis	Mesangio-MPGN Tubular necrosis	Proteinuria Mild renal failure
Babesia bovis, Babesia divergens, Babesia microti	Tubular necrosis	Acute renal failure
Echinococcus granulosus (hydatid disease)	Cyst (usually solitary) Membranous GP (rare)	Mass effect Nephrotic syndrome

Continued

Table 15-5 Selected Infectious Diseases and Their Renal Glomerular and Other Manifestations—cont'd

Organism	Pattern of Injury	Presentation and Comments
Loa loa, *Wuchereria bancrofti, Brugia malayi* (lymphatic filariasis), *Onchocerca volvulus* (river blindness)	Interstitial nephritis Amyloidosis (rare) Mesanigo-MPGN	Renal failure Nephrotic syndrome Proteinuria or even nephritic syndrome
Wuchereria bancrofti	Acute GN (rare)	Nephritic syndrome
Loa loa	Membranous GP FSGS (rare)	Nephrotic syndrome

CGN, collapsing glomerulopathy; CMV, cytomegalovirus; FSGS, focal segmental glomerulosclerosis; GN, glomerulonephritis; GP, glomerulopathy; HIV, human immunodeficiency virus; HIVAN, HIV-associated nephropathy; Ig, immunoglobulin; MPGN, membranoproliferative glomerulonephritis; MRSA, methicillin-resistant *Staphylococcus aureus.*
Data from: Weiss M, Liapis H, Tomaszewski JE, Arend LJ: Pyelonephritis and other infections, reflux nephropathy, hydronephrosis, and nephrolithiasis. In Jennette JC, Olson JL, Schwartz MM, Silva FG (eds): Heptinstall's Pathology of the Kidney, vol 2, 6th ed. Philadelphia, Lippincott Williams & Wilkins, 2007:991; van Velthuysen ML, Florquin S: Glomerulopathy associated with parasitic infections. Clin Microbiol Rev 2000;13:55-66; and Barisoni L, Meehan S, Arend LJ: Introduction to renal biopsy. In Zhou M (ed): Genitourinary Pathology. Philadelphia, Churchill Livingstone Elsevier, 2007.

Table 15-6 Patterns of Glomerular Injury in Selected Infectious Diseases

Pattern	Light Microscopy	Immunofluorescence Microscopy	Electron Microscopy
Minimal change disease	Normal; lipid in tubules	Negative	Loss (effacement) of foot processes; no deposits
Focal segmental glomerulosclerosis	Focal and segmental sclerosis and hyalinosis	Focal; IgM and C3	Loss (effacement) of foot processes; epithelial denudation
Membranoproliferative GN	Mesangial proliferation; BM thickening; splitting ("tram tracks")	IgG + C3; C1 + C4	Subendothelial deposits
Mesangioproliferative GN	Expanded mesangial matrix and proliferation of mesangial cells	Immunoglobulins in mesangium	Deposits in mesangium
Diffuse proliferative GN	Diffuse proliferation; leukocytic infiltration	Granular IgG and C3 in glomerular BM and mesangium	Subepithelial humps
Membranous GP	Diffuse capillary wall thickening with "spikes"	Granular IgG and C3; diffuse	Subepithelial deposits
IgA Nephropathy	Focal proliferative GN; mesangial expansion/widening	IgA + IgG, IgM, and C3 in mesangium	Mesangial and paramesangial dense deposits, often closely apposed to mesangial cells

BM, basement membrane; GN, glomerulonephritis; GP, glomerulopathy; Ig, immunoglobulin.
Data from Haas M: IgA nephropathy and Henoch Schönlein purpura. In Jennette JC, Olson JL, Schwartz MM, Silva FG (eds): Heptinstall's Pathology of the Kidney, vol 1, 6th ed. Philadelphia, Lippincott Williams & Wilkins, 2007, p 424; van Velthuysen ML, Florquin S: Glomerulopathy associated with parasitic infections. Clin Microbiol Rev 2000;13:55-66; Nadasdy T, Sedmak D: Acute and chronic tubulointerstitial nephritis. In Jennette JC, Olson JL, Schwartz MM, Silva FG (eds): Heptinstall's Pathology of the Kidney, vol 2, 6th ed. Philadelphia, Lippincott Williams & Wilkins, 2007, p 322; and Barisoni L, Meehan S, Arend LJ: Introduction to renal biopsy. In Zhou M (ed): Genitourinary Pathology. Philadelphia, Churchill Livingstone Elsevier, 2007.

Postinfectious glomerulonephritis (PSGN) usually occurs after exposure to group A β-streptococcus type 12, 4, or 1, such as after an upper respiratory tract infection, although other organisms may account for the glomerulonephritis. Clinically, in addition to hematuria and the nephritic syndrome, patients with PSGN have elevated anti–streptolysin-O (ASO) titers and low levels of serum complement. The pediatric population is the most commonly affected age group. Approximately 90% of cases resolve within a few weeks, but adults may have

a less favorable prognosis. Histologically, there is typically a diffuse proliferative glomerulonephritis, often with prominent intracapillary neutrophils (Fig. 15-19). One of the most useful diagnostic features is the presence of amorphous subepithelial, electron-dense deposits on electron microscopy. The deposits are also known as subepithelial humps. In addition, immunofluorescence shows the presence of IgG and C3 in a granular, "starry sky" pattern in the mesangium and capillary walls.[73,163-165]

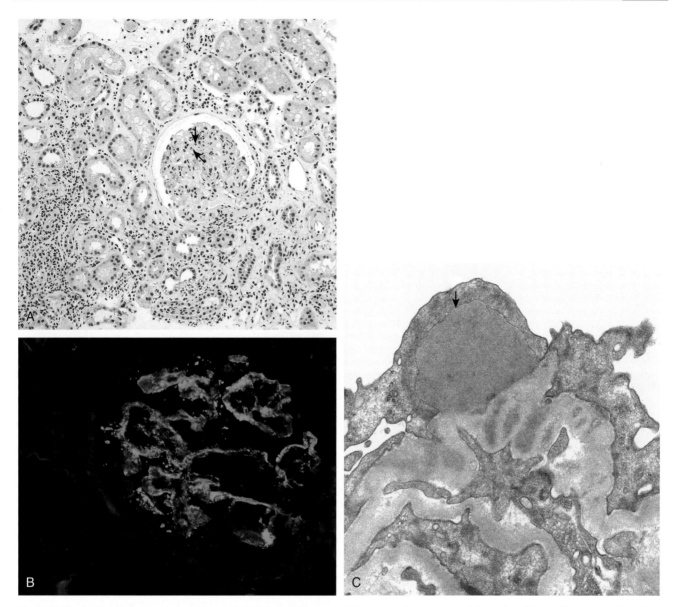

Figure 15-19. Acute poststreptococcal glomerulonephritis (PSGN). **A,** Light microscopic appearance showing increased glomerular cellularity with numerous intracapillary neutrophils *(arrows).* **B,** Immunofluorescence microscopy showing granular positivity for immunoglobulin G, primarily along the periphery of capillary loops. **C,** Electron microscopy showing subepithelial amorphous, electron-dense deposits *(arrow),* also known as subepithelial humps.

Membranoproliferative Glomerulonephritis

Membranoproliferative glomerulonephritis (MPGN) is a pathologic pattern of injury that may appear in association with a number of infectious disorders. One of the most important infectious associations with a MPGN-type pattern occurs in hepatitis virus infections. Hepatitis viruses can produce a number of patterns of injury, but MPGN and cryoglobulinemic glomerulonephritis are some of the most noteworthy. MPGN is characterized by "tram-tracking" or "double contours" of the glomerular basement membrane (GBM). Immune deposits (C3 in all cases and also usually IgG and IgM) are recognized by immunofluorescence, and frequently by IgG and IgM. Ultrastructurally, it can be appreciated that the double contours of the GBM are caused by mesangial matrix and cellular interposition and basement membrane duplication. Subendothelial, electron-dense deposits are appreciated on electron microscopy, and deposits may also sometimes be subepithelial.[73,163,166-171]

At times, a MPGN-like pattern can be associated with cryoglobulins, particularly in cases of hepatitis C; and in these special cases the glomerulonephritis is referred to as a cryoglobulinemic glomerulonephritis. In cryoglobulinemic glomerulonephritis, "pseudothrombi" composed of the cryoglobulin can be recognized in glomerular capillary lumens, particularly with PAS stains. Glomeruli also have intraluminal hypercellularity, and many of these cells can be identified as monocyte-macrophages with a CD68 immunohistochemical stain. Deposits with a somewhat granular, "wormy" substructure can be seen on electron microscopy (Fig. 15-20).[73,163,166-171]

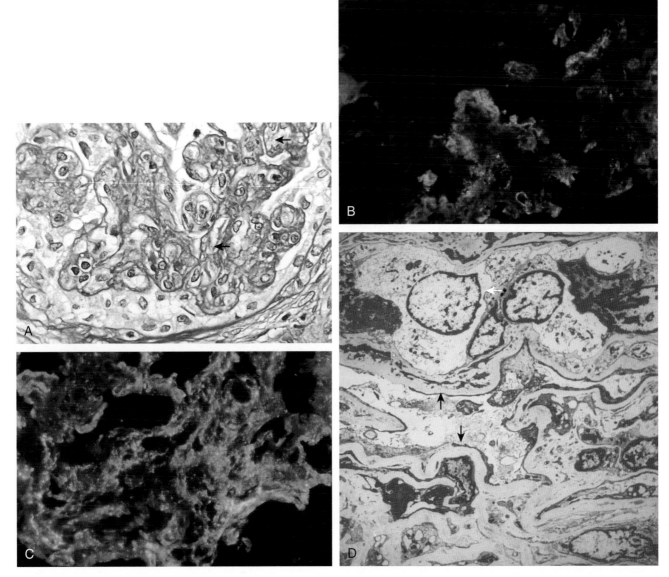

Figure 15-20. Membranoproliferative glomerulonephritis (MPGN) associated with hepatitis C. **A,** Light microscopic appearance of MPGN (type I). There is a lobulated, hypercellular glomerulus with basement membrane duplication *(arrows)*, best appreciated on PAS stains (as shown here) or on silver stains such as the Jones stain. **B,** Immunofluorescence microscopy showing positivity for immunoglobulin (IgM) in a granular pattern, primarily along the periphery of capillary loops but also in the mesangium. Immunofluorescence is typically positive for IgG and C3, but IgM may also be present. **C,** Immunofluorescence microscopy showing positivity for C3 in a granular pattern, primarily in the mesangium. **D,** Electron microscopy shows intracapillary hypercellularity *(white arrow)* and areas of basement membrane duplication with mesangial matrix and cellular interposition *(black arrows)*, corresponding to the areas of duplication seen on the PAS stain.

Bladder Infections

Bacterial Cystitis

The most common population affected by bacterial cystitis includes women of reproductive age (particularly sexually active women 20 to 40 years old). These infections result most commonly from ascending bacterial infections of the distal urethra and introitus. Recurrent cystitis may occur in patients with structural (e.g., bladder exstrophy) or physiologic abnormalities or systemic disease (e.g., diabetes, immunosuppression). Symptoms include frequency, urgency, dysuria, and abdominal and supra-

pubic pain. Common organisms include gram-negative enteric bacteria: *E. coli*, followed by *Proteus* (especially *Proteus mirabilis*), *Enterobacter,* and *Klebsiella* and then by various organisms such as *Staphylococcus saprophyticus* and enterococci. Rare cases are caused by mycobacteria and *Actinomyces.* Typically, there is a chronic inflammatory background, although acute inflammation may predominate. Many special histologic patterns, some of which are discussed later in this chapter, may be present. Of note is granulomatous cystitis, which can occur in a number of situations, notably after BCG treatment of transitional cell (i.e., urothelial) carcinoma of the bladder, although concurrent infections with other mycobacteria cannot be excluded (Figs. 15-21 and 15-22).[3,70,172]

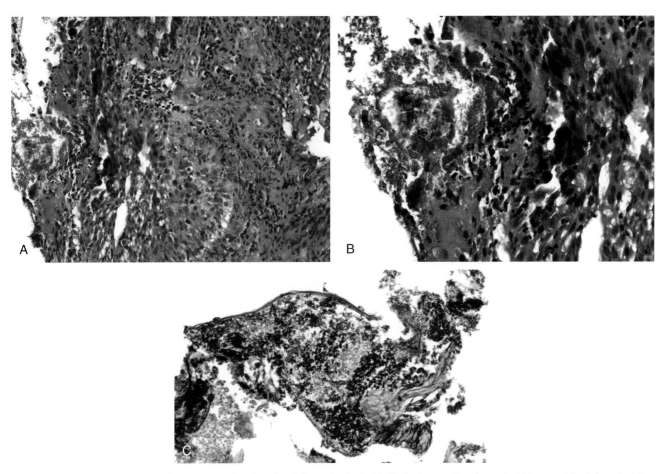

Figure 15-21. Encrusted cystitis. **A** and **B,** H&E-stained sections show inflammation in the bladder lamina propria and necrotic debris covered by fibrin and calcium. **C,** Brown-Hopps tissue Gram stain highlights bacteria in the necrotic debris.

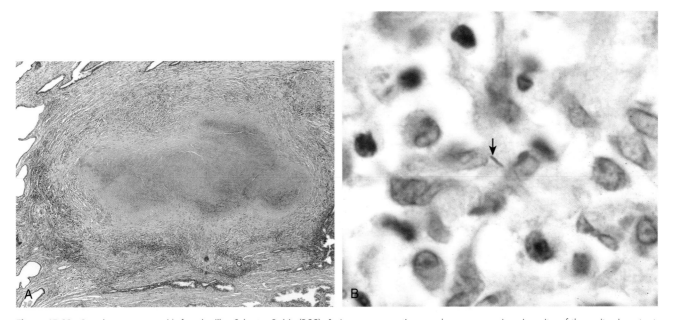

Figure 15-22. Granulomatous prostatitis from bacillus Calmette-Guérin (BCG). **A,** Loose, noncaseating granulomas are seen in various sites of the genitourinary tract, including the bladder, and, as shown here, the prostate. **B,** Acid-fast bacilli *(arrow)* stain positive in a granuloma of the bladder. These would be consistent with BCG infection, with the appropriate history of BCG treatment; however, mycobacterial infection of the bladder (e.g., *Mycobacterium tuberculosis*) cannot be excluded.

Fungal Cystitis

Fungal cystitis occurs in patients with immunosuppression (including those on steroid therapy), indwelling catheters, diabetes, or bladder outlet obstruction. Urinalysis may show pyuria and microhematuria. *C. albicans* is the most common cause. Fungus balls from *Candida* causing obstructive uropathy have been reported. Candiduria may result from noninvasive colonization, low-grade infection, or extensive urinary tract infection. Fungal cystitis occurs less commonly from *Aspergillus, Mucor, Blastomyces, Histoplasma, Cryptococcus,* and *Coccidioides*. Microscopically, there is inflammation in the lamina propria, and there may even be ulceration with identifiable fungal forms.[3,70] Special stains such as silver and PAS stains may be helpful in identifying fungal pseudohyphae and yeast forms. *Cryptococcus* may have large, clear capsules surrounding yeast forms, which can be seen most readily with India ink preparations or mucicarmine stains.[3,70]

Viral Infections

Cystitis caused by viral pathogens is rare. HSV (notably type 2), CMV, and polyomavirus are DNA viruses that affect the urinary tract most commonly. Adenovirus (specifically types 11 and 21) may lead to a hemorrhagic cystitis, particularly in patients receiving chemotherapy or after bone marrow transplantation.[3,57,70] Hemorrhagic cystitis may also be caused by polyomavirus (BK), CMV, human herpesvirus 6 (HHV-6), HSV, or *Strongyloides*. Viruses that can be detected in the urine, sometimes by cytologic or molecular methods, include polyomavirus, papillomavirus, and adenovirus type 2. Viral inclusions are more frequently identifiable by cytology than on tissue sections. RNA viruses and oncogenic RNA viruses (Retroviridae) are not thought to be important pathogens.[3,70]

Herpes Simplex Virus

HSV can lead to hemorrhagic cystitis, particularly in patients with genital herpes, and there have also been reports of this condition in immunocompetent patients, although it is more common in the immunocompromised. Cell enlargement, multinucleation, nuclear molding, and ground glass nuclei are present in a background of acute inflammation, and Cowdry A, eosinophilic, irregular nuclear inclusions may be present. Concurrent BK polyomavirus and acyclovir-resistant HSV infections leading to hemorrhagic cystitis have been reported.[3,173]

Cytomegalovirus

CMV, a member of the herpesvirus family of double-stranded linear DNA viruses, can lead to hemorrhagic cystitis in patients who are immunosuppressed, such as AIDS patients and those receiving chemotherapy for bone marrow transplantation. Urine culture is not sensitive for the diagnosis of CMV in this setting. CMV-infected cells may appear like the infected renal tubular cells shown in Figure 15-5. Intracytoplasmic inclusions can also occasionally be found.[3,51]

BK Polyomavirus

Polyomavirus, the renal disease manifestations of which have already been discussed, is usually acquired at an early age. Clinical manifestations of polyomavirus occur only with immunosuppression, such as after bone marrow transplantation, and can include cystitis and hematuria. Urine cytology can detect polyomavirus, and the cytopathic effect may persist for several months after cessation of symptoms. Recognition of polyomavirus cytopathic effect in routine surgical pathology histologic sections is more difficult than on cytology. Polyomavirus is implicated in BK nephropathy, which typically occurs in the setting of transplantation or immunosuppression and is discussed later.[3,174-176]

Human Papillomavirus

HPV leads to many types of lesions, both neoplastic and nonneoplastic (see Table 15-2). In men, it is the causative agent of condyloma acuminatum. Bladder condylomas may occur when anogenital condylomas extend into the urethra and bladder. Bladder condylomas are more common in women. HPV types 6 and 11 have been found in bladder condylomas. Despite the well-known role of HPV in cervical carcinogenesis, it is controversial whether HPV contributes to all urothelial carcinomas[177,178]; however, it is possible that it plays a role in urothelial carcinogenesis, particularly in the immunosuppressed. Grossly, lesions may be exophytic and may give rise to squamous cell carcinoma (Fig. 15-23). Histologically, condyloma in the bladder consists of papillary fronds of thickened squamous epithelium that may be hyperkeratotic. Koilocytes with perinuclear halos are often present in many of the epithelial cells. Koilocytes can be detected in urine samples. Cytology of condylomas obtained through such methods as brush cytology show a higher yield than urine cytology; however, condylomas of the external genitalia and urethra should be excluded before a diagnosis of a bladder condyloma is made.[3,176]

Parasitic Infections

Schistosomiasis

S. hematobium is endemic to Mediterranean Asia and Africa. It inhabits the pelvic veins and sheds its eggs into the urinary bladder, causing hematuria or chronic cystitis. Urinary egg excretion has diurnal periodicity: shedding is most prominent at midday. *S. hematobium* is recognized by its terminal spine (Fig. 15-24). Rarely, adult "worm" forms may be recognized. These forms usually are paired male and female organisms and usually reside in the venous plexus of the bladder (Fig. 15-25). Histologically, there is typically a chronic inflammatory background. Bladder biopsies may show urothelial squamous and intestinal metaplasia, mural granulomas, fibrosis, and calcified eggs. Chronic infection may eventually lead to fibrosis and calcification of the lower ureters, with resultant renal parenchymal damage and kidney failure. Urothelial squamous cell carcinoma may eventually develop, and this is particularly a problem in certain parts of the world where the infection is endemic, notably Egypt and other areas of Africa. Although they are typically found in the stool, *S. mansoni* eggs (identified by their characteristic lateral spines) may also sometimes be found in the urine.[3,157]

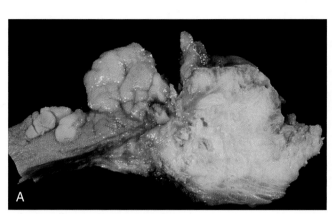
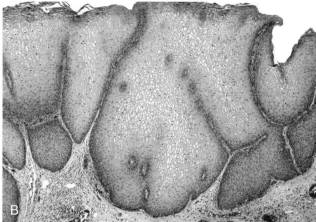

Figure 15-23. Bladder condyloma. **A,** Bladder condyloma with urothelial hyperplasia and koilocytic change. **B,** Squamous cell carcinoma showing an exophytic growth pattern, arising in bladder condyloma. (Images courtesy of Dr. Robert H. Young.)

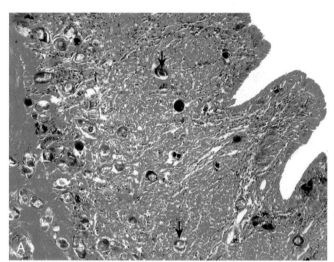
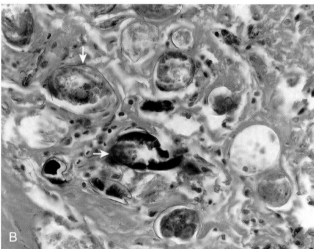

Figure 15-24. Schistosomiasis of the urinary bladder. **A,** Medium-power image shows schistosomal eggs *(arrows)* in the lamina propria of the bladder with a chronic inflammatory background. **B,** High-power view of schistosomal eggs *(arrows)*.

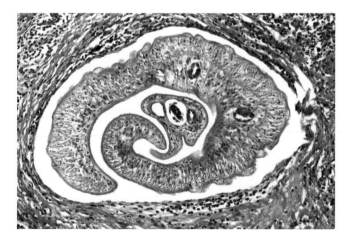

Figure 15-25. Schistosomiasis of the urinary bladder in worm form. The schistosomal organisms in this form usually reside in the venous plexus of the bladder and are present paired as adult male and female worms. (Images courtesy of Dr. Robert H. Young.)

Trichomoniasis

Trichomonas can cause urethritis and cystitis, particularly if there is a coexisting genital trichomoniasis. After HPV, *Trichomonas* is probably the most common sexually transmitted infection in the United States, so recognizing this entity is important. *Trichomoniasis* is increasingly being acknowledged as a cause of nongonococcal urethritis and as a contributor to male factor infertility. Diagnosis is typically established by urine cytology.[3,179-184]

Special Bladder Conditions with an Infectious Association

Malakoplakia

Malakoplakia is a vaguely granulomatous, chronic inflammatory disease that primarily affects the urinary tract, particularly the bladder and ureters, but also other organ systems. Middle-aged women are most commonly affected. Urine culture often isolates *E. coli.* Submucosal aggregates of large histiocytes (von Hansemann cells) containing cytoplasmic Michaelis-Gutmann bodies, thought to consist of mineralized bacterial fragments, are present.[3,185]

Encrusted Cystitis

Encrusted cystitis is a condition in which inorganic salts (e.g., calcium) are deposited in the urinary bladder in areas of urothelial mucosal injury from urea-splitting bacteria, which alkalinize the urine. Necrotic debris covered with fibrin and calcium is deposited in the lamina propria (see Fig. 15-21).[70] Common causative organisms include bacteria with potent urease activity, such as *Corynebacterium* (particularly group D2, now known as *Corynebacterium urealyticum*), but many organisms have been reported. A substantial number of patients have been immunocompromised, particularly after renal transplantation. Urine may contain abundant calcified, mucopurulent debris. The main therapy is antibiotic treatment, as well as acidification of the urine. Excision of the encrusted plaques may be required. Graft nephrectomy has been required in some cases.[186,187]

Emphysematous Cystitis

Emphysematous cystitis is an inflammatory condition of the urinary bladder in which gas-filled cystic spaces (called pockets or blebs) are formed in the wall of the bladder. These can be appreciated grossly or by cystoscopy. This condition is more common in women and diabetics and is usually caused by the *E. coli. Enterobacter aerogenes* (formerly called *Aerobacter aerogenes*), *K. pneumoniae, Enterococcus, Candida,* and *Clostridium perfringens* are other offending organisms. Predisposing conditions include neurogenic bladder, chronic urinary infection, trauma, instrumentation, urinary stasis, and fistula formation. Microscopically, there are empty cavities in the lamina propria lined by attenuated cells, including foreign body giant cells.[70,188,189] Urinary obstruction may result, requiring surgical intervention.[188,190]

Infections of the Urethra

Infections that affect the urinary bladder can affect both the male and female urethra, and vice versa. Infections often ascend the urethra to affect the bladder, particularly in women of reproductive age. In this process, bacterial cystitis usually results from bacterial infection that ascends from the introitus and distal urethra. The most common organisms are gram-negative enteric bacteria (*E. coli,* followed by *Proteus, Enterobacter,* and *Klebsiella*).[3]

Gonorrhea, caused by *Neisseria gonorrhoeae,* is the second most commonly reported notifiable disease that is an important cause of urethritis.[191] Nongonococcal urethritis is typically due to *Chlamydia* or *Mycoplasma* infection.[192,193] Malakoplakia can rarely involve the urethra.[194]

Urethritis is part of the classic triad—urethritis, conjunctivitis, and arthritis—that is seen in Reiter syndrome, also known as reactive arthritis, a condition of uncertain pathogenesis.

Infections of the Male Genitourinary System

Prostate

Acute and chronic prostatitis are both relatively common clinical problems in routine urologic practice, but they rarely require surgery and are usually treated empirically with antibiotics.[195,196] Histologically, acute bacterial prostatitis usually shows abundant neutrophils surrounding acini, desquamated cellular debris, hyperemia, stromal edema, and sometimes microabscess formation.[195] It is impossible to distinguish chronic infectious prostatitis from nonspecific chronic inflammation seen in benign prostatic hyperplasia.[195] In the case of diffuse lymphocytic infiltrate of the prostate, the possibility of chronic lymphocytic lymphoma should be considered. Malakoplakia rarely involves the prostate; its appearance is similar to malakoplakia seen in other areas of the urinary tract.[102,195,197,198]

Mycotic prostatitis is usually caused by blastomycosis, coccidioidomycosis,[199] or cryptococcosis. Histoplasmosis, paracoccidioidomycosis, aspergillosis, and candidiasis have also been reported. The most common setting is the infection of an immunocompromised patient via a hematogenous route.[195,200]

Tuberculous prostatitis occurs in 3% to 12% of patients with disseminated tuberculosis. More than 90% of patients with tuberculous prostatitis have lung involvement. Surgical pathology specimens of tuberculous prostatitis are not seen as frequently as they once were, primarily because the incidence of tuberculosis has decreased. Tuberculous involvement may still be seen in the setting of BCG immunotherapy for superficial transitional cell carcinoma of the bladder. Granulomas from BCG may show positivity with acid-fast stains, as in the bladder (see Fig. 15-22); they diffusely involve the prostate, may be small and noncaseating, but can also be large and caseating.[172,195] Abscesses may occur.[201] Patients may have abnormal digital rectal examination findings or increased prostate-specific antigen levels, or both, after BCG therapy.[202] Acid-fast stains can be used to demonstrate the bacteria, but the use of stains to identify the organisms is not typically recommended.[172,195,201,203-205] *Mycobacterium* other than tuberculosis (MOTT) and atypical mycobacteria such as *Mycobacterium fortuitum, M. kansasii,* and *M. avium* complex may also infect the prostate. Histologically, these mycobacteria give rise to a granulomatous prostatitis similar to that seen with other mycobacteria. Acid-fast bacterial stains may be useful in establishing the diagnosis, although the concurrent presence of BCG or other mycobacterial organisms cannot always be excluded.[172,195,206-209]

Other infections that affect the prostate include brucellosis,[210] syphilis, actinomycosis,[211] *Cryptococcus,*[212] amebic prostatitis,[213] schistosomiasis (which has been associated with cases of prostatic adenocarcinoma),[214-217] echinococcosis,[218] cytomegalovirus,[219] and herpes zoster.[220]

The topic of prostatitis and its relationship to neoplasia has been the subject of a great deal of research.[221-226]

Epididymis

Epididymitis is said to be the most common intrascrotal inflammatory process.[227] *C. trachomatis* and *N. gonorrhoeae* are the most frequent causes of scrotal swelling due to epididymitis in sexually active men younger than 35 years of age. Epididymitis is associated with urinary tract infections, and in that setting bacterial infections ascend via the urinary tract or lymphatics. Infections may also be spread hematogenously, leading to a number of bacterial infections of the epididymis and testis.[196,228]

Acute epididymitis consists of an enlarged epididymis that microscopically shows suppurative inflammation with fibrin covering. The epididymal duct may contain pus and may rupture, producing sperm granulomas, as classically described by Glassy and Mostofi.[229] Chronic epididymitis consists of a fibrotic process with a narrowed epididymal duct and a variable number of chronic inflammatory cells.[230]

Cytomegalovirus epididymitis has been reported in an immunosuppressed patient after renal transplantation and in patients with AIDS. Cytologic changes were similar to those typically seen with cytomegalovirus.[231,232]

Testis

Bacterial

Bacterial infections usually spread to the testis from the epididymis, leading to epididymo-orchitis. Hematogenous and lymphatic orchitis can be caused by *E. coli, Staphylococcus, Streptococcus, Klebsiella, Salmonella,*[233-235] *Pseudomonas aeruginosa, Brucella, Listeria monocytogenes,* and *Actinomyces.* Significant destruction of the testicular parenchyma may occur. Infections in neonates can occur, and mixed anaerobic and aerobic abscesses in neonates have been reported. There are a number of histologic patterns, including malakoplakia, which has virtually the same histologic appearance as in other sites (Fig. 15-26).[228,236-239]

Mycobacterial

M. tuberculosis infection can secondarily infect the testis, leading to a granulomatous orchitis. Spread to the testis is hematogenous or via the epididymis, which can be enlarged and dilated. There is usually bilateral involvement. Scrotal fistulas may occur. Grossly (Fig. 15-27) and microscopically, caseating or noncaseating granulomas are observed, similar to those seen in other parts of the body; however, granulomatous orchitis (Fig. 15-28) has a number of causes, including autoimmune disorders and nonspecific granulomatous orchitis, a disorder of unknown but probably infectious etiology.[240-242] An infiltrate of mononuclear lymphoid cells may be present. Acid-fast bacilli can be identified with the aid of special stains. The testis may also be infected by nontuberculous organisms such as *M. avium-intracellulare* and *M. kansasii.*[228,242-247]

Testicular infection by *M. leprae* is more common in other parts of the world than in the United States. The infection can be divided into three phases. First, there is a vascular phase, in which cells packed with acid-fast bacilli, known as lepra cells, are observed in the interstitium and blood vessels. Second, there is an interstitial phase, with interstitial fibrosis, obliterative endarteritis, Leydig cell clusters, and variable numbers of histiocytes containing acid-fast bacilli (Fig. 15-29). Spermatogenesis may be reduced. Third, there is an obliterative phase, with complete fibrosis, severe reduction to complete loss of seminiferous tubules, diminished vascularity, and rare acid-fast bacilli. Fite stains can be useful to identify the organisms.[228,248-250] Cytology of semen or testicular aspirates may be useful in the diagnosis of testicular leprosy.[251] Involvement of the testis by leprosy can lead to reduction in testicular volume and hypogonadism, gynecomastia, oligospermia or azoospermia, and infertility.[228,248,252]

Fungal

Fungal infections can result in epididymo-orchitis. Organisms such as *Candida, Blastomyces, Actinomyces, Aspergillus, H. capsulatum, Trichophyton mentagrophytes,* and *C. immitis* have been implicated. Notably, *Aspergillus* has been reported in a renal transplant recipient.[253] The histologic appearance can be variable and usually is that typical of the fungal infection; however, the histologic findings can be unique.[228,252-255] A case of *H. capsulatum* has been reported that gave the appearance of sperm granulomas.[255]

Viral

A number of viral infections can involve the testis, including mumps, variola, varicella, EBV, echovirus, lymphocytic choriomeningitis virus, group B arbovirus, influenza, West Nile virus, Dengue fever, sandfly fever, and Cocksackie B virus.[228,256-258] A case of West Nile virus orchitis has been reported in a renal transplant recipient.[258]

Mumps

Mumps is a member of the paramyxovirus group, which are spherical, single-stranded RNA viruses. It was once an important cause of orchitis, with 20% of postpubertal males infected with the virus developing orchitis, usually unilaterally. Mumps orchitis is now rare in developed countries due to immunization[51,259,260]; however, cases still persist among patients who have not been immunized, and there have been recent outbreaks in the United States and the United Kingdom.[261] Rare cases of orchitis have been reported with immunization.[196,227,262-264] Histologically (Fig. 15-30), edema and inflammation of the tunica albuginea, edema and inflammation with lymphoid aggregation of the interstitium, and congestion of the tunica vasculosa are observed. Inflammation is usually mixed, with lymphocytes, histiocytes, plasma cells, and neutrophils. Necrosis of spermatogenic cells occurs, leaving only Sertoli cells, which may also eventually disappear from the tubules. Infertility may result. Orchitis rarely occurs prepubertally. Atrophy develops in approximately one third of patients, but infertility in only about 2%.[228,265,266] Healed orchitis usually shows little or no inflammation, with foci of tubular sclerosis and decreased numbers of germ and Sertoli cells.[228]

Human Immunodeficiency Virus

The testes are noticeably affected in AIDS. Although the effects may not be appreciated clinically, autopsy studies have demonstrated a generalized atrophy with decreased spermatogenesis, tunica propria thickening, interstitial fibrosis, tubular hyalinization, and interstitial inflammation with reduced numbers of germ and Leydig cells.[267-271] It has been suggested that prolonged survival with antiviral therapy has resulted in a shift toward greater loss of germ cells. Characterization and quantitation of

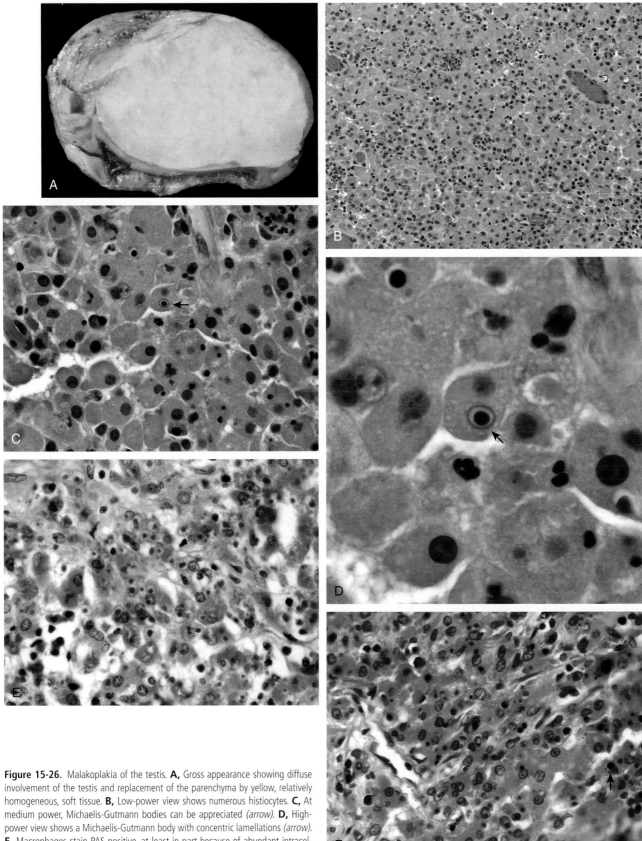

Figure 15-26. Malakoplakia of the testis. **A,** Gross appearance showing diffuse involvement of the testis and replacement of the parenchyma by yellow, relatively homogeneous, soft tissue. **B,** Low-power view shows numerous histiocytes. **C,** At medium power, Michaelis-Gutmann bodies can be appreciated *(arrow)*. **D,** High-power view shows a Michaelis-Gutmann body with concentric lamellations *(arrow)*. **E,** Macrophages stain PAS positive, at least in part because of abundant intracellular glycogen. **F,** Iron stain highlights the Michaelis-Gutmann bodies *(arrow)*.

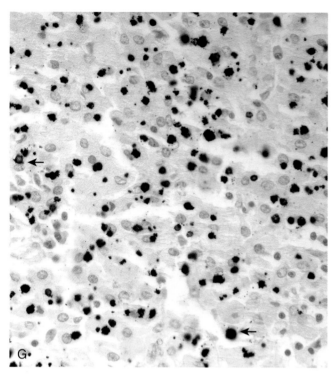

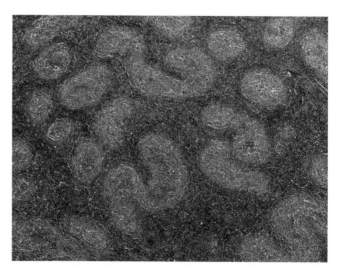

Figure 15-28. Granulomatous orchitis. This pattern can be seen in a number of conditions, including mycobacterial infections of the testis. Granulomas can be caseating or noncaseating.

Figure 15-26, cont'd. G, von Kossa stain, which is a stain for phosphate salts (including notably calcium salts), also stains the Michaelis-Gutmann bodies. (Images courtesy of Dr. Robert H. Young.)

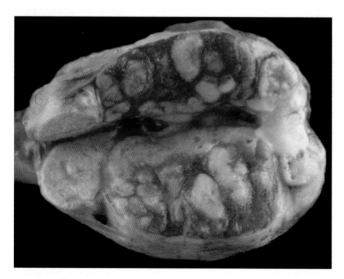

Figure 15-27. Tuberculous orchitis. Gross image of tuberculous orchitis heterogeneously replacing the testis parenchyma with areas of caseous necrosis. (Image courtesy of Dr. Robert H. Young.)

the testicular cells, particularly the germ cells, is thought to be important, because the testis is believed to be an important location for sexual transmission of the virus.[270,271]

Additionally, the testis can be involved by numerous opportunistic organisms in AIDS patients, including *M. tuberculosis*[272] and *Toxoplasma*. AIDS is also a predisposing factor for testicular neoplasia.[273-282]

Other Diseases

Orchitis has been described in patients with Q fever or typhus.[228,283] Typhus usually displays a vasculitis composed of swollen capillary endothelial cells containing large numbers of organisms and accompanying vascular thrombi.[228]

Syphilis can lead to orchitis. Fibromatous and gummatous stages have been described. An enlarged, irregular, nodular testis is usually present in the gummatous form, and discrete gummas can be seen grossly. The gummas (Fig. 15-31) contain coagulative necrosis with a peripheral zone containing a mixed inflammatory infiltrate of lymphocytes, plasma cells, and occasional histiocytes, some of which may be the giant cell form.[284] An obliterative endarteritis may be present. The fibromatous form consists of a painless, enlarged testis with peritubular inflammation and fibrosis with decreased numbers of germ cells.[228,285] Spirochetes cannot usually be identified in the fibromatous stage, but they may be present in the gummatous stage. PCR on tissue may be required to make the diagnosis.[286]

Penis and Scrotum

The penis and scrotum may be affected by genitourinary cutaneous infections, as previously discussed. In addition, there are some special infections of this region.

Bacterial Infection

The population most affected by bacterial infection of the penis and scrotum is uncircumcised male newborns, who develop inflammation of the mucosa of the glands (balanitis) and prepuce (posthitis).[3,29,287] Bacteria can more readily adhere to and colonize the mucosal surface of the prepuce, making balanoposthitis more common in uncircumcised men.[29,287] A nonspecific inflammatory infiltrate is usually found. Uncommonly, balanoposthitis may be caused by *Gardnerella vaginalis* or *Trichomonas*, and gonococcal infections have been reported to cause median raphe

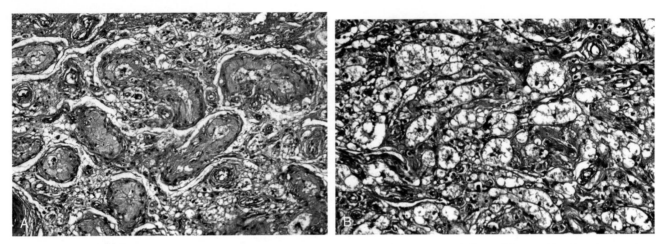

Figure 15-29. Testis with leprosy. **A,** Medium power shows atrophy and obliteration of the seminiferous tubules with fibrosis of the interstitium. **B,** High power shows obliteration and loss of the seminiferous tubules and histiocytes, which may contain acid-fast bacilli. (Images courtesy of Dr. Robert H. Young.)

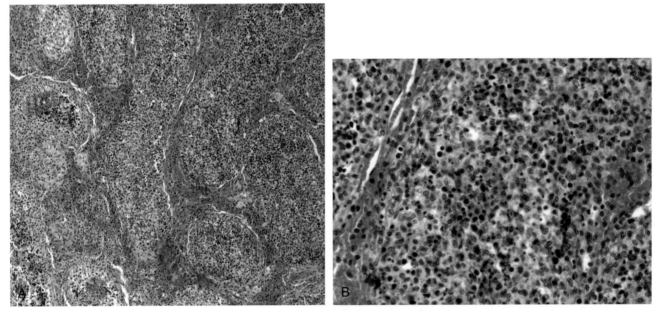

Figure 15-30. Mumps orchitis. **A,** Low-power view shows necroinflammatory debris in the seminiferous tubules. **B,** Medium power shows degeneration of the seminiferous tubular epithelium and vascular congestion. (Images courtesy of Dr. Robert H. Young.)

cysts and deeper soft tissue infections of the penis. These infections are usually transmitted sexually. Pediatric cases are caused by chronic, mixed bacterial infections, and perianal infections can occur, leading to perianal streptococcal cellulitis. Localized infections can spread and result in cellulitis, which usually is caused by streptococcal organisms. Severe cases may lead to necrotizing fasciitis, which in this region is referred to as Fournier gangrene and often involves the dartos and penile fascia. Previous trauma, burns, diabetes, leukemia, and alcoholic cirrhosis may be predisposing conditions.[3,29]

The penis is often the site of primary syphilis in males, which manifests as a solitary papule that typically ulcerates and forms an indurated base, known as the chancre. The chancre is usually on the inner prepuce, coronal sulcus, penile shaft, or penile base. Additional details of primary, secondary (condyloma lata), and tertiary syphilis were described earlier in this chapter.[29]

Mycobacterial infections can affect the penis; however, this is now rare. Tuberculosis involving the penis can result from direct spread from adjacent infection or from hematogenous dissemination. Microscopically, the appearance is that of mycobacterial infections in other sites.[29]

As previously discussed, granuloma inguinale (*K. granulomatis*) (see Fig. 15-1) and chancroid (*H. ducreyi*) may affect the penis in the same manner as in the genitourinary skin.[29] Granuloma inguinale is usually present on the prepuce, glans, penile

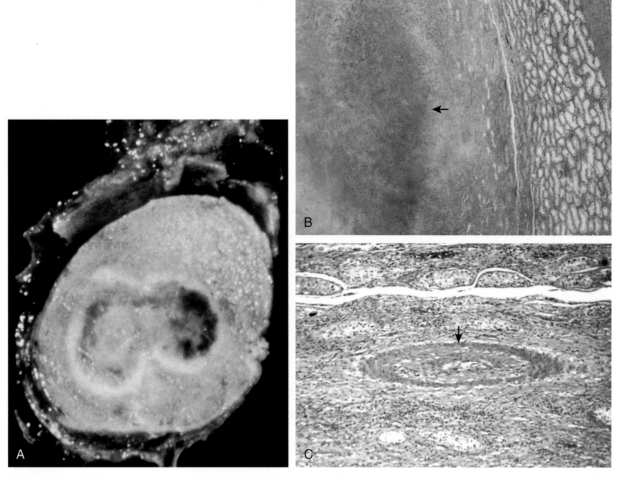

Figure 15-31. Syphilis involving the testis. **A,** Gross image of testis involved by syphilis, showing a characteristic gumma with caseating necrosis. **B,** Medium-power image of syphilitic gumma showing caseating necrosis *(arrow).* **C,** Medium-power image of vasculitis caused by syphilis involving the testis. (Images courtesy of Dr. Robert H. Young.)

shaft, or scrotum. Satellite lesions may be present and are referred to as pseudobuboes.[29]

Fungal Infection

Superficial fungal (mycotic) infections of the penis are the most common mycotic infections. Dermatophytes commonly affect the penis and often spread from other areas of the groin. Another common superficial mycotic organism that affects the penis is *C. albicans,* which is present in 15% to 20% of men. This infection is considered to be sexually transmitted and may be a source of infection and reinfection in candidal vaginosis.[29,288]

Deep penile mycotic infections are rare. An example causative organism is *C. neoformans.*[29,288]

Parasitic Infection

Lymphogranuloma venereum, caused by an obligate intracellular parasite, was discussed previously. It may also be present with lymphadenitis with bubo formation. Scabies can also affect the penis.[29]

Viral Infection

As previously discussed in the section on infections of the genitourinary skin, the penis can be affected by herpes, molluscum contagiosum, and HPV or HPV-associated lesions (see Table 15-1).

REFERENCES

1. Sherris JC, Ryan KJ, Ray CG, et al. (eds): Medical Microbiology: An Introduction to Infectious Diseases. New York, Elsevier Science, 1984.
2. Weedon D, Strutton G: Skin Pathology. 2nd ed. Edinburgh, Churchill Livingstone, 2002.
3. Tannenbaum M, Madden JF (eds): Diagnostic Atlas of Genitourinary Pathology. Philadelphia, Churchill Livingstone Elsevier, 2006.

4. Stoler MH, Mills SE, Frierson HF Jr: The vulva and vagina. In Mills SE, Carter D, Greenson JK, et al. (eds): Sternberg's Diagnostic Surgical Pathology, vol 2, 4th ed. Philadelphia, Lippincott Williams & Wilkins, 2004, p 2333.

5. Shelley WB, Shelley ED: Coexistent erythrasma, trichomycosis axillaris, and pitted keratolysis: An overlooked corynebacterial triad? J Am Acad Dermatol 1982;7:752-757.

6. Leyden JJ, McGinley KJ, Holzle E, et al: The microbiology of the human axilla and its relationship to axillary odor. J Invest Dermatol 1981;77:413-416.

7. White SW, Smith J: Trichomycosis pubis. Arch Dermatol 1979;115:444-445.

8. Shelley WB, Miller MA: Electron microscopy, histochemistry, and microbiology of bacterial adhesion in trichomycosis axillaris. J Am Acad Dermatol 1984;10:1005-1014.

9. Duhra P, Ilchyshyn A: Perianal streptococcal cellulitis with penile involvement. Br J Dermatol 1990;123:793-796.

10. Acay MC, Oral ET, Yenigun M, Sahin A: *Pasteurella multocida* ulceration on the penis. Int J Dermatol 1993;32:519-520.

11. Lapins J, Jarstrand C, Emtestam L: Coagulase-negative staphylococci are the most common bacteria found in cultures from the deep portions of hidradenitis suppurativa lesions, as obtained by carbon dioxide laser surgery. Br J Dermatol 1999;140:90-95.

12. Jansen T, Plewig G: What's new in acne inversa (alias hidradenitis suppurativa)? J Eur Acad Dermatol Venereol 2000;14:342-343.

13. Jemec GB: Medical treatment of hidradenitis suppurativa. Expert Opin Pharmacother 2004;5:1767-1770.

14. Slade DE, Powell BW, Mortimer PS: Hidradenitis suppurativa: Pathogenesis and management. Br J Plast Surg 2003;56:451-461.

15. Brozna JP: Shwartzman reaction. Semin Thromb Hemost 1990;16:326-332.

16. Roca B, Cunat E, Simon E: HIV infection presenting with fournier's gangrene. Neth J Med 1998;53:168-171.

17. Roca B, Soler S, Saez-Royuela A, Simon E: Fournier's gangrene: A case report. An Med Interna 1997;14:651-652.

18. Kearney GP, Carling PC: Fournier's gangrene: An approach to its management. J Urol 1983;130:695-698.

19. Basoglu M, Gul O, Yildirgan I, et al: Fournier's gangrene: Review of fifteen cases. Am Surg 1997;63:1019-1021.

20. Mouraviev VB, Pautler SE, Hayman WP: Fournier's gangrene following penile self-injection with cocaine. Scand J Urol Nephrol 2002;36:317-318.

21. Cunningham DL, Persky L: Penile ecthyma gangrenosum: Complication of drug addiction. Urology 1989;34:109-110.

22. Rabinowitz R, Lewin EB: Gangrene of the genitalia in children with pseudomonas sepsis. J Urol 1980;124:431-432.

23. Manian FA, Alford RH: Nosocomial infectious balanoposthitis in neutropenic patients. South Med J 1987;80:909-911.

24. Dahl DM, Klein D, Morgentaler A: Penile mass caused by the newly described organism *Mycobacterium celatum*. Urology 1996;47:266-268.

25. Wise GJ, Marella VK: Genitourinary manifestations of tuberculosis. Urol Clin North Am 2003;30:111-121.

26. Erol A, Ozgur S, Tahtali N, et al: Bacillus Calmette-Guerin (BCG) balanitis as a complication of intravesical BCG immunotherapy: A case report. Int Urol Nephrol 1995;27:307-310.

27. Beckett JH, Bigbee JW: Immunoperoxidase localization of *Treponema pallidum*: Its use in formaldehyde-fixed and paraffin-embedded tissue sections. Arch Pathol Lab Med 1979;103:135-138.

28. Lee WS, Lee MG, Chung KY, Lee JB: Detection of *Treponema pallidum* in tissue: A comparative study of the avidin-biotin-peroxidase complex, indirect immunoperoxidase, FTA-ABS complement techniques and the darkfield method. Yonsei Med J 1991;32:335-341.

29. Cubilla AL, Velazquez EF, Barreto J, Ayala G: The penis. In Mills SE, Carter D, Greenson JK, et al. (eds): Sternberg's Diagnostic Surgical Pathology, vol 2, 4th ed. Philadelphia, Lippincott Williams & Wilkins, 2004.

30. Margolis RJ, Hood AF: Chancroid: Diagnosis and treatment. J Am Acad Dermatol 1982;6:493-499.

31. Winkler B, Crum CP: *Chlamydia trachomatis* infection of the female genital tract: Pathogenetic and clinicopathologic correlations. Pathol Annu 1987;22(Pt 1):193-223.

32. Gray Y, Libbey NP: Xanthogranulomatous salpingitis and oophoritis: A case report and review of the literature. Arch Pathol Lab Med 2001;125:260-263.

33. Kuberski T: Granuloma inguinale (donovanosis). Sex Transm Dis 1980;7:29-36.

34. Kuberski T, Papadimitriou JM, Phillips P: Ultrastructure of *Calymmatobacterium granulomatis* in lesions of granuloma inguinale. J Infect Dis 1980;142:744-749.

35. Lynch PJ: Sexually transmitted diseases: Granuloma inguinale, lymphogranuloma venereum, chancroid, and infectious syphilis. Clin Obstet Gynecol 1978;21:1041-1052.

36. Davis CM: Granuloma inguinale: A clinical, histological and ultrastructural study. JAMA 1970;211:632-636.

37. de Boer AL, de Boer F, Van der Merwe JV: Cytologic identification of donovan bodies in granuloma inguinale. Acta Cytol 1984;28:126-128.

38. Clement PB, Young RH: Atlas of Gynecologic Surgical Pathology, 2nd ed. Philadelphia, Saunders Elsevier, 2008.

39. Alexander LJ, Shields TL: Squamous cell carcinoma of the vulva secondary to granuloma inguinale. AMA Arch Derm Syphilol 1953;67:395-402.

40. Saltzstein SL, Woodruff JD, Novak ER: Postgranulomatous carcinoma of the vulva. Obstet Gynecol 1956;7:80-90.

41. Scott RA, Gallis HA, Livengood CH: Phycomycosis of the vulva. Am J Obstet Gynecol 1985;153:675-676.

42. Winn W Jr, Allen S, Janda W, et al. (eds): Koneman's Color Atlas and Textbook of Diagnostic Microbiology, 6th ed. Philadelphia, Lippincott Williams & Wilkins, 1997.

43. Blumenthal HL: Tinea versicolor of penis. Arch Dermatol 1971;103:461-462.

44. Nia AK, Smith EL: Pityriasis versicolor of the glans penis. Br J Vener Dis 1979;55:230.

45. Mayser P: Mycotic infections of the penis. Andrologia 1999;31(Suppl 1):13-16.

46. Watanabe T, Nakamura K, Wakugawa M, et al: Antibodies to molluscum contagiosum virus in the general population and susceptible patients. Arch Dermatol 2000;136:1518-1522.

47. Tyring SK: Molluscum contagiosum: The importance of early diagnosis and treatment. Am J Obstet Gynecol 2003;189:S12-S16.

48. Gur I: The epidemiology of molluscum contagiosum in HIV-seropositive patients: A unique entity or insignificant finding? Int J STD AIDS 2008;19:503-506.

49. Mulugeta A: Giant molluscum contagiosum presenting as a tumour in an HIV-infected patient: Case report. Ethiop Med J 2000;38:125-130.

50. Pereira B, Fernandes C, Nachiambo E, et al: Exuberant molluscum contagiosum as a manifestation of the immune reconstitution inflammatory syndrome. Dermatol Online J 2007;13:6.

51. Brooks GF, Butel JF, Morse SA: Jawetz, Melnick, and Adelberg's Medical Microbiology, 22nd ed. New York, Appleton and Lange/Lange Medical Books/McGraw-Hill, 2001.

52. Gupta R, Warren T, Wald A: Genital herpes. Lancet 2007;370:2127-2137.

53. Nikkels AF, Delvenne P, Sadzot-Delvaux C, et al: Distribution of varicella zoster virus and herpes simplex virus in disseminated fatal infections. J Clin Pathol 1996;49:243-248.

54. Nikkels AF, Debrus S, Sadzot-Delvaux C, et al: Comparative immunohistochemical study of herpes simplex and varicella-zoster infections. Virchows Arch A Pathol Anat Histopathol. 1993;422:121-126.

55. Cohen PR: Tests for detecting herpes simplex virus and varicella-zoster virus infections. Dermatol Clin 1994;12:51-68.

56. Eyzaguirre EJ, Walker DH, Zaki SR: Immunohistology of infectious diseases. In Dabbs D (ed): Diagnostic Immunohistochemistry, 2nd ed. Philadelphia, Churchill Livingstone Elsevier, 2006, p 43.

57. Mais DD: Quick Compendium of Clinical Pathology, 2nd ed. Chicago, American Society of Clinical Pathology Press, 2008.

58. Cubilla AL, Velazques EF, Reuter VE, et al: Warty (condylomatous) squamous cell carcinoma of the penis: A report of 11 cases and proposed classification of "verruciform" penile tumors. Am J Surg Pathol 2000;24:505-512.

59. Bezerra AL, Lopes A, Santiago GH, et al: Human papillomavirus as a prognostic factor in carcinoma of the penis: Analysis of 82 patients treated with amputation and bilateral lymphadenectomy. Cancer 2001;91:2315-2321.

60. Bezerra AL, Lopes A, Landman G, et al: Clinicopathologic features and human papillomavirus DNA prevalence of warty and squamous cell carcinoma of the penis. Am J Surg Pathol 2001;25:673-678.

61. Delvenne P, Fontaine MA, Delvenne C, et al: Detection of human papillomaviruses in paraffin-embedded biopsies of cervical intraepithelial lesions: Analysis by immunohistochemistry, in situ hybridization, and the polymerase chain reaction. Mod Pathol 1994;7:113-119.

62. Lopez-Beltran A, Escudero AL, Carrasco-Aznar JC, Vicioso-Recio L: Human papillomavirus infection and transitional cell carcinoma of the bladder: Immunohistochemistry and in situ hybridization. Pathol Res Pract 1996;192:154-159.

63. Meyer MP, Markiw CA, Matuscak RR, et al: Detection of human papillomavirus DNA in genital lesions by using a modified commercially available in situ hybridization assay. J Clin Microbiol 1991;29:1308-1311.

64. Wilbur DC, Reichman RC, Stoler MH: Detection of infection by human papillomavirus in genital condylomata: A comparison study using immunocytochemistry and in situ nucleic acid hybridization. Am J Clin Pathol 1988;89:505-510.

65. Rodrigue RB: Amebic balanitis. JAMA 1978;239:109.

66. Lu S, Tran TA, Jones DM, et al: Localized lymphedema (elephantiasis): A case series and review of the literature. J Cutan Pathol 2008;36:1-20.

67. McKee PH, Wright E, Hutt MS: Vulval schistosomiasis. Clin Exp Dermatol 1983;8:189-194.

68. Councilman WT: Acute interstitial nephritis. J Exp Med 1898;3:393-420.

69. Rossert J: Drug-induced acute interstitial nephritis. Kidney Int 2001;60:804-817.

70. Zhou M, Magi-Galluzzi C (eds): Genitourinary Pathology. Philadelphia, Churchill Livingstone Elsevier, 2007.

71. Michel DM, Kelly CJ: Acute interstitial nephritis. J Am Soc Nephrol 1998;9:506-515.

72. Rastegar A, Kashgarian M: The clinical spectrum of tubulointerstitial nephritis. Kidney Int 1998;54:313-327.

73. Weiss M, Liapis H, Tomaszewski JE, Arend LJ: Pyelonephritis and other infections, reflux nephropathy, hydronephrosis, and nephrolithiasis. In Jennette JC, Olson JL, Schwartz MM, Silva FG (eds): Heptinstall's Pathology of the Kidney, vol 2, 6th ed. Philadelphia, Lippincott Williams & Wilkins, 2007:991.

74. Colvin RB, Fang LST: Interstitial nephritis. In Tisher CC, Brenner BM (eds): Renal Pathology with Clinical and Functional Correlations, vol 2, 2nd ed. Philadelphia, JB Lippincott, 1994.

75. Nasr SH, Koscica J, Markowitz GS, D'Agati VD: Granulomatous interstitial nephritis. Am J Kidney Dis 2003;41:714-719.

76. Ito M, Hirabayashi N, Uno Y, et al: Necrotizing tubulointerstitial nephritis associated with adenovirus infection. Hum Pathol 1991;22:1225-1231.

77. Mazoyer E, Daugas E, Verine J, et al: A case report of adenovirus-related acute interstitial nephritis in a patient with AIDS. Am J Kidney Dis 2008;51:121-126.

78. Alsaad KO, Tobar A, Belanger E, et al: Late-onset acute haemorrhagic necrotizing granulomatous adenovirus tubulointerstitial nephritis in a renal allograft. Nephrol Dial Transplant 2007;22:1257-1260.

79. Lim AK, Parsons S, Ierino F: Adenovirus tubulointerstitial nephritis presenting as a renal allograft space occupying lesion. Am J Transplant 2005;5:2062-2066.

80. Asim M, Chong-Lopez A, Nickeleit V: Adenovirus infection of a renal allograft. Am J Kidney Dis 2003;41:696-701.

81. Platt JL, Sibley RK, Michael AF: Interstitial nephritis associated with cytomegalovirus infection. Kidney Int 1985;28:550-552.

82. Cameron J, Rigby RJ, van Deth AG, Petrie JJ: Severe tubulointerstitial disease in a renal allograft due to cytomegalovirus infection. Clin Nephrol 1982;18:321-325.

83. Trimarchi H, Jordan R, Iotti A, et al: Late-onset cytomegalovirus-associated interstitial nephritis in a kidney transplant. Nephron 2002;92:490-494.

84. Cataudella JA, Young ID, Iliescu EA: Epstein-barr virus-associated acute interstitial nephritis: Infection or immunologic phenomenon? Nephron 2002;92:437-439.

85. Bonsib SM: Non-neoplastic disease of the kidney. In Bostwick DG, Eble JN (eds): Urologic Surgical Pathology. St. Louis, Mosby, 1997.

86. Nadasdy T, Sedmak D: Acute and chronic tubulointerstitial nephritis. In Jennette JC, Olson JL, Schwartz MM, Silva FG (eds): Heptinstall's Pathology of the Kidney, vol 2, 6th ed. Philadelphia, Lippincott Williams & Wilkins, 2007, p 1084.

87. Talner LB, Davidson AJ, Lebowitz RL, et al: Acute pyelonephritis: Can we agree on terminology? Radiology 1994;192:297-305.

88. Craig WD, Wagner BJ, Travis MD: Pyelonephritis: Radiologic-pathologic review. Radiographics 2008;28:255-277; quiz 327-328.

89. Kumar PD, Brown LA: Focal bacterial nephritis (lobar nephronia) presenting as renal mass. Am J Med Sci 2000;320:209-211.

90. Rosenfield AT, Glickman MG, Taylor KJ, et al: Acute focal bacterial nephritis (acute lobar nephronia). Radiology 1979;132:553-561.

91. McDonough WD, Sandler CM, Benson GS: Acute focal bacterial nephritis: Focal pyelonephritis that may simulate renal abscess. J Urol 1981;126:670-673.

92. Tai HC, Yang PJ, Lee PH, et al: Acute lobar nephronia in a renal allograft: A case report and literature review. Transplant Proc 2008;40:1737-1740.

93. Yang CW, Kim YS, Yang KH, et al: Acute focal bacterial nephritis presented as acute renal failure and hepatic dysfunction in a renal transplant recipient. Am J Nephrol 1994;14:72-75.

94. Michaeli J, Mogle P, Perlberg S, et al: Emphysematous pyelonephritis. J Urol 1984;131:203-208.

95. Evanoff GV, Thompson CS, Foley R, Weinman EJ: Spectrum of gas within the kidney: Emphysematous pyelonephritis and emphysematous pyelitis. Am J Med 1987;83:149-154.

96. Huang JJ, Tseng CC: Emphysematous pyelonephritis: Clinicoradiological classification, management, prognosis, and pathogenesis. Arch Intern Med 2000;160:797-805.

97. Wang MC, Tseng CC, Lan RR, et al: Double cancers of the kidney and ureter complicated with emphysematous pyelonephritis within the parenchyma of the renal tumour. Scand J Urol Nephrol 1999;33:420-422.

98. McClure J: Malakoplakia. J Pathol 1983;140:275-330.

99. McClure J: Malakoplakia of the urinary tract. Br J Urol 1982;54:181-185.

100. McClure J, Cameron CH, Garrett R: The ultrastructural features of malakoplakia. J Pathol 1981;134:13-25.

101. Stevens S, McClure J: The histochemical features of the Michaelis-Gutmann body and a consideration of the pathophysiological mechanisms of its formation. J Pathol 1982;137:119-127.

102. McClure J: Malakoplakia of the prostate: A report of two cases and a review of the literature. J Clin Pathol 1979;32:629-632.

103. McClure J: Malakoplakia of the testis and its relationship to granulomatous orchitis. J Clin Pathol 1980;33:670-678.

104. McClure J: Malakoplakia of the gastrointestinal tract. Postgrad Med J 1981;57:95-103.

105. Von Hansemann D: Über malakoplaie der harnblase. Virchows Arch A Pathol Anat Histopathol 1903;173:302.

106. Michaelis L, Gutmann C: Über einschlüsse in blastentumoren. Z Klin Med 1903;47:208.

107. Garrett IR, McClure J: Renal malakoplakia: Experimental production and evidence of a link with interstitial megalocytic nephritis. J Pathol 1982;136:111-122.

108. Tam VK, Kung WH, Li R, Chan KW: Renal parenchymal malacoplakia: A rare cause of ARF with a review of recent literature. Am J Kidney Dis 2003;41:E13-E17.

109. Stanton MJ, Maxted W: Malacoplakia: A study of the literature and current concepts of pathogenesis, diagnosis and treatment. J Urol 1981;125:139-146.

110. Dobyan DC, Truong LD, Eknoyan G: Renal malacoplakia reappraised. Am J Kidney Dis 1993;22:243-252.

111. Saleem MA, Milford DV, Raafat F, White RH: Renal parenchymal malakoplakia: A case report and review of the literature. Pediatr Nephrol 1993;7:256-258.

112. Hartman DS, Davis CJ Jr, Lichtenstein JE, Goldman SM: Renal parenchymal malacoplakia. Radiology 1980;136:33-42.

113. Esparza AR, McKay DB, Cronan JJ, Chazan JA: Renal parenchymal malakoplakia: Histologic spectrum and its relationship to megalocytic interstitial nephritis and xanthogranulomatous pyelonephritis. Am J Surg Pathol 1989;13:225-236.

114. Fishman JA: Infection in solid-organ transplant recipients. N Engl J Med 2007;357:2601-2614.

115. Thamboo TP, Jeffery KJ, Friend PJ, et al: Urine cytology screening for polyoma virus infection following renal transplantation: The Oxford experience. J Clin Pathol 2007;60:927-930.

116. Nickeleit V, Mihatsch MJ: Polyomavirus nephropathy in native kidneys and renal allografts: An update on an escalating threat. Transpl Int 2006;19:960-973.

117. Mischitelli M, Bellizzi A, Anzivino E, et al: Complications post renal transplantation: Literature focus on BK virus nephropathy and diagnostic tools actually available. Virol J 2008;5:38.

118. Matlosz B, Durlik M: Polyoma virus BK nephropathy in kidney allograft recipients. Przegl Epidemiol 2006;60:133-140.

119. Jevnikar AM, Mannon RB: Late kidney allograft loss: What we know about it, and what we can do about it. Clin J Am Soc Nephrol 2008;3(Suppl 2):S56-S67.

120. Egli A, Binggeli S, Bodaghi S, et al: Cytomegalovirus and polyomavirus BK posttransplant. Nephrol Dial Transplant 2007;22(Suppl 8):viii72-viii82.

121. Drachenberg CB, Papadimitriou JC, Ramos E: Histologic versus molecular diagnosis of BK polyomavirus-associated nephropathy: A shifting paradigm? Clin J Am Soc Nephrol 2006;1:374-379.

122. Bonvoisin C, Weekers L, Xhignesse P, et al: Polyomavirus in renal transplantation: A hot problem. Transplantation 2008;85:S42-S48.

123. Bohl DL, Brennan DC: BK virus nephropathy and kidney transplantation. Clin J Am Soc Nephrol 2007;2(Suppl 1):S36-S46.

124. Blanckaert K, De Vriese AS: Current recommendations for diagnosis and management of polyoma BK virus nephropathy in renal transplant recipients. Nephrol Dial Transplant 2006;21:3364-3367.

125. Beimler J, Sommerer C, Zeier M: The influence of immunosuppression on the development of BK virus nephropathy: Does it matter? Nephrol Dial Transplant 2007;22(Suppl 8):viii66-viii71.

126. Colvin RB: Calcineurin inhibitor toxicity, polyoma virus, and recurrent disease. In Fogo AB, Bruijn JA, Cohen AH, et al (eds): Fundamentals of Renal Pathology. New York, Springer, 2006, p 201.

127. Pappo O, Demetris AJ, Raikow RB, Randhawa PS: Human polyoma virus infection of renal allografts: Histopathologic diagnosis, clinical significance, and literature review. Mod Pathol 1996;9:105-109.

128. Nebuloni M, Tosoni A, Boldorini R, et al: BK virus renal infection in a patient with the acquired immunodeficiency syndrome. Arch Pathol Lab Med 1999;123:807-811.

129. Elli A, Banfi G, Fogazzi GB, et al: BK polyomavirus interstitial nephritis in a renal transplant patient with no previous acute rejection episodes. J Nephrol 2002;15:313-316.

130. Boldorini R, Omodeo-Zorini E, Suno A, et al: Molecular characterization and sequence analysis of polyomavirus strains isolated from needle biopsy specimens of kidney allograft recipients. Am J Clin Pathol 2001;116:489-494.

131. Boldorini R, Zorini EO, Fortunato M, et al: Molecular characterization and sequence analysis of polyomavirus BKV-strain in a renal-allograft recipient. Hum Pathol 2001;32:656-659.

132. Colvin RB, Nickeleit V: Renal transplant pathology. In Jennette JC, Olson JL, Schwartz MM, Silva FG (eds): Heptinstall's Pathology of the Kidney, vol 2, 6th ed. Philadelphia, Lippincott Williams & Wilkins, 2007, p 1347.

133. Oertel SH, Verschuuren E, Reinke P, et al: Effect of anti-CD 20 antibody rituximab in patients with post-transplant lymphoproliferative disorder (PTLD). Am J Transplant 2005;5:2901-2906.

134. Eastwood JB, Corbishley CM, Grange JM: Tuberculosis and the kidney. J Am Soc Nephrol 2001;12:1307-1314.

135. Simon HB, Weinstein AJ, Pasternak MS, et al: Genitourinary tuberculosis: Clinical features in a general hospital population. Am J Med 1977;63:410-420.

136. Njeh M, Jemni M, Abid R, et al: Renal tuberculosis with pseudotumoral form: Apropos of a case. J Urol (Paris) 1993;99:150-152.

137. Benn JJ, Scoble JE, Thomas AC, Eastwood JB: Cryptogenic tuberculosis as a preventable cause of end-stage renal failure. Am J Nephrol 1988;8:306-308.

138. Nakayama EE, Ura S, Fleury RN, Soares V: Renal lesions in leprosy: A retrospective study of 199 autopsies. Am J Kidney Dis 2001;38:26-30.

139. Mandell GL, Bennett JE, Dolin R (eds): Mandell, Douglas, and Bennett's Principles and Practice of Infectious Diseases, 6th ed. Philadelphia, Elsevier, 2005.

140. Fukuzawa M, Inaba H, Hayama M, et al: Improved detection of medically important fungi by immunoperoxidase staining with polyclonal antibodies. Virchows Arch 1995;427:407-414.

141. Reed JA, Hemann BA, Alexander JL, Brigati DJ: Immunomycology: Rapid and specific immunocytochemical identification of fungi in formalin-fixed, paraffin-embedded material. J Histochem Cytochem 1993;41:1217-1221.

142. Jensen HE, Schonheyder HC, Hotchi M, Kaufman L: Diagnosis of systemic mycoses by specific immunohistochemical tests. APMIS 1996;104:241-258.

143. Verweij PE, Smedts F, Poot T, et al: Immunoperoxidase staining for identification of Aspergillus species in routinely processed tissue sections. J Clin Pathol 1996;49:798-801.

144. Choi JK, Mauger J, McGowan KL: Immunohistochemical detection of aspergillus species in pediatric tissue samples. Am J Clin Pathol 2004;121:18-25.

145. Sinniah R, Churg J, Sobin LH (eds): Renal Disease: Classification and Atlas of Infectious and Tropical Diseases. Chicago, ASCP Press, 1988.

146. Burke DG, Emancipator SN, Smith MC, Salata RA: Histoplasmosis and kidney disease in patients with AIDS. Clin Infect Dis 1997;25:281-284.

147. Rich AR: The pathology of nineteen cases of a peculiar and specific form of nephritis associated with acquired syphilis. Bull Johns Hopkins Hosp 1932;50:357.

148. Dumler JS, Walker DH: Diagnostic tests for Rocky Mountain spotted fever and other rickettsial diseases. Dermatol Clin 1994; 12:25-36.

149. White WL, Patrick JD, Miller LR: Evaluation of immunoperoxidase techniques to detect *Rickettsia rickettsii* in fixed tissue sections. Am J Clin Pathol 1994;101:747-752.

150. Procop GW, Burchette JL Jr, Howell DN, Sexton DJ: Immunoperoxidase and immunofluorescent staining of *Rickettsia rickettsii* in skin biopsies: A comparative study. Arch Pathol Lab Med 1997;121:894-899.

151. Paddock CD, Greer PW, Ferebee TL, et al: Hidden mortality attributable to Rocky Mountain spotted fever: Immunohistochemical detection of fatal, serologically unconfirmed disease. J Infect Dis 1999;179:1469-1476.

152. Zamora J, Riedemann S, Cabezas X, Vega S: Comparison of 4 microscopy techniques for the diagnosis of leptospirosis in wild rodents in a rural area of Valdivia, Chile. Rev Latinoam Microbiol 1995;37:267-272.

153. Collins WE, Jeffery GM: *Plasmodium malariae:* Parasite and disease. Clin Microbiol Rev 2007;20:579-592.

154. Eiam-Ong S: Malarial nephropathy. Semin Nephrol 2003;23:21-33.

155. Elsheikha HM, Sheashaa HA: Epidemiology, pathophysiology, management and outcome of renal dysfunction associated with plasmodia infection. Parasitol Res 2007;101:1183-1190.

156. Barsoum RS: Malarial acute renal failure. J Am Soc Nephrol 2000;11:2147-2154.

157. Gryseels B, Polman K, Clerinx J, Kestens L: Human schistosomiasis. Lancet 2006;368:1106-1118.

158. Barsoum RS: Schistosomiasis and the kidney. Semin Nephrol 2003;23:34-41.

159. Gogus C, Safak M, Baltaci S, Turkolmez K: Isolated renal hydatidosis: Experience with 20 cases. J Urol 2003;169:186-189.

160. Angulo JC, Escribano J, Diego A, Sanchez-Chapado M: Isolated retrovesical and extrarenal retroperitoneal hydatidosis: Clinical study of 10 cases and literature review. J Urol 1998;159: 76-82.

161. Haas M: IgA nephropathy and Henoch Schönlein purpura. In Jennette JC, Olson JL, Schwartz MM, Silva FG (eds): Heptinstall's Pathology of the Kidney, vol 1, 6th ed. Philadelphia, Lippincott Williams & Wilkins, 2007, p 424.

162. Schwartz MM: Membranous glomerulonephritis. In Jennette JC, Olson JL, Schwartz MM, Silva FG (eds): Heptinstall's Pathology of the Kidney, vol 1, 6th ed. Philadelphia, Lippincott Williams & Wilkins, 2007, p 205.

163. van Velthuysen ML, Florquin S: Glomerulopathy associated with parasitic infections. Clin Microbiol Rev 2000;13:55-66.

164. Nadasdy T, Silva FG: Acute postinfectious glomerulonephritis and glomerulonephritis caused by persistent bacterial infection. In Jennette JC, Olson JL, Schwartz MM, Silva FG (eds): Heptinstall's Pathology of the Kidney, vol 1, 6th ed. Philadelphia, Lippincott Williams & Wilkins, 2007, p 322.

165. Bright R: Cases and observations illustrative of renal disease accompanied with the secretion of albuminous urine. Guy's Hosp Rep 1836;1:338.

166. Barisoni L, Meehan S, Arend LJ: Introduction to renal biopsy. In Zhou M (ed): Genitourinary Pathology. Philadelphia, Churchill Livingstone Elsevier, 2007.

167. Levy M, Chen N: Worldwide perspective of hepatitis B-associated glomerulonephritis in the 80s. Kidney Int Suppl 1991;35:S24-S33.

168. Lhotta K: Beyond hepatorenal syndrome: Glomerulonephritis in patients with liver disease. Semin Nephrol 2002;22:302-308.

169. Pucillo LP, Agnello V: Membranoproliferative glomerulonephritis associated with hepatitis B and C viral infections: From viruslike particles in the cryoprecipitate to viral localization in paramesangial deposits, problematic investigations prone to artifacts. Curr Opin Nephrol Hypertens 1994;3:465-470.

170. Takekoshi Y, Tochimaru H, Nagata Y, Itami N: Immunopathogenetic mechanisms of hepatitis B virus-related glomerulopathy. Kidney Int Suppl 1991;35:S34-S39.

171. Kern WF, Silva FG, Laszik ZG, et al (eds): The Atlas of Renal Pathology. Philadelphia, WB Saunders, 1999.

172. Gonzalez JA, Marcol BR, Wolf MC: Complications of intravesical bacillus Calmette-Guerin: A case report. J Urol 1992;148:1892-1893.

173. Andrei G, Fiten P, Goubau P, et al: Dual infection with polyomavirus BK and acyclovir-resistant herpes simplex virus successfully treated with cidofovir in a bone marrow transplant recipient. Transpl Infect Dis 2007;9:126-131.

174. Harkensee C, Vasdev N, Gennery AR, et al: Prevention and management of BK-virus associated haemorrhagic cystitis in children following haematopoietic stem cell transplantation: A systematic review and evidence-based guidance for clinical management. Br J Haematol 2008;142:717-731.

175. Hirsch HH, Steiger J: Polyomavirus BK. Lancet Infect Dis 2003;3:611-623.

176. Leung AY, Yuen KY, Kwong YL: Polyoma BK virus and haemorrhagic cystitis in haematopoietic stem cell transplantation: A changing paradigm. Bone Marrow Transplant 2005;36:929-937.

177. Mvula M, Iwasaka T, Iguchi A, et al: Do human papillomaviruses have a role in the pathogenesis of bladder carcinoma? J Urol 1996;155:471-474.

178. Youshya S, Purdie K, Breuer J, et al: Does human papillomavirus play a role in the development of bladder transitional cell carcinoma? A comparison of PCR and immunohistochemical analysis. J Clin Pathol 2005;58:207-210.

179. Soper D: Trichomoniasis: Under control or undercontrolled? Am J Obstet Gynecol 2004;190:281-290.

180. Burstein GR, Zenilman JM: Nongonococcal urethritis: A new paradigm. Clin Infect Dis 1999;28(Suppl 1):S66-S73.

181. Erbelding EJ, Quinn TC: Urethritis treatment. Dermatol Clin 1998;16:735-738, xi-xii.

182. Schwartz MA, Hooton TM: Etiology of nongonococcal nonchlamydial urethritis. Dermatol Clin 1998;16:727-733, xi.

183. Krieger JN: Trichomoniasis in men: Old issues and new data. Sex Transm Dis 1995;22:83-96.

184. Giacomini G, Bianchi G, Moretti D: Detection of sexually transmitted diseases by urethral cytology, the ignored male counterpart of cervical cytology. Acta Cytol 1989;33:11-15.

185. Long JP Jr, Althausen AF: Malacoplakia: A 25-year experience with a review of the literature. J Urol 1989;141:1328-1331.

186. Meria P, Desgrippes A, Arfi C, Le Duc A: Encrusted cystitis and pyelitis. J Urol 1998;160:3-9.

187. Soriano F, Tauch A: Microbiological and clinical features of *Corynebacterium urealyticum*: Urinary tract stones and genomics as the rosetta stone. Clin Microbiol Infect 2008;14:632-643.

188. Quint HJ, Drach GW, Rappaport WD, Hoffmann CJ: Emphysematous cystitis: A review of the spectrum of disease. J Urol 1992; 147:134-137.

189. Grupper M, Kravtsov A, Potasman I: Emphysematous cystitis: Illustrative case report and review of the literature. Medicine (Baltimore) 2007;86:47-53.

190. Patel NP, Lavengood RW, Fernandes M, et al: Gas-forming infections in genitourinary tract. Urology 1992;39:341-345.

191. Newman LM, Moran JS, Workowski KA: Update on the management of gonorrhea in adults in the United States. Clin Infect Dis 2007;44(Suppl 3):S84-S101.

192. Galadari I, Galadari H: Nonspecific urethritis and reactive arthritis. Clin Dermatol 2004;22:469-475.

193. Wagenlehner FM, Weidner W, Naber KG: Chlamydial infections in urology. World J Urol 2006;24:4-12.

194. Sharma TC, Kagan HN, Sheils JP: Malacoplakia of the male urethra. J Urol 1981;125:885-886.

195. Epstein JI: The prostate and seminal vesicles. In Mills SE, Carter D, Greenson JK, et al. (eds): Sternberg's Diagnostic Surgical Pathology, vol 2, 4th ed. Philadelphia, Lippincott Williams & Wilkins, 2004, p 2083.

196. Ludwig M: Diagnosis and therapy of acute prostatitis, epididymitis and orchitis. Andrologia 2008;40:76-80.

197. Srigley JR: Benign mimickers of prostatic adenocarcinoma. Mod Pathol 2004;17:328-348.

198. Wagner D, Joseph J, Huang J, Xu H: Malakoplakia of the prostate on needle core biopsy: A case report and review of the literature. Int J Surg Pathol 2007;15:86-89.

199. Yurkanin JP, Ahmann F, Dalkin BL: Coccidioidomycosis of the prostate: A determination of incidence, report of 4 cases, and treatment recommendations. J Infect 2006;52:e19-e25.

200. Wise GJ, Silver DA: Fungal infections of the genitourinary system. J Urol 1993;149:1377-1388.

201. Matlaga BR, Veys JA, Thacker CC, Assimos DG: Prostate abscess following intravesical bacillus Calmette-Guerin treatment. J Urol 2002;167:251.

202. Leibovici D, Zisman A, Chen-Levyi Z, et al: Elevated prostate specific antigen serum levels after intravesical instillation of bacillus Calmette-Guerin. J Urol 2000;164:1546-1549.

203. Mukamel E, Konichezky M, Engelstein D, et al: Clinical and pathological findings in prostates following intravesical bacillus Calmette-Guerin instillations. J Urol 1990;144:1399-1400.

204. Oates RD, Stilmant MM, Freedlund MC, Siroky MB: Granulomatous prostatitis following bacillus Calmette-Guerin immunotherapy of bladder cancer. J Urol 1988;140:751-754.

205. Oppenheimer JR, Kahane H, Epstein JI: Granulomatous prostatitis on needle biopsy. Arch Pathol Lab Med 1997;121:724-729.

206. Sporer A, Auerbach O: Tuberculosis of prostate. Urology 1978;11:362-365.

207. Lee LW, Burgher LW, Price EB Jr, Cassidy E: Granulomatous prostatitis: Association with isolation of *Mycobacterium kansasii* and *Mycobacterium fortuitum*. JAMA 1977;237:2408-2409.

208. Phillips P, Bonner S, Gataric N, et al: Nontuberculous mycobacterial immune reconstitution syndrome in HIV-infected patients: Spectrum of disease and long-term follow-up. Clin Infect Dis 2005;41:1483-1497.

209. Mikolich DJ, Mates SM: Granulomatous prostatitis due to *Mycobacterium avium* complex. Clin Infect Dis 1992;14:589-591.

210. Kelalis PP, Greene LF, Weed LA: Brucellosis of the urogenital tract: A mimic of tuberculosis. J Urol 1962;88:347-353.

211. de Souza E, Katz DA, Dworzack DL, Longo G: Actinomycosis of the prostate. J Urol 1985;133:290-291.

212. de Lima MA, dos Santos JA, Lazo J, et al: Cryptococcus infection limited to the prostate in an AIDS patient with disseminated mycobacteriosis: A necropsy report. Rev Soc Bras Med Trop 1997;30:501-505.

213. Goff DA, Davidson RA: Amebic prostatitis. South Med J 1984;77:1053-1054.

214. Alexis R, Domingo J: Schistosomiasis and adenocarcinoma of prostate: A morphologic study. Hum Pathol 1986;17:757-760.

215. Lambertucci JR, Voieta I, Barbosa AJ: *Schistosomiasis mansoni* of the prostate. Rev Soc Bras Med Trop 2006;39:233-234.

216. Ma TK, Srigley JR: Adenocarcinoma of prostate and schistosomiasis: A rare association. Histopathology 1995;27:187-189.

217. Arean VM: Lesions caused by *Schistosoma mansoni* in the genitourinary tract of men. Am J Clin Pathol 1956;26:1010-1021.

218. Houston W: Primary hydatid cyst of the prostate gland. J Urol 1975;113:732-733.

219. Clason AE, McGeorge A, Garland C, Abel BJ: Urinary retention and granulomatous prostatitis following sacral herpes zoster infection: A report of 2 cases with a review of the literature. Br J Urol 1982;54:166-169.

220. Benson PJ, Smith CS: Cytomegalovirus prostatitis. Urology 1992;40:165-167.

221. De Marzo AM, Platz EA, Sutcliffe S, et al: Inflammation in prostate carcinogenesis. Nat Rev Cancer 2007;7:256-269.

222. Kramer G, Marberger M: Could inflammation be a key component in the progression of benign prostatic hyperplasia? Curr Opin Urol 2006;16:25-29.

223. Platz EA, De Marzo AM: Epidemiology of inflammation and prostate cancer. J Urol 2004;171:S36-S40.

224. Nelson WG, De Marzo AM, DeWeese TL, Isaacs WB: The role of inflammation in the pathogenesis of prostate cancer. J Urol 2004;172:S6-S11; discussion S11-S12.

225. De Marzo AM, Meeker AK, Zha S, et al: Human prostate cancer precursors and pathobiology. Urology 2003;62:55-62.

226. Schaeffer AJ: Epidemiology and demographics of prostatitis. Andrologia 2003;35:252-257.

227. Krieger JN: Epididymitis, orchitis, and related conditions. Sex Transm Dis 1984;11:173-181.

228. Levin HS: Nonneoplastic diseases of the testis. In Mills SE, Carter D, Greenson JK, et al. (eds): Sternberg's Diagnostic Surgical Pathology, vol 2, 4th ed. Philadelphia, Lippincott Williams & Wilkins, 2004, p 2133.

229. Glassy FJ, Mostofi FK: Spermatic granulomas of the epididymis. Am J Clin Pathol 1956;26:1303-1313.

230. Mikuz G, Damjanov I: Inflammation of the testis, epididymis, peritesticular membranes, and scrotum. Pathol Annu 1982;17(Pt 1):101-128.

231. McCarthy JM, McLoughlin MG, Shackleton CR, et al: Cytomegalovirus epididymitis following renal transplantation. J Urol 1991;146:417-419.

232. Dalton AD, Harcourt-Webster JN: The histopathology of the testis and epididymis in AIDS: A post-mortem study. J Pathol 1991;163:47-52.

233. Lalitha MK, John R: Unusual manifestations of salmonellosis: A surgical problem. Q J Med 1994;87:301-309.

234. Huth RG, Goldstein E: Testicular abscess caused by *Salmonella typhi*. South Med J 1991;84:1156-1157.

235. Desche P, Benoit G, Pocheville M, et al: Extradigestive forms of nontyphoid salmonellosis in renal transplant patients: 5 Cases. Ann Med Interne (Paris) 1983;134:545-548.

236. von Schnakenburg C, Hinrichs B, Fuchs J, Kardorff R: Post-transplant epididymitis and orchitis following *Listeria monocytogenes* septicaemia. Pediatr Transplant 2000;4:156-158.

237. Navarro-Martinez A, Solera J, Corredoira J, et al: Epididymoorchitis due to *Brucella mellitensis*: A retrospective study of 59 patients. Clin Infect Dis 2001;33:2017-2022.

238. Hunt AC, Bothwell PW: Histological findings in human brucellosis. J Clin Pathol 1967;20:267-272.

239. Singh D, Dutta S, Kumar P, Narang A: Mixed anaerobic and aerobic testicular abscess in a neonate. Indian J Pediatr 2001;68:561-562.

240. Ulbright TM: The most common, clinically significant misdiagnoses in testicular tumor pathology, and how to avoid them. Adv Anat Pathol 2008;15:18-27.

241. Aitchison M, Mufti GR, Farrell J, et al: Granulomatous orchitis: Review of 15 cases. Br J Urol 1990;66:312-314.

242. Kahn RI, McAninch JW: Granulomatous disease of the testis. J Urol 1980;123:868-871.

243. Hepper NG, Karlson AG, Leary FJ, Soule EH: Genitourinary infection due to *Mycobacterium kansasii*. Mayo Clin Proc 1971;46:387-390.

244. De Paepe ME, Guerrieri C, Waxman M: Opportunistic infections of the testis in the acquired immunodeficiency syndrome. Mt Sinai J Med 1990;57:25-29.

245. Garbyal RS, Gupta P, Kumar S, Bohra A: Diagnosis of isolated tuberculous orchitis by fine-needle aspiration cytology. Diagn Cytopathol 2006;34:698-700.

246. Jacob JT, Nguyen TM, Ray SM: Male genital tuberculosis. Lancet Infect Dis 2008;8:335-342.

247. Ludwig M, Velcovsky HG, Weidner W: Tuberculous epididymo-orchitis and prostatitis: A case report. Andrologia 2008;40:81-83.

248. Akhtar M, Ali MA, Mackey DM: Lepromatous leprosy presenting as orchitis. Am J Clin Pathol 1980;73:712-715.

249. Grabstald H, Swan LL: Genitourinary lesions in leprosy, with special reference to the problem of atrophy of the testes. J Am Med Assoc 1952;119:1287-1291.

250. El-Beheiry A, Abou Zeid S, El-Ghazzawi E, et al: The leprous testis. Arch Androl 1979;3:173-176.

251. Singh N, Arora VK, Jain A, et al: Cytology of testicular changes in leprosy. Acta Cytol 2002;46:659-663.

252. Saporta L, Yuksel A: Androgenic status in patients with lepromatous leprosy. Br J Urol 1994;74:221-224.

253. Singer AJ, Kubak B, Anders KH: Aspergillosis of the testis in a renal transplant recipient. Urology 1998;51:119-121.

254. Schuster TG, Hollenbeck BK, Kauffman CA, et al: Testicular histoplasmosis. J Urol 2000;164:1652.

255. Monroe M: Proceedings: Granulomatous orchitis due to *Histoplasma capsulatum* masquerading as sperm granuloma. J Clin Pathol 1974;27:929-930.

256. Riggs S, Sanford JP: Viral orchitis. N Engl J Med 1962;266:990-993.

257. Craighead JE, Mahoney EM, Carver DH, et al: Orchitis due to coxsackie virus group B, type 5: Report of a case with isolation of virus from the testis. N Engl J Med 1962;267:498-500.

258. Smith RD, Konoplev S, DeCourten-Myers G, Brown T: West nile virus encephalitis with myositis and orchitis. Hum Pathol 2004;35:254-258.

259. Gall EA: The histopathology of acute mumps orchitis. Am J Pathol 1947;23:637.

260. Singh R, Mostafid H, Hindley RG: Measles, mumps and rubella: The urologist's perspective. Int J Clin Pract 2006;60:335-339.

261. Hviid A, Rubin S, Muhlemann K: Mumps. Lancet 2008;371:932-944.

262. Abdelbaky AM, Channappa DB, Islam S: Unilateral epididymo-orchitis: A rare complication of MMR vaccine. Ann R Coll Surg Engl 2008;90:336-337.

263. Wong TW, Straus FH 2nd, Warner NE: Testicular biopsy in the study of male infertility. Arch Pathol 1973;95:151-159.

264. Masarani M, Wazait H, Dinneen M: Mumps orchitis. J R Soc Med 2006;99:573-575.

265. Werner CA: Mumps orchitis and testicular atrophy: A factor in male sterility. Ann Intern Med 1950;32:1075-1086.

266. Werner CA: Mumps orchitis and testicular atrophy: Occurrence. Ann Intern Med 1950;32:1066-1074.

267. Welch K, Finkbeiner W, Alpers CE, et al: Autopsy findings in the acquired immune deficiency syndrome. JAMA 1984;252:1152-1159.

268. Reichert CM, O'Leary TJ, Levens DL, et al: Autopsy pathology in the acquired immune deficiency syndrome. Am J Pathol 1983;112:357-382.

269. Mhawech P, Onorato M, Uchida T, Borucki MJ: Testicular atrophy in 80 HIV-positive patients: A multivariate statistical analysis. Int J STD AIDS 2001;12:221-224.

270. Shevchuk MM, Nuovo GJ, Khalife G: HIV in testis: Quantitative histology and HIV localization in germ cells. J Reprod Immunol 1998;41:69-79.

271. Shevchuk MM, Pigato JB, Khalife G, et al: Changing testicular histology in AIDS: Its implication for sexual transmission of HIV. Urology 1999;53:203-208.

272. Bannur HB, Malur PR, Dhorigol VM: Tubercular orchitis in a patient with AIDS: Report of a case with fine needle aspiration diagnosis. Acta Cytol 2007;51:459-460.

273. Leibovitch I, Baniel J, Rowland RG, et al: Malignant testicular neoplasms in immunosuppressed patients. J Urol 1996;155:1938-1942.

274. Ramadan A, Naab T, Frederick W, Green W: Testicular plasmacytoma in a patient with the acquired immunodeficiency syndrome. Tumori 2000;86:480-482.

275. Wilson WT, Frenkel E, Vuitch F, Sagalowsky AI: Testicular tumors in men with human immunodeficiency virus. J Urol 1992;147:1038-1040.

276. Roehrborn CG, Worrell JT, Wiley EL: Bilateral synchronous testis tumors of different histology in a patient with the acquired immunodeficiency syndrome related complex. J Urol 1990;144:353-355.

277. Tessler AN, Catanese A: AIDS and germ cell tumors of testis. Urology 1987;30:203-204.

278. Ikematsu H, Cerutti A, Zan H, et al: Ongoing hypermutation in the ig V(D)J gene segments and c-myc proto-oncogene of an AIDS lymphoma segregates with neoplastic B cells at different sites: Implications for clonal evolution. Hum Immunol 2000;61:1242-1253.

279. Siskin GP, Haller JO, Miller S, Sundaram R: AIDS-related lymphoma: Radiologic features in pediatric patients. Radiology 1995;196:63-66.

280. Leibovitch I, Goldwasser B: The spectrum of acquired immune deficiency syndrome-associated testicular disorders. Urology 1994;44:818-824.

281. Buzelin F, Karam G, Moreau A, et al: Testicular tumor and the acquired immunodeficiency syndrome. Eur Urol 1994;26:71-76.

282. Armenakas NA, Schevchuk MM, Brodherson M, Fracchia JA: AIDS presenting as primary testicular lymphoma. Urology 1992;40:162-164.

283. Wolback SB, Todd JC, Palfrey FW: The Etiology and Pathology of Typhus. Cambridge, Mass., Harvard University Press, 1922, pp 13-14.

284. Dao AH, Adkins RB: Bilateral gummatous orchitis. South Med J 1980;73:954-955.

285. Terao T, Kura N, Ohashi H, et al: Syphilitic orchitis: Report of a case. Hinyokika Kiyo 1993;39:973-976.

286. Nakano Y, Chokyu H, Inaba Y, et al: Syphilitic orchitis: A case report. Hinyokika Kiyo 1999;45:289-291.

287. Fussell EN, Kaack MB, Cherry R, Roberts JA: Adherence of bacteria to human foreskins. J Urol 1988;140:997-1001.

288. Perfect JR, Seaworth BA: Penile cryptococcosis with review of mycotic infections of penis. Urology 1985;25:528-531.

Gynecologic Infections

Rosemary Tambouret

Because the female genital tract comprises both cutaneous and mucosal surfaces in contact with the external environment, exposure to a significant number of infectious agents, either commensal or pathogenic, is the norm. And because the lower genital tract is in communication with the normally sterile peritoneal cavity, ascending infections can be treacherous. In addition, close physical contact with sexual partners can lead to infectious sexually transmitted disease (STD), especially if the woman is exposed to multiple sexual partners. The external genitalia and the lower female genital tract are the sites of the majority of infections, which are often transitory and without serious sequelae. Most of these infections are recognized clinically without need of biopsy and are treated on the basis of the clinical presentation. However, biopsy is warranted if the prescribed treatment is not effective or if the presentation is atypical. Also, routine cervical cytology specimens (the Pap smear), used to screen for malignant and premalignant lesions, regularly identify a limited number of potential pathogens.

The upper genital tract can be the site of silent infections with serious secondary effects such as infertility. In the case of suspected infection, the endometrium is readily amenable to biopsy, but the fallopian tubes and ovaries are usually examined only if significant disease is present.

Immunocompromised patients often experience more severe infections or infections due to organisms not previously associated with disease. The patients most affected include transplant recipients, oncology patients, and patients with acquired immunodeficiency syndrome (AIDS).

Most clinical reviews of infections of the female genital tract emphasize the anatomic site and clinical manifestations, with an added emphasis on the clinical appearance of lesions arising in the lower genital tract and the appearance on radiologic imaging for infections in the upper genital tract. For example, herpes infection of the cervix often causes small vesicles that evolve into shallow ulcers. Where appropriate, the clinical or radiologic appearance of the lesion is mentioned in the text here.

Lower Genital Tract

Vulva and Vagina

Viral Infections

Genital infection by human papillomavirus (HPV) produces exophytic genital warts or condyloma acuminata, usually found on the perineum and labia and, with less frequency, on the vagina, cervix, and anal region. Cervical and vaginal lesions caused by HPV infection are common but are usually flat condylomata. More than 100 HPV types have been identified, at least 31 of which infect the genital tract.[1] A subset of the genital HPV types confer a high risk to the infected epithelium for development of cancer. All HPV types are epitheliotropic obligate intracellular viruses that promote cell proliferation in normally quiescent, more differentiated epithelial cells. HPV infection produces a hyperplastic epithelial lesion. On the external genitalia, condyloma acuminata appear as exophytic, smooth to somewhat rough, flesh-colored papules, either single or multiple, that are not usually biopsied before treatment.[2] However, because cervical or vaginal lesions often accompany condyloma acuminata of the external genitalia, a careful vaginal and cervical examination should be done, usually with a speculum examination after application of acetic acid, which causes an aceto-white appearance of

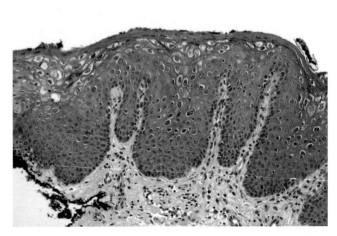

Figure 16-1. Condylomatous lesion of the vulva with viral cytopathic effect (koilocytosis) of human papillomavirus infection (H&E, ×40).

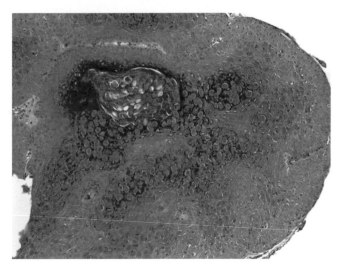

Figure 16-2. Molluscum contagiosum viral cytopathic effect on squamous epithelium of the vulva (H&E, ×40).

the HPV-induced lesions due to coagulation of cytokeratins of infected squamous cells.[3] If the condyloma acuminatum is biopsied, the histologic findings include acanthosis, parakeratosis, and hyperkeratosis which may be associated with a branching papillomatous architecture with fibrovascular cores (Fig. 16-1).[4] But the hallmark is the HPV viral cytopathic effect, known as koilocytosis, which corresponds to a cavitation of the cytoplasm of the infected cell along with nuclear hyperchromasia and enlargement with membrane irregularity. Koilocytosis occurs as a result of the vegetative cycle of the HPV and is due to the accumulation of infective virions in the nucleus with disruption of cytoplasmic keratin in infected squamous cells.[5,6] Koilocytosis is less pronounced in lesions of the perineum, vulva, and vagina than in lesions of the cervix.[3,7,8]

Molluscum contagiosum is caused by a chronic, localized infection with poxvirus that causes flesh-colored, rounded, raised papules with an umbilicated center.[9] Diagnosis is usually based on the clinical appearance, but if a biopsy is performed to rule out other clinically similar lesions, such as those caused by cryptococcosis or histoplasmosis, the keratinocytes are found to contain large, eosinophilic cytoplasmic viral inclusions (Fig. 16-2).[10,11]

Herpes simplex virus (HSV) is common and often subclinical (manifested only by the serum antibody response), so the incidence of disease is difficult to determine.[12] Both HSV type 1 and type 2 cause genital HSV infection. HSV infections are categorized as primary if the patient has no preexisting antibodies to HSV-1 or HSV-2; as nonprimary if a new infection arises in a patient with antibody evidence of the other HSV type; or as recurrent if there is serologic evidence of the same type as found in the reactivated infection. In a survey of adults in New York City, 28% were found to be infected with HSV-2 but only 12% were aware that they were infected.[13] The most severe symptoms tend to occur during primary infection and include genital vesicles with subsequent ulcer formation, fever, and regional lymphadenopathy. Clinical diagnosis of HSV infection is confirmed by viral culture, polymerase chain reaction (PCR), direct fluorescence antibody, and type-specific serologic tests.[14]

Figure 16-3. Tzanck-stained smear of vulvar ulcer showing ground glass nuclear herpes simplex virus cytopathic effect in epithelial cells (Papanicolaou stain, ×100).

PCR and serology are more sensitive than culture.[15,16] If need be, a genital ulcer can be scraped to obtain material for cytology (Tzanck preparation) or biopsied. The Tzanck smear, reported to have a low sensitivity and specificity for HSV cytopathic effect, is prepared by scraping the base of a fresh ulcer (Fig. 16-3).[17] The slide may be air dried and stained with Wright-Giemsa stain, or the cells may be fixed with alcohol and stained with Papanicolaou stain. HSV-infected epithelial cells show either a homogenization of the chromatin, with a termed ground glass appearance, or clumping of the chromatin on the nuclear membrane and in the center of the nucleus. The infected cells are often multinucleated. Biopsy is most informative if an intact vesicle is sampled. The intraepidermal vesicle shows degenerating keratinocytes; intranuclear viral cytopathic changes are most easily found on the margin of the vesicle. With ulceration, the changes are less specific and include chronic inflammation and granulation tissue (Fig. 16-4).

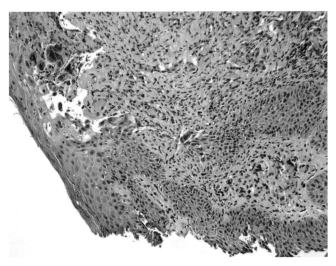

Figure 16-4. Vulvar biopsy with vesicle secondary to herpes simplex virus cytopathic effect in squamous cells (H&E, ×20).

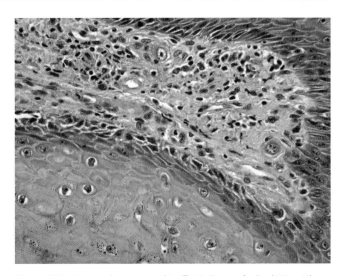

Figure 16-5. Cytomegalovirus cytopathic effect in biopsy of vulva (H&E, ×40).

Table 16-1 Genital Infections Presenting as Ulcers

Organism (Disease)	Gross Characteristics
Herpes simplex virus	Shallow painful ulcers, initially pruritic focus evolves to blister
Epstein-Barr virus	Ulcer similar to herpes
Cytomegalovirus	Ulcer similar to herpes
Treponema pallidum (chancre of primary syphilis)	Painless ulcers
Chlamydia trachomatis (lymphogranuloma venereum)	Shallow, painless ulcer
Haemophilus ducreyi (chancroid)	Begins as nodule, evolves to pustule, then to painful ulcer
Klebsiella granulomatis (granuloma inguinale)	Painless ulcers evolve to hidradenitis
Escherichia coli (malakoplakia)	Papule or plaque evolving to ulcer

HSV-2 infection in HIV-infected women may produce hypertrophic vulvar lesions that may mimic a neoplasm.[18] Biopsies to demonstrate viral cytopathic effect and culture are necessary to diagnose this uncommon condition.

Rarely, primary infection with Epstein-Barr virus (EBV) can be accompanied by genital ulcers that clinically mimic the more common ulceration caused by HSV (Table 16-1).[19,20] Ulceration due to EBV should be considered in young patients who have painful ulcers, lymphadenopathy in a region distant from the ulcer, and systemic symptoms. An EBV etiology should be considered if bacterial and viral cultures, as well as the results of syphilis serology studies, are negative.

Cytomegalovirus (CMV) infection of the vulva manifests with ulceration.[21] Characteristic viral intranuclear and intracytoplasmic inclusions are identified in epithelial cells and endothelial cells (Fig. 16-5).

Bacterial Infections

Erythrasma, an uncommon infection of the vulva caused by *Corynebacterium minutissimum*, is usually diagnosed by fluorescence of the bacteria under the Wood lamp.[22] Rarely, Wood lamp examination is negative, but the diagnosis can be made histologically.[23] The clinical presentation is similar to vulvar candidiasis, but, on biopsy, filamentous bacteria are present in the stratum corneum.[23]

The chancre, the primary lesion of syphilis caused by the spirochete *Treponema pallidum*, is a nontender ulcer with a clean base.[24] *T. pallidum* cannot be cultured. Dark-field microscopy or direct fluorescent antibody is used on scrapings from the ulcer bed to diagnosis primary infection.[25] The epidermis is acanthotic along the rim and thinned or eroded in the center of the lesion. A dense lymphoplasmacytic infiltrate is found in the dermis surrounding blood vessels with swollen endothelial cells. Silver stains, such as Warthin-Starry stain, demonstrate many 8- to 15-μm spirochetes within the epidermis and around blood vessels.[4]

Condyloma lata, the lesions of secondary syphilis that arise 1 to 6 months after healing of the primary chancre, appear clinically raised, somewhat flattened, and velvety.[26] On biopsy, condyloma lata show epidermal hyperplasia and lymphoplasmacytic infiltration of dermal vessels with endothelial hyperplasia, dilatation of the vascular lumens, and thickening of their walls. Interface dermatitis and scattered epithelioid granulomas may be seen. Silver stain highlights spirochetes in a minority of cases, usually around blood vessels and within the epidermis.[4]

Bacillary angiomatosis of the vulva and cervix has been reported in a patient with AIDS; it manifested as red-purple nodules that microscopically comprised a lobular epithelioid vascular proliferation with neutrophils and aggregates of bacterial organisms (Table 16-2).[27] The responsible gram-negative bacterium, *Bartonella henselae*, can be demonstrated by blood cultures and histologically with Warthin-Starry stain.[28] The differential diagnosis in an immunocompromised patient is Kaposi sarcoma secondary to human herpesvirus 8 (HHV-8) infection.[29]

Acute inflammation or folliculitis of the hair follicles of the vulva produces an erythematous papule that evolves into a

Table 16-2 Genital Infections Manifesting as Raised Nodules

Organism (Disease)	Characteristics
Human papillomavirus	Smooth to rough, flesh-colored papules
Molluscum contagiosum	Nodule with central crater
Cryptococcus neoformans	Nodules can evolve to painless ulcer
Histoplasma capsulatum	Nodules can evolve to ulcers
Treponema pallidum (condyloma lata of secondary syphilis)	
Bartonella henselae (bacillary angiomatosis)	Red-purple papules
Human herpesvirus 8 (Kaposi sarcoma)	Red-purple papules
Mycobacterium tuberculosis	Dermal or lamina propria nodules
Trichophyton spp. (Majocchi granuloma)	Erythematous raised plaque with prominent border
Myiasis	Dome-shaped lesion with central pore

pustule, then a carbuncle through coalescence of several pustules, and even a furuncle or boil if the abscess extends into the subcutaneous tissue.[30,31] The most common causative species is *Staphylococcus aureus*, but other bacteria may be the cause, such as *Pseudomonas aeruginosa* secondary to hot-tub or swimming-pool contamination.[32] Less common causative agents include non-tuberculous mycobacteria, *Klebsiella oxytoca*, and *Acinetobacter baumannii*.

Recurrent abscess formation leading to scarring and sinus formation is termed hidradenitis suppurativa; it is a relatively common condition, occurring in 1% to 4% of the population.[33,34] It is probably caused by obstruction of a hair follicle followed by secondary bacterial infection.[35] The condition affects more women than men and primarily the intertriginous skin, including the perianal and perineal regions. Clinically, hidradenitis suppurativa is characterized by recurrent deep, painful nodules that ultimately drain malodorous, purulent material and that often lead to scarring and sinus formation or even fistulas to contiguous organs such as the bladder.[36,37] Central necrosis, characteristic of a furuncle, is not a feature of hidradenitis suppurativa. The lesion is excised if malignancy is suspected or to remove scarred tissue harboring sinuses. The differential diagnosis includes Crohn disease of the vulva and chronic granuloma inguinale, which is distinguished by involvement of the vagina and cervix as well as the external genitalia.

Chancroid, although rarely encountered in the United States, is a common cause of genital ulcers in sub-Saharan Africa, Latin America, and Asia.[38] The cause is *Haemophilus ducreyi*, a small, gram-negative rod that requires special hemin-containing medium in a high CO_2 atmosphere at 33° to 35° C for culture.[39] Gram staining of the culture shows a parallel array of bacteria resembling a school of fish. This sexually transmitted infection produces a papule that progresses to a pustule and finally to a

painful ulcer with a gray, purulent base, usually associated with painful inguinal lymph node swelling.[40] Biopsy of the lesion shows acute inflammation in the epidermis and a perivascular mononuclear infiltrate or granulomatous response within the dermis; gram-negative bacteria can sometimes be found in the tissue with special staining techniques.[4] Clinical diagnosis and Gram staining of a sample of the exudate from the bed of the ulcer have low sensitivity; culture is more sensitive, but the culture medium is not widely available. The most sensitive method of diagnosis is muliplex PCR.[41]

Lymphogranuloma venereum, rare in the United States, is found in Asia, Africa, and South America. It is caused by the L serovars of *Chlamydia trachomatis*, which cause a painless, shallow, solitary ulcer on the vulva, vagina, or perianal region.[42] The ulcer is often missed. If it is left untreated, painful regional lymphadenopathy of the secondary, or inguinal, stage ensues.[43] If the disease continues to progress, fistulas, labial scarring, and even labial elephantiasis can develop. Diagnosis is primarily serologic, but recently a PCR test has been developed.[44] Biopsy findings show nonspecific, chronic inflammation or granulomatous inflammation.

Granuloma inguinale is rare in the United States but is common in the tropical regions of Asia and South America. Despite the name, it causes genital ulcers.[45] More men are infected than women. Initially, a papule that ulcerates forms on the vulva, vagina, or cervix; if left untreated, granuloma inguinale can lead to scarring similar to hidradenitis suppurativa. Granuloma inguinale, or donovanosis, is caused by the gram-negative rod, *K. granulomatis* (formerly called *Donovania granulomatis* or *Calymmatobacterium granulomatis* but reclassified by means of 16S ribosomal RNA analysis). The infection is rarely seen outside endemic areas that include India, Papua New Guinea, Australia, Brazil, and South Africa; sporadic cases occur in other areas of South Africa, the West Indies, and South America.[46] Clinically, the infection manifests as a papule or a nontender, red ulcer that can easily bleed and can evolve into secondary ulcers with necrosis and subsequent scarring. The ulcer may be verrucous. Besides the labia, the cervix and upper genital tract can be involved. *K. granulomatosis* can be cultured only with difficulty,[47] so diagnosis relies on demonstration of the bacteria on cytology or histology by special stain. Romanowsky-stained air-dried smears from the ulcer bed demonstrate numerous intracytoplasmic, short bacilli within macrophages.[46] Biopsy of the ulcer base, performed for smear-negative cases, should be stained with Giemsa or Warthin-Starry stain.[48] A PCR test has been developed for granuloma inguinale.[49] Ulcers caused by multiple infectious agents have been reported.[50,51]

Tuberculosis of the vulva is the rarest form of genital tuberculosis and is usually associated with foci of infection elsewhere in the genital tract.[52] Hypertrophic lesions with sinus formation may develop.[53,54] Surgery may be necessary in conjunction with anti-tuberculosis drugs.[55] Necrotizing granulomas are found on biopsy. PCR is increasingly used to diagnose *Mycobacterium tuberculosis* in clinical samples[56] and on fixed paraffin-embedded tissue to identify the strain of *M. tuberculosis* complex.[57,58]

Malakoplakia, a chronic histiocytic inflammatory response characterized by calcified Michaelis-Gutmann bodies, usually occurs in the urinary tract, more often in women than in men. Malakoplakia has been reported on rare occasions in the female genital tract, including the vulva[59,60] and, more often, the

Table 16-3 Genital Infections Presenting as Flat Lesions

Organism (Disease)	Characteristics
Candida albicans	Erythematous swelling
Schistosoma haematobium	"Sandy patches" appear as tiny rice grains beneath skin; also ulcers and polyps
Sarcoptes scabiei	Pruritic, erythematous, scaly tracts; also blisters and pustules
Corynebacterium minutissimum (erythrasma)	Erythematous lesion similar to candidiasis
Malassezia furfur (pityriasis or tinea versicolor)	Oval or irregular, flat, hypopigmented or hyperpigmented, 0.5- to 2.5-cm lesions

vagina.[61,62] Diagnosis of vaginal malakoplakia has been made by cytology, including fine-needle aspiration cytology.[63,64]

Fungal Infections

Candida is found in the vaginal tract of up to 50% of asymptomatic women; before menopause, the majority of women will have at least one episode of *Candida* vulvovaginitis, which is not considered to be an STD.[65-67] *Candida albicans* accounts for up to 90% of infections; *Candida glabrata* and *Candida parapsilosis* are less commonly the cause.[68,69] *Candida* vulvovaginitis manifests as a pruritic, erythematous swelling of the vulva with a thick, white vaginal exudate.[70,71] Diagnosis is usually achieved in the clinic by means of microscopic demonstration of yeast forms, with pseudohyphae in the case of *C. albicans*, after application of 10% potassium hydroxide to vaginal secretions (to disaggregate squamous cells) with a normal vaginal pH of less than 4.5. Biopsy occasionally is performed on long-standing, chronically pruritic, hyperkeratotic lesions; often, only a few organisms are found in the stratum corneum. Periodic acid–Schiff (PAS) with diastase or Grocott methenamine silver (GMS) stain can be used to highlight the yeast and pseudohyphae.[72] *Candida* spp. can cause pustular lesions in immunocompromised patients (Table 16-3).[31]

A recent marked nationwide increase in incidence of coccidioidomycosis has occurred in the United States, most particularly in endemic regions including Arizona and California.[73] Infection, which is four times more prevalent in men than in women, occurs after inhalation of spores. Most infections (60%) are asymptomatic, but flulike symptoms can occur; fewer than 1% of patients develop disseminated disease. Although vulvar lesions have not been reported, scrotal lesions have been described.[74]

Histoplasma capsulatum is a dimorphic fungus that is found worldwide but is most common in North and Central America.[75] In the United States, the fungus is endemic to the Mississippi and Ohio River valleys. Soil and caves contaminated by bird or bat guano are especially rich in this fungus. Infection, usually asymptomatic, occurs by the respiratory route. Fewer than 1% of patients develop clinically recognized symptoms, mainly pulmonary. Disseminated histoplasmosis usually occurs in immunocompromised patients, such as patients with AIDS or transplant recipients.[76] The liver, spleen, bone marrow, gastrointestinal tract, skin, and mucous membranes are involved. Ulcers of the female genital tract due to *H. capsulatum* have only rarely been described.[76,77] Disseminated histoplasmosis can also occur in non-immunocompromised elderly patients, in whom the slow disease progression is usually fatal. Disease in the elderly is not always accompanied by constitutional symptoms. A case of venereal spread provoking an isolated vulvar ulcer has been described.[78]

Cryptococcus neoformans, an encapsulated yeast, is found worldwide, especially in soil harboring pigeon guano, but infection usually causes symptoms only in immunocompromised patients.[79,80] With symptomatic infection, a granulomatous response develops. The fungus occurs as a yeast form in tissue and can be recognized on routine staining by its more variable size compared with other fungi (2-20 μm in diameter). Special stains used to highlight *Cryptococcus* include PAS and methenamine silver. The capsule can be seen in negative relief on smears with India ink and is demonstrated in tissue sections with mucicarmine stain. *Cryptococcus* contains phenol oxidase, which is involved in the metabolism of phenolic compounds to melanin. Phenol oxidase is a virulence factor, and the melanin that is produced can be detected by the Fontana-Masson stain on histologic sections.[81] Isolated lesions of the female genital tract have rarely been reported. A vaginal nodular lesion was found in a 20-year-old, non-immunocompromised woman,[82] and a painless ulcer of the labia major occurred in a 60-year-old renal transplant recipient.[83] In both instances, biopsy was performed because the lesions were clinically suspected to be carcinoma, and in both cases, granulomatous inflammation with mucin-positive fungi was found.

Trichophyton mentagrophytes has been reported to cause a case of Majocchi granuloma of the vulva in a young woman.[84] Majocchi granuloma, or nodular granulomatous perifolliculitis, is an uncommon intradermal infection by dermatophytes that usually cause follicular lesions.

Parasitic Infections

Genital schistosomiasis, usually caused by the bladder trematode, *Schistosoma haematobium*, which is endemic to Africa, has been reported to involve the vulva of women living in endemic areas such as Malawi[85,86] and in travelers.[87] The eggs gain access to the stromal tissue of the vulva via the venous drainage from the bladder and engender granulomatous inflammation.[88] A variety of lesions are associated with genital schistosomiasis, including polyps and ulcers, but the most common lesion is the "sandy patch," which appears as an aggregate of tiny rice grains beneath smooth mucosa.[89,90] Regional lymphadenopathy often accompanies the genital lesions.[91] The diagnosis relies on demonstration of the characteristic egg with a terminal spine in tissue biopsy.[86,92] It can be seen with routine hematoxylin and eosin (H&E) stain, but silver stains highlight the egg. *Schistosoma mansoni*, the cause of intestinal schistosomiasis, is found in many of the same regions of Africa as *S. haematobium*, as well as in South America and the Caribbean, and has also been associated with genital disease, although the incidence is less certain.[86,90,93] The ova of *S. mansoni* are differentiated from those of *S. haematobium* by the presence of a lateral spine; both are about 60 μm wide by 160 μm long (Fig. 16-6).

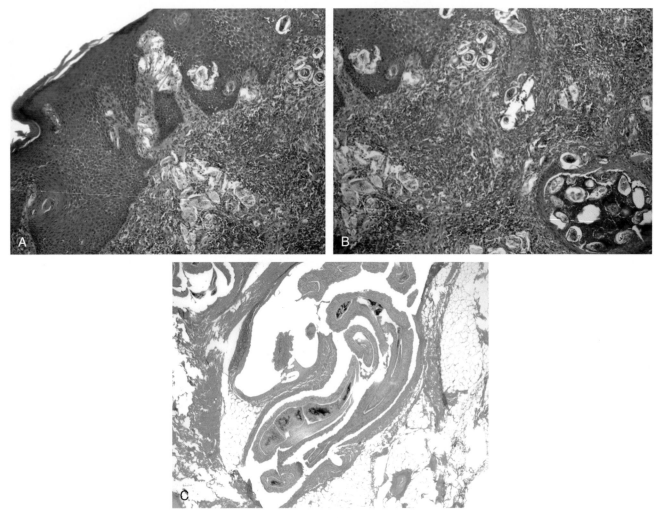

Figure 16-6. Vulvar biopsy of 7-year-old with swelling of the vulva. No purulent exudate was obtained on incision and drainage, so a biopsy was performed. It showed an intact, albeit acanthotic squamous epidermis **(A)**. Within the dermis were numerous, mostly embryonated, schistosome eggs, a few of which showed the terminal spine of *Schistosoma haematobium* **(B)**. Within the subcutis, a distended vein contained a pair of *Schistosoma* worms (male and female) (H&E). (Courtesy James Kitinya, MD, Tanzania.)

Vulvovaginitis secondary to *Enterobiasis vermicularis* has been reported in prepubertal girls and, rarely, in older women.[94]

Scabies is caused by the mite *Sarcoptes scabiei*, which is spread by fomites such as bed linens or as an STD, producing genital scabies. The mites burrow into the epidermis to lay eggs. Clinically, the burrow is linear and intensely pruritic. The mites and eggs are found in the epidermis, and a polymorphous inflammatory infiltrate is present in the dermis.[95,96]

Larval Infestations

Myiasis is the cutaneous infestation by larvae of several fly species. The larvae can infest devitalized tissue of open wounds or burrow into healthy skin of the vulva, resulting in furuncular myiasis. The lesion is dome-shaped, with a central pore from which a variable number of larvae exit. The infestation occurs mainly in tropical climates and is associated with poor hygiene, diabetes, and travel.[97-99]

Noninfectious Lesions in the Differential Diagnosis of Vulvar and Vaginal Infections

Fixed drug eruptions are circumscribed erythematous plaques that are usually located on the hands, feet, and external genitalia; the lesions recur in the same site with repeated exposure to the drug.[21,72] A central vesicle may develop. Biopsy of a vulvar lesion may be necessary, if the association with the offending drug is not recognized, to exclude similar-appearing infectious lesions such as HSV or secondary syphilis.[100] The histologic appearance of a fixed drug eruption consists of basal cell hydropic change, interface lymphoid infiltrate occasionally with eosinophils, and individual keratinocyte necrosis.[92]

Behçet disease, a rare cause of vulvar ulcers, occurs in Japan and Eastern Mediterranean countries. The diagnosis is made in the presence of recurrent oral ulcers and at least one of the following: genital ulcers, skin pustules or nodules, and uveitis/retinitis.[101] Herpetiform or aphthous vulvar ulcers show necrotizing vasculitis of all calibers of vessels, with acute or chronic

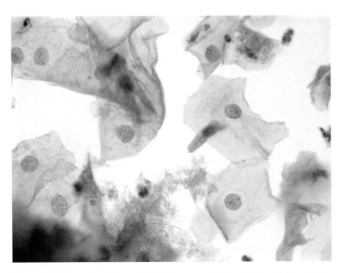

Figure 16-7. Lactobacilli in cervical cytology sample (Papanicolaou stain, ×100).

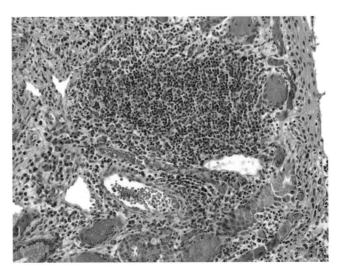

Figure 16-8. Follicular cervicitis: germinal center in the lamina propria of a cervical biopsy specimen.

inflammation.[92,102] The diagnosis is one of exclusion; ulcerative lesions of the vulva may be the presenting symptom.[103]

The differential diagnosis of vulvar and perianal abscesses, sinus tracts, and fistula formation includes Crohn disease. Crohn disease can be particularly challenging to diagnose if the genital manifestations precede the gastrointestinal lesions, in which case a diagnosis of granulomatous vulvitis may be made.[104] Sarcoidosis of the vulva has been reported.[105]

Cervix and Vagina

Normal Cervical and Vaginal Flora

The normal cervical-vaginal milieu is moist and acidic (pH 4-4.5), with a relatively large assortment of bacteria, the variety of which changes with the hormonal state of the woman. The predominant bacteria under normal conditions are lactobacillus, diphtheroids, and *Staphylococcus epidermidis.*

Lactobacillus acidophilus, a facultative anaerobic, gram-positive bacterium, predominates in the normal vaginal flora and produces an acidic vaginal pH due to the production of lactic acid from intracellular glycogen. During the normal female reproductive cycle, glycogen gradually accumulates in the squamous cells of the vagina and cervix. By the end of the luteal phase, in the absence of pregnancy, abundant lactobacilli will be found on cervical cytology preparations amid marked cytolysis or cytoplasmic debris and naked nuclei resulting from the action of the bacteria on the glycogen of the squamous cells (Fig. 16-7).

Cervicitis and Vaginitis

Symptoms of vaginitis and cervicitis are very common and consist of increased and malodorous vaginal discharge, pruritus, burning, and dyspareunia. The diagnosis is usually made clinically based on the presence of an abnormal discharge and erythema of the mucosa of the vagina, the cervix, or both. In the case of vaginitis, the diagnostic workup consists of assessment of the vaginal pH in women of reproductive age. A pH greater than 4.5 suggests bacterial vaginosis or *Trichomonas* infection and tends to

exclude candidiasis. In premenarchal and postmenopausal women, assessment of the pH is less helpful, because it is generally higher in these age groups. A saline wet preparation of vaginal-cervical secretions may demonstrate increased polymorphonuclear leukocytes, motile trichomonads, candidal yeast or pseudohyphae or clue cells (squamous cells covered by a blanket of coccobacilli) representing bacterial vaginosis. Culture or molecular tests should be performed for bacterial vaginosis, *Candida* vaginitis, and trichomoniasis, because clinical diagnosis and saline microscopy are poorly sensitive for these organisms.[71,106] Likewise, for *C. trachomatis* and *Neisseria gonorrhoeae* molecular tests should be performed.[107]

Varying degrees of acute and chronic inflammation including a mixture of lymphocytes, neutrophils, plasma cells, eosinophils, and histiocytes are commonly found in the mucosa of the cervix as an incidental finding on cervical biopsy specimens obtained at colposcopy as part of the workup of an abnormal cytology finding. Chronic cervicitis is diagnosed if the inflammation is marked and can be caused by a variety of organisms. Well-formed germinal cells are present in follicular cervicitis (Fig. 16-8).

On clinical examination, acute cervicitis is often recognized by erythema and a mucopurulent exudate. Microorganisms, chemical injury (spermaticides), or local trauma (intrauterine device [IUD], pessary, tampons) may be the cause. Acute inflammation is exceedingly common in cervical cytology samples obtained to screen for cancer, and the underlying cause is not usually evident.

Common Causes of Symptomatic Cervicitis and Vaginitis
Tissue biopsy is rarely performed in this setting, but a cervical-vaginal cytology sample may be obtained. A number of organisms are routinely identified on cervical cytology as incidental findings. In contrast to surgical pathology, special stains are not usually used on cervical cytology samples to highlight microorganisms. However, molecular tests, either alone or in conjunction with cytologic analysis, are commonly employed.

The most common causes of mucopurulent cervicitis are *C. trachomatis* and *N. gonorrhoeae. C. trachomatis is* a small, obligate intracellular, gram-negative bacterium that is transmitted by sexual contact. The life cycle of *C. trachomatis* comprises two phases. Infection begins with penetration of the small elementary body form of the bacterium into the cell, where the bacterium converts to the larger, metabolically active, reticular form, creating intracytoplasmic vacuoles. After 48 to 72 hours the cell ruptures, releasing infectious elementary bodies. The prevalence of *C. trachomatis* is 3% to 5% in asymptomatic women and as high as 20% in women attending STD clinics.[108] These figures probably reflect the successful use of screening texts, although most cases of *C. trachomatis* are not reported to the Centers for Disease Control and Prevention (CDC) from STD clinics. Reported cases are about three times more frequent in women than in men.[109] *Chlamydia* infection induces weak immunity and can lead to pelvic inflammatory disease (PID) in 30% of untreated patients. If untreated during pregnancy, infection can lead to early rupture of the membranes and risk of conjunctivitis and pneumonia in the newborn. Diagnosis is made primarily by nucleic acid amplification tests (NAATs) that include PCR. Samples for NAATs can be obtained from urine or from self-collected vaginal swabs. Screening programs for sexually active women younger than 25 years of age have been instituted in various health care settings. Although the cytopathic effect of *C. trachomatis* has been described as cytoplasmic vacuoles containing small eosinophilic coccoid bodies with epithelial cells,[110-114] the morphologic recognition of *Chlamydia* inclusions within epithelial cells is unreliable on both cytology and histology.[115-118] However, immunocytochemical staining has been shown to be sensitive for chlamydial infection.[117]

A shift in vaginal flora to a predominance of mainly anaerobic coccobacilli, including *Gardnerella vaginalis* and *Mobiluncus* species, is known as bacterial vaginosis, a condition that was formerly thought to be innocuous but in recent years has been found to be associated with an increased susceptibility to STDs and with preterm birth. Women with bacterial vaginosis are often asymptomatic but may present with a fishy-smelling vaginal discharge. On cervical cytology, the presence of a film of small coccobacilli covering the background of the smear as well as the entire surface of squamous cells is suggestive of bacterial vaginosis but must be correlated with the clinical findings (Fig. 16-9). The cytologist may choose to report the shift in vaginal flora, but this will probably have little impact on the treatment of the patient, because cervical cytology, by virtue of being a screening test, usually has a certain delay in being reported. The columnar epithelium of the endocervix is more susceptible to both bacterial and chlamydial infections, and this is thought to explain why young women and pregnant women with large ectropions are more susceptible to the development of acute endocervicitis.[108,119]

Trichomonas vaginalis infection is an STD that may be asymptomatic or may cause a thin, malodorous vaginal discharge accompanied by pruritus, dysuria, and other symptoms. Trichomoniasis is associated with premature rupture of membranes in the pregnant patient. On cervical cytology, the trichomonads assume a round, ovoid, or pear shape ranging from 15 to 30 µm. The cytoplasm is gray-blue, and the lancet-shaped nucleus is only slightly darker than the cytoplasm (Fig. 16-10). Occasionally, eosinophilic flagellae and cytoplasmic granules may be appreciated. The organisms occur singly or in clusters. A filamentous bacterium, *Leptothrix,* may accompany the trichomonads. The

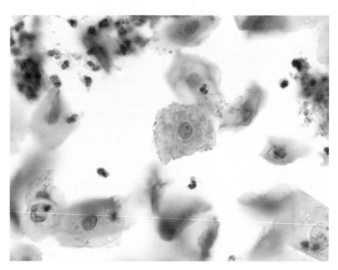

Figure 16-9. A film of coccobacilli covers squamous cells in a cervical cytology sample. This aspect is commonly referred to as "clue cells" and is associated with bacterial vaginosis (Papanicolaou stain, ×100).

squamous cells often show small, perinuclear halos that may be the first clue to the presence of *Trichomonas* infection. Cervicovaginitis emphysematosa, a rare condition in which blue-gray subepithelial cysts form in the vagina, has been associated with trichomoniasis.[120]

Candida species are identified on cervical cytology as small yeast forms; in the case of *C. albicans*, pseudohyphae are also present. The squamous cells often have inflammatory changes consisting of pseudoparakeratosis (small, superficial squamous cells with pyknotic nuclei and orangeophilic cytoplasm) and perinuclear halos. On liquid-based preparations, the pseudohyphae may appear to have skewered stacks of squamous cells (Fig. 16-11).

Actinomyces israelii are finely filamentous bacteria that manifest as fuzzy, densely tangled, dark blue masses easily recognized at low magnification on a cervical cytology slide (Fig. 16-12). *Actinomyces* has been determined to be commensal in the vagina.[121] The presence of aggregates of *Actinomyces* is most often associated with an IUD and has rarely led to pelvic abscess formation,[122] but usually cultures of removed IUD do not grow *Actinomyces*.[123,124] Pseudo-sulfur granules have been described and are sometimes, but not always, associated with IUD devices.[125-128] The pseudo-sulfur granules, also known as pseudoactinomycotic radiate granules (PAMRAGs), are recognized by their more crystalline appearance and failure to stain with special stains for microorganisms (Fig. 16-13).

Although in the United States serologic prevalence of HSV-1 and HSV-2 is 67% and 26%, respectively; only a fraction of seropositive patients are diagnosed with genital HSV infections.[129] Detection of the viral cytopathic effect of HSV in cervical cytology is even less common, 1% or less.[130,131] Breakdown of the primary vesicles can lead to acute, sometimes severe and necrotizing, inflammation.[132] Both squamous cells and endocervical cells show ground glass nuclei with chromatin marginated as a thin rim beneath the nuclear membrane. Clustering of multiple nuclei is common (Fig. 16-14).[133] Alternatively, a large eosinophilic inclusion appears in the nucleus surrounded by a clear halo.

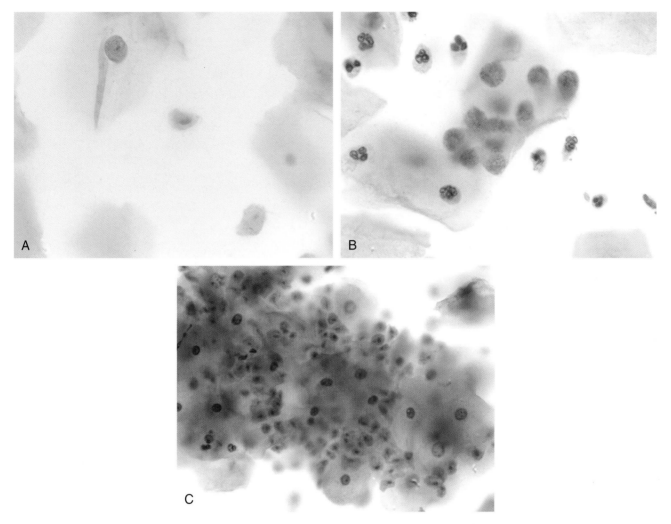

Figure 16-10. A, *Trichomonas* organisms are pear shaped and have a lancet-shaped nucleus. **B,** The organisms often demonstrate red cytoplasmic granules. **C,** The organisms may, on occasion, be so numerous as to form sheets (Papanicolaou stain, ×100).

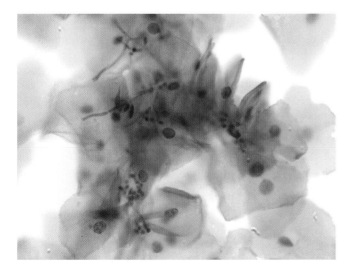

Figure 16-11. *Candida* species are present as yeast forms and pseudohyphae in association with squamous cells on cervical cytology samples (Papanicolaou stain, ×100).

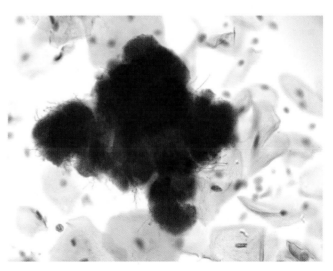

Figure 16-12. A mass of filamentous *Actinomyces* bacteria, known as sulfur granules, is identified in a cervical cytology sample from a woman with an intra-uterine device (Papanicolaou stain, ×100).

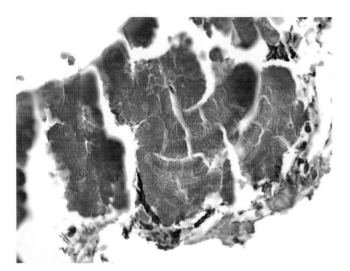

Figure 16-13. Pseudoactinomycotic radiate granules (PAMRAGS) are seen in an endometrial biopsy specimen (H&E, ×60).

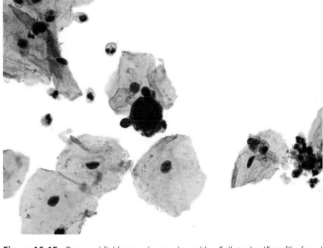

Figure 16-15. Paracoccidioidomycosis organism with a "pilot-wheel" profile, found in a cervical cytology sample (Papanicolaou stain, ×100).

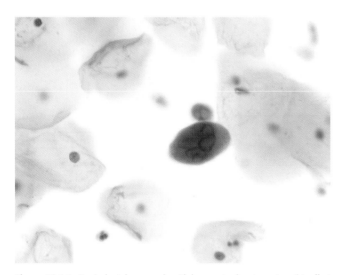

Figure 16-14. Cervical cytology sample with herpes simplex virus cytopathic effect in a multinucleated endocervical cell. Papanicolaou stain ×100.

Uncommon Causes of Cervicitis and Vaginitis

CMV is less common but produces cytologic changes that are difficult to distinguish from those of HSV; it infects not only epithelial cells but also endothelial cells and stromal cells. A recent report of five cases of CMV cervicitis noted that all cervical biopsies were performed for atypical cells seen on cervical cytology. The biopsies showed a dense, mixed, acute and chronic inflammatory infiltrate. CMV inclusions were identified on routine stain and mainly in endocervical cells.[134] CMV infection of the cervix is more commonly determined by culture than identified by its viral cytopathic effects on cytology or histology samples.[135-138]

Similarly, certain fungi are rarely reported as true pathogens in cervical samples. Included among this group are *Aspergillus, Fusarium, Blastomyces, Coccidioides, Cryptococcus,* and *Paracoccidioides.*[139-145] In the case of *Paracoccidioides,* the organism

appears in cervical cytology samples as yeast, 30-μm in diameter, with multiple budding daughter yeast forms protruding from the periphery, appearing like a "pilot's wheel." The offspring are 2 to 10 μm in diameter (Fig. 16-15). To confirm the fungal nature of the organisms, a cell block from the liquid-based cytology preparation can be obtained; special stains for fungi (PAS and GMS) are performed on the cell block to highlight the yeast.[145]

Tuberculous cervicitis is rare and usually occurs secondary to tuberculosis of the upper female genital tract. Some, but not all, patients have a history of pulmonary disease.[146] The cervix may grossly appear ulcerated or may have many small lesions or larger, tumor-like lesions.[147] Microscopically, granulomatous inflammation, often with necrosis, is present. Demonstration of the mycobacteria can be achieved by acid-fast stain or by PCR.[148] Nested PCR has been used on cells from a cervical cytology sample to confirm the diagnosis of tuberculous cervicitis.[149]

Although the external genitalia is the usual site of granuloma inguinale (donovanosis), the cervix is occasionally infected.[46] As noted in the discussion of granuloma inguinale in the vulva, multiple methods of diagnosis are possible, including special stains on smears or biopsies and PCR. Granuloma inguinale has been recognized on Papanicolaou-stained cervical cytology samples. Many short rods (Donovan bodies) are aggregated within histiocytes.[150] Granuloma inguinale of the cervix can be mistaken grossly for carcinoma.[151]

Schistosomiasis, where endemic, is a cause of cervicitis and may even be common, but, because women in countries where schistosomiasis is endemic may never get physical examinations, documentation may be poor.[90,152] In a study of women in Malawi who had ova of *S. haematobium* in their urine, more than 60% were found to have cytologic crush preparation or histologic evidence of ova in the vagina or cervix as well.[89] Cervical infection may be present in the absence of urinary egg excretion.[153] Infection by *S. haematobium* causes ulcers or nodular lesions.[154] Histologically, non-necrotizing granulomas with fibrosis are seen.[108,132] Other, rare parasitic infections

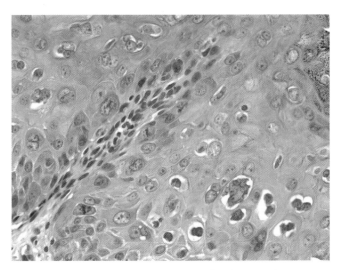

Figure 16-16. Human papillomavirus cytopathic effect (koilocytosis) in squamous dysplasia identified on a cervical biopsy specimen (H&E, ×40).

of the cervix include *Echinococcus,* amebiasis, and Chagas disease.[155-158]

Cervical and Vaginal Infections Causing Scant Inflammation

Productive infections by HPV can be recognized in cytologic preparations by the viral cytopathic effect in squamous cells. After the initial infection of the basal cell, viral replication is dependent on maturation of squamous cells. As the superficial squamous cells are sloughed, thousands of intact virions, present in the nucleus of the squamous cell, are released into the environment. The infected superficial squamous cell is characterized by the viral cytopathic effect of koilocytosis or cytoplasmic cavitation, nuclear enlargement, irregularity, hyperchromasia, and multinucleation. Although exophytic condyloma acuminatum (most often caused by HPV-6 or HPV-11) can occur on the cervix, the more usual lesion is a flat condyloma, which is caused in most cases by the high-risk types of HPV. The flat condyloma requires the magnification by the colposcope for visualization, which is enhanced by the application of acetic acid or Lugol solution. Associated inflammation is not a feature of HPV infection. Whereas many low-grade HPV lesions regress without treatment, guidelines for treatment recommend colposcopy with ablative treatment because of the risk of association with or progression to a higher-grade HPV–associated premalignant lesion (Fig. 16-16).[159]

Malakoplakia has been reported to occur in the cervix.[59,160] In certain cases, the initial recognition of the disease has been on cervical cytology.[161-163]

Noninfectious Lesions Mimicking Infections

Rarely, the cervix can harbor a lymphoid infiltrate so dense as to suggest the presence of lymphoma. Although lymphomas of the genital tract are uncommon, many of these cases are primary to the cervix.[164] A few cases of non-neoplastic, lymphoma-like lesions of the cervix have been described.[165]

Pemphigus vulgaris is a dermatosis that produces vesicles that mimic those produced by HSV.[166] Evidence of pemphigus can be found on cervical cytology.[167]

Upper Genital Tract

Pelvic Inflammatory Disease

PID is acute inflammation of the upper female genital tract and includes endometritis, salpingitis, pelvic peritonitis, and tubo-ovarian abscess. In 2005, approximately 45,000 women were hospitalized for treatment of PID, although the number of initial visits to the physician for PID declined by more than 50% from 1997 to 2005.[109] The disease is thought to have peaked in 1982.[168] The decline is thought to be the result of increased screening and treatment of *C. trachomatis,* one of the main causative agents of PID. The normal vaginal flora is polymicrobial but is dominated by *Lactobacillus,* which, along with the barrier of the endocervical canal, protects against more potentially pathogenic bacteria. Widening of the endocervical canal with menses or immediately after IUD insertion increases the risk for PID. Another risk factor is sexual activity at a young age, with one study finding the highest rates in the 20-to-24-year-old group.[169] Additional factors include multiple sex partners, neglecting to use a barrier method of contraception, intercourse during menses, and sexually transmitted infections with *C. trachomatis* or *N. gonorrhoeae.* In more than 50% of PID cases, *C. trachomatis* or *N. gonorrhoeae,* or both, are cultured.[170] *Mycoplasma genitalium,* a common sexually transmitted pathogen, has been increasingly implicated in PID.[171,172]

Although patients are often asymptomatic, the main symptom of PID is lower abdominal pain, usually of recent onset and worsened by coitus or during menses. Vaginal discharge and fever may be present; the uterus and adnexa are tender on physical examination. PID can be associated with perihepatitis inflammation (Fitzhugh-Curtis syndrome) leading to right upper quadrant pain. There is no gold standard test to diagnose PID; cases are considered confirmed with certain positive findings, including demonstration of acute or chronic endometritis on biopsy. The CDC has issued guidelines for diagnosis of PID that include histologic evidence of endometritis, radiologic images of thickened, fluid-filled fallopian tubes, and laparoscopic abnormalities indicating PID.[173] Gram staining of vaginal discharge that shows gram-negative, intracellular diplococci suggestive of *N. gonorrhoeae* is highly suggestive of PID. In practice, a constellation of clinical findings is used to diagnose PID. Empirical antibiotic treatment is given even in the face of minimal findings, because, if left untreated, PID can lead to infertility.

Endometrium

In women of reproductive age, certain types of inflammatory cells can be found in the endometrium, depending on the time of the woman's monthly cycle. Neutrophils are abundant in menstrual endometrium.[174] Lymphocytes, also known as large granular lymphocytes, are present, either singly or in aggregates, throughout the cycle but increase in number in the luteal phase.[175-178] Immunohistochemical studies have found that most of the lymphocytes are T cells.[179]

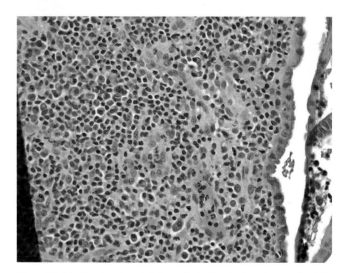

Figure 16-17. Chronic endometritis is manifested by abundant plasma cells within the endometrial stroma of an endometrial biopsy (H&E, ×60).

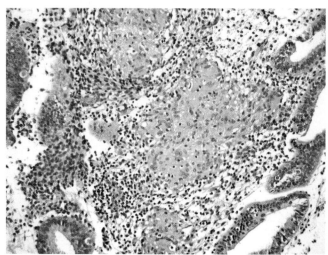

Figure 16-18. Granulomatous endometritis is characterized by well-formed, non-necrotizing granulomas found within the stroma of an endometrial biopsy sample (H&E, ×60).

Endometritis

Endometritis usually results from ascending infection secondary to unobstructed passage via the normally blocked endocervical canal during menstruation, parturition, or instrumentation permitting retrograde spread of microorganisms to the endometrial cavity.

Purely acute endometritis is the presence of microabscesses involving the endometrial glands and stroma, which is a rarely reported finding outside obstetrically related endometritis. The endometritis most often associated with PID is chronic or plasma cell endometritis, although lymphocytes and neutrophils are also present.[180,181] Low-power clues to the presence of endometritis are the presence of spindled stromal cells arranged in a swirling pattern or difficulty in dating the endometrium. Histologic findings of chronic endometritis include plasma cells within the stroma near surface epithelium, glands, blood vessels, and lymphoid infiltrates (Fig. 16-17). The plasma cells may not be numerous and may be interspersed singly among lymphocytes and neutrophils. Primary or secondary lymphoid follicles may be present. Neutrophils are present in the surface and glandular epithelium and may even form microabscesses. The endometrial glands may appear inactive, and the stroma may take on a spindled appearance. Although histochemical staining with methyl green pyronin and immunohistochemical staining with syndecan-1 have been advocated for increased sensitivity in identification of plasma cells, special stains to highlight plasma cells are not recommended, because the cases so identified are not always associated with PID.[182] If the finding of a rare plasma cell is the only finding in an endometrial sample, the diagnosis of chronic endometritis may not be warranted, because a minority of control subjects in several studies of endometritis have been found to have plasma cells in their endometrial samples.[182-185]

Granulomatous Endometritis

Granulomatous endometritis is uncommon and may result from a variety of diseases, including reaction to a foreign body, or as a manifestation of sarcoidosis (Fig. 16-18). Granulomatous endometritis, either non-necrotizing or necrotizing, resulting from systemic *M. tuberculosis* infection, has rarely been reported in the United States in recent years but is not uncommon in Asia and Africa.[186-190]

An incidental case of uterine coccidioidomycosis was diagnosed at the time of hysterectomy for squamous carcinoma of the cervix.[191] In another case, an endometrial curettage performed for irregular vaginal bleeding in a 33-year-old contained well-formed granulomas, some with spherules, identified within the endometrium on routine stain.[192] Endometrial coccidioidomycosis was reported in a woman who had undergone chemotherapy for Hodgkin disease.[193] A rare case of chronic endometritis with giant cell formation and necrosis secondary to *C. neoformans* infection occurred in an immunocompromised patient (Fig. 16-19) (personal communication, Blaise Clarke, MD). *Blastomyces dermatitidis* has been reported to produce granulomatous endometritis as part of disseminated infection.[194] *E. vermicularis* ova were found in endometrium examined in the workup of postmenopausal bleeding.[195,196] Coccidiosis, a rare protozoan infection that usually produces disease in the gastrointestinal tract, has been reported in endometrium.[197] The 20- to 30-μm cysts of coccidiosis were identified within the endometrial glandular cells, and non-necrotizing granulomas were present in the endometrium. Other unusual parasitic infections of the endometrium include *Echinococcus granulosus*, *Schistosoma*, and *Toxoplasma gondii*.[198-200] Malakoplakia, an uncommon reaction to bacterial infection, has been reported to occur in the endometrium (Fig. 16-20).[201]

Fallopian Tube and Ovary

Acute Salpingitis

The fallopian tube may be the site of physiologic endosalpingitis at the time of menses, presumably due to reflux of blood, but the neutrophilic response is sparse compared with an infectious process. Acute salpingitis occurs most frequently in young, sexually active women, the majority of whom are younger than 25

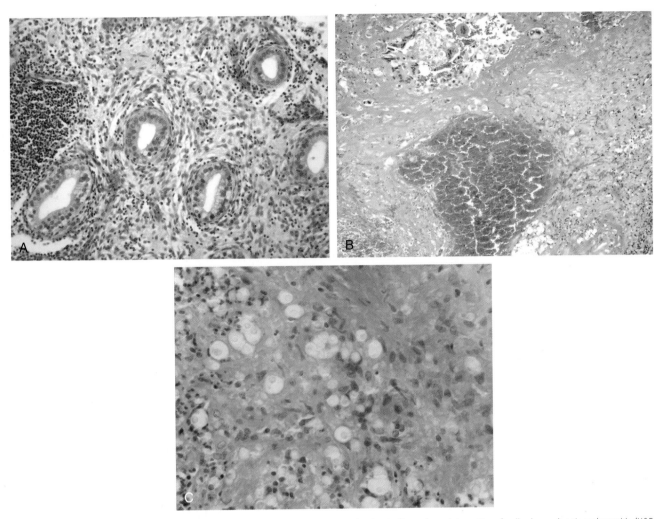

Figure 16-19. An immunocompromised woman presented with pelvic pain and menorrhagia. **A,** The endometrial curettage focally shows chronic endometritis (H&E, ×20). **B,** Elsewhere, the tissue is necrotic with granulomatous response and giant cells at low power (H&E, ×10). **C,** On high power, the pale round yeast-forms of *Cryptococcus neoformans,* surrounded by a clear halo, are found embedded within the granulomatous inflammation (H&E, ×40). (Courtesy of Blaise Clarke, MD, University of Toronto).

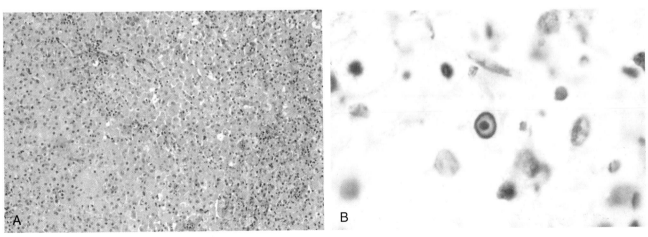

Figure 16-20. A, An endometrial biopsy sample shows marked histiocytic inflammation characteristic of malakoplakia. **B,** High-power view of the biopsy sample shows Michaelis-Gutmann bodies (H&E).

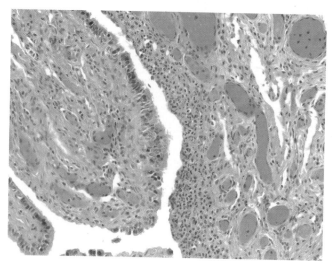

Figure 16-21. In acute salpingitis, neutrophils predominate. In this case, there is an impressive amount of eosinophilic infiltration of the wall of the fallopian tube (H&E, ×20).

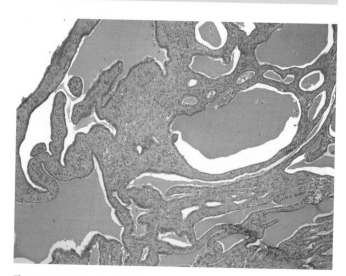

Figure 16-22. Chronic salpingitis with marked chronic inflammation in the distorted plical mucosa (H&E, ×20).

years of age.[202] Factors other than age that increase the risk include instrumentation and abortion.[203] As discussed in the section on PID, the bacteria most often responsible for primary acute salpingitis are *N. gonorrhoeae* and *C. trachomatis,* but cultures usually demonstrate a polymicrobial infection (facultative and anaerobic) which dictates the treatment.[204,205] In acute salpingitis, the fallopian tube is grossly edematous. Histologically, the plicae initially become edematous and infiltrated by polymorphonuclear leukocytes (Fig. 16-21) and tend to adhere to one another. With more severe infection, inflammation extends through the entire wall, producing a fibrinopurulent exudate within the lumen (pyosalpinx) and beyond the tube to the ovary, resulting in tubo-ovarian adhesions and abscess. The epithelium may show reactive changes such as loss of cilia.[202] If the infection progresses so far as to produce pyosalpinx, surgery may be necessary. Culture of surgical tissue specimens, obtained either by the operating room team or by the pathologist, is the standard. A case of *Enterobiasis* infection resulting in isolated acute salpingitis has been described.[206]

Actinomycosis may occur secondary to IUD contraception, although most PID cases secondary to IUD use are not due to actinomycosis,[124] and can produce a marked acute salpingitis or tubo-ovarian abscess.[207] Rarely, sulfur granules, the grossly apparent colonies of actinomycosis, similar to those seen in tonsils, may be present within the abscess cavity. Sulfur granules identified on endometrial curettage or in cervicovaginal smears are often associated with actinomycosis of the upper genital tract. A mimic of actinomycotic granules is the noninfectious PAMRAGs, which can be distinguished by the absence of coloration with histologic stains for microorganisms (Brown and Brenn, Gomori methenamine silver, or acid-fast bacillus stain).[128]

Chronic Salpingitis

As acute salpingitis resolves, the fallopian tube may become distorted, with occlusion of the fimbriated end of the tube, dilation of the lumen, and accumulation of serous fluid creating a hydrosalpinx. Microscopically, there is, at first, chronic inflam-

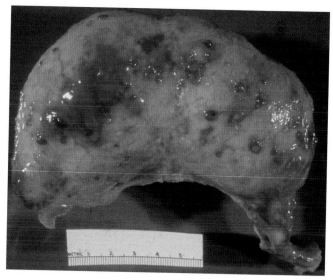

Figure 16-23. This massively distorted fallopian tube was found to be infected with *Mycobacterium tuberculosis.*

mation with shortening, blunting, fusion, and fibrosis of the plicae, which may result in pseudoglandular spaces, a condition also referred to as chronic follicular salpingitis (Fig. 16-22). Pseudocarcinomatous hyperplasia of the epithelium of the fallopian tube can occur in chronic salpingitis.[208] Persistent hydrosalpinx leads to attenuation of the fallopian tube plicae. A large hydrosalpinx may obscure the adjacent ovary and may be mistaken for an ovarian cyst. A case of *Entamoeba histolytica* associated with hydrosalpinx has been reported.[209]

Granulomatous Salpingitis and Oophoritis

Mycobacterial disease is the most common cause of granulomatous salpingitis, which is present in 80% to 90% of women with genital tuberculosis. There is bilateral involvement in 90% of cases (Fig. 16-23). With time, the fallopian tube becomes grossly

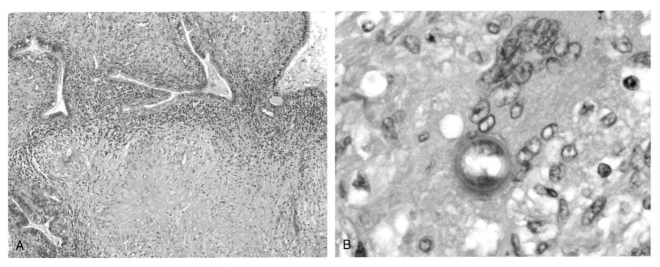

Figure 16-24. A, Low-power view of granulomatous salpingitis due to coccidioidomycosis (H&E, ×10). **B,** Higher-power demonstrates the budding yeast forms within granulomatous inflammation (H&E, ×40). (Courtesy of Drs. Sarah Chiang and John Carpenter, Tucson, AZ.)

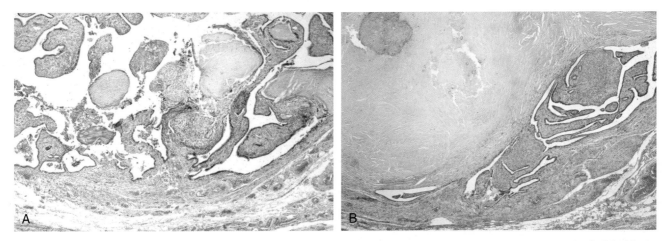

Figure 16-25. A, Granulomatous salpingitis secondary to *Enterobius vermicularis* (pinworm) is characterized by granulomas within the plicae and wall of the fallopian tube. **B,** High-power view demonstrates the organisms (H&E, ×40).

nodular, mimicking salpingitis isthmica nodosa.[207] Often, dense tubo-ovarian adhesions form.[210] However, the lumen and fimbria may remain patent, a sign considered by some to be characteristic of tuberculous salpingitis.[211] Microscopically, there is prominent granulomatous inflammation, often with necrosis, which begins in the mucosa but eventually engulfs the wall and can extend into surrounding tissues. As in other forms of chronic salpingitis, fusion of plicae can produce a cribriform pattern, which should not be mistaken for adenocarcinoma.

Rarely, fungal or parasitic disease provokes granulomatous salpingitis. Coccidioidomycosis can lead to chronic granulomatous salpingitis.[142,193] Granulomatous salpingitis secondary to schistosomiasis is common in regions endemic for *S. haematobium*. Grossly, the fallopian tube may be nodular or scarred. Microscopically, there may be a granulomatous reaction to ova, which may be identified amid the inflammation.[207] Tubal schistosomiasis may lead to ectopic pregnancy.[212,213] Cysticerci associated with endometriosis have been reported to cause focal granulomatous salpingitis containing partially calcified

cestode larvae.[214] *E. vermicularis* (pinworm) can cause chronic salpingitis (Fig. 16-24).

Noninfectious causes of salpingitis include sarcoidosis and Crohn disease.[207,215] Pseudoxanthomatous salpingitis secondary to pelvic endometriosis shows edematous plicae with chronic inflammation and abundant foamy macrophages.[216,217]

Granulomas can be found in the ovary and often are secondary to exposure to foreign material (e.g., sutures, keratin). The granulomas may be associated with multinucleated giant cells, or they may be palisading granulomas (Fig. 16-25).

Tubo-ovarian Abscess

Bacterial infection of the ovary usually occurs as a consequence of salpingitis and PID. Ovarian involvement is typically bilateral but may be unilateral in the rare case of extension from the gastrointestinal tract (appendicitis, diverticulitis). During the acute phase, in addition to purulent exudates, tubo-ovarian adhesions are usually present (Fig. 16-26). Tubo-ovarian

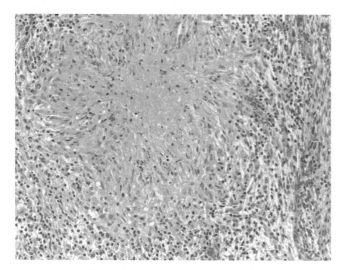

Figure 16-26. Incidentally found palisading granuloma within an otherwise normal ovary. Special stains for acid-fast bacilli and fungi were negative (H&E, ×20).

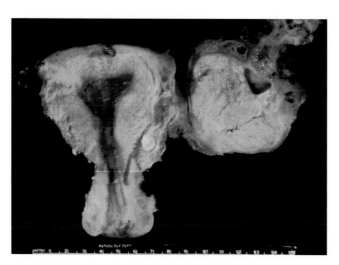

Figure 16-27. Gross image of an actinomycotic tubo-ovarian abscess.

abscesses may heal, forming cysts, which may mimic cystic ovarian lesions.[218] Rarely, a chronic abscess develops, producing a solid, yellow, xanthogranulomatous mass.[219] A clue to the inflammatory nature of the cystic change is the presence of entrapped inflamed fallopian tubal plicae. Tubo-ovarian inflammatory disease may produce changes similar to those observed in polycystic ovarian disease.[220]

The bacteria responsible for tubo-ovarian abscesses are most commonly *C. trachomatis* and *N. gonorrhoeae,* but *M. genitalium* is increasingly recognized as a culprit.[170-172] Other, less commonly encountered bacteria include non–sexually transmitted organisms such as anaerobes (*Prevotella, Bacteroides,* and *Peptostreptococcus*), *Nocardia, Streptococcus pneumoniae,* and *S. aureus*).

Actinomycotic tubo-ovarian abscesses are associated with IUD use (Fig. 16-27).[221] Actinomycotic granules are only rarely grossly visible. The inflammatory infiltrate may be intense, mainly neutrophils and histiocytes; a specific diagnosis is made

by microscopic identification of actinomycotic granules, which comprise gram-positive, argyrophilic, filamentous bacteria radially arranged. Occasionally, a preoperative diagnosis can be achieved by recognition of actinomycotic granules on cervical cytology or endometrial curettage.[222,223]

In about 10% of cases of tuberculous salpingitis, the ovary is also involved, producing tubo-ovarian adhesions and granulomatous inflammation.[224] The granulomas are usually within the cortex of the ovary.[221] *Mycobacterium leprae* has been reported to infect the ovary.[221,225] The resulting leprous oophoritis shows chronic inflammation, fibrosis, and acid-fast–positive bacilli.

As in the fallopian tube, fungal and parasitic infections can lead to tubo-ovarian abscesses. Coccidioidomycosis can cause considerable granulomatous inflammation in the female genital tract, including the ovaries, secondary to systemic disease.[142,226] A tubo-ovarian abscess due to *Blastomyces dermatitidis* manifested as an abdominal mass and was initially diagnosed on cervical cytology.[227] The first evidence of disseminated cryptococcosis was as a tubo-ovarian abscess in a 25-year-old, HIV-positive woman.[228]

Enterobiasis has rarely been implicated in tubo-ovarian abscess formation.[196,229,230] Infection by *Taenia* spp. has been reported to cause a tubo-ovarian abscess.[231] Ovarian schistosomiasis is encountered in endemic areas, along with involvement of the fallopian tube.[232]

Rarely, oophoritis results from a viral infection. CMV viral cytopathic effect may be found in stromal cells and endothelial cells of the ovary, usually as a part of systemic infection.[221,233,234] Mumps oophoritis occurs much less commonly than mumps orchitis.[221]

Malakoplakia has been reported to involve the ovary[61,235-237] and can manifest as a tubo-ovarian abscess.[238] The ovaries are transformed into friable, yellow masses.[221]

Noninfectious inflammatory processes in the ovaries that must be distinguished from infectious oophoritis include foreign body granulomas, necrobiotic granulomas, sarcoidosis, Crohn disease, and incidental cortical granulomas.[221]

REFERENCES

1. Castellsague X: Natural history and epidemiology of HPV infection and cervical cancer. Gynecol Oncol 2008;110(3 Suppl 2):S4-S7.
2. Kennedy CM, Boardman LA: New approaches to external genital warts and vulvar intraepithelial neoplasia. Clin Obstet Gynecol 2008;51:518-526.
3. Sonnex C: Human papillomavirus infection with particular reference to genital disease. J Clin Pathol 1998;51:643-648.
4. Wilkinson EJ, Hassanein AM: The vulva and vagina. In Silverberg SG (ed): Silverberg's Principles and Practice of Surgical Pathology and Cytopathology, vol 2, 4th ed. Philadelphia, Elsevier, 2006, pp 1885-1932.
5. Casas-Cordero M, Morin C, Roy M, et al: Origin of the koilocyte in condylomata of the human cervix: Ultrastructural study. Acta Cytol 1981;25:383-392.
6. Koss LG, Melamed MR: Squamous carcinoma of the uterine cervix and its precursors. In Koss LG, Melamed MR (eds): Koss' Diagnostic Cytology and its Histopathologic Bases, 5th ed. Philadelphia, JB Lippincott, 2006, pp 282-394.
7. Sonnex C, Scholefield JH, Kocjan G, et al: Anal human papillomavirus infection: A comparative study of cytology, colposcopy and DNA hybridisation as methods of detection. Genitourin Med 1991;67:21-25.

8. Longacre TA, Kong CS, Welton ML: Diagnostic problems in anal pathology. Adv Anat Pathol 2008;15:263-278.

9. Brown TJ, Yen-Moore A, Tyring SK: An overview of sexually transmitted diseases: Part II. J Am Acad Dermatol 1999;41(5 Pt 1):661-677; quiz 678-680.

10. Cotell SL, Roholt NS: Images in clinical medicine: Molluscum contagiosum in a patient with the acquired immunodeficiency syndrome. N Engl J Med 1998;338:888.

11. Blanco P, Viallard JF, Beylot-Barry M, et al: Cutaneous cryptococcosis resembling molluscum contagiosum in a patient with non-Hodgkin's lymphoma. Clin Infect Dis 1999;29:683-684.

12. Benedetti J, Corey L, Ashley R: Recurrence rates in genital herpes after symptomatic first-episode infection. Ann Intern Med 1994;121:847-854.

13. Schillinger JA, McKinney CM, Garg R, et al: Seroprevalence of herpes simplex virus type 2 and characteristics associated with undiagnosed infection: New York City, 2004. Sex Transm Dis 2008;35:599-606.

14. Gupta R, Warren T, Wald A: Genital herpes. Lancet 2007;370:2127-2137.

15. Schomogyi M, Wald A, Corey L: Herpes simplex virus-2 infection: An emerging disease? Infect Dis Clin North Am 1998;12:47-61.

16. Ramaswamy M, McDonald C, Smith M, et al: Diagnosis of genital herpes by real time PCR in routine clinical practice. Sex Transm Infect 2004;80:406-410.

17. Sen P, Barton SE: Genital herpes and its management. BMJ 2007;334:1048-1052.

18. Yudin MH, Kaul R: Progressive hypertrophic genital herpes in an HIV-infected woman despite immune recovery on antiretroviral therapy. Infect Dis Obstet Gynecol 2008, vol. 2008, Article ID 592532, 4 pages.

19. Taylor S, Drake SM, Dedicoat M, Wood MJ: Genital ulcers associated with acute Epstein-Barr virus infection. Sex Transm Infect 1998;74:296-297.

20. Cheng SX, Chapman MS, Margesson LJ, Birenbaum D: Genital ulcers caused by Epstein-Barr virus. J Am Acad Dermatol 2004;51:824-826.

21. Wilkinson EJ, Xie D-L: Benign diseases of the vulva. In Kurman RJ (ed): Blaustein's Pathology of the Female Genital Tract, 5th ed. New York, Springer-Verlag, 2002, pp 37-98.

22. Marks R, Ramnarain ND, Bhogal B, Moore NT: The erythrasma microorganism in situ: Studies using the skin surface biopsy technique. J Clin Pathol 1972;25:799-803.

23. Mattox TF, Rutgers J, Yoshimori RN, Bhatia NN: Nonfluorescent erythrasma of the vulva. Obstet Gynecol 1993;81(5 Pt 2):862-864.

24. Singh AE, Romanowski B: Syphilis: Review with emphasis on clinical, epidemiologic, and some biologic features. Clin Microbiol Rev 1999;12:187-209.

25. Larsen SA, Steiner BM, Rudolph AH: Laboratory diagnosis and interpretation of tests for syphilis. Clin Microbiol Rev 1995;8:1-21.

26. Brown TJ, Yen-Moore A, Tyring SK: An overview of sexually transmitted diseases: Part I. J Am Acad Dermatol 1999;41:511-532.

27. Long SR, Whitfeld MJ, Eades C, et al: Bacillary angiomatosis of the cervix and vulva in a patient with AIDS. Obstet Gynecol 1996;88(4 Pt 2):709-711.

28. Gasquet S, Maurin M, Brouqui P, et al: Bacillary angiomatosis in immunocompromised patients. AIDS 1998;12:1793-1803.

29. Schwartz EJ, Dorfman RF, Kohler S: Human herpesvirus-8 latent nuclear antigen-1 expression in endemic Kaposi sarcoma: An immunohistochemical study of 16 cases. Am J Surg Pathol 2003;27:1546-1550.

30. Bernard P: Management of common bacterial infections of the skin. Curr Opin Infect Dis 2008;21:122-128.

31. Stevens DL, Bisno AL, Chambers HF, et al: Practice guidelines for the diagnosis and management of skin and soft-tissue infections. Clin Infect Dis 2005;41:1373-1406.

32. Ratnam S, Hogan K, March SB, Butler RW: Whirlpool-associated folliculitis caused by *Pseudomonas aeruginosa*: Report of an outbreak and review. J Clin Microbiol 1986;23:655-659.

33. Jemec GB, Heidenheim M, Nielsen NH: The prevalence of hidradenitis suppurativa and its potential precursor lesions. J Am Acad Dermatol 1996;35(2 Pt 1):191-194.

34. Revuz JE, Canoui-Poitrine F, Wolkenstein P, et al: Prevalence and factors associated with hidradenitis suppurativa: Results from two case-control studies. J Am Acad Dermatol 2008;59:596-601.

35. Jemec GB, Hansen U: Histology of hidradenitis suppurativa. J Am Acad Dermatol 1996;34:994-999.

36. Wiseman MC: Hidradenitis suppurativa: A review. Dermatol Ther 2004;17:50-54.

37. Wolkenstein P, Loundou A, Barrau K, et al: Quality of life impairment in hidradenitis suppurativa: A study of 61 cases. J Am Acad Dermatol 2007;56:621-623.

38. Al-Tawfiq JA, Spinola SM: *Haemophilus ducreyi*: Clinical disease and pathogenesis. Curr Opin Infect Dis 2002;15:43-47.

39. Trees DL, Morse SA: Chancroid and *Haemophilus ducreyi*: An update. Clin Microbiol Rev 1995;8:357-375.

40. Lewis DA: Chancroid: Clinical manifestations, diagnosis, and management. Sex Transm Infect 2003;79:68-71.

41. Orle KA, Gates CA, Martin DH, et al: Simultaneous PCR detection of *Haemophilus ducreyi*, *Treponema pallidum*, and herpes simplex virus types 1 and 2 from genital ulcers. J Clin Microbiol 1996;34:49-54.

42. Mabey D, Peeling RW: Lymphogranuloma venereum. Sex Transm Infect 2002;78:90-92.

43. Rosen T, Brown TJ: Cutaneous manifestations of sexually transmitted diseases. Med Clin North Am 1998;82:1081-1104, vi.

44. Hampton T: Lymphogranuloma venereum targeted: Those at risk identified; diagnostic test developed. JAMA 2006;295:2592.

45. Carter JS, Bowden FJ, Bastian I, et al: Phylogenetic evidence for reclassification of *Calymmatobacterium granulomatis* as *Klebsiella granulomatis* comb. nov. Int J Syst Bacteriol 1999;49(Pt 4):1695-1700.

46. O'Farrell N: Donovanosis. Sex Transm Infect 2002;78:452-457.

47. Carter J, Hutton S, Sriprakash KS, et al: Culture of the causative organism of donovanosis (*Calymmatobacterium granulomatis*) in HEp-2 cells. J Clin Microbiol 1997;35:2915-2917.

48. Richens J: Donovanosis (granuloma inguinale). Sex Transm Infect 2006;82(Suppl 4):iv21-22.

49. Carter J, Bowden FJ, Sriprakash KS, et al: Diagnostic polymerase chain reaction for donovanosis. Clin Infect Dis 1999;28:1168-1169.

50. Samuel M, Aderogba K, Dutt N, et al: A hat trick of ulcerating pathogens in a single genital lesion. Int J STD AIDS 2007;18:65-66.

51. Suntoke TR, Hardick A, Tobian AA, et al: Evaluation of multiplex real-time PCR for detection of *H. ducreyi*, *T. pallidum*, HSV-1, and HSV-2 in the diagnosis of genital ulcer disease in Rakai District, Uganda. Sex Transm Infect 2009;85:97-101.

52. Saracoglu OF, Mungan T, Tanzer F: Pelvic tuberculosis. Int J Gynaecol Obstet 1992;37:115-120.

53. Bhattacharya P: Hypertrophic tuberculosis of the vulva. Obstet Gynecol 1978;51(1 Suppl):21s-22s.

54. Manoj K, Soma M, Ajay L, et al: Tubercular sinus of labia majora: Rare case report. Infect Dis Obstet Gynecol 2008, vol. 2008, Article ID 817515, 3 pages.

55. Chowdhury NN: Overview of tuberculosis of the female genital tract. J Indian Med Assoc 1996;94:345-346, 361.

56. Updated guidelines for the use of nucleic acid amplification tests in the diagnosis of tuberculosis. MMWR Morb Mortal Wkly Rep 2009;58:7-10.

57. Ghossein RA, Ross DG, Salomon RN, Rabson AR: Rapid detection and species identification of mycobacteria in paraffin-embedded tissues by polymerase chain reaction. Diagn Mol Pathol 1992;1:185-191.

58. van der Zanden AG, Hoentjen AH, Heilmann FG, et al: Simultaneous detection and strain differentiation of *Mycobacterium tuberculosis* complex in paraffin wax embedded tissues and in stained microscopic preparations. Mol Pathol 1998;51:209-214.

59. Agnarsdottir M, Hahn L, Sellgren U, Willen R: Malacoplakia of the cervix uteri and vulva. Acta Obstet Gynecol Scand 2004;83:214-216.

60. Teeters JC, Betts R, Ryan C, et al: Rectal and cutaneous malakoplakia in an orthotopic cardiac transplant recipient. J Heart Lung Transplant 2007;26:411-413.

61. Chalvardjian A, Picard L, Shaw R, et al: Malacoplakia of the female genital tract. Am J Obstet Gynecol 1980;138:391-394.

62. Fishman A, Ortega E, Girtanner RE, Kaplan AL: Malacoplakia of the vagina presenting as a pelvic mass. Gynecol Oncol 1993;49:380-382.

63. Saad AJ, Donovan TM, Truong LD: Malakoplakia of the vagina diagnosed by fine-needle aspiration cytology. Diagn Cytopathol 1993;9:559-561.

64. Chalvardjian A, Carydis B, Cohen S: Cytologic diagnosis of extravesical malacoplakia. Diagn Cytopathol 1985;1:216-220.

65. Goldacre MJ, Watt B, Loudon N, et al: Vaginal microbial flora in normal young women. BMJ 1979;1:1450-1455.

66. Geiger AM, Foxman B, Gillespie BW: The epidemiology of vulvovaginal candidiasis among university students. Am J Public Health 1995;85(8 Pt 1):1146-1148.

67. Geiger AM, Foxman B: Risk factors for vulvovaginal candidiasis: A case-control study among university students. Epidemiology 1996;7:182-187.

68. Horowitz BJ, Giaquinta D, Ito S: Evolving pathogens in vulvovaginal candidiasis: Implications for patient care. J Clin Pharmacol 1992;32:248-255.

69. Vermitsky JP, Self MJ, Chadwick SG, et al: Survey of vaginal-flora *Candida* species isolates from women of different age groups by use of species-specific PCR detection. J Clin Microbiol 2008;46:1501-1503.

70. Anderson MR, Klink K, Cohrssen A: Evaluation of vaginal complaints. JAMA 2004;291:1368-1379.

71. Landers DV, Wiesenfeld HC, Heine RP, et al: Predictive value of the clinical diagnosis of lower genital tract infection in women. Am J Obstet Gynecol 2004;190:1004-1010.

72. Selim M, Smoller B, Shea C, et al: Vulvar dermatoses and infections. In Robboy S, Mutter G, Prat J, et al. (eds): Robboy's Pathology of the Female Reproductive Tract, 2nd ed. Philadelphia, Churchill Livingstone Elsevier, 2009, pp 23-58.

73. Increase in coccidioidomycosis—California, 2000-2007. MMWR Morb Mortal Wkly Rep 2009;58:105-109.

74. Weyrauch HM, Norman FW, Bassett JB: Coccidioidomycosis of the genital tract. Calif Med 1950;72:465-468.

75. Kauffman CA: Histoplasmosis: A clinical and laboratory update. Clin Microbiol Rev 2007;20:115-132.

76. Smith MB, Schnadig VJ, Zaharopoulos P, Van Hook C: Disseminated *Histoplasma capsulatum* infection presenting as genital ulcerations. Obstet Gynecol 1997;89(5 Pt 2):842-844.

77. Gass M, Kobayashi GS: Histoplasmosis: An illustrative case with unusual vaginal and joint involvement. Arch Dermatol 1969;100:724-727.

78. Sills M, Schwartz A, Weg JG: Conjugal histoplasmosis: A consequence of progressive dissemination in the index case after steroid therapy. Ann Intern Med 1973;79:221-224.

79. Emmons CW: Saprophytic sources of *Cryptococcus neoformans* associated with the pigeon (*Columba livia*). Am J Hyg 1955;62:227-232.

80. Hajjeh RA, Brandt ME, Pinner RW: Emergence of cryptococcal disease: Epidemiologic perspectives 100 years after its discovery. Epidemiol Rev 1995;17:303-320.

81. Wang Y, Aisen P, Casadevall A: *Cryptococcus neoformans* melanin and virulence: Mechanism of action. Infect Immun 1995;63:3131-3136.

82. Ranganathan S, Moosa F, Kamarulzaman A, Looi LM: MRI and CT findings of cryptococcal vaginitis. Br J Radiol 2005;78:353-354.

83. Blocher KS, Weeks JA, Noble RC: Cutaneous cryptococcal infection presenting as vulvar lesion. Genitourin Med 1987;63:341-343.

84. Chang SE, Lee DK, Choi JH, et al: Majocchi's granuloma of the vulva caused by *Trichophyton mentagrophytes*. Mycoses 2005;48:382-384.

85. Wright ED, Chiphangwi J, Hutt MS: Schistosomiasis of the female genital tract: A histopathological study of 176 cases from Malawi. Trans R Soc Trop Med Hyg 1982;76:822-829.

86. Helling-Giese G, Sjaastad A, Poggensee G, et al: Female genital schistosomiasis (FGS): Relationship between gynecological and histopathological findings. Acta Trop 1996;62:257-267.

87. Carey FM, Quah SP, Hedderwick S, et al: Genital schistosomiasis. Int J STD AIDS 2001;12:609-611.

88. Laven JS, Vleugels MP, Dofferhoff AS, Bloembergen P: Schistosomiasis haematobium as a cause of vulvar hypertrophy. Eur J Obstet Gynecol Reprod Biol 1998;79:213-216.

89. Kjetland EF, Poggensee G, Helling-Giese G, et al: Female genital schistosomiasis due to *Schistosoma haematobium*: Clinical and parasitological findings in women in rural Malawi. Acta Trop 1996;62:239-255.

90. Kjetland EF, Ndhlovu PD, Mduluza T, et al: Simple clinical manifestations of genital *Schistosoma haematobium* infection in rural Zimbabwean women. Am J Trop Med Hyg 2005;72:311-319.

91. Attili VR, Hira SK, Dube MK: Schistosomal genital granulomas: A report of 10 cases. Br J Vener Dis 1983;59:269-272.

92. Calonje E, Neill S: Diseases of the genital skin. In McKee P, Calonje E, Granter S (eds): Pathology of the Skin, vol 1, 3rd ed. St. Louis, Elsevier Mosby, 2005, pp 473-538.

93. Mohammed AZ, Edino ST, Samaila AA: Surgical pathology of schistosomiasis. J Natl Med Assoc 2007;99:570-574.

94. Paradise JE, Campos JM, Friedman HM, Frishmuth G: Vulvovaginitis in premenarcheal girls: Clinical features and diagnostic evaluation. Pediatrics 1982;70:193-198.

95. Grayson W, Calonje E, McKee P: Infectious diseases of the skin. In McKee P, Calonje E, Granter S (eds): Pathology of the Skin, vol 1, 3rd ed. St. Louis, Elseiver Mosby, 2005, pp 838-992.

96. Falk ES, Eide TJ: Histologic and clinical findings in human scabies. Int J Dermatol 1981;20:600-605.

97. Yazar S, Ozcan H, Dincer S, Sahin I: Vulvar myiasis. Yonsei Med J 2002;43:553-555.

98. Jelinek T, Nothdurft HD, Rieder N, Loscher T: Cutaneous myiasis: Review of 13 cases in travelers returning from tropical countries. Int J Dermatol 1995;34:624-626.

99. Passos MR, Varella RQ, Tavares RR, et al: Vulvar myiasis during pregnancy. Infect Dis Obstet Gynecol 2002;10:153-158.

100. Sehgal VH, Gangwani OP: Genital fixed drug eruptions. Genitourin Med 1986;62:56-58.

101. Sakane T, Takeno M, Suzuki N, Inaba G: Behcet's disease. N Engl J Med 1999;341:1284-1291.

102. Balabanova M, Calamia KT, Perniciaro C, O'Duffy JD: A study of the cutaneous manifestations of Behcet's disease in patients from the United States. J Am Acad Dermatol 1999;41:540-545.

103. Haidopoulos D, Rodolakis A, Stefanidis K, et al: Behcet's disease: Part of the differential diagnosis of the ulcerative vulva. Clin Exp Obstet Gynecol 2002;29:219-221.

104. Guerrieri C, Ohlsson E, Ryden G, Westermark P: Vulvitis granulomatosa: A cryptogenic chronic inflammatory hypertrophy of vulvar labia related to cheilitis granulomatosa and Crohn's disease. Int J Gynecol Pathol 1995;14:352-359.

105. Klein PA, Appel J, Callen JP: Sarcoidosis of the vulva: A rare cutaneous manifestation. J Am Acad Dermatol 1998;39(2 Pt 1):281-283.

106. Lowe NK, Neal JL, Ryan-Wenger NA: Accuracy of the clinical diagnosis of vaginitis compared with a DNA probe laboratory standard. Obstet Gynecol 2009;113:89-95.

107. Frenkl TL, Potts J: Sexually transmitted infections. Urol Clin North Am 2008;35:33-46; vi.

108. Wright T, Ferenczy A: Benign diseases of the cervix. In Kurman R (ed): Blaustein's Pathology of the Female Genital Tract, 5th ed. New York, Springer-Verlag, 2002, pp 225-252.

109. Centers for Disease Control and Prevention: Sexually Transmitted Disease Surveillance, 2006. Atlanta: Department of Health and Human Services, November 2007.

110. Oriel JD, Powis PA, Reeve P, et al: Chlamydial infections of the cervix. Br J Vener Dis 1974;50:11-16.

111. Bartlett JG, Onderdonk AB, Drude E, et al: Quantitative bacteriology of the vaginal flora. J Infect Dis 1977;136:271-277.

112. Carr MC, Hanna L, Jawetz E: Chlamydiae, cervicitis, and abnormal Papanicolaou smears. Obstet Gynecol 1979;53:27-30.

113. Gupta PK, Lee EF, Erozan YS, et al: Cytologic investigations in Chlamydia infection. Acta Cytol 1979;23:315-320.

114. Hilton AL, Richmond SJ, Milne JD, et al: Chlamydia A in the female genital tract. Br J Vener Dis 1974;50:1-10.

115. Giampaolo C, Murphy J, Benes S, McCormack WM: How sensitive is the Papanicolaou smear in the diagnosis of infections with Chlamydia trachomatis? Am J Clin Pathol 1983;80:844-849.

116. Henry MR, de Mesy Jensen KL, Skoglund CD, Armstrong DW 3rd: Chlamydia trachomatis in routine cervical smears: A microscopic and ultrastructural analysis. Acta Cytol 1993;37:343-352.

117. Edwards JM, Campbell AR, Tait A, Lusher M: Demonstration of Chlamydia trachomatis in colposcopic cervical biopsy specimens by an immunoperoxidase method. J Clin Pathol 1991;44:1027-1029.

118. Winkler B, Crum CP: Chlamydia trachomatis infection of the female genital tract: Pathogenetic and clinicopathologic correlations. Pathol Annu 1987;22(Pt 1):193-223.

119. Critchlow CW, Wolner-Hanssen P, Eschenbach DA, et al: Determinants of cervical ectopia and of cervicitis: Age, oral contraception, specific cervical infection, smoking, and douching. Am J Obstet Gynecol 1995;173:534-543.

120. Gardner HL, Fernet P: Etiology of vaginitis emphysematosa: Report of ten cases and review of literature. Am J Obstet Gynecol 1964;88:680-694.

121. Persson E: Genital actinomycosis and Actinomyces israelii in the female genital tract. Adv Contracept 1987;3:115-123.

122. Fiorino AS: Intrauterine contraceptive device-associated actinomycotic abscess and Actinomyces detection on cervical smear. Obstet Gynecol 1996;87:142-149.

123. Lippes J: Infection and the IUD: A preliminary report. Contraception 1975;12:103-106.

124. Tsanadis G, Kalantaridou SN, Kaponis A, et al: Bacteriological cultures of removed intrauterine devices and pelvic inflammatory disease. Contraception 2002;65:339-342.

125. O'Brien PK, Roth-Moyo LA, Davis BA: Pseudo-sulfur granules associated with intrauterine contraceptive devices. Am J Clin Pathol 1981;75:822-825.

126. O'Brien PK, Roth-Moyo LA: Real and pseudo sulfur granules. Hum Pathol 1983;14:829.

127. Bhagavan BS, Ruffier J, Shinn B: Pseudoactinomycotic radiate granules in the lower female genital tract: Relationship to the Splendore-Hoeppli phenomenon. Hum Pathol 1982;13:898-904.

128. Pritt B, Mount SL, Cooper K, Blaszyk H: Pseudoactinomycotic radiate granules of the gynaecological tract: Review of a diagnostic pitfall. J Clin Pathol 2006;59:17-20.

129. Gynecologic herpes simplex virus infections. ACOG Practice Bulletin No. 57. American College of Obstetricians and Gynecologists. Obstet Gynecol 2004;104:1111-1117.

130. Naib ZM, Nahmias AJ, Josey WE: Cytology and histopathology of cervical herpes simplex infection. Cancer 1966;19:1026-1031.

131. Nahmias A, DelBuono I, Pipkin J, et al: Rapid identification and typing of herpes simplex virus types 1 and 2 by a direct immunofluorescence technique. Appl Microbiol 1971;22:455-458.

132. Malpica A, Robboy S: Cervical benign and non-neoplastic conditions. In Robboy S, Mutter G, Prat J, et al. (eds): Robboy's Pathology of the Female Reproductive Tract. Philadelphia, Churchill Livingstone Elsevier, 2009, pp 141-172.

133. Meisels A, Morin C: Infections and other benign changes. In Meisels A, Morin C (eds): Modern Uterine Cytopathology. Chicago, ASCP Press, 2007, pp 31-62.

134. McGalie CE, McBride HA, McCluggage WG: Cytomegalovirus infection of the cervix: Morphological observations in five cases of a possibly under-recognised condition. J Clin Pathol 2004;57:691-694.

135. Chiang WT, Chen HM, Hsieh CY, et al: Cytomegalovirus infection of the uterine cervix: Local cervical infection and antibody response. Int J Gynaecol Obstet 1981;19:177-180.

136. Hunt JL, Baloch Z, Judkins A, et al: Unique cytomegalovirus intracytoplasmic inclusions in ectocervical cells on a cervical/endocervical smear. Diagn Cytopathol 1998;18:110-112.

137. Oei AL, Salet-van de Pol MR, Borst SM, et al: "Owl's eye" cells in a cervical smear of a transplant recipient: Don't forget to inform the referring physician. Diagn Cytopathol 2007;35:227-229.

138. Byard RW, Mikhael NZ, Orlando G, et al: The clinicopathological significance of cytomegalovirus inclusions demonstrated by endocervical biopsy. Pathology 1991;23:318-321.

139. Hoda RS, Colello C, Roddy M, Houser PM: "Fruiting body" of Aspergillus species in a routine cervico-vaginal smear (Pap test). Diagn Cytopathol 2005;33:244-245.

140. Gupta S, Sodhani P, Jain S: Macroconidia of Fusarium species: An unusual finding in cervical smears. Acta Cytol 2003;47:41-44.

141. Dyer ML, Young TL, Kattine AA, Wilson DD: Blastomycosis in a Papanicolaou smear: Report of a case with possible venereal transmission. Acta Cytol 1983;27:285-287.

142. Saw EC, Smale LE, Einstein H, Huntington RW Jr: Female genital coccidioidomycosis. Obstet Gynecol 1975;45:199-202.

143. Chen CK, Chang DY, Chang SC, et al: Cryptococcal infection of the vagina. Obstet Gynecol 1993;81(5 Pt 2):867-869.

144. Sheyn I, Mira JL, Thompson MB: Paracoccidioides brasiliensis in a postpartum Pap smear: A case report. Acta Cytol 2001;45:79-81.

145. Alsharif M, Martin AU, Shelton JB Jr, Pambuccian SE: Paracoccidioides brasiliensis in a liquid-based Papanicolaou test from a pregnant woman: Report of a case. Diagn Cytopathol 2008;36:557-560.

146. Chakraborty P, Roy A, Bhattacharya S, et al: Tuberculous cervicitis: A clinicopathological and bacteriological study. J Indian Med Assoc 1995;93:167-168.

147. Lamba H, Byrne M, Goldin R, Jenkins C: Tuberculosis of the cervix: Case presentation and a review of the literature. Sex Transm Infect 2002;78:62-63.

148. Schulz S, Cabras AD, Kremer M, et al: Species identification of mycobacteria in paraffin-embedded tissues: Frequent detection of nontuberculous mycobacteria. Mod Pathol 2005;18:274-282.

149. Ferrara G, Cannone M, Guadagnino A, et al: Nested polymerase chain reaction on vaginal smears of tuberculous cervicitis: A case report. Acta Cytol 1999;43:308-312.

150. de Boer AL, de Boer F, Van der Merwe JV: Cytologic identification of Donovan bodies in granuloma inguinale. Acta Cytol 1984;28:126-128.

151. Hoosen AA, Draper G, Moodley J, Cooper K: Granuloma inguinale of the cervix: A carcinoma look-alike. Genitourin Med 1990;66:380-382.

152. Rand RJ, Lowe JW: Schistosomiasis of the uterine cervix. Br J Obstet Gynaecol 1998;105:1329-1331.

153. Poggensee G, Kiwelu I, Saria M, et al: Schistosomiasis of the lower reproductive tract without egg excretion in urine. Am J Trop Med Hyg 1998;59:782-783.

154. Poggensee G, Sahebali S, Van Marck E, et al: Diagnosis of genital cervical schistosomiasis: Comparison of cytological, histopathological and parasitological examination. Am J Trop Med Hyg 2001;65:233-236.

155. Destombes P: [Parasitic disease of the female genital tract: Histopathological aspects]. Rev Fr Gynecol Obstet 1973;68:167-171.

156. Veliath AJ, Bansal R, Sankaran V, et al: Genital amebiasis. Int J Gynaecol Obstet 1987;25:249-256.

157. Nopdonrattakoon L: Amoebiasis of the female genital tract: A case report. J Obstet Gynaecol Res 1996;22:235-238.

158. Concetti H, Retegui M, Perez G, Perez H: Chagas' disease of the cervix uteri in a patient with acquired immunodeficiency syndrome. Hum Pathol 2000;31:120-122.

159. Wright TC Jr, Massad LS, Dunton CJ, et al: 2006 Consensus guidelines for the management of women with abnormal cervical cancer screening tests. Am J Obstet Gynecol 2007;197:346-355.

160. Willén R, Stendahl U, Willén H, Tropé C: Malacoplakia of the cervix and corpus uteri: A light microscopic, electron microscopic, and X-ray microprobe analysis of a case. Int J Gynecol Pathol 1983;2:201-208.

161. Wahl RW: Malacoplakia of the uterine cervix: Report of two cases. Acta Cytol 1982;26:691-694.

162. Stewart CJ, Thomas MA: Malacoplakia of the uterine cervix and endometrium. Cytopathology 1991;2:271-275.

163. Falcon-Escobedo R, Mora-Tiscareno A, Pueblitz-Peredo S: Malacoplakia of the uterine cervix: Histologic, cytologic and ultrastructural study of a case. Acta Cytol 1986;30:281-284.

164. Kosari F, Daneshbod Y, Parwaresch R, et al: Lymphomas of the female genital tract: A study of 186 cases and review of the literature. Am J Surg Pathol 2005;29:1512-1520.

165. Young RH, Harris NL, Scully RE: Lymphoma-like lesions of the lower female genital tract: A report of 16 cases. Int J Gynecol Pathol 1985;4:289-299.

166. Kaufman RH, Watts JM, Gardner H: Pemphigus vulgaris: Genital involvement. Report of two cases. Obstet Gynecol 1969;33:264-266.

167. Akhyani M, Chams-Davatchi C, Naraghi Z, et al: Cervicovaginal involvement in pemphigus vulgaris: A clinical study of 77 cases. Br J Dermatol 2008;158:478-482.

168. Aral SO, Mosher WD, Cates W Jr: Self-reported pelvic inflammatory disease in the United States, 1988. JAMA 1991;266:2570-2573.

169. Westrom L: Incidence, prevalence, and trends of acute pelvic inflammatory disease and its consequences in industrialized countries. Am J Obstet Gynecol 1980;138(7 Pt 2):880-892.

170. Lareau SM, Beigi RH: Pelvic inflammatory disease and tubo-ovarian abscess. Infect Dis Clin North Am 2008;22:693-708, vii.

171. Haggerty CL, Ness RB: Diagnosis and treatment of pelvic inflammatory disease. Womens Health (Lond) 2008;4:383-397.

172. Ross J: Pelvic inflammatory disease. Clin Evid 2006:2176-2182.

173. Workowski KA, Berman SM: Sexually transmitted diseases treatment guidelines, 2006. MMWR 2006;55(RR-11):1-94.

174. Poropatich C, Rojas M, Silverberg SG: Polymorphonuclear leukocytes in the endometrium during the normal menstrual cycle. Int J Gynecol Pathol 1987;6:230-234.

175. Geppert M, Geppert J: Lymphocytes in the epithelial layers of decidua and normal or abnormal endometrium. Arch Gynecol 1982;233:47-51.

176. Morris H, Edwards J, Tiltman A, Emms M: Endometrial lymphoid tissue: An immunohistological study. J Clin Pathol 1985;38:644-652.

177. Bulmer JN, Morrison L, Longfellow M, et al: Granulated lymphocytes in human endometrium: Histochemical and immunohistochemical studies. Hum Reprod 1991;6:791-798.

178. Klentzeris LD, Bulmer JN, Warren A, et al: Endometrial lymphoid tissue in the timed endometrial biopsy: Morphometric and immunohistochemical aspects. Am J Obstet Gynecol 1992;167:667-674.

179. Searle RF, Jones RK, Bulmer JN: Phenotypic analysis and proliferative responses of human endometrial granulated lymphocytes during the menstrual cycle. Biol Reprod 1999;60:871-878.

180. Eckert LO, Hawes SE, Wolner-Hanssen PK, et al: Endometritis: The clinical-pathologic syndrome. Am J Obstet Gynecol 2002;186:690-695.

181. Kiviat NB, Wolner-Hanssen P, Eschenbach DA, et al: Endometrial histopathology in patients with culture-proved upper genital tract infection and laparoscopically diagnosed acute salpingitis. Am J Surg Pathol 1990;14:167-175.

182. Gilmore H, Fleischhacker D, Hecht JL: Diagnosis of chronic endometritis in biopsies with stromal breakdown. Hum Pathol 2007;38:581-584.

183. Korn AP, Hessol N, Padian N, et al: Commonly used diagnostic criteria for pelvic inflammatory disease have poor sensitivity for plasma cell endometritis. Sex Transm Dis 1995;22:335-341.

184. Korn AP, Bolan G, Padian N, et al: Plasma cell endometritis in women with symptomatic bacterial vaginosis. Obstet Gynecol 1995;85:387-390.

185. Sherman ME, Mazur MT, Kurman RJ: Benign diseases of the endometrium. In Kurman R (ed): Blaustein's Pathology of the Female Genital Tract, 5th ed. New York, Springer-Verlag, 2002, pp 421-466.

186. Kumar P, Shah NP, Singhal A, et al: Association of tuberculous endometritis with infertility and other gynecological complaints of women in India. J Clin Microbiol 2008;46:4068-4070.

187. Ojo BA, Akanbi AA, Odimayo MS, Jimoh AK: Endometrial tuberculosis in the Nigerian middle belt: An eight-year review. Trop Doct 2008;38:3-4.

188. Gupta N, Sharma JB, Mittal S, et al: Genital tuberculosis in Indian infertility patients. Int J Gynaecol Obstet 2007;97:135-138.

189. Hassoun A, Jacquette G, Huang A, et al: Female genital tuberculosis: Uncommon presentation of tuberculosis in the United States. Am J Med 2005;118:1295-1296.

190. Rivasi F, Curatola C, Garagnani L, Negri G: Detection of *Mycobacterium tuberculosis* DNA by polymerase chain reaction from paraffin samples of chronic granulomatous endometritis. Histopathology 2007;51:574-578.

191. Hart WR, Prins RP, Tsai JC: Isolated coccidioidomycosis of the uterus. Hum Pathol 1976;7:235-239.

192. Salgia K, Bhatia L, Rajashekaraiah KR, et al: Coccidioidomycosis of the uterus. South Med J 1982;75:614-616.

193. Bylund DJ, Nanfro JJ, Marsh WL Jr: Coccidioidomycosis of the female genital tract. Arch Pathol Lab Med 1986;110:232-235.

194. Farber ER, Leahy MS, Meadows TR: Endometrial blastomycosis acquired by sexual contact. Obstet Gynecol 1968;32:195-199.

195. al-Rufaie HK, Rix GH, Perez Clemente MP, al-Shawaf T: Pinworms and postmenopausal bleeding. J Clin Pathol 1998;51:401-402.

196. Khabir A, Makni S, Khmiri H, et al: [Enterobiasis of the female pelvi-genital tract: A report of three cases]. J Gynecol Obstet Biol Reprod (Paris) 2005;34:162-165.

197. de Otazu RD, Garcia-Nieto L, Izaguirre-Gondra E, et al: Endometrial coccidiosis. J Clin Pathol 2004;57:1104-1105.

198. Okumus Y, Tayyar M, Patiroglu T, Aygen E: Uterine hydatid cyst. Int J Gynaecol Obstet 1994;45:51-53.

199. Billy-Brissac R, Foucan L, Gallais A, et al: [Genital *Schistosoma mansoni* bilharziasis in women: Apropos of 2 cases in Guadeloupe.] Med Trop (Mars) 1994;54:345-348.

200. Stray-Pedersen B, Lorentzen-Styr AM: Uterine toxoplasma infections and repeated abortions. Am J Obstet Gynecol 1977;128:716-721.

201. Kawai K, Fukuda K, Tsuchiyama H: Malacoplakia of the endometrium: An unusual case studied by electron microscopy and a review of the literature. Acta Pathol Jpn 1988;38:531-540.

202. Zheng W, Robboy S: Fallopian tube. In Robboy S, Mutter G, Prat J, et al. (eds): Robboy's Pathology of the Female Reproductive Tract. Philadelphia, Churchill Livingstone Elsevier, 2009, pp 485-514.

203. Yip L, Sweeny PJ, Bock BF: Acute suppurative salpingitis with concomitant intrauterine pregnancy. Am J Emerg Med 1993;11:476-479.

204. Soper DE, Brockwell NJ, Dalton HP, Johnson D: Observations concerning the microbial etiology of acute salpingitis. Am J Obstet Gynecol 1994;170:1008-1014; discussion 1014-1017.

205. Heinonen PK, Miettinen A: Laparoscopic study on the microbiology and severity of acute pelvic inflammatory disease. Eur J Obstet Gynecol Reprod Biol 1994;57:85-89.

206. Erhan Y, Zekioglu O, Ozdemir N, Sen S: Unilateral salpingitis due to *Enterobius vermicularis*. Int J Gynecol Pathol 2000;19:188-189.

207. Wheeler J: Diseases of the fallopian tube. In Kurman R (ed): Blaustein's Pathology of the Female Genital Tract, 5th ed. New York, Springer-Verlag, 2002, pp 617-648.

208. Cheung AN, Young RH, Scully RE: Pseudocarcinomatous hyperplasia of the fallopian tube associated with salpingitis: A report of 14 cases. Am J Surg Pathol 1994;18:1125-1130.

209. Calore EE, Calore NM, Cavaliere MJ: Salpingitis due to *Entamoeba histolytica*. Braz J Infect Dis 2002;6:97-99.

210. Haines M: Tuberculous salpingitis as seen by the pathologist and the surgeon. Am J Obstet Gynecol 1958;75:472-481.

211. Schaefer G: Tuberculosis of the female genital tract. Clin Obstet Gynecol 1970;13:965-998.

212. Ekoukou D, Luzolo-Lukanu A, Mulard C, et al: [Peritoneal and tubal *Schistosoma haematobium* bilharziasis: Two case reports]. J Gynecol Obstet Biol Reprod (Paris) 1995;24:819-824.

213. Ville Y, Leruez M, Picaud A, et al: Tubal schistosomiasis as a cause of ectopic pregnancy in endemic areas? A report of three cases. Eur J Obstet Gynecol Reprod Biol 1991;42:77-79.

214. Abraham JL, Spore WW, Benirschke K: Cysticercosis of the fallopian tube: Histology and microanalysis. Hum Pathol 1982;13:665-670.

215. Boakye K, Omalu B, Thomas L: Fallopian tube and pulmonary sarcoidosis: A case report. J Reprod Med 1997;42:533-535.

216. Franco V, Florena AM, Guarneri G, Gargano G: Xanthogranulomatous salpingitis: Case report and review of the literature. Acta Eur Fertil 1990;21:197-199.

217. Seidman JD, Oberer S, Bitterman P, Aisner SC: Pathogenesis of pseudoxanthomatous salpingiosis. Mod Pathol 1993;6:53-55.

218. Clement P, Young R: Tumor-like lesions of the ovary. In Clement P, Young R (eds): Atlas of Gynecologic Surgical Pathology, 2nd ed. Philadelphia, Saunders Elsevier, 2008, pp 283-303.

219. Ladefoged C, Lorentzen M: Xanthogranulomatous inflammation of the female genital tract. Histopathology 1988;13:541-551.

220. Quan A, Charles D, Craig JM: Histologic and functional consequences of periovarian adhesions. Obstet Gynecol 1963;22:96-101.

221. Clement P: Nonneoplastic lesions of the ovary. In Kurman R (ed): Blaustein's Pathology of the Female Genital Tract, 5th ed. New York, Springer-Verlag, 2002, pp 675-728.

222. Burkman R, Schlesselman S, McCaffrey L, et al: The relationship of genital tract actinomycetes and the development of pelvic inflammatory disease. Am J Obstet Gynecol 1 1982;143:585-589.

223. Keebler C, Chatwani A, Schwartz R: Actinomycosis infection associated with intrauterine contraceptive devices. Am J Obstet Gynecol 1983;145:596-599.

224. Nogales-Ortiz F, Tarancon I, Nogales FF Jr: The pathology of female genital tuberculosis: A 31-year study of 1436 cases. Obstet Gynecol 1979;53:422-428.

225. Bonar BE, Rabson AS: Gynecologic aspects of leprosy. Obstet Gynecol 1957;9:33-43.

226. Chowfin A, Tight R: Female genital coccidioidomycosis (FGC), Addison's disease and sigmoid loop abscess due to *Coccidioides immites*. Case report and review of literature on FGC. Mycopathologia 1999;145:121-126.

227. Murray JJ, Clark CA, Lands RH, et al: Reactivation blastomycosis presenting as a tuboovarian abscess. Obstet Gynecol 1984;64:828-830.

228. Sing Y, Ramdial PK: Cryptococcal inflammatory pseudotumors. Am J Surg Pathol 2007;31:1521-1527.

229. Smolyakov R, Talalay B, Yanai-Inbar I, et al: *Enterobius vermicularis* infection of female genital tract: A report of three cases and review of literature. Eur J Obstet Gynecol Reprod Biol 2003;107:220-222.

230. McMahon JN, Connolly CE, Long SV, Meehan FP: *Enterobius* granulomas of the uterus, ovary and pelvic peritoneum: Two case reports. Br J Obstet Gynaecol 1984;91:289-290.

231. Pairwuti S, Ratanawichitrasin A, Koetsawang A, Robertson DI: Tubo-ovarian abscess containing tapeworm proglottids and ova: A case report. Asia Oceania J Obstet Gynaecol 1993;19:285-290.

232. Mahmood K: Granulomatous oophoritis due to *Schistosoma mansoni*. Am J Obstet Gynecol 1975;123:919-920.

233. Subietas A, Deppisch LM, Astarloa J: Cytomegalovirus oophoritis: Ovarian cortical necrosis. Hum Pathol 1977;8:285-292.

234. Williams DJ, Connor P, Ironside JW: Pre-menopausal cytomegalovirus oophoritis. Histopathology 1990;16:405-407.

235. Aikat BK, Radhakrishnan VV, Rao MS: Malakoplakia: A report of two cases with review of the literature. Indian J Pathol Bacteriol 1973;16:64-70.

236. Klempner LB, Giglio PG, Niebles A: Malacoplakia of the ovary. Obstet Gynecol 1987;69(3 Pt 2):537-540.

237. van der Voort HJ, ten Velden JA, Wassenaar RP, Silberbusch J: Malacoplakia: Two case reports and a comparison of treatment modalities based on a literature review. Arch Intern Med 1996;156:577-583.

238. Chou SC, Wang JS, Tseng HH: Malacoplakia of the ovary, fallopian tube and uterus: A case associated with diabetes mellitus. Pathol Int 2002;52:789-793.

17

Perinatal Infections

Drucilla J. Roberts

The placenta is a fetally derived organ present in the maternal uterus; it has many different functions, including serving as a barrier to infection. Maternal infectious diseases and vaginal colonization can lead to congenital infections if the placental barrier is breached. The fetus develops in a fluid-filled space surrounded by membranes composed of two epithelial-mesodermal layers, the amnion and chorion (Fig. 17-1). These membranes generally cover the endocervical os. The fetus and its fluid environment are thus isolated from the microorganisms in the cervicovaginal vault by only four layers of tissue and the cervical mucus. The human placental disk adheres to the maternal uterus via direct colonization of the uterine vascular bed beneath and is directly exposed to maternal blood. Organisms can gain entry into the placenta by direct hematogenous spread or by breaching the membranes over the endocervix, resulting in ascending infection. Fetal infection can follow, but this depends on many factors, including the type and number of microorganisms and the maturity of the fetal immunologic response.

Ascending Infections

The histologic hallmark of ascending infections is acute chorioamnionitis (ACA). Organisms reach the amniotic fluid, where they multiply and stimulate an inflammatory response from the mother and the fetus. Histologically, presence of inflammatory cells within the fetal membranes (Fig. 17-2) represents the maternal inflammatory response to microorganisms in the amniotic fluid. The fetal response is diagnosed by the presence of inflammatory cells derived from the fetus in the umbilical cord or chorionic plate vessels, or both (Fig. 17-3). The diagnosis of histologic ACA should be made if there is sufficient inflammation to warrant it and should be staged as to the anatomic location and source of the inflammation. Redline and colleagues[1] have provided a grading and staging system that is summarized in Table 17-1.

The diagnosis of ACA is established clinically when one or more of the following features is present: maternal fever, fetal tachycardia, uterine tenderness, pus per cervical os. The most common use of the diagnosis is with maternal fever in labor. The histologic confirmation of this clinical diagnosis is poor, with less than a 25% concordance rate.

The clinical significance of ACA is, first, that it is one of the most common causes of preterm labor.[2-5] Also, the presence of ACA stimulates the common practice of culturing a tissue sample from the neonate and treating for a presumption of infection pending results of the culture.[5,6] Newer literature suggests that the presence of a fetal response to the chorioamnionitis is associated with neurocompromise in the neonate.[7-10]

Although it is largely believed that ACA is diagnostic of amniotic fluid infection, this is still not proven. In preterm chorioamnionitis, the association with infection is well substantiated.[11-15] Organisms responsible can be single species, such as a group G streptococcus,[12] but most cases of ACA are polymicrobial.[13,14,16-18] In third-trimester cases of ACA, and especially at term, the incidence of chorioamnionitis falls, as does the association with documented infection.[6,15,19,20]

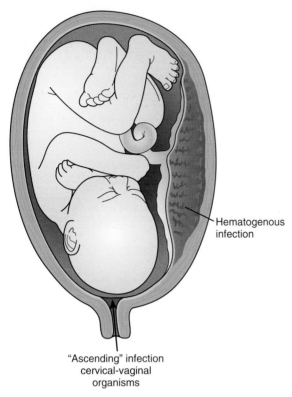

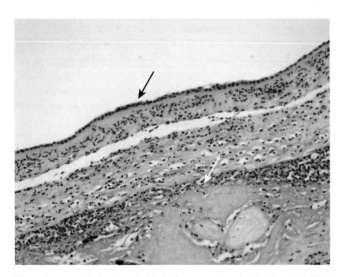

Figure 17-1. The routes of fetal infection. (Modified from Netter Anatomy Illustration Collection, © Elsevier Inc. All Rights Reserved.)

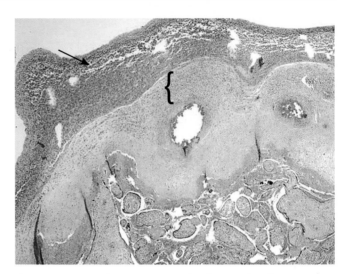

Figure 17-3. Acute chorioamnionitis on the chorionic plate (*arrow* points to neutrophils in chorionic plate mesoderm). This is maternal stage 3 grade 2, fetal stage 1 (*bracket*) grade 2.

Figure 17-2. Acute chorioamnionitis, in this case maternal stage 2 grade 2. *Black arrow* points to the amniotic epithelium and *white arrow* to the chorionic epithelium.

Hematogenously Spread Infections

Maternal infection can spread directly to the placenta. The hallmark of this type of placental infection is villitis, an inflammatory infiltrate of the placental villi (Fig. 17-4). The dominant cell type depends on the type of organism. The most common infections that occur during pregnancy and lead to sepsis are bacterial infec-

tions of the urinary tract,[21] although these rarely cause placental infections via sepsis. The two bacterial groups that most commonly infect the placenta and result in villitis are group B streptococci (GBS)[22] and *Listeria monocytogenes*.[23-29] The villitis associated with these infections is termed *acute villitis* because the infiltrate shows a predominance of neutrophils. The classic infections that are hematogenously spread to the placenta are not bacterial but viral or parasitic and lead to *chronic villitis*, with a predominance of lymphocytes and plasma cells in the villous infiltrate.[30]

Although chronic villitis is the most common pathologic manifestation of hematogenously spread infections to the placenta, it is not specific. Chronic villitis at term is common but is very rarely caused by infection.[31,32] Most cases have an unknown etiology and are thought to represent a manifestation of an immunologically based host-versus-graft reaction; therefore, a recurrence risk is present, and the infection can potentially result in placental rejection with fetal sequelae.[33-35] In noninfectious chronic villitis, maternal lymphocytes invade the villi.[36] If infection is the cause of chronic villitis, it usually has distinctive features that help distinguish it from the noninfectious type (Table 17-2). The source of the inflammatory cells in infectious chronic villitis has not been studied. The pathologic workup of chronic villitis should be based on the clinical history and the presence of any of the features listed in Table 17-2.

Specific Infectious Organisms

Bacterial Infections

Group B Streptococci

GBS infection is typically due to colonization, usually asymptomatic, of the genital and/or gastrointestinal tract. These bacteria infect the placenta either by ascending through the cervix into the amniotic cavity or via the urinary tract resulting in urinary

Table 17-1 Grading and Staging of Acute Chorioamnionitis

Diagnostic Category	Definition
Maternal Inflammatory Response	
Stage (location)	
1 (Early)	Neutrophils in subchorionic fibrin, in chorionic plate, or in chorionic epithelial layer of membranes
2 (Intermediate)	Neutrophils within chorionic or amnionic mesoderm
3 (Advanced)	Stage 2 plus necrosis of amnionic epithelium and/or neutrophils
Grade (severity)	
1 (Mild to moderate)	Anything less than severe (grade 2)
2 (Severe)	Confluent or more than three foci ≥200 cells
Fetal Inflammatory Response	
Stage	
1 (Early)	Fetal inflammatory cells within chorionic plate vessel walls or umbilical vein vessel wall or both
2 (Intermediate)	Fetal inflammatory cells within umbilical arteries ± vein
3 (Advanced)	Necrotizing funisitis
Grade	
1 (Mild to moderate)	Not severe (grade 2)
2 (Severe)	Confluent fetal inflammatory cells with attenuation/degeneration of smooth muscle

From Redline RW, Faye-Petersen O, Heller D, et al: Amniotic infection syndrome: Nosology and reproducibility of placental reaction patterns. Pediatr Dev Pathol 2003;6:435-448.

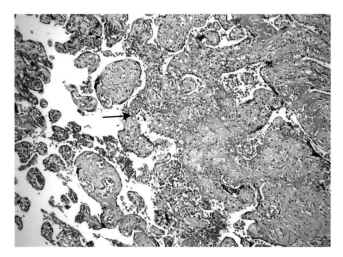

Figure 17-4. Chronic villitis. *Black arrow* points to region of clustered villi with increased intravillous and intervillous inflammatory cells and decreased to absent villous vessels.

Table 17-2 Features Suggesting Infectious Chronic Villitis

Clinical Features
Prematurity
Stillbirth
NICU admission
Hydrops fetalis or placentalis
Trimmed placental weight <5th percentile
Positive HIV status in mother
Suspected or confirmed maternal illness or exposure
Pathologic Features
Marked and diffuse stromal expansion of villi
Diffuse chronic villitis with any of the following:
Plasma cells
Giant cells
Hemosiderin
Fetal normoblastemia (if >20 wk gestational age)
Chorionic plate vascular thrombi

HIV, human immunodeficiency virus; NICU, neonatal intensive care unit.

tract infection and bacteremia.[22] GBS infection is particularly lethal to the fetus, because it can cause pneumonia and sepsis. For this reason, it was the focus of a recent late pregnancy screening and treatment protocol in the United States.[37-39] Infection during pregnancy can occur in the absence of ruptured membranes.[12] Classically, GBS causes a necrotizing chorioamnionitis of high maternal and fetal stage (Fig. 17-5A).[40,41] Rapid bacterial growth often allows the organisms to be readily visualized on the placental membranes (see Fig. 17-5B). In cases of retained stillbirth, especially in the second trimester, one can occasionally see organisms filling the villous vascular spaces (see Fig. 17-5C). The usual histology of ACA due to GBS amnionic fluid infection is nonspecific, but if necrotizing ACA is present, GBS should be strongly suspected, especially if there is high fetal and maternal stage. Umbilical cord involvement is usually limited to the vessels, but in some cases, small surface abscesses may be present (see Fig. 17-5D), different from the larger abscesses seen with candidal omphalitis (discussed later).

Hematogenously spread GBS can also result in acute villitis. The histology is usually an isolated villitis without necrosis or abscess formation (see Fig. 17-5E), which helps in differentiating it from listerial placentitis (discussed later).

Fusobacterium

Fusobacterium species of filamentous gram-negative, anaerobic bacilli are the cause of ACA in approximately 10% of all cultured cases but in a much higher percentage of preterm ACA.[42-44] They cause necrotizing ACA (Fig. 17-6) comparable to that associated with GBS. The overgrowth of organisms makes them easy to identify on routine hematoxylin and eosin (H&E) staining (see Fig. 17-6). Silver stains or immunohistochemical studies can be used to confirm the diagnosis. The organism does not cause

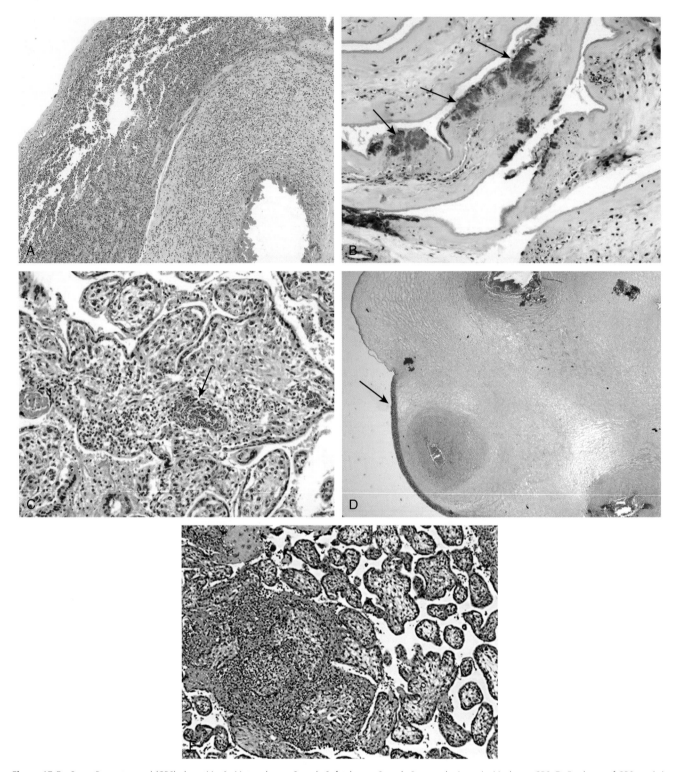

Figure 17-5. Group B streptococcal (GBS) placentitis. **A,** Maternal stage 3 grade 2, fetal stage 3 grade 2 acute chorioamnionitis due to GBS. **B,** Fatal case of GBS sepsis in utero with placental membranes showing overgrowth of the bacteria *(black arrows)*. **C,** Fatal case of GBS sepsis with bacteria present in chorionic villous vessels *(arrow)* and acute villitis. **D,** GBS "phlebitis" with abscess on the surface of the umbilical cord *(arrow)*. **E,** GBS acute villitis.

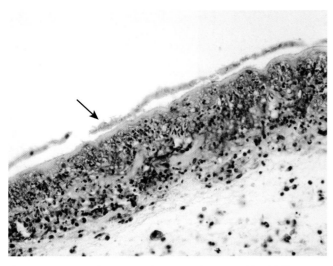

Figure 17-6. Maternal stage 3 grade 2 acute chorioamnionitis with filamentous rods on amniotic surface *(arrow)*, typical for fusobacteria.

infection in the neonate or fetus but is associated with premature delivery due to preterm ACA.[42-44]

Listeria monocytogenes

Listeria monocytogenes, a gram-positive motile bacterium, is a well-known perinatal pathogen. It is a common cause of septic abortion in cattle and sheep, and infection occurs in a wide variety of mammals including humans. The organism is ubiquitous and is present in soil, water, and animal feces. Human infections result from consumption of contaminated foods, most commonly processed meats.[45] Miniepidemics of infections have been reported as a result of the consumption of cole slaw and dairy products that were improperly pasteurized or unpasteurized.[46-50]

Listeria typically produces gastrointestinal illnesses or an influenza-type disease that is self-limited. In immunocompromised hosts, the elderly, and pregnant women, the infection can be serious and life-threatening. In pregnancy, a mild maternal gastrointestinal syndrome or flu-like symptoms may be all that is observed, yet a marked placentitis with congenital infection can occur. Congenital listeriosis is fatal in 40% to 50% of cases. Other known complications include abortion, prematurity, and stillbirth.[24-29]

The placental findings are striking and can be made grossly. The placenta often grossly shows infected yellow membranes (ACA) that emanate a characteristic fruity odor. Parenchymal abscesses may be large enough to be grossly diagnosed (Fig. 17-7A). The presence of placental abscesses should be considered evidence for the diagnosis of listerial placentitis until proven otherwise. The clinicians for the mother and infant should be immediately notified, and the microbiology laboratory alerted, because specific culture methods may be needed to identify the organism, which grows best at slightly cooler temperatures.

Histologically, both microabscesses and macroabscesses are present, with acute suppurative villitis (see Fig. 17-7B) and necrotizing ACA. The organisms can be identified by silver staining or by immunohistochemistry, and they are located in the center of the abscess or in the amniotic epithelium (see Fig. 17-7C).[51]

Mycobacterium tuberculosis

Mycobacterium tuberculosis is currently causing a worldwide epidemic of tuberculosis, facilitated by human immunodeficiency virus (HIV) infection, resistant strains, and poverty. Women, whether pregnant or not, are at risk for common pulmonary tuberculosis but can also be infected genitally. Congenital infections result from direct extension from an infected endomyometrium[52] or from hematogenous spread that seeds the placenta. The fetus becomes infected by hematogenous infection in the fetal blood[53,54] or by rupture of a caseous lesion into the amniotic fluid and aspiration of the fluid in utero.[55]

The placental pathology in congenital tuberculosis is the same as for infection elsewhere, with caseating granulomas and miliary tubercles involving the villi, intervillous space, or basal plate (Fig. 17-8).

Fungal Infections

Candida

Candida species are the most frequent cause of fungal infections of the placenta,. Whereas most *Candida* infections are benign and produce no clinical sequelae in mother or infant, systemic congenital candidiasis is associated with a high fetal mortality rate.[10,56-58] The risk factors for candidal placentitis include maternal glucose intolerance, maternal sickle cell disease or trait, the presence of a foreign object (e.g., intrauterine device, cerclage), and HIV infection.

The hallmark of candidal placentitis is abscesses along the surfaces of the umbilical cord that are visible grossly (Fig. 17-9A).[59-61] Microscopic examination reveals multiple abscesses on the cord, with hyphae often visible on routine H&E staining (see Fig. 17-9B). The presence of hyphae invading into the Wharton jelly is thought to increase the risk of true congenital infection,[60] although that has not been my personal experience.

Other *Candida* species can infect the placenta, most commonly *Candida glabrata*.[62] The placental lesions include the presence of the organism in the membranes (see Fig. 17-9C),[63] although the placenta can be uninvolved despite congenital infection.[61] The risk factors for this type of infection include those for *Candida albicans* infection and immunosuppression.[62]

Other yeast infections have been reported in placentas, although extremely rarely and in exceptional circumstances. They manifest as yeast forms present in the intervillous space associated with maternal sepsis.[64]

Parasitic Infections

Plasmodium falciparum

Malarial infections are a devastating reality to the developing world, with a high mortality rate among children. Congenital infections are also common and lead to morbidity and mortality for both mother and infant. The fetus, in cases of maternal malarial infection, is at increased risk for prematurity, low birth weight, and death.[65,66] Maternal mortality is also increased.[66] Pregnancy increases the parasite burden in all species of malaria, irrespective of parity and maternal age.[67]

Placental pathology in malaria can be striking, because the pigment-laden maternal red blood cells aggregate in the intervil-

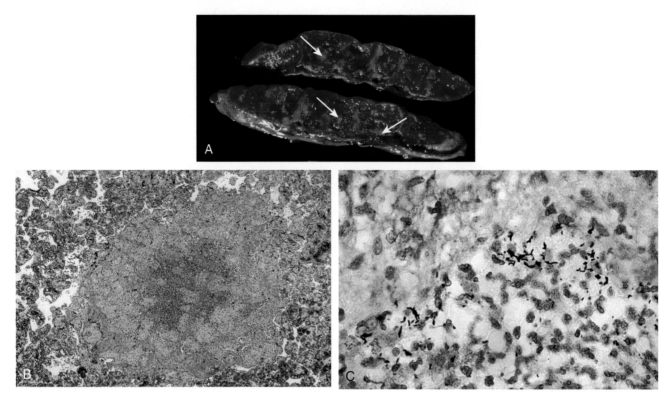

Figure 17-7. Listerial placentitis. **A,** Gross photograph of a term placenta with multiple yellow, soft lesions in the parenchyma *(arrows)* which are the microabscesses and macroabscesses typical of listerial placentitis. **B,** Histologic specimen of placental abscess. **C.** Steiner silver stain demonstrates the rod-shaped listerial organisms.

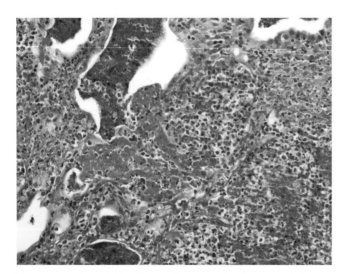

Figure 17-8. Placenta infected by *Mycobacterium tuberculosis*. A 30-week gestational age placenta with two granulomatous giant cells in a confirmed case of tuberculosis involving the placenta. (Used with permission from Wong RMS, Wong KY, Lam BCC: Atypical presentation of congenital tuberculosis in a preterm infant. Hong Kong J Paediatr 2007;12:133-136.)

lous space, as do macrophages with large granules of pigment. In some cases, the placenta "sequesters" the organisms, giving the appearance of a malarial "abscess" (Fig. 17-10).[68,69] This infiltrate affects placental function by interfering with oxygen delivery by the infected red blood cells.[70,71] The whole effect is exacerbated by the concurrent maternal anemia caused by the infection.

Congenital malaria can be diagnosed on placental examination by the presence of the infected red blood cells or malarial pigment in hematopoietic cells in the placental circulation. Clinically, the onset of disease is often delayed by several days and up to months.[72] There is a good association between placental malarial sequestration and congenital malarial infection.[73]

Schistosomiasis

Although infection by most *Schistosoma* species has been reported in animal species, only *Schistosoma mansoni* has been documented as a congenital infection in humans.[74] *S. mansoni* is prevalent in many regions of the world, yet placental involvement has only rarely been described. Reports of *S. mansoni* eggs[75] and adult worms[76,77] in the placenta in the fetal circulation have been published (Fig. 17-11). The sources include direct extension from the involved female genital tract[78] or backward migration of eggs or worms into the dilated uterine venous system.[75]

Toxoplasma gondii

The apicomplexan parasite *Toxoplasma gondii* can infect any warm-blooded animal. Its preferred host is the domesticated cat. Infections in immunocompetent adults are typically silent and result in protective antibodies, although it has been estimated that only 15% of women of reproductive age in the United States have antibodies.[79] The parasite infects the placenta with a trans-

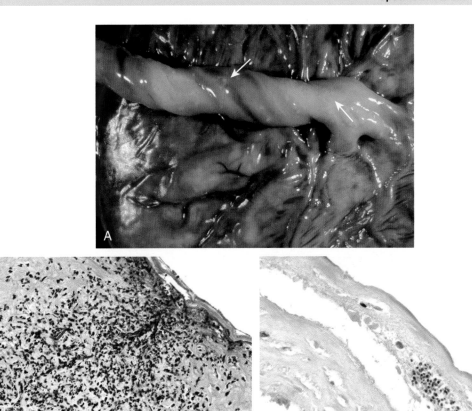

Figure 17-9. Candidal placentitis. **A,** Green, discolored placenta and cord with candidal abscesses (*white arrows*) on umbilical cord. **B,** Histologic examination of the abscesses from **A** showed deep involvement of Wharton jelly. Pseudohyphae are easily seen. **C,** *Candida glabrata* organisms within membranes with relatively little acute chorioamnionitis.

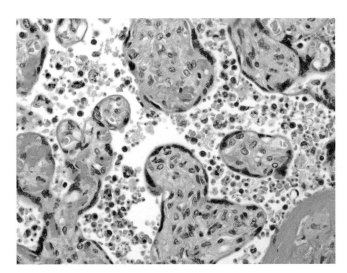

Figure 17-10. Malaria sequestration. Pigment and organisms are present in maternal red blood cells in the intervillous space.

mission rate of about 40% and is especially lethal to the fetus, although the lethality is lessened closer to term.[80,81] The organism adheres to and infects the villous trophoblast via migration.[82,83] *T. gondii* trophozoites and cysts can be identified in the umbilical cord in Wharton jelly (Fig. 17-12A) and within the chorionic plate amniocytes (see Fig. 17-12B), although even in documented cases of toxoplasmosis these are difficult to find. The characteristic placental finding is a granulomatous villitis (see Fig. 17-12C)[84,85] or hydrops placentalis.[86] The difficulty in finding the organism has led to molecular techniques for improved diagnosis.[79]

It is known that the "visibility" of the organism in the placenta relates to the fetal/neonatal outcome: easily identifiable cysts and pseudocysts are present in severely affected cases.[87] The severity of congenital infection and its associated morbidity and mortality are dictated by the timing of the infection in relationship to gestational age; death is most common with first-trimester infections, but infectious transmission is more common in the third trimester.[71,88] There appears to be a latency period in congenital toxoplasmosis infection, such that placental infection is present for some time before fetal infection occurs—the

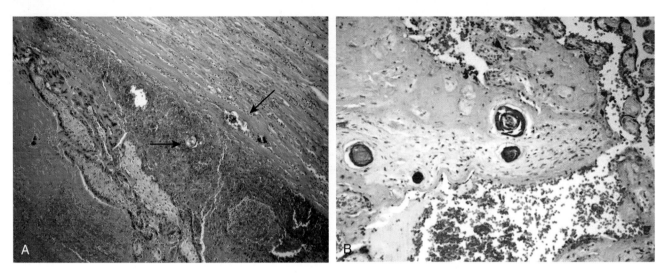

Figure 17-11. Schistosomiasis in the placenta. *Schistosoma* eggs are present in the villi *(arrows)* of a preterm placenta **(A)** and in the wall and intervillous space of a tubal ectopic pregnancy **(B)**. (**A,** Courtesy of Dr. A. L. Bittencourt. **B,** Courtesy of Dr. J. N. Kitinya.)

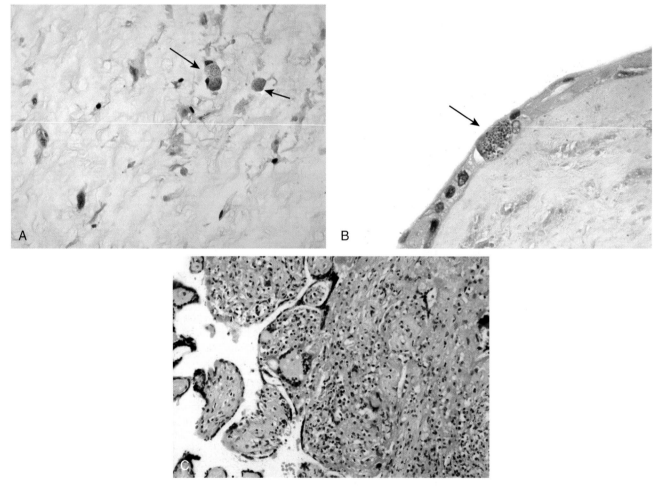

Figure 17-12. Toxoplasmosis. Cyst forms *(arrows)* are seen in Wharton jelly **(A)** and in amniotic epithelium *(arrow)* **(B)**. **C,** A giant cell chronic villitis is present in a hydropic stillbirth at 28 weeks' gestational age.

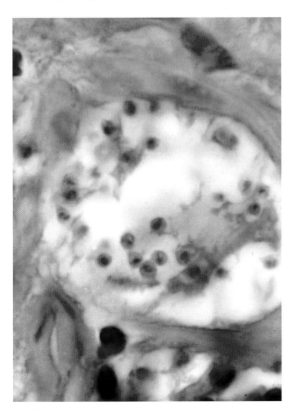

Figure 17-13. Chagas disease. The parasites are present in the chorionic villi. (Courtesy of Dr. A. L. Bittencourt.)

so-called prenatal incubation period.[89] As a result, the greatest risk to the fetus for severely damaging infection occurs during the gestational age of 10 to 24 weeks.[71]

Trypanosoma cruzi

Chagas disease, caused by infection with the protozoan *Trypanosoma cruzi*, affects millions of people worldwide and has been shown to be vertically transmitted.[71] Hematogenous spread of the organism can lead to infection of the trophoblast. Following differentiation into amastigotes, the organisms then spread to the Hofbauer cells, from which they are released into the fetal circulation. The parasites can be present in the villi or membranes[90] (Fig. 17-13); when present, they are usually associated with intrauterine fetal demise.[91,92] Hematogenously spread placental infection occurs most often in the chronic form of the disease, and the mother is often asymptomatic.[71]

Mycoplasmal and Ureaplasmal Infections

The prokaryotes *Mycoplasma* and *Ureaplasma* are both commonly present in the flora of the lower female genital tract in sexually active women, often without causing symptoms. They have been documented in 30% to 80% of sexually active women, either singly or together.[71] Therefore, these organisms and cultures of amniotic fluid or the chorionic plate are commonly

associated with histologic ACA.[13,14,93-96] Although the association is much better with preterm ACA, *Mycoplasma* and *Ureaplasma* are still cultured frequently in term ACA. There are no specific histopathologic features for *Mycoplasma hominis* or *Ureaplasma urealyticum,* although they are one of the few documented infections of the amniotic cavity that can occur despite intact membranes.[95,97,98]

Syphilis

Treponema pallidum, a member of the family Spirochaetaceae, has a long and fascinating medical history[99] and still causes congenital infections worldwide. The morbidity of syphilis infection in pregnancy depends on the treatment the mother has received and on the stage of her disease. Untreated disease carries a high risk of fetal mortality (at any gestational age), with early syphilis being the most lethal.[100,101]

The placental findings in congenital syphilis are very subtle. There is a diffuse thickening and pallor of the disk grossly. Histologically, the hallmarks include relative immaturity of the villi, very mild mixed inflammatory villitis, thickening of the villous perivascular tissues and endothelium ("onion skinning"; Fig. 17-14A), persistent normoblastemia, and a mild ACA (see Fig. 17-14B).[102,103] In the older literature, necrotizing funisitis (a distinctive pattern of umbilical cord inflammation in which the inflammatory cells cluster and break down in a mid–Wharton jelly location; see Fig. 17-14C) was considered to be specific for congenital syphilis,[104,105] but this has not proved to be true; however, the etiology has remained elusive.[106,107] Despite the details of pathologic findings associated with maternal syphilis, placental pathology in syphilis is not correlated with congenital infection.[103,108]

Viral Infections

Cytomegalovirus

The most common congenital viral infection in humans is cytomegalovirus (CMV). As with other viral infections, placental involvement is a function of viral load and therefore occurs almost exclusively in primary infection or with immunocompromise. Reinfection or reactivation has been shown to have perinatal sequelae.[109-112] Although the CMV transmission rate is high (approximately 40%[113]), most congenital infections are asymptomatic or mild. However, CMV is one of the most common infectious causes of intrauterine growth restriction, intrauterine fetal demise, neurocompromise, blindness, and deafness.[113-116] Between 1% and 2% of all pregnancies are complicated by congenital CMV, and 10% to 20% of those will have clinical sequelae.[113-116]

CMV placentitis is typified by a thick placental disk, often visualized by antenatal ultrasound.[117] The histopathologic findings include large, "pink" villi caused by stromal expansion and a mild lymphoplasmacytic villitis (Fig. 17-15A). The villi often have focal surface necrosis with intervillositis (see Fig. 17-15B). Chorionic plate vascular thromboses are also common. In active infections, the cytoplasmic and nuclear inclusions are numerous and include villous stromal and endothelial cells (see Fig. 17-15C). Plasma cell deciduitis is common.[30]

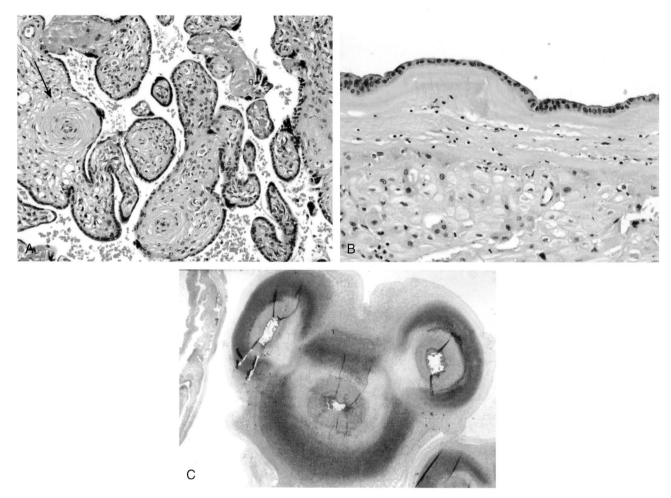

Figure 17-14. Syphilitic placentitis. Mild hypertrophy of the vessel wall **(A)** is often seen with congenital syphilis. Other nonspecific findings that are common in syphilitic placentitis include a mild acute or chronic chorioamnionitis **(B)** and a necrotizing funisitis **(C)**.

Herpes Simplex Virus

Maternal herpes simplex virus (HSV) infection can involve the fetus or neonate transplacentally or during or after delivery.[118] The transmission rate in primary infection is high, greater than 50%. These infections characteristically occur in asymptomatic women and may occur with either viral type (HSV-1 or HSV-2). Congenital infections are frequently lethal and, if not lethal, are associated with prematurity, intrauterine growth restriction, and severe neurosequelae. Because most of these infections are not clinically apparent, the diagnosis rests on placental pathology or the obvious presence of fetal or neonatal disease (discussed later).

Placental findings are not diagnostic but include severe chronic villitis (Fig. 17-16A) with plasma cell deciduitis.[119] In one case of fetal death at term and unsuspected maternal primary HSV, the placental infection included a marked chorionic plate plasma cell infiltrate (see Fig. 17-16B).

Human Immunodeficiency Virus

Although it is clear that the HIV virus can infect the chorionic villi (trophoblast, stroma, and Hofbauer cells all can be shown to have viral DNA),[120] there appear to be no specific histopatho-logic findings predictive of transmission.[121-124] There are reports that the incidence of ACA in HIV-positive mothers may be increased in some populations, but this has not been established.[125-127] What is clear is that coinfections are increased with maternal HIV infection and that there is an increased morbidity due to congenital toxoplasmosis,[128] malaria,[129,130] CMV,[112] syphilis,[131] and other infections.[132] Because of the rarity of these infections in the United States, in practice I encourage clinical consideration for HIV evaluation whenever any placental infection is demonstrated or suspected to be transplacental.

Parvovirus

Parvovirus is a relatively common pediatric pathogen that can cause significant morbidity in the fetus if a pregnant woman becomes infected. The virus preferentially infects rapidly dividing cells, and the fetal hematopoietic system is a prime target. Mortality is high if infection occurs during the first or early second trimester, when fetal red blood cell mass is low. From midgestation on, the mortality rate declines, but significant fetal anemia and hydrops fetalis can still occur. The virus easily traverses through the villi into the fetal bloodstream, where it infects hematopoietic precursors. Infected cells are unable to

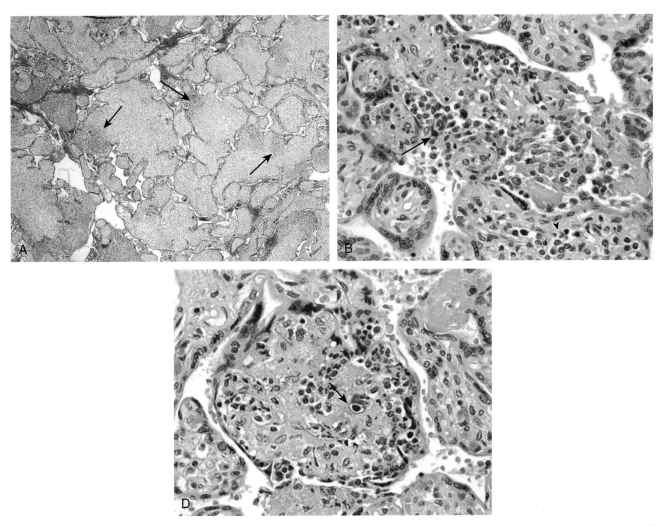

Figure 17-15. Cytomegalovirus (CMV) placentitis. **A,** Low-power photomicrograph of a 28-week placenta infected with CMV shows the expanded villi with necrosis of their surfaces *(arrows)*. **B,** Higher-power image shows nonspecific lymphohistiocytic intervillositis *(arrow)* and chronic villitis *(arrowhead)*. **C,** CMV virus in a villous stromal cell *(arrow)*.

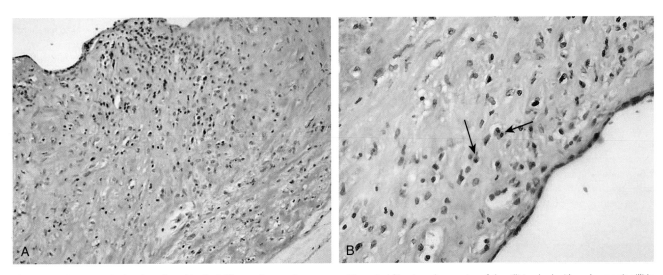

Figure 17-16. Herpes simplex virus placentitis. **A,** Stillborn twin gestation at term with marked fibrosis and expansion of the villi involved with a plasmacytic villitis. **B,** The chorionic plate was also involved and showed numerous plasma cells *(arrows)*.

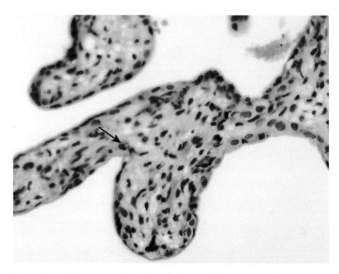

Figure 17-17. Term gestation with nonfatal congenital parvovirus infection. Notice the inclusion in a red blood cell circulating within the villous vessels *(arrow)*.

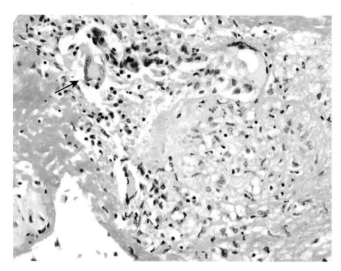

Figure 17-19. Varicella placentitis. Granulomatous villitis with giant cells *(arrow)* in a stillborn at term with maternal varicella pneumonia.

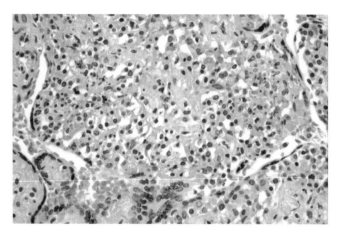

Figure 17-18. Congenital rubella. Necrotizing chronic villitis in a term placenta complicated with maternal and congenital rubella. (Courtesy of H. Rosenberg.)

carry oxygen well and therefore lyse easily, causing anemia and hypoxemia. The placenta does not become directly infected, and the pathology is limited to the infected fetal erythroid cells (Fig. 17-17); the hypoxic and anemic effects on the fetus include hydrops placentalis and chorangiosis.[133-135]

Rubella

Congenital rubella is rare in developed countries but is still a risk among nonimmunized pregnant women in the developing world.[136,137] The congenital syndrome is devastating and well described. Placental findings are nonspecific and depend on gestational age.[138] Chronic villitis, with or without necrosis and fibrin agglutination, has been described (Fig. 17-18). Occasionally, inclusions are present, which can assist in the differential diagnosis.[138]

Rubeola

Congenital measles is extraordinarily rare. Transplacental transmission has been reported to occur, but placental findings have

only rarely been described.[139,140] In one report, it appeared that the viral particles could be identified in the trophoblast cells.[140]

Varicella

Varicella-zoster infection during pregnancy often results in significant maternal morbidity.[141,142] Fetal morbidity includes congenital varicella syndrome, when maternal infection occurs during the first 20 weeks of gestation,[143] and fetal death.[144,145] Transmission is low after 20 weeks' gestation but can be associated with both fetal and neonatal morbidity.[146] Placental findings are uncommon but characteristic; they include marked granulomatous villitis with multinucleated giant cells (Fig. 17-19).[145-147]

Pregnancy-Associated Uterine Infections

Endomyometritis is a complication of pregnancy that can lead to sepsis, iatrogenic perforation of the uterus during manipulation, gravid hysterectomy, and death. The risk factors include pregnancy complicated by infection (typically bacterial), ACA, retained placenta, and uterine cavity exploration, either manually or with curettage. The pathologist may receive a curettage specimen or the gravid uterus for evaluation, and this may occur immediately or up to several days after delivery.

The histologic features of endomyometritis include inflammation with a predominance of either neutrophils and eosinophils (acute endomyometritis) or chronic inflammatory cells. Inflammation may be associated with necrosis and hemorrhage of the endometrium and myometrium. In the immediate postpartum period, these features may be confused with those resulting from normal labor and delivery. Acute endometritis with hemorrhage and necrosis is a common finding of the labored endometrium. A diagnosis of either acute or chronic endomyometritis requires the presence of myometrial inflammation.

Most cases of endomyometritis are caused by bacterial infections that are common in pregnancy and have no specific histo-

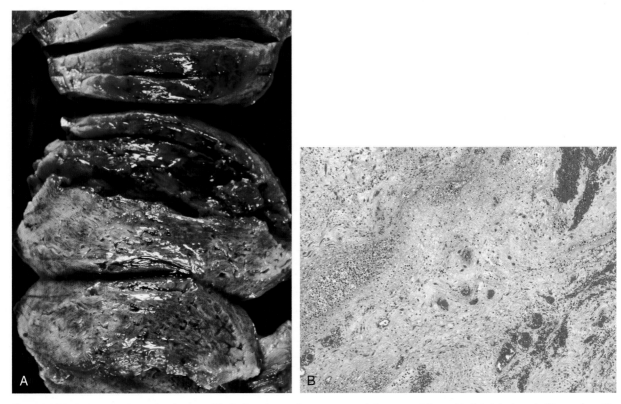

Figure 17-20. Group A streptococcal endomyometritis. **A,** Gross image of a uterus resected after a term delivery with clinical chorioamnionitis complicated by postpartum hemorrhage and septic shock. **B,** Histopathology of the uterus from the same patient as in **A,** showing diffuse hemorrhagic and inflammatory necrosis of the myometrium.

pathologic features other than those listed previously. However, group A streptococcal infection causes a specific infectious endomyometritis that is especially lethal.[148-151] The infection is often fulminant and can occur in the third trimester,[152] during labor,[153] and through the puerperium.[154] The course is rapid and follows an upper respiratory tract infection but causes relatively mild symptoms initially, other than fever.[154] However, multiorgan failure ensues, leading to both maternal and fetal or infant death. The histopathology shows necrotizing endomyometritis (Fig. 17-20).

Fetal and Congenital Infections

Congenital infections occur in transplacental and ascending infections and are often lethal. The histopathologic features mirror the route of infection.

Infected amniotic fluid involves the fetus by so-called aspiration, leading to aspiration pneumonia due to the presence of maternal neutrophils, with or without organisms, in the developing airways or, rarely, a true congenital pneumonia due to a response by the fetus. Both can result in sepsis (Fig. 17-21A). The fetus also may become infected by "swallowing" the contents of the amniotic fluid; this fills the lumen of the gastrointestinal tract (see Fig. 17-21B) with swallowed inflammatory cells and organisms, leading to sepsis. In addition, the fetus can become directly infected by exposure of the skin, ear canals, or eyes to the infected amniotic fluid.

The presence of ACA and intrauterine fetal demise or neonatal death (especially in prematurity) should raise the suspicion for an amniotic fluid infection–related death. Samples for microbiologic culture should be taken from the placenta (by peeling back the amnion and swabbing the exposed chorionic plate) and from the fetus at autopsy (by exposing the thoracic cavity and obtaining a small piece of lung using sterile tools). Both aerobic and anaerobic cultures should be requested. In addition, the microbiology laboratory should be alerted for directed culture techniques if there is suspicion of *L. monocytogenes, M. hominis,* or *U. urealyticum* infection clinically or based on the gross examination of the placenta or fetus.

Hematogenous spread of maternal infection results in congenital infection through involvement of the villous stroma and endothelium, and access to the fetal blood results in fetal sepsis.

Each organism has tropism for specific organs, which it preferentially infects, although liver, lungs, and kidneys are most commonly involved. Specific patterns of infection are a function of the route of congenital infection and the tropism of the organism. For example, parvovirus preferentially infects the most rapidly dividing cells in the fetus, typically the hematopoietic elements, leading to the presence of circulating infected fetal nucleated red blood cells (see Fig. 17-17). Congenital bacterial infections from ACA typically lead to congenital pneumonia and sepsis. Most hematogenously spread congenital infections infect the fetal liver initially and then show some level of tropism to other organs. For example, HSV infects the lung and liver, yielding geographic necrosis, and can also infect the central nervous

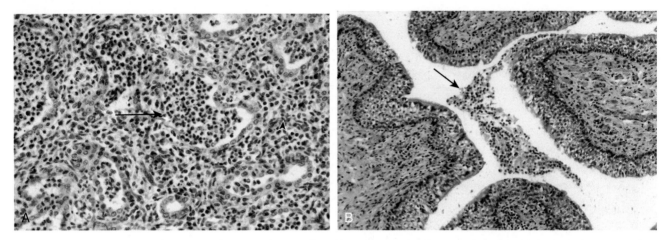

Figure 17-21. Congenital pneumonia. **A,** Specimen from a second-trimester fetus delivered prematurely with amniotic fluid infection (acute chorioamnionitis). The fetus died during labor. Maternal inflammatory cells were "aspirated" in utero and were found to be present in the developing airways *(arrow).* The fetal response in the interstitium *(arrowhead)* documents infection before death. **B,** Mature (maternal) inflammatory cells in the lumen of the fetal esophagus *(arrow).*

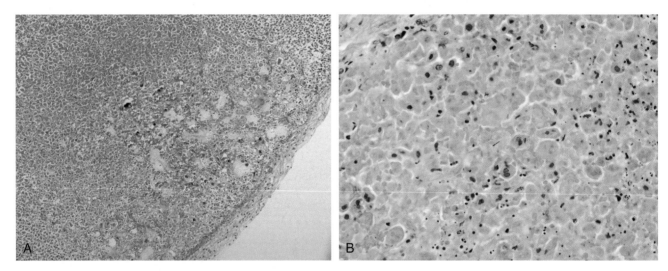

Figure 17-22. Congenital herpes simplex virus (HSV) infection. **A,** Autolyzed stillbirth at term with congenital HSV, showing classic wedge-shaped adrenal cortical infarct with calcifications. **B,** Typical HSV viral inclusions are seen in hepatic geographic necrosis.

system and the cranial nerve ganglia. It produces a characteristic pattern of infection in the developing adrenal gland, targeting the subcapsular cortical regions of both the definitive and the fetal cortex, and producing a wedge-shaped infarct, often with dystrophic calcifications (Fig. 17-22A), which can be identified even in the most autolyzed cases. The inclusions are often present in the center of the necrotic area and may be recognized on routine H&E staining (see Fig. 17-22B). *T. pallidum* can be demonstrated by special stains in the liver even in very autolyzed stillbirths[155] and in my experience is easy to find in the vitreous of the eye. Parvovirus infects bone marrow and hematopoietic precursors in the liver. CMV is often disseminated diffusely but is unique in its preference for infecting the islets in the pancreas. Coxsackievirus targets myocardium.

In general, hematogenously spread infections result in non-specific findings of intrauterine growth restriction, hydrops fetalis, normoblastemia, hepatosplenomegaly, calcifications in the central nervous system, and intrauterine fetal demise. Suspi-

cion for such a congenital infection should be increased if two or more of these features are present, and maternal antibody status should be evaluated. Molecular or virologic studies can also be performed on placental or fetal tissue, if needed for the diagnosis, although usually the histopathology is definitive.

REFERENCES

1. Redline RW, Faye-Petersen O, Heller D, et al: Amniotic infection syndrome: Nosology and reproducibility of placental reaction patterns. Pediatr Dev Pathol 2003;6:435-448.
2. Odibo AO, Rodis JF, Sanders MM, et al: Relationship of amniotic fluid markers of intra-amniotic infection with histopathology in cases of preterm labor with intact membranes. J Perinatol 1999;19:407-412.
3. Salafia CM, Pezzullo JC, Lopez-Zeno JA, et al: Placental pathologic features of preterm preeclampsia. Am J Obstet Gynecol 1995;173:1097-1105.

4. Romero R, Gotsch F, Pineles B, Kusanovic JP: Inflammation in pregnancy: Its roles in reproductive physiology, obstetrical complications, and fetal injury. Nutr Rev 2007;65:S194-S202.

5. Newton ER: Preterm labor, preterm premature rupture of membranes, and chorioamnionitis. Clin Perinatol 2005;32:571-600.

6. Edwards RK: Chorioamnionitis and labor. Obstet Gynecol Clin North Am 2005;32:287-296.

7. Redline RW, Minich N, Taylor HG, Hack M: Placental lesions as predictors of cerebral palsy and abnormal neurocognitive function at school age in extremely low birth weight infants (<1 kg). Pediatr Dev Pathol 2007;10:282-292.

8. Folkerth RD: The neuropathology of acquired pre- and perinatal brain injuries. Semin Diagn Pathol 2007;24:48-57.

9. Wu YW, Lynch JK, Nelson KB: Perinatal arterial stroke: Understanding mechanisms and outcomes. Semin Neurol 2005;25:424-434.

10. Redline RW: Severe fetal placental vascular lesions in term infants with neurologic impairment. Am J Obstet Gynecol 2005;192:452-457.

11. Joste NE, Kundsin RB, Genest DR: Histology and *Ureaplasma urealyticum* culture in 63 cases of first trimester abortion. Am J Clin Pathol 1994;102:729-732.

12. Gibbs RS, Schrag S, Schuchat A: Perinatal infections due to group B streptococci. Obstet Gynecol 2004;104:1062-1076.

13. Hillier SL, Martius J, Krohn M, et al: A case-control study of chorioamnionic infection and histologic chorioamnionitis in prematurity. N Engl J Med 1988;319:972-978.

14. Hecht JL, Onderdonk A, Delaney M, et al: Characterization of chorioamnionitis in 2nd-trimester C-section placentas and correlation with microorganism recovery from subamniotic tissues. Pediatr Dev Pathol 2008;11:15-22.

15. Onderdonk AB, Hecht JL, McElrath TF, et al: Colonization of second-trimester placenta parenchyma. Am J Obstet Gynecol 2008;199:52.31-52.310.

16. Casey BM, Cox SM: Chorioamnionitis and endometritis. Infect Dis Clin North Am 1997;11:203-222.

17. Duff P: Antibiotic selection in obstetric patients. Infect Dis Clin North Am 1997;11:1-12.

18. Newton ER: Chorioamnionitis and intraamniotic infection. Clin Obstet Gynecol 1993;36:795-808.

19. Romero R, Nores J, Mazor M, et al: Microbial invasion of the amniotic cavity during term labor: Prevalence and clinical significance. J Reprod Med 1993;38:543-548.

20. Salafia CM, Mangam HE, Weigl CA, et al: Abnormal fetal heart rate patterns and placental inflammation. Am J Obstet Gynecol 1989;160:140-147.

21. Chapman ST: Prescribing in pregnancy: Bacterial infections in pregnancy. Clin Obstet Gynaecol 1986;13:397-416.

22. Winn HN: Group B streptococcus infection in pregnancy. Clin Perinatol 2007;34:387-392.

23. Cito G, Luisi S, Faldini E, et al: Listeriosis in pregnancy: A case report. J Matern Fetal Neonatal Med 2005;18:367-368.

24. Cruikshank DP, Warenski JC: First-trimester maternal *Listeria monocytogenes* sepsis and chorioamnionitis with normal neonatal outcome. Obstet Gynecol 1989;73:469-471.

25. Fan YD, Pastorek JG 2nd, Janney FA, Sanders CV: Listeriosis as an obstetric complication in an immunocompromised patient. South Med J 1989;82:1044-1045.

26. Frederiksen B, Samuelsson S: Feto-maternal listeriosis in Denmark 1981-1988. J Infect 1992;24:277-287.

27. Khong TY, Frappell JM, Steel HM, et al: Perinatal listeriosis: A report of six cases. Br J Obstet Gynaecol 1986;93:1083-1087.

28. Svare J, Andersen LF, Langhoff-Roos J, et al: Maternal-fetal listeriosis: Two case reports. Gynecol Obstet Invest 1991;31:179-181.

29. Wagner M, Allerberger F: Characterization of *Listeria monocytogenes* recovered from 41 cases of sporadic listeriosis in Austria by

30. serotyping and pulsed-field gel electrophoresis. FEMS Immunol Med Microbiol 2003;35:227-234.

30. Altshuler G, Russell P: The human placental villitides: A review of chronic intrauterine infection. Curr Top Pathol 1975;60:64-112.

31. Gersell DJ: Chronic villitis, chronic chorioamnionitis, and maternal floor infarction. Semin Diagn Pathol 1993;10:251-266.

32. Redline RW: Villitis of unknown etiology: Noninfectious chronic villitis in the placenta. Hum Pathol 2007;38:1439-1446.

33. Boog G: Chronic villitis of unknown etiology. Eur J Obstet Gynecol Reprod Biol 2008;136:9-15.

34. Redline RW: Inflammatory responses in the placenta and umbilical cord. Semin Fetal Neonatal Med 2006;11:296-301.

35. Redline RW: Infections and other inflammatory conditions. Semin Diagn Pathol 2007;24:5-13.

36. Redline RW, Patterson P: Villitis of unknown etiology is associated with major infiltration of fetal tissue by maternal inflammatory cells. Am J Pathol 1993;143:473-479.

37. American College of Obstetrics and Gynecologists, Committee on Obstetric Practice: ACOG committee opinion: Prevention of early-onset group B streptococcal disease in newborns. Number 173, June 1996. Int J Gynaecol Obstet 1996;54:197-205.

38. Centers for Disease Control and Prevention: Prevention of perinatal group B streptococcal disease: A public health perspective. MMWR Recomm Rep 1996;45:1-24.

39. Steele RW: A revised strategy for the prevention of group B streptococcal infection in pregnant women and their newborns. Medscape Womens Health 1996;1:2.

40. De Paepe ME, Friedman RM, Gundogan F, et al: The histologic fetoplacental inflammatory response in fatal perinatal group B-streptococcus infection. J Perinatol 2004;24:441-445.

41. Winram SB, Jonas M, Chi E, Rubens CE: Characterization of group B streptococcal invasion of human chorion and amnion epithelial cells in vitro. Infect Immun 1998;66:4932-4941.

42. Altshuler G, Hyde S: Clinicopathologic considerations of fusobacteria chorioamnionitis. Acta Obstet Gynecol Scand 1988;67:513-517.

43. Altshuler G, Hyde S: Fusobacteria: An important cause of chorioamnionitis. Arch Pathol Lab Med 1985;109:739-743.

44. Chaim W, Mazor M: Intraamniotic infection with fusobacteria. Arch Gynecol Obstet 1992;251:1-7.

45. Gottlieb SL, Newbern EC, Griffin PM, et al: Multistate outbreak of listeriosis linked to turkey deli meat and subsequent changes in US regulatory policy. Clin Infect Dis 2006;42:29-36.

46. Rocourt J, Jacquet C, Reilly A: Epidemiology of human listeriosis and seafoods. Int J Food Microbiol 2000;62:197-209.

47. Kiss R, Tirczka T, Szita G, et al: *Listeria monocytogenes* food monitoring data and incidence of human listeriosis in Hungary, 2004. Int J Food Microbiol 2006;112:71-74.

48. Wagner M, Melzner D, Bago Z, et al: Outbreak of clinical listeriosis in sheep: Evaluation from possible contamination routes from feed to raw produce and humans. J Vet Med B Infect Dis Vet Public Health 2005;52:278-283.

49. Danielsson-Tham ML, Eriksson E, Helmersson S, et al: Causes behind a human cheese-borne outbreak of gastrointestinal listeriosis. Foodborne Pathog Dis 2004;1:153-159.

50. Heisick JE, Wagner DE, Nierman ML, Peeler JT: *Listeria* spp. found on fresh market produce. Appl Environ Microbiol 1989;55:1925-1927.

51. Parkash V, Morotti RA, Joshi V, et al: Immunohistochemical detection of *Listeria* antigens in the placenta in perinatal listeriosis. Int J Gynecol Pathol 1998;17:343-350.

52. Surve TY, Malkani M, Mhatre A, Samdani VP: Congenital TB associated with asymptomatic maternal endometrial TB. Trop Doct 2006;36:59-61.

53. Chen S: Maternal and fetal infection with *Mycobacterium tuberculosis*. Arch Dis Child Fetal Neonatal Ed 1997;77:F77-F78.

54. Kaplan C, Benirschke K, Tarzy B: Placental tuberculosis in early and late pregnancy. Am J Obstet Gynecol 1980;137:858-860.

55. Hertzog AJ, Chapman S, Herring J: Congenital pulmonary aspiration-tuberculosis: Report of a case. Am J Clin Pathol 1949;19:1139-1142.

56. Gerberding KM, Eisenhut CC, Engle WA, Cohen MD: Congenital candida pneumonia and sepsis: A case report and review of the literature. J Perinatol 1989;9:159-161.

57. Levy I, Shalit I, Birk E, et al: Candida endocarditis in neonates: Report of five cases and review of the literature. Mycoses 2006;49:43-48.

58. Reed BD: Risk factors for Candida vulvovaginitis. Obstet Gynecol Surv 1992;47:551-560.

59. Qureshi F, Jacques SM, Bendon RW, et al: Candida funisitis: A clinicopathologic study of 32 cases. Pediatr Dev Pathol 1998;1:118-124.

60. Schwartz DA, Reef S: Candida albicans placentitis and funisitis: Early diagnosis of congenital candidemia by histopathologic examination of umbilical cord vessels. Pediatr Infect Dis J 1990;9:661-665.

61. Matsuzawa S, Ohyama M, Kawataki M, et al: Congenital Candida glabrata infection without specific nodules on the placenta and umbilical cord. Pediatr Infect Dis J 2005;24:744-745.

62. Fidel PL Jr, Vazquez JA, Sobel JD: Candida glabrata: Review of epidemiology, pathogenesis, and clinical disease with comparison to C. albicans. Clin Microbiol Rev 1999;12:80-96.

63. Quirke P, Hwang WS, Validen CC: Congenital Torulopsis glabrata infection in man. Am J Clin Pathol 1980;73:137-140.

64. Molnar-Nadasdy G, Haesly I, Reed J, Altshuler G: Placental cryptococcosis in a mother with systemic lupus erythematosus. Arch Pathol Lab Med 1994;118:757-759.

65. Steketee RW, Nahlen BL, Parise ME, Menendez C: The burden of malaria in pregnancy in malaria-endemic areas. Am J Trop Med Hyg 2001;64:28-35.

66. Shulman CE, Dorman EK: Importance and prevention of malaria in pregnancy. Trans R Soc Trop Med Hyg 2003;97:30-35.

67. Bray RS, Anderson MJ: Falciparum malaria and pregnancy. Trans R Soc Trop Med Hyg 1979;73:427-431.

68. Ordi J, Ismail MR, Ventura PJ, et al: Massive chronic intervillositis of the placenta associated with malaria infection. Am J Surg Pathol 1998;22:1006-1011.

69. Galbraith RM, Fox H, Hsi B, et al: The human materno-foetal relationship in malaria: II. Histological, ultrastructural and immunopathological studies of the placenta. Trans R Soc Trop Med Hyg 1980;74:61-72.

70. Muthusamy A, Achur RN, Bhavanandan VP, et al: Plasmodium falciparum-infected erythrocytes adhere both in the intervillous space and on the villous surface of human placenta by binding to the low-sulfated chondroitin sulfate proteoglycan receptor. Am J Pathol 2004;164:2013-2025.

71. Remington JS, Klein JO: Infectious Diseases of the Fetus and Newborn Infant, 6th ed. Philadelphia, Elsevier Saunders, 2006.

72. Hindi RD, Azimi P: Congenital malaria due to Plasmodium falciparum. Pediatrics 1980;66:977-979.

73. Uneke CJ: Impact of placental Plasmodium falciparum malaria on pregnancy and perinatal outcome in sub-Saharan Africa: I. Introduction to placental malaria. Yale J Biol Med 2007;80:39-50.

74. Friedman JF, Mital P, Kanzaria HK, et al: Schistosomiasis and pregnancy. Trends Parasitol 2007;23:159-164.

75. Peres LC: Schistosoma mansoni eggs in the placenta: An unusual finding. Rev Hosp Sao Paulo Esc Paul Med 1994;5:44-47.

76. Bittencourt AL, Mott K: Placental schistosomiasis. Gaz Med Bahia 1969;69:113-117.

77. Bittencourt AL, Cardoso de Almeida MA, Iunes MA, Casulari da Motta LD: Placental involvement in schistosomiasis mansoni: Report of four cases. Am J Trop Med Hyg 1980;29:571-575.

78. Swai B, Poggensee G, Mtweve S, Krantz I: Female genital schistosomiasis as an evidence of a neglected cause for reproductive ill-health: A retrospective histopathological study from Tanzania. BMC Infect Dis 2006;6:134.

79. Fricker-Hidalgo H, Brenier-Pinchart MP, Schaal JP, et al: Value of Toxoplasma gondii detection in one hundred thirty-three placentas for the diagnosis of congenital toxoplasmosis. Pediatr Infect Dis J 2007;26:845-846.

80. Elliott WG: Placental toxoplasmosis: Report of a case. Am J Clin Pathol 1970;53:413-417.

81. Dische MR, Gooch WM 3rd: Congenital toxoplasmosis. Perspect Pediatr Pathol 1981;6:83-113.

82. Barragan A, Sibley LD: Migration of Toxoplasma gondii across biological barriers. Trends Microbiol 2003;11:426-430.

83. Abbasi M, Kowalewska-Grochowska K, Bahar MA, et al: Infection of placental trophoblasts by Toxoplasma gondii. J Infect Dis 2003;188:608-616.

84. Popek EJ: Granulomatous villitis due to Toxoplasma gondii. Pediatr Pathol 1992;12:281-288.

85. Yavuz E, Aydin F, Seyhan A, et al: Granulomatous villitis formed by inflammatory cells with maternal origin: A rare manifestation type of placental toxoplasmosis. Placenta 2006;27:780-782.

86. Abdel Salam AM, Eissa MH, Mangoud AM, et al: Pathologic examination of the placenta in human cases of toxoplasmosis. J Egypt Soc Parasitol 1990;20:549-554.

87. Sarrut S: [Histological study of the placenta in congenital toxoplasmosis]. Ann Pediatr (Paris) 1967;14:2429-2435.

88. Desmonts G, Couvreur J: Congenital toxoplasmosis: A prospective study of 378 pregnancies. N Engl J Med 1974;290:1110-1116.

89. Thalhammer O: [Prenatal incubation period (author's transl)]. Padiatr Padol 1972;7:14-19.

90. Bittencourt AL: Congenital Chagas disease. Am J Dis Child 1976;130:97-103.

91. Bittencourt AL, Sadigursky M, Barbosa HS: [Congenital Chagas' disease: Study of 29 cases]. Rev Inst Med Trop Sao Paulo 1975;17:146-159.

92. Teruel JR, Nogueira JL: [Fetal losses in a high prevalence area of chronic Chagas' disease]. Rev Inst Med Trop Sao Paulo 1970;12:239-244.

93. Quinn PA, Butany J, Taylor J, Hannah W: Chorioamnionitis: Its association with pregnancy outcome and microbial infection. Am J Obstet Gynecol 1987;156:379-387.

94. Cassell GH, Davis JK, Waites KB, et al: Pathogenesis and significance of urogenital mycoplasmal infections. Adv Exp Med Biol 1987;224:93-115.

95. Cassell GH, Davis RO, Waites KB, et al: Isolation of Mycoplasma hominis and Ureaplasma urealyticum from amniotic fluid at 16-20 weeks of gestation: Potential effect on outcome of pregnancy. Sex Transm Dis 1983;10:294-302.

96. Kundsin RB, Driscoll SG, Monson RR, et al: Association of Ureaplasma urealyticum in the placenta with perinatal morbidity and mortality. N Engl J Med 1984;310:941-945.

97. Foulon W, Naessens A, Dewaele M, et al: Chronic Ureaplasma urealyticum amnionitis associated with abruptio placentae. Obstet Gynecol 1986;68:280.

98. Gray DJ, Robinson HB Jr, Malone J, Thomsom RB: Adverse outcome in pregnancy following amniotic fluid isolation of Ureaplasma urealyticum. Prenat Diagn 1992;12:111-117.

99. Rosebury T: Microbes and Morals: The Strange Story of Venereal Diseases. Cambridge, Harvard University Press, 1971.

100. American Academy of Pediatrics: Syphilis. In Pickering LK (ed): Report of the Committee on Infectious Deseases (Red Book), 27th ed. Elk Grove Village, Ill., American Academy of Pediatrics, 2006.

101. Sheffield J, Wendel GD Jr, Zeray F, et al: Congenital syphilis: The influence of maternal stage of syphilis on vertical transmission. Am J Obstet Gynecol 1999;180:85S.

102. Genest DR, Choi-Hong SR, Tate JE, et al: Diagnosis of congenital syphilis from placental examination: Comparison of histopathology, Steiner stain, and polymerase chain reaction for *Treponema pallidum* DNA. Hum Pathol 1996;27:366-372.

103. Sheffield JS, Sanchez PJ, Wendel GD Jr, et al: Placental histopathology of congenital syphilis. Obstet Gynecol 2002;100:126-133.

104. Benirschke K: Congenital syphilis and necrotizing funisitis. JAMA 1989;262:904.

105. Navarro C, Blanc WA: Subacute necrotizing funisitis: A variant of cord inflammation with a high rate of perinatal infection. J Pediatr 1974;85:689-697.

106. Craver RD, Baldwin VJ: Necrotizing funisitis. Obstet Gynecol 1992;79:64-70.

107. Jacques SM, Qureshi F: Necrotizing funisitis: A study of 45 cases. Hum Pathol 1992;23:1278-1283.

108. Qureshi F, Jacques SM, Reyes MP: Placental histopathology in syphilis. Hum Pathol 1993;24:779-784.

109. Huang ES, Huong SM, Tegtmeier GE, Alford C: Cytomegalovirus: Genetic variation of viral genomes. Ann N Y Acad Sci 1980;354:332-346.

110. Kenneson A, Cannon MJ: Review and meta-analysis of the epidemiology of congenital cytomegalovirus (CMV) infection. Rev Med Virol 2007;17:253-276.

111. Gaytant MA, Rours GI, Steegers EA, et al: Congenital cytomegalovirus infection after recurrent infection: Case reports and review of the literature. Eur J Pediatr 2003;162:248-2453.

112. Boppana SB, Fowler KB, Britt WJ, et al: Symptomatic congenital cytomegalovirus infection in infants born to mothers with preexisting immunity to cytomegalovirus. Pediatrics 1999;104:55-60.

113. Nelson DT, Demmler GJ: Cytomegalovirus infection in the pregnant mother, fetus, and newborn infant. In Stoll GJ, Weisman LE (eds): Infections in Perinatology, vol 24. Philadelphia, WB Saunders, 1999:151-160.

114. Kylat RI, Kelly EN, Ford-Jones EL: Clinical findings and adverse outcome in neonates with symptomatic congenital cytomegalovirus (SCCMV) infection. Eur J Pediatr 2006;165:773-778.

115. Ahlfors K, Ivarsson SA, Harris S: Report on a long-term study of maternal and congenital cytomegalovirus infection in Sweden: Review of prospective studies available in the literature. Scand J Infect Dis 1999;31:443-457.

116. Raynor BD: Cytomegalovirus infection in pregnancy. Semin Perinatol 1993;17:394-402.

117. La Torre R, Nigro G, Mazzocco M, et al: Placental enlargement in women with primary maternal cytomegalovirus infection is associated with fetal and neonatal disease. Clin Infect Dis 2006;43:994-1000.

118. Kohl S: Neonatal herpes simplex virus infection. In Stoll GJ, Weisman LE (eds): Infections in Perinatology. Philadelphia, WB Saunders, 1997:129-150.

119. Kaplan C: The placenta and viral infections. Semin Diagn Pathol 1993;10:232-250.

120. Wabwire-Mangen F, Gray RH, Mmiro FA, et al: Placental membrane inflammation and risks of maternal-to-child transmission of HIV-1 in Uganda. J Acquir Immune Defic Syndr 1999;22:379-385.

121. Anderson VM: The placental barrier to maternal HIV infection. Obstet Gynecol Clin North Am 1997;24:797-820.

122. Kesson AM, Fear WR, Williams L, et al: HIV infection of placental macrophages: Their potential role in vertical transmission. J Leukoc Biol 1994;56:241-246.

123. Backe E, Jimenez E, Unger M, et al: Demonstration of HIV-1 infected cells in human placenta by in situ hybridisation and immunostaining. J Clin Pathol 1992;45:871-874.

124. Lewis SH, Reynolds-Kohler C, Fox HE, Nelson JA: HIV-1 in trophoblastic and villous Hofbauer cells, and haematological precursors in eight-week fetuses. Lancet 1990;335:565-568.

125. Ladner J, Leroy V, Hoffman P, et al: Chorioamnionitis and pregnancy outcome in HIV-infected African women. Pregnancy and HIV Study Group. J Acquir Immune Defic Syndr Hum Retrovirol 1998;18:293-298.

126. Bhoopat L, Khunamornpong S, Sirivatanapa P, et al: Chorioamnionitis is associated with placental transmission of human immunodeficiency virus-1 subtype E in the early gestational period. Mod Pathol 2005;18:1357-1364.

127. Mwanyumba F, Gaillard P, Inion I, et al: Placental inflammation and perinatal transmission of HIV-1. J Acquir Immune Defic Syndr 2002;29:262-269.

128. Biedermann K, Flepp M, Fierz W, et al: Pregnancy, immunosuppression and reactivation of latent toxoplasmosis. J Perinat Med 1995;23:191-203.

129. Cumberland P, Shulman CE, Maple PA, et al: Maternal HIV infection and placental malaria reduce transplacental antibody transfer and tetanus antibody levels in newborns in Kenya. J Infect Dis 2007;196:550-557.

130. van Eijk AM, Ayisi JG, Ter Kuile FO, et al: HIV, malaria, and infant anemia as risk factors for postneonatal infant mortality among HIV-seropositive women in Kisumu, Kenya. J Infect Dis 2007;196:30-37.

131. Mwapasa V, Rogerson SJ, Kwiek JJ, et al: Maternal syphilis infection is associated with increased risk of mother-to-child transmission of HIV in Malawi. AIDS 2006;20:1869-1877.

132. Nisida IV, Amato Neto V, Braz LM, et al: A survey of congenital Chagas' disease, carried out at three health institutions in Sao Paulo City, Brazil. Rev Inst Med Trop Sao Paulo 1999;41:305-311.

133. Rodis JF: Parvovirus infection. Clin Obstet Gynecol 1999;42:107-120; quiz 174-175.

134. Schwarz TF, Nerlich A, Hottentrager B, et al: Parvovirus B19 infection of the fetus: Histology and in situ hybridization. Am J Clin Pathol 1991;96:121-126.

135. Satosar A, Ramirez NC, Bartholomew D, et al: Histologic correlates of viral and bacterial infection of the placenta associated with severe morbidity and mortality in the newborn. Hum Pathol 2004;35:536-545.

136. De Santis M, Cavaliere AF, Straface G, Caruso A: Rubella infection in pregnancy. Reprod Toxicol 2006;21:390-398.

137. Robinson JL, Lee BE, Preiksaitis JK, et al: Prevention of congenital rubella syndrome: What makes sense in 2006? Epidemiol Rev 2006;28:81-87.

138. Garcia AG, Marques RL, Lobato YY, et al: Placental pathology in congenital rubella. Placenta 1985;6:281-295.

139. Kobayashi K, Tajima M, Toishi S, et al: Fetal growth restriction associated with measles virus infection during pregnancy. J Perinat Med 2005;33:67-68.

140. Ohyama M, Fukui T, Tanaka Y, et al: Measles virus infection in the placenta of monozygotic twins. Mod Pathol 2001;14:1300-1303.

141. Sauerbrei A, Wutzler P: Herpes simplex and varicella-zoster virus infections during pregnancy: Current concepts of prevention, diagnosis and therapy. Part 2: Varicella-zoster virus infections. Med Microbiol Immunol 2007;196:95-102.

142. Tan MP, Koren G: Chickenpox in pregnancy: Revisited. Reprod Toxicol 2006;21:410-420.

143. Sauerbrei A, Wutzler P: The congenital varicella syndrome. J Perinatol 2000;20:548-554.

144. Oyer CE, Cai R, Coughlin JJ, Singer DB: First trimester pregnancy loss associated with varicella zoster virus infection: Histological definition of a case. Hum Pathol 1998;29:94-95.

145. Robertson NJ, McKeever PA: Fetal and placental pathology in two cases of maternal varicella infection. Pediatr Pathol 1992;12:545-550.

146. Blanc WA: Pathology of the placenta and cord in ascending and in haematogenous infection. Ciba Found Symp 1979;77:17-38.

147. Qureshi F, Jacques SM: Maternal varicella during pregnancy: Correlation of maternal history and fetal outcome with placental histopathology. Hum Pathol 1996;27:191-195.

148. Ooe K, Udagawa H: A new type of fulminant group A streptococcal infection in obstetric patients: Report of two cases. Hum Pathol 1997;28:509-512.

149. Margin CJ: Streptococcus group A maternal death: An important message for readers. Aust N Z J Obstet Gynaecol 1995;35:227.

150. Castagnola DE, Hoffman MK, Carlson J, Flynn C: Necrotizing cervical and uterine infection in the postpartum period caused by group A streptococcus. Obstet Gynecol 2008;111:533-535.

151. Udagawa H, Oshio Y, Shimizu Y: Serious group A streptococcal infection around delivery. Obstet Gynecol 1999;94:153-157.

152. Crum NF, Chun HM, Gaylord TG, Hale BR: Group A streptococcal toxic shock syndrome developing in the third trimester of pregnancy. Infect Dis Obstet Gynecol 2002;10:209-216.

153. Panaro NR, Lutwick LI, Chapnick EK: Intrapartum transmission of group A streptococcus. Clin Infect Dis 1993;17:79-81.

154. Lee VH, Sulis C, Sayegh RA: Puerperal group A Streptococcus infection: A case report. J Reprod Med 2005;50:621-623.

155. Braunstein H: Congenital syphilis in aborted second trimester fetus: Diagnosis by histological study. J Clin Pathol 1978;31:265-267.

18

Infections of the Nervous System

Sandra Camelo-Piragua and E. Tessa Hedley-Whyte

CHAPTER

describes noninfectious causes that can produce the same type of reaction and should be considered in the differential diagnosis.

The brain has a limited number of ways in which it can respond to infections. There can be an acute inflammatory response, such as is seen in other organ systems of the body. This is usually generated by bacterial organisms but can occur in some viral infections, particularly herpes simplex. Some infectious organisms have a specific tropism in the CNS. In particular, viruses can be neurotropic (i.e., specifically targeting neurons) or pantropic (i.e., affecting the entire neuropil). Some of the neurotropic viruses, particularly rabies, may result in no or only minimal inflammatory response. Acute inflammatory reactions need to be differentiated from acute infarction, which can on occasion resemble an acute cerebritis (Fig. 18-1). Some infections generate a chronic inflammatory response including lymphocytes and plasma cells. Perivascular lymphocytic cuffing is a characteristic feature of infection of the brain (Fig. 18-2). A unique response to infection in the brain is the appearance of rod-shaped microglial cells in gray matter structures (Fig. 18-3). Specific examples are viral spirochetal infections and subacute sclerosing panencephalitis (SSPE).

Introduction

The central nervous system (CNS) is well protected and separated from the rest of the body by a thick physical barrier, the skull and the spine, and by a more fine blood-brain barrier. Therefore, infections of the CNS occur either by trauma, by hematogenous spread with disruption of the blood-brain barrier, or by direct spread in more vulnerable areas such as the olfactory nerve.

If an infection of the CNS is suspected, the most common approach is to analyze the cerebrospinal fluid (CSF) for cell count and microorganisms or to examine blood cultures if a systemic disease is suspected. This will not likely be a challenge for the surgical pathologist. The challenge occurs when infection is not suspected and a brain biopsy is performed for other reasons, such as imaging abnormalities with no clear etiology. It is important to remember that, radiologically, infections can mimic primary brain tumors, metastases, or even lymphomas.

Because infection may not be among the possibilities being considered by the clinical team, it is important for surgical pathologists to recognize or suspect an infectious etiology in certain circumstances. The objective of this chapter is to approach the various infectious entities by pattern of nervous system inflammation rather than by specific organism. The chapter also

Acute Inflammatory Response

Infectious

Bacterial

Meningitis

Bacterial meningitis is an important cause of morbidity and mortality. It is usually caused by hematogenous dissemination of bacteria from another source, although other routes of entry are also seen, such as direct extension from the skin after trauma or developmental anomalies (e.g., myelomeningoceles, congenital sinuses) that can be found in the sacral region. The most common etiologic agents of meningitis are *Haemophilus influenzae* type B, *Neisseria meningitidis*, and *Streptococcus pneumoniae*. However, since the development of vaccination, the incidence of *Haemophilus* has decreased by more than 90% in developed countries.[1-3] These organisms tend to affect specific age groups. For instance β-hemolytic streptococci and *Escherichia coli* are most commonly seen in the neonatal period, whereas *S. pneumoniae* is seen at the extremes of life, both infants and the elderly. *N. meningitidis* is primarily a disease of children and young adults (Table 18-1). Patients present with severe headache, neck stiffness, and high fever.[4] Acute meningitis shows a massive number of neutrophils in the leptomeninges, with spread

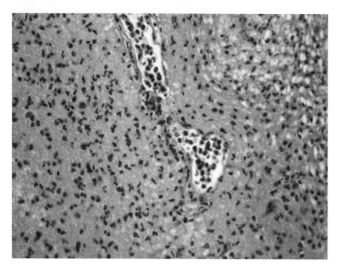

Figure 18-1. Cerebral infarct. Acute inflammation in the brain parenchyma of a recent infarct resembling a cerebritis. Note the neutrophils in the vessel lumen and in the brain parenchyma.

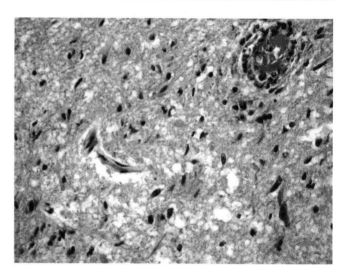

Figure 18-3. Microglia distributed throughout the neuropil. Note the small, necrotic vessel with lymphocytic infiltration of its wall.

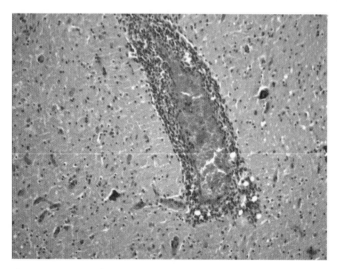

Figure 18-2. Brain with perivascular lymphocytic inflammation, a common indicator of an infectious etiology.

Table 18-1 Bacterial Meningitis Pathogens by Age Group Affected

Pathogen	<1 Mo	1-3 Mo	3 Mo to 50 Yr	>50 Yr
Group B streptococcus	X	X		
Escherichia coli	X	X		X
Listeria monocytogenes	X			
Haemophilus influenzae		X	X	
Streptococcus pneumoniae		X	X	X
Neisseria meningitidis		X	X	X

throughout the Virchow-Robin spaces. Bacteria can be found within the neutrophils or outside them, in the inflammatory infiltrate (Fig. 18-4). The neutrophilic infiltrate can invade leptomeningeal vessels, leading to a vasculitis with subsequent thrombosis and infarcts (Fig. 18-5). After 2 or 3 days, the inflammatory infiltrate changes to lymphocytes, plasma cells, and macrophages; eventually, it becomes an organized exudate, leading to fibrosis of the subarachnoid space that obstructs the CSF flow and causes hydrocephalus. (Fig. 18-6).

Abscess

Another acute inflammatory process that is seen by the surgical pathologist is a brain abscess. Abscesses begin as a focus of acute cerebritis and progress to a sharply circumscribed, encapsulated, necrotic mass with prominent neutrophilic exudate surrounded by a fibrous capsule (Fig. 18-7). The only other cause of fibrosis

within the brain is trauma, either accidental or surgical. The fibrous capsule is easily demonstrated by use of a trichrome stain (Fig. 18-8). Most brain abscesses are caused by infections with mixed flora, such as those present in the oral cavity. Patients with cyanotic congenital heart disease or a history of drug abuse are particularly susceptible to brain abscesses after dental work.[5,6] On imaging, an abscess may be hard to differentiate from a malignant tumor.[7]

Tuberculous abscesses can be seen in immunocompromised patients. Under such circumstances, there is no granulomatous response. These lesions are characterized by a fibrous wall surrounding caseous material with neutrophils. The fibrous capsule forms 10 to 13 days after the initial abscess formation and isolates the necrotic and infected tissue from the rest of the brain parenchyma (Fig. 18-9). Dense granulation tissue with new vessel formation, lymphocytes, macrophages, and plasma cells admixed with fibroblasts start the capsule formation. A well-encapsulated abscess has a necrotic center with surrounding macrophages, vessels, and a rim of lymphocytes and plasma cells with dense fibrous tissue around it (Fig. 18-10). The brain parenchyma around the abscess is densely gliotic and may exhibit Rosenthal fibers. At this point, the abscess can be drained or excised from the brain parenchyma.

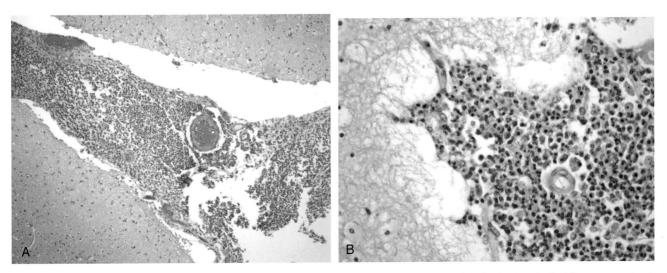

Figure 18-4. Bacterial meningitis. **A,** Pus is present in the subarachnoid space. Note the mild astrocytic reaction in the subpial regions. **B,** The inflammatory exudate is composed of numerous neutrophils with rare eosinophils.

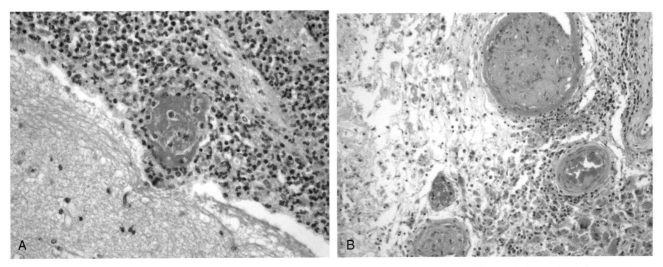

Figure 18-5. Bacterial meningitis. Neutrophils invading blood vessel walls can lead to vasculitis **(A)** and thrombosis **(B)**. Note the hemosiderin-laden macrophages, indicating prior hemorrhage, accompanying the inflammatory response.

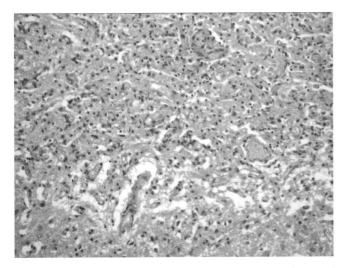

Figure 18-6. Bacterial meningitis, showing organizing exudate leading to fibrosis with an inflammatory infiltrate composed of lymphocytes, plasma cells, and macrophages. Note adjacent brain parenchyma with reactive astrocytes at the base of the picture.

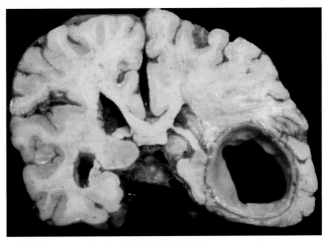

Figure 18-7. Abscess. Coronal section of the brain demonstrates an abscess cavity in the right temporal lobe. Note the fibrous capsule that separates the abscess from the surrounding brain parenchyma. The pus has drained out of the cavity.

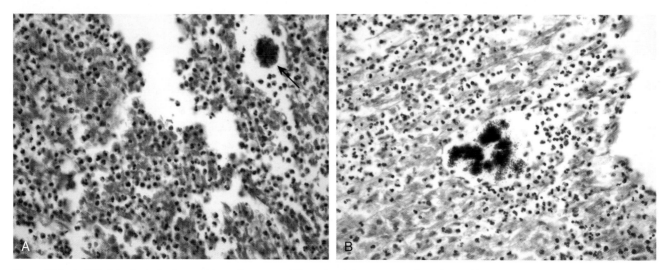

Figure 18-8. A, H&E stain of a brain abscess with prominent neutrophilic exudate in its center as well as clumps of bacteria. **B,** Gram stain highlights a colony of gram-positive cocci.

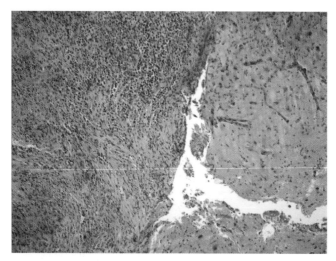

Figure 18-9. Abscess at 10 to 13 days. The dense fibrous capsule delineates the abscess from the inflammatory infiltrate consisting of lymphocytes and plasma cells. Note the reactive astrocytes and proliferation of capillaries in the adjacent brain.

Figure 18-10. Abscess. The fibrous capsule is highlighted by Masson's trichrome stain.

Viral

Herpes Simplex Virus

The prototypic herpes encephalitis is caused by herpes simplex type 1 (HSV-1). The primary infection involves the mucocutaneous and oropharyngeal mucosa. The route of entry to the CNS is controversial, but it is believed that the virus can travel by retrograde transport from the olfactory bulbs to the posterior orbital, frontal, and limbic regions or via the peripheral trigeminal sensory fibers innervating the face and dura to the trigeminal ganglion and then into the brainstem.[8-9] Up to 15% of infections occur via the olfactory nerve after a primary nasopharyngeal infection.[10]

HSV manifests as an asymmetric hemorrhagic mass of the temporal lobe or, less often, the insula, cingulate, or posterior orbital frontal cortex, accompanied by marked swelling of the temporal lobes (Figs. 18-11 and 18-12). It can be unilateral or bilateral. The earliest changes are lymphocytes and macrophages in the leptomeninges with mild parenchymal inflammation. The disease progresses from the meninges to the gray and white matter, leading to hemorrhagic necrosis of the gray and white matter with a neutrophilic reaction (Fig. 18-13). The neurons lose their nuclear outlines and their Nissl substance with dense eosinophilic cytoplasm, and there may be neuronophagia and microglial nodule formation (Fig. 18-14). Viral inclusions are best identified at the edge of the lesion and consist of eosinophilic intranuclear inclusions with marginated chromatin in neurons, ganglion cells, and glial cells (Fig. 18-15). At a later stage, the tissue collapses and the brain is left with a cystic glial scar not unlike that seen after an infarct (Fig. 18-16). Although the reaction can resemble ischemia, the differential point here is that the lesion does not fall into a vascular territory. The chronic inflammatory response can remain in the damaged tissue for many years. The virus can be demonstrated by immunohistochemistry and viral antigens can be detected for up to 3 weeks after the onset of the encephalitis.[11] Alternative methods of detection include DNA in situ hybridization of frozen or paraffin tissue with PCR amplification.[12,13]

HSV encephalitis is usually a fatal condition if not treated. If the patient survives, severe sequelae persist, such as behavioral and memory disturbances.

Neonatal HSV encephalitis is caused predominantly by HSV-2 and is acquired during delivery when the fetus is in contact with genital lesions. The herpes encephalitis in neonates is a panencephalitis with no predilection for any particular anatomic area of the brain; it can affect cerebrum, the cerebellum, and rarely, the brainstem.[14] A similar distribution of herpes encephalitis is seen in immunocompromised people.

Varicella-Zoster Virus

Several patterns of infection are related to varicella-zoster virus, the most common being dorsal root ganglionitis leading to shingles. Other patterns include vasculitis, myeloradiculitis, brainstem encephalitis, and encephalitis involving the visual system, ventriculitis, and, in the immunosuppressed, multifocal lesions of the white matter (Figs. 18-17 and 18-18).[15,16] The white matter lesions are characterized by large areas of necrotizing inflammation, particularly of blood vessels, with perivascular and interstitial infiltration by lymphocytes and macrophages

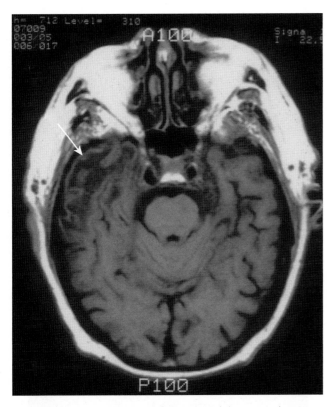

Figure 18-11. Herpes simplex virus infection. This radiologic image demonstrates involvement of the right temporal lobe by herpes encephalitis *(arrow)*. The disease is frequently asymmetric.

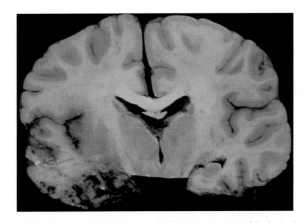

Figure 18-12. Herpes simplex virus encephalitis. Coronal section of the brain shows a large hemorrhagic area in the left temporal lobe, with surrounding edema, and minor hemorrhagic necroses in the right temporal lobe and left cingulate gyrus.

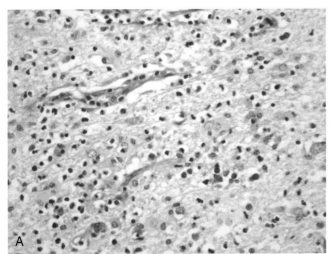
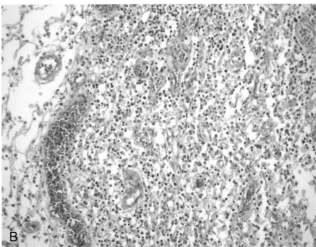

Figure 18-13. Herpes simplex virus encephalitis. **A,** Brain parenchyma with neutrophils, lymphocytes, capillary proliferation, and few reactive astrocytes. **B,** Note the almost total destruction of the brain tissue, with acute and chronic inflammation, rare macrophages, and vascular proliferation.

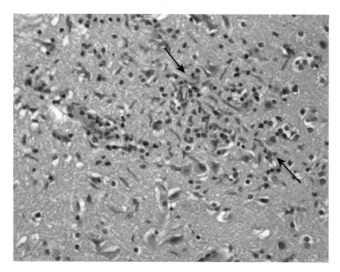

Figure 18-14. Herpes simplex virus encephalitis. Brain parenchyma with numerous rod-shaped microglia (between arrows), forming a nodule and surrounding neurons.

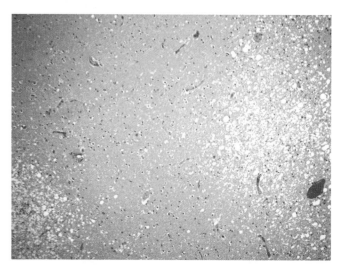

Figure 18-16. Herpes simplex virus encephalitis. Note acute infarction in adjacent brain.

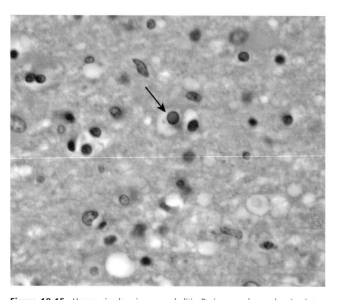

Figure 18-15. Herpes simplex virus encephalitis. Brain parenchyma showing intranuclear viral inclusion *(arrow)* with glassy chromatin and marginated chromatin.

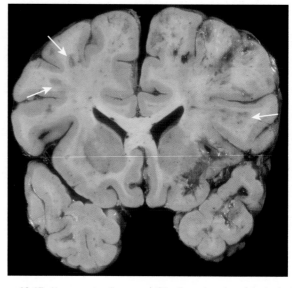

Figure 18-17. Herpes zoster virus encephalitis. Coronal section of the brain demonstrating multiple hemorrhagic cavities as well as sharply defined but pale round areas in the deep white matter.

(Fig. 18-19A). Intranuclear inclusions can be detected with hematoxylin and eosin (H&E) staining and immunohistochemistry, particularly around the borders of the white matter lesions (see Fig. 18-19B). Brainstem encephalitis is characterized by prominent neuronophagia and microglial nodules. Brain biopsies are performed for the diagnosis of cerebral vasculitis. Many cases of CNS vasculitis are due to varicella-zoster.[17] The vasculitis is characterized by a lymphocytic infiltrate of the arterial wall, with occasional giant cells but no fibrinoid change (Fig. 18-20). The elastic lamina is disrupted by the transgression of inflammatory cells through the vessel wall (Fig. 18-21). In this situation, viral inclusions are rarely recognized, and the diagnosis is confirmed by immunohistochemistry for varicella or PCR from paraffin-embedded tissue.

Eastern Equine Encephalitis Virus

Eastern equine encephalitis (EEE) virus belongs to the arbovirus family. Encephalitis due to EEE virus has its highest incidence during the late summer. EEE is seen most commonly on the eastern and Gulf coasts of the United States, in Caribbean countries, and in South America. It affects predominantly children and elderly people. It is a severe disease with a mortality rate that ranges from 50% to 80%. Patients who survive are left with significant neurologic sequelae.[18] The most severely affected parts of the CNS are the basal ganglia, thalamus, and brainstem.[19] Unlike most viral encephalitides, EEE has a prominent acute neutrophilic infiltrate (Fig. 18-22). Vasculitis with marked endothelial swelling and thrombosis is also characteristic. Necrosis is abundant and may extend to the white matter with small microabscesses (Fig. 18-23). The diagnosis is made by reverse transcriptase PCR on CSF.[20,21]

Protozoal

Toxoplasmosis

Toxoplasma are parasites which can infect the CNS in two different age groups. *Toxoplasma* as an in utero infection causes a necrotizing leukoencephalitis with a predilection for the periventricular white matter, whereas in adults *Toxoplasma* has a predilection for the basal ganglia, the thalamus, and the gray-white matter junction (Fig. 18-24).[22] In the adult, toxoplasmosis is most commonly thought to represent reactivation in an immunocompromised host.[23] It was a rare event until the onset of the AIDS epidemic, when it became one of the AIDS-defining diseases. Clinically, toxoplasmosis manifests with focal or nonspe-

cific clinical signs, depending on the location of the lesions. Radiologically in the adult, it is characterized by multiple enhancing parenchymal lesions. The differential diagnosis includes CNS lymphoma or neoplasm.[24,25] The diagnosis is confirmed by biopsy or autopsy or by response to specific treatment with pyrimethamine. If the lesions disappear, the assumption is that they were due to *Toxoplasma*.[26,27] Histologically, the lesions are characterized by a cerebritis with lymphocytes and plasma cells or by abscess formation with an eosinophilic acellular necrotic center surrounded by an inflammatory reaction, which can have a vaguely granulomatous appearance (Fig. 18-25). Necrotizing abscesses are poorly circumscribed, with varying degrees of associated hemorrhage. Typically, there is coagulative necrosis with abundant cellular debris. Parasites may be found in vessel walls, causing vasculitis, thrombotic occlusion, and subsequent hemorrhages. The parasites may be seen within pseudocysts (bradyzoites) or as free forms (tachyzoites 2 μm in diameter) (Fig. 18-26). The latter may be difficult to recognize on H&E, because the organisms resemble cellular debris, but they are easily identified with immunohistochemistry.

Fungal

Aspergillus

Aspergillosis of the CNS is predominantly an opportunistic disease of the immunocompromised host.[28,29] *Aspergillus* usually disseminates by hematogenous spread from the lungs or gastrointestinal tract. *Aspergillus* is an angioinvasive organism that transgresses vessels, producing hemorrhages, necrosis, and dense acute inflammation (Fig. 18-27). The inflammatory response, the hemorrhage and ischemia, is so intense that there is destruction of the parenchyma. *Aspergillus* in tissue is an acute-branching, septated, hyphal organism (Fig. 18-28). The diagnosis of aspergillosis of the brain is usually made on postmortem examination. It is rare that a biopsy of the brain is done for diagnosis. The diagnosis is usually made by biopsy of another organ or by isolation of the fungus from the lung.

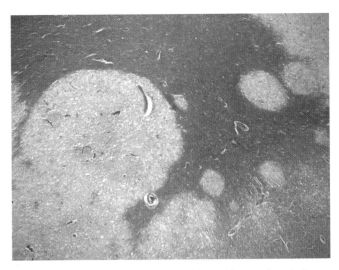

Figure 18-18. Herpes zoster virus. Luxol fast blue and hematoxylin stain demonstrate sharply circumscribed areas of white matter damage in a patient with AIDS.

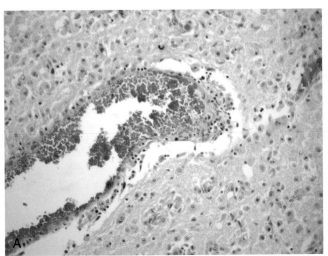
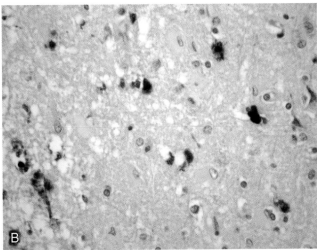

Figure 18-19. Herpes zoster virus. **A,** Necrotic blood vessel with a few perivascular lymphocytes and many macrophages in the white matter surrounding the necrotic areas. **B,** Immunohistochemistry using an anti-HZV antibody highlights the viral inclusions.

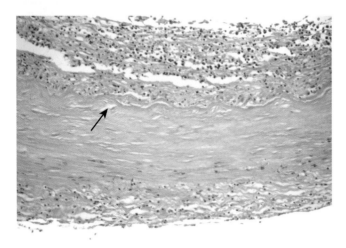

Figure 18-20. Herpes zoster virus. Zoster vasculitis with arterial wall invaded by inflammatory cells, predominantly lymphocytes, with no evidence of fibrinoid necrosis. Note partially destroyed elastic lamina *(arrow)*.

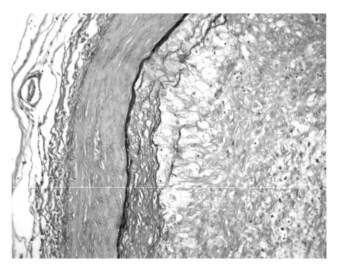

Figure 18-21. Herpes zoster virus. Elastic stain demonstrates disruption of the internal elastic lamina by the inflammatory infiltrate of the vessel wall.

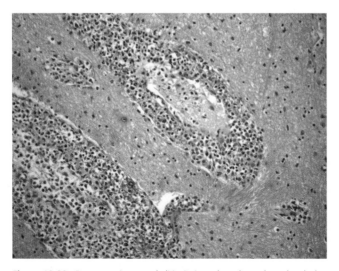

Figure 18-22. Eastern equine encephalitis. Perivascular polymorphonuclear leukocytes and lymphocytes with migration from the vessel lumens. A few neutrophils are present also in the parenchyma.

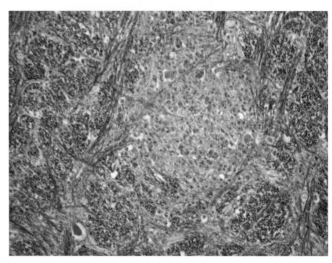

Figure 18-23. Eastern equine encephalitis. Luxol fast blue and hematoxylin stain. Note the microabscess in the white matter.

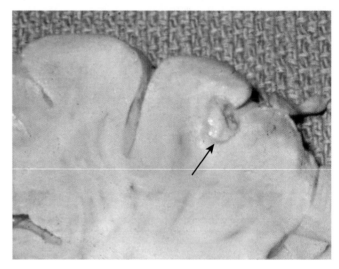

Figure 18-24. Toxoplasmosis. Healed toxoplasmic abscess *(arrow)* demonstrating predilection of *Toxoplasma* for the gray-white junction. Note the well-defined cyst with a necrotic center.

Mucormycosis

Rhinocerebral mucormycosis is an entity seen primarily in diabetic patients with ketoacidosis, as a consequence of direct extension of the fungal organism from the nasal sinuses to the brain, with predilection for the base of the brain and the basal ganglia. Histologically, this is a vascular destructive and invasive organism that produces poorly defined ischemic areas with necrosis and hemorrhage. Brisk neutrophilic infiltrate and areas of necrosis are common (Fig. 18-29). The course from infection to death is usually a matter of days or weeks.[30] The diagnosis can be made by biopsy of the nasal sinus. Brain biopsy is only rarely used for diagnosis. The fungus can be seen with H&E staining as a nonseptated, broad, gray-blue, ribbon-like hyphal organism, 10 μm thick, with right-angle branching (Fig. 18-30). *Mucor* can also produce an aneurysm of the circle of Willis removed from the primary site of infection in the nasal sinuses. Carotid artery involvement and cavernous sinus thrombosis are common.[31,32]

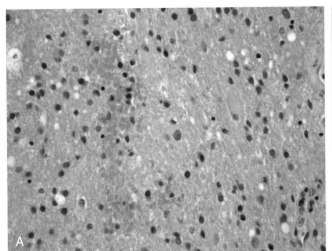
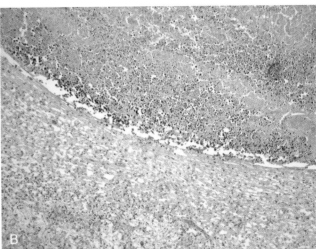

Figure 18-25. Toxoplasmosis. **A,** Cerebritis with multifocal infiltration by lymphocytes and plasma cells. **B,** Abscess formation with an eosinophilic, acellular, necrotic center surrounded by an inflammatory reaction with lymphocytes and reactive astrocytes.

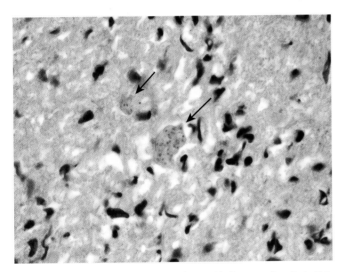

Figure 18-26. Toxoplasmosis. Brain parenchyma with dense reactive gliosis. Note two bradyzoites in the center *(arrows)* filled with microorganisms.

Amebic

The three most common amebas involving the CNS are *Naegleria fowleri*, *Acanthamoeba*, and *Balamuthia*. *Naegleria* is typically found in warm fresh water and invades the CNS through the nasal mucosa. *Naegleria* is a free-swimming, nonencapsulated ameba. *Naegleria* produces an acute meningoencephalitis in immunocompetent people. It produces hemorrhagic necrosis of the fronto-orbital cortex and the olfactory bulbs. The inflammation is composed of a dense neutrophilic infiltrate with variable degree of mononuclear cells. The inflammation tends to extend through the Virchow–Robin spaces to the gray-white matter junction and produces hemorrhagic necrosis (Fig. 18-31).[33] The diagnosis is made by finding the free-swimming ameba in the CSF. *Naegleria* is very sensitive to amphotericin B, but delay in diagnosis carries a high mortality, up to 95%.[34,35]

Acanthamoeba and *Balamuthia mandrillaris* are ubiquitous free-living, soil-dwelling, encapsulated amebas. *Acanthamoeba* can produce keratitis or encephalitis. It has been found in non-

sterile lens solutions, and it can also enter the CNS through lesions in the skin or the upper respiratory tract or via inhalation of airborne cysts. Patients present with signs and symptoms of a brain mass with surrounding edema. Brain biopsy is the only way to make the diagnosis before death. Even so, the diagnosis is often missed, as the organisms strongly resemble macrophages and may not be numerous in the biopsied material. The pathologic findings of *Acanthamoeba* consist of multiple areas of hemorrhagic, granulomatous inflammation that can become confluent. The initial lesion can have a necrotic center. The tissue reaction is a mixed inflammatory infiltrate with neutrophils, lymphocytes, plasma cells, and fibroblasts. The lesions are usually angiocentric. The vessels are inflamed, with areas of fibrinoid necrosis (Fig. 18-32).[36,37] Sometimes, a skin ulcer or nodule, if present, can be biopsied and the diagnosis can reflect the process in the brain.[38] The organism can be typed by PCR or immunofluorescence, although these tests may not be available in all institutions, and samples may need to be sent to the Centers for Disease Control and Prevention (CDC).

Combinations of amphotericin B with rifampin or imidazole agents may be tried. However, the mortality rate is very high, even with appropriate treatment, when the CNS is involved.[39] In rare instances, patients with granulomatous amebic encephalitis have survived, usually in cases manifesting with a single lesion that could be excised surgically.[40] Distinctive features of the most common amebas involving the CNS that can be helpful in the diagnosis are highlighted in Table 18-2.[41]

Noninfectious

Infarct

Acute cerebral infarction, between 24 and 48 hours old, can have the appearance of an acute cerebritis, with numerous polymorphonuclear leukocytes permeating the tissue and margination of neutrophils around blood vessels, but special stains fail to reveal any organisms, and cultures are sterile (Fig. 18-33). The presence of intravascular thrombi can be helpful in making the diagnosis (Fig. 18-34). The surrounding brain parenchyma can show other signs of early ischemia, such as red neurons with shrunken

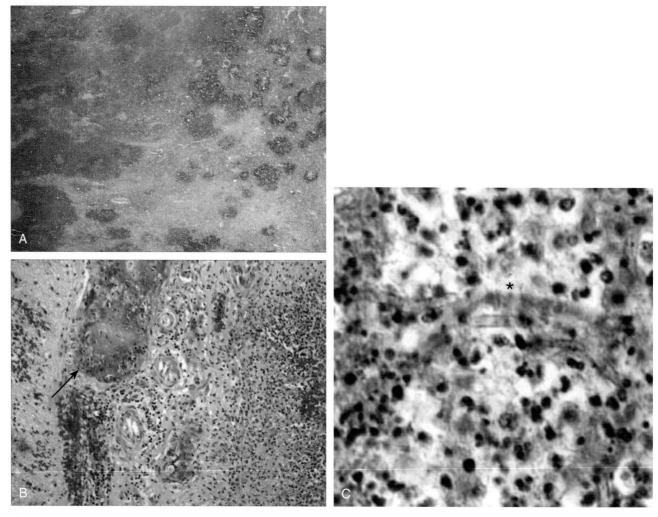

Figure 18-27. Aspergillosis. **A,** Note the dense hemorrhagic and necrotic areas in the white matter (Luxol fast blue, H&E). **B,** Angioinvasion with blood vessel destruction *(arrow)*. Note the purulent exudate on the right side of the picture. **C,** Note the hyphal organism intermixed with macrophages and polymorphonuclear leukocytes *(asterisk)*.

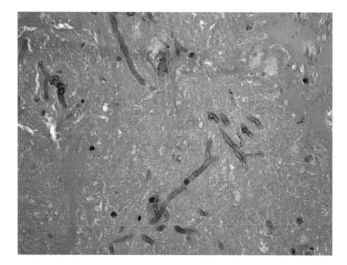

Figure 18-28. Aspergillosis. The organism is identified by its acute branching with septated hyphae.

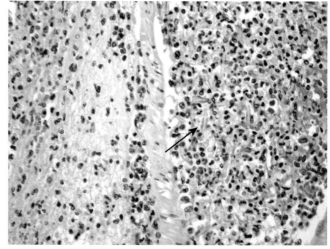

Figure 18-29. Mucormycosis. Note the blue hyphal forms surrounded by neutrophils *(arrow)*. The adjacent brain is infiltrated by neutrophils and lymphocytes.

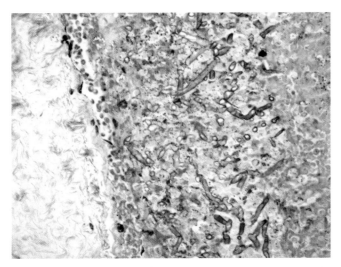

Figure 18-30. Mucormycosis. GMS stain highlights the broad, nonseptated hyphae.

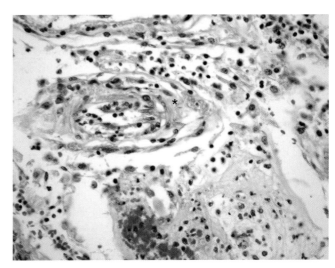

Figure 18-32. Amebic encephalitis. Angiocentric inflammation with fibrinoid necrosis of the vessels *(asterisk)*.

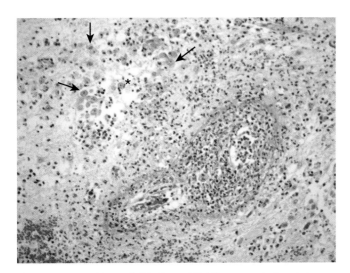

Figure 18-31. Amebic encephalitis. Neutrophilic infiltrate extends through the arterial wall into the Virchow–Robin spaces *(arrows)*. There is surrounded hemorrhagic necrosis and acute inflammation with multiple clusters of encapsulated amebas in the surrounding parenchyma. The amebas have a prominent nucleolus *(asterisk)*.

nuclei, hyperchromatic nuclei, loss of nucleoli, eosinophilic cytoplasm with loss of the Nissl substance, and damaged glial parenchyma with a more clear eosinophilic and granular texture (Fig. 18-35).

Chronic Inflammatory Response

Infectious

Bacterial

Syphilis
Symptomatic neurosyphilis can occur as the secondary (early neurosyphilis) or tertiary (late neurosyphilis) stage of the disease.

Table 18-2 Clinical and Pathologic Features of Free-Living Amebas Involving the CNS

Feature	Acanthamoeba spp. and Balamuthia mandrillaris	Naegleria fowleri
Predisposition	Immunodeficient patients and those with chronic debilitating diseases	Healthy individuals; associated with exposure to contaminated water
Route of entry	Upper respiratory tract, conjunctiva, or injury to the skin; infection of CNS through the bloodstream	Nasal mucosa, traveling along olfactory nerves
Histopathologic features	Angiocentric lesions with parasites clustered around vessels, perivascular inflammation, fibrinoid necrosis, and granulomatous inflammation	Hemorrhagic necrosis of the fronto-orbital cortex and olfactory bulbs with dense neutrophilic infiltrate and variable mononuclear cells; no granulomas formed
Forms present	*Cysts*: Thick cell wall, PAS positive *Trophozoites* (14-40 μm): Pale eosinophilic granular cytoplasm with prominent nucleoli	*Only trophozoites* (<10 μm): Vacuolated cytoplasm; nuclei with prominent nucleoli
Clinical progression	Progression from infection to CNS involvement may take months; after this, there is a rapid fatal progression (about 1 mo)	Incubation is 1-14 days, followed by rapidly fatal progressive course

CNS, central nervous system; PAS, periodic acid–Schiff stain.

The most common clinical presentation is aseptic meningitis, but syphilis can also manifest with iritis or uveitis or, less commonly, with cranial nerve paralysis and hydrocephalus. It involves meninges, blood vessels, and the CSF. Patients with vascular involvement can present with stroke. A rarer syndrome occurs if there is parenchymal involvement and can include progressive personality changes, psychiatric disorders, or dementia (also known as general paralysis of the insane).

In general, syphilis manifests as a gumma or as chronic meningitis, composed predominantly of plasma cells and lymphocytes, usually leading to fibrosis of the meninges that leads to CSF obstruction. The meningitis may be accompanied by an arteritis characterized by invasion of the arterial walls by lymphocytes and plasma cells (Heubner arteritis), which induces intimal proliferation, and thinning of the media with intact elastic lamina (Fig. 18-36). The vasa vasorum are surrounded by inflammatory cells, which may lead to ischemic lesions (Fig. 18-37).

Viral

Most viral meningitides are culture-negative and are characterized by a chronic inflammatory response with a mild lymphocytic infiltrate in the subarachnoid space. The diagnosis is made by examination of the CSF and serology.

West Nile Virus

West Nile virus causes an arthropod-related encephalitis of late summer and early fall. Most of the infections occur through a mosquito bite, although the virus can also be acquired through breast milk, transplacentally, or via organ transplantation.[42-44] Fewer than 15% of the human infections result in aseptic meningitis or encephalitis.[45,46] Most cases of West Nile viral infection are subclinical, but in a few patients a polio-like syndrome or parkinsonism occurs.[47,48] The CDC has strong programs for reporting, control, and prevention of the disease,

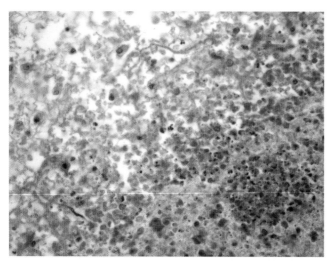

Figure 18-33. Infarct. Necrotic center of an infarct with scattered inflammatory cells that can be mistaken for an abscess.

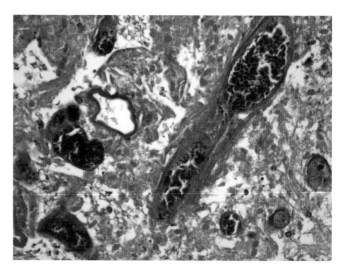

Figure 18-34. Edge of infarct with phosphotungstic acid hematoxylin (PTAH) staining highlighting the intravascular thrombi.

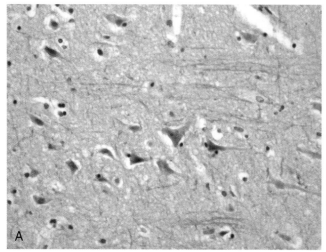

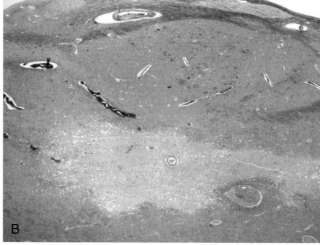

Figure 18-35. Infarct. **A,** Brain parenchyma with shrunken red neurons, a common sign of irreversible ischemia. **B,** Acute infarct. Sharply delineated area of pallor with scalloped edges and "spongy" center defines the acutely infarcted thalamus.

because West Nile virus can cause many fatalities (Table 18-3). This is manifested histologically by the presence of non-necrotizing inflammation involving particularly motor neurons in the spinal cord, neurons of the substantia nigra, and Purkinje cells. There is an infiltration of CD3-positive lymphocytes, macrophages, and microglial nodules, associated with chromatolytic neurons and neuronophagia.[49-52] Viral inclusions are not seen by light microscopy, but on some occasions, the presence of the virus can be detected by immunohistochemistry in the remaining neurons involved (Fig. 18-38). The CSF has an elevated protein content and a high white blood cell count, predominantly neutrophils.[53] The diagnosis is made mainly by the detection of antibodies in CSF, although in some cases PCR of CSF is required.[54]

Progressive Multifocal Leukoencephalopathy

Progressive multifocal leukoencephalopathy (PML) is a subacute demyelinating disease of immunocompromised patients, including patients with human immunodeficiency virus (HIV) infection, leukemia, lymphoma, renal transplants, or chronic immunosuppression.[55] PML is caused by the polyomavirus known as JC virus, which was first cultured from brain tissue in 1971.[56] The clinical and radiologic appearance can mimic that of tumor (Fig. 18-39). The histologic features are characterized by multifocal, poorly delineated areas of demyelination with some loss of axons and many foamy macrophages (Fig. 18-40). In most cases, there is no or only mild perivascular lymphocytic infiltrate, but occasionally there is a striking inflammatory reaction with many perivascular and parenchymal lymphocytes and plasma cells. This reaction has been seen particularly in some patients with AIDS, especially after initiation of highly active antiretroviral therapy (HAART).[57,58] It has been posited that this is a sign of immune reconstitution.[59] The inflammatory response can be so intense as to raise the possibility of a second infectious agent, particularly *Toxoplasma*.[60] It is therefore necessary to perform special stains for bacteria and fungi as well as immunohistochemistry for *Toxoplasma*. Reactive astrocytes are usually present and can be very large and bizarre; care should be taken not to misinterpret these bizarre large astrocytes as a high-grade astrocytoma on frozen sections (Fig. 18-41).

The pathognomonic feature of PML is the presence of enlarged, glassy, dark-staining viral inclusions in oligodendrocytes, seen particularly at the edges of the demyelinating process (see Fig. 18-41). Occasionally, inclusions may be seen in the granular cells of the cerebellum.[61] Electron microscopic examination of biopsy specimens reveals the characteristic morphologic

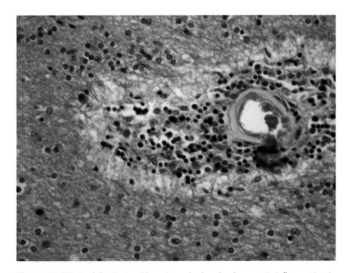

Figure 18-36. Syphilis. Brain with perivascular lymphoplasmacytic inflammation in a case of syphilis.

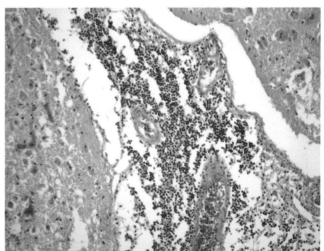

Figure 18-37. Syphilis. Dense chronic inflammation of the leptomeninges with involvement of the vessels, surrounded by infarction with macrophages and reactive astrocytes.

Table 18-3 Total Human Cases of West Nile Virus Infection Reported to the CDC from 2000 to 2008

Cases	2000	2001	2002	2003	2004	2005	2006	2007	2008
Total no. reported	21	66	4156	9862	2539	3000	4269	3630	1370
No. fatalities	2	10	284	264	100	119	177	124	37
No. of states with reported cases	3*	10	46	46	41	44	44	43	42

CDC, Centers for Disease Control and Prevention.
*New York, New Jersey, and Connecticut.
Adapted from Centers for Disease Control and Prevention, Division of Vector-Borne Infectious Diseases: West Nile Virus: Statistics, Surveillance and Control, 2008. Available at http://www.cdc.gov/ncidod/dvbid/westnile/mapsactivity/surv&control08maps.htm (accessed August 6, 2009).

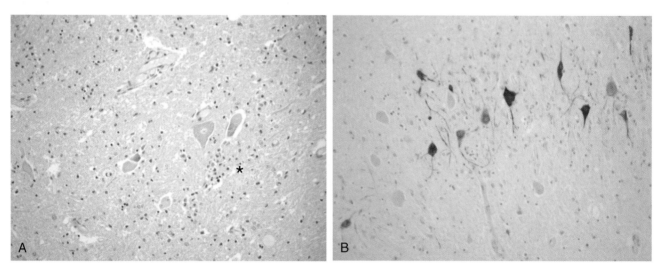

Figure 18-38. West Nile virus infection. **A,** Anterior horn of the spinal cord with necrotic motor neurons. Lymphocytic infiltration, occasional macrophages, and microglial nodules *(asterisk)* are present. **B,** Immunohistochemical analysis with an antibody to West Nile virus demonstrates intense immunoreaction in the neuronal cell bodies and dendrites in the hippocampus.

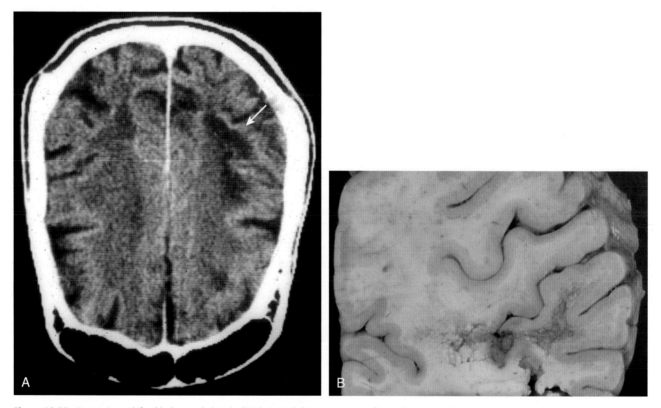

Figure 18-39. Progressive multifocal leukoencephalopathy (PML). **A,** Radiologic appearance of PML, showing a white matter–based lesion *(arrow).* **B,** Coronal section of brain with white matter–based lesion.

appearance of JC virus (Fig. 18-42).[62] The diagnosis is most often confirmed with the use of immunohistochemistry against BK virus or polyomavirus (Fig. 18-43).

Human Immunodeficiency Virus

In the CNS, HIV infects microglia and T lymphocytes. The CNS involvement and pattern of inflammation vary, from a diffuse, low-grade, perivascular lymphocytic infiltrate with microglial

nodules to demyelination and diffuse gliosis of the deep gray matter. Multinucleated cells surrounding capillaries with scant or sometimes abundant cytoplasm can aggregate in a granulomatous fashion and are helpful in the diagnosis (Fig. 18-44).[63-64] When faced with a brain biopsy of a patient with HIV/AIDS, it is important to remember associated infections or diseases such as mycobacterial (especially with atypical mycobacteria), parasitic (*Toxoplasma*), viral (cytomegalovirus, PML, herpes zoster virus), and fungal (*Cryptococcus, Aspergillus, Coccidioides, Histoplasma*) infections, as well as primary CNS lymphomas.[65] Biopsy of the brain may reveal only mild perivascular lymphocytic cuffing and a microglial response (Fig. 18-45).

Cytomegalovirus
Cytomegalovirus (CMV) infection of the nervous system occurs in neonates and immunocompromised patients. The virus primarily infects endothelial and ependymal cells. There are several reaction patterns, ranging from microglial nodules with cytomegalic cells and otherwise minimal inflammation to severe necrotizing encephalitis with cystic changes resembling infarcts in perinates (Fig. 18-46).[66] A common pattern of injury in immunocompromised adults is ventriculoencephalomyelitis with

enlargement of the ventricles and hemorrhagic necrosis of the surrounding parenchyma.[67] CMV can also affect the peripheral nervous system with a vasculopathy and microvascular thrombi around nerve roots, producing a meningoradiculitis and myelitis. The diagnosis is made on tissue examination by the presence of enlarged cells with large intranuclear inclusions and less conspicuous cytoplasmic inclusions (Fig. 18-47).

Subacute Sclerosing Panencephalitis
SSPE is a chronic progressive panencephalitis that occurs several years after exposure to measles. Most patients have a history of measles in the first 2 years of life. The onset of disease usually occurs between 5 and 15 years of age, but the disease has also been reported in adults.[68-70] Clinically, patients progress from intellectual and behavioral changes to myoclonus, dystonias, spasticity, stupor, coma, dysautonomia, and, finally, death.[71] The diagnosis is usually made by the finding of high anti-measles titers in the CSF. However in the rare instances of adult onset of disease, the diagnosis has been made by brain biopsy.

The gray matter shows perivascular inflammation with lymphocytes and macrophages, gliosis, loss of neurons with occasional neuronophagia, and eosinophilic intranuclear inclusions in neurons (Fig. 18-48). The latter are very sharply defined eosinophilic inclusions with a surrounding halo. The white matter exhibits abundant gliosis, perivascular inflammation, and patchy demyelination. A striking feature in chronic cases is the presence of classic neurofibrillary tangles in the cerebral cortex, hippocampus, nucleus basalis of Meynert, hypothalamus, and raphe nuclei of the brainstem (Fig. 18-49).[72]

Fungal

Candida
CNS involvement by *Candida* occurs mainly in patients with alteration of the immune defenses or mechanical barriers, such as patients with diabetes, lymphoma, HIV infection, IV drug use,

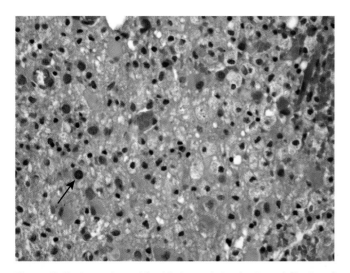

Figure 18-40. Progressive multifocal leukoencephalopathy. Dense infiltration of foamy macrophages, reactive astrocytes, and numerous oligodendroglial cells with intranuclear inclusions *(arrow)* are seen (Luxol fast blue stain).

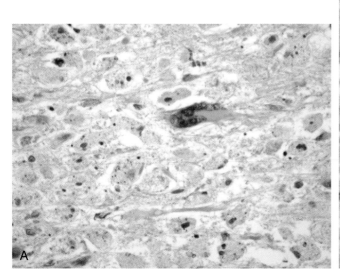
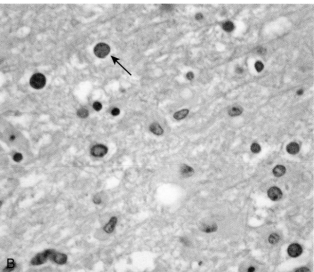

Figure 18-41. Progressive multifocal leukoencephalopathy (PML). **A,** A large, bizarre astrocyte is seen in PML and could be misinterpreted as a primary high-grade malignant neoplasm in the frozen section. **B,** High-power view of oligodendroglial cells with intranuclear inclusions *(arrow)*, marginated chromatin, and glassy nuclear appearance.

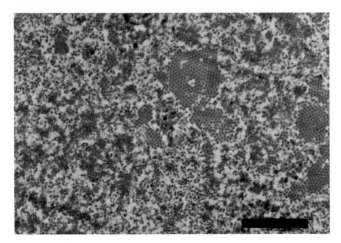

Figure 18-42. Progressive multifocal leukoencephalopathy. Electron microscopic appearance of the virus.

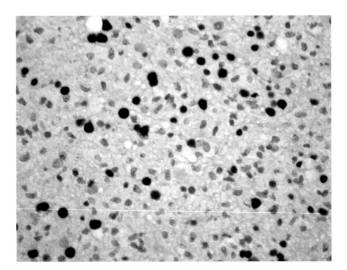

Figure 18-43. Progressive multifocal leukoencephalopathy. Immunohistochemistry with antibodies against simian virus 40 (SV40), which cross-reacts with polyomavirus, highlights the cells infected with the virus.

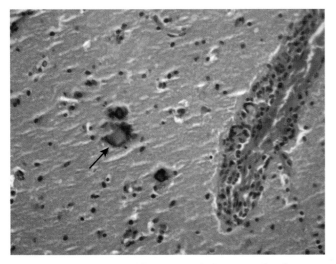

Figure 18-44. Human immunodeficiency virus infection. Perivascular inflammation with surrounding multinucleated giant cells *(arrow)* and focal mineral deposition in the adjacent white matter.

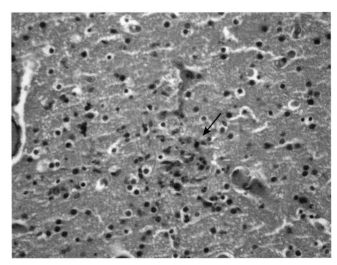

Figure 18-45. Human immunodeficiency virus infection. Subacute encephalitis with microglial nodules *(arrow)*.

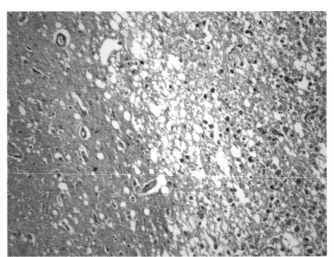

Figure 18-46. Cytomegalovirus. Spongy changes in white matter resemble an early infarct.

ventriculoperitoneal shunt, neurosurgery, or lumbar puncture. *Candida* infections of the brain result in tiny microabscesses with chronic inflammation, necrosis, and vasculitis with thrombus formation. *Candida* is identified by the presence of budding yeasts 2 μm in diameter and pseudohyphae. The organism can be seen with H&E staining and is highlighted by Grocott methenamine silver (GMS) and periodic acid–Schiff (PAS) stains (Fig. 18-50).

Helminthic

Cysticercosis

Cysticercus is the most common parasitic infection of the CNS. It is caused by ingestion of the egg of the pig tapeworm (*Taenia solium*) from contaminated water or undercooked meat. The egg loses its capsule when it comes into contact with the acid pH of the stomach. The larvae enter the bloodstream and spread to

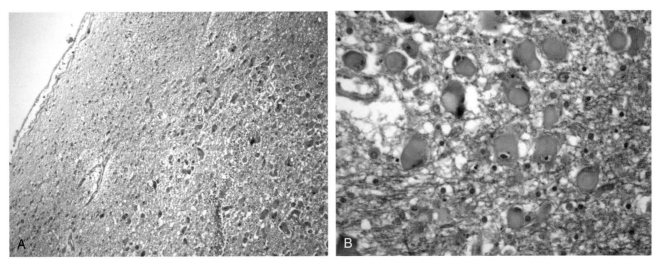

Figure 18-47. Cytomegalovirus ventriculitis. **A,** Cytomegalic cells with nuclear and cytoplasmic inclusions in the subependymal astrocytes. **B,** Note the large size of the inclusion-bearing cells compared with the normal oligodendrocytes and astrocytes in the background.

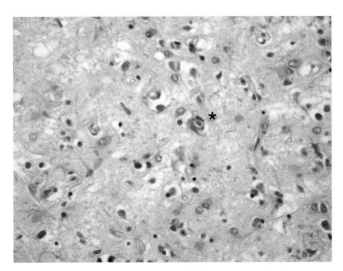

Figure 18-48. Subacute sclerosing panencephalitis. Gray matter with lymphocytes, macrophages, loss of neurons, and numerous fibrous astrocytes. Note the intranuclear viral inclusion in a neuron *(asterisk)*.

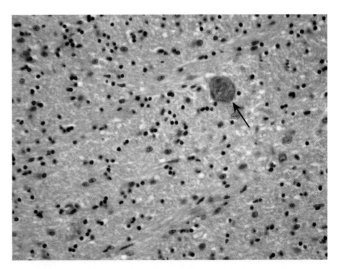

Figure 18-49. Subacute sclerosing panencephalitis (SSPE). Intraneuronal globose neurofibrillary tangle *(arrow)* is present in a chronic case of SSPE.

various organs, including the CNS, where they encyst (Fig. 18-51). In this environment, they cannot grow to adult worms, so they remain as cysts indefinitely. Initially, the cyst produces minimal response, and the infestation may remain silent for years. The cysts are usually found in the cerebral cortex but can occur in the meninges of the base of the brain, in the ventricles, and, rarely, in the spinal cord (Fig. 18-52).[73] Symptoms occur when the worm dies, the cyst ruptures, and the contents leak, producing a dense inflammatory response composed of lymphocytes, eosinophils, and plasma cells. With time, a fibrous capsule forms (Fig. 18-53). Patients usually present with seizures or hydrocephalus, and brain imaging reveals the calcified cyst.[74,75] The cysts may also be found incidentally when the patient has a brain computed tomography scan for a different reason. To make the definitive diagnosis histologically, one must see the parasite. The live parasite has a single scolex with four suckers and a double row of hooklets. The cyst wall has an outer cuticular layer, a

middle pseudoepithelial cellular layer, and an inner reticular layer. However, in excisions or biopsies of *Cysticercus*, only the cuticular layer of the dead worm is seen with H&E stain (Fig. 18-54).

Rickettsial

Rickettsia are intracellular microorganisms that are transmitted by ticks or mites. Once in the bloodstream, they transgress the vessels, damaging the endothelial and smooth muscle vascular cells. In fact, vessel wall damage is one of the hallmarks of rickettsial infections. There is usually angiocentric inflammation composed of lymphocytes and macrophages, with thrombosis and microinfarcts but without fibrinoid necrosis of the vessels (Fig. 18-55).[76] The organisms can be very difficult to find but can be seen as gram-negative coccobacilli inside macrophages with the use of Brown-Hopps stain. The disease is severe and

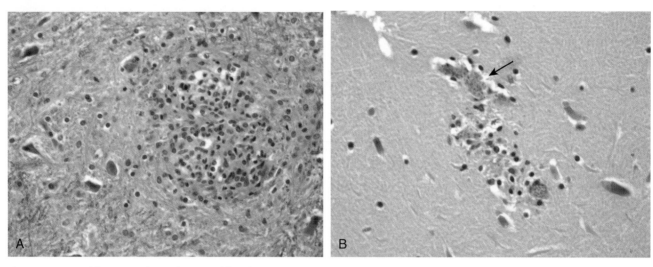

Figure 18-50. *Candida.* **A,** Microabscess due to *Candida* in the cerebral cortex. **B,** Arrow shows small yeasts in a blood vessel in the center of a microglial nodule in the molecular layer of cerebellum.

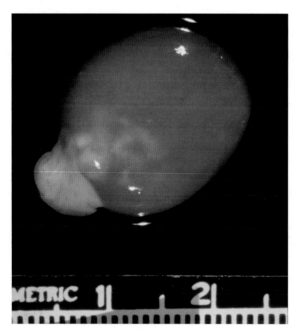

Figure 18-51. Cysticercosis. Intact *Cysticercus* cyst surgically removed from the fourth ventricle of the brain.

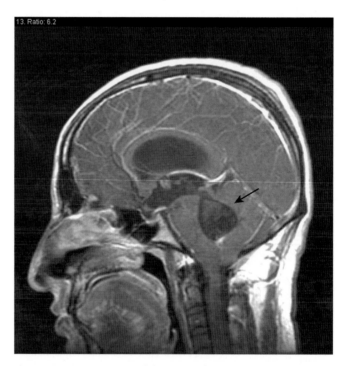

Figure 18-52. Cysticercosis. Radiologic image demonstrates a cyst in the fourth ventricle *(arrow)*, with obstruction of the cerebrospinal fluid flow and hydrocephalus.

may be fatal in the elderly, in patients with alcohol abuse, and in those with glucose-6-phosphate dehydrogenase (G6PD) deficiency. The diagnosis is made by serology and PCR.[77]

Noninfectious

Vasculitis

CNS vasculitis is a rare disorder that can be primary or secondary. Most frequently, it is part of a systemic disorder such as systemic lupus erythematosus (SLE), Sjögren's syndrome, Wegener granulomatosis, or polyarteritis nodosa, but giant cell arteritis and granulomatous small-vessel vasculitis limited to the brain also

occur. The main histologic findings are vascular fibrinoid necrosis with inflammatory infiltration of the vessel wall and rupture of the elastic lamina.[78] The degree of inflammation varies depending on previous treatment and the chronicity of the process (Fig. 18-56).

Paraneoplastic Limbic Encephalitis

Paraneoplastic encephalomyelitis is typically encountered as a complication of small cell carcinoma of the lung, but it is also associated with non–small cell cancer of the lung, ovarian tumors,

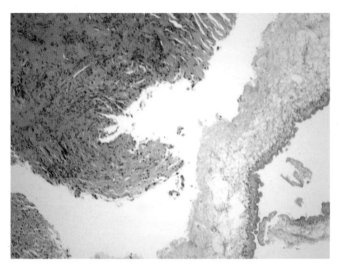

Figure 18-53. Cysticercosis. Wall of dead worm, with cyst wall, lymphoplasmacytic infiltrate, and dense fibrous tissue.

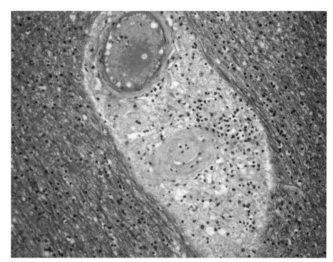

Figure 18-55. *Rickettsia.* Angiocentric inflammation composed of lymphocytes and macrophages, with thrombosis but no fibrinoid necrosis of the vessels.

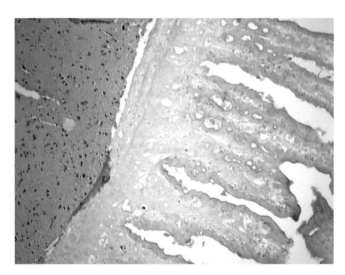

Figure 18-54. Cysticercosis. Cuticular layer that helped to identify the dead worm in an excisional biopsy.

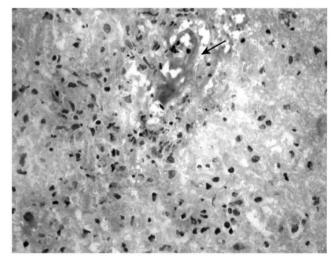

Figure 18-56. Vasculitis. Fibrinoid necrosis of a vessel wall *(arrow)*, showing moderate inflammatory infiltrate and reactive gliosis in adjacent tissue (frozen section, H&E).

Hodgkin lymphoma, breast carcinoma, and testicular germ cell tumors.[79] Clinically, the patients presents with short-memory loss; complex, partial or generalized seizures; confusion; and personality disturbances. Magnetic resonance imaging often shows a T2-hyperintense lesion of the medial temporal lobe, involving the amygdala, hippocampus, and entorhinal cortex.[80,81]

Histologic examination shows a florid reactive astrocytosis, perivascular lymphoid cuffing, and neuronophagia with microglial nodules suggestive of viral encephalitis. Occasionally, the detection of autoantibodies in the CSF (e.g., anti-Hu, anti-Yo, anti-Tr) is helpful in the diagnosis (Fig. 18-57).[82]

Lymphoma

Lymphoma can mimic an infectious process in the brain. The most common lymphoma involving the CNS is the diffuse large B-cell lymphoma. It diffusely involves the brain parenchyma with a perivascular pattern of growth. Histologically, the cells are dyshesive with usually large, prominent nucleoli, prominent mitoses and apoptosis, and occasional macrophages. The diagnosis can be made on H&E but is confirmed with immunohistochemistry, which reveals a predominantly B cell (CD20-positive) population with occasional T cells (CD3-positive). In situ hybridization for κ and λ light chains can demonstrate monoclonality, although some large B-cell lymphomas have limited light-chain expression (Fig. 18-58). At the margins of the lymphoma, the diagnosis may be difficult because of the often atypical T-cell reaction to the presence of the lymphoma in the neuropil. Pretreatment with steroids can also abolish the B-cell neoplastic population, making the diagnosis difficult. In such cases, the diagnosis can be made from the immunohistochemical profile of the invading cells and the lack of infectious organisms on special stains. T-cell lymphomas are much rarer in the CNS.[83,84]

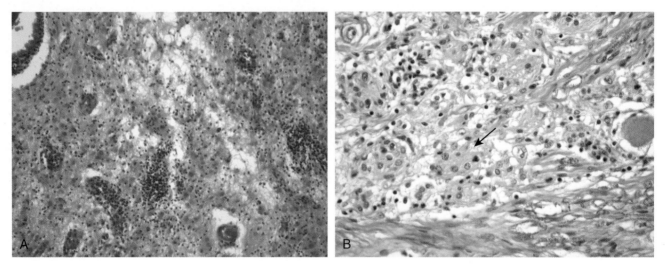

Figure 18-57. Paraneoplastic encephalomyelitis. **A,** Marked destruction of the medial temporal lobe with microglial nodules, gliosis, loss of neurons, and collections of lymphocytes. **B,** Note the loss of ganglion cells and the lymphocytic infiltrates (arrow).

Patients with AIDS have a 50 to 60 times greater risk of developing primary CNS lymphoma than the general population. In the AIDS population, the lymphoma is usually Epstein-Barr virus–driven, and this can be demonstrated by in situ hybridization (see Fig. 18-58).[85,86]

Lymphomas can also manifest as dural-based masses mimicking meningiomas. Immunohistochemical characterization may be less helpful here, because the lymphomas tend to be of the more indolent type, with a mixed population of T and B cells. Therefore, infectious causes have to be ruled out with stains for bacteria, spirochetes, mycobacteria, and fungi.

Extramedullary Plasmacytoma

The most common location of extramedullary plasmacytoma in the CNS is the suprasellar region, although other sites, such as the meninges, can be involved. The lesions are usually attached to the dura and radiographically resemble meningioma. Histologically, they are composed of a dense infiltrate of plasma cells. The plasma cells can have a normal mature morphology with eccentric nuclei, clock face chromatin, and a perinuclear halo. Binucleated forms, eosinophilic intranuclear inclusions (Dutcher bodies), or cytoplasmic inclusions (Russell bodies) can be seen (Fig. 18-59). Monoclonality can be proved with ancillary studies, such as immunohistochemistry or flow cytometry. Occasionally, extramedullary plasmacytoma can manifest as a pituitary adenoma, in which case immunohistochemical studies are helpful for identifying hormonal activity or demonstrating plasma cell markers.[87,88]

Idiopathic Hypertrophic Pachymeningitis

Idiopathic hypertrophic pachymeningitis is an inflammatory fibrosing process of the dura mater. It manifests clinically with headache, progressive cranial neuropathy, and cerebellar ataxia.[89,90] Radiologically, there is a multifocal and diffuse thickening of the dura, often involving the tentorium, the falx, peribulbar meninges, and even the spine at the exit of peripheral

nerves, causing peripheral neuropathies or compressing the spinal cord itself. Biopsies reveal dense fibrosis as the hallmark, with a mixed lymphoplasmacytic infiltrate; in some instances, necrosis and granuloma formation are present (Fig. 18-60). Note that this is a diagnosis of exclusion; other processes, such as tuberculosis, Wegener granulomatosis, sarcoidosis, rheumatoid meningitis, and other specific causes of a fibrous meningitis should be considered. Appropriate special stains, including those for infectious organisms, need to be performed.

Acute Disseminated Encephalomyelitis

Acute disseminated encephalomyelitis is an entity that usually follows an infection or recent vaccination. It may be associated with a preceding skin rash. Clinically, its manifestations can include hemiparesis, seizures, encephalopathy, visual disturbances, ataxia, cranial nerve palsies, and psychosis. The lesions are characterized by small, perivenous inflammatory infiltrates and demyelination with relative sparing of the axons. The inflammation is composed of lymphocytes, plasma cells, and some macrophages. The density of macrophages is low, and they are confined to the perivascular spaces. Frequently, perivascular hemorrhages are also present. A Luxol fast blue stain demonstrates the perivenular demyelination (Fig. 18-61). In general, these patients have a single episode with no recurrences and no or only minor neurologic sequelae.[91,92]

Germinoma

Germinomas occur in the midline and involve predominantly the pituitary and pineal regions in the CNS. The challenge of this entity is that the appearance on a biopsy specimen may resemble an infectious process, because it usually consists of a dense lymphocytic infiltrate with only rare scattered large cells with clear cytoplasm and prominent nucleoli (germ cells). Smear preparations from frozen section can be helpful in identifying the neoplastic germ cell population. This is a diagnosis to keep in mind when encountering a midline inflammatory lesion, especially in

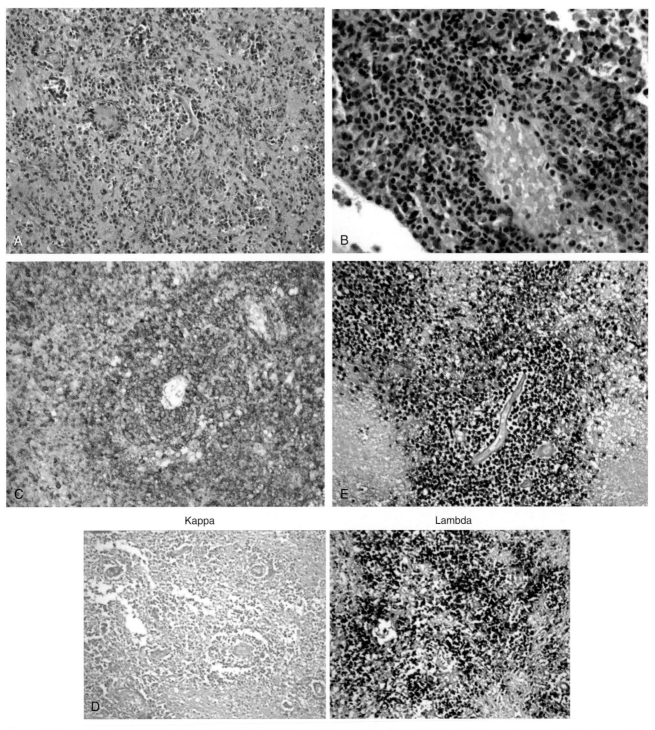

Kappa   Lambda

Figure 18-58. Lymphoma. **A,** Brain with dense, atypical lymphocytic infiltrate with some perivascular predilection. **B,** High power demonstrates dyshesive population of large cells with high nuclear-cytoplasmic ratio and prominent nucleoli. **C,** Immunohistochemical staining for CD20 shows a predominant neoplastic B-cell population. **D,** The κ and λ light chains are demonstrated by in situ hybridization. The monoclonality of the λ light chain supports the diagnosis of diffuse large B-cell lymphoma. **E,** Positive Epstein-Barr virus in situ hybridization in a patient with human immunodeficiency virus infection.

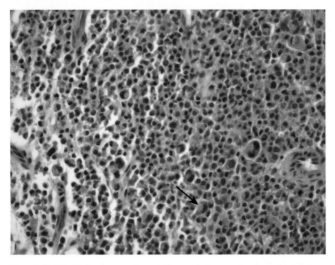

Figure 18-59. Plasmacytoma. Dense infiltrate of plasma cells, some of which have dense intracytoplasmic eosinophilic inclusions, known as Russell bodies *(arrow)*.

adolescents and young adults, because the peak incidence is between 10 and 14 years of age. Ancillary studies are helpful in arriving at the diagnosis and may include CSF germ cell markers and stains for C-kit (KIT), placental alkaline phosphatase (PLAP), and the homeobox transcription factors NANOG and Oct-4 (POU5F1) (Fig. 18-62).[93,94]

Granulomatous or Predominantly Histiocytic Inflammatory Pattern

Infectious Etiologies

Bacteria

Tuberculosis
Mycobacterium tuberculosis causes meningitis and parenchymal caseous granulomas. Tuberculous meningitis is usually due to hematogenous dissemination of the tubercle bacillus. The men-

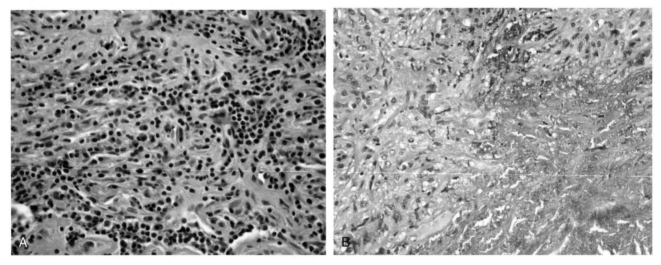

Figure 18-60. Pachymeningitis. **A,** Dura with dense fibrosis and lymphoplasmacytic infiltrate. **B,** Dura with chronic inflammation surrounding an area of necrosis.

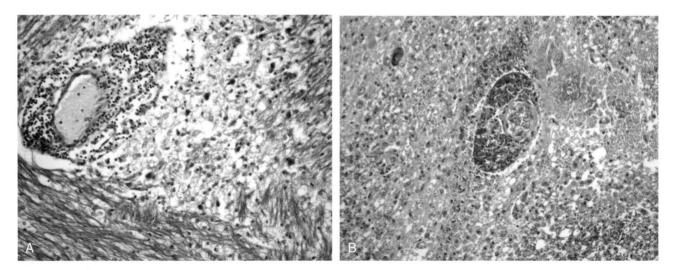

Figure 18-61. Acute disseminated encephalomyelitis. **A,** Luxol fast blue and H&E staining of white matter emphasizes the perivenular lymphocytic infiltrate and the perivenular demyelination. **B,** Perivascular hemorrhage and demyelination.

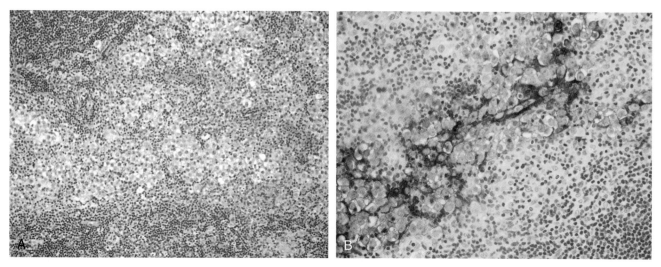

Figure 18-62. Germinoma. **A,** Dense lymphocytic infiltrate surrounding admixed large cells with clear cytoplasm, large nucleus, and prominent nucleoli (germ cells). **B,** Immunostaining for placental alkaline phosphatase (PLAP) highlights the germ cells.

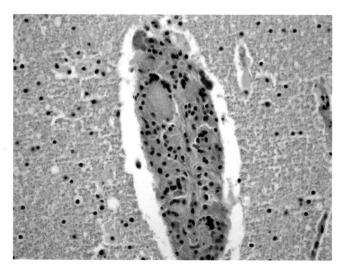

Figure 18-63. Tuberculosis. A dense perivascular granulomatous infiltrate involves the Virchow-Robin space.

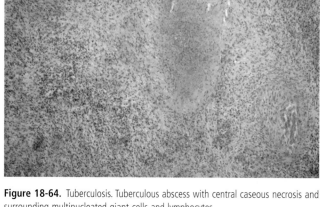

Figure 18-64. Tuberculosis. Tuberculous abscess with central caseous necrosis and surrounding multinucleated giant cells and lymphocytes.

ingitis predominantly involves the base of the brain but extends throughout the subarachnoid space. The inflammatory infiltrate extends into the subpial region, the ventricles, and subependymal parenchyma (Fig. 18-63). The viscous nature of the inflammatory exudate leads to the rapid development of hydrocephalus. The inflammatory infiltrate is composed of lymphocytes, mononuclear cells, epithelioid histiocytes, and occasional multinucleated giant cells (Fig. 18-64). Granulomas with epithelioid histiocytes and lymphocytes surrounding central caseous necrosis can be seen. Frequently, arterial lesions with endarteritis obliterans are present and are responsible for the development of ischemic infarcts.

Tuberculomas are the most common brain tumors in India and other areas of the world where tuberculosis is still a common infection. Tuberculomas can be multiple and can involve any lobe of the brain. Histologically, they are multiloculated, with a fibrous capsule and a caseous center surrounded by epithelioid macrophages and lymphocytes (Fig. 18-65). Old tuberculomas

may become cystic or calcified with minimal inflammatory infiltrate.

If tuberculosis is suspected, an acid-fast bacterial stain should be performed and carefully examined (Fig. 18-66), keeping in mind that a negative stain does not exclude the diagnosis. If tuberculosis is clinically suspected, CSF cultures and PCR nucleic amplification should be performed.[95,96]

Whipple Disease
Whipple disease usually manifests as a systemic disease, although it may be confined to the CNS. Clinically, patients present with arthralgia, abdominal pain, malabsorption, and progressive weight loss. CNS involvement is characterized by confusion, memory loss, cranial nerve abnormalities, nystagmus, and ophthalmoplegia.[97,98] There are usually small lesions throughout the CNS, with special predilection for the subpial regions of the cortex, basal ganglia, hypothalamus, brainstem, and dentate. The response is characterized by infiltrates of foamy macrophages

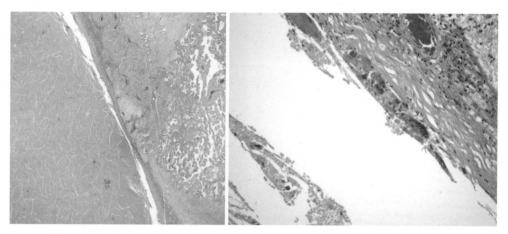

Figure 18-65. Tuberculoma. Low- and high-power views of a tuberculoma with a fibrous capsule and a caseous center surrounded by epithelioid macrophages and lymphocytes.

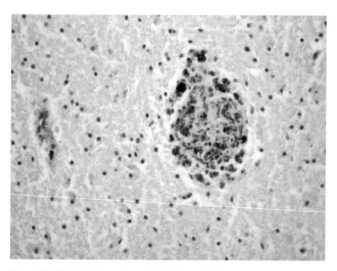

Figure 18-66. Atypical mycobacteria. Acid-fast stain demonstrates numerous mycobacteria. Numerous organisms are more likely to be seen in infections with atypical mycobacteria in immunosuppressed hosts.

filled with bacilli of *Tropheryma whippelii*, which may have a gray-blue appearance on H&E staining and can be confirmed by PAS stain (Fig. 18-67). This dense macrophage infiltrate is associated with a dense reactive astrocytosis and parenchymal lymphocytes. Diagnosis of the disease in the brain in the absence of a systemic diagnosis is done by biopsy and demonstration of the bacilli on PAS staining, electron microscopic examination, or PCR analysis.[99,100]

Cerebral Syphilitic Gummas

Cerebral syphilitic gummas are seen less and less commonly in clinical practice, although one must be aware of the possibility. Syphilitic gummas can be confused clinically and radiologically with brain tumors.[101] They are firm, necrotic nodules that extend from the brain parenchyma to the leptomeninges. Microscopically, there is a central area of necrosis with ghost cells surrounded by a granulomatous reaction of epithelioid macrophages, fibroblasts, and multinucleated giant cells (Figs. 18-68 and 18-69). It is usually not possible to identify the spirochetes.

Fungal

Dimorphic Fungi

The fungi that elicit granulomatous inflammation in the CNS are some of the dimorphic fungi, including *Blastomyces, Histoplasma, Coccidioides,* and *Paracoccidioides.* All of these manifest with primary lung infection and secondary dissemination to other organs including the CNS. However, CNS involvement is rare and is more commonly seen in immunosuppressed patients.

Blastomycosis can manifest with single or multiple parenchymal abscesses or as a dural-based mass. Morphologically, *Blastomyces* is an 8- to 15-μm yeast that divides by broad-based budding (Fig. 18-70). It is usually found within macrophages, although extracellular forms are also present (Fig. 18-71).[102,103]

Histoplasmosis is most frequently seen as a basal meningitis with a gray-yellow exudate. Histologically, this consists of a large granulomatous lesion with caseous necrosis, giant cells, and surrounding fibrosis. As in tuberculosis, endarteritis obliterans with areas of ischemic necrosis is frequently seen. *Histoplasma* is an obligate intracellular microorganism that can be seen within macrophages. The yeasts are small, with an average diameter of 2 to 5 μm (Fig. 18-72).[104]

Coccidioides infection of the CNS manifests as a basal meningitis, although paravertebral abscess formation with spinal cord compression is also common. Histologically, it produces a granulomatous inflammation with mixed acute and chronic inflammation and, typically, numerous eosinophils. Chronic lesions form nodules with central caseous necrosis surrounded by granulomas and fibrosis. *Coccidioides* is a large yeast that measures up to 40 μm in diameter.[105]

Paracoccidioides infection of the CNS usually involves the cerebral hemispheres, although dural meningitis and spinal cord involvement have also been reported. The fungus elicits a granulomatous response and is identified by the presence of multiple small yeasts budding from a central medium-size yeast, the so called steering wheel pattern.[106-108]

Parasitic

Schistosomiasis

Schistosomiasis is uncommon in the United States, but is endemic in South America, the Middle East, and Africa. *Schisto-*

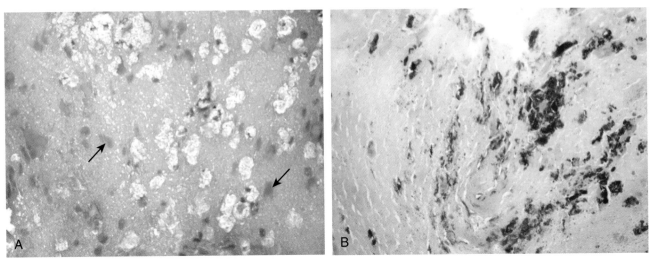

Figure 18-67. Whipple disease. **A,** Dense infiltrate of macrophages with foamy blue cytoplasm. **B,** The microorganisms can be highlighted by PAS staining.

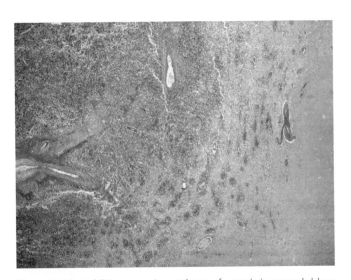

Figure 18-68. Syphilitic gumma. A central area of necrosis is surrounded by a granulomatous reaction of epithelioid macrophages, fibroblasts, and multinucleated giant cells.

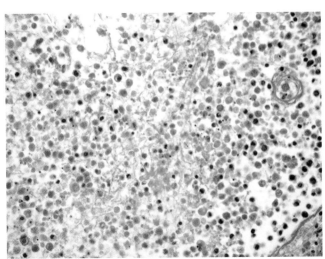

Figure 18-69. Syphilitic gumma. Higher magnification demonstrates the ghost cells.

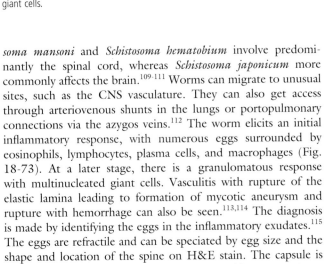

soma mansoni and *Schistosoma hematobium* involve predominantly the spinal cord, whereas *Schistosoma japonicum* more commonly affects the brain.[109-111] Worms can migrate to unusual sites, such as the CNS vasculature. They can also get access through arteriovenous shunts in the lungs or portopulmonary connections via the azygos veins.[112] The worm elicits an initial inflammatory response, with numerous eggs surrounded by eosinophils, lymphocytes, plasma cells, and macrophages (Fig. 18-73). At a later stage, there is a granulomatous response with multinucleated giant cells. Vasculitis with rupture of the elastic lamina leading to formation of mycotic aneurysm and rupture with hemorrhage can also be seen.[113,114] The diagnosis is made by identifying the eggs in the inflammatory exudates.[115] The eggs are refractile and can be speciated by egg size and the shape and location of the spine on H&E stain. The capsule is acid-fast with Ziehl-Nielsen stain. *S. mansoni* has a prominent lateral spine.

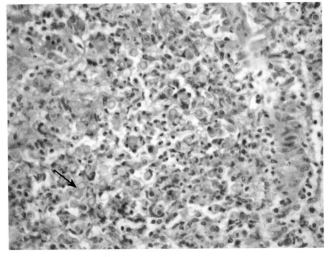

Figure 18-70. Blastomycosis. Brain tissue with extensive destruction and invasion by medium-sized (8-15 μm) yeast *(arrow)*, scattered lymphocytes, and macrophages.

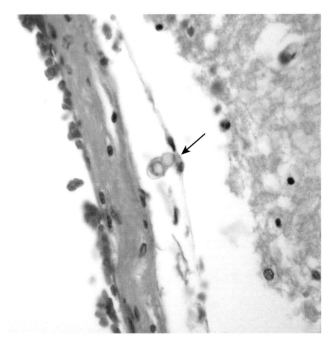

Figure 18-71. Blastomycosis. Higher magnification demonstrates broad-based budding *(arrow)*, characteristic of this organism.

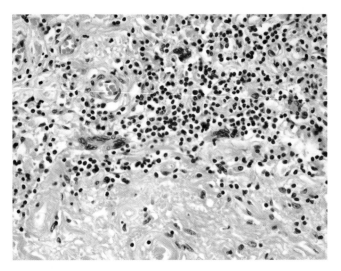

Figure 18-72. Histoplasmosis. Wall of caseous granuloma in the spinal cord, with multinucleated giant cells and mild chronic inflammation.

Noninfectious Etiologies

Demyelination

Demyelination is a clinical and pathologic challenge, because acute inflammatory demyelination can mimic a primary CNS neoplasm radiologically, and the dense inflammatory reaction may lead the pathologist to confuse it with an infectious disease or an infarct.[116]

By far the most common demyelinating process of the CNS is multiple sclerosis. Acute inflammatory multiple sclerosis can manifest as a mass lesion and may be biopsied with a preoperative diagnosis of neoplasm.

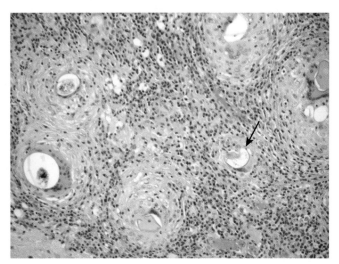

Figure 18-73. Schistosomiasis. Numerous eggs *(arrow)* are surrounded by eosinophils, lymphocytes, plasma cells, and macrophages.

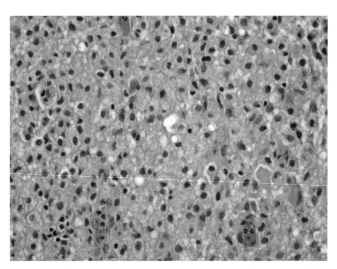

Figure 18-74. Acute inflammatory demyelination. Luxol fast blue stains myelin blue. In this picture, one can appreciate the edge of the demyelinating lesions where the parenchyma is devoid of myelin (Luxol fast blue and H&E stain).

The active plaque of multiple sclerosis is sharply demarcated from the surrounding parenchyma; however, stereotactic biopsies may sample only the center of the demyelinating area. Affected tissue displays abundant foamy macrophages (resulting in a hypercellular appearance), mixed reactive astrocytosis, perivascular lymphocytes (predominantly T cells), and occasional plasma cells (Figs. 18-74 and 18-75). The definitive diagnosis can be made by demonstration of loss of myelin (Luxol fast blue or immunostains for myelin basic protein) with relative preservation of axons (immunostain for neurofilament or silver preparation for axons such as Bielschowsky) (Fig. 18-76). The remnants of myelin can be seen as a phagocytized element in the macrophages.[117-119] Caution is recommended with this entity, because many mistakes can be made if the lesions are misinterpreted as neoplasms such as oligodendrogliomas, due to the abundant clear cytoplasm of the macrophages, or astrocytomas, due to the

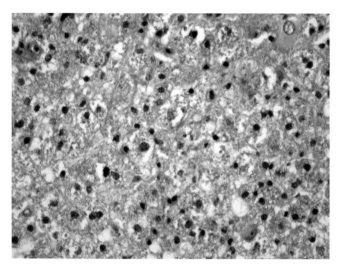

Figure 18-75. Demyelination. High power demonstrates that the lesion is rich in macrophages that contain myelin debris (Luxol fast blue and H&E stain).

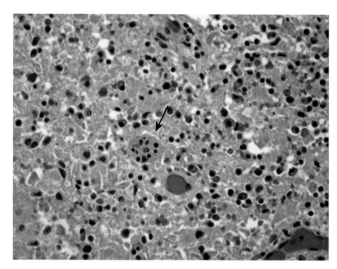

Figure 18-77. Rosai-Dorfman disease. Dura with mixed lymphoplasmacytic inflammatory infiltrate and variable numbers of pale-staining histiocytes. The histiocytes display the characteristic emperipolesis (*arrow*).

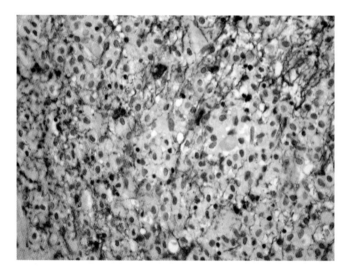

Figure 18-76. Demyelination. Immunostaining with an antibody to neurofilament demonstrates relative preservation of the axons in a background of numerous macrophages (immunoperoxidase reaction).

prominent reactive astrocytes, which can be atypical and may display numerous mitotic figures. Correct diagnosis for appropriate treatment is imperative to avoid the devastating consequences of irradiating a "tumor" that is no more than a demyelinating process. Diffuse infiltration of macrophages is a rare feature of untreated gliomas and practically excludes the diagnosis of glioma.

Of note, steroid-treated lymphomas also can have abundant macrophages, lymphocytes, and plasma cells without evidence of demyelination. This is an entity that must be kept in mind.[120]

Rosai-Dorfman Disease

Also known as sinus histiocytosis with massive lymphadenopathy, Rosai-Dorfman disease (RDD) is an idiopathic histiocytic proliferation, usually affecting lymph nodes, that can be misin-

terpreted as an infection. The most common clinical presentation is painless cervical lymphadenopathy. The disease occurs most often in the third and fourth decades and may be accompanied by leukocytosis, elevated erythrocyte sedimentation rate (ESR), weight loss, and possibly hypergammaglobulinemia. Whereas lymph node involvement often dominates the clinical presentation, other anatomic sites are involved in 30% to 40% of cases, most commonly skin, upper respiratory tract, orbit, or testes.

RDD is uncommon in the CNS (<5% of cases) but can masquerade as a meningioma, manifesting as a dural-based lesion with contrast enhancement and with vasogenic edema in the underlying cerebral cortex and white matter, leading to a biopsy.[121,122] The dural involvement may be the only manifestation, or it may be part of multifocal disease. Approximately 75% of the CNS RDD cases are intracranial, whereas only 20% involve the spine.[123]

Histologically, the lesions consist of a mixed lymphoplasmacytic inflammatory infiltrate with occasional neutrophils and eosinophils and variable numbers of pale-staining histiocytes. The histiocytes display the characteristic emperipolesis (Fig. 18-77). Binucleate plasma cells and intracytoplasmic eosinophilic inclusions (Russell bodies) are commonly observed. There is usually a dense fibrous proliferation in the background. Special stains for organisms are necessary to rule out an infectious etiology and are generally negative. The large histiocytes are positive for S-100 protein and CD68, but negative for CD1a. Examination of immunostained sections can facilitate the recognition of emperipolesis (Fig. 18-78).[124] Necrosis, well-formed granulomas, and eosinophilia are not present.

The etiology of RDD is not known, but it has been suggested that it is an autoimmune disease. There has been no definitive evidence of any infectious agent. Currently, it is considered a benign, idiopathic histiocytosis.[125]

Meningiomas with Dense Lymphoplasmacytic Response

Some meningiomas may be largely replaced by a pronounced chronic inflammatory reaction of lymphocytes and plasma cells

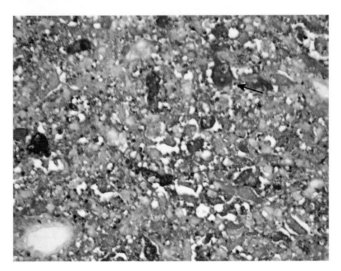

Figure 18-78. Rosai-Dorfman disease. Immunostaining with antibodies to S-100 highlights the macrophages in dark brown, with negative staining of the "passing by" cells (emperipolesis) (immunoperoxidase reaction).

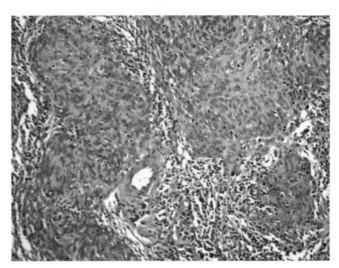

Figure 18-79. Meningioma with dense lymphoplasmacytic response. Although it can be confused with an infectious etiology, areas of meningothelial growth reveal the nature of the process.

(Fig. 18-79). However, classic areas of meningioma can be identified. Confirmatory immunostaining for epithelial membrane antigen (EMA) may be helpful in the diagnosis, to avoid confusion with an infectious process.[126]

Langerhans Cell Histiocytosis

Langerhans cell histiocytosis primarily affects children. It can manifest as a single lesion (eosinophilic granuloma), as multiple lesions with disseminated disease and involvement of lymph nodes, skin, liver, and pancreas (Letterer-Siwe disease), or as multiple lytic lesions involving the calvarium and base of the skull with clinical diabetes insipidus or exophthalmos (Hand-Schüller-Christian disease).[127]

Langerhans histiocytosis can also manifest as discrete histiocytic nodules attached to the dura.

Histologically, Langerhans cells are histiocytes with characteristic cytologic features consistent with moderate to abundant clear cytoplasm and a reniform nucleus with longitudinal nuclear grooves and lobulations. Numerous eosinophils are often present and are helpful in the diagnosis. Other inflammatory cells, such as plasma cells and neutrophils, may be seen, although in a lower proportion than eosinophils. Langerhans histiocytes are CD1a and S-100 positive (Fig. 18-80). Ultrastructural studies demonstrate the classic Birbeck granules.[128,129]

Sarcoidosis

Sarcoidosis is a systemic granulomatous disorder of unknown etiology. The lungs are the usual site of disease, but the meninges, skeletal muscle, and peripheral nerves can also be involved. Sarcoidosis of the nervous system is usually a basilar meningitis manifesting as multiple cranial nerve or spinal root palsies. The CSF generally shows elevation of angiotensin-converting enzyme (ACE).[130,131] Occasionally, the hypothalamus is involved, leading to diabetes insipidus. Histologically, the lesions are composed of compact, noncaseating, epithelioid granulomas surrounded by

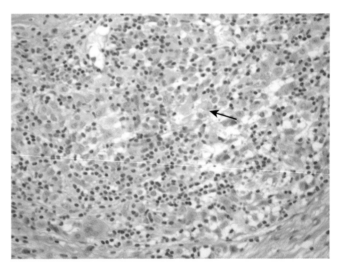

Figure 18-80. Langerhans histiocytosis. Dense chronic inflammation is present, with occasional eosinophils admixed with Langerhans cells, which have characteristic reniform or cleaved nuclei *(arrow)*.

lymphocytes and monocytes. They may coalesce and form large masses simulating neoplasms (Fig. 18-81).[132] The granulomas tend to be located around blood vessels and follow the Virchow-Robin spaces (Fig. 18-82). Occasionally, granulomas can be seen intraparenchymally around blood vessels, surrounded by a dense reactive gliosis; they can also be found around the third ventricle or in the choroid plexus.[133,134] This is a diagnosis of exclusion, and special stains to rule out an infectious etiology (e.g., fungal infection, tuberculosis) must be done.

Rheumatoid Meningitis

Another cause of chronic pachymeningitis or leptomeningitis is rheumatoid arthritis. Rheumatoid nodules in the meninges manifest as localized masses in the dura or the subarachnoid space.

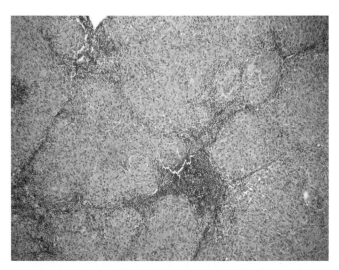

Figure 18-81. Sarcoid. Multiple, tightly packed, noncaseating granulomas coalesce and mimic a mass. The granulomas are surrounded by lymphocytic infiltrate.

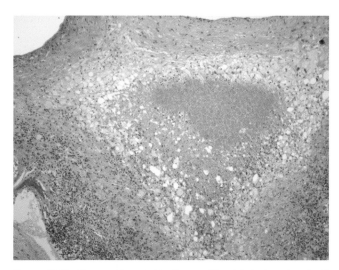

Figure 18-83. Rheumatoid meningitis. Rheumatoid nodule in the subarachnoid space consists of a lymphoplasmacytic infiltrate with a necrotic center.

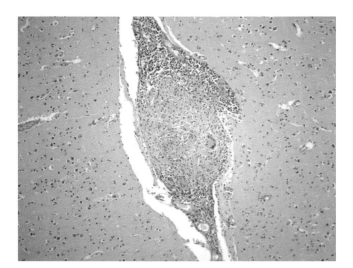

Figure 18-82. Sarcoid. A granuloma around a blood vessel is present in the subarachnoid space. The granulomas can also be found in the Virchow-Robin spaces.

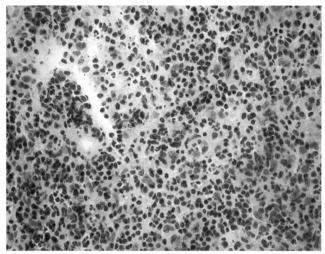

Figure 18-84. Granulomatous hypophysitis. Large collection of histiocytes admixed with lymphoplasmacytic infiltrate and normal anterior pituitary cells.

They consist of a lymphoplasmacytic infiltrate with a necrotic center and the typical radial arrangement of fibroblasts and inflammatory cells seen in peripheral rheumatoid nodules, but they are not usually as well defined as those in the periphery (Fig. 18-83).[135,136] This is a diagnosis of exclusion, because a gumma or tuberculous granuloma has to be ruled out. Special stains for bacteria, fungi, and other infectious organisms are negative.

Granulomatous Hypophysitis

Granulomatous hypophysitis is a rare condition of unknown etiology that usually causes hormonal imbalance, hyperprolactinemia, diabetes insipidus, headache, and nausea. Imaging reveals a contrast-enhancing mass in the pituitary, and the diagnosis is made by biopsy. Although the biopsy is performed to rule out an adenoma, it is very rare for a pituitary adenoma to manifest with diabetes insipidus. Microscopically, large collections of histiocytes admixed with lymphocytes and plasma cells, with occasional multinucleated giant cells, almost obliterate the normal anterior pituitary architecture (Fig. 18-84). Recognizing the presence of embedded anterior pituitary cells is the first clue to the diagnosis. Special stains for microorganisms are required to eliminate an infectious etiology, and tests for lymphocytic markers are needed to rule out lymphoma. Stains for the pituitary hormones reveal the scattered remaining anterior pituitary cells in the background of the inflammatory reaction (see Fig. 18-84).[137,138] Lymphocytic hypophysitis is thought to be an autoimmune disorder, because it can be accompanied by other endocrine autoimmune disorders such as Hashimoto thyroiditis or adrenalitis.[139]

Foreign Body

Patients with prior surgery, trauma, or embolization treatments may develop a focal, dense, chronic inflammatory response with a mixed lymphoid and plasma cell infiltrate and foreign body giant cell reaction. Usually, the foreign material can be identified by light microscopy or by polarization.

Minimal or No Inflammatory Response

Fungi

Cryptococcus

Cryptococcus is the most common mycosis of the CNS. It often affects immunocompromised patients. *Cryptococcus* usually causes minimal inflammatory response or a mild chronic meningitis in both immunocompetent and immunocompromised individuals. The symptoms are severe headache with or without neck stiffness. The pattern of inflammation varies depending on the host response. Because of the mucoid capsule that protects the organism from being recognized by the immune system, dissemination through the meninges is fast, producing a gelatinous or mucoid surface to the brain and a honeycomb-like appearance with multiple cyst-like spaces where the organism floats in a mucin background in the brain parenchyma (Fig. 18-85). On the other hand, patients who elicit a strong immune response may have sclerotic and granulomatous masses containing only a few yeast forms. *Cryptococcus* is a round budding yeast that varies in size from 2 to 15 μm in diameter. The bud has a narrow neck, in contrast to the broad-base budding yeast of blastomycosis (Fig. 18-86).[140,141] The microorganism is highlighted by PAS and GMS staining. The yeast is surrounded by a polysaccharide capsule that can be identified by mucicarmine or Alcian blue stains.

Caution should be taken not to confuse corpora amylacea in the brain with *Cryptococcus*. Corpora amylacea are the same size as *Cryptococcus* and also stain positively with PAS and GMS. The distinction can be made by examination of the CSF using India ink, which allows one to see the cryptococcal budding yeasts surrounded by clear halos. Although the sensitivity of this test is only 25%, it increases to 53% when multiple samples are used.[142] Currently, a combination of capsular antigen detection in CSF (sensitivity, 60-95%) and culture is used for the diagnosis.

Hyphal Organisms in the Immunocompromised Host

This category includes pathogens such as *Aspergillus*, *Mucor*, *Pseudallescheria*, *Fusarium,* and *Penicillium* species. These organisms usually affect persons who are at risk of systemic

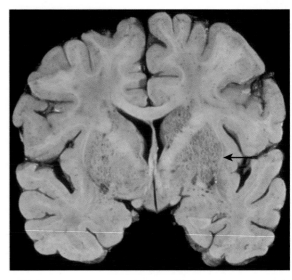

Figure 18-85. *Cryptococcus.* Coronal section of the brain demonstrates the honeycomb-like appearance, with multiple cyst-like spaces where the organism floats in a mucinous background *(arrow).*

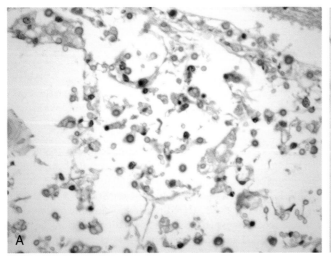
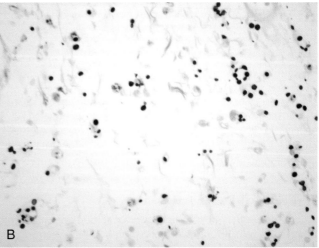

Figure 18-86. *Cryptococcus.* **A,** Mucicarmine staining highlights the polysaccharide capsule around the yeasts in the subarachnoid space. **B,** GMS staining shows small yeasts (2 μm) in the subarachnoid space with narrow budding.

mycosis, such as chronic alcoholics, intravenous drug abusers, and patients who are immunosuppressed therapeutically. The organisms often spread by direct intracranial extension from adjacent structures. Although in immunocompetent hosts they may cause a strong inflammatory response, as addressed earlier, in the immunocompromised host these organisms may be primarily intraparenchymal with minimal host inflammatory response.[143,144]

Viruses

Rabies

Most human rabies infections result from introduction of the virus through saliva from a rabid animal bite. Rabies is endemic particularly in raccoons and bats in the United States, as well as in other mammals in the Americas, Europe, Africa, and Asia.

The virus replicates within the skeletal muscle, then reaches the neuromuscular junction and is transported via the axon centrally to the CNS, where it spreads rapidly between neurons in the spinal cord, brainstem, cerebrum, and cerebellum.[145,146] Once the infection has reached the CNS, the virus spreads peripherally through axons to salivary and lacrimal glands, skin, heart, lungs, gastrointestinal tract, adrenal glands, kidneys, and bladder. The incubation period ranges from 1 to 3 months but can be as long as 1 year. Early postexposure prophylaxis virtually eliminates the disease. The disease course is inexorable once clinical signs appear.

In general, inflammation is minimal and there is usually a discrepancy between the viral load and the degree of inflammation. Leptomeningeal inflammation with perivascular lymphocytic infiltration and neuronophagia can be seen. Rabies is an RNA virus that replicates in the cytoplasm, forming what corresponds to Negri bodies.[147] Negri bodies are sharply delineated, round to oval, eosinophilic cytoplasmic inclusions found in most parts of the CNS, although they are easiest to identify in Purkinje cells (Fig. 18-87), hippocampal pyramidal cells, and brainstem

nuclei. Ultrastructurally, rabies virus has a characteristic bullet shape, 70 to 85 nm in diameter and 180 nm in length (see Chapter 5).

Prions

Creutzfeldt-Jakob Disease

Creutzfeldt-Jakob disease (CJD) is a rare transmissible spongiform encephalopathy that is associated with the accumulation of an abnormal prion protein in neuronal processes and neuropil, which leads to destruction of the neurons with a striking reactive astrocytosis. In most cases. there is no obvious inflammatory reaction. The patient presents with a clinical picture of a rapidly progressive dementia associated with neurologic findings such as ataxia, visual abnormalities, myoclonus, and extrapyramidal signs, among others.[148,149] Magnetic resonance imaging often shows an increased signal in the basal ganglia, with variable degrees of signal intensity changes in the cerebral cortex.[150,151]

The characteristic histologic feature is the development of a spongiform appearance of the tissue, with multiple tiny vacuoles confined to the gray matter, accompanied by neuronal loss and reactive gliosis without an inflammatory infiltrate (Fig. 18-88). The severity of the changes varies within different regions of the brain.[152,153] The abnormal prion protein can be demonstrated by immunohistochemistry and/or by Western blot analysis, which in the United States is performed at the National Prion Disease Surveillance Center at Case Western Reserve University.[154,155] The definitive diagnosis can be made only from brain tissue, but the characteristic clinical course and the presence of protein 14-3-3 in CSF leads to a high suspicion. The presence of protein 14-3-3 in the CSF can also be found in other neuronal destructive diseases and in stroke.[156-158] If the diagnosis is suspected and surgery is necessary, disposable instruments should be used, because the disease has been transmitted by the use of contaminated surgical instruments and by dural and corneal transplants.[159] There is little or no justification for brain

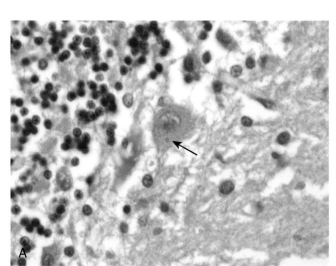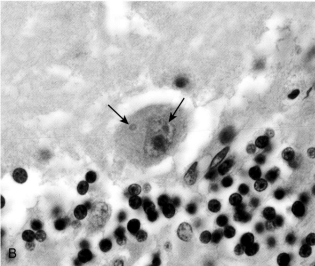

Figure 18-87. Rabies. Purkinje cells show well-circumscribed, eosinophilic intracytoplasmic inclusions (Negri bodies) in **A** *(arrow)* and **B** *(arrow on the left)*; **B** also demonstrates an intranuclear inclusion *(arrow on the right)*.

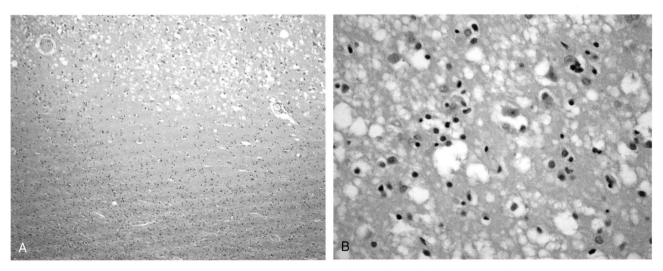

Figure 18-88. Creutzfeldt-Jakob disease. **A,** Brain with spongiform changes, composed of multiple vacuoles of varying size, confined to the gray matter. Some of the vacuoles are contained within the thickness of the section. **B,** Higher magnification reveals neuronal loss and reactive gliosis without any inflammatory response.

biopsy. The abnormal prion protein is highly resistant to most decontaminating agents, and tissue can remain infectious unless it is treated according to a precise protocol.[160] Any tissue block coming from a patient with suspected CJD should be fixed in formalin for 24 hours and then soaked in 90% formic acid for 1 hour before returning it to formalin for routine histologic processing.[160]

REFERENCES

1. Gold R: Epidemiology of bacterial meningitis. Infect Dis Clin North Am 1999;13:515-525.
2. Centers for Disease Control and Prevention: Decline in *Haemophilus influenzae* type b meningitis—Seattle-King County, Washington, 1984-1989. MMWR Morb Mortal Wkly Rep 1990; 39:924-925.
3. Centers for Disease Control and Prevention: Progress toward introduction of *Haemophilus influenzae* type b vaccine in low-income countries—Worldwide, 2004-2007. MMWR Morb Mortal Wkly Rep 2008;57:148-151.
4. van de Beek D, de Gans J, Spanjaard L, et al: Clinical features and prognostic factors in adults with bacterial meningitis. N Engl J Med 2004;351:1849-1859.
5. Lu CH, Chang WN, Lui CC: Strategies for the management of bacterial brain abscess. J Clin Neurosci 2006;13:979-985.
6. Sennaroglu L, Sozeri B: Otogenic brain abscess: Review of 41 cases. Otolaryngol Head Neck Surg 2000;123:751-755.
7. Kastrup O, Wanke I, Maschke M: Neuroimaging of infections. NeuroRx 2005;2:324-332.
8. Baringer JR, Swoveland P: Recovery of herpes-simplex virus from human trigeminal ganglions. N Engl J Med 1973;288:548-550.
9. Stevens JG, Haar L, Poter DD, et al: Prominence of the herpes simplex virus latency-associated transcript in trigeminal ganglia from seropositive humans. J Infect Dis 1988;188:117-123.
10. Liedtke W, Opalka B, Zimmermann CW, Lignitz E: Age distribution of latent herpes simplex 1 and varicella-zoster virus genome in human nervous tissue. J Neurol Sci 1993;116:6-11.
11. Esiri MM: Herpes simplex encephalitis: An immunohistochemical study of the distribution of viral antigen within the brain. J Neurol Sci 1982;54:209-226.
12. Lakeman FD, Whitley RJ: Diagnosis of herpes simplex encephalitis: Application of polymerase chain reaction to cerebrospinal fluid from brain-biopsied patients and correlation with disease. National Institute of Allergy and Infectious Diseases Collaborative Antiviral Study Group. J Infect Dis 1995;171:857-863.
13. Hausfater P, Fillet AM, Rozember F, et al: Prevalence of viral infectious markers by polymerase chain reaction amplification and interferon-alpha measurements among patients undergoing lumbar puncture in an emergency department. J Med Virol 2004;73:137-146.
14. Pelligra G, Lynch N, Miller SP, et al: Brainstem involvement in neonatal herpes simplex virus type 2 encephalitis. Pediatrics 2007;120:e442-e446.
15. Doyle PW, Gibson G, Dolman CL: Herpes zoster ophthalmicus with contralateral hemiplegia: Identification of the cause. Ann Neurol 1983;14:84-85.
16. Gray F, Chrétien F, Vallat-Decouvelaere AV, Scaravilli F: The changing pattern of HIV neuropathology in the HAART era. J Neuropathol Exp Neurol 2003;62:429-440.
17. Gilden DH, Kleinschmidt-DeMasters BK, LaGuardia JJ, et al: Neurologic complications of the reactivation of varicella-zoster virus. N Engl J Med 2000;342:635-644.
18. Deresiewicz RL, Thaler SJ, Hsu L, Zamani AA: Clinical and neuroradiographic manifestations of eastern equine encephalitis. N Engl J Med 1997;336:1867-1874.
19. Bastian FO, Wende RD, Singer BD, et al: Eastern equine encephalomyelitis: Histopathologic and ultrastructural changes with isolation of the virus in a human case. Am J Clin Pathol 1975;64:10-13.
20. Jacques J, Carquin J, Brodard V, et al: New reverse transcription-PCR assay for rapid and sensitive detection of enterovirus genomes in cerebrospinal fluid specimens of patients with aseptic meningitis. J Clin Microbiol 2003;41:5726-5728.
21. Kares S, Lonnrot M, Vuorinen P, et al: Real-time PCR for rapid diagnosis of entero- and rhinovirus infections using LightCycler. J Clin Virol 2004;29:99-104.
22. Sell M, Klingebiel R, Di Iorio G, Sampaolo S: Primary cerebral toxoplasmosis: A rare case of ventriculitis and hydrocephalus in AIDS. Clin Neuropathol 2005;24:106-111.
23. Chimelli L, Rosemberg S, Hann MD, et al: Pathology of the central nervous system in patients infected with the human immunodeficiency virus (HIV): A report of 252 autopsy cases from Brazil. Neuropathol Appl Neurobiol 1992;18:478-488.

24. Offiah CE, Turnbull IW: The imaging appearances of intracranial CNS infections in adult HIV and AIDS patients. Clin Radiol 2006;61:393-401.

25. Scaravilli F, Gray F, Mikol J, et al: Pathology of the nervous system. In Scaravilli F (ed): The Neuropathology of AIDS. London, Springer, 1983, pp 99-169.

26. Luft BJ, Hafner R, Korzun AH, et al: Toxoplasmic encephalitis in patients with the acquired immunodeficiency syndrome. Members of the ACTG 077p/ANRS 009 Study Team. N Engl J Med 1993;329:995-1000.

27. Katlama C, De Wit S, O'Doherty E, et al: Pyrimethamine-clindamycin vs. pyrimethamine-sulfadiazine as acute and long-term therapy for toxoplasmic encephalitis in patients with AIDS. Clin Infect Dis 1996;22:268-275.

28. Lang W, Miklossy J, Deruaz JP, et al: Neuropathology of the acquired immune deficiency syndrome (AIDS): A report of 135 consecutive autopsy cases from Switzerland. Acta Neuropathol 1989;77:379-390.

29. Singh N: Fungal infections in the recipients of solid organ transplantation. Infect Dis Clin North Am 2003;17:113-134.

30. Yohai RA, Bullock JD, Aziz AA, et al: Survival factors in rhino-orbital-cerebral mucormycosis. Surv Ophthalmol 1994;39:3-22.

31. Ellis CJ, Daniel SE, Kennedy PG: Rhino-orbital zygomycosis. J Neurol Neurosurg Psychiatry 1985;48:455-458.

32. Seton M, Pless M, Fishman JA, et al: Case records of the Massachusetts General Hospital. Case 18-2008: A 68-year-old man with headache and visual changes after liver transplantation. N Engl J Med 2008;358:2619-2628.

33. Martinez AJ, Visvesvara GS: Free-living, amphizoic and opportunistic amebas. Brain Pathol 1997;7:583-598.

34. Seidel JS, Harmatz P, Visvesvara GS, et al: Successful treatment of primary amebic meningoencephalitis. N Engl J Med 1982;306:346-348.

35. Schuster FL, Visvesvara GS: Opportunistic amoebae: Challenges in prophylaxis and treatment. Drug Resist Updat 2004;7:41-51.

36. Murakawa GJ, McCalmont T, Altman J, et al: Disseminated acanthamebiasis in patients with AIDS: A report of five cases and a review of the literature. Arch Dermatol 1995;131:1291-1296.

37. Sissons J, Kim KS, Stins M, et al: Acanthamoeba castellanii induces host cell death via a phosphatidylinositol 3-kinase-dependent mechanism. Infect Immun 2005;73:2704-2708.

38. White JM, Barker RD, Salisbury JR, et al: Granulomatous amoebic encephalitis. Lancet 2004;364:220.

39. Cha JHJ, Furie K, Kay J, et al: Case records of the Massachusetts General Hospital. Case 39-2006: A 24-year-old woman with systemic lupus erythematosus, seizures, and right arm weakness. N Engl J Med 2006;355:2678-2689.

40. Deetz TR, Sawyer MH, Billman G, et al: Successful treatment of Balamuthia amoebic encephalitis: Presentation of 2 cases. Clin Infect Dis 2003;37:1304-1312.

41. Lucas S, Bell J, Chimelli L: Parasitic and fungal infections infections. In Love S, Louis D, Ellison D: Greenfield's Neuropathology, 8th ed. London, Hodder Arnold, 2008, pp 1468-1472.

42. Iwamoto M, Jernigan DB, Guasch A, et al: Transmission of West Nile virus from an organ donor to four transplant recipients. N Engl J Med 2003;348:2196-2203.

43. Harrington T, Kuehnert MJ, Kamel H, et al: West Nile virus infection transmitted by blood transfusion. Transfusion 2003;43:1018-1022.

44. Center for Disease Control and Prevention: Interim guidelines for the evaluation of infants born to mothers infected with West Nile virus during pregnancy. MMWR Morb Mortal Wkly Rep 2004:53:154-157.

45. Petersen LR, Marfin AA: West Nile virus: A primer for the clinician. Ann Intern Med 2002;137:173-179.

46. Sejvar JJ, Haddad MB, Tierney BC, et al: Neurologic manifestations and outcome of West Nile virus infection. JAMA 2003;290:511-515.

47. Gradoth N, Wiitzman S, Lehmann EE: Acute anterior myelitis complicating West Nile fever. Arch Neurol 1979:36:172-173.

48. Jeha LE, Sila CA, Lederman RJ, et al: West Nile virus infection: A new acute paralytic illness. Neurology 2003;61:55-59.

49. Fratkin JD, Leis AA, Stokic DS, et al: Spinal cord neuropathology in human West Nile virus infection. Arch Pathol Lab Med 2004;128:533-537.

50. Bosanko CM, Gilroy J, Wang AM, et al: West Nile virus encephalitis involving the substantia nigra: Neuroimaging and pathologic findings with literature review. Arch Neurol 2003;60:1448-1452.

51. Omalu BI, Shakir AA, Wang G, et al: Fatal fulminant pan-meningo-polioencephalitis due to West Nile virus. Brain Pathol 2003;13:465-472.

52. Hollander H, Schaefer PW, Hedley-Whyte ET: Case records of the Massachusetts General Hospital. Case 22-2005: An 81-year-old man with cough, fever, and altered mental status. N Engl J Med 2005;353:287-295.

53. Rawal A, Gavin PJ, Sturgis CD: Cerebrospinal fluid cytology in seasonal epidemic West Nile virus meningo-encephalitis. Diagn Cytopathol 2006;34:127-129.

54. Rondini S, Pingle MR, Das S, et al: Development of multiplex PCR-ligase detection reaction assay for detection of West Nile virus. J Clin Microbiol 2008;46:2269-2279.

55. Berger JR: Progressive multifocal leukoencephalopathy in acquired immunodeficiency syndrome: Explaining the high incidence and disproportionate frequency of the illness relative to other immunosuppressive conditions. J Neurovirol 2003;9(Suppl 1):38-41.

56. Padgett BL, Walker DL, ZuRhein GM, et al: Cultivation of papova-like virus from human brain with progressive multifocal leukoencephalopathy. Lancet 1971;1:1257-1260.

57. Cinque P, Bossolasco S, Brambilla AM, et al: The effect of highly active antiretroviral therapy-induced immune reconstitution on development and outcome of progressive multifocal leukoencephalopathy: Study of 43 cases with review of the literature. J Neurovirol 2003;9(Suppl 1):73-80.

58. Miralles P, Berenguer J, García de Viedma D, et al: Treatment of AIDS-associated progressive multifocal leukoencephalopathy with highly active antiretroviral therapy. AIDS 1998;12:2467-2472.

59. Vendrely A, Bienvenu B, Gasnault J, et al: Fulminant inflammatory leukoencephalopathy associated with HAART-induced immune restoration in AIDS-related progressive multifocal leukoencephalopathy. Acta Neuropathol 2005;109:449-455.

60. Bertrand E, Lewandowska E, Nerurkar V, et al: Progressive multifocal leukoencephalopathy (PML) and cerebral toxoplasmosis in an adult patient, with no symptoms of underlying immunosuppressing illness. Folia Neuropathol 1998;36:229-234.

61. Wüthrich C, Cheng YM, Joseph JT, et al: Frequent infection of cerebellar granule cell neurons by polyomavirus JC in progressive multifocal leukoencephalopathy. J Neuropathol Exp Neurol 2009;68:15-25.

62. Silberman L, Rubenstein LJ: Electron microscopic observations on a case of progressive multifocal leukoencphalopathy. Acta Neuropathol 1965;5:215-224.

63. Budka H, Costanzi G, Cristina S, et al: Brain pathology induced by infection with the human immunodeficiency virus (HIV): A histological, immunocytochemical, and electron microscopical study of 100 autopsy cases. Acta Neuropathol 1987;75:185-198.

64. Budka H, Wiley CA, Kleihues P, et al: HIV-associated disease of the nervous system: Review of nomenclature and proposal for neuropathology-based terminology. Brain Pathol 1991;1:143-152.

65. Bell JE: An update on the neuropathology of HIV in the HAART era. Histopathology 2004;45:549-559.

66. Vinters HV, Kwok MK, Ho HW, et al: Cytomegalovirus in the nervous system of patients with the acquired immune deficiency syndrome. Brain 1989;112:245-268.

67. Seo SK, Regan A, Cihlar T, et al: Cytomegalovirus ventriculoencephalitis in a bone marrow transplant recipient receiving antiviral maintenance: Clinical and molecular evidence of drug resistance. Clin Infect Dis 2001;33:e105-e108.

68. Singer C, Lang AE, Suchowersky O: Adult-onset subacute sclerosing panencephalitis: Case reports and review of the literature. Mov Disord 1997;12:342-353.

69. Gagnon A, Bouchard RW: Fulminating adult-onset subacute sclerosing panencephalitis in a 49-year-old man. Arch Neurol 2003;60:1160-1161.

70. Prashanth LK, Taly AB, Ravi V, et al: Adult onset subacute sclerosing panencephalitis: Clinical profile of 39 patients from a tertiary care centre. J Neurol Neurosurg Psychiatry 2006;77:630-633.

71. Jabbour JT, Garcia JH, Lemmi H, et al: Subacute sclerosing panencephalitis: A multidisciplinary study of eight cases. JAMA 1969;207:2248-2254.

72. Mandybur TI: The distribution of Alzheimer's neurofibrillary tangles and gliosis in chronic subacute sclerosing panencephalitis. Acta Neuropathol 1990;80:307-310.

73. Case records of the Massachusetts General Hospital: Weekly clinicopathological exercises. Case 24-2000: A 23-year-old man with seizures and a lesion in the left temporal lobe. N Engl J Med 2000;343:420-427.

74. Pittella JE: Neurocysticercosis. Brain Pathol 1997;7:681-693.

75. Zee CS, Go JL, Kim PE, et al: Imaging of neurocysticercosis. Neuroimaging Clin North Am 2000;10:391-407.

76. Walker DH, Hawkins HK, Hudson P: Fulminant Rocky Mountain spotted fever: Its pathologic characteristics associated with glucose-6-phosphate dehydrogenase deficiency. Arch Pathol Lab Med 1983;107:121-125.

77. Paddock CD, Finley RW, Wright CS, et al: *Rickettsia parkeri* rickettsiosis and its clinical distinction from Rocky Mountain spotted fever. Clin Infect Dis 2008;47:1188-1196.

78. Goel D, Reddy SR, Sundaram C, et al: Active necrotizing cerebral vasculitis in systemic lupus erythematosus. Neuropathology 2007;27:561-565.

79. Bataller L, Dalmau JO: Paraneoplastic disorders of the central nervous system: Update on diagnostic criteria and treatment. Semin Neurol 2004;24:461-467.

80. Younes-Mhenni S, Janier MF, Cinotti L, et al: FDG-PET improves tumour detection in patients with paraneoplastic neurological syndromes. Brain 2004;127:2331-2338.

81. Ances BM, Vitaliani R, Taylor RA, et al: Treatment-responsive limbic encephalitis identified by neuropil antibodies: MRI and PET correlates. Brain 2005;128:1764-1777.

82. Vitaliani R, Zoccarato M, Giometto B: Diagnosis and treatment of paraneoplastic neurological syndromes. Curr Clin Pharmacol 2008;3:46-50.

83. Braaten KM, Betensky RA, de Leval L, et al: BCL-6 expression predicts improved survival in patients with primary central nervous system lymphoma. Clin Cancer Res 2003;9:1063-1069.

84. Schlegel U, Schmidt-Wolf IG, Deckert M: Primary CNS lymphoma: Clinical presentation, pathological classification, molecular pathogenesis and treatment. J Neurol Sci 2000;181:1-12.

85. Ambinder RF: Epstein-Barr virus associated lymphoproliferations in the AIDS setting. Eur J Cancer 2001;37:1209-1216.

86. Hamilton-Dutoit SJ, Raphael M, Audouin J, et al: In situ demonstration of Epstein-Barr virus small RNAs (EBER 1) in acquired immunodeficiency syndrome-related lymphomas: Correlation with tumor morphology and primary site. Blood 1993;82:619-624.

87. Yaman E, Benekli M, Coskun U, et al: Intrasellar plasmacytoma: An unusual presentation of multiple myeloma. Acta Neurochir (Wien) 2008;150:921-924.

88. Pitini V, Arrigo C, Alafaci C, et al: Extramedullary plasmacytoma presented as a non-functional invasive pituitary macro-adenoma. J Neurooncol 2008;88:227-229.

89. Kupersmith MJ, Martin V, Heller G, et al: Idiopathic hypertrophic pachymeningitis. Neurology 2004;62:686-694.

90. Rudnik A, Larysz D, Gamrot J, et al: Idiopathic hypertrophic pachymeningitis: Case report and literature review. Folia Neuropathol 2007;45:36-42.

91. Menge T, Kieseier BC, Nessrler S, et al: Acute disseminated encephalomyelitis: An acute hit against the brain. Curr Opin Neurol 2007;20:247-254.

92. Tenembaum S, Chitnis T, Ness J, et al: Acute disseminated encephalomyelitis. Neurology 2007;68(16 Suppl 2):S23-S36.

93. Ngan KW, Jung SM, Lee LY, et al: Immunohistochemical expression of OCT4 in primary central nervous system germ cell tumours. J Clin Neurosci 2008;15:149-152.

94. Santagata S, Hornick JL, Ligon KL: Comparative analysis of germ cell transcription factors in CNS germinoma reveals diagnostic utility of NANOG. Am J Surg Pathol 2006;30:1613-1618.

95. Lin JJ, Harn HJ, Hsu YD, et al: Rapid diagnosis of tuberculous meningitis by polymerase chain reaction assay of cerebrospinal fluid. J Neurol 1995;242:147-152.

96. Desai MM, Pal RB: Polymerase chain reaction for the rapid diagnosis of tuberculous meningitis. Indian J Med Sci 2002;56:546-552.

97. Deriban G, Marth T: Current concepts of immunopathogenesis, diagnosis and therapy in Whipple's disease. Curr Med Chem 2006;13:2921-2926.

98. Louis ED, Lynch T, Kaufmann P, et al: Diagnostic guidelines in central nervous system Whipple's disease. Ann Neurol 1996;40:561-568.

99. Powers JM, Rawe SE: A neuropathologic study of Whipple's disease. Acta Neuropathol 1979;48:223-226.

100. Yogi T, Hokama A, Kinjo F, et al. Whipple's disease: The first Japanese case diagnosed by electron microscopy and polymerase chain reaction. Intern Med 2004;43:566-570.

101. Darwish BS, Fowler A, Ong M, et al: Intracranial syphilitic gumma resembling malignant brain tumour. J Clin Neurosci 2008;15:308-310.

102. Chapman SW, Lin AC, Hendricks KA, et al: Endemic blastomycosis in Mississippi: Epidemiological and clinical studies. Semin Respir Infect 1997;12:219-228.

103. Pappas PG, Pottage JC, Powderly WG, et al: Blastomycosis in patients with the acquired immunodeficiency syndrome. Ann Intern Med 1992;116:847-853.

104. Klein CJ, Dinapoli RP, Temesgen Z, et al: Central nervous system histoplasmosis mimicking a brain tumor: Difficulties in diagnosis and treatment. Mayo Clin Proc 1999;74:803-807.

105. Bañuelos AF, Williams PL, Johnson RH, et al: Central nervous system abscesses due to *Coccidioides* species. Clin Infect Dis 1996;22:240-250.

106. de Almeida SM: Central nervous system paracoccidioidomycosis: An overview. Braz J Infect Dis 2005;9:126-133.

107. Plá MP, Hartung C, Mendoza P, et al: Neuroparacoccidioidomycosis: Case reports and review. Mycopathologia 1994;127:139-144.

108. Elias J Jr, dos Santos AC, Carlotti CG Jr, et al: Central nervous system paracoccidioidomycosis: Diagnosis and treatment. Surg Neurol 2005;63(Suppl 1):S13-S21.

109. Nascimento-Carvalho CM, Moreno-Carvalho OA: Neuroschistosomiasis due to *Schistosoma mansoni*: A review of pathogenesis, clinical syndromes and diagnostic approaches. Rev Inst Med Trop Sao Paulo 2005;47:179-184.

110. Pollner JH, Schwartz A, Kobrine A, et al: Cerebral schistosomiasis caused by *Schistosoma haematobium*: Case report. Clin Infect Dis 1994;18:354-357.

111. Zhou J, Li G, Xia J, et al: Cerebral schistosomiasis japonica without gastrointestinal system involvement. Surg Neurol 2009;71:481-486.

112. Calabresi P, Abelmann WH: Porto-caval and porto-pulmonary anastomoses in Laennec's cirrhosis and in heart failure. J Clin Invest 1957;36:1257-1265.

113. Pompeu F, Sampaio de Lacerda PR: Subarachnoid hemorrhage due to *S. mansoni*: A rare etiology. J Neurol 1979;221:203-207.

114. Case records of the Massachusetts General Hospital: Weekly clinicopathological exercises. Case 21-2001: A 31-year-old man with an apparent seizure and a mass in the right parietal lobe. N Engl J Med 2001;345:126-131.

115. Pittella JE, Lana-Peixoto MA: Brain involvement in hepatosplenic schistosomiasis mansoni. Brain 1981;104:621-632.

116. Cunliffe CH, Fischer I, Monoky D, et al: Intracranial lesions mimicking neoplasms. Arch Pathol Lab Med 2009;133:101-123.

117. Lucchinetti CF, Parisi J, Bruck W: The pathology of multiple sclerosis. Neurol Clin 2005;23:77-105.

118. Annesley-Williams D, Farrell MA, Staunton H, et al: Acute demyelination, neuropathological diagnosis, and clinical evolution. J Neuropathol Exp Neurol 2000;59:477-489.

119. Pittock SJ, McClelland RL, Achenbach SJ, et al: Clinical course, pathological correlations, and outcome of biopsy proved inflammatory demyelinating disease. Neurol Neurosurg Psychiatry 2005; 76:1693-1697.

120. Omuro AM, Leite CC, Mokhtari K, et al: Pitfalls in the diagnosis of brain tumours. Lancet Neurol 2006;5:937-948.

121. Simos M, Dimitrios P, Philip T: A new clinical entity mimicking meningioma diagnosed pathologically as Rosai-Dorfman disease. Skull Base Surg 1998;8:87-92.

122. Gupta DK, Suri A, Mahapatra AK, et al: Intracranial Rosai-Dorfman disease in a child mimicking bilateral giant petroclival meningiomas: A case report and review of literature. Childs Nerv Syst 2006;22:1194-1200.

123. Bhandari A, Patel PR, Patel MP: Extranodal Rosai-Dorfman disease with multiple spinal lesions: A rare presentation. Surg Neurol 2006;65:308-311.

124. Lopez P, Estes ML: Immunohistochemical characterization of the histiocytes in sinus histiocytosis with massive lymphadenopathy: Analysis of an extranodal case. Hum Pathol 1989;20:711-715.

125. Gaitonde S: Multifocal, extranodal sinus histiocytosis with massive lymphadenopathy: An overview. Arch Pathol Lab Med 2007; 131:1117-1121.

126. Bruno MC, Ginguené C, Santangelo M, et al: Lymphoplasmacyte rich meningioma: A case report and review of the literature. J Neurosurg Sci 2004;48:117-124.

127. Favara BE, Feller AC, Pauli M, et al: Contemporary classification of histiocytic disorders: The WHO Committee on Histiocytic/Reticulum Cell Proliferations, Reclassification Working Group of the Histiocyte Society. Med Pediatr Oncol 1997;29:157-166.

128. Favara BE, Jaffe R: The histopathology of Langerhans cell histiocytosis. Br J Cancer Suppl 1994;23:S17-S23.

129. Favara BE: Langerhans' cell histiocytosis pathobiology and pathogenesis. Semin Oncol 1991;18:3-7.

130. Oksanen V, Fyhrquist F, Somer H, et al: Angiotensin converting enzyme in cerebrospinal fluid: A new assay. Neurology 1985; 35:1220-1223.

131. Baudin B: [Angiotensin 1-converting enzyme (ACE) for sarcoidosis diagnosis]. Pathol Biol (Paris) 2005;53:183-188.

132. Cahill DW, Salcman M: Neurosarcoidosis: A review of the rarer manifestations. Surg Neurol 1981;15:204-211.

133. Scott TF: Neurosarcoidosis: Progress and clinical aspects. Neurology 1993;43:8-12.

134. Stern BJ, Krumholz A, Johns C, et al: Sarcoidosis and its neurological manifestations. Arch Neurol 1985;42:909-917.

135. Kato T, Hoshi K, Sekijima Y, et al: Rheumatoid meningitis: An autopsy report and review of the literature. Clin Rheumatol 2003;22:475-480.

136. Starosta MA, Brandwein SR: Clinical manifestations and treatment of rheumatoid pachymeningitis. Neurology 2007;68:1079-1080.

137. Gutenberg A, Hans V, Puchner MJ, et al: Primary hypophysitis: Clinical-pathological correlations. Eur J Endocrinol 2006;155:101-107.

138. Gutenberg A, Buslei R, Fahlbusch R, et al: Immunopathology of primary hypophysitis: Implications for pathogenesis. Am J Surg Pathol 2005;29:329-338.

139. Kiaer W, Norgaard JO: Granulomatous hypophysitis and thyroiditis with lymphocytic adrenalitis. Acta Pathol Microbiol Scand 1969;76:229-238.

140. Perfect JR, Casadevall A: Cryptococcosis. Infect Dis Clin North Am 2002;16:837-874.

141. Marton KI Gean AD: The spinal tap: A new look at an old test. Ann Intern Med 1986;104:840-848.

142. Shen CC, Cheng WY, Yang MY: Isolated intramedullary cryptococcal granuloma of the conus medullaris: Case report and review of the literature. Scand J Infect Dis 2006;38:562-565.

143. Black KE, Baden LR: Fungal infections of the CNS: Treatment strategies for the immunocompromised patient. CNS Drugs 2007;21:293-318.

144. Schmidt-Hieber M, Zweigner J, Uharek L, et al: Central nervous system infections in immunocompromised patients: Update on diagnostics and therapy. Leuk Lymphoma 2009;50:24-36.

145. Jackson AC: Rabies virus infection: An update. J Neurovirol 2003;9:253-258.

146. Mark RE, Young L: Rabies encephalitis in humans: Pathology pathogenesis and pathophysiology. J Neuropathol Exp Neurol 1994;53:1-10.

147. Kristensson K, Dastur DK, Manghani DK, et al: Rabies—Interaction between neurons and viruses: A review of the history of Negri inclusion bodies. Nauropathol Appl Neurobiol 1996; 22:179-187.

148. Johnson RT, Gibbs CJ Jr: Creutzfeldt-Jakob disease and related transmissible spongiform encephalopathies. N Engl J Med 1998;339:1994-2004.

149. Will RG, Ward HJ: Clinical features of variant Creutzfeldt-Jakob disease. Curr Top Microbiol Immunol 2004;284:121-132.

150. Mittal S, Farmer P, Kalina P, et al: Correlation of diffusion-weighted magnetic resonance imaging with neuropathology in Creutzfeldt-Jakob disease. Arch Neurol 2002;59:128-134.

151. Ukisu R, Kushihashi T, Kitanosono T, et al: Serial diffusion-weighted MRI of Creutzfeldt-Jakob disease. AJR Am J Roentgenol 2005;184:560-566.

152. Peden AH, Ironside JW: Review: Pathology of variant Creutzfeldt-Jakob disease. Folia Neuropathol 2004;42(Suppl A):85-91.

153. Will R: Variant Creutzfeldt-Jakob disease. Folia Neuropathol 2004;42(Suppl A):77-83.

154. Parchi P, Giese A, Capellari S, et al: Classification of sporadic Creutzfeldt-Jakob disease based on molecular and phenotypic analysis of 300 subjects. Ann Neurol 1999;46:224-233.

155. Ironside JW, Head MW, Bell JE, et al:. Laboratory diagnosis of variant Creutzfeldt-Jakob disease. Histopathology 2000;37:1-9.

156. Castellani RJ, Colucci M, Xie Z, et al: Sensitivity of 14-3-3 protein test varies in subtypes of sporadic Creutzfeldt-Jakob disease. Neurology 2004;63:436-442.

157. Zeidler M, Green A: Advances in diagnosing Creutzfeldt-Jakob disease with MRI and CSF 14-3-3 protein analysis. Neurology 2004;63:410-411.

158. Siman R, McIntosh TK, Soltesz KM, et al: Proteins released from degenerating neurons are surrogate markers for acute brain damage. Neurobiol Dis 2004;16:311-320.

159. Brown P, Preece M, Brandel JP, et al: Iatrogenic Creutzfeldt-Jakob disease at the millennium. Neurology 2000;55:1075-1081.

160. Brown P, Wolff A, Gajdusek DC: A simple and effective method for inactivating virus infectivity in formalin-fixed tissue samples from patients with Creutzfeldt-Jakob disease. Neurology 1990; 40:887-890.

Skin Infections

Carlos Nicolas Prieto-Granada, Alice Z. C. Lobo, and
Martin C. Mihm, Jr.

19

CHAPTER

Cutaneous infections are very common and can be caused by a variety of different organisms.[1,2] In certain circumstances, more than one organism can be involved. Since the onset of the era of transplantation and the human immunodeficiency virus (HIV) epidemic, many infections have appeared that are novel to humans. In some instances, infections with multiple organisms have occurred, posing a major therapeutic challenge to the infectious disease expert. Furthermore, it is now understood that the skin may exhibit a reaction to different parts of an organism, or display a hypersensitivity reaction to an organism, even without direct infection. This has helped to explain many rashes of previously unknown etiology and also has led to an understanding of the mechanisms of cutaneous disease. Another revelation has been the role of certain viral diseases with endotheliotropic propensity to exacerbate connective tissue diseases. This discovery has helped in the management of patients with idiopathic pulmonary fibrosis and in those with lupus erythematosus who faced devastating consequences from parvovirus B19 infection, among others. Their response in some instances to intravenous immunoglobulin G (IgG) has been remarkable.

Therefore, it is clear that a chapter on infectious diseases cannot be simply a descriptive iteration of a disease, its clinical features, and pathogenic agents, but must also illuminate the significance of the infectious agents in the pathogenic hierarchy of the host organism and the host's response to assault by microbes. In each of the following sections, the disorder is described in terms of clinical features, then histopathology, and then etiology and pathogenesis.

Diagnostic Approach

The approach to the patient with a suspected infection, no matter how trivial it may seem, requires a complete history and physical examination to rule out an underlying condition that may exacerbate or lead to the infection. An example is the patient with undiscovered diabetes who has persistent folliculitis. Much less obvious is the patient who is taking one of the newer antipsoriasis medications that lowers resistance to infection. Even more enigmatic is the patient presenting with recurrent diarrhea who is a carrier of an enterovirus and is intermittently symptomatic. After this background work has been performed, one can begin to make a clinical diagnosis and go on to work up the infection. The remainder of this chapter addresses the various types of cutaneous infections.

Bacterial Infections of the Skin

Once an appropriate inquiry and examination has taken place and an infection is established, the next step is to try to identify the organism. The easiest method for pathologists is to stain the tissue and look for organisms. However, one must be careful in evaluating the skin for bacterial organisms because of the resident flora of the skin. For example, in a hair follicle, one can find not only *Demodex folliculorum* mites but also yeast forms of *Pityrosporum*, gram-positive cocci, and coccobacilli that are normal corynebacterial and staphylococcal organisms in these structures. On the other hand, the presence of gram-positive cocci outside the follicles in the dermis or fat can be evidence of a very serious infection such as cellulitis or even fasciitis. Bacterial infections can be secondary to another, underlying infection or to a non-infectious condition of the skin. As the clinician must also think of underlying causes or other infections, so must the pathologist be aware of how widespread secondary bacterial infections are. For example, a Majocchi granuloma caused principally by a dermatophyte can become secondarily infected and be mistaken for a bacterial folliculitis. In the scalp, persons with seborrheic dermatitis can develop secondary bacterial infections that render the dermatitis more difficult to treat. In patients with immunosuppression, one must always suspect infections with multiple organisms.

Although stains can be very helpful, the most reliable way to make a definitive diagnosis of a skin infection is by culture. However, culture, by itself, is not always reliable. As stated by Rapini, fewer than 10% of cultures are positive in infectious cellulitis.[1] Swab cultures should be used only for the most superficial types of bacterial infections, such as impetigo or ecthyma. They are useless in deep infections such as cellulitis or panniculitis. In these instances, the best approach is to culture the tissue directly. Optimally, a biopsy should be taken, with at least half of the specimen saved for routine processing and diagnostic microscopy. The other half should be transported immediately to the laboratory, where it will be appropriately dissected into small pieces and placed on the culture medium. Desiccation of the tissue ensures a negative culture. If there is a chance of delay in getting tissue to the laboratory, the tissue may be transported on sterile, normal saline–soaked gauze.

Touch preparations may be used in special cases. For example, in chancroid or in granuloma inguinale, positivity is very infrequently found in tissue-stained samples. Touch preparations are extremely useful in infections with acid-fast organisms. In expert hands, touch preparations of traumatized ear lobe from patients with lepromatous or borderline lepromatous leprosy can yield a very good estimate of the number of beaded bacteria. The Fite stain is particularly useful in identifying the Hansen bacillus (Fig. 19-1). Auramine fluorescence is also useful.

More recent methods using immunoperoxidase stains and molecular biologic techniques, such as evaluation of tissue by the polymerase chain reaction (PCR) and in situ hybridization, have proved to be very useful. Their use is not yet widespread but can be obtained in many instances by contacting the U.S. Centers for Disease Control and Prevention (CDC). Many of the academic centers in the United States are also developing at least the immunoperoxidase techniques for identifying organisms.

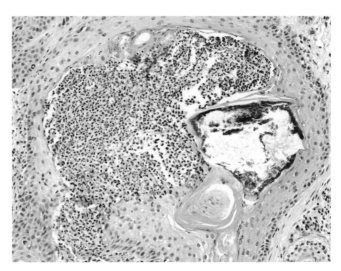

Figure 19-1. Bacterial folliculitis. There is a marked accumulation of neutrophils in response to proliferation of gram-positive bacteria in the follicular infundibulum.

Reaction Patterns in Bacterial Skin Infections

The overwhelming number of bacterial infections produce a neutrophilic infiltrate (see Fig. 19-1). If they are subcorneal, they are designated as subcorneal abscesses, the most common cause of which is impetigo. If they form abscesses that replace the epidermis, they are called ecthyma. If they are in the dermis, they are called cellulitis; in the panniculus, a suppurative reaction or panniculitis; and in the fascia, neutrophilic, suppurative, or necrotizing fasciitis, depending on the extent and the clinical presentation.

As neutrophilic infections become more chronic, they exhibit plasma cells. Very rarely do infections, except for syphilis and other treponemal infections, cause a predominantly plasma cell infiltrate. Infiltrates may be superficial and deep, involving vessels with prominent endothelial swelling and showing perineural inflammation. Only a few bacteria are associated with lymphocytes, the principal one being the agent of Lyme disease. There are admixed plasma cells with this infiltrate, which is also superficial and deep and can show involvement of nerves. In addition, one must always remember that 40% of early secondary lues is associated with lymphocytes.

Some bacteria induce the formation of granulomas, *Mycobacterium tuberculosis* being an excellent example. However, *M. tuberculosis* infection begins as a neutrophilic cellulitis that goes on gradually to be infiltrated by lymphocytes and, finally, by monocyte-macrophages that form a granuloma, resulting from a type IV hypersensitivity response.

Specific Disorders

Impetigo

Impetigo affects mainly children, commonly around the mouth, the nose, and the groin, often after trauma. The lesions occur acutely. They are most commonly crusted and have been described as exhibiting a honey-colored crust.[3] There is a bullous form in which lesions 1 to 2 cm in size appear, especially below

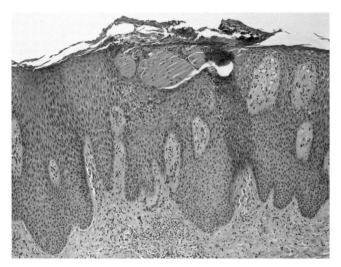

Figure 19-2. Impetiginized eczema. There is prominent spongiosis and a scale crust that shows evidence of superinfection and corneal microabscess formation.

the nose and in the groin and upper thighs.[4] These lesions are not pustular but are clearly bullous.

Impetigo frequently occurs in a setting of other dermatoses. For example, eczematous dermatitis commonly becomes infected, especially when weeping begins. Honey-colored crusts are the hallmark of this complication.

The acute lesion consists of a subcorneal blister in which there are varying numbers of neutrophils. Wherever neutrophils appear in a subcorneal bulla, there are always variable numbers of acantholytic cells. Especially if there are acantholytic dendritic cells, the diagnosis of pemphigus foliaceus must be excluded. A Gram stain can demonstrate the presence of organisms confirming the diagnosis of impetigo. If doubt persists, immunofluorescence studies may be necessary to resolve the diagnostic dilemma. If there has been a preceding eczematous response, the eczematized tissue will reveal a prominent scale crust (Fig 19-2). There are no spongiform pustules to help rule out the diagnosis of pustular psoriasis. Rather, the neutrophils infiltrate in scattered fashion below the crusted area.

The etiology of impetigo includes, in many instances, a prior trauma. Poor hygiene in children, hot and humid weather, and occlusive clothing with sweating all appear to contribute to the process. The organisms most commonly involved are *Staphylococcus aureus* and *Streptococcus pyogenes*. Each of these can cause the lesion,[5] but the most common cause of bullous impetigo is the phage group II of *S. aureus*.

Strains have been proven to elaborate the A and B types of exfoliative toxins that result in the subcorneal bulla. These toxins act on desmoglein 1, the target of antibodies in pemphigus foliaceus, rather than desmoglein 3.[6,7] The streptococcus-induced forms have been associated with glomerulonephritis in rare instances. For this reason, many clinicians treat impetigo with oral antibiotics in addition to topical care.

Staphylococcal Scalded-Skin Syndrome

The staphylococcal scalded-skin syndrome (SSSS) begins with the appearance of bright red skin around the head and neck, which most commonly goes on to blister.[8] This disorder affects

children mainly before 5 years of age and can appear perinatally. The bright erythema of the head and neck gradually spreads to the trunk, the axillae, the groin, and then the extremities. The source of infection is usually occult; conjunctivitis, groin or nostril infection, or even gastrointestinal or urinary tract infection may be the origin. Patients develop constitutional symptoms as the lesions progress. Mortality in children is usually low, except in neonates. In adults, mortality can be as high as 60%, and the disorder is often associated with kidney failure or other debilitating illness.[9,10] Clinically, adults with SSSS present with desquamation of the skin, not blistering.[9]

This condition differs from a disease called staphylococcal scarlet fever, in which there is severe desquamation without blistering. The latter disorder also has circulating enterotoxins and may represent a form of toxic shock syndrome.[11]

The major differential diagnostic consideration is toxic epidermal necrolysis (TEN). In this disorder, there is sloughing of the skin due to full-thickness necrosis of the epidermis. It can involve the entire skin and the oral, conjunctival, and genital mucosae. Frozen-section diagnosis is usually conclusive. One need only take a Q tip and roll up the sloughed skin. In SSSS, one sees only stratum corneum with a rare keratinocyte, as opposed to the full-thickness necrotic skin observed in TEN. Bullous impetigo is probably a localized form of SSSS. In this instance, the bacteria proliferate at the site. In SSSS, the proliferation is at a distant site.

The pathologic changes are minimal but distinctive. Because there has been enzymatic dissection of the stratum corneum, there is a very regular, smooth surface of keratinocytes that is associated with a rare acantholytic cell. There is no hint of dyskeratosis to suggest pemphigus foliaceus, nor of inflammation to indicate impetigo.

The causative agent of toxic SSSS can be bacterial or viral. Even varicella and measles have been known to give rise to this syndrome. The syndrome is caused by the production of exfoliative exotoxins A or B and is frequently associated with a specific strain of *S. aureus*, namely the phage type II group, especially type 71.[12] These toxins target desmoglein 1, the same antigen targeted by autoantibodies in bullous impetigo and in pemphigus foliaceus.[7]

The toxin is not excreted by the kidneys in children until they mature. In adults, there must be at least some impairment of kidney function or other debilitating disease that impedes release of the toxin.[10]

Toxic Shock Syndrome

In toxic shock syndrome, a strikingly ill patient presents acutely high fever and a very diffuse rash with brightly erythematous patches that resembles sunburn. This rash subsequently desquamates, and marked desquamation of the palms and soles may occur. The patient also experiences nausea with vomiting and diarrhea, headache, and possibly vertigo. Marked hypotension is usually present as another indication of multiple system involvement. This syndrome was first described in association with tampon use.[13] The causative organisms grew in the vagina in the proteinaceous menstruum.[13,14] To date, a significant number of cases have been associated with other infections, including abscesses, wound infections, and other systemic infections.[15] Culture typically reveals a phage group I strain of *S. aureus*, although other staphylococcal organisms may be involved. Streptococcal disease can also cause this reaction, in which case it is called streptococcal toxic shock syndrome (STSS).[5,16,17]

Skin changes vary and include, at first, a mild, spongiotic reaction, with intraepidermal lymphocytes and neutrophils overlying dermal edema, and a perivenular lymphoid infiltrate with scattered neutrophils and red blood cells. The presence of a few aggregates of neutrophils in the epidermis, with dyskeratotic cells, may indicate TSS as the correct diagnosis. In the most florid reaction, there is a pustular vasculitis, with a neutrophilic abscess in the subcorneal space, in the epidermis, beneath the epidermis, or in the follicular orifice or the sweat gland pore. In addition, in the dermis, either necrotizing vasculitis with focal fibrinoid necrosis of vessels or a Sweet-like reaction may take place. The latter exhibits endothelial cell swelling and a perivascular lymphocytic infiltrate admixed with occasional neutrophils and eosinophils. There is no evidence of fibrinoid necrosis, but there is definite extravasation of red blood cells. Pustular vasculitis may be seen in other septic conditions, including deep fungal infections as well as connective tissue diseases, Behçet disease, and other infections. Drug eruptions can also manifest with similar histologic changes.

As mentioned earlier, the causative agent was originally described as an *S. aureus* of the phage group I, the toxin of which causes the syndrome. Other types of staphylococcal and streptococcal organisms have also been described. The causative toxin or endotoxin is definitely different from the one that causes SSSS. It is clear that the toxins represent a class of superantigens. These protein molecules do not react with a focal receptor, as is the case with most antigens, and as is seen in the typical major histochemical complex (MHC) class II presentation; rather, they react with the entire variable (V) portion of the T-cell β-receptors.[18,19] This interaction results in a florid immunologic response including secretion of many cytokines. Particularly noteworthy is the release of interleukin 1 and tumor necrosis factor (TNF).[19] This massive release of active cytokines results in TSS and also explains the success of intravenous IgG therapy in some cases.[20]

Ecthyma

Ecthyma, like impetigo, favors children and can similarly affect the occlusive areas of the body. It appears as a well-demarcated ulcer filled with purulent material. There is often a crust overlying the lesion. Ecthyma resembles any type of inflamed, infected skin lesion with crusting. Culture is the best manner of diagnosing the exact cause of the lesion.

The lesion usually has a sharply demarcated border in which aggregates of neutrophils are present in the center of the lesion and diffusely throughout the superficial dermis. There is frequently a neutrophil-impregnated crust (Fig. 19-3). Bacteria can often be visualized using tissue Gram stain.

Ecthyma has features similar to those of impetigo as far as the organisms and pathogenesis are concerned. However, the causative organism is usually *S. pyogenes*. Often, culture reveals mixed staphylococcal and streptococcal infections.

Ecthyma Gangrenosum

This lesion begins with a red macule or papule and progresses rapidly to a pustule or bulla in a very sick, often immunosup-

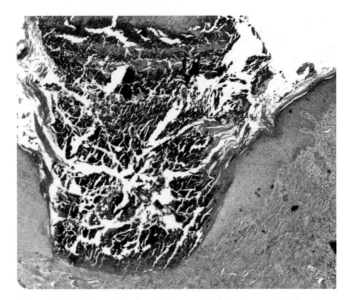

Figure 19-3. Ecthyma. This sharply demarcated ulcer, characteristic of ecthyma, contains purulent material and bacterial colonies.

pressed patient. It then progresses to become a bulla and/or directly ulcerates, with formation of a black eschar. In some patients, multiple lesions develop. The involved infecting organism is classically *Pseudomonas aeruginosa*.[21] The history and physical features are classic and are considered to portend a serious prognosis unless treated adequately and promptly. Even with proper treatment, the mortality rate is high.

The histologic changes are quite characteristic in the classic case. They include an ulcerated, necrotic epidermis with a fibrin-laden base filled with debris overlying a pauci-inflammatory vasculopathy or vasculitis with minimal perivascular neutrophils and sometimes lymphocytes. In addition, one may see clusters of gram-negative rods in the vessel wall and surrounding the vessels. The principal differential is indicated by the presence of a fungal organism, such as *Zygomycetes* spp., that can also cause necrosis and vasculitis. Appropriate stains aid in diagnosis.

The lesion usually appears in a severely debilitated or immunosuppressed patient who is septic. The offending organism in the classic case is *P. aeruginosa*.[22] Other organisms have been implicated. Usually, these patients have an underlying mild coagulopathy that sets the stage for the thrombotic septic changes that occur. The lesional history is characteristic, with lesions appearing in 12 hours or less. The eschar or crust has been referred to as a sphacelus.

Erysipelas

The infection known as erysipelas was recognized by the ancient Greeks. It manifests with a characteristic rapid swelling almost always affecting the face.[23,24] It is bright red and markedly edematous, with a well-demarcated, advancing border. In some areas, the swelling is so marked that blisters or bullae appear. Caused most commonly by *S. pyogenes*, it is associated with marked symptoms of malaise, fever, vomiting, and high temperatures. Cultures are only rarely positive.[23] Detection of elevated anti-streptolysin O or anti-DNAase B in the patient's

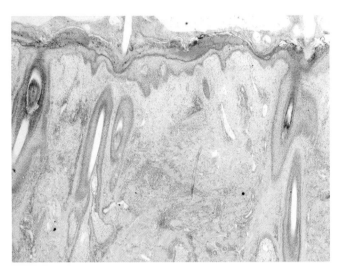

Figure 19-4. Erysipelas. Note the diffuse edema of the papillary and reticular dermis with extensive diffuse infiltration by neutrophils.

serum is useful; however, the clinical symptomatology is so striking and characteristic. Prompt treatment is necessary, because a small percentage of patients develop bacteremia. Erysipelas can be recurrent and can be associated with diabetes.

Other diseases, such as a severe contact dermatitis, photoallergy, or even lupus erythematosus, may resemble this infection, but the lesions of erysipelas have a more specific distribution pattern; in contrast to contact dermatitis or photoallergy, patients usually lack severe fever and constitutional symptoms.

This lesion is a classic example of severe cellulitis. There is marked edema in all compartments of the skin (Fig. 19-4). At the least, there is epidermal intercellular edema, but in more severe cases, subepidermal bullae can appear. The papillary and reticular dermal fibers are markedly separated and, due to fibrin exudation, may have a more bluish, less refractory character. Lymphatics are dilated. There is also edema of the subcutis, with small zones of fat necrosis caused by a relative ischemia. Scattered throughout the edematous areas are neutrophils and neutrophilic debris. There is no particular perivascular localization. Bacteria are difficult to observe in this lesion. In cellulitis of other types, bacteria may be easily demonstrable with Gram staining, especially in the presence of immunosuppression.

As indicated, the pathogenic agent is a streptococcal organism. The streptolysin elaborated by the bacteria results in dissection of the tissue.

Erysipeloid Lesion

The erysipeloid lesion was so named because it resembles erysipelas, with prominent edema and a well-demarcated border. However, it is less severe and affects mainly the fingers. It occurs principally in fishermen and in persons who handle fish or other animal tissues. The infectious agent is *Erysipelothrix rhusiopathiae*, also known as *Erysipelothrix insidiosa*. Usually, a bluish or erythematous macule appears and then extends. As the lesion gradually increases in size, it develops a well-defined border. With slow extension, there tends to be central clearing. In con-

trast to erysipelas, the lesion is much less edematous and erythematous, and there are less marked constitutional symptoms. If the clinician suspects the diagnosis, an attempt should be made to culture the lesion. The use of minced tissue guarantees the best return. Other types of cellulitis may resemble this infection on the hands, especially those caused by staphylococcal and streptococcal organisms. Brucellosis also affects the hands of persons who are in contact with animal tissues, but it is clinically different, with multiple papules and pustules. Anthrax and tularemia both ulcerate. Because other organisms can cause hand infections, culture of the tissue is imperative. Cultures of *E. rhusiopathiae* can resemble other gram-positive infections, so it is important to communicate the suspected diagnosis to the laboratory personnel.

The changes of the erysipeloid lesion include marked dermal edema with scattered neutrophils infiltrating between the collagen bundles. Lymphatics are dilated. The changes are much less severe than in erysipelas. In this disorder, lymphocytes and plasma cells can be frequently observed. There is no vasculitis and no perivascular prominence of the infiltrate. The organisms are very difficult, if not impossible, to recognize in tissue with Gram stain.

The causative organism grows in decaying animal tissues and causes infection after an injury. The causative organism *E. rhusiopathiae* grows in ordinary culture medium. Culture is most successful if a biopsy of the border of the lesion is submitted after mincing of the tissue.

Cellulitis, Including Perianal Streptococcal Dermatitis

Clinical Features

Cellulitis is a general term that refers to an inflammation of the skin that manifests as a red, brightly erythematous macule or plaque or as an indurated nodule or plaque that is warm and usually tender. It thus qualifies for the ancient definition of infection: tumor, dolor, calor, and rubor. As the lesions become more chronic, scaling, bullae, and even ulceration may appear. Lymphangitis and even lymphadenopathy are sometimes present. The most common causative organisms in the immunocompetent patient are *S. aureus* and group A streptococci. In the immune-suppressed patient, there are many other possible causative organisms. A distinctive type of perianal cellulitis that exhibits the characteristic features of cellulitis is termed perianal streptococcal "dermatitis" or "cellulitis." In human or animal bites, unusual oral flora can cause disease.

Histology

The previous description of cellulitis summarizes the findings. There is diffuse dermal and subcuticular edema with a diffuse infiltrate of neutrophils. Depending on the degree of edema, there can be vascular ectasia with extravasation of red blood cells. Dilated lymphatics are also observed and are a clue to the nature of the process. Organisms are almost impossible to observe, even with appropriate stains.

In the more chronic lesions, the epidermis may show spongiosis with intraepidermal vesicles and even ulceration and necrosis. Likewise, intraepidermal pustules may be noted. In extensive disease, neutrophil-rich areas may give the appearance of vasculitis; such vascular involvement is considered secondary to the cellulitis. In very chronic lesions, fibrosis may also be noted in reaction to the zones of necrosis. Culture of tissue is necessary to identify the organisms.

In cases of marked cellulitis with neutrophils, the question of neutrophilic dermatoses is raised. The latter lesions differ by their clinical presentation, often by the patterns of neutrophilic infiltration, and by negativity of tissue cultures.

Etiology and Pathogenesis

As indicated earlier, the most common causes of cellulitis are *S. aureus* and group A streptococci. However, in the immunosuppressed patient one may find acid-fast organisms, fungi, and a variety of bacteria, including *Klebsiella*, *Proteus*, *Clostridium*, cryptococcal organisms, other yeasts, and even amebas. The pathologist must be aware of the possibility of finding these many diverse organisms. Immunosuppressed patients may have multiple infections, presenting a challenge to pathologist and clinician.

One pediatric type of cellulitis that should be emphasized is the facial or periorbital cellulitis that is caused by *Hemophilus influenzae* type B. This infection occurs in the first years of life.

Necrotizing Fasciitis

Necrotizing fasciitis is an often extremely destructive infection that occurs acutely in the fascia and the soft tissues, with a very rapid course, resulting in extensive necrosis of the tissue. It usually occurs in a background of peripheral vascular disease, diabetes, chronic alcoholism, or drug abuse[25] but can occur spontaneously in otherwise healthy young patients. There is often a history of injury.

Three types of necrotizing fasciitis have been described. Type I is a mixed infection.[25,26] Type II is caused by either *S. aureus* or group A streptococci.[16,26,27] Type III is the most destructive type and often occurs after an injury or puncture wound. Its cause is the *Vibrio* group of organisms, such as *Vibrio vulnificans*.[27] Because these infections are all so virulent, intense antibiotic therapy and radical surgical débridement are often necessary to save the life of the patient.[28] Clinically, the lesions manifest as rapidly progressive, painful areas of marked induration and erythema. Blisters and ulceration develop quickly with the extensive necrosis. The mortality rate is approximately 50%.

In contrast to the other types of cellulitis, this process involves the dermis and subcutis, but the most necrotizing areas are in the fascia and deep soft tissues, where extensive hemorrhage, necrosis, thrombosis, and secondary vasculitis are observed.

Numerous organisms can cause necrotizing fasciitis in addition to *S. aureus* and group A streptococci. These include *Proteus* spp. and, very importantly, anaerobes such as the clostridial organisms, *Bacteroides* spp., *Peptostreptococcus* spp., and the marine group of *Vibrio* species.[26,27]

Pyoderma Vegetans (Blastomycosis-Like Pyoderma)

The lesion of pyoderma vegetans manifests as one or more verrucous plaques that are studded with pustules and exhibit sinus tracts. The most common sites of involvement are the axillae and groin and the lower extremities. There is a facial variant that can be markedly disfiguring. The most common infectious cause of this disorder is considered to be *S. aureus*, although a few other bacteria have been described.[29,30] It also occurs as a variant of

pyoderma gangrenosum associated with inflammatory bowel disease.[31]

Marked pseudoepitheliomatous hyperplasia is associated with hyperkeratosis and parakeratosis and multiple intraepidermal abscesses. There are also dermal abscesses. A perivenular infiltrate of lymphocytes, histiocytes, neutrophils, and occasional eosinophils is present. Scattered granulomas may also be observed.

There are two important differential diagnoses: infection, especially deep fungal infection, and pemphigus vegetans. The former is ruled out by the absence of organisms; the latter, by the absence of acantholysis.

This lesion was originally confused with pemphigus vegetans. Pyoderma vegetans exhibits histologically unequivocal acantholysis, often only in the deeper regions of the proliferated epidermis. It is clear that staphylococcal organisms play some role, at least in the variant not associated with inflammatory bowel disease. Further work must be carried out to understand the pathogenic role of the microorganism.

Corynebacterial Infections

The bacteria of the genus *Corynebacterium* are rodlike or coccobacillary and may form filaments. These lesions are relatively uncommon but have important distinctive features.[32,33]

Diphtheria

Once common in the United States, diphtheria has virtually disappeared because of the immunization program that is required of almost all children and adults. The rare cases that occur may be a result of altered immunity in older persons or infection acquired during surgery. The infection is localized to the skin and mucosae or to a wound site. Recent epidemics have occurred among older people.

The very characteristic, gray-colored pseudomembrane on the tonsils and pharynx is the most common sign of the infection. Any systemic involvement is associated with the production of toxin by the bacteria. When diphtheria appears in the skin elsewhere, it is usually as a superinfection of preexisting disorders such as eczema or scabies or as a secondary infection of a wound. The wound site shows a membrane, and there is hypesthesia of the area around the wound due to the toxin. Similar changes occur in areas of eczema or scabetic nodules that have been superinfected by the bacteria. The differential diagnosis includes other lesions with a membrane (e.g., anthrax), some ischemic ulcers, and ulcers caused by vasculitis or nodular lymphomatous infiltrates, as well as the primary lesion of typhus.

The principal change noted is an ulcer covered by a dense fibrin mesh that contains a foreign material and debris. Neutrophils may be present on the surface of the ulcer. If the diphtheria occurs secondary to another infection or lesion, evidence of the prior dermatosis will also be seen. The diagnosis is histologically confirmed by the identification of gram-positive rods of *C. diphtheriae*.

One should consider diphtheria in the presence of any ulcer covered by an apparent sphacelus or densely adherent membrane. The toxin has a neurologic effect, with diminution of sensation in the area bathed by it. Appropriate cultures can be done only if the laboratory is alerted to the possible diagnosis and uses the appropriate medium (i.e., Löffler medium).

Erythrasma

Erythrasma is associated with a variety of corynebacteria, the most common being *Corynebacterium minutissimum*.[34,35] These organisms can also cause trichomycosis and pitted keratolysis. This interesting entity is associated with the presence of characteristic patches of brown, dusky discoloration in the groin, the axillae, and the inframammary regions. Sometimes they also are found between the toes. There may be scaling. A diagnostic test involves a Wood light examination, which reveals a characteristic coral-red fluorescence.

A very characteristic picture is seen in which there is virtually no host response but the changes are limited to the stratum corneum. One can often see the coccobacillary and filamentous bacterial structures on hematoxylin and eosin (H&E) examination. The cells are gram positive and also stain with periodic acid–Schiff (PAS), Grocott methenamine silver (GMS), and Giemsa stains.[36]

These organisms require moist areas of the body, where they infect the stratum corneum. Other disorders that should be considered include superficial fungal infections, yeast infections, and intertrigo. However, the coral-red color induced by the Wood light is specific for erythrasma. On light microscopy, the yeast and dermatophyte organisms are much larger than the bacteria.

Trichomycosis

Trichomycosis is caused by a variety of bacteria. The most commonly implicated organism is *Corynebacterium tenuis*. The appearance of yellow to white or even black and red nodules on axillary and pubic hairs is characteristic.[37] These concretions appear to be caused by substances from the organism or by aggregation and drying of apocrine sweat. The diagnosis of this lesion is made clinically.

Filamentous and coccobacillary corynebacteria are present within the nodules on the hair. They are visible with H&E but are best seen with Giemsa stain.

As indicated earlier, the concretions are formed as a combination of secreted material from the organism or drying and aggregation of contents of apocrine sweat. Other concretions on the hairs include the so-called white and black piedra. Black piedra occurs on the scalp. It is caused by *Piedraia hortae*. White piedra occurs on the scalp, mustache, and groin hair. The causative organism is *Trichosporum cutaneum*.

Pitted Keratolysis

Species of *Corynebacterium* as well as other organisms, including *Actinomyces* spp., can result in the superficial disorder of the skin known as pitted keratolysis.[38,39] The stratum corneum on the soles appears macerated and exhibits small (1.0-2.0 mm) pits. These also are odoriphores.

Numerous coccobacillary and filamentous forms are found in the stratum corneum. They can be seen with H&E staining but are best observed with Gram, PAS, GMS, or Giemsa stain. There is no host response.

Prolonged occlusion of the feet associated with heat and subsequent moisture accumulation is the background necessary for this disorder to occur. The organisms produce an enzyme that is responsible for the formation of the pits by protein digestion. Because of the location on the feet, the maceration, and the odoriferous quality of the lesion, pitted keratolysis can usually be distinguished from pits on the palms and soles caused by Darier disease or possibly basal cell nevus syndrome.

Neisserial Infections

Neisserial organisms are responsible for two relatively common and potentially debilitating and fatal infections. Both organisms can be associated with epidemics. *Neisseria meningitidis* is associated with meningitis that occurs more commonly in children, and *Neisseria gonorrhoeae* is associated with a venereal disease.

Meningococcal Infection

N. meningitidis can be found in the throats of a small number of asymptomatic persons who are carriers.[40] The disease is spread by the respiratory route. It may occur as isolated cases or in sporadic epidemics. Patients who develop meningococcal septicemia are usually severely ill with high fever and exhibit a variety of skin lesions, including papules, nodules, and ecchymoses. The earliest lesions may be petechial and can lead to a correct diagnosis clinically.[41,42] A devastating complication of the disease is associated with adrenocortical insufficiency and shock. This symptom complex is known as the Waterhouse-Friderichsen syndrome. The organism can be identified easily in patients with meningitis from the blood and spinal fluid as well as from the skin in a significant number of patients. Chronic meningococcemia is associated with recurrent episodes of fever and arthritis. Especially noteworthy is the presence of petechiae and papulopustules that occur on the lower extremities during these episodes.[43,44]

The histopathology varies according to the stage of the disease. In patients with the fulminant form, microthrombi are almost always present in dermal vessels. At times, one can also find necrotizing vasculitis with or without thrombi and pustular thrombi. Pustular vasculitis includes an intraepidermal or intrafollicular or subepidermal abscess with extensive vasculopathy and vasculitis of vessels throughout the dermis. The picture of microthrombi with necrotizing vasculitis must always raise the possibility of a septic process as well. The chronic form of meningococcemia exhibits a relatively paucicellular type of vasculitis associated with perivascular neutrophils and lymphocytes and debris. There is also necrotizing fibrinoid necrosis.

The pathogenesis of the Waterhouse-Friderichsen syndrome is usually associated with disseminated intravascular coagulation leading to vasomotor collapse. Also, the bacterial wall glycoproteins serve as antigens, leading to immune complex formation. The organisms may be found in the cytoplasm of infected endothelial cells, in the neutrophils, and in extracellular locations. The shock-like events appear to be a result of specific thrombosis of the pulmonary microvasculature. The thrombi appear to be due to the effect of toxins elaborated by the bacteria, which cause aggregation of fibrin and neutrophils. The pulmonary infection and vascular compromise result in cor pulmonale. This event does not respond to heparinization. On the other hand, another meningococcal endotoxin may result in disseminated intravascular coagulation in which one finds pure fibrin thrombi. This form of the disease is treatable by heparin. The acute phase of meningococcemia can resemble the effects of other infective agents, such as viruses, gonococcemia, and other gram-negative organisms. Evaluation with appropriate cultures is indicated. The chronic form requires ruling out other causes of necrotizing vasculitis such as Henoch-Schönlein syndrome, Still disease, and connective tissue diseases.

Gonococcal Infection

The venereal disease called gonorrhea manifests differently in men than in women. Women most commonly have endocervicitis, whereas men develop an acute urethritis with definite painful micturition. They also can develop proctitis or oral pharyngitis.[45]

A common presentation of gonococcal septicemia includes the presence of scattered hemorrhagic pustules that are usually few in number but sometimes manifest as a folliculitis or even with bullae formation. This lesion is therefore one of the causes of the dermatitis arthritis syndromes. The *Neisseria* species are incapable of invading intact skin, so the presence of pustules and vasculitis implies disseminated disease. The classic gonococcal picture in the skin is a pustule surrounded by an erythematous ring associated with arthritis and tendonitis.[46,47] The differential diagnosis includes, importantly, Reiter syndrome, because of the urethritis, as well as meningococcemia and other bacteremias.

The histopathology of the characteristic pustule is that of pustular vasculitis with intraepidermal subcorneal intrafollicular or subepidermal abscesses associated with diffuse vasculitis and vasculopathy throughout the dermis. Lesions that resemble cellulitis have a much more diffuse picture without vascular prominence. A simple test to confirm the diagnosis involves performing a Gram stain on a smear of one of the pustular lesions.

As indicated, neisserial organisms cannot invade the intact skin. Therefore, the presence of skin lesions definitely implies a systemic disorder. The pustular event and development of vasculitis can be similar to those described for meningococcemia.

Mycobacterial Infections

The mycobacteria can be divided into two major groups based on their culture growth and biochemical characteristics. The slow growers include *M. tuberculosis, Mycobacterium avium* and related organisms, *Mycobacterium kansasii, Mycobacterium marinum,* and *Mycobacterium ulcerans.* The rapid growers include *Mycobacterium fortuitum* and *Mycobacterium chelonei.* Another slow grower, *Mycobacterium haemophilum,* has special requirements. Totally separate from this classification is *Mycobacterium leprae,* because it cannot be grown in culture. The bacilli of tuberculosis and leprosy are intracellular parasites. Because they are limited to the tissues of humans and animals, they are transmitted by exposure to afflicted hosts.

The other mycobacteria are present in soil and water. The exposure of persons to these bacteria is widespread but usually is not associated with significant clinical disease. As far as staining characteristics are concerned, these organisms are weakly gram positive and are best identified by techniques that show that they are acid-fast.[2]

Tuberculosis

Primary Inoculation, Tuberculosis Verrucosa Cutis, and Miliary Tuberculosis

M. tuberculosis infection had been well controlled in recent years in North America and Europe, but it has remained a prominent problem in resource-poor countries. Lately, there has been a surge in incidence in developed countries, mainly due to increase in migration of persons from Asia and Africa, where tuberculosis is endemic, as well as increased poverty, increased numbers of refugees from Third World countries, and the HIV pandemic.[48] Although the pulmonary route of infection is the most common, *M. tuberculosis* can also infect the skin.

There are three ways in which the skin can be affected by *M. tuberculosis.*[49] First is direct inoculation, which results in a primary nodule or chancre-like lesion, a verrucous response (so-called tuberculosis verrucosa cutis), or inoculation of the mucosae resulting in tuberculosis cutis orificialis. Second, the infection can be spread from an internal focus, such as the lung, to the skin by a hematogenous route, which results in lesions such as lupus vulgaris or gumma. Finally, infection can occur by direct extension from an underlying infected lymph node that has broken down and caused cutaneous ulceration. This form of tuberculosis is relatively rare in the skin and can occur, for example, as a result of a needle stick injury,[50] by accidental inoculation during an autopsy[51] or a surgical procedure, or even during mouth-to-mouth resuscitation.[52]

In primary inoculation, a nodule usually appears within 2 to 4 weeks and then becomes ulcerated with an overlying crust. The draining lymph nodes become affected and may suppurate. This is the classic chancriform complex that includes an ulcerated nodule with draining lymph nodes. Often, pus can be expressed from the surface. The most common sites of involvement are the hands in adults, but in children the lesions may occur especially in the lower extremities.[49] Tuberculosis verrucosa cutis, which occurs frequently due to needle inoculation during an autopsy, results in an isolated lesion that is verrucous and surrounded by an inflammatory border. Miliary tuberculosis describes infection of the skin by the hematogenous route; it consists of a generalized cutaneous eruption including papules and pustules a few millimeters in diameter.

Inoculated human tissues show a specific series of reactions. First, there is an acute, neutrophil-mediated infiltrate produced while the bacilli are rapidly multiplying. Next, macrophages migrate to the area and phagocytize the bacteria. As the T cells become sensitized, the tuberculous antigens result in cytokine release, which causes activation of macrophages to become epithelioid cells and giant cells. As the host delayed hypersensitivity reaction becomes stronger, necrosis of the aggregates of macrophages occurs and inactivates or indeed kills the offending organisms. A necrotic granuloma is the final picture.[49]

The course after primary inoculation depends on a variety of factors, including the quantity of bacteria, the manner in which the infection occurred, and the patient's immune response. HIV infection or the acquired immunodeficiency syndrome (AIDS), debilitating therapy, and immune dysregulatory drugs, particularly the new TNF inhibitors, can all affect the outcome.[2] Histology of the primary lesion exhibits epidermal ulceration, in the base of which is fibrin and neutrophilic debris. In the dermis, depending on the age of the lesion, there may be only diffuse neutrophils, but as the delayed hypersensitivity response becomes stronger, granulomas form randomly in the dermis. Acid-fast bacilli are usually present and easily demonstrable by special stains.[51]

In tuberculosis verrucosa cutis, there is marked epidermal hyperplasia with prominent hyperkeratosis and papillomatosis. In early lesions, dermal abscesses may be observed, but as the infection progresses, well-formed granulomas with variable necrosis are present. Miliary tuberculosis regularly exhibits a central area of abscess formation in the dermis containing neutrophils, debris, and easily visible tuberculosis bacilli.[1,2,53]

Cutis Orificialis

The lesions of cutis orificialis can occur by direct inoculation of the skin or mucosa or secondarily, in patients who have extensive tuberculosis, for example in the bowel, and are actively excreting bacilli. Patients with disseminated tuberculosis, for example in the colon with lesions that are pouring bacilli into the feces, can eventually develop perianal or perineal ulcers.[54,55]

A superficial ulcer is often present in association with well-formed granulomas; the lesions are profoundly necrotic and extend deep into the skin. Tubercle bacilli are easily demonstrable with appropriate stains.[1,2]

Lupus Vulgaris, Scrofuloderma, and Tuberculous Gumma

The lesions of lupus vulgaris commonly occur on or adjacent to the nose,[1,2,56] and almost always in the head and neck region. The lesions consist of well-formed patches or plaques that on palpation reveal a prominent nodule. The individual lesions may vary from 1.0 mm to a few centimeters. As the lesions progress, areas of atrophy appear. Other areas at the same time may become raised or verrucous. Ulceration occurs in approximately 20% of the lesions and rarely may be associated with squamous cell carcinoma.[57] Scrofuloderma refers to an ulceration of the skin overlying a tuberculous lymph node or bone. The lesion, at first a nodule, becomes fistulized and ulcerated and exudes purulent material at times. Tuberculous gumma results from hematogenous spread of organisms to the skin. A large dermal and subcutaneous nodule that is partially necrotic gradually appears and can often ulcerate the skin.

Lupus vulgaris characteristically produces numerous granulomas in the upper third to upper half of the dermis, where they abut the dermal epidermal interface. Caseation necrosis is focal and sometimes absent.[56] The granulomas contain Langhans giant cells. The inflammation can also extend along hair follicles into the subcutis. The overlying epidermis exhibits atrophy, alternating often with hyperplasia and papillomatosis. Occasionally, squamous cell carcinoma can supervene in areas of hyperplasia.[57] Tubercle bacilli are present in very small numbers and are rarely demonstrable. Patients with this manifestation usually have very intense delayed hypersensitivity reactions to the purified protein derivative (PPD) test.[1,2,49] Scrofuloderma produces a large cutaneous ulcer with abscesses and areas of small, well-formed but edematous granulomas with prominent necrosis. Tubercle bacilli are easily found. Tuberculous gumma exhibits massive caseation necrosis with a rim of tubercles and epithelioid cells and giant cells. There are also often lymphocytes and plasma cells admixed with the giant cells.

Etiology and Pathogenesis of Tuberculosis

Pathogenesis of these lesions directly relates to the degree of immunity of the host. In the naïve host, the first sign of infection is the presence of neutrophils.[2,49] As the delayed hypersensitivity reaction progresses, granulomas occur. The clinical features also reflect hypersensitivity, so that, for example, a person with a fairly established immune response will exhibit a papillary epidermal hyperplasia with a very prominent lymphogranulomatous and neutrophilic infiltrate.

There are many disorders that must be considered in the differential diagnosis because of the variety of different reactions that tuberculosis may cause. One of the most important is sarcoidosis. This disorder usually manifests with so-called naked tubercles without inflammation. However, inflammation can occur in sarcoidosis, so one must be certain of the etiology of the granuloma. Necrosis can also be seen in sarcoidosis, but it is usually fibrinoid rather than the caseating granular type seen in tuberculosis. Silica granulomas and zirconium granulomas can look very much like sarcoidosis. A polarizing light examination of the granulomatous infiltrate should always be performed to rule out a foreign body as the cause of the inflammation. Special stains, including acid-fast stain, PAS, and GMS, must also be performed to rule out other infections.[1,2]

PCR has now been shown to be very useful in demonstrating evidence of tuberculosis bacilli in tissue.[58] Of course, culture should also be performed.[1]

Atypical Mycobacterial Infections

Atypical mycobacteria are acquired by direct inoculation or by bloodborne spread from another infected site.[1,2,59-61] Because these organisms are present in soil, water, and the natural environment, they are found throughout the world.[61] Also, the immunosuppressed states associated with AIDS[62] and iatrogenic causes lead to more frequent infection by these agents. In general, the histopathology of these lesions shares virtually the same spectrum as that of the tuberculosis organism.[63,64] Only a few of these atypical mycobacteria are highlighted here.

Mycobacterium kansasii

The most common presentation after infection by *M. kansasii* is with pulmonary and nodal infections.[65] Skin lesions are rare but can be inoculated.[66] A resultant ulceronodule appears, and multiple lesions may spread along the extremity, similar to sporotrichosis.[67] Histologically, the lesions show acute inflammation associated with some granulomatous response and numerous acid-fast bacilli.[2]

Mycobacterium avium-intracellulare

M. avium-intracellulare infection can occur in children, manifesting as a swollen cervical lymph node or as a cause of pulmonary infection in lungs that have been previously injured or damaged.[68] The onset of HIV/AIDS has led to rather common infections with this organism, manifesting as a variety of cutaneous papules and nodules.[69] The histology varies according to the immune competence of the patient. There may be an acute inflammatory response, a mixed acute and chronic inflammatory response, or a histiocytic infiltrate suggestive of lepromatous leprosy. There are also, at times, lesions that have virtually no inflammation but are teeming with organisms.[70] The index of suspicion of possible infection with these organisms should be very high in patients with HIV/AIDS.

Mycobacterium marinum

The most common cause of infection by *M. marinum* is trauma, typically a minor abrasion incurred while bathing in a swimming pool, lake, or the ocean. However, documented cases have occurred in patients after they cleaned an aquarium in their home.[71] Epidemics can occur if a swimming pool is affected.[72] About 3 weeks after inoculation, rather reddish, sometimes hyperkeratotic, sometimes papillomatous, papulonodules and plaques can occur. Occasionally, ulceration is noted. Prominences of the extremities, hands, and feet are the most affected sites. A sporotrichosis-like spread can occur.[73] Histopathologically, the changes resemble the evolution of tuberculosis infection. In the early lesions, neutrophils and macrophages are found, but as the lesions mature, multinucleate giant cells with small granulomas are noted. In the well-formed lesion, verrucous hyperplasia can be associated with tubercle formation.[74] Acid-fast bacilli are too difficult to observe after the very early infection. The late lesions show virtually no bacilli and must be cultured.

Mycobacterium ulcerans

The Buruli ulcer occurs after direct inoculation or a bite by an aquatic insect. The organism is found near inland lakes and rivers, predominantly in West and Central Africa, Central America, and South Australia.[75-77] The lesion begins as a papulonodule that relatively rapidly progresses to ulceration of the skin, with resultant large subcutaneous effects that undermine the epidermis and extend into fascia and bone.[78] The lesions are usually painless. More rarely, ulcers occur on the trunk or even on the face.[77]

Histopathologically, the first change results in an ischemic alteration of fat and collagen with prominent collagen necrobiosis. There are large aggregates of mycobacteria in the necrotic fat zones. Eventually, there is some neutrophilic infiltration at sites of necrosis, and the vessels exhibit thrombosis. Granulation tissue can be observed in more chronic lesions in the borders of the necrotic fat. If treatment is successful, healing results in scar formation with re-epithelialization. Clumps of bacteria are present in the areas of necrosis.[76,79] This unique organism has a pathogenesis related to a toxin that is a polyketide mycolactone and causes direct extensive necrosis.[80] Healing is associated with the presence of a lymphocyte host response as evidence of delayed hypersensitivity reaction. A recent study showed a correlation between the presence of granulomas, a high expression of interferon-γ, and prognosis.[81] Because these organisms live best in nonoxygenated tissue, hyperbaric chamber therapy has been successful.

Mycobacterium fortuitum-chelonei

Cutaneous infections with unusual features caused by rapidly growing mycobacteria have recently been reported.[82] These lesions manifest as nodules in the dermis and subcutaneous fat. They may be mistaken for erythema nodosum when on the extremities. The patients usually have some immunosuppressive feature, such as prednisone therapy or another immunodeficient state. The dermis and subcutis exhibit mainly a suppurative inflammatory response with focal necrosis and marked karyorrhexis. Pseudocyst formation has also been noted. There is usually little, if any, granulomatous formation. The lesions can be mistaken for a Sweet-like reaction pattern. Organisms are easily visible after staining with acid-fast stains. The Fite stain is sometimes more consistently positive. Reportedly, the organisms are characteristically focally gram-positive. Culture must be performed to rule out other causes of the infection.[1,82]

Leprosy or Hansen Disease

Leprosy, more commonly referred to now as Hansen disease, is worldwide in distribution and affects millions of people.[1,2] It is a disease principally of the skin and the peripheral nerves. The disease is endemic mainly in the sub-Saharan countries in Africa, Brazil, the Indian subcontinent, and Southeast Asia.[83] In the United States, most cases are seen in immigrants. However, cases have been detected in Louisiana[84] and Texas.[85] It is possible that the armadillo (*Dasypus novemcinctus*) is the source of infection for these patients.[86,87]

The mode of transmission in leprosy is unclear. It is hypothesized that the leprosy bacillus enters the environment from the nasal passages, sebum, and saliva of an infected person with limited immunity in whom it has proliferated. Another source may be the soil. There is no evidence that skin-to-skin contact produces infection. Inhalation of the bacteria discharged into the atmosphere from an infected patient results in spread to various organs, particularly the skin and nerves, where the organism then induces a reaction. The extent of the reaction determines the course of leprosy in the patient.[83]

Clinical Features

The Ridley-Jopling classification divides leprosy according to the immune status of the patient. The tuberculoid form occurs in persons who have strong immunity.[88,89] In patients with limited immunity and in those who are anergic, the lepromatous form appears with extensive cutaneous lesions.

In the tuberculoid form, patients have intact immunity and usually exhibit a single lesion or a small cluster of lesions (Fig. 19-5). The anergic patient has diffuse involvement of the skin, which can lead to hypopigmented or erythematous papules, macules, and plaques. The so-called leonine facies, in which there is edema of the face with loss of eyebrows and eyelashes, is an example of severe lepromatous leprosy.

Borderline leprosy is subdivided into borderline lepromatous, borderline tuberculoid, and pure borderline forms, in direct relation to the degree of possible immunity. As immunity improves, the lesions become less widespread, so that, for example, a borderline or borderline tuberculoid lesion would occur.

Indeterminate leprosy refers to the very earliest manifestation of the disease. It consists of a few hypopigmented macules with varying degrees of loss of sensation. Indeterminate leprosy can be associated with healing and eradication of the disease, or it can evolve into one of the subtypes of leprosy.

A variant of lepromatous leprosy is the so-called histoid leprosy, characterized by firm nodules resembling a dermatofibroma.[2]

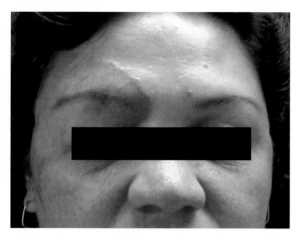

Figure 19-5. Tuberculoid leprosy. There is a plaque with raised, irregular, erythematous borders and a flat, hypopigmented center. These lesions cause sensory impairment due to the neurotropism of the mycobacteria and the host response. (Courtesy of Mirian Sotto, MD, PhD, Department of Dermatology, Hospital das Clinicas, University of Sao Paulo.)

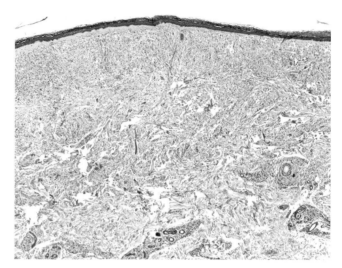

Figure 19-6. Lepromatous leprosy. At low magnification, one sees a diffuse dermal infiltrate composed of histiocytes with a foamy appearance and a scant lymphoid infiltrate. Granulomas are absent. Note the characteristic grenz zone. (Courtesy of Mirian Sotto, MD, PhD, Department of Dermatology, Hospital das Clinicas, University of Sao Paulo.)

Types of Reactional Leprosy

There are basically three types of reactions that occur in leprosy. They occur both with and without treatment and are directly related to the immune status of the patient, which can wax and wane.[90-93]

In the first of the so-called type I reactions, also known as the Lepra reaction, the patient has shifted during therapy from a lepromatous pattern toward a tuberculoid pattern. This change, called the reversal reaction, is directly related to an increase in the immune response of the patient. There is also a downgrading reaction that occurs when a patient who is not under therapy progressively becomes more anergic and begins to show changes of lepromatous leprosy. These are the two manifestations of the so-called type I reaction, which can result in systemic symptoms with a change in the size of the lesions and the peripheral nerves.[2,91]

The type II reactions, which are known as erythema nodosum leprosum, occur principally in borderline lepromatous patients. This type of reaction is also associated with changes in immune response and may occur with treatment or spontaneously. It is characterized by the formation of immune complexes resulting in a vasculitis or vasculopathy. The lesions evolve as very tender, red papules, plaques, and nodules that occur in normal skin.[2,94]

The third type of reaction, also called Lucio phenomenon, is associated only with lepromatous leprosy.[92] The patient develops a striking, diffuse skin edema, which tends to efface the age-related wrinkles on the face and gave rise to the historic term, "la belle femme." However, hemorrhagic plaques can occur suddenly on the arms, legs, and buttocks, and these eventually lead to widespread severe ulcerations.

Clinical Pathologic Correlation

Early Indeterminate Leprosy In early indeterminate leprosy, clinically sparse lesions that are hypopigmented macules can be associated with hypesthesia. These sometimes resemble an eczematous patch. They may disappear completely if there is eradication of the disease by the host response, or they may persist with development of one of the types of leprosy. The Mitsuda test is a delayed hypersensitivity reaction test to the lepromatous bacilli; it can help predict the evolution of the indeterminate lesion. If the Mitsuda test is negative, the patient will usually go on to lepromatous or borderline lepromatous leprosy. If the Mitsuda test is positive, the patient will more likely develop tuberculoid leprosy or have a spontaneous remission of the lesion.[91]

The changes can be very subtle and include a very slight lymphohistiocytic infiltrate. These cells are present particularly around neurovascular bundles and affect both superficial and deep venular plexuses, as well as the sweat glands and the arrector pili muscle. One may observe infiltration into the epidermis and may actually see lymphocytic inflammation of dermal nerves. Careful observation reveals a few acid-fast bacilli, and the diagnosis is made if the bacilli are found in the nerve or in the arrector pili muscle, just under the dermis, or in a perivascular monocyte-macrophage cell. If bacilli are not demonstrated, then the diagnosis is considered presumptive.[1,2,83,93]

Lepromatous Leprosy In lepromatous leprosy, there are diffuse lesions throughout the body. These may be macular, poorly defined, and either slightly hypopigmented or erythematous. They are frequently infiltrative, so that they become plaque-like. The most common type, the infiltrative nodular type, usually develops from a macule. These lesions are often dull red; they affect the forehead and cheeks, resulting in the leonine facies, and also affect hair follicles, resulting in loss of eyebrows and eyelashes. As the lesions progress, the nerves become involved, swollen, and very prominent. These changes are associated with some dysesthesias and nerve paralyses. The most commonly involved nerves are the ulnar, radial, and common perineal nerves.[1,2,94]

The histopathology of the lepromatous lesion includes an extensive, diffuse cellular infiltrate. This infiltrate involves the entire dermis but is clearly separated from the epidermis by a

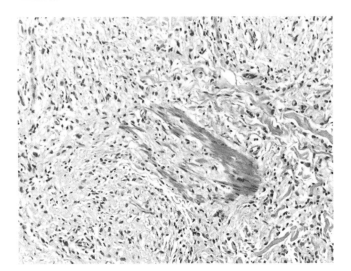

Figure 19-7. Lepromatous leprosy. In this example, diffuse infiltration of the arrector pili muscles is seen. (Courtesy of Mirian Sotto, MD, PhD, Department of Dermatology, Hospital das Clinicas, University of Sao Paulo.)

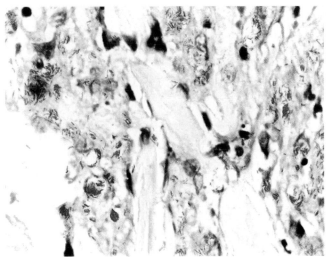

Figure 19-9. Lepromatous leprosy (Wade-Fite stain). The foamy histiocytes contain thick aggregates of mycobacteria, known as globi. Note the relationship between the bacilli and the vessels. (Courtesy of Mirian Sotto, MD, PhD, Department of Dermatology, Hospital das Clinicas, University of Sao Paulo.)

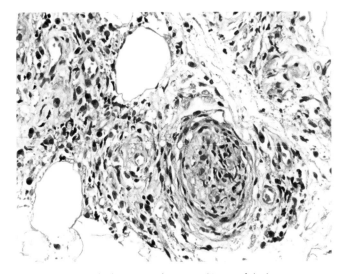

Figure 19-8. Subpolar lepromatous leprosy. In this part of the leprosy spectrum, one can find plasma cells and the classic "onion skin" pattern of perineural fibroblastic proliferation. (Courtesy of Mirian Sotto, MD, PhD, Department of Dermatology, Hospital das Clinicas, University of Sao Paulo.)

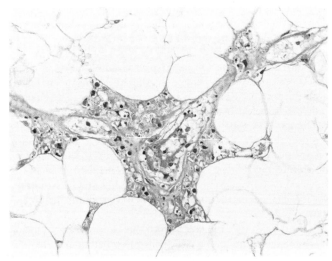

Figure 19-10. Lucio phenomenon. Severe vascular involvement is seen in this example that exhibits thrombogenic vasculitis. (Courtesy of Mirian Sotto, MD, PhD, Department of Dermatology, Hospital das Clinicas, University of Sao Paulo.)

small grenz zone of collagen (Fig. 19-6). The infiltrate causes destruction of the appendages and also extends into the subcutaneous fat (Fig. 19-7). The involved monocyte-macrophages exhibit a rather eosinophilic cytoplasm in which one can observe bacilli, many of which are fragmented. In these chronically persistent lesions, one can observe clumps of bacteria and bacterial fragments that are called globi.[2,91]

There is no evidence of any formation of epithelioid cells, and there are few lymphocytes, which are found percolating amidst the infiltrate. Plasma cells are frequently found in and peripheral to the infiltrate, especially in the transition to the borderline lepromatous form (subpolar lepromatous leprosy) (Fig. 19-8). As the lesions persist, one can observe vacuoles in the macrophages that contain quite prominent lipid associated

with fragmentation of the bacteria. The Fite stain is useful in identifying the mycobacteria under these circumstances. Nerves exhibit very prominent bacilli in the lepromatous lesion (Fig. 19-9).[91]

In the Lucio phenomenon, the lesions are associated with perivascular prominence of the bacilli, especially around the small dermal vessels (Figs. 19-10 and 19-11). The histiocytoid variant of lepromatous leprosy is associated with cells that have a fusiform shape and may be arranged in a storiform pattern (Fig. 19-12). These fibrohistiocytic cells usually have a basophilic or amphophilic cytoplasm that is laden with mycobacteria (Figs. 19-13 and 19-14).[91-93]

Borderline Lepromatous Leprosy The lesions in borderline lepromatous leprosy are fewer in number and are not symmetri-

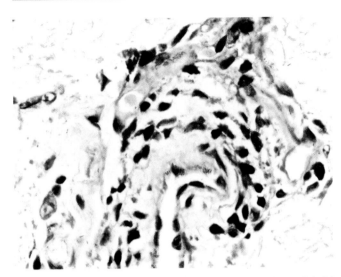

Figure 19-11. Lucio phenomenon (Wade-Fite stain). Colonization of the endothelial cells by the mycobacteria is characteristic. (Courtesy of Mirian Sotto, MD, PhD, Department of Dermatology, Hospital das Clinicas, University of Sao Paulo.)

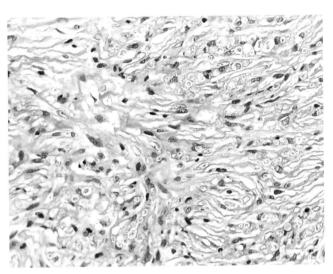

Figure 19-13. Histoid leprosy. The spindle cells show an amphophilic cytoplasm that is filled with mycobacteria. (Courtesy of Mirian Sotto, MD, PhD, Department of Dermatology, Hospital das Clinicas, University of Sao Paulo.)

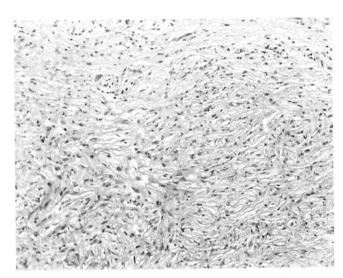

Figure 19-12. Histoid leprosy. This variant manifests as a prominent proliferation of spindle cells that can be confused with a fibrohistiocytic neoplasm. (Courtesy of Mirian Sotto, MD, PhD, Department of Dermatology, Hospital das Clinicas, University of Sao Paulo.)

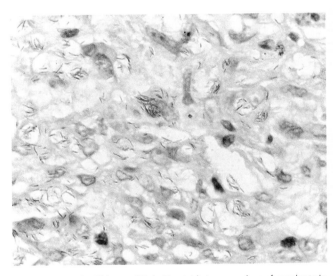

Figure 19-14. Histoid leprosy (Wade-Fite stain). Large numbers of mycobacteria, arranged in bundles, are seen within the histoid cells. (Courtesy of Mirian Sotto, MD, PhD, Department of Dermatology, Hospital das Clinicas, University of Sao Paulo.)

cally disposed. They often have a central delve or dimple. The lesions vary in number according to the degree of host response. In borderline lesions with poor host response, they are more numerous. As the host response becomes stronger, fewer lesions appear and form plaques, designated as borderline tuberculoid leprosy.

In the histopathology of this lesion, there are lymphocytes and some areas of possibly very early, poor granuloma formation (Fig. 19-15). Interestingly, there can be an "onion skin" appearance to some of the nerves because of perineural fibroblastic proliferation (Fig. 19-16). Foamy cells are much less prominent, and one does not see globi in this form.[91]

Mid-borderline Leprosy The lesions of mid-borderline leprosy are very irregularly dispersed and plaque-like but have what

appear to be prominent central depressions. These lesions are also quite edematous and have been referred to as saucer-like lesions.[89,91]

Histopathologically, the monocyte-macrophages now begin to form epithelioid cells that are scattered but display no true granuloma formation (Fig. 19-17). There are also scanty lymphocytes and scattered Langhans giant cells.[2,91]

Borderline Tuberculoid Leprosy Borderline tuberculoid leprosy is associated clinically with a few scattered plaques with central hypopigmentation. These plaques are also hairless. Clinically, nerve enlargement is very marked.

The histopathology of these lesions includes granulomas associated with peripheral lymphocytes that follow along the neurovascular bundles. Occasional Langhans giant cells are

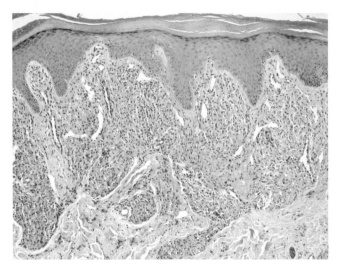

Figure 19-15. Borderline lepromatous leprosy. The infiltrate is somewhat more circumscribed, and there are more lymphocytes and even a tendency to form granulomas. Note the accentuation of the neurovascular bundles by the infiltrate. (Courtesy of Mirian Sotto, MD, PhD, Department of Dermatology, Hospital das Clinicas, University of Sao Paulo.)

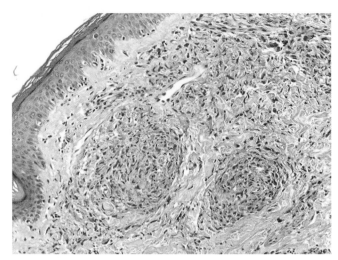

Figure 19-17. Mid-borderline leprosy. Poorly formed granulomas are seen scattered in the dermis. (Courtesy of Mirian Sotto, MD, PhD, Department of Dermatology, Hospital das Clinicas, University of Sao Paulo.)

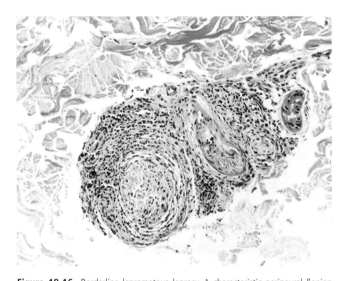

Figure 19-16. Borderline lepromatous leprosy. A characteristic perineural "onion skin" fibroblastic proliferation can be often found. (Courtesy of Mirian Sotto, MD, PhD, Department of Dermatology, Hospital das Clinicas, University of Sao Paulo.)

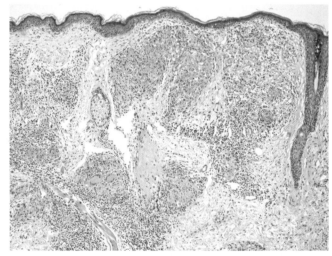

Figure 19-18. Borderline tuberculoid leprosy. The granulomas are better formed and exhibit occasional Langhans giant cells and a lymphocytic cuff. (Courtesy of Mirian Sotto, MD, PhD, Department of Dermatology, Hospital das Clinicas, University of Sao Paulo.)

noted (Fig. 19-18). Accumulation of granulomas along the superficial vascular plexuses is often observed (Fig. 19-19), but there is no evidence of infiltration of the epidermis itself. Bacteria are scant in number.[1,2,89,91]

Tuberculoid Leprosy   Tuberculoid leprosy is associated with the most striking immune response and manifests as very dry, scaly, hypopigmented patches or plaques with very sharply defined edges. The plaques are usually anesthetic except those on the face. The number of lesions ranges from one to five. Peripheral nerves can be very prominent.[91,95]

The histopathology of this lesion exhibits true epithelioid cell granulomas following along the neurovascular bundles

(Figs. 19-20 and 19-21). Langhans giant cells usually are not found, but in some cases they can be prominent (Fig. 19-22). The granulomas are associated with a dense lymphocytic cuff (Fig. 19-23). Acid-fast bacilli are rarely, if ever, found. The lesion is very similar to sarcoidosis or silicosis, except that the nerves show a very marked destructive appearance.[91]

Reactions in Leprosy   The type I reactions in leprosy have not been very well characterized. The type II reaction, erythema nodosum leprosum, clinically has some features that are more akin to erythema multiforme in the reaction state; this reaction occurs only in lepromatous or borderline lepromatous patients. One can observe rather tender plaques and nodules scattered over the skin surface. There are usually marked constitutional symptoms, especially malaise and arthralgias. There are

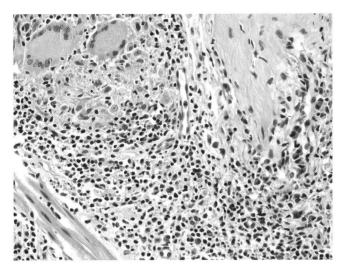

Figure 19-19. Borderline tuberculoid leprosy. The Langhans giant cells are surrounded by an exuberant lymphocytic infiltrate. (Courtesy of Mirian Sotto, MD, PhD, Department of Dermatology, Hospital das Clinicas, University of Sao Paulo.)

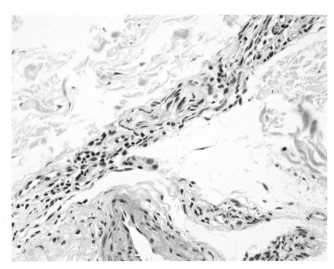

Figure 19-21. Tuberculoid leprosy. The early perineural lymphoid infiltrate will progress into a granulomatous infiltrate. (Courtesy of Mirian Sotto, MD, PhD, Department of Dermatology, Hospital das Clinicas, University of Sao Paulo.)

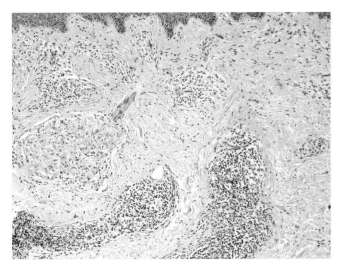

Figure 19-20. Tuberculoid leprosy. Well-formed granulomas are seen throughout the dermis. (Courtesy of Mirian Sotto, MD, PhD, Department of Dermatology, Hospital das Clinicas, University of Sao Paulo.)

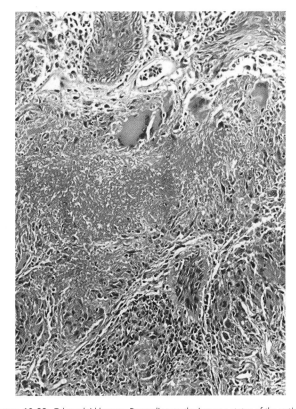

Figure 19-22. Tuberculoid leprosy. Depending on the immune status of the patient, central necrosis may be found in the granulomas. (Courtesy of Mirian Sotto, MD, PhD, Department of Dermatology, Hospital das Clinicas, University of Sao Paulo.)

numerous neutrophils scattered in the sea of infected monocyte-macrophages, and even dermal abscesses may be noted (Figs. 19-24 and 19-25). There is a perivascular infiltrate that may vary from neutrophils to neutrophils and lymphocytes with evidence of vasculitis (Fig. 19-26).[94]

The type III or Lucio reaction is again confined to patients with lepromatous leprosy who have had no treatment or inadequate treatment. The systemic symptoms are not present, but the lesions show striking, irregularly shaped, hemorrhagic plaques that can ulcerate. The histopathology differs in that there is striking luminal obliteration of medium-sized vessels by endothelial cell proliferation, with variable thrombosis (see Fig. 19-10). There is a sparse lymphohistiocytic infiltrate, but acid-fast bacilli are very prominent in the walls and endothelium of normal vessels, as well as in those vessels showing the proliferative

changes (see Fig. 19-11). The resultant ischemic necrosis leads to ulceration in many patients.

The basic pathogenetic mechanism of leprosy is a defect in T cell activation against the mycobacteria.[1,2,85] This failure of reaction leads to an inability of macrophages to destroy the

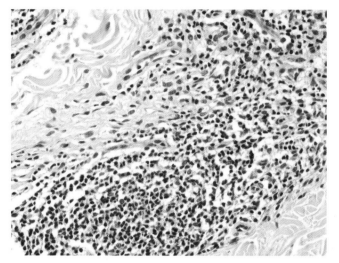

Figure 19-23. Tuberculoid leprosy. A prominent lymphocytic cuff is seen around the granulomas. (Courtesy of Mirian Sotto, MD, PhD, Department of Dermatology, Hospital das Clinicas, University of Sao Paulo.)

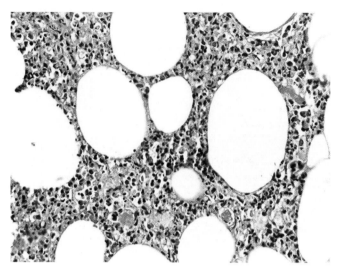

Figure 19-25. Erythema nodosum leprosum. Note the involvement of the micro-vasculature and the abundance in neutrophils. (Courtesy of Mirian Sotto, MD, PhD, Department of Dermatology, Hospital das Clinicas, University of Sao Paulo.)

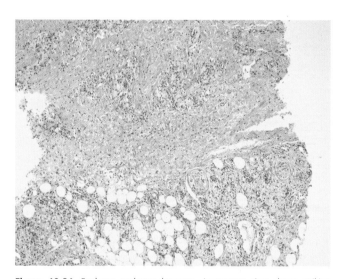

Figure 19-24. Erythema nodosum leprosum. Low-power view shows striking resemblance to ordinary erythema nodosum. (Courtesy of Mirian Sotto, MD, PhD, Department of Dermatology, Hospital das Clinicas, University of Sao Paulo.)

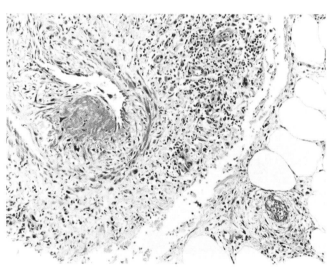

Figure 19-26. Erythema nodosum leprosum. Striking vasculopathy with thrombosis and perivascular inflammatory infiltrate are seen. (Courtesy of Mirian Sotto, MD, PhD, Department of Dermatology, Hospital das Clinicas, University of Sao Paulo.)

bacilli. The specificity of the defect is demonstrated by the fact that patients with lepromatous leprosy can react to other immunologic stimuli. Lymphocytes from lepromatous patients do not produce macrophage migration-inhibiting factors (MIF) after incubation with lepromin. On the other hand, patients with tuberculoid leprosy produce MIF after such exposure. Patients with tuberculoid leprosy have the ability to produce Th1 reactions, whereas those with lepromatous leprosy produce Th2 reactions. The Th2 reactions give rise to humoral immunity, which is ineffective against leprosy.[95,96] In those patients who have either erythema nodosum leprosum or Lucio reaction, one can find IgG and C3 in the vessel walls, indicating the probable role of immune complexes in the patho-genesis of these reactions (i.e., they are apparently type III reactions).[97]

Miscellaneous Bacterial Infections

Anthrax

The causative organism of anthrax is *Bacillus anthracis*. The incidence of anthrax is low in the United States, but in some parts of the world the disease is much more common.[98] The exposed skin is characteristically involved. In adults, the lesion is more common on the hands due to contact with infected animals such as rabbits, goats, and sheep. A gastrointestinal form can occur after ingestion of infected meat. In children, the head and neck are the common sites, where they have been bitten by insects carrying the organism. The initial lesion is a red macule that rapidly goes through a papular, vesicular, and ulcerative phase with the formation of a black adherent eschar, also known

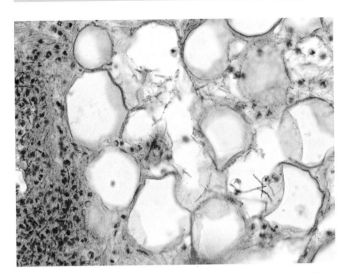

Figure 19-27. Cutaneous anthrax. There is a prominent inflammatory infiltrate comprised mostly of polymorphonuclear leukocytes. The elongated gram-positive bacilli are readily identified.

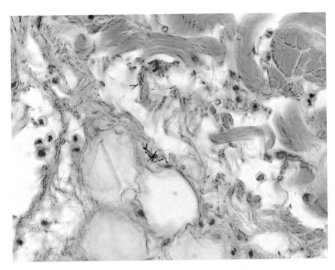

Figure 19-28. Cutaneous anthrax. The process often extends into the subcutaneous fat, and there is prominent edema.

as a sphacelus. Although the initial lesion may be pruritic, the well-formed ulcer is not symptomatic. As the lesion evolves, there can be severe, striking edema with blisters. Regional lymphadenopathy is found in association with fever and chills. Lesions heal in 1 to 2 weeks in most cases; however, death has been reported in 20% of untreated cutaneous cases. Gastrointestinal anthrax is associated with vomiting, bloody diarrhea, acute abdominal pain, and carbuncles and shows much higher mortality if not treated appropriately with antibiotics.[1,2]

Biopsy of the lesion exhibits marked, severe dermal edema with necrosis and ulceration of the epidermis, hemorrhage, and a diffuse lymphocytic and neutrophilic infiltrate. The eschar is represented by a dense necrotic zone of tissue. Beneath, there is striking neutrophilic infiltration that can be associated with vasculitis. In addition to the necrotic debris, one can see marked foci of chronic inflammation. The organism is usually easily demonstrated as gram-positive rods that range up to 10 μm in size. They are especially present in the necrotic debris and beneath in the inflamed dermis (Figs. 19-27 and 19-28).[2]

The route of infection is threefold. The first route is primary inoculation of the skin by direct contact with herbivores. A small percentage of cases are due to the inhalation of anthrax, as in wool sorters' disease. Finally, there is the gastrointestinal type of anthrax that is acquired from eating infected meat. The differential diagnosis includes other infectious disorders such as staphylococcal pyoderma, sporotrichosis, tularemia, and orf. At times, insect bites with secondary infection may resemble this lesion. The differential diagnosis of sphacelus includes the membrane of diphtheria, the eschar of ecthyma gangrenosum, tularemia, the dense crust of diabetic ulcers or ischemic ulcers associated with an arterial vasculitis, and the dark-crusted center of ulcerated lymphoma nodules.[10]

Brucellosis

Brucellosis occurs after ingestion of contaminated food or following direct inhalation of organisms. The incubation period is usually 30 to 60 days but can be as short as 5 days. A small percentage of patients have a polymorphous rash that may include macules, eczema, a measles-like appearance, erythema multiforme, or even blistering disorder and petechiae. Other symptoms include severe headache, nausea, vomiting, and possibly associated arthritis or arthropathy. There is an inoculation type of brucellosis that results in redness, papules, and pustules in workers who deal with animals, especially veterinarians.[99]

The eczematous rash is associated with dyskeratotic cells and some extravasation of red blood cells. The erythema multiforme–like rash is associated with a superficial and deep lymphohistiocytic infiltration. Inoculation brucellosis may be associated with eosinophils. Both septal and lobular panniculitis may be observed, and sometimes they are associated with necrosis.[1,2]

The lesions of brucellosis may be caused by *Brucella melitensis*, *Brucella suis*, *Brucella abortus*, or *Brucella canis*.[99,100] This gram-negative coccobacillus is usually found in milk or animal products. Serologic diagnosis is preferred because of the long delay in culture.

Yersiniosis and Plague

Yersinia is a gram-negative bacillus; the medically relevant species, which are zoonotic, include *Yersinia pestis*, *Yersinia enterocolitica*, and *Yersinia pseudotuberculosis*. The normal hosts are wild rodents and their fleas; humans are sporadically involved.[101] Untreated, the resultant plague is 100% lethal, but with appropriate rapid treatment, approximately 50% of patients can be saved.

Patients may develop mild or severe symptoms. Fever is characteristic, with generalized malaise associated with regional lymph node involvement in bubonic plague or with pneumonia in pneumonic plague. These symptoms are followed by generalized infection and septicemia with shock and death. An important clinical sign is that pustules or carbuncles may exhibit centrifugal vesicles around the central inflammation, usually at the site of a bite or a bubo. Diffuse erythema is common, but one may also find petechiae and purpura. The organism that causes plague is *Y. pestis*; infection with *Y. enterocolitica* or

Y. pseudotuberculosis leads to a reactive polyarthritis associated with fever, gastrointestinal symptoms, and signs of erythema nodosum.[102-104] Appropriate cultures of blood and stools, throat, sputum, or aspirated fluid from buboes lead to the correct diagnosis. Serologic tests are also available, and a Gram stain of tissue or fluid from infected sites may reveal the organisms.

The histopathology of the various lesions depends on their clinical presentation. The lesions of erythema nodosum have a septal panniculitis. The morbilliform rash is associated with a perivenular lymphoid infiltrate. In lesions with petechiae and purpura, and especially in those associated with shock, there is usually evidence of disseminated intravascular coagulation.

Granuloma Inguinale

Granuloma inguinale is a disorder associated with intracellular obligate parasites, including the organisms that cause rhinoscleroma, histoplasmosis, and leishmaniasis. The causative agent of granuloma inguinale is *Calymmatobacterium granulomatis*.[105,106] The diagnosis is made via smears of tissue stained with either Giemsa or Warthin-Starry reagents.[104] The lesions manifest as painless ulcers affecting the genitalia or the perianal area that develop marked granulation tissue. These lesions spread in an unusual serpiginous pattern. Lymphadenopathy is common. Large unattended ulcers can result in prominent destruction of tissue.

The differential diagnosis includes chancroid, syphilis, and lymphogranuloma venereum; herpes simplex virus (HSV) infection can at times resemble this disorder. Lesions with pseudo-epitheliomatous hyperplasia can be confused with squamous cell carcinoma.

Lesions show granulation tissue with reactive epidermal hyperplasia adjacent to the ulcers. Away from ulcerated areas, one may see lymphocytes and macrophages as well as small abscesses. The abscesses are associated with macrophages up to 20 μm in diameter that contain the organisms. The organisms are 1 to 2 μm in size and exhibit a characteristic "safety pin" appearance in sections stained with Giemsa or Warthin-Starry. Smears made from biopsy samples may be crushed or cut into 1-μm sections and prepared for electron microscopy after staining with toluidine blue to allow for identification of the organisms. Culture can be performed, although appropriate techniques are not widely available.[1,10,107]

Chancroid

Chancroid is a rather common sexually transmitted disorder that may occur alone or as part of mixed infection with other venereal organisms. Mixed infections are less common in the United States but may be found in travelers returning from some Third World countries. The cause of this infection is *Haemophilus ducreyi*.[105]

The lesion of chancroid exhibits a very shallow, minimally indurated ulcer. Sometimes several ulcers are observed. The ulcers have a yellow to grayish exudate on their surface and can be exquisitely tender. Secondary lymphadenitis can occur unilaterally or bilaterally.[1,2,10] The differential diagnosis includes the multiple tender ulcers of herpes simplex. Smears can help differentiate this lesion. The ulcer of granuloma inguinale may

resemble this lesion but is nontender and does not show undermining at the margin.

The histologic picture is distinctive and essentially includes three zones of alteration. At the surface of the lesion, the exudate contains fibrin, neutrophils, neutrophilic debris, and red blood cells. The middle zone is broad and exhibits a generous granulation tissue. At times, thrombi are observed in association with focal necrosis. The third layer at the base exhibits a dense, prominent infiltrate of lymphocytes and plasma cells. However, typical zonation is not present in all cases.[10,108] The bacillus is a small gram-negative coccobacillus that is ~1.5 μm in length and ~0.2-μm in width. They often occur in chains and can be seen amidst the cells of the surface-most portion of the lesion with Gram Giemsa stains. Smears taken from the edge of the ulcer also show the bacillus. Confirmation of the diagnosis by culture requires blood-enriched agar.

Rhinoscleroma

Rhinoscleroma is a disorder that was found originally in central Europe. In recent years, more cases have appeared in Central America and Africa. It is caused by *Klebsiella rhinoscleromatis*.[109,110] This lesion begins in the nose but can spread to the pharynx and the upper respiratory passages, including larynx and trachea. In some patients, it extends onto the lip, which is then markedly indurated with granulomatous inflammation.

The histopathology of this lesion includes a prominent plasma cellular infiltrate with scattered lymphocytes in a setting of proliferated vessels. There are prominent Russell bodies and occasional polymorphonuclear cells. Careful inspection reveals large histiocytes, measuring 10 to 100 μm in diameter, with markedly vacuolated cytoplasm. These cells are called Mikulicz cells. In the vacuoles, the organism is best seen after Giemsa or Warthin-Starry stain. They are faintly visible on H&E staining. This bacterium is gram-negative and measures 2 to 3 μm in size. There are clusters organized in the vacuoles. The best clue to the Mikulicz cell is that it has a foamy appearance, and the bacteria can be appreciated on high-power microscopy. This bacterium is also PAS-positive. Electron microscopy likewise reveals bacilli with a filamentous coat of mucopolysaccharides.

On a purely histologic basis, this lesion can resemble granuloma annulare and must be differentiated from other infections and disorders that contain vacuolated macrophages, including the mycoses, leishmania, and Hansen disease.[108,109]

Tularemia

Like plague, tularemia is a zoonotic infection. The cause is a gram-negative coccobacillus, *Francisella tularensis*.[111] Reservoirs for this disease include wild rabbits, deer flies, and the feces of ticks, but the infection can result from direct contact with other animals.[112] The characteristic presentation of this disease is the so-called ulceroglandular presentation. Usually, the finger or hand is the first site of the inoculation, where a rapidly growing papulonodule ulcerates.[113] A black eschar or sphacelus appears within 3 to 5 days after contact.[10] Culture of the organism is problematic and could result in infection of laboratory personnel; serologic diagnosis is safer and more effective. PCR studies are likewise diagnostic.[114] Other important forms of tularemia include gastrointestinal and pulmonary types, with high mortality rates especially in tularemic pneumonia.[115]

Dense fibrin necrotic debris–laden exudate overlies an ulcer bed in which there is dermal necrosis with palisading neutrophils and even suppurative granulomatous response. The organisms are gram-negative and difficult to observe, but the Dieterle stain may be helpful. Usually, the history is very helpful in the differential diagnosis, especially if there has been contact with an animal. Lesions that can resemble tularemia include atypical acid-fast infections and sporotrichosis. Cat scratch disease also must be considered in the differential diagnosis, however, the skin lesion with eschar is quite different from these other infections.[116]

Cat Scratch Disease

After much investigation, *Bartonella henselae*, a gram-negative bacillus, is now thought to be the cause of this disease.[101,116,117] Because of problems in culture of the organism, a skin test (Hanger-Rose test) and PCR are used for diagnosis. A small papule or macule resembling an insect bite is the first sign of the disorder and usually occurs at the site of a cat scratch or bite. The lesions usually occur in children, often on the hand or forearm, and are nonpruritic.[118] After 10 to 14 days, the small (5.0 mm wide) maculopapules resolve spontaneously. However, some patients develop fever or other constitutional symptoms as well as other skin lesions. Morbilliform and even erythema multiforme–like rashes have been reported. The chief problem in the patients who develop a reaction to the bite is regional lymphadenopathy, which appears several weeks after the original trauma. The node may suppurate and break down. The conjunctiva is the site of entry in Parinaud oculoglandular syndrome, with patients exhibiting conjunctivitis, retrotarsal granulation tissue, and preauricular lymphadenopathy.[1]

The characteristic picture of the site of inoculation includes a palisading granulomatous response resembling granuloma annulare around zones of necrobiosis. Included in the palisading inflammation are lymphocytes, eosinophils, and sometimes giant cells. The morbilliform rashes that can occur show interface dermatitis microscopically, with a perivascular lymphoid and plasmacellular infiltrate both superficial and deep, and may even include a lymphocytic panniculitis. The small (0.2-0.5 μm), gram-negative rods can also be seen with the Warthin-Starry stain. The lymph node histology includes stellate microabscesses with inflammation surrounding foci of necrosis. As the lesions become more chronic, a more granulomatous response appears. Organisms can be identified in this area. Because the lesion exhibits a palisaded appearance histologically, one must consider other lesions in the differential diagnosis. The clinical presentation and history should be helpful. The stellate abscesses of lymph nodes can be seen also in tularemia, lymphogranuloma venereum, sporotrichosis, and yersiniosis. Likewise, some acid-fast infections as well as Kawasaki disease and Kikuchi disease must also be considered.[1,2]

Bacillary Angiomatosis

Bacillary angiomatosis has been described mainly in immunocompromised patients, many of whom have AIDS,[119-122] but has also been seen in patients who have undergone organ transplan-tation or are immunosuppressed due to chemotherapy.[123] It has also rarely been described in patients with no known immunosuppressive disorder.[124] Although *B. henselae* and in some cases *Bartonella quintana* have been described as the main organisms that cause this disorder, there is still debate about the etiology as the various manifestations of the disease have become apparent. The angiomatosis variant refers to papulonodules of the skin that have a granulation tissue–like appearance. If the liver or spleen is affected, the disorder is called bacillary peliosis. It has been known to occur also in the gastrointestinal tract, lungs, soft tissues, and even bone.

Clinically, pyogenic granuloma-like nodules appear in the skin. In some instances, they are related to a cat scratch. Rarely, the lesions manifest as subcutaneous nodules or even fungating ulcerated lesions.[121] In patients with AIDS, the disorder appears when CD4-positive T-lymphocyte counts are low and can go on to systemic disease with death. Antibiotics, especially erythromycin, are effective in early disease.[122] But in some AIDS patients, the course is intractable, leading to death.[125]

In the dermis, single or multiple vascular proliferative nodules are associated with an inflammatory infiltrate in which there are both neutrophils and mononuclear cells. On low power, the changes resemble granulation tissue.[121] On higher-power examination, one can appreciate extracellular smudgy areas that are bluish to amphophilic, but actually represent masses of bacilli. There are scattered neutrophils with debris around the pale, amphophilic, amorphous, and smudged areas. These organisms can also be identified by tissue Gram stain as gram-negative bacilli. Other useful stains are the Warthin-Starry and the GMS stain. Electron microscopy can be used in difficult cases.[123]

As far as differential diagnosis is concerned, the most important consideration is to rule out Kaposi sarcoma, but one must also consider pyogenic granuloma and epithelioid hemangioma. The most useful and helpful clue is an appreciation of the pale blue or amphophilic granular smudged areas that abut vessels and are not seen in other neoplastic or infectious diseases except for verruga peruana (Carrión disease, caused by *Bartonella bacilliformis.*). The clinical lesions of verruga peruana can be compared to those of bacillary angiomatosis. Patients develop nodules and papules, some fungating. The vector is *Phlebotomus verrucarum,* the sand fly. Three weeks after a fly bite, an acute illness with hemolysis occurs, followed in 3 to 6 months by nodules similar to those of bacillary angiomatosis.[1,2,10]

Malacoplakia

Malacoplakia is commonly found in the urinary tract and the gastrointestinal tract, as well as other organs, and rarely affects the skin. *Escherichia coli* is the most common causative organism, but *S. aureus* and *Pseudomonas* spp. can also cause the lesion.[126-128] Very nondescript red nodules or papules are present in the lower abdomen and the area of the groin, often around follicles. In some cases, abscesses and sinus tracks develop.

Numerous macrophages containing discrete eosinophilic cytoplasmic granules exhibit small, eccentric nuclei. The granules stain with eosin. These have been designated as von Hanseman cells. There are also very large phagolysosomes that stain basophilic in the cytoplasm of some cells, and these 5- to 15-μm structures are called Michaelis-Gutmann bodies. These bodies are composed of iron and bacterial products; they are focally calcified and therefore stain with PAS, von Kossa, and Perl stains. Because there are portions of bacteria in the cytoplasm of the macrophages, the Gram stain can be positive focally. There is a quite striking infiltrate of lymphocytes and plasma cells amidst the infiltrative macrophages.[1,2,126,128]

Nocardiosis

Human infection by microorganisms of the *Nocardia* genus is usually related to an immunosuppressed status,[129] in patients with HIV/AIDS, or in those receiving immunosuppressive medications such as corticosteroids or TNF inhibitors (infliximab).[130]

Nocardia is an aerobic, branching, gram-positive, weakly acid-fast bacterium that was first classified as belonging to the Fungi Kingdom. It is ubiquitous and can be isolated from soil, water, and organic matter.[131] The most common species associated with skin involvement are *Nocardia asteroides*[129] and *Nocardia brasiliensis*.[132-134] Other clinically relevant species are *Nocardia farcinica* and *Nocardia nova*.[135]

The classic route of infection is via the respiratory tract (inhalation), with pulmonary infection and subsequent systemic dissemination, mainly to the central nervous system (CNS) and to the skin. This mechanism is usually seen in immunocompromised patients.[129,130,136] Immunocompetent individuals acquire cutaneous lesions through traumatic percutaneous inoculation, usually through contaminated thorns.[134,137] However, secondary hematogenous nocardiosis skin lesions may be indistinguishable to the primary cutaneous form, so it is always important to evaluate affected patients for pulmonary lesions.[138]

Cutaneous involvement by *Nocardia* appears clinically as a lymphocutaneous infection[133] that has a chancriform[139] or sporotrichoid[140] morphology. This presentation can be found in children as the cervicofacial variant.[141] The infections can appear also as mycetoma or other common superficial cutaneous infections such as abscesses, ulcers, or cellulitis.[142-144]

Microscopically, lesions can appear as abscesses surrounded by a dense neutrophilic infiltrate, which can extend from the dermis to the subcutis and can exhibit necrosis, hemorrhage, and ulceration. A fibrous capsule surrounded by chronic inflammatory lesions is seen in chronic cases.[145-147] Lesions can also manifest atypically, such as a pseudoepitheliomatous hyperplasia with an extensive lymphohistiocytic infiltrate containing epithelioid and giant cells (Fig. 19-29). One can also find sulfur granules, which can be indistinguishable from the ones found in actinomycosis (see later discussion). However, the granules contain bacterial forms that are positive for acid-fast staining techniques. In addition, one can find evidence of eosinophilic crystalline structures in a starburst pattern as part of the Splendore-Hoeppli phenomenon.[148]

The bacteria cannot be visualized on routine H&E-stained sections. One must rely on Gram stain or acid-fast stains, which reveal fine, branched, filamentous bacteria that break up into coccobacillary forms. The silver methenamine method is also useful to highlight the organisms.[147] Also, a GMS stain can reveal the presence of the bacteria. In addition, acid-fast stains are weakly positive, whereas a Fite stain is much more positive (Figs. 19-30 and 19-31).[2] If organisms are not visualized morphological, PCR methods or culture can be used to identify the agent.

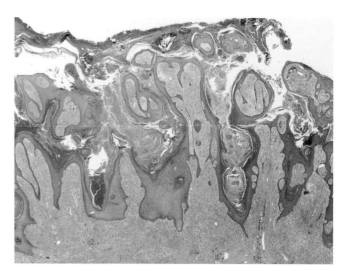

Figure 19-29. Cutaneous nocardiosis. Prominent epidermal hyperplasia and a diffuse lymphohistiocytic infiltrate with scattered giant cells can be found, especially in immunocompromised individuals. This patient was a renal transplant recipient.

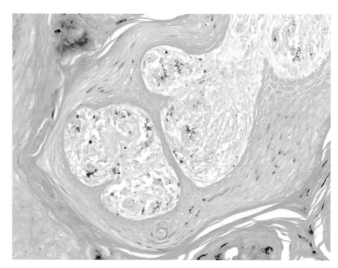

Figure 19-30. Cutaneous nocardiosis. GMS stain highlights the bacteria, which grow by forming branching filaments.

Actinomycosis

Actinomyces are anaerobic, nonvirulent organisms that are usually present in the oropharynx, gastrointestinal tract, and female genitalia as part of the resident microbial flora. The four clinically important species are *Actinomyces israelii*, *Actinomyces naeslundii*, *Actinomyces viscosus*, and *Actinomyces odontolyticus*.[149] Infection by these organisms requires either a disruption of the natural barriers, from trauma or iatrogenic instrumentation, or an alteration of the normal microbial flora.[150] The classic clinical forms are cervicofacial (55%), abdominopelvic (20%), thoracic (15%), and disseminated (10%). The disseminated form can involve multiple organs, such as the CNS, skin, pericardium, and the extremities.[149] Infection can be found in immunocompromised patients. However, the risk of actinomycosis does not vary between immunocompetent patients and those in an immunosuppressed state.[150,151]

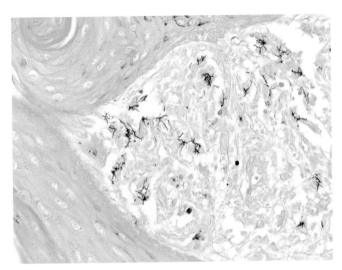

Figure 19-31. Cutaneous nocardiosis. Branching filamentous forms of *Nocardia* are best seen with the GMS stain at high power.

Cutaneous actinomycosis is a rare event and can be the product of either direct inoculation or hematogenous seeding.[149] Clinically, the lesions show soft, painless nodules usually with multiple sinus tracts and fistulas with discharge of purulent material and sulfur granules. These granules are represented macroscopically by firm, yellowish grains.[150,152]

The histologic picture is dominated by the presence of abscesses and sinus tracts surrounded by granulation tissue and an outer fibrous capsule with a diffuse, mixed inflammatory infiltrate composed of foamy histiocytes, lymphocytes, and plasma cells. The sulfur granules are readily identified as discrete multilobulated granules of basophilic material, which are tangled bacterial colonies. These bodies can measure from 300 μm up to 1 to 2 mm in diameter and are surrounded by a crown of closely attached neutrophils.[152,153] Sometimes, one can also see an eosinophilic, loose rim around the granules, which is known as the Splendore effect, part of the Splendore-Hoeppli phenomenon.[148] The bacteria are highlighted by Gram stain and PAS stain with diastase, and they are negative for acid-fast stains. With the specific stains, the microorganisms are visualized as filamentous, branching mycelia that sometimes adopt a "V" shape.[150]

Botryomycosis

Botryomycosis is a chronic bacterial infection that manifests clinically as tumors or plaques that are often ulcerated and have discharging sinuses draining small whitish granules; hence, they closely mimic mycetoma or other fungal infection.[154-156] The granules are also found within the abscesses, and they can be disposed in clusters shaped as a bunch of grapes (*botrys* is the Greek term for "cluster of grapes").[157]

The lesions usually involve the head and neck region and the extremities.[158] The causative agents are usually pyogenic, grampositive bacteria such as *S. aureus*. However, gram-negative organisms such as *P. aeruginosa*,[159] *Proteus* spp., and *Actinobacillus lignieresii*, among others, have also been implicated.[154,160]

There is a clear relationship between botryomycosis and immune suppressive states such as diabetes mellitus,[161] HIV/ AIDS,[162,163] cystic fibrosis,[164] and other conditions.[157,158] However, only a small portion of the cutaneous staphylococcal infections in these immune-compromised individuals manifest as botryomycosis. Also, there have been reports of botryomycosis occurring in otherwise healthy individuals.[164,165] These facts suggest that there are other factors, besides immune dysregulation, behind the genesis of these lesions with a chronic fungal infection–like morphology.[157]

Culture is determinant, not only to definitely identify the agent but to provide appropriate antibiotic therapy.

The histologic picture closely resembles that of mycetoma lesions. It is composed of an abscess cavity filled with purulent material which contains the variably sized, irregularly shaped basophilic granules. The granules are composed of massive colonies of bacteria, which can be gram-positive or gram-negative.[154] One can occasionally find a surrounding eosinophilic rim as part of the Splendore-Hoeppli phenomenon.[148] The organisms are negative with acid-fast stains, PAS, and silver stains. Transepidermal elimination of granules can occasionally be found.

Treponemal Diseases

The treponemal group consists of disorders have been classified as venereal and nonvenereal, as reviewed in the treatise by A. N. Crowson and colleagues.[166] The etiologic agents are elongated, motile bacteria that belong to the Spirochaetaceae family, among which are the *Borrelia* and *Leptospira* genera.[167] Yaws, pinta, and endemic syphilis are the nonvenereal treponematoses. The first recorded case of venereal treponeme infection, namely acquired syphilis, occurred in the 15th century, and syphilis became a dreaded disease with high mortality.[168] High rates of mortality and morbidity continued into the 20th century, when increased public health awareness and the advent of antibiotics, especially penicillin, greatly reduced the incidence.[169] Of late, especially with the spread of HIV, the incidence has been increasing. Transmission usually occurs by contact of an infected site with an abrasion or minor injury. *Treponema pallidum*, the causative agent, has a transmission rate of 10% to 60%.

Venereal Syphilis

Primary and Secondary Syphilis
Clinical Features The primary lesion of venereal syphilis appears within 21 days after exposure and manifests as a redbrown, indurated nodule or plaque 1 to 2 cm in size. It is frequently ulcerated and is painless. With the appearance of a swollen, draining lymph node, the so-called chancriform complex is complete. Lesions may appear on the tongue and be mistaken for squamous cell carcinoma. The primary lesion may disappear spontaneously, but it always responds to appropriate therapy.

After a few weeks, a generalized eruption of reddish-brown, scaly, often oval plaques—the secondary eruption—disseminates all over the body. It may resemble pityriasis rosea or psoriasis, or, rarely, may be pustular.[170] The palms and soles are characteristically affected. Involvement of the scalp may lead to alopecia. Involvement of the anogenital or axillary areas can result in a confluence of papillomatous papules (e.g., in perianal array). These lesions are known as condyloma lata. In late secondary lues, the eruption may have a serpiginous appearance and can appear as annular lesions. These lesions, if left untreated, may persist for some time or recur, as may partially treated syphilis.

The tertiary phase appears after the primary and secondary phases go into a latency period, or latent phase, which has been defined by the CDC to be early if present for less than 1 year or late if present for more than 1 year. The World Health Organization (WHO) uses 2 years as the cutoff between early and late latent phase.[166] Meningovascular syphilis can occur during the late secondary phase or in the tertiary phase.[171] The other manifestations include skin nodules and cardiovascular and neurologic disorders.[172,173] The skin and mucosal lesions are nodules referred to as gummas.

Congenital syphilis should be suspected in the child born of a mother with active or inadequately treated syphilis, or in the event of a reactive serologic test for syphilis, a positive test of the cerebrospinal fluid, elevated cerebrospinal fluid protein, or an elevated white blood cell count of unknown cause.[174] The clinical features include so-called sniffles or rhinitis, chancres, or a widely disseminated rash of unknown cause.[175] Transplacental infection occurs and is more common in mothers with secondary syphilis (about 50%) and less common in mothers with early (40%) or late (10%) latent syphilis.[174]

Histopathology   Two very important histologic observations in any lesion of syphilis are the presence of endothelial swelling, often with obliteration of the vessel lumen, and the presence of a perivascular lymphocytic and plasmacellular infiltrate. The organism can be seen by dark-field microscopic examination, especially in material obtained from the chancre. Staining with a Warthin-Starry or Steiner stain, both of which are silver stains, is also helpful in highlighting organisms. The organism is 8 to 16 μm in length and 0.10 to 0.18 μm in width.[166,176]

The chancre exhibits a markedly hyperplastic epidermis that is often ulcerated. Beneath the epidermis is a dense infiltrate of mainly lymphocytes with mononuclear cells and plasma cells. A striking endarteritis obliterans is present, with lymphoid cells and plasma cells infiltrating the walls of the vessels. Spirochetes can be identified with appropriate silver stains or by electron microscopy. Organisms are found between the keratinocytes, at the basement membrane zone, and in the dermis in perivascular array.[177-179] The infiltrate is so dense and activated that lymphoma is sometimes considered in differential diagnosis.

The draining lymph node exhibits reactive changes, with numerous plasma cells associated with follicular hyperplasia. Careful inspection reveals the prominent endothelial cell changes already discussed. Occasionally, poorly formed granulomas may be observed. Spirochetes are plentiful and can be seen with proper staining.[180]

The main differential diagnosis of cutaneous primary syphilis is chancroid. However, in that disorder, the ulcer is superficial; numerous capillaries are proliferated, and the lymphoplasmacellular infiltrate is at the base. Giemsa staining reveals the numerous coccobacillary forms between keratinocytes and along the basement membrane zone.

Cutaneous lesions in secondary syphilis can be psoriasiform, lichenoid, annular, papular, or nodular, and they commonly affect the palms and soles, as well as the oral mucosa and scalp. There is usually epidermal hyperplasia overlying a band-like infiltrate of lymphocytes and plasma cells (Fig. 19-32). There may

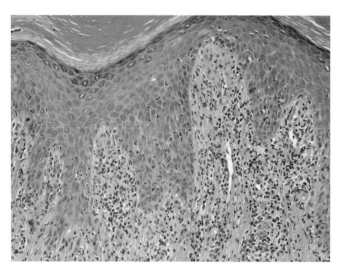

Figure 19-32. Secondary syphilis. Medium-power view of the characteristic band-like interface of lymphoplasmacytic infiltrate of secondary lues. Note endothelial cell swelling.

be rare neutrophils with debris. Beneath is a superficial and deep perivascular infiltrate with mononuclear cells that form almost granuloma-like aggregates. Endothelial swelling is prominent and may in part lead to the granulomatous appearance.[181,182] In some cases, however, the infiltrate is focal and slight, and the endothelial swelling is the clue to the diagnosis in the presence of the plasma cells. In other cases, the infiltrate may be so dense and associated with activated lymphoid cells as to suggest mycosis fungoides.[183]

In late stages of secondary syphilis, granulomas are invariably present[182] and may even suggest sarcoidosis. In 25% to 40% of early secondary syphilis, lymphocytes predominate, with the plasma cells entering later. As far as vascular changes are concerned, one may find fibrinoid necrosis in some cases of syphilis, especially in so-called lues maligna, in which thrombotic vasculitic changes are present.[184-186]

With regard to luetic alopecia, the hair follicles are infiltrated by lymphocytes and plasma cells, and perifollicular fibrosis is present.[175] A lichenoid and perivascular lymphoplasmacellular infiltrate is also noted.

Appropriate silver stains demonstrate the spirochete in about one third of cases (Figs. 19-33 and 19-34). They are best visualized in the epidermis.[186] Fluorescent antibody studies are positive in almost 100% of cases.

Tertiary Syphilis

The tertiary phase of syphilis is classified as nodular tertiary syphilis in skin or gummatous tertiary syphilis, mainly in skin, bone, and liver. Other types include cardiovascular syphilis, hepatic syphilitic cirrhosis, and neurosyphilis, and the reader is referred to classic pathology textbooks to learn their extent in these organs.

Nodular tertiary syphilis exhibits small nodules with scattered giant cells, rare granulomas, and scattered lymphocytes and plasma cells. In gummatous tertiary syphilis, there is quite prominent necrosis that is acellular. It is associated with striking plasmacellular vascular changes that extend into the dermis.[187]

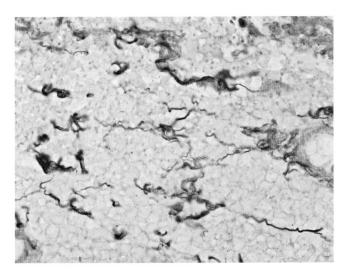

Figure 19-33. Secondary syphilis (Steiner stain). Numerous spirochetes can be found in secondary syphilis lesions.

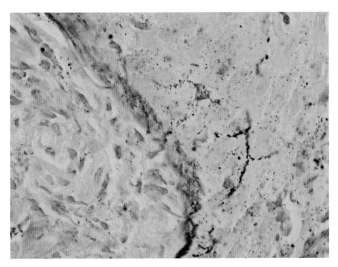

Figure 19-34. Primary syphilis (Steiner stain). High-power view of *Treponema pallidum* reveals its characteristic helicoidal structure.

Yaws

Yaws is caused by *Treponema pertenue*, a subspecies of *T. pallidum*. It varies by substitution of a single nucleotide in its DNA.[188] It also is spread by contact. It is found in warm climates.[189] Twenty-one days after inoculation, a nodule appears at the site; it enlarges centrifugally to a lesion 1 to 5 cm in size, with a reddish, crusted appearance, surrounded by pustules. The lesion is said to resemble a raspberry and therefore has been dubbed "frambesiform." Lesions can spontaneously disappear and leave a scar. Fever and constitutional symptoms may be present. Weeks to months later, constitutional symptoms reappear, associated with the onset of a widespread eruption of smaller lesions that resemble the first and have been designated "daughter yaws." The lesions can be annular and thereby resemble syphilis, and they can, in the same way as syphilis, affect the axillae and groin areas. As annular lesions, they can appear in the

orifacial area. Pustular lesions may be noted. Hyperkeratotic lesions also can occur; when present on the feet, they result in an awkward gait known as "yaws gait." Lesions can recur for up to 5 years and affect mainly the perioral areas and the axillae. Secondary bone lesions may result in periosteal nodules and thickening.

Tertiary yaws occurs in about 10% of cases and in the skin produces nodules, ulcers, and serpiginous tracts, as well as scars and keloids. In some cases, there is keratoderma and even palmar-plantar hyperkeratosis. Involvement of other organs is characteristic. The bone and joint lesions can include osteomyelitis and sometimes hypertrophic periostitis; chronic tibial disease can give rise to "saber shin." The facial bones can be involved with bilateral hypertrophy of the nasal component of the maxilla, an obstructive lesion known as goundou. Yaws is another disease that can cause ulceration of the nasal septum or palate, called gangosa. These complications can all be averted by proper antibiotic therapy.

The primary lesion exhibits hyperplasia of the epidermis with intercellular edema and intraepidermal abscesses with focal papillomatosis. In the dermis, there is a striking infiltrate of lymphoid cells, with histiocytes and plasma cells and scattered neutrophils and eosinophils. The prominent vascular change seen in syphilis is not present.[190] The secondary form is associated with epidermal hyperplasia and papillomatosis, and the infiltrate is again diffuse without vasculopathy. The tertiary yaws cutaneous lesions resemble the ulcerative granulomatous lesions of syphilis.

One can demonstrate the organisms by dark-field microscopy in the first two phases. Silver stains reveal the organisms to be present between keratinocytes, but they do not appear in the dermis.[190,191]

Pinta

Pinta is the only treponemal condition that affects the skin only. The disease occurs endemically in Central America and is not found outside the Western Hemisphere. It is caused by *Treponema carateum*. Transmission is also by contact, often among family members.[192]

This disease is limited to the skin and is associated with abnormalities of pigmentation. The primary lesion is a small, reddish to reddish-brown papule surrounded by a halo. The lesion gradually spreads and may reach a size of 10 to 12 cm with a psoriasiform appearance. The secondary lesions, called pintids, are small, scaly papules that coalesce into psoriasiform plaques. The primary and secondary lesions are highly infectious. The third stage consists of hypopigmentation over the ankles, wrists, knees, and elbows. These areas are mixed with areas of hyperpigmented or hypopigmented skin. The hypopigmentation is often symmetric and, in late achromic stages, has a stocking- or glove-like appearance. Both atrophic and hyperkeratotic areas may be present in a given lesion.

Histologically, irregular epidermal hyperplasia with a sparse infiltrate of lymphocytes, plasma cells, and neutrophils around dilated vessels is characteristic of both the first and second stages,[193] with melanophages more prominent in the second stage. In the third stage, there is either marked hyperpigmentation with numerous melanophages or profound depigmentation with a scattered lymphocytic and plasma cellular infiltration. The organisms are present in all but the very late tertiary-stage lesions.[190,194]

Endemic Syphilis

Endemic syphilis is caused by another of the subspecies of *T. pallidum*, namely *Treponema endemicum*. This particular organism is also limited in its geographic location, to the southern border of the Sahara Desert and the Arabian peninsula.[191] It is caused by contact and affects mainly children up to 15 years of age. It is also spread by common use of pipes or drinking cups. It is known as *bejel* in the language of the nomadic tribes of the areas affected. The primary lesions are rare and sometimes manifest as papules or ulcerated lesions of the oropharynx. Rarely, an infected infant can give the disease to a nursing mother, with a resultant nipple lesion occurring.

On the other hand, secondary lesions are common and may be the first sign of the disease. Small, painless papules and shallow ulcers appear on the lips, mouth, pharynx, and even larynx, with resultant hoarseness. Regional adenopathy is common. Less commonly, one can find condyloma lata–like lesions in the axillae and the groin.

The tertiary phase can manifest as gummatous lesions that form ulcers that scar and affect skin, nasopharynx, larynx, and bone. The bony lesions can greatly resemble those of yaws, in which one can find marked periosteal thickening. In addition, there can be perforation of the nasopharynx or the palate.

The histology of the lesions has not been well characterized but has been described in the ulcerated stage as showing epidermal and epithelial hyperplasia with a loosely arrayed lymphohistiocytic and plasmacellular infiltrate. Spirochetes are present in the early lesions, with prominent intraepidermal involvement.

Borrelioses

Lyme Disease

Lyme disease derives its name from the city of Lyme, Connecticut, where the first epidemic of the disease was described.[195] The lesion is caused by the spirochete *Borrelia burgdorferi*. It is transmitted by the tick *Ixodes dammini*, and other soft ticks of the species *Ornithodoros* have also been implicated.[196] The disease has been identified in 32 states and elsewhere in the world, including Europe, Africa and Asia.[197]

There are three phases of the disease. The first is associated with a lesion at the site of inoculation: Erythema chronicum migrans appears 3 to 30 days after the tick bite as a red papule that then spreads centrifugally with central clearing. The lesion can reach a size of 25 cm in diameter.[198] Some variants of the presentation include hemorrhagic vesicles and linear lesions. This component lasts for about 1 month in the American variant and 2 to 3 months in the European variant. The lesion may be associated with hematogenous spread and can result in multiple cutaneous lesions, orchitis, pneumonia, and arthritis, all associated with fever. The second phase of the lesion involves mainly the cardiac and neural systems. The nervous system changes can include meningitis, neuritis, radiculoneuritis, and even cerebritis. Heart involvement includes heart block and arrhythmias associated with myocarditis. The third phase of the disease shows predominantly chronic neural symptoms in European

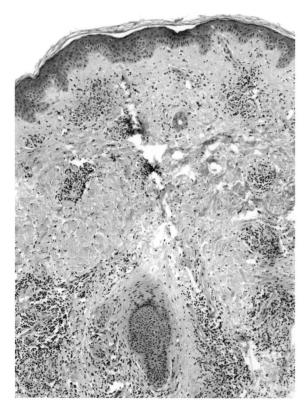

Figure 19-35. Lyme disease. Note the superficial and deep perivascular lymphocytic and plasmacellular infiltrate.

patients and musculoskeletal symptoms in patients in the United States.[199]

The lesion resembles a prominent delayed hypersensitivity reaction, as seen especially in association with an arthropod bite or drug reaction. One must also consider a connective tissue disease. Other figurate erythemas can also give a similar picture.

The primary lesion is associated with full-thickness involvement of the skin by a prominent lymphoplasmacellular infiltrate with rare eosinophils that is superficial and deep. The lesion is angiocentric with a vasculopathy, neurotropic, and eccrinotropic (Fig. 19-35). The vessel involvement includes transmural infiltration of lymphocytes and plasma cells, with a dissecting effect on the vessel architecture (Figs. 19-36 and 19-37). There is often a granulomatous component to the vasculitis and neuritis and, at times, a thrombogenic vasculopathy. An interstitial infiltrate is associated with a sclerosing reaction. Plasma cells are more intensely seen in the periphery of the lesions, with eosinophils more in the center.[200] A reactive psoriasiform hyperplasia with spongiosis is commonly observed. The spirochetes can be seen in almost half of the lesions in the advancing border, where they manifest as scattered organisms measuring 10 to 25 μm by 0.2 μm. Myocardial biopsy specimens show an interstitial lymphoplasmacellular infiltrate with a band-like infiltration beneath the endocardium. Acute myocarditis can also be seen.

Chlamydial Infections

There are two disorders that belong in this group. One is an infection transmitted by birds that is caused by *Chlamydia*

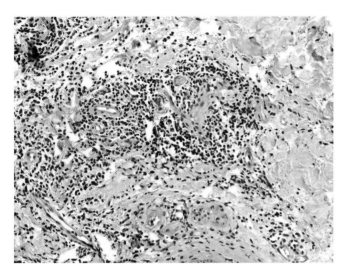

Figure 19-36. Lyme disease. The infiltrate is characteristically neurotropic.

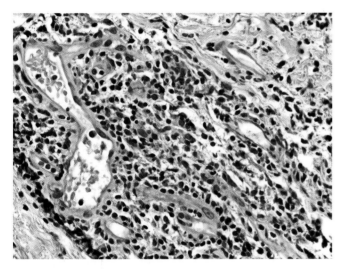

Figure 19-37. Lyme disease. The infiltrate is composed predominantly of lymphocytes and plasma cells. Note infiltration of the vascular walls without the prominent endothelial swelling seen in secondary syphilis.

psittaci, now known as *Chlamydophila psittaci*. The other is a venereal disease caused by *Chlamydia trachomatis*. The bird infection is known as psittacosis, and the venereal disease as lymphogranuloma venereum.

Psittacosis

Psittacosis affects parrots predominantly, but also other birds. Its name comes from the Latin word for parrot, *psittacines*. It is caused by *C. psittaci*. Human infection occurs through the respiratory root and results in a systemic disease that includes fever and pneumonitis. The diagnosis is usually based on serologic studies.[201-204] This illness can vary from mild to very severe and, rarely, can cause death. There is total systemic involvement, with fever, pneumonitis, and pleurisy, even pericarditis and myocarditis. There are a variety of cutaneous symptoms and signs. First, there are red macular lesions called Horder spots. These spots

occur on the abdomen and trunk and can resemble typhoid fever. However, hypersensitivity reactions, including urticaria, erythema nodosum, and erythema multiforme, have been reported. In severe cases with disseminated disease, intravascular coagulation and purpura can be observed. Differential diagnosis clinically includes the spectrum of viral, deep fungal, and bacterial pneumonias that can cause systemic disease.

The morphology of the lesions is that of the clinical type. The rose spots apparently show a mild, perivenular lymphoid infiltrate.

Lymphogranuloma Venereum

The sexually transmitted disease called lymphogranuloma venereum is more common in African Americans and occurs more frequently in areas of warm climate. The causative organism, *Chlamydia trachomatis*, is an intracellular obligate.[3,205] The genital lesions appear an average of 7 days after contact and manifest as small (2-3 mm) papules or ulcers. This lesion heals rapidly and may be associated with a nonspecific urethritis. Within 10 days to 2 weeks after the initial lesion appears, inguinal adenopathy appears in men and is associated with the so-called groove sign, which results from enlargement of lymph nodes surrounding the Poupart ligament. Inguinal involvement can also occur in women, but at times, because of infection of the lower vagina, the affected nodes are the iliac and anal rectal. Such nodal involvement can lead to rectal stricture. As late complications, massive edema of the penis and scrotum can occur in men, and marked vulvar edema in women.

In the differential diagnosis, the lesions of chancroid are larger than those of lymphogranuloma venereum and very painful, but swollen nodes can be found in both disorders. The culture of *Chlamydia* and serologic studies, as well as smears for *H. ducreyi*, are very helpful in differentiating these lesions. Granuloma inguinale has much larger ulcers with prominent granulation tissue.

The cutaneous lesions have a granulomatous inflammation associated with endothelial cell swelling, histiocytes, activated lymphocytes, and plasma cells. Only rarely are the organisms visible by Giemsa stain. Both organisms can be cultured, and serologic studies are available. The lymph nodes, on the other hand, have stellate microabscesses in which necrotic debris is surrounded by granulomatous inflammation.[10]

Rickettsia and Rickettsia-like Organisms

Like the *Chlamydia* group, these unusual bacteria known as rickettsia are obligate intracellular parasites and are somewhat midway between bacteria and viruses.[3] Because their habitat is the nutrient-rich cytosol of parasitized cells, these organisms have a unique genome which lacks portions that encode diverse enzymes related to sugar, amino acid, and lipid metabolism.[206] In the past, they were classified as part of the *Rickettsia* group. The well-known taxonomic conundrum with regard to these organisms has since been partially resolved through phylogenetic studies.[206,207] Today, we know that organisms such as *Coxiella burnetii* are part of the *Legionella* group.[208] Also, the agent of the scrub typhus, formerly designated *Rickettsia tsutsugamushi*, is now called *Orientia tsutsugamushi* and is part of the *Orientia* group.[209] New species and new strains of existing species are being characterized, and there is also re-emergence of "older" organisms.[206,207] The *Rickettsia* organisms are divided into the spotted fever group and the typhus group.

Spotted Fever Group

Rocky Mountain Spotted Fever

The first organism to be considered in the spotted fever group is *Rickettsia rickettsii*, the agent of Rocky Mountain spotted fever (RMSF), which is the most common tickborne disease in the United States.[210] RMSF is considered to be one of the most virulent infections in humans. This bacterium is a small (0.2-0.5 μm) fastidious, gram-negative, pleomorphic coccobacillus that infects vascular endothelial cells causing severe systemic manifestations.[3] Ticks from the hard tick family (Ixodidae) act as both reservoirs and vectors of this organism.[211] Other mechanisms of infection include blood transfusion and inhalation of contaminated aerosol, the latter occurring almost exclusively in laboratories. The disease is distributed mainly in countries of the Western Hemisphere.[212]

The mean incubation period of RMSF is 7 days, and multiple systems and organs are characteristically affected.[213] The early manifestations include sudden onset of fever, malaise, and severe headache.[212-214] A rash is present in only 3% of the cases in this phase.[215] Rather, the cutaneous lesions typically appear 2 to 5 days after the onset of the fever, thereby completing the classic triad of fever, headache, and rash.[212,214] The rash is composed initially of 1- to 5-mm, blanching erythematous macules on the wrists and ankles. These lesions extend first centrifugally to the palms and soles, and then centripetally to the trunk.[212,216] In severe infections, skin necrosis and gangrene may be present and may even require amputation.[217] The rash is absent in 9% to 12% of cases, and this phenomenon is related to fatal cases, older patients, and African-American patients.[212]

The diagnosis of RMSF is always troublesome for the clinicians, because the clinical manifestations depend on the organs and systems affected. Serologic tests are of limited help, because antibodies do not appear until 7 to 10 days after disease onset.[218] The Weil-Felix test has become obsolete and is falling into disuse.[212,219] Enzyme-linked immunosorbent assays (ELISA) can be useful.[212] The gold standard is the indirect fluorescence antibody test, which is highly sensitive.[218,220] However, it cannot distinguish among *R. rickettsia* and other spotted fever *Rickettsia* species.[221] There are now available more sensitive methods, such as newer quantitative PCR assays, that solve this problem.[222] The differential diagnosis is quite broad and includes conditions exhibiting small-vessel vasculitis, such as insect bites or drug reactions, and diseases associated with leukocytoclastic vasculitis.[223]

Because the infection is targeted toward endothelial cells, it is not surprising to find prominent lymphohistiocytic and sometimes neutrophilic small-vessel vasculitis.[3] There is a spectrum of histologic findings according to the stage of the disease and the severity of the infection. In the acute phase, maculopapular lesions exhibit a tight perivascular infiltrate that extends into the vessel walls, causing endothelial cell swelling, extravasation of red blood cells, and edema. More advanced lesions show a clinical presentation with hemorrhage and petechiae caused by a leukocytoclastic vasculitis with endothelial necrosis. Focal fibrin thrombi and an interface dermatitis also appear at this stage. Rare findings represent an eccrine hidradenitis and acute lobular panniculitis.[223]

Rickettsial antigens can be demonstrated in paraffin-embedded sections with immunohistochemical stains. This can be useful in making the diagnosis, especially when a rash is biopsied in its acute phase.[224]

Other Rickettsia Species from the Spotted Fever Group

The other rickettsial organisms that form the spotted fever group cause conditions that clinically are similar to RSMF but with the main difference that an eschar is formed at the site of the tick's bite (inoculation eschar).

One of the principal members of this group is *Rickettsia conorii*, which has numerous strains and is distributed in the Mediterranean area. The various strains of the organism cause the disease known as Mediterranean spotted fever, which has some regional characteristics.[225]

Another recently characterized disease that is part of the spotted fever group is African tick bite fever. This condition, caused by *Rickettsia africae*, has been found predominantly in sub-Saharan Africa, and recently in the Caribbean.[226]

Typhus Group

The name typhus is derived from *tuphos*, the Greek word for "smoke," because it affects the sensorium. Typhus is a disease related to poor sanitary conditions (e.g., wars, famines) that was probably first identified as early as in 1083 in Spain. However, clinical overlap of this disease with typhoid fever is common.[227] Two organisms comprise this group, *Rickettsia typhi* and *Rickettsia prowazekii*. *R. typhi* is transmitted by fleas and causes the murine typhus; it is more common in warm climates. *R. prowazekii* is transmitted by body lice (*Pediculus humanus corporis*), with a peak in transmission during cold months.[228]

The incubation period is usually 10 to 14 days.[227] The clinical course is dominated by high fever, as well as debilitating headaches and myalgias.[228] Dermatologic manifestations are also quite common. They manifest first as a nonconfluent, blanching, erythematous rash on the trunk, which evolves into a nonblanching petechial and even purpuric rash with centrifugal spread to the extremities.[228,229] Severe cases may exhibit symmetric gangrene of fingers and toes.[227]

The Brill-Zinsser clinical form of typhus is a reactivation of the disease which can occur years after the primary episode. This reactivation phenomenon is unique to this group of rickettsial diseases and produces as a milder and shorter episode in comparison to the original infection. However, it can be fatal in some cases.[228,230]

As is characteristic of this type of organisms, the clinical diagnosis can be quite troublesome. Several methods can aid the clinician, including culture and PCR.[228]

Common to all rickettsial infections, a massive injury of endothelial cells is seen. This results in a widespread vasculitis with concomitant edema, extravasation of red blood cells, and activation of the coagulation cascade with formation of thrombi. These thrombi are accompanied by inflammatory infiltrates composed of macrophages, lymphocytes, and plasma cells.[228]

Rickettsia-like Organisms

Scrub Typhus

Caused by the organism recently named *Orientia tsutsugamushi*, scrub typhus is a systemic disease that is distributed among Asian countries. It is transmitted by mites of the *Leptotrombidium* genus ("chiggers").[231] Early in the disease, one finds the triad of a cutaneous eschar at the site of inoculation, regional lymphadenectomy, and a maculopapular rash. The disease then becomes systemic and affects multiple organs.[231] The eschar is one of the most useful tools to make the diagnosis clinically, and it is most frequently found where clothes and skin meet, namely in the axillae, groin, neck, waist, and inguinal areas.[232] Eschars usually begin as a small papule which evolves into a necrotic lesion with a black crust and an erythematous halo.

Histologically, there is dermal vasculitis with a lymphohistiocytic perivascular infiltrate and necrosis.[231,233] Immunohistochemical identification of the parasites in biopsy samples taken from the eschars can be helpful.[233] Molecular and serologic tests are available to aid diagnosis.

Q Fever

Q fever, a zoonosis caused by *Coxiella burnetii*, has a worldwide distribution with the exception of New Zealand.[208] It can be acquired through inhalation of contaminated aerosols, which makes this organism highly infective and a potential biological weapon.[234,235] Another possible means of contamination is consumption of unpasteurized dairy products.[236] Known reservoirs of the organism include cattle, sheep, and goats.[237] This parasite infects human macrophages and also can infect free-living amebas such as *Acanthamoeba* spp., which serve as "microscopic reservoirs."[238]

The clinical course can vary from an asymptomatic infection to a systemic disease with prominent involvement of the myocardium and the lungs. The clinical manifestations in the acute phase depend on host factors (e.g., sex, age, immune status), inoculum size, strain specificity, and route of infection.[208] The cutaneous manifestations of Q fever are not specific and are usually represented by transient punctiform rashes, maculopapular eruptions, and, rarely, erythema nodosum.[239,240]

Viral Infections of the Skin

Diseases caused by viruses are common, and many of them affect the skin.[241] With the onset of immunotherapy and the HIV epidemic, many viruses have been found to have much more serious sequelae in immunocompromised patients. This situation has led to more intensive studies of viruses, especially of therapeutic means to block the viral sequelae. Viruses are intracellular obligates with a genome composed of either DNA or RNA and no replication machinery. They replicate within the host cells by taking over the ribosomes and mitochondria of the cell. The process of infection includes, first, attachment of the infecting agent to specific cell surface receptors. The virus then enters the cell cytoplasm via endocytosis, during which the virus becomes covered with part of the plasmomembrane. This mode of entry is associated with coating of the virus by glycolipoproteins. Digestion of the outer coat of plasmomembrane takes place in the cytoplasm, whereupon the viral material or nucleoids lose their structural framework. At this point, the viruses are considered to be in an "eclipse phase," virtually disappearing within the cell. They reappear only after sufficient replication of new virions has occurred. The proteins that are produced after viral infection of a cell are characteristic of the virus rather than the cell. The release of new virions to the exterior occurs by lysis of the cell or by budding from the cell surface.

Viruses can be observed by light microscopy when they are gathered to form an inclusion body. Although the size of the individual virus ranges from 10 nm in the case of echoviruses to 300 nm for viruses of the pox family, 7 μm is the average size of the viral inclusion body. Most of them occur in the nucleus, particularly in DNA viruses. The inclusion bodies are found by light microscopy in only three groups of viruses: herpesviruses, papillomaviruses and poxviruses.[241]

The viruses that most commonly affect the skin are members of the family Herpesviridae, including HSV, varicella-zoster virus (VZV), cytomegalovirus (CMV), *Roseolovirus* (human herpesvirus 6, or HHV-6), *Lymphocryptovirus* (Epstein-Barr virus, or EBV), HHV-7, and HHV-8. These viruses proliferate in the nucleus of an infected cell. Another common viral group, which multiplies in the cytoplasm, is the Poxviridae. Members of this family cause smallpox, milker's nodules, orf, and molluscum contagiosum. The third family of dermotropic viruses that affect the skin is the Papillomaviridae. These viruses, which contain DNA and replicate in the nucleus, include the various genotypes of human papillomavirus (HPV). A fourth type of virus is the Picornaviridae, which contain RNA. The so-called hand-foot-and-mouth disease is caused by coxsackievirus A16. The fifth group is the Retroviridae, which are also genetically composed of RNA. This group's most prominent member is HIV, the cause of AIDS.[241]

Many other virus families can infect the skin, such as Adenoviridae, Togaviridae, Reoviridae, Parvoviridae, Paramyxoviridae, Flaviviridae, and Hepadnaviridae. The lesions from the first three DNA virus families discussed in this section (i.e., Papillomaviridae, Herpesviridae, and Poxviridae) contain diagnostic viral inclusions. The other groups of viruses result often in a superficial perivascular lymphoid infiltrate, sometimes with exocytosis directed above the inflamed venules and sometimes with a mild extravasation of red blood cells and debris. In some cases, such as parvovirus B19 infection, there can be changes that resemble other dermatoses, such as erythema nodosum or erythema multiforme. There may also be apoptotic cells noted in the epidermis with cytoid bodies in the dermis.[241]

As far as confirming histologic changes by other methods, one can perform viral cultures. Other routes are immunohistochemistry and electron microscopy. With the use of the PCR amplification technique, one can detect the presence of the specific viral DNA. In addition, there are now probes that can be used for this detection. As far as the serologic approaches are concerned, one examines acute and convalescent sera to detect whether there has been a greater than fourfold rise in antiviral IgG. The detection of virus-specific IgM in a single acute or early recovery phase sample is very useful. This technique is currently used for certain types of infection, such as infectious mononucleosis, viral hepatitis, and parvovirus B19 infection, among others.[241]

In any case, the specimen must be obtained directly at the site of the infection during early eruption. Specimens must be kept at 4° C in the refrigerator or on wet ice. If the material must be stored for later use, one must use a freezer at −7° C.[241]

Papillomaviridae

The HPV family contains more than 80 genotypes of non-enveloped, double-stranded DNA viruses with molecular heterogeneity.[242] The clinical manifestations usually arise 1 to 8 months after infection by the virus. The HPV viruses target cutaneous or mucosal squamous epithelial cells mainly from the oral, the cervical, or the anogenital area. Initially, they were considered to be sexually transmitted, but they have also been implicated in cancers of the oropharynx,[243] esophagus,[244] lung,[245] and skin.[246] HPV clinical manifestations are also related to immunosuppression.[247]

Some genotypes (i.e., HPV-16, -18, -31, -33, and -51) are considered to carry a high risk for carcinogenesis, and a close follow-up of patients with a clinical history of exposure to them is recommended.[247] Molecular pathology has contributed greatly to identification of this group of patients with the help of DNA hybridization or amplification by PCR of HPV genomic material. However, clinical practice has shown that a positive result is not absolutely predictive of future carcinogenesis.

Verruca Vulgaris

Verruca vulgaris is a common wart, related to the 1, 2, 4, 7, and 49 genotypes of HPV, that has been associated with defective cell-mediated immunity and immunosuppression. The viral particles are 50-nm spherical bodies, easily recognized as basophilic spherules in histologic sections stained with H&E. In situ hybridization and PCR techniques can be used for definitive identification of the virus.[241] Verruca vulgaris commonly manifests on the dorsal aspect of the hands and fingers of children and adults, with a great predilection in butchers and slaughterhouse workers. The palms, soles, face, and scalp are less commonly affected, whereas the oral mucosa is an exceptional site of development. The verrucae occur usually as painless, sometimes tender, whitish or pink, single lesions 1 to 10 mm in diameter. They may also occur in groups. They are well circumscribed, firm, and elevated, with a papillomatous hyperkeratotic surface. Spontaneous regression has been reported. Recurrences and appearance of new warts at sites of trauma have been documented.[241]

Verruca vulgaris is easily differentiated from other papillomatous lesions of the skin, especially with the use of epiluminescence microscopy. The differential diagnosis is based on the presence of koilocytosis, parakeratotic tiers, and foci of coarse keratohyaline granules. In old lesions where no basophilic nuclei indicative of the presence of the virus are seen, the architecture of the lesion is especially helpful for making the correct diagnosis.

Acanthosis, papillomatosis, hyperkeratosis, tiers of parakeratotic cells, and foci of clumped keratohyaline granules are features of verruca vulgaris, combined with a characteristic architecture of elongated peripheral rete ridges oriented toward the center of the lesion. Foci of koilocytosis in the upper portion of the hyperplastic epidermis, together with small, round, intensely basophilic nuclei and pale-staining cytoplasm surrounded by a clear halo, are characteristic and prominent in young lesions but can be absent in old ones. The parakeratotic cells have large, intensively basophilic nuclei; they overlie the tips of the papillomatous projections, often accompanied by foci of

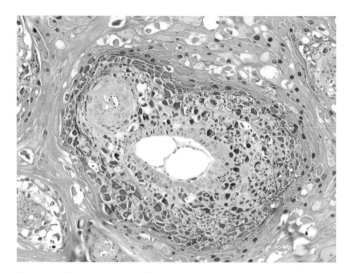

Figure 19-38. Verruca vulgaris. This example of a plantar verruca exhibits severe viral cytopathic effect with koilocytosis and prominent basophilic inclusions.

hemorrhage, and granular cells with heavy, irregular clumps of keratohyaline are located in the intervening valleys (Fig. 19-38). Slender papillomatous projections and intense hyperkeratosis are characteristic of the filiform type of verruca vulgaris, which is often seen in the face and scalp area.

In regressing lesions, lymphocytes are present in the hyperplastic epithelium in conjunction with basal cell liquefaction, epidermal degeneration, and vessel thrombosis in the upper dermis. Verruca vulgaris may be found in combination with a cutaneous horn; it is only exceptionally related to an in situ or infiltrative squamous cell carcinoma.

Verruca Plana

Verruca plana is usually related to the HPV-2, -3, or -10 genotype. It appears as flat, grayish-yellow, possibly hyperpigmented, and slightly elevated papules of a few millimeters in diameter, with a smooth surface; they are usually located on the face, shins, and dorsal area of the hands. Verruca plana is common in childhood. In adult life, it can be found in women and men with HIV-related immunodeficiency. The lesions are usually few in number, but in children who have a coexistent familial incidence, they may be multiple, distributed on the extremities and the trunk. Regression can spontaneously take place, and multiple lesions may appear in areas of scratching. Multiple verrucae planae in young patients with a familial distribution can bring up problems in differentiating this disease from epidermodysplasia verruciformis (EV, discussed in the next section). The absence of red, tinea versicolor–like lesions is helpful for the correct diagnosis. In progressively regressed lesions, the presence of cells with koilocytic appearance is helpful for making the correct diagnosis.

Verruca plana shares with verruca vulgaris the presence of acanthosis, hyperkeratosis, and koilocytic-appearing cells, but there is no parakeratosis or papillomatosis. Hypergranulosis is prominent throughout the lesion, and a basket-weave appearance of hyperkeratotic material is considered to be characteristic (Fig. 19-39). Regressed lesions have apoptotic cells and foci of exocytosis in the epidermis and a lymphocytic infiltrate with extravasation of red blood cells in the upper dermis.

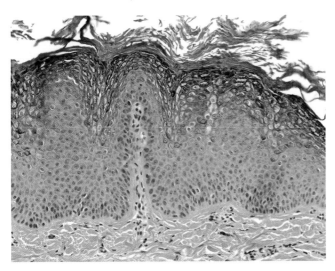

Figure 19-39. Verruca plana. There is prominent hyperkeratosis and acanthosis with numerous vacuolated keratinocytes in the granular layer.

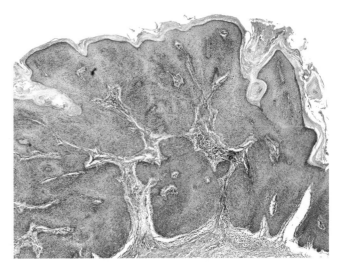

Figure 19-40. Condyloma acuminatum. Arborescent keratinocytic proliferation with pronounced acanthosis.

Epidermodysplasia Verruciformis

EV is a rare genetic disease that is related to a wide range of HPV genotypes, some of them considered to be specific for the lesion.[249] It usually manifests in childhood and has two different clinical settings. The first one is related to the HPV-3 and HPV-10 genotypes, is sometimes familial, has no tendency toward malignant transformation, and manifests with a widespread eruption reminiscent of disseminated verrucae planae. The second one is primarily related to HPV-5 and secondarily to HPV-8. It is often familial, with an autosomal recessive or X-linked recessive character of inheritance. In approximately one fourth of the patients, it is associated with the development of squamous cutaneous carcinoma, mostly of the intraepidermal Bowen type and occasionally with an invasive pattern.

Immunosuppression related to HIV infection[250] or other causes[251] can be the underlying factor in a patient with an EV-like dermatologic picture. EV can be misdiagnosed as a verruca plana if the clinician does not focus on the more extensive and prominent character of the epidermal hyperplasia in EV. The abundance of coarse keratohyaline granules and the clear appearance of the nuclei of the keratinocytes also point to the correct diagnosis.

EV in non-immunocompromised patients exhibits extensive and prominent epidermal hyperplasia that is reminiscent of a verruca plana. One sees hyperkeratosis, relatively mild acanthosis, and swollen squamous cells with large clear or pyknotic nuclei and with abundant intracytoplasmic presence of coarse basophilic keratohyaline granules. Vacuolated cells can be seen in the upper portion of the epidermis, and dyskeratotic cells are found in the lower part of the hyperplastic epithelium. In immunosuppressed patients, the histology differs, with focal thickening of the granular layer being the most characteristic finding in a slightly hyperplastic epidermis. Squamous dysplasia is a common finding.[252]

Condyloma Acuminatum

Condyloma acuminatum is a mostly asymptomatic anogenital warty lesion, related to HPV infection and specifically to both low-risk (HPV-6, HPV-11) and high-risk (HPV-16, -18, -31 through -33, -35, -39, -42, and -51 through -54) genotypes of the virus, affecting the anal and genital area. It is considered to be a sexually transmitted disease that can affect both genders. It is often present in young adults but it is rare in childhood. Condyloma acuminatum, especially when related to high-risk HPV genotypes, can progress to in situ squamous cell carcinoma of the Bowen or common type, or to invasive squamous cell carcinoma of the genital area in both sexes, with the vagina and cervix of women in reproductive age being primarily affected.[253] Local recurrence is quite common in the anal area, although spontaneous regression often reported in childhood is independent of the low- or high-risk nature of the genotype of the virus.[254]

Giant condyloma acuminatum of Buschke and Loewenstein is a large, cauliflower-like lesion, frequently located in the glans penis and foreskin of men, with resemblance to condyloma acuminatum in early stage of development. It is locally destructive, with a tendency for ulceration and recurrence. It is related to HPV genotypes 6, 11, and 16 and can undergo malignant transformation with low metastatic potentiality. In the absence of koilocytosis, condyloma acuminatum can mimic seborrheic keratosis. In situ hybridization or PCR techniques can be helpful in detection of the virus. In fact, a great percentage of vulvar seborrheic keratoses may represent senescent condylomas.[255]

Giant condyloma acuminatum of Buschke and Loewenstein needs to be thoroughly examined to exclude a squamous cell carcinoma of the verrucous subtype. Detailed examination of morphology, especially in the lower portion of the lesion, is helpful in the establishment of the correct diagnosis. Increased mitoses, nuclear atypia, and foci of dermal microinvasion in conjunction with immunohistochemical overexpression of Ki67 proliferation index and Rb or p53 oncoprotein throughout the hyperplastic epithelium, are evidence of malignant transformation.[256,257]

Condyloma acuminatum is a papillomatous epidermal lesion exhibiting acanthosis, hyperkeratosis, and parakeratosis (Fig. 19-40). Coarse keratohyaline granules can be seen in the superficial part of the lesion. Vacuolated keratinocytes with

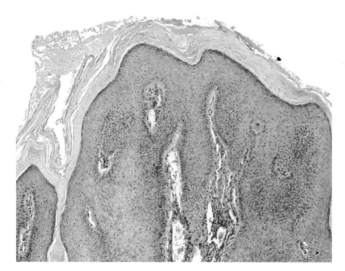

Figure 19-41. Condyloma acuminatum. Note the fine fibrovascular papillae characteristic of this virus-induced proliferation.

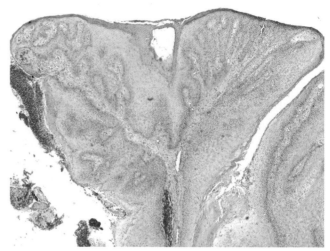

Figure 19-43. Giant condyloma (Buschke-Loewenstein stain). Prominent papillomatous growth with marked epithelial hyperplasia and hyperkeratosis.

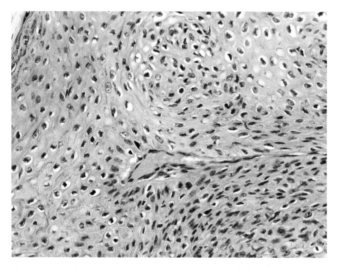

Figure 19-42. Condyloma acuminatum. High-power view of the lesions reveals the koilocytic viral change of the cells.

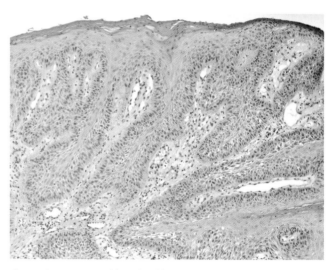

Figure 19-44. Giant condyloma (Buschke-Loewenstein stain). Medium-power view exhibiting a well-developed basal cell layer.

morphologic characteristics of koilocytosis are diagnostic when found in both upper and lower portions of the hyperplastic epidermis (Figs. 19-41 and 19-42). Numerous mitoses and necrotic keratinocytes at the bottom of the epithelium may be seen in lesions previously treated with podophyllin. In giant condyloma acuminatum of Buschke and Loewenstein, the vacuolized keratinocytes may be few or absent, and the endophytic deep part of the lesion has a well-developed basal cell layer (Figs. 19-43 and 19-44).

Bowenoid Papulosis

Bowenoid papulosis is a mostly papular and exceptionally verrucous, small, red or red-brown, discrete lesion of approximately 4 mm in diameter that can be related to HPV, mainly the HPV-16 and HPV-18 genotypes. It develops in the genitalia of sexually active young men or women (glans and shaft of penis,

vulva) and in the perineal or the perianal area in the form of multiple lesions, partially forming a plaque. Exceptionally, it may be found on the face, neck, or fingers. Spontaneous regression and rare development of carcinoma are reported in bowenoid papulosis. Bowenoid papulosis can be differentiated from Bowen disease on the basis of circumscription, slight elevation, and size of the lesion, as well as the multiplicity and the young age of the patients.

Bowenoid papulosis has microscopic features reminiscent of Bowen disease. There is acanthosis with full-thickness atypia of keratinocytes and nuclei partially dyskeratotic, pleomorphic, or multinucleated. There are multiple mitoses, some of them atypical. Hyperkeratosis and vacuolated keratinocytes can be seen in the superficial portion of the lesion. True koilocytosis is uncommon. An increased number of apoptotic keratinocytes and atypical mitotic figures is reported to be related to recent treatment with podophyllin resin.

Herpesviridae

There are three families in this classification, all of which are double-stranded DNA viruses. The first family includes HSV-1 and -2, VSV, CMV, EBV, and HHV-6, -7, and -8.

Herpes Simplex

Herpes simplex can be caused by HSV-1 (orofacial type) or HSV-2 (genital type). The infection with HSV-1 can occur at any time in life and is thought to be usually first acquired in childhood with a subclinical infection. However, 10% of cases can demonstrate an acute gingivostomatitis, more commonly in children than in adults. There are some very unusual presentations, including a respiratory infection, Kaposi varicelliform eruption, and keratoconjunctivitis. There is also a fatal widespread disease in children that is visceral and affects most organs in the body. HSV-2 infection usually occurs after the onset of sexual activity.[258] The exception is HSV-2 acquired during gestation or during birth, when the child comes into contact with an herpetic infection of the birth canal.[259] In addition, HSV-1 can affect the genital area in some cases. As far as recurrent herpes is concerned, the most common manifestation is that of cold sores on the vermilion border of the lips. However, any part of the body can be affected by HSV-1. For example, herpes gladiatorum may occur in athletes such as wrestlers if infected material is transferred from the lips to the mat and from there to other parts of the body.

Clinical Features

Primary and recurrent herpes simplex in the earliest stages causes slight erythema with discomfort, followed by the rapid appearance of groups of tiny, clear vesicles. These lesions occur most commonly around the lips but can occur anywhere on the body, as described earlier. Triggering factors include emotional or physical stress, the onset of menses, hot or cold temperature changes, and sunlight. In some patients, the lesions are triggered by fever and are called "fever blisters."[260] The primary infection of herpes usually manifests with a sense of dysesthesia and the appearance of very clear, small vesicles grouped on an edematous, erythematous base. The lesions may break down rapidly or become pustular; they eventually heal within a few days without scarring, unless there is a superimposed bacterial infection. However, in children and rarely in adults, the primary infection can be associated with a severe gingivostomatosis, keratoconjunctivitis, Kaposi varicelliform eruption, or even a fatal visceral disease.

Eczema herpeticum, also known as Kaposi varicelliform eruption, represents a complication in patients with atopic eczema but also occurs sometimes in association with seborrheic dermatitis, pityriasis rubra pilaris, pemphigus foliaceus, or Darier disease.[261,262] It is usually caused by HSV-1, and rarely by HSV-2, but also can be caused by Coxsackie A16 virus and vaccinia. The primary type occurs mainly in infants and children and may result from external infection or from reactivation of the virus. Primary eczema herpeticum is a serious disease, especially in children, and can spread to the entire system. Secondary (recurrent) infection is less severe and is not associated with internal organ disease unless the patient is immunocompromised. Death sometimes ensues because of bacterial superinfection or in cases of impaired

immunity. Ten percent of immunocompromised patients succumb. The characteristic rash is an extensive vesiculation of the skin with small pustules associated with high fever. The vesiculopustules are scattered especially on skin affected by the dermatitic disorder.

Herpetic folliculitis is an unusual variant of herpes simplex that manifests as a small area of grouped, painful papules that have a follicular orifice in the center which may or may not be associated with a vesicle. These usually heal within a few weeks.[263] Deep infection of the nail results in painful paronychia or pain on the volar surface of the fingers. This disorder, so-called herpetic whitlow, is very common in physicians and dentists and their assistants.[264] Another unusual type of herpes is hyperplastic herpes. It manifests as a nodule, usually in the area of the lips, and can be mistaken for squamous cell carcinoma or keratoacanthoma. Other primary herpetic infections result in keratoconjunctivitis, which can cause blindness.[265] Herpetic balanitis, pneumonia, encephalitis, and even herpetic proctitis can also be encountered. Herpetic encephalitis is often associated with recurrent herpes of the external ear.

Congenital herpes simplex usually is transmitted from a mother with an active infection in the vagina or vulva and hence is usually caused by recurrent HSV-2 viral infection. In cases of primary HSV-2 infection in pregnancy, the timing of the exposure is very important. Marked congenital malformations of the fetus can result if the infection occurs during the first 8 weeks of gestation.[266] With later infections, the effects on the fetus are less severe and can include even a generalized vesicular eruption. In the case of recurrent maternal herpes, the eruption is localized to the skin, but transplacental herpetic infection can affect many organs and may result in pneumonia or even encephalitis.[259,263]

Finally, one must consider the various types of herpes that occur in immunocompromised patients. These include a chronic ulcerative disorder that begins on the face or perineum and gradually spreads (Fig. 19-45).[267] A second type of infection is acute mucocutaneous herpes simplex that becomes generalized after a localized vesicular eruption.[268] Generalized systemic HSV infection can result in infection of many organs and can cause marked hepatorenal necrosis, pancreas necrosis, encephalitis, and brain necrosis.

Histopathology

The first changes that occur in herpes infection affect the basilar layer and result in nuclear swelling. The earliest change is the margination of nuclear chromatin in the periphery of the nucleus in small nodules—the so-called Cowdry type B bodies. The changes gradually involve the entire epidermis. As the virus proliferates in the nucleus, a slight gray coloration occurs in the nuclei. During this time, two changes can occur with the keratinocytes. One, termed ballooning degeneration, is a swelling of the keratinocytes, and the other is reticular degeneration. After the nuclei become infected by the virus, there is cell fusion resulting in multinucleate giant cells. As the cells swell more, they become separated from one another and exhibit acantholysis. As far as the progressive nuclear changes are concerned, the virus passes into the nucleus and leaves behind a prominent eosinophilic body that is surrounded by a halo or clear space. The eosinophilic body is 3 to 8 μm in diameter (Figs. 19-46 and 19-47). The reticular degeneration occurs because of rupture of ballooning cells. The reticular degeneration resembles vesicles in

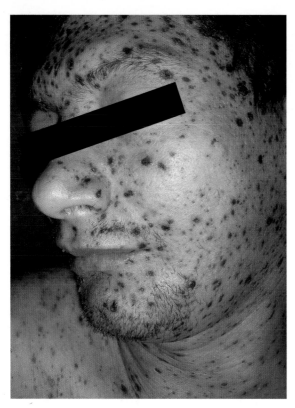

Figure 19-45. Herpes simplex infection in a patient with HIV/AIDS. Note the generalized distribution of the lesions.

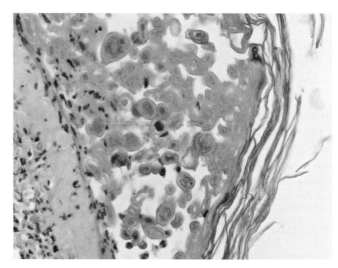

Figure 19-46. Herpes simplex infection. Note the intraepidermal vesicle, in which the keratinocytes exhibit acantholysis and prominent ballooning degeneration. In addition, there are multinucleated cells with nuclear molding.

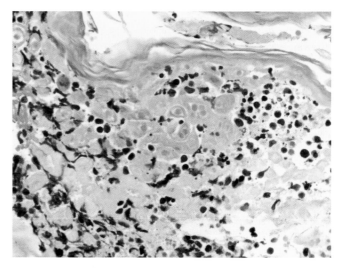

Figure 19-47. Herpes simplex infection. Numerous keratinocytes exhibit eosinophilic intranuclear inclusions also known as Cowdry A bodies.

eczema, but often one can see the cell membranes intact focally, the cytoplasmic contents having been evacuated from the cell due to focal rupture of the membranes. The nuclear changes are seen predominantly in the basal cells, but multinucleate cells can be seen extensively in the acantholytic areas, as can cells with the characteristic inclusions. These nuclear changes can also be observed in endothelial cells, sebaceous gland cells, and cells of the hair follicle and eccrine ducts. One of the first changes in herpetic infection is necrosis of sebaceous glands (Figs. 19-48 and 19-49). Any time one observes interface dermatitis along the epidermis and hair follicle that is associated with eosinophilic necrosis of a sebaceous gland, the first diagnostic consideration should be HSV infection.[269]

In summary, keratinocytes undergo ballooning degeneration beginning at the base of the vesicle. At first, there is margination of the nuclear chromatin; this becomes associated with replacement of the nucleus by gunmetal-gray or blue-gray coloration as the cells balloon, and fusion and multinucleation, as well as acanthosis, occur. At that point, the nuclei begin to lose their basophilia and are left with an eosinophilic inclusion body 3 to 8 μm in diameter. This inclusion body is nonviral and is composed of RNA and non–histone-containing nuclear protein (Fig. 19-50). It is called the Cowdry A body. As the cells become more inflated, they rupture their membranes and give rise to reticular degeneration, which resembles spongiosis. In contrast to spongiosis, one may find membranes relatively intact but without any evidence of cytosol or other cytoplasmic contents.

Varicella and Herpes Zoster

Varicella and herpes zoster are caused by the same virus, VZV. Varicella is contracted by a person who was not exposed to the virus before. Herpes zoster occurs in persons who previously experienced varicella. Ganglia of major sensitive nerves, such as the spinal cord sensory ganglia or the ganglia of the fifth cranial nerve, are the sites where VZV remains latent after the initial (varicella) infection. When reactivation occurs, VZV spreads along the sensory nerve tracts into the skin, manifesting clinically as herpes zoster, or "shingles."

Varicella

VZV is a lymphotropic virus that especially affects T cells. During the initial infection with the virus, usually 2 weeks after contact, there is a viremia, which is followed by a dissemination of the virus through infected mononuclear cells to the epithelial cells.

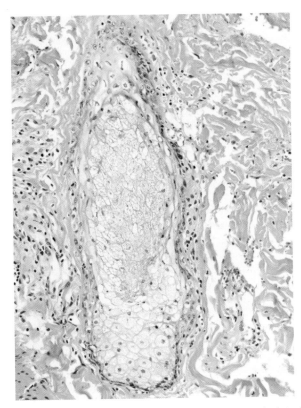

Figure 19-48. Herpes simplex infection. Necrosis of the sebaceous glands is often observed in herpes simplex virus infection and can be a useful clue for the diagnosis.

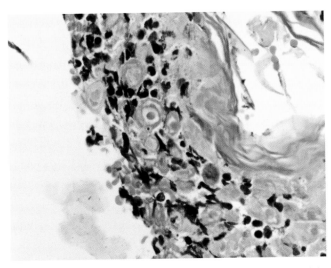

Figure 19-50. Herpes simplex infection. Prominent intranuclear inclusions of the keratinocytes induced by proliferation of the herpes simplex virus.

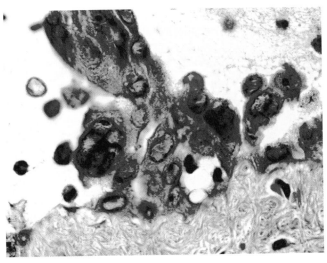

Figure 19-49. Herpes simplex infection. Some keratinocytes exhibit Cowdry B inclusions, which are more nodular clumps of basophilic staining material dispersed along the nuclear membranes. Note the Cowdry A bodies that are also present in other nuclei.

From there, the virus spreads to the tissues, resulting in the clinical features of varicella. After the varicella lesions have cleared, the late phase of the process occurs, with the virus entering the ganglia of sensory nerves. Reactivation of latent virus, which causes herpes zoster, may be triggered by fever, trauma, or immunosuppression.

After the incubation period of 2 weeks, the patient suffers with the symptoms of a viremia with fever and malaise. This is followed by a cutaneous eruption that consists of erythematous macules that become vesicular; in some of the more severe cases, there are pustules as well. The picture of vesicles on an erythematous base has been poetically described as a "nude drop on a rose petal." Over the course of several days, more lesions arise, resulting in numerous lesions at various stages of eruption and healing. Usually, these lesions do not leave scars unless they become superinfected or are traumatized in some manner.

Most cases of primary varicella occur in children of 14 years of age or younger.[270] If varicella occurs as a primary event in adults, serious complications may ensue, including pneumonia and death. Three specific complications associated with varicella must be mentioned: primary varicella pneumonia, Reye syndrome (which is also associated with other viral diseases), and varicella affecting the fetus and the newborn. Approximately one fifth of adults with this condition develop varicella pneumonia, which is associated with increased mortality. Reye syndrome is an acute, severe, and usually fatal encephalopathy that is associated with fatty degeneration of the liver and other organs. It occurs more commonly in children but it can occur in adults.[271] Varicella occurring during the first 20 weeks of pregnancy carries a small risk (<5%) of congenital malformations.[272] Varicella occurring in late pregnancy can be transmitted to the fetus, either transplacentally or during passage through the birth canal. If varicella occurs in immunosuppressed persons, there is a more prolonged course, and there are more severe complications which can include a usually fatal viral pneumonia. Cutaneous lesions in immunosuppressed patients consist of large, vegetating, and usually necrotic lesions with ulceration.[273]

Herpes Zoster

As indicated earlier, herpes zoster (shingles) occurs as a result of reactivation of VZV previously acquired as varicella that remains latent in the sensory ganglia of sensitive nerves. This reactivation may occur many years after the original varicella eruption and involves spread of the virus along sensitive cutaneous nerves into the skin, usually demarcating the nerve's dermatome. The mechanisms that lead to the interruption of the dormant state include trauma, stress, older age, underlying immunosuppressive conditions such as lymphoma, and iatrogenic-induced immunosuppression caused by various types of therapy. The incidence of herpes zoster increases with age.[274] A very small percentage of zoster cases occur in children younger than 15 years of age.

The typical lesions of zoster are clustered vesicles, often on a hemorrhagic base and following along a dermatome. In addition, there may be scattered lesions on the skin and even occasionally in the oral cavity. The most commonly involved sensitive ganglia are the ones from the thoracolumbar and facial regions. The result of the viral reactivation is usually severe pain due to neuritis. This occurs along with dysesthesia and prominent hyperesthesia. The symptoms appear to be worse in people older than 50 years of age and in those who have an immunocompromised status. Herpes zoster does not pose a problem in pregnancy, and there has been no documented transplacental infection of a fetus. In immunocompromised hosts, the incidence of herpes zoster is higher, especially in patients with advanced Hodgkin disease and in those infected with HIV. In the setting of HIV infection, herpes zoster lesions can become chronic and painful, exhibiting a vegetating, hyperplastic appearance with ulceration.[275] A fatal result is much more common in immunocompromised patients.

The histologic pictures of herpes zoster and herpes simplex, as far as the viral lesions are concerned, are indistinguishable by routine microscopy. However, in herpes zoster, one usually finds more evidence of vasculopathy, including vasculitis in some instances, and a thrombogenic vasculopathy as well. Although this can occur rarely in herpes simplex, it is more common in herpes zoster.[276] In very severe cases of either herpes zoster or varicella, usually seen in immunocompromised hosts, nuclear inclusions can be observed in endothelial cells and even in nerves.

There are monoclonal antibodies that allow for a separation between VZV and HSV.[277] HSV will grow in ordinary tissue cultures, whereas VZV grows only in human fetal diploid kidney cells or fibroblasts of human foreskin. Culture is the gold standard for identification. Electron microscopic examination of VZV lesions show viruses in the capillary endothelium and sometimes in the dermal nerves. HSV and VZV cannot be distinguished on the basis of ultrastructure examination.

Cytomegalovirus

CMV infection is very common throughout the world. It is considered that approximately 1% of newborns are infected transplacentally, and as many as 5% acquire the infection during passage through the birth canal. Antibodies to the virus continue to increase throughout life, but especially during adolescence.[278] CMV can be sexually transmitted. The virus is lymphotropic, and for this reason, it can also be transmitted through blood transfusions.

The initial infection is associated with a mild malaise and flu-like symptoms. Subsequently, the virus becomes latent, persisting in a variety of tissues. For this reason, patients with HIV infection or another immunosuppressive state can exhibit involvement of the virus in almost any organ.[279] Cutaneous manifestations of CMV infection are usually only seen in patients who have an immunocompromised status. The lesions vary and can produce ulceration of the genitalia or other areas of the skin. Maculopapular rashes have been described, as have urticaria and lesions with hyperkeratosis and even bullous disorders. Neonatal CMV infection can result in a variety of lesions, including petechiae and purpura, papules, plaques, and nodules with bluish discoloration due to hemorrhage—a "blueberry muffin baby." The so-called TORCH syndrome comprises a congenital infection caused by a variety of organisms, including *Toxoplasma gondii*, CMV, rubella virus and herpesvirus. This particular syndrome results in damage to the fetus' brain, chorioretinitis, and pneumonitis.[280]

The first clue to CMV infection is the presence of dilated dermal vessels exhibiting large (approximately 10 μm), very basophilic, and hyperchromatic intranuclear inclusions. There are also some small, intracytoplasmic, basophilic inclusions 3 μm in size. The very large, basophilic nucleus is the most characteristic feature and the one that draws the most attention. One may also see a vasculitis associated with a mixed inflammatory infiltrate or a vasculopathy.

CMV culture again is the gold standard and can be successfully accomplished by the use of human fibroblasts. As far as molecular techniques are concerned, PCR is useful in diagnosing CMV, and there are polyclonal and monoclonal antibodies to CMV antigens that allow for identification of the virus in paraffin-embedded sections. Electron microscopic examination reveals large intranuclear particles that are approximately 100 nm in diameter and resemble herpesvirus inclusions.

Epstein-Barr Virus

EBV has been implicated in the etiology of infectious mononucleosis, oral hairy leukoplakia, lymphoproliferative disorders including Burkitt lymphoma, and nasopharyngeal carcinoma.[281] Infections with EBV begin in the salivary glands, and for this reason, the virus is easily spread from one person to another through the saliva. After the initial infection, the virus remains present, apparently for life, in the host's mononuclear cells. The infection is often acquired in Third World countries, and more than 75% of the population in developing countries are infected.[282] The infection usually occurs in childhood and it is asymptomatic. However, if it is acquired in adolescence or adult life, there is a high possibility of developing infectious mononucleosis.[283]

As mentioned, the three entities that are more common in this infection are infectious mononucleosis, oral hairy leukoplakia, and lymphoproliferative disorders. Infectious mononucleosis manifests with a transient maculopapular rash, usually located on the trunk and upper extremities. Occasionally, the palms, soles, and oral mucosa can be involved. Oral hairy leukoplakia is a finding associated with immunosuppressive states. Usually in the setting of HIV/AIDS, it occurs as a more severe and disseminated disease. The lesions are white patches that typically occur on the lateral surfaces of the tongue and may be unilateral or bilateral. There is usually a verrucous filiform surface that can be scraped off. Patients complain of dysesthesia and burning, but this is probably associated with coinfection with *Candida* species.[284] EBV is also known to induce lymphoproliferative disorders, including cutaneous T-cell lymphoma. These conditions may manifest with lesions such as nodules or papulovesicles. In some instances, there are multiple nodules on the legs, which may be evidence of a cutaneous angiocentric disorder.[285]

The histology of the eruption in infectious mononucleosis is usually that of an "id"-like reaction to a virus, which includes interface dermatitis with a perivascular lymphoid infiltrate that extends into the deep dermis. There may be a palisading infiltrate resembling granuloma annulare in some cases; in others, the dermis is clear. The histopathology of oral hairy leukoplakia shows an irregular epithelial hyperplasia with striking associated parakeratosis. The keratinocytes show ballooning degeneration and very small pyknotic nuclei with intranuclear inclusions; these intranuclear inclusions are deeply basophilic and have halos around them. The cytoplasm may have a glass-like appearance. Hyphae of *Candida* species can be easily observed in the superficial epithelium and in the keratin layer. There is a mixed lymphohistiocytic infiltrate beneath the epithelium. Occasionally, a cutaneous necrotizing vasculitis can also be observed in association with EBV infection and in lesions of perioral leukoplakia.

Other Human Herpesviruses

These viruses are quite widespread and have been known to cause primary infections as well as chronic persistent infections. They may remain in a state of latency for many years, until some change in the immune status of the patient leads to reactivation.

Human Herpesvirus 6
HHV-6 has been classified into two variants, HHV-6A and HHV-6B. This virus is the causative agent of exanthema subitum. Almost all children show antibodies against HHV-6 in their sera. The primary infection may go unnoticed, or it may manifest with the classic clinical picture of exanthema subitum.

Reactivation of the virus is often triggered after allogeneic bone marrow transplantation (in the first month). It can exhibit a skin rash or even a generalized vesiculobullous disorder. The palpable purpura, the "gloves-and-socks" syndrome, the papular acrodermatitis of childhood, the so-called Gianotti-Crosti syndrome, and pityriasis rosea have also been linked to HHV-6 infection.[286-289]

The exanthem subitum exhibits a perivascular lymphoid infiltrate and focal interface dermatitis with exocytosis of lymphocytes. Herpes-like inclusions usually are not seen. However, one can detect degenerative changes in the nuclei of the endothelial cells.

Human Herpesvirus 7
HHV-7 is considered to be a lymphotropic herpesvirus that is also shed into the saliva. Children are infected at a young age. As with all herpesviruses, there is a latent phase of the infection. The latent phase takes place in the peripheral blood T cells. Pityriasis rosea has also been linked to HHV-7, but this association is still controversial.[286]

Human Herpesvirus 8
HHV-8 has been identified in patients with AIDS and Kaposi sarcoma. In contrast to the other herpesviruses, HHV-8 is not widely disseminated but seems to be concentrated in the areas where Kaposi sarcoma appears. However, HHV-8 is also found latent in mononuclear cells in the peripheral blood. This virus is shed into the saliva and is transmitted during sexual activity. HHV-8 is found in all types of Kaposi sarcoma and is present in

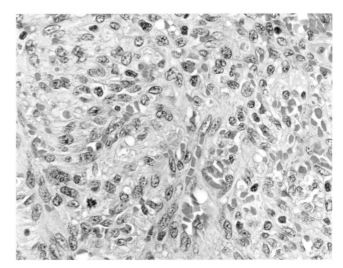

Figure 19-51. Kaposi sarcoma. High-power view of this viral-induced neoplasm shows the typical features, namely vascular channels surrounded by spindle cells, "box-car" disposition of the red blood cells, and the classic eosinophilic bodies.

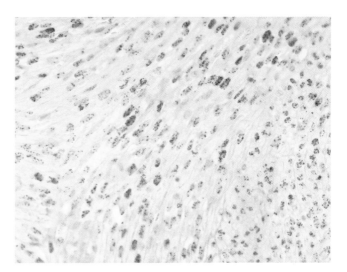

Figure 19-52. Kaposi sarcoma. A human herpes virus 8 immunoperoxidase stain reveals the characteristic dotted nuclear pattern.

the nuclei of the spindle cells and endothelial cells comprising the lesion (Figs. 19-51 and 19-52). Kaposi sarcoma can occur in patients with or without HIV/AIDS.

HHV-8 has also been associated with multicentric Castleman disease and the so-called primary infusion lymphoma.[290]

Poxviridae

The poxvirus group is composed of relatively large (300 × 250 × 200 nm), brick-shaped to oval (parapoxvirus), enveloped DNA viruses. The medically important members are part of the Chordopoxvirinae group, which includes the *Orthopoxvirus, Parapoxvirus, Yatapoxvirus,* and *Molluscipoxvirus* genera. There is a great deal of genetic homology among these viruses, ranging from 90% homology among smallpox, cowpox, and vaccinia to 70% homology between smallpox and molluscum contagiosum virus.[291] Most of the conditions produced by these viruses are zoonoses, with only the smallpox and molluscum contagiosum viruses being obligate human pathogens.[292] The smallpox virus remains a latent danger for humans, and the CDC considers it a high-priority bioterrorism agent (class A).[293] On the other hand, the use of other virulent poxviruses (e.g., monkeypox, camelpox) in biowarfare is also feasible.[294] In addition, the rising popularity of exotic pets, which are usually wild animals imported directly from their original habitats, can give rise to outbreaks of virulent imported poxvirus zoonoses[290] The term "pox" relates to the formation of pocks in the skin, with subsequent scarring and formation of pockmarks, a classic finding among smallpox survivors.

Orthopoxvirus

Variola (Smallpox)

Smallpox was officially declared eradicated from the world by the WHO in 1980, and the last recorded case occurred in 1977 in Somalia. This condition, historically denominated as "smallpox" (with syphilis being "the Great Pox"), has been known to affect humans since the time of the ancient Egyptians (3000 BC).[295] Recent retrospective studies revealed that the epidemics followed a seasonal pattern and were usually associated with dry weather conditions.[296]

Because vaccination against this virus has not been performed worldwide since 1982, there is a large population of susceptible persons. Furthermore, it is believed that only 20% of vaccinated individuals still retain immunity against smallpox. Therefore, the potential re-emergence of the smallpox virus in the form of a biological weapon justifies the constant reminder of this condition's characteristics and efforts in obtaining better vaccines and treatment.[297] A new smallpox vaccine was recently approved by the U.S. Food and Drug Administration and can be massively produced in case of an epidemic.[298]

Transmission of the virus occurs usually through respiratory droplets, with subsequent invasion of the mucous membranes and the lymphatic system. Percutaneous inoculation has also been described, as well as rare cases of conjunctival and transplacental transmission.[295] After a latent period of 4 to 14 days, during which the virus massively multiplies in the reticuloendothelial system, a prodromal period begins with sudden fever, vomiting, and body aches. Enanthematous lesions appear on the mouth and oropharynx 1 day before the cutaneous rash is established. The rash is caused by viral invasion of the capillary endothelium in the dermis. The characteristic skin lesions begin as small, reddish macules that become 2- to 3-mm papules and then 4- to 6-mm pustules, all in a period of 3 or 4 days. The rash occurs first on the face and extremities, and then spreads generally throughout the body in a centrifugal manner. Usually, all of the lesions are in the same state of evolution; they last for a total of 5 to 8 days with umbilication and crusting.[298]

Death from smallpox results mainly from the cytopathic effects of the virus in the target organs[299]—contrary to the classic literature, which attributed the demise of smallpox patients mainly to sepsis with massive immune complex formation and hypotension. Recent studies using molecular engineering revealed the presence of a protein complex termed smallpox inhibitor of complement enzymes (SPICE), which specifically inhibits the human C3b and C4b components of complement.

This virulence factor is absent in the other orthopoxviruses such as vaccinia and molluscum contagiosum virus.[300]

Classically, the most common cutaneous complication of smallpox was the presence of numerous pockmarks or pitted lesions, which appear predominantly on the face and were caused by infection of the large sebaceous glands. These lesions can sometimes be identified in portraits of historical characters. Other, more grave complications among survivors included encephalitis, panophthalmitis with subsequent blindness, and arthritis. The classic WHO classification of smallpox encompasses five variants[253]: variola major (90% of cases), which had a mortality rate of 30%; the modified variant; hemorrhagic smallpox; a flat or malignant type; and the "variola sine eruptione" variant.[295,297]

Vaccinia

The vaccinia virus (VACV) is antigenically very similar to smallpox virus, with both viruses presumably being derived from a common ancestor, a feature that led to the extensive use of VACV as a vaccine against smallpox. Vaccination with VACV confers immunity against several viruses from the *Orthopoxvirus* genus. Inoculation with VACV leads to cutaneous lesions similar to those seen in smallpox. The inoculation site evolves to a vesicle that becomes pustular, crusts, and finally heals, leaving a scar. Adverse reactions do occur with vaccination, especially in immunocompromised or atopic patients.[301,302]

Since 1999, there have been reports of outbreaks involving strains of VACV, particularly in rural areas of Brazil.[303-306] In these cases, the clinical picture and transmission mechanisms bear a striking resemblance to cowpox infection (discussed later), including acquisition of the infection from cows through udder lesions and the presence of umbilicated papular lesions with lymphangitis and regional lymphadenopathy.[305,306] However, several molecular studies have characterized the causative virus as VACV.[303,306] The possible origin, mechanisms of circulation, and reservoirs of these zoonotic VACV infections are largely unknown. It is speculated that VACV could have remained latent in unknown animal reservoirs for decades, because it was relatively common for domestic animals to become infected with VACV from recently vaccinated individuals during the massive smallpox vaccination campaigns of the past.[303,307]

Laboratory-acquired infection is also possible, because VACV is extensively used in laboratory-based research in the study of virology, immunology, and vaccine development. Because VACV remains pathogenic to unvaccinated individuals, laboratory workers who handle VACV strains that are not highly attenuated must receive the appropriate vaccine.[308]

Cowpox

The primary reservoirs of cowpox virus are wild rodents, especially bank voles (*Clethrionomys glareolus*) and wood mice (*Apodemus sylvaticus*).[309] The vectors that spread the virus are the rodents' predators, which are usually domestic cats.[310] The disease is known as cowpox because it usually infects humans through lesions in the teats and udders of infected cows. It is also transmitted by direct contact with infected cats.[310,311] Through his pioneering observations, Edward Jenner reached the conclusion that cowpox infection, when induced by inoculation in healthy persons, would reduce the severity of subsequent smallpox disease.[312]

Cowpox infection is seen almost exclusively in European countries, especially in the United Kingdom.[313] The disease was almost forgotten after the eradication of smallpox in the late 1970s. However, because of the loss of immunity in the population against orthopoxviruses resulting from the interruption of smallpox vaccination, cowpox is now acting as a re-emergent disease, one that poses a considerable threat especially to immunocompromised and atopic patients.[314,315] The route of infection is almost always a skin lesion, but some cases of mucosal transmission have been reported.[316,317] After inoculation, there is a incubation period that varies from 7 to 12 days, after which an inflamed macule appears that successively changes to a papule, a vesicle, and a pustule, which is usually hemorrhagic. Finally, this pustule ulcerates and gives rise to the characteristic black eschar surrounded by erythema and edema.[313,316,318] The eschars are usually painless, can show adherence to the underlying tissues, and heal in approximately 2 weeks, sometimes leaving a scar.[319] Usually, a regional tender lymphadenopathy is present.[313] Systemic manifestations, such as malaise and flu-like symptoms, are often seen.[313,318] In immunosuppressed patients and in atopic individuals, the infection tends to have a much more severe course. In these patients, one can see a generalized, partly confluent poxvirus exanthema comprising hemorrhagic pustules with central necrosis that evolve to deep-seated, black eschars. This occurs along with severe systemic manifestations that can lead to a lethal outcome.[314,315]

The suspicion of cowpox virus is usually raised after failure of empirical antibiotic treatment of a skin lesion. Various methods are available to confirm the diagnosis, and they usually require extraction of material from the pustules. Electron microscopy is the first-line approach and reveals the brick-shaped viral particles.[318] Molecular methods such as PCR are also useful in characterizing this agent.[320] Culture is another option, and a variety of cell culture lines can be used.[313,316] The important differential diagnostic considerations are herpesvirus infection, orf, and anthrax.[319] If the port of entry is a mucous membrane such as the conjunctiva or the nasal mucosa, the infection can mimic an *H. influenzae* phlegmon or erysipelas due to the massive edema that is usually seen in these cases.[317]

Regarding the molecular aspects of cowpox virus pathology, there are some recent data showing that these viruses have the ability to interfere with MHC class I intracellular transport. This would help the viruses avoid the antiviral responses of CD8+ T lymphocytes.[321]

Monkeypox

Monkeypox virus is a rare zoonosis that occurs mainly in West Africa and the Congo basin.[322] This virus and variola (smallpox) virus are the two members of the orthopoxvirus group that can produce a severe systemic illness with widespread vesiculopustular rash in humans. In its final report on smallpox eradication, the WHO considered monkeypox virus to be the most medically important orthopoxvirus in the post-smallpox era.[323] It has one great advantage in comparison to variola: the existence of a wide range of hosts,[324,325] which would preclude worldwide eradication through a massive vaccination program. However, experiences in a recent human monkeypox outbreak showed that human-to-human transmission of this virus is quite difficult, in contrast to variola.[325-327] Some recent findings have revealed the presence of mechanisms of immune evasion that allow the virus to spread systemically and sometimes to remain dormant for long periods. These mechanisms, which may be present in variola as well, cause the induction of a state of unresponsiveness in CD4+ and CD8+ T cells when they interact with monkeypox virus–infected cells. The process seems to be MHC-independent.[328]

The route of infection can be percutaneous, through bites or scratches of infected animals or during manipulation of infected material, or via respiratory or mucosal routes. In African endemic regions, spread of the infection is related to the hunting, skinning, preparing, and eating of infected rodents and monkeys.[325]

Recently, an outbreak of monkeypox virus in the United States was produced by the importation of infected prairie dogs to be commercialized as pets.[329] This raised concern and awareness of the possibility that this agent could spread worldwide, either through the practice of importing wild animals as exotic pets, as a consequence of the ever-increasing volume of international travel, or as a component of biological weapons in terrorist attacks.[325]

The clinical manifestations of monkeypox infection are strikingly similar to those found in smallpox, including an incubation period of roughly 14 days and a 2-day prodrome with fever and malaise. However, during the prodrome phase, there is a feature that is present only in monkeypox infection: a severe lymphadenopathy that can become generalized. The rash usually has a centrifugal distribution, lasts for 14 to 21 days, and shows the typical maculopapular-papular-vesicular-pustular progression before sloughing and leaving dyspigmented scars.[330-332] The clinical differential diagnostic considerations are chickenpox, drug eruption, eczema herpeticum, dermatitis herpetiformis, rickettsial infection, and molluscum contagiosum. Also, smallpox would be an important diagnostic consideration in the unfortunate case of a re-emergence.[325]

Histopathology of Cutaneous Orthopoxvirus Infections

The microscopic characteristics of cutaneous lesions caused by orthopoxviruses are quite similar. The changes bear some resemblance to those seen in herpes simplex, herpes zoster, and varicella and include massive intraepidermal vesiculation with ballooning degeneration and apoptosis of keratinocytes, serous exudation, and formation of multinucleated cells.[298,397,333] The distinctive feature is that orthopoxviruses replicate in the cytoplasm of the infected cells, thus creating intracytoplasmic inclusion bodies, rather than intranuclear inclusions as seen in the herpesvirus group. These intracytoplasmic inclusions have been classified into two types.[334] Type A inclusions are formed early in the viral replication cycle and are represented by cytoplasmic basophilic corpuscles that are usually located near the nuclei and have a halo around them. These structures appear in all poxvirus infections and were known as Guarnieri bodies when seen in smallpox lesions (Figs. 19-53 and 19-54). The type B inclusions, which are much smaller proteinaceous particles, are associated with certain types of poxvirus infections, such as cowpox.[335]

Electron microscopy is an extremely helpful diagnostic tool. It can be used on a variety of materials, such as touch preparations of material from the lesions or ordinary skin biopsy specimens. It usually reveals the classic brick-shaped morphology of the viral particles, especially with the use of

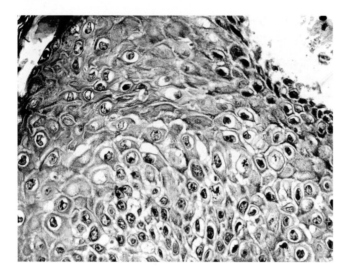

Figure 19-53. Variola (smallpox). The infected keratinocytes show severe intracellular edema and cytoplasmic inclusion bodies known as Guarnieri bodies.

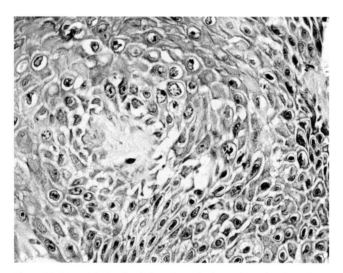

Figure 19-54. Variola (smallpox). The inclusion bodies are located in close relation to the nuclei and are surrounded by a clear halo.

negative-stain technique in thin sections.[333] However, for a definitive diagnosis as to which type of poxvirus is the infecting agent, one must rely on molecular techniques such as PCR amplification.[336,337]

Parapoxvirus

Paravaccinia (Milker's Nodule)

Milker's nodule is a zoonosis that characteristically affects ungulates, such as cows. It is transmitted to humans through direct contact during manipulation of an infected cow's udders.[338,339] Indirect transmission through fomites has also been reported.[340]

The usual clinical presentation involves a solitary lesion on the hands, although other areas of the body can be affected, and sometimes multiple lesions are seen. The lesions usually are 0.5- to 2-cm, red-violaceous nodules that sometimes show crusting or ulceration.[339]

Ecthyma Contagiosum (Orf)

Orf affects primarily young sheep and goats in the form of perioral lesions, and it is transmitted to humans who have contact with these lesions.[341-344] Transmission through trauma inflicted by contaminated fomites has been described.[345] The lesions are usually on the hands and forearms, but they can appear on the scalp, on the face, and in other locations.[346] They are represented by 1- to 3-cm nodules that usually show umbilication and an erythematous halo. The lesions last for 7 days until regression occurs.[343,344] They can be complicated by painful regional lymphadenitis, impetiginization, and even a widespread varicelliform eruption.[344] Other cutaneous disorders that can be associated with orf are bullous pemphigoid, erythema multiforme, and toxic erythema.[347,348]

Histopathology of Cutaneous Parapoxvirus Infections

Paravaccinia and ecthyma contagiosum lesions are considered to be microscopically indistinguishable.[341] Their histopathologic features depend on the stage of the lesion.[339,341] Early lesions show prominent moderate acanthosis and severe vacuolization with ballooning degeneration of keratinocytes in the upper third of the epidermis.[341,349] This ballooning degeneration, especially when it occurs in follicular structures, has been termed "spongiform degeneration" and can lead to vesicle formation.[341] Intracytoplasmic viral inclusions are usually readily identified and can rarely be intranuclear.[342]

As the lesions progress, epidermal necrosis can be found; it can be quite extensive, especially in orf lesions. Extensive epidermal necrosis is usually associated with ulceration and crusting. In the papillary dermis, one sees prominent edema with ectatic vessels which can become quite prominent and simulate a vascular proliferation.[350] A prominent inflammatory infiltrate, composed of lymphocytes, histiocytes, plasma cells, and occasional eosinophils, is seen in the papillary and mid-dermal regions.[344] Neutrophils can be observed in the epidermis when epidermal necrosis occurs. Regressing and more advanced lesions exhibit prominent reduction of the acanthosis and of the inflammatory infiltrate.[341,343]

As with all poxviruses, electron microscopy is quite useful for rapid diagnosis when the crusts of early lesions are examined, revealing the classic brick-shaped viral particles.[351,352] Immunoperoxidase techniques are useful if it is necessary to discern between the two species.

Molluscipoxvirus

Molluscum Contagiosum

Molluscum contagiosum virus infection is a relatively common skin condition in both immunocompetent and immunocompromised patients. Transmission of the infection can be through direct skin-to-skin contact, through fomites, or during sexual activity.[353] Cases involving vertical transmission have been also described.[354] The disease is more commonly found among adolescents and young adults. Persons with an immunocompromised status are frequently affected by this virus.[355,356] The lesions of molluscum contagiosum have a predilection for the head and neck region, the flexural areas, and the genitalia. They may be solitary or may appear in crops, sometimes forming plaques. They consist of dome-shaped papules and nodules that are flesh-colored, have a waxy consistency, and exhibit a

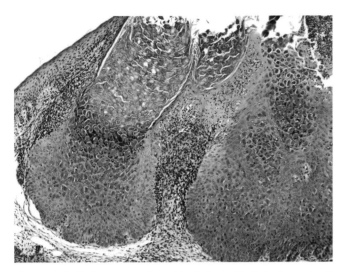

Figure 19-55. Molluscum contagiosum. The distinctive histologic picture of molluscum contagiosum, with its well-circumscribed, lobulated endophytic hyperplasia, makes the lesion instantly recognizable. Note that this lesion is arising in the midst of a nevus.

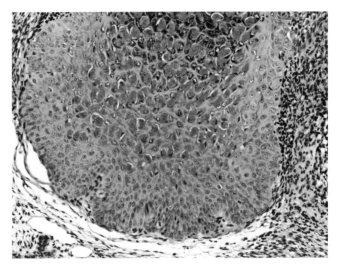

Figure 19-56. Molluscum contagiosum. The intracytoplasmic viral inclusion bodies arise near the basal layer and displace the nuclei of the keratinocytes.

dell or umbilication in the center.[353,357] These lesions measure 2 to 8 mm on average, although solitary lesions can be larger.[358]

In immunocompetent persons, the infection is self-limited and spontaneously regresses in approximately 1 year. However, in atopic individuals, untreated lesions tend to become chronic and sometimes manifest with complications such as pitted scarring.[359,360] In immunosuppressed individuals, the clinical course is typically complicated with large and extensive lesions that usually require antiviral treatment with physical ablation and cidofovir.[361,362]

Clinically, molluscum contagiosum is usually readily identified. However, the clinical presentation can be quite atypical, especially in patients with HIV/AIDS.[356] Under these circumstances, the differential diagnostic considerations include basal cell carcinoma, keratoacanthoma, and infections by other organisms such as *Histoplasma* and *Cryptococcus*.[356,363]

The molluscum contagiosum virus, along with variola virus and vaccinia virus (VACV), are the only members of the poxvirus group that are not zoonoses and infect exclusively humans. Like other poxviruses, molluscum contagiosum virus has several mechanisms to evade the immune system, which involve blockade of MHC type I processes and secretion of nonfunctional analogues of the CC chemokines, among others.[357]

The microscopic features of molluscum contagiosum infection usually involve an inverted expansile growth of lobules composed of hyperplastic basal cells and hypertrophic keratinocytes. These nodules compress the intermingled dermis to fine fibrovascular septa (Fig. 19-55). The infected epithelial cells contain the characteristic intracytoplasmic viral inclusions, which are called molluscum bodies or Henderson-Patterson bodies. The viral particles appear as minute, eosinophilic particles in the keratinocytes forming the Malpighi layer. As these granules ascend, they increase in size, up to 35 μm in diameter, and they become intensely basophilic (Fig. 19-56). As they reach to the stratum corneum, these infected cells disintegrate into a mixture of keratinaceous debris and molluscum bodies that are eliminated

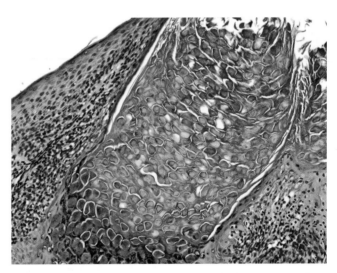

Figure 19-57. Molluscum contagiosum. The inclusion bodies acquire strong basophilic tinctorial properties as they ascend toward the stratum corneum to their final elimination through the central pore of the lesion. The basophilic staining is due to DNA that has been uncovered by an enzyme that digests the RNA, which stains pink.

through the central pore of the lesion (Fig. 19-57). This central crater with its extruding material represents the umbilication seen in clinical lesions.[363,364]

The dermis surrounding the lesions can show a variety of inflammatory patterns. In early processes, there is usually no or minimal inflammatory infiltrate; a variable chronic inflammatory response is found in regressing lesions (Fig. 19-58). Foreign-body giant cell response and even flame figures[365] can be seen in response to intrusion of infected keratinocytes or molluscum bodies. Rarely, one can find a pseudolymphomatous CD8+ lymphoid infiltrate with scattered CD30+ cells.[366] Molluscum contagiosum lesions can be found associated with a variety of cutaneous processes such as melanocytic lesions and epidermal cysts, among others.[364] Cutaneous involvement by *Cryptococcus*

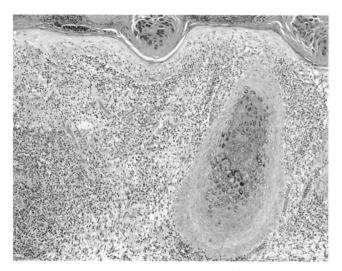

Figure 19-58. Molluscum contagiosum. Some cases can show an exuberant, almost pseudolymphomatous host response, as is seen in this regressing lesion.

neoformans can even manifest as a molluscum-like variant with a histopathologic aspect similar to molluscum contagiosum.[363]

Picornaviridae

Hand-Foot-and-Mouth Disease

The condition known as hand-foot-and-mouth disease, caused by the Coxsackie A16 virus and enterovirus 71, usually affects children[367] and rarely affects healthy adults.[368,369] It typically manifests as small community outbreaks, but severe epidemics have been reported in Taiwan[369,370] and in continental China.[371] The disease is transmitted through direct contact with nasal secretions, feces, and blood. The incubation period ranges from 3 to 7 days and is followed by a prodrome of fever, malaise, headache, abdominal pain, and diarrhea. After this prodromal period, painful blisters and ulcers appear on the buccal mucosa, tongue, and lips. A self-limited eruption follows, first as small, erythematous papules that erupt on the palms and soles, fingers and toes.[368,370] These papules progress to gray-colored vesicles with an erythematous halo.

Although complications of hand-foot-and-mouth disease caused by Coxsackie A16 virus are rarely seen, severe sequelae have been described in enterovirus 71–related cases, including myocarditis, encephalitis, aseptic meningitis, and a poliomyelitis-like disease.[372,373] The mortality rate with enterovirus 71–induced disease is approximately 8%, and deaths are usually related to cardiorespiratory failure with pulmonary edema.[370,372]

Histologically, the lesions show intraepidermal vesiculation with prominent reticular degeneration and ballooned cells. Epidermal necrosis and dyskeratosis can be observed, along with prominent edema of the papillary dermis and a mild perivascular infiltrate.[367]

Parvoviridae

Parvovirus

The parvovirus group is composed of non-enveloped, 22- to 25-nm DNA viruses.[374] The only member of this group known to be pathogenic to humans is the B19 type. Parvovirus B19 is ubiquitous, with a reported seropositivity of 90% in elderly persons.[375] Seroprevalence tends to increase with age, because individuals are exposed to the virus throughout life.[375,376] The infection is acquired mainly through the respiratory route[377] but can be transmitted through blood products, particularly factor VIII and factor IX concentrates.[378] Transplacental transmission of parvovirus B19 is an important cause of fetal demise during the second trimester.[379]

The pathogenic action of this virus is targeted toward the erythroid precursors, erythrocytes, and endothelial cells. This distinct tropism is caused by the presence of the P antigen, a globoside (neutral glycosphingolipid) that is also referred to as the blood group P antigen, which acts as the virus receptor.[380] It has been found that individuals lacking this antigen are resistant to parvovirus B19 infection.[381]

Infections with parvovirus B19 in immunocompetent individuals tend to be asymptomatic.[382] However, polyarthritis and polyarthralgias[383] may appear, sometimes accompanied by a mild transient anemia. The presence of an underlying hemoglobinopathy (e.g., sickle cell disease) or an immunosuppressed state can give rise to a severe pure aplastic anemia.[384] Parvovirus B19 infection in a pregnant woman and subsequent infection of the fetus can lead to miscarriage or hydrops fetalis.[385] Two clinical presentations of parvovirus B19 are represented by the "gloves and socks" papular-purpuric syndrome and erythema infectiosum (fifth disease), which is mostly seen in children. The gloves-and-socks syndrome features erythematous, pruritic papules with petechiae and edema involving the hands and feet.[386] Systemic symptoms such as fever and arthralgias may be present. The disease usually has a self-limited course in immunocompetent individuals. Erythema infectiosum of infancy manifests initially with the classic "slapped cheek" sign, which is usually unilateral. This localized rash is followed by perioral pallor and a subsequent diffuse reticular erythema of the extremities. A petechial rash may also be seen in acral surfaces. A prodrome of fever, sore throat, myalgia, and arthralgias usually precedes these symptoms.[387]

Parvovirus B19 produces an immune-based microvascular injury through upregulation of the TNF-α pathway, which leads to accelerated apoptosis of endothelial cells with subsequent release of numerous nuclear and cytoplasmic antigens (e.g., Ro, La, RNP) that later trigger further autoimmune phenomena.[388,389] This mechanism suggests a possible relationship between B19 infection and the development of several autoimmune conditions, including scleroderma[389] and dermatomyositis.[390] Also, idiopathic pulmonary fibrosis[391] and some cases of multiorgan vasculitis syndromes (e.g., Henoch-Schönlein purpura)[392] have been related to parvovirus B19 infection. The presence of the virus genome in endothelial cells, fibroblasts, and sometimes keratinocytes can be demonstrated by in situ PCR.[389,393] The treatment of choice for parvovirus B19 is intravenous immune globulin, which seems to modulate the immune response through autoantibody neutralization and reduction of Fc-mediated phagocytosis, among other mechanisms.[394,395]

The histologic features of cutaneous parvovirus B19 lesions, regardless of the clinical presentation, usually comprise an interstitial histiocytic infiltrate, which can be reminiscent of interstitial granuloma annulare.[396] This is accompanied by a tight perivascular lymphohistiocytic infiltrate located in postcapillary venules. These vessels can be focally infiltrated by lymphocytes. The inflammatory infiltrate is overlaid by an epidermis showing mild vacuolar change, some exocytosis of lymphocytes, and a rare apoptotic keratinocyte. Chronic lesions can exhibit a prominent granuloma annulare–like picture along with a hypercellular dermis with mucin deposition.[396,397]

Measles

The measles (rubeola) virus, an enveloped, single-strand RNA virus that is part of the paramyxovirus group of the *Morbillivirus* genus, causes a systemic infection with a characteristic generalized cutaneous maculopapular erythematous eruption. The histologic examination reveals a spongiotic epidermis with keratinocytes showing degenerative changes such as cytoplasmic swelling and dyskeratosis.[398] Epidermal vesiculation is also seen (Fig. 19-59). Multinucleated cells may occasionally be seen in the upper epidermis, in hair follicles, and in the acrosyringium.[399,400]

Human Immunodeficiency Virus

Clinical Features

Infection with HIV, an RNA virus from the Retroviridae family, and subsequent development of AIDS, is accompanied by myriad cutaneous processes of an infectious, inflammatory, or neoplastic nature.[275] The HIV/AIDS-related dermatologic infectious conditions are mostly caused by atypical and opportunistic agents, including viruses, bacteria, fungi, and protozoa. Ectoparasitic infestations (e.g., scabies, demodicosis) are also seen in these patients and are reviewed later in this chapter.

HIV-Related Dermatoses

Dermatologic conditions that are commonly found in the general population manifest in HIV/AIDS patients with atypical and aggressive features. An explosive episode of psoriasis or seborrheic dermatitis may be the first manifestation of HIV infection. Such manifestations are thought to be a product of the profound HIV-induced immune dysregulation and immune suppression. However, some of the lesions may be related solely to the direct action of HIV as a pathogen. The presence of these dermatoses in a patient who presents with a suspicious clinical picture provides a useful clue to the correct diagnosis. The following sections describe some of these HIV/AIDS-related inflammatory manifestations.

HIV Seroconversion-Related Rash

The maculopapular rash seen in the acute phase of HIV infection, also known as acute exanthem[401] of HIV infection, is present in roughly 70% of cases.[402,403] The histopathologic picture is similar to that seen in most viral exanthems, consisting of a tight, superficial perivascular, lymphohistiocytic infiltrate. A variety of mild changes are seen in the epidermis, including spongiosis, vacuolar alteration, scattered dyskeratotic cells, and sometimes epidermal necrosis.[404-406]

Immune Reconstitution Inflammatory Syndrome

With the advent of highly active antiretroviral therapy (HAART), a tremendous reduction of HIV-related morbidity and mortality

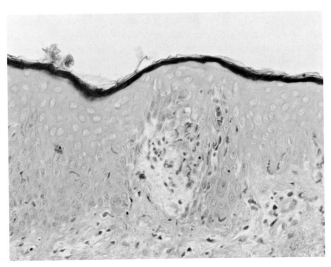

Figure 19-59. Measles. The cutaneous histologic features of this systemic viral infection are composed mainly of spongiosis and vesiculation of the epidermis. Note the multinucleated cells.

has been achieved. However, along with the drug-related complications, a subset of patients undergoing treatment with HAART develop a paradoxical worsening of opportunistic infections and inflammatory conditions. This condition is known as immune reconstitution inflammatory syndrome (IRIS).[407] It can appear days or months after the initiation of HAART and is thought to be produced by immune dysregulation and redistribution of various populations of T cells.[408]

Pruritic Papular Eruption in HIV Disease

A pruritic papular eruption (PPE) is the most common cutaneous condition in HIV patients, with a prevalence ranging from 11% to 46%. Some authors consider PPE a manifestation of primary HIV infection of the skin. However, it can also be found in non-HIV patients with CD4+ lymphocytopenia. Clinically, PPE is characterized by multiple pruritic, discrete, skin-colored papules on the extremities, face, and trunk. The condition tends to be chronic and waxes and wanes.[409]

Microscopic examination of PPE lesions reveals basically a dense, superficial and deep, perivascular, lymphoeosinophilic infiltrate associated with epidermal hyperplasia with hyperkeratosis, acanthosis, and focal dyskeratosis. Dermal fibrosis with a proliferation of factor XIIIa+ cells and a dermal infiltrate composed of lymphocytes, plasma cells, eosinophils, and mast cells have also been described.[409]

Eosinophilic Folliculitis

Eosinophilic folliculitis appears in advanced HIV cases and can also occur as part of IRIS. Clinically, it manifests as intensely pruritic, erythematous and folliculocentric papules that can evolve to pustules. The lesions appear most commonly on the forehead, neck, shoulders, trunk, and upper arms.[410,411] Microscopically, the lesions are composed of folliculocentric aggregates of eosinophils and lymphocytes, often with necrosis of sebaceous glands.[411]

Seborrheic Dermatitis

Seborrheic dermatitis affects approximately 4% of the general population and 85% of the HIV-positive population.[275] The clinical picture is similar to that seen in the general population, but the lesions tend to be much more exuberant, sometimes with an erythroderma-like presentation.[411] AIDS-related seborrheic dermatitis biopsy specimens show an atypical histopathologic picture including marked hyperkeratosis with confluent parakeratosis, follicular plugging, acanthosis, and slight spongiosis. Exocytosis of lymphocytes and neutrophils, along with dyskeratosis, is also seen.[412]

Other important inflammatory dermatoses that are present more exuberantly in HIV/AIDS patients include xerosis, atopic dermatitis, pruritus, Reiter syndrome, and psoriasis. Excellent reviews are available on these subjects.[275,411]

Fungal Skin Infections

Superficial Mycoses

The superficial mycoses are caused by fungi that invade only fully keratinized tissues, including the stratum corneum, hair, and nails. They are usually divided into two groups: noninflammatory and inflammatory superficial mycoses (Table 19-1).

Pityriasis Versicolor

Pityriasis versicolor, or tinea versicolor, is caused by lipophilic yeasts grouped in the genus *Malassezia*.[413] It has worldwide distribution but is significantly more common in humid and tropical climates.[414] Most cases occur during adolescence and young adulthood, with no clear gender predilection.[414,415] The infection, which is not considered contagious, follows a chronic and recurrent course.[414] Skin lesions manifest as macules and patches, which tend to become confluent, involving large areas of the chest, neck, upper arms, and back.[414] Involvement of the face is unusual in temperate climates but seems to be common in tropical and subtropical regions.[413] These lesions typically show fine scaling when scratched.[414] The macules and patches are yellowish-brown, pale yellow, or dark brown, sometimes reddish or pinkish, appearing hypopigmented or hyperpigmented.[415]

The genus *Malassezia* includes 10 anthropophilic and obligatory lipophilic species (*globosa, restricta, slooffiae, obtusa, furfur, sympodialis, japonica, yamatoensis, dermatis,* and *nana*) and three zoophilic species (*pachydermatis, caprae,* and *equina*).[416] *Malassezia globosa* seems to be the predominant species found in the lesions of pityriasis versicolor.[413,417-419] *Malassezia* yeasts are considered part of the normal flora of the skin, being particularly common on the scalp, face, and trunk.[420] Under certain predisposing conditions, the yeast form undergoes a dynamic change to a pathogenic mycelial form associated with clinical disease.[414] Heat and humidity, oily skin, hyperhidrosis, heredity, and immunosuppression (including AIDS) are thought to be predisposing factors.[414]

The pathogenesis of the hypopigmentation observed in pityriasis versicolor has not been fully elucidated.[421] Dicarboxylic acids produced by the fungi (e.g., azelaic acid) might inhibit the dopa-tyrosine reaction to induce hypopigmentation.[415,422,423] In addition, the size and distribution of melanosomes within melanocytes and keratinocytes might also be modified, producing hypopigmentation or hyperpigmentation, respectively, when the melanosomes are abnormally small or abnormally large.[415,424]

Histologically, there is mild hyperkeratosis and acanthosis. Short, septate hyphae and round budding yeasts are present in the stratum corneum, in a pattern resembling "spaghetti and meatballs."[415] The organisms can be highlighted with special stains, such as PAS, methenamine silver nitrate, or Giemsa stains.[414] Occasionally, a mild, chronic, superficial perivascular inflammatory reaction is observed in the dermis. Hyperpigmented lesions can show pigment incontinence, and, when compared with hypopigmented lesions, they display a thicker keratin layer containing more organisms, along with a more intense perivascular infiltrate.[414,422,425,426]

Pityrosporum Folliculitis

Pityrosporum folliculitis is a form of chronic folliculitis caused by *Malassezia* yeasts.[427] It has a worldwide distribution, although it is more commonly found in tropical climates.[428] The condition is seen in adults, who present with erythematous follicular papules and pustules located mainly on the trunk, neck, and upper arms. These lesions may be asymptomatic or pruritic.[427] Predisposing factors for *Pityrosporum* folliculitis include exposure to heat and humidity, use of systemic and topical steroids, and immunosuppression.[428] Follicular occlusion is thought to be the primary event in the development of this condition, with yeast overgrowth being a secondary occurrence.[429] Increased conversion of triglycerides in sebum to free fatty acids by the fungi may promote a free fatty acid–mediated inflammation within the follicle.[430]

Histopathologic examination shows a chronic inflammatory infiltrate around the infundibular region of the pilosebaceous follicles.[414] These follicles are usually plugged and dilated, containing keratinous debris.[430] Clusters of round to oval budding yeast forms are observed within the hair follicle infundibulum.[430,431] The organisms are PAS-positive and measure 2 to 4 μm.[430] Unlike pityriasis versicolor, hyphae are rarely seen.[414] Furthermore, a lymphohistiocytic perivascular inflammatory infiltrate is observed in the superficial dermis; it is composed primarily of CD4+ T cells associated with an increased number of Langerhans cells.[414,432,433] Intradermal rupture of the follicular epithelium can lead to an intense folliculocentric, neutrophilic inflammatory response with a perifollicular foreign body giant cell reaction.[428,431] Intrafollicular deposits of mucin are sometimes present.[428,432]

Table 19-1 Superficial Skin Mycoses

Clinical Presentations	Etiologic Agents
Noninflammatory (producing little or no tissue reaction)	
Pityriasis versicolor	*Malassezia* spp.
Tinea nigra	*Hortaea werneckii*
White piedra	*Trichosporon* spp.
Black piedra	*Piedraia hortae*
Inflammatory (commonly leading to inflammatory response)	
Dermatophytoses	*Trichophyton, Microsporum, Epidermophyton* spp.
Cutaneous candidiasis	*Candida* spp.

Malassezia yeasts as nonpathogenic saprophytes can be seen occasionally in the infundibular portion of a hair follicle and are not associated with inflammatory changes in the hair follicle.[428]

Tinea Nigra

Tinea nigra is caused by the dematiaceous fungus *Hortaea werneckii* (formerly known as *Phaeoannellomyces werneckii, Exophiala werneckii,* and *Cladosporium werneckii*).[415,434] Another dematiaceous fungus, *Stenella araguata,* which occurs in Venezuela, produces a similar clinical picture.[414,415] Tinea nigra typically occurs in children and young adults, with female predominance.[434] It is observed in patients living in warm countries and in those who have lived in or visited the tropics or subtropics.[434] It is presumed that the mycosis is acquired from sandy soil.[435] The organism's attachment to the skin surface is probably facilitated by minor trauma and moisture.[436] *H. werneckii* can be found in soil, compost, and sewage; on wood; in house dust, on salted dried fish; and even on clinically normal-appearing skin.[436] *S. araguata* has not been isolated from the environment to date.[437]

Tinea nigra is clinically characterized by a sharply marginated, light-brown to black, nonscaly, oval-shaped macule. In some patients, this macule is mottled and might be irregular in shape.[415] The lesion is usually single and asymptomatic. It is mainly observed on the palmar surface.[434] However, involvement of the plantar surface, neck, or trunk can also occur.[434] Hyperhidrosis could be a risk factor.[416] Lesions of tinea nigra are quite characteristic, but they can be misdiagnosed as junctional melanocytic nevus or malignant melanoma.[435,437]

Dark-colored, branching, septate hyphae and round to oval yeast forms are present in the superficial layers of the stratum corneum. As a result of pigmented cell walls, these fungi are usually evident on routine staining with hematoxylin and eosin.[415] There is generally no inflammatory response.

White Piedra and Trichosporonosis

White piedra is a *fungal* infection of the hair shaft caused by fungi in the *Trichosporon* genus, class Basidiomycetes. This condition was previously thought to be caused by *Trichosporon beigelii* (now called *Trichosporon cutaneum*).[438] However, recent molecular studies have shown that the *Trichosporon* genus includes several pathogenic species, including *T. cutaneum, Trichosporon asahii, Trichosporon mucoides, Trichosporon ovoides, Trichosporon asteroides,* and *Trichosporon inkin.*[439,440] White piedra is most prevalent in temperate and subtropical climates.[414] The natural habitats of *Trichosporon* species are soil, lake water, and plants, and such fungi are occasionally seen as normal flora of the human skin and mouth.[434] White piedra is not considered contagious; instead, it is probably acquired from the environment by susceptible individuals under appropriate conditions.[414]

White piedra is characterized by small, white to tan, irregular nodules that encircle the hair shaft.[438] These nodules are soft and can be easily detached from the hair shaft; the affected hairs may be split or broken.[434] A variety of hairy areas may be affected, including the scalp, beard, moustache, genitals, axillae, eyebrows, and eyelashes. Typically, only one area is involved.[414] In genital white piedra, a synergistic coinfection, usually with coryneform bacteria, might occur.[415-442] *Trichosporon* species can

also cause onychomycosis, visceral infection, and summer-type hypersensitivity pneumonitis.[415] Disseminated trichosporonosis is seen primarily in immunosuppressed patients, especially those with hematologic malignancies and neutropenia.[443,444] Disseminated infection can also occur in relatively immunocompetent individuals, such as intravenous drug users, patients with prosthetic devices, and patients with severe burn injuries.[443] Cutaneous involvement occurs in approximately 30% of these patients and most frequently manifests as purpuric papules and nodules with central necrosis or ulceration.[445]

In white piedra, potassium hydroxide mounting of an affected hair reveals sleevelike concretions that are composed of loosely arranged hyphae, blastoconidia, and arthroconidia.[434] The use of a fungal stain such as chlorazol black E can highlight these elements.[446] In some patients, bacteria coexist, typically at the periphery of the nodules of white piedra.[415] In systemic infections, hyphae and budding yeasts can be observed in the walls of blood vessels and in the dermis.[445,447,448] In neutropenic patients, the inflammatory infiltrate is usually sparse.[447]

Black Piedra

Black piedra is an infection of the hair produced by the ascomycete *P. hortae.*[449] The condition is usually seen in the tropics worldwide, where it is hot and humid, and sporadically in other regions as a result of international travel.[415,450] *P. hortae* is present in soil; however, stagnant water and crops can also contain it.[415]

Black piedra is characterized by stone-hard black nodules, measuring 1 to 2 mm, that are tightly adherent to the hair shafts.[414] This infection usually affects scalp hair, whereas facial and pubic hair typically are not affected.[415] A single hair shaft may have one or multiple nodules scattered along its entire length.[414] This fungus has been shown to have keratinolytic activity, with the capacity to damage the cuticle and hair cortex.[450]

Direct microscopic examination of affected hair shafts shows tightly packed, darkly pigmented hyphae, asci, and ascospores within the black nodules.[434] Each asci contains two to eight crescent-shaped ascospores.[414] The periphery of the nodule has regularly aligned hyphae and arthroconidia.[415] Both sexual and asexual reproduction occur. Sexual reproduction gives rise to ascospores and asexual reproduction to arthrospores.[451]

Dermatophytoses

Dermatophytes are keratinophilic fungi associated with infections of the skin, hair, and nails. They belong to three genera: *Trichophyton, Microsporum,* and *Epidermophyton.*[452] The incidence of dermatophyte infections and their epidemiologic characteristics depend on social, geographic, and environmental factors and may change over time.[453-459]

Dermatophytes are spread by direct contact from other people (anthropophilic organisms), animals (zoophilic organisms), and soil (geophilic organisms), as well as indirectly from fomites.[460] Zoophilic and geophilic dermatophytes in general tend to form lesions that are more inflammatory than those formed by anthropophilic dermatophytes, and those lesions are also more likely to resolve spontaneously.[452]

The clinical manifestations vary depending on the infecting fungus, the body site infected and the keratinization at that site, as well as the immune status of the host.[461] The dermatophytoses are

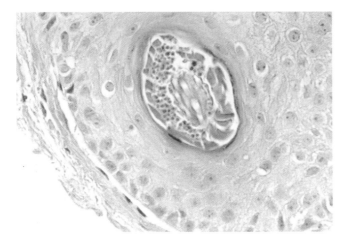

Figure 19-60. Tinea capitis. An example of the ectothrix pattern of infection, which results in fungal proliferation outside the hair shaft in addition to the hyphal forms in the hair itself. This pattern is mostly seen with *Microsporum audouinii, Microsporum canis, Trichophyton verrucosum,* and *Trichophyton mentagrophytes* infection, among others.

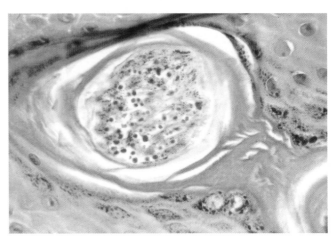

Figure 19-61. Tinea capitis. The endothrix pattern of infection, which is seen mainly in infection with *Trichophyton tonsurans* and *Trichophyton violaceum.*

traditionally divided according to the site infected. Several anatomic sites may be infected by a single dermatophyte species, and different species may produce clinically identical lesions. The major etiologic agents (e.g., *Trichophyton rubrum*) are globally distributed, whereas the distribution of others varies geographically.[452]

Clinical Types

Tinea Barbae   Tinea barbae is a dermatophytic infection that is limited to the coarse hair-bearing beard and mustache areas in men.[462] Clinically, it ranges from mild and superficial to a severe inflammatory pustular folliculitis.[452] In inflammatory cases, the zoophilic ectothrix dermatophytes *Trichophyton verrucosum* and *Trichophyton mentagrophytes* are most frequently responsible for the infection.[461,463]

Tinea Capitis (Scalp Ringworm)   Tinea capitis can be located on the scalp, eyebrows, or eyelashes and is caused by members of the genera *Microsporum* and *Trichophyton*.[461] Both the skin surface and hairs are involved. The clinical presentation can vary, from scaly and erythematous inflammatory lesions with or without alopecia, to noninflamed lesions resembling seborrheic dermatitis, to large inflamed kerions that may resemble an abscess.[464] Infection of the hair may be ectothrix (sheath of arthroconidia formed on the outside of the hair shaft) (Fig. 19-60) or endothrix (arthroconidia formed within the hair shaft) (Fig. 19-61).[464] Since the 1950s, *Trichophyton tonsurans* has been observed to be the most frequent cause of tinea capitis in the United States and the United Kingdom.[464,465]

Tinea Favosa   Tinea favosa, usually caused by *Trichophyton schoenleinii*, is characterized by the presence of yellow, cup-shaped crusts called scutula on the scalp and glabrous skin.[452,465] Direct microscopic examination of hairs in potassium hydroxide shows an endothrix invasion, with hyphae and air spaces in the hair shafts.[466] *T. schoenleinii* was a widespread trigger of family epidemics in Europe in the 18th century.[467] Currently, it has almost disappeared from developed European countries, although it is found in areas of Africa.[467]

Kerion Celsi   Kerion celsi is the inflammatory, suppurative type of tinea capitis. It produces a painful, inflammatory, crusted mass that can be associated with purulent discharge and regional lymphadenopathy.[468] Kerions are mainly caused by zoophilic dermatophytes.

Tinea Corporis   The ringworm tinea corporis is the typical infection of the exposed glabrous skin and can be caused by any dermatophyte.[461] Patients typically present with an annular patch or plaque with an advancing, raised, scaling border and central clearing.[469]

Tinea Cruris   Tinea cruris is an infection of the groin most commonly seen in adult men.[461] *T. rubrum* and *Epidermophyton floccosum* are the most frequent etiologic agents.[452] Lesions are usually bilateral, erythematous to reddish-brown, and sharply demarcated. The periphery of these lesions shows fine scaling, with papules and pustules being seen in more inflammatory cases.[461,469]

Tinea Imbricata (Tokelau)   Tinea imbricata is a chronic dermatophytosis that affects glabrous skin and is exclusively caused by the anthropophilic *Trichophyton concentricum*.[470] Skin lesions are characteristically concentric and lamellar plaques of scale resembling erythema gyratum repens.[461] The infection is geographically restricted to Southeast Asia, India, Central America, and Southwest Polynesia.[461]

Tinea Manuum   In tinea manuum, the palmar and interdigital areas of the hand are affected, most commonly showing unilateral diffuse hyperkeratosis with accentuation of the flexural creases.[452] *T. rubrum* is the most frequent infecting dermatophyte.[461]

Tinea Pedis (Foot Ringworm, Athlete's Foot)   Tinea pedis involves the feet, especially the soles and web spaces. In the interdigital form, the web spaces of the feet show maceration, scaling, and fissuring. The spaces between the fourth and fifth toes are the most commonly affected.[462] Another common presentation is the chronic squamous, hyperkeratotic form, in which fine silvery scales cover the pinkish skin of the soles, heels, and sides of the foot.[452] Additionally, there is an acute inflammatory form, in which vesicles, pustules, and sometimes bullae are observed. Infections due to *T. mentagrophytes* var. *interdigitale* often lead to inflammatory lesions.[461] *T. rubrum* is usually associated with chronic, noninflammatory lesions, whereas *E. floccosum* may produce either type of reaction.[461]

Tinea Unguium   Tinea unguium is caused by invasion of the nail plate by a dermatophyte. The term *onychomycosis* also includes infection of the nail by nondermatophytic fungi. There are three main types of nail involvement: distal-lateral subungual onychomycosis, superficial white onychomycosis, and proximal white subungual onychomycosis.[471] Proximal white subungual onychomycosis occurs almost exclusively in immunodeficient patients.[472] The most commonly detected dermatophyte in tinea unguium is *T. rubrum*, followed by *T. mentagrophytes*.[473]

Majocchi Granuloma Majocchi granuloma, or nodular granulomatous perifolliculitis, is a dermatophytic infection in which the lesions clinically manifest as nodules or plaques and histologically show granulomatous perifolliculitis. This presentation is commonly seen in immunocompromised individuals.

Immunology
Cell-mediated immunity seems to be the major immunologic defense in clearing dermatophyte infections.[452] The majority of chronic and recurrent dermatophyte infections are caused by *T. rubrum*; these patients often fail to express a delayed-type hypersensitivity reaction to trichophytin when it is injected intradermally.[474]

Histopathology
In tinea corporis, cruris, manuum, and pedis, the epidermis usually shows parakeratosis with neutrophils and variable acanthosis and spongiosis. In the acute forms, there is more dermal edema. Chronic forms usually display epidermal hyperplasia and hyperkeratosis. Subcorneal pustules are sometimes present. The underlying dermis shows mild perivascular inflammation, with lymphocytes and occasionally neutrophils or eosinophils. If there is follicular involvement, the dermal inflammation is heavier. The fungal septate hyphae are found in the stratum corneum and are highlighted by the PAS stain.

Folliculitis caused by dermatophytes is characterized by the presence of fungal elements in follicles and signs of a foreign body reaction, with foreign-body giant cells in the dermal inflammatory infiltrate.[452] Granuloma formation may occur.

In kerion, parakeratosis, intraepidermal collections of neutrophils, acanthosis, and spongiosis are present. The tissue reaction is suppurative with formation of abscesses, which may discharge via sinuses. A chronic inflammatory infiltrate with multinucleated giant cells may be present in the vicinity of disrupted hair follicles.[468] Ultimately, the process may resolve with fibrosis.

In Majocchi granuloma, there is a dense perifollicular mixed inflammatory infiltrate, with granulomatous features. Hyphae and arthrospores are present within hair follicles and in the dermis.

In tinea favosa of the scalp, hyphae, often empty or vacuolated, are observed within infected hairs, while the scalp shows cup-shaped areas of densely interwoven mycelium, scales, and debris referred to as scutula.[452] A chronic inflammatory infiltrate is seen in the underlying dermis. Affected hair follicles tend to atrophy.

In onychomycosis, fungal filaments and rounded arthroconidia are present between the cells of the nail plate.[475]

Candidosis

Candidoses, or candidiases, are infections of the skin, mucous membranes, or internal organs caused by yeasts of the genus *Candida*.[476] This genus includes many species, with *Candida albicans* being the major pathogenic species.[477,478] *C. albicans* is a human commensal inhabiting the gastrointestinal tract, oral cavity, vagina, and skin in a significant proportion of healthy individuals; therefore, the source of infection is usually endogenous.[477] Candidoses are considered opportunistic infections.[476] Disease occurs in the presence of local or systemic predisposing factors.[479] Local predisposing factors include occlusion, increased skin moisture, maceration, and topical corticosteroid use.[476] Systemic predisposing factors include immunosuppression (including AIDS), age (infancy, old age), pregnancy, endocrinopathies (diabetes mellitus, Cushing syndrome), drugs (corticosteroids, broad-spectrum antibiotics, immunosuppressors), and indwelling catheters.[476,479,480]

The candidoses range from relatively trivial superficial infections to life-threatening disseminated disease.[478] The superficial infections mainly include cutaneous, oral, and genital candidosis. *Candida* species may also enter the bloodstream (candidemia), and they can penetrate almost any organ of the body, causing systemic or disseminated candidosis.[480]

Clinical Types
Oral Mucous Membrane Infections Oral mucous membrane infection can have various clinical presentations. The three major clinical variants are the pseudomembranous, erythematous, and hyperplastic types.[481] Pseudomembranous candidiasis (thrush) is characterized by curd-like white plaques that can be removed by scraping, leaving an erythematous base.[482,483] The white plaque consists of a tangled mass of fungal hyphae, blastospores, bacteria, inflammatory cells, fibrin, and desquamated epithelial cells.[481] Erythematous candidiasis is the most common variant seen in HIV infection.[481] The clinical presentation consists of a red patch, often on the midposterior dorsum of the tongue, palate, or buccal mucosa.[481,483] Lesions on the tongue manifest as depapillated areas.[481] Hyperplastic candidiasis, or candidal leukoplakia, manifests as palpable whitish plaques or nodules that cannot be removed by scraping.[481,484] These lesions usually occur on the inside surface of one or both cheeks at the commissural areas, and less frequently on the lateral surfaces of the tongue.[481] Candidal leukoplakia is associated with an increased risk of malignant transformation.[485]

In addition to these clinical variants, there are several other oral lesions associated with *Candida* in which the fungus is not considered the sole etiologic agent.[481] This category includes denture stomatitis, angular cheilitis, median rhomboid glossitis, and linear gingival erythema.[481]

Genital Infections Vulvovaginal candidosis is one of the most common vaginal infections, representing 40% to 50% of all cases of infectious vulvovaginitis.[486] Between 70% and 75% of sexually active women will experience at least one episode of vulvovaginal candidosis in their lifetime, and 5% to 8% of adult women have recurrent disease, defined as four or more episodes per year.[486]

Infection with *Candida* species, usually *C. albicans*, is the most common cause of balanitis.[487] Candidal balanitis manifests with erythema, papules, and pustules that are easily ruptured on the glans.

Cutaneous Infections Cutaneous infection with *Candida* species is commonly seen in intertriginous areas, such as the submammary region, inguinal folds, intergluteal crease, and finger spaces. The affected sites present shiny, erosive erythema that is typically accompanied by satellite pustules. This infection is also common in the diaper area of infants (napkin candidosis).

Decubital candidosis is a particular form of cutaneous candidosis that occurs on the dorsal skin of chronically bedridden patients.[476] The skin lesions are clinically similar to the ones observed in intertriginous and napkin candidosis.[476]

Candida Onychomycosis   *Candida* onychomycosis is a rare condition that exclusively affects immunocompromised individuals, including patients with chronic mucocutaneous candidiasis, patients with HIV infection, and patients receiving immunosuppressive drugs.[488] Nail invasion by *Candida* produces primary total onychomycosis associated with periungual swelling.[488]

Congenital Cutaneous Candidosis   Congenital cutaneous candidosis appears to be acquired in utero by the ascension of organisms from an infected vagina into the uterine cavity.[489] It manifests within the first 6 days of life.[489] Clinically, there are generalized erythematous macules, papules, vesicles, pustules, or some combination of these.[490] Although all infants are at risk for disseminated disease, this risk seems to be higher in preterm infants.[489,490]

Neonatal Candidosis   Neonatal candidosis is acquired during passage through the birth canal or later from nursery contacts.[490] It usually appears after the fifth day of life and commonly manifests as oral thrush.[490] Diaper dermatitis can also be seen.

The incidence of neonatal candidemia or disseminated candidiasis in extremely low-birth-weight infants (<1000 g) is higher than in neonates with a birth weight greater than 1500 g.[491]

Infantile Gluteal Granuloma   *Infantile gluteal granuloma* is a term applied to a condition that is seen in the anogenital region of infants as a complication of diaper dermatitis.[492] Clinically, erythematous to violaceous nodules and plaques, usually oval in shape, are observed on the buttocks, vulva, perianal region, and scrotum. Predisposing factors include prolonged topical corticosteroid use, long-term diarrhea, occlusive plastic pants, detergents, and *C. albicans* infection.[493]

Chronic Mucocutaneous Candidiasis   Chronic mucocutaneous candidiasis is not a single entity but a heterogeneous group of immunologic disorders characterized by persistent or recurrent infections of the skin, nails, and mucous membranes by organisms of the genus *Candida*, usually *C. albicans*.[494,495] Impaired cellular immunity to *Candida* species has been reported in patients with chronic mucocutaneous candidiasis.[495] In some individuals, the defect is specific to *Candida*, but in others the immunologic response to other organisms is also defective.[494] The associated findings include autoimmune disorders, polyendocrinopathies, thymoma, interstitial keratitis, alopecia, and vitiligo, among others.[496,497]

The age at onset and the clinical spectrum of candidal infections are variable.[496] The affected nails are dystrophic and can be associated with paronychia. In some patients, the skin lesions are markedly thick and keratotic, forming cutaneous horns, usually on the face and scalp.[494,495] Esophageal stricture formation has been described in some patients.[498]

Disseminated or Systemic Candidosis   *Candida* is one of the 10 leading causes of bloodstream infections in developed countries.[499] Approximately 33% to 55% of all episodes of candidemia occur in intensive care units (ICU), with associated mortality rates of up to 71%.[499] *Candida* fungemia may have an endogenous or an exogenous origin.[499]

Predisposing factors to candidemia and systemic candidosis include intravascular catheters, neutropenia, acute renal failure, parenteral nutrition, broad-spectrum antibiotics, a prolonged ICU stay, use of corticosteroids, mucosal colonization with *Candida*, chemotherapy, bone marrow transplantation, underlying cancer, and immunosuppression.[479,499,500] Involvement of multiple organs can occur, with cutaneous lesions being observed in 13% of patients with systemic candidosis.[500] Cutaneous lesions include erythematous macules, papules, pustules, nodules, and petechiae on the trunk and extremities.[500,501] Lesions resembling ecthyma gangrenosum have been reported.[502]

Systemic candidosis has been described in heroin addicts.[503,504] These patients present with cutaneous, ocular, and osteoarticular involvement.[504] The cutaneous lesions are painful nodules and pustules that occur mainly on the scalp and beard area.[504]

Histopathology

The histopathologic features are similar in cutaneous and mucous membrane infections.[505,506] Typically, in candidal lesions, the epidermis (or epithelium) is infiltrated by large numbers of neutrophils (Fig. 19-62).[483] Occasionally, subcorneal or spongiform pustules can be seen.[476] The former should be differentiated from impetigo and the latter from psoriasis. The epidermis displays acanthosis and focal spongiosis. Usually, a chronic inflammatory infiltrate is seen in the underlying connective tissue.[476,483] Yeast forms and pseudohyphae can be found in the stratum corneum with the use of standard H&E preparations, but visualization is easier with a fungal stain such as PAS (Fig. 19-63). The organisms may show budding (Fig. 19-64).[507] The yeast form can be seen in the oral mucosa and does not necessarily indicate pathogenicity.

In chronic mucocutaneous candidiasis, the histologic features resemble the ones described earlier, but the lesions are usually more acanthotic and hyperkeratotic.[494,508] Yeast forms and pseudohyphae are often numerous and easy to visualize with the PAS stain.

In systemic candidosis, the fungi are located within the dermis, indicating hematogenous spread.[501] Often, the organ-

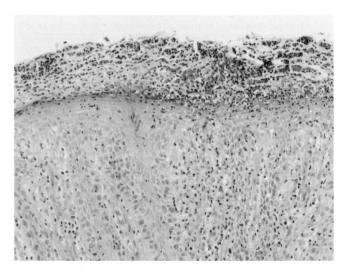

Figure 19-62. Cutaneous candidiasis (PAS stain). Note the prominent acanthotic and spongiotic epidermis associated with a heavy infiltration by neutrophils, especially in the superficial layers.

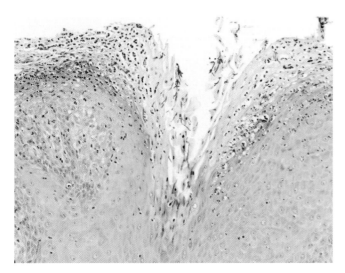

Figure 19-63. Cutaneous candidiasis (PAS stain). Yeast and pseudohyphal forms are readily identified with a PAS stain.

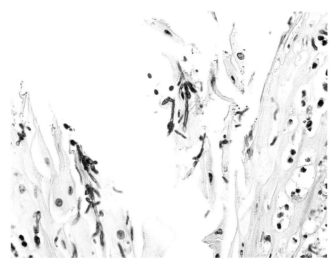

Figure 19-64. Cutaneous candidiasis (PAS stain). High-power view of the organism exhibits both yeast and pseudohyphal forms, resulting from germ tube formation.

isms are located at sites of vascular damage.[500] Focal dermal necrosis, hemorrhage, and perivascular lymphocytic infiltration are also seen.[500] Features of leukocytoclastic vasculitis have been described in disseminated infection.[507] In lesions that resemble ecthyma gangrenosum, the papillary dermis displays edema and a large number of pseudohyphae, which may extend into vessels.[502] Ulceration is also observed.

In heroin addicts, dermal abscesses with abundant neutrophils, surrounded by lymphocytes, histiocytes, and giant cells, are seen.[504] In some cases, yeasts and pseudohyphae are seen invading the hair shafts.[504]

Etiology and Pathogenesis

C. albicans is a polymorphic microorganism that exists in three basic morphologic entities; namely, yeasts, pseudohyphal, and hyphal forms.[478]

In recent years, a shift in the relative prevalence of species has occurred, with a decrease in prevalence of *C. albicans* as a cause of infection and an increase in non-*albicans Candida*, such as *Candida glabrata*, *Candida tropicalis*, *Candida krusei*, and *Candida parapsilosis*.[477,505]

Attributes that contribute to *C. albicans* virulence include adhesion, hyphal formation, phenotypic switching, and extracellular hydrolytic enzyme production.[506] The ability to undergo phenotypic switching is thought to aid survival in different microenvironments and evasion of the immune response.[480]

Systemic Mycoses

Systemic mycoses are caused by truly pathogenic fungi, which are capable of causing infection in otherwise healthy individuals. The fungi traditionally included in this group are *Blastomyces dermatitidis*, *Coccidioides immitis*, *Histoplasma capsulatum* (var. *capsulatum* and var. *duboisii*), and *Paracoccidioides brasiliensis*. They are thermally dimorphic, growing as mycelia in their natural state and converting to yeast form in tissues. The infection is usually acquired through the respiratory tract, and the organisms

can disseminate hematogenously to reach the skin and other sites. The severity of infection is determined both by the extent of the exposure to the organism and by the immune status of the patient. The systemic mycoses have always been a significant health problem, but they have gained importance due to the growing immunosuppressed population.

Blastomycosis

Clinical Features

Blastomycosis, or North American blastomycosis, is caused by *Blastomyces dermatitidis*. It is mostly seen in North America, but cases have also been documented in India, Africa, and Central and South America.[509] There are three forms: pulmonary, systemic, and primary cutaneous blastomycosis. The disease is more common in adult men. Almost all cases of blastomycosis begin as a primary pulmonary infection resulting from inhalation of conidia. The primary infection may progress or resolve spontaneously.[510] Hematogenous spread to other organs may occur, with the skin being the most common extrapulmonary site (40-80%).[511]

Cutaneous blastomycosis causes a variety of skin lesions, which are typically divided into ulcerative or verrucous.[512] The verrucous type has a serpiginous, advancing, raised border and may reach many centimeters in diameter.[512] The center of the lesion is usually atrophic and crusted. Ulcerative-type skin lesions begin as a small pustule that progresses to an ulcer with heaped borders.[513] The cutaneous lesions tend to occur on the face and other exposed areas. The mucous membranes may also be affected. A widespread pustular eruption has been described.[514] A case with lesions that were clinically and histologically reminiscent of Sweet syndrome was reported in 2003.[515]

The primary cutaneous form is rare and results from direct inoculation of organisms into the skin. It usually is reported after autopsy, laboratory accidents, dog bites, infection of open wounds, or outdoor trauma.[512] Lymphangitic lesions, similar to those of sporotrichosis, can occur.

Immunologically compromised patients with blastomycosis are more commonly diabetic, receiving long-term corticosteroid therapy, or undergoing cytotoxic therapy for malignancy.[516] The infection is relatively uncommon in patients with HIV infection.[516]

Histopathology

Initial lesions of blastomycosis show a dermal inflammatory infiltrate of polymorphonuclear leukocytes with numerous organisms. After a few weeks, occasional giant cells may be seen.[516] Later, the lesion becomes fully developed, with a verrucous appearance. The skin biopsy from the advancing edge of these lesions displays downward proliferation of the epidermis, often progressing to pseudocarcinomatous hyperplasia. Intraepidermal aggregates of neutrophils forming microabscesses are common.[511] There is a polymorphous dermal inflammatory cell infiltrate, usually with numerous neutrophils and abscesses. Within the dermal infiltrate, there are scattered multinucleate giant cells.[511] Occasionally, tuberculoid granulomas are seen, but without caseation necrosis. The histologic features of ulcerative lesions are the same as in the verrucous form, except for the absent epidermis.[517]

The yeasts are usually found in the center of the abscesses and in the giant cells. Occasionally, broad-based budding forms are seen. Bud attachment bases are characteristically 4 to 5 μm, which is a broader base in comparison to *P. brasiliensis, H. capsulatum,* or other spherical yeasts.[518,519] In well-fixed tissue, the multiple nuclei of the yeast forms can be seen.[518,519] The PAS or the GMS stains allow better visualization of the fungi.[519] The histopathologic findings in the primary inoculation form are the same as in secondary forms of cutaneous disease.[519]

The diagnosis of blastomycosis is often made by morphologic examination of cytologic or tissue samples.[516] In this context, two other organisms should be distinguished from *B. dermatitidis: P. brasiliensis* and *Cryptococcus.* The former exhibits more polymorphic shapes, thinner cell walls, and multiple small buds surrounding the large parent yeasts.[516] *Cryptococcus* has a thick, mucicarmine-positive, mucoid capsule, as opposed to the thin, incomplete, mucicarmine-positive layer occasionally seen in *Blastomyces* yeast forms.[516]

A positive culture renders a definite diagnosis, but requires a 2- to 4-week incubation period.[517] Culture at body temperature yields a slow-growing, white or light brown yeast colony.[517] Tissue culture on Sabouraud dextrose agar at room temperature produces a fluffy white colony.[519]

Etiology and Pathogenesis

B. dermatitidis is a dimorphic fungus that exists in the yeast phase in tissues (37° C) and in the mycelial phase in nature (25° C).[517] In endemic areas of the United States, the organism has been isolated from soil.[513,518] The yeasts have thick, refractile cell walls and measure 8 to 15 μm in diameter. They reproduce by a single broad-based bud, with the daughter cell often as large as the mother cell before detachment.[517]

Some variation in size, shape, staining, and wall thickness of yeast forms of *B. dermatitidis* can occur in different fields of the same specimen in immunocompetent hosts.[518-520] However, the greatest variation in yeast forms is found in immunosuppressed patients, in whom hyphal forms may also be observed.[518,521,524,525] Giant yeast forms (>40 μm in diameter) are very rare but have been reported and can cause confusion with *C. immitis.*[518,520,522]

Coccidioidomycosis

Clinical Features

Coccidioidomycosis, caused by *C. immitis,* is found in the southwestern United States, in northern Mexico, and in some areas of South America (mainly in Argentina and Paraguay).[526] It is usually an acute, self-limited pulmonary infection resulting from inhalation of airborne arthrospores from the soil. Dissemination of the infection is rare, occurring in approximately 1% of the cases.[527] HIV-infected persons, organ transplant recipients, other immunocompromised patients, and pregnant women have an increased risk of severe disease and dissemination.[527] African Americans and Filipinos also have a greater risk of disseminated disease.[528]

Cutaneous involvement in most cases results from dissemination from a primary pulmonary focus. The skin is the most common extrapulmonary site in coccidioidomycosis.[529] The joints, bones, and CNS are also frequently involved in disseminated disease.[526,527] Cutaneous manifestations are variable and may consist of verrucous papules, nodules, or plaques or of subcutaneous abscesses, which may form draining sinuses.[509,530] Skin lesions resembling mycosis fungoides[531] or lepromatous leprosy[532] have been described. Multiple papulopustular lesions can occur and probably indicate acute hematogenous dissemination.[530]

Primary cutaneous coccidioidomycosis is very rare and results from inoculation of the organisms at sites of minor trauma. It usually consists of an ulcerated nodule on an extremity or other exposed area. Secondary nodules in a linear distribution along the lymphatic pathways, similar to sporotrichosis, can be seen.[533] Regional lymphadenopathy may be associated, and the affected lymph nodes may ulcerate.[527]

Reactive skin eruptions, which contain no viable organisms, are common and include erythema nodosum, an acute generalized exanthem, erythema multiforme, Sweet syndrome, and reactive interstitial granulomatous dermatitis.[527,534]

Histopathology

Established cutaneous lesions show pseudoepitheliomatous hyperplasia with intraepidermal microabscesses. A diffuse infiltrate of neutrophils, lymphocytes, eosinophils, plasma cells, histiocytes, and giant cells is present in the dermis. There may be abscess formation, with surrounding granulomatous response. These histologic features resemble those of blastomycosis, but in coccidioidomycosis, caseation necrosis may occur.[523]

Vascular changes include plump endothelial cells proliferated in capillary masses with an admixture of eosinophils, lymphocytes, and plasma cells, suggesting the possibility of vasculitis. However, no evidence of vasculitis (e.g., fibrinoid change, vessel necrosis) is present.[530]

Eosinophils are usually prominent.[530] They can be present in the perivascular inflammation or form eosinophilic abscesses. Small flame figures have been described.[530]

The spherules are observed in the dermis, both free and within giant cells. Endospores (sporangiospores) are seen within the spherules (sporangia) (Fig. 19-65). In some cases, the organisms are few, and meticulous examination is required to see them.[530] Extrusion through the epidermis (perforation) of inflammatory tissue together with the organisms has been described.[530] They can be identified in H&E-stained slides but

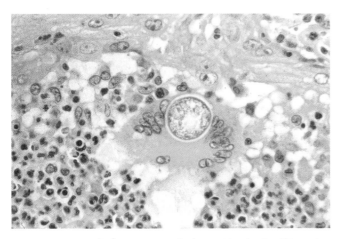

Figure 19-65. Coccidioidomycosis. *Coccidioides immitis* spherule within a giant cell. These characteristic fungal structures are usually difficult to find.

are demonstrated best by methenamine silver stain. The endospores are PAS-positive, but the spherules are negative.[523]

The histopathologic features in the skin are similar in disseminated infection and in primary cutaneous infection.[527]

The spherules found in tissue are much larger than the yeast forms of other fungi, such as *Blastomyces* or *Cryptococcus*. On the other hand, the spherules and endospores of coccidioidomycosis are much smaller than those of rhinosporidiosis.

Skin biopsies of the acute generalized exanthem or "toxic erythema" associated with coccidioidomycosis show a nonspecific pattern of spongiotic dermatitis and/or interface dermatitis with a mild perivascular inflammatory infiltrate including lymphocytes, neutrophils, eosinophils, and karyorrhectic debris.[527,534] Necrotic keratinocytes are rare.

On rare occasions, atypical morphologic forms of *C. immitis* in tissues from humans have been described, including morula-like, broad-based yeast-like, moniliform, and true hyphae types.[535] This could lead to confusion with the tissue forms of other pathogenic fungi. For this reason, culture remains the most reliable means to establish a definite diagnosis.[535]

Aggregates of altered blood cells can, albeit rarely, mimic the appearance of an endosporulating fungus such as *C. immitis*. This artifact has been referred to as "subcutaneous myospherulosis."[536]

Etiology and Pathogenesis
C. immitis is a dimorphic fungus that exists as a mold in the soil. As the soil dries or nutrients become limiting, the fungus reproduces asexually by disarticulating the hyphae into small, environmentally resistant arthroconidia.[537] These are easily dispersed into the air when the soil is disturbed by wind or human activities. After inhalation by the host, the arthroconidia become spherules, which have thick walls and measure 10 to 80 μm in diameter. The spherules then grow larger and contain hundreds to thousands of endospores.[526] After rupture into the tissues, the endospores grow to form new spherules, thereby repeating the growth cycle in the host.[526]

In coccidioidomycosis, cell-mediated immunity is important in generating an effective response to the infection.[527] On the other hand, antibodies do not appear to confer protection against the organisms.[537]

A second species, *Coccidioides posadasii*, has been identified as the predominant organism outside California.[40,526,538] These two species of fungi are genetically different but are phenotypically undistinguishable at this time.[537] The disease and the immune response to the organisms are also the same.[537]

Paracoccidioidomycosis

Clinical Features
Paracoccidioidomycosis, also known as South American blastomycosis or Lutz-Splendore-Almeida disease, is caused by *P. brasiliensis*. The disease is confined to Latin America, with endemic areas in Brazil, Argentina, Colombia, and Venezuela.[523,539,540] The incidence of the disease before 12 years of age is similar in boys and in girls. However, after this age, the incidence increases progressively in males. Up to 90% of affected individuals are men between 29 and 40 years old, predominantly rural workers.[541]

The respiratory tract is the usual portal of entry; from there, hematogenous dissemination to other parts of the body occurs. Paracoccidioidomycosis is usually classified as acute/subacute or chronic.[132] The acute/subacute form usually affects children, teenagers, and young adults and is also called "juvenile type."[542] This form mainly involves the spleen, liver, lymph nodes, intestinal tract, and bones.[543] On the other hand, lung and mucosal lesions are rare. The chronic form, or adult type, is much more common and generally affects individuals older than 30 years of age. This form is characterized by involvement of the lungs, mucosa, and skin.[543] Oropharyngeal mucous membrane ulcerations are frequent; they have a characteristic appearance, showing hemorrhagic dots over a granulomatous base, and are known as Aguiar-Pupo stomatitis.[544] Skin lesions can manifest as crusted papules and nodules, ulcers, or verrucous plaques. They can also exhibit hemorrhagic dots, similar to the lesions in mucous membranes.[131] Primary cutaneous infections are rare.[545,546]

Paracoccidioidomycosis in AIDS patients usually manifests in a form similar to severe acute/subacute cases; however, the incidence of coinfected individuals is low.[541,546]

Histopathology
The lesions of paracoccidioidomycosis are characterized by a granulomatous inflammatory response with formation of epithelioid granulomas with giant cells.[543] These granulomas range from well-organized to poorly organized, probably reflecting the degree of cellular immune response (Fig. 19-66).[540] Epidermal changes include hyperkeratosis, parakeratosis, acanthosis, and pseudocarcinomatous hyperplasia (Figs. 19-67 and 19-68).[540] Epidermal microabscesses can also be seen, sometimes with fungi among the polymorphonuclear cells (Fig. 19-69).[540] In addition to the granulomatous reaction, the dermis also shows a perivascular inflammatory infiltrate with lymphocytes, plasma cells, and macrophages.[540] Neutrophils and eosinophils are commonly present, but dermal necrosis and fibrosis are unusual.[540] Vascular alterations are characterized by swelling of endothelial cells.[540]

The fungi are seen in the cytoplasm of macrophages and giant cells in routinely stained sections (Fig. 19-70).[540] They are highlighted by the PAS or GMS stains (Figs. 19-71 and 19-72).[547,548] *P. brasiliensis* can be confused with *B. dermatitidis* if only single budding is observed; however, the former organism has thinner cell walls and narrow-based buds. *Cryptococcus* can

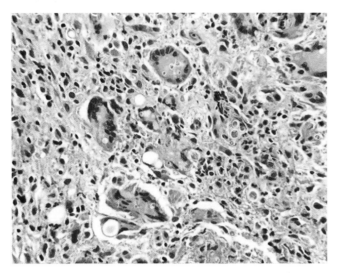

Figure 19-66. Paracoccidioidomycosis. There is usually a prominent chronic inflammatory infiltrate which is rich in giant cells containing fungal organisms. (Courtesy of Mirian Sotto, MD, PhD, Department of Dermatology, Hospital das Clinicas, University of Sao Paulo.)

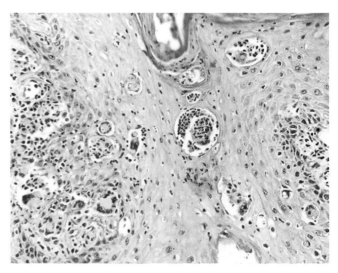

Figure 19-68. Paracoccidioidomycosis. The intraepidermal inflammatory infiltrate is quite prominent in this example. Organisms are frequently found in the intraepidermal abscesses. (Courtesy of Mirian Sotto, MD, PhD, Department of Dermatology, Hospital das Clinicas, University of Sao Paulo.)

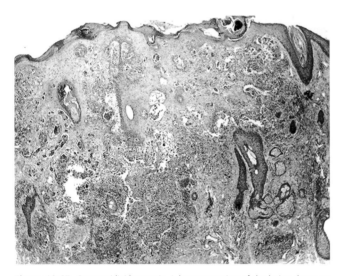

Figure 19-67. Paracoccidioidomycosis. A low-power view of the lesion shows an exuberant pseudoepitheliomatous hyperplasia with intraepidermal neutrophilic abscesses overlying a dermal granulomatous and suppurative inflammatory infiltrate. (Courtesy of Mirian Sotto, MD, PhD, Department of Dermatology, Hospital das Clinicas, University of Sao Paulo.)

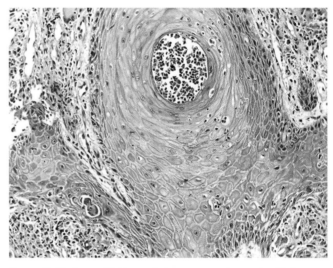

Figure 19-69. Paracoccidioidomycosis. In some cases, the pseudoepitheliomatous epidermal hyperplasia is striking and can be confused with squamous cell carcinoma. (Courtesy of Mirian Sotto, MD, PhD, Department of Dermatology, Hospital das Clinicas, University of Sao Paulo.)

show similar variation in yeast size but has the characteristic mucicarmine-positive mucinous capsule.[539]

Etiology and Pathogenesis
P. brasiliensis is a dimorphic fungus that appears in tissues as small and large budding yeasts that measure 2 to 30 μm in diameter.[544] They are round to oval and have a birefringent capsule.[547] The diagnostic organisms have multiple buds resembling a "steering wheel" or a "Mickey Mouse head," with narrow points of attachment of buds to mother cells.[537,544]

The presence of β-estradiol receptors in the cytoplasm of the mycelium and yeast forms of *P. brasiliensis* suggests that this

hormone is capable of inhibiting the transformation of the mycelium to the yeast form.[509,537,539] This could be one reason for the lower incidence of cases in adult women.

Histoplasmosis

Clinical Features
Histoplasmosis, or Darling disease, results from infection with *H. capsulatum* var. *capsulatum*. The disease has a worldwide distribution, but the largest endemic focus is in the central eastern United States, especially the Ohio, Mississippi, and Missouri River valleys.[549]

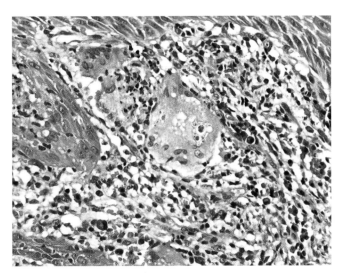

Figure 19-70. Paracoccidioidomycosis. The budding yeast form of the fungus, with the classic "steering wheel" morphology, can be recognized even without the use of special stains. In this excellent example, the organisms are outlined by the cytoplasm of the giant cell. (Courtesy of Mirian Sotto, MD, PhD, Department of Dermatology, Hospital das Clinicas, University of Sao Paulo.)

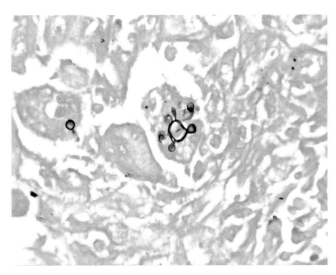

Figure 19-72. Paracoccidioidomycosis (GMS stain). The classic "steering wheel" configuration of *Paracoccidioides brasiliensis*. (Courtesy of Mirian Sotto, MD, PhD, Department of Dermatology, Hospital das Clinicas, University of Sao Paulo.)

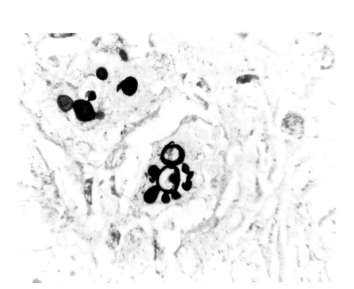

Figure 19-71. Paracoccidioidomycosis (Grocott's methenamine silver stain). The budding yeast form is highlighted by this special stain. (Courtesy of Mirian Sotto, MD, PhD, Department of Dermatology, Hospital das Clinicas, University of Sao Paulo.)

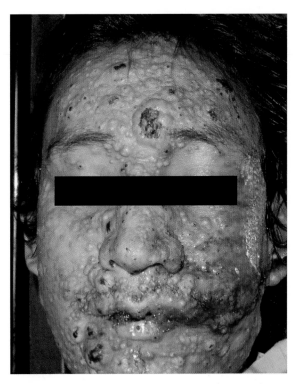

Figure 19-73. Histoplasmosis. This HIV/AIDS patient presented with disseminated disease with extensive cutaneous involvement. Note the disfiguring lesions ranging from papules to ulcerated plaques.

Microconidia (mold form) inhalation is the main form of infection. In 99% of cases, the pulmonary infection is self-limited and asymptomatic.[550] Symptomatic disseminated disease is usually seen in infants and immunosuppressed patients, particularly those with AIDS.[551] Acute life-threatening histoplasmosis may complicate immunotherapy with TNF-α antagonists, particularly infliximab.[535]

Mucous membrane lesions are common in disseminated histoplasmosis, usually manifesting as oral ulcerations.[549] Cutaneous involvement occurs in approximately 6% of patients with disseminated disease.[552] Skin lesions are variable and are not considered characteristic. They may manifest as papules, nodules, pustules, ulcers, cellulitis-like areas, acneiform lesions, or molluscum-like papules (Fig. 19-73).[509,549,550] Erythroderma has also been described in these patients.[552]

The primary cutaneous form is rare and usually manifests as a solitary, self-limited, ulcerated nodule at the site of fungal inoculation.[553] Erythema nodosum and erythema multiforme can occur as hypersensitivity manifestations.[509]

Histopathology

Cutaneous lesions show a granulomatous infiltrate in the dermis, sometimes extending into the subcutaneous tissue, with numerous macrophages (Figs. 19-74 and 19-75). Tiny oval yeast forms (2-4 μm), surrounded by a clear halo (pseudocapsule), are seen in the cytoplasm of both macrophages and multinucleated giant cells (Fig. 19-76).[547] An infiltrate containing lymphocytes, plasma cells, and giant cells is usually present. However, in acute disseminated cases, parasitized macrophages predominate.[552] Extracellular organisms are occasionally seen (Fig. 19-77).[549,550] The PAS or the GMS stains can be used to better visualize the fungi (Fig. 19-78).

In patients with AIDS, there is a sparse inflammatory cell infiltrate.[509] Leukocytoclasia and dermal necrosis can also be observed.[554] *H. capsulatum* within cutaneous nerves has been described in disseminated histoplasmosis in patients with AIDS.[555]

The differential diagnosis includes other conditions in which parasitized macrophages are seen, especially leishmaniasis and *Penicillium marneffei* infections.[549] The parasites in leishmaniasis lack the clear halo seen in *H. capsulatum* and have a tendency to aggregate at the periphery of the macrophage (marquee sign).[549] The *P. marneffei* yeast forms replicate by binary division and have a septate appearance, whereas *H. capsulatum* divides by budding.[549]

Etiology and Pathogenesis

The mycelial form of *H. capsulatum* (var. *capsulatum*) is found in the soil, especially in areas contaminated with bird or bat droppings, which provide added nutrients for growth.[535] The microconidia are inhaled and deposited in the alveoli of the infected individual. At body temperature, they convert into

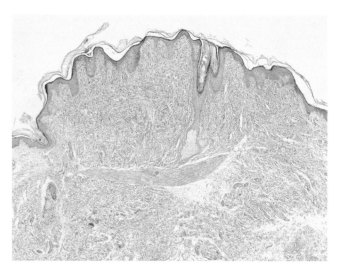

Figure 19-74. Histoplasmosis. There is a diffuse infiltration of the papillary and reticular dermis by histiocytes filled with organisms, with little or no lymphocytes. Note the absence of grenz zone. This skin biopsy specimen is from the same patient as in Figure 19-73.

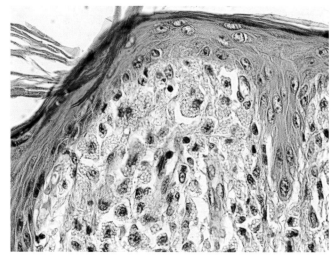

Figure 19-76. Histoplasmosis. High-power view of the same lesion as in Figure 19-74 reveals the presence of intracellular round structures within the histiocytes.

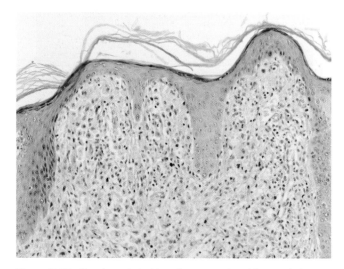

Figure 19-75. Histoplasmosis. In this medium-power view of the same lesion as in Figure 19-74, one can identify the fungi-laden histiocytic population.

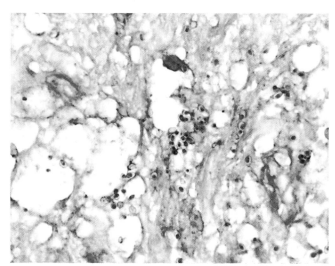

Figure 19-77. Histoplasmosis (PAS stain). In immunosuppressed patients, "free" fungal forms can be found in the midst of the inflammatory infiltrate. (Courtesy of Mirian Sotto, MD, PhD, Department of Dermatology, Hospital das Clinicas, University of Sao Paulo.)

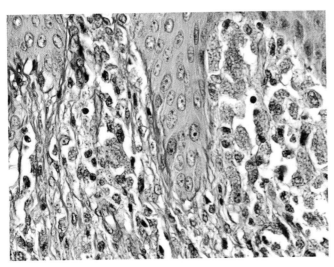

Figure 19-78. Histoplasmosis (PAS stain). *Histoplasma capsulatum* is strongly PAS-positive and can be differentiated from other intracellular parasites, such as *Leishmania* spp., by the absence of a kinetoplast and the presence of a capsule.

the yeast form and are ingested by macrophages. The yeasts multiply within these cells and gain access to the blood circulation, disseminating throughout the body.[535] If adequate cellular immunity ensues, macrophages become fungicidal and control the infection.[535] The organism is not encapsulated, but in tissues it appears to be surrounded by a clear halo that was misinterpreted by Darling as being a capsule.[509,550]

African Histoplasmosis

African histoplasmosis is caused by *Histoplasma capsulatum* var. *duboisii*. It is endemic in Central and West Africa and in the island of Madagascar.[556] Rare cases have been reported in Europe, but were all imported.[550] This form of histoplasmosis is characterized by the presence of granulomatous and suppurative lesions on the skin, subcutaneous tissues, lymph nodes, and bones.[556] In contrast to *H. capsulatum* var. *capsulatum*, pulmonary disease is rare.[557] Although HIV infection and *H. capsulatum* var. *duboisii* coexist in Africa, this coinfection seems to be rare.[550] HIV-infected patients have substantially more disseminated disease than HIV-negative individuals.[558]

The histopathology is different from that of classic histoplasmosis. Characteristic lesions show a granulomatous inflammatory reaction with numerous giant cells of foreign body and Langhans type, most of them containing numerous oval yeast cells (8-15 µm in diameter).[559] The yeast cells may sometimes occur in chains of four or five cells.[556] Necrosis and suppuration are commonly present.[558] The organisms can also be observed extracellularly in clusters.[559] The fungus is visible in H&E-stained sections, but is better demonstrated by silver methenamine or PAS stain.[556]

The pathogenesis of African histoplasmosis remains unclear. The exact portal of entry into the body is unknown, but inhalation into lungs and direct inoculation in the skin have been incriminated.[556] *H. capsulatum* var. *duboisii* has much larger yeasts than *H. capsulatum* var. *capsulatum*, measuring from 8 to 15 µm in diameter.[556] They have thick walls and are lemon-shaped, with narrow budding.[558] In cultures grown at 25° C, the

mycelia from the two *H. capsulatum* varieties cannot be distinguished, either macroscopically or microscopically.[557]

Penicilliosis

Clinical Features

Penicilliosis, caused by *P. marneffei*, is endemic in tropical Asia, especially Thailand, northeastern India, China, Hong Kong, Vietnam, and Taiwan.[560] The organism was discovered in 1956 as an infection of bamboo rats.[561] However, the importance of *P. marneffei* as a human pathogen was recognized only after the HIV pandemic arrived in Asia and the prevalence of infection increased in local populations among visitors from areas where the infection is not endemic.[559,562] After tuberculosis and cryptococcosis, penicilliosis is the third most common opportunistic infection in patients with AIDS in northern Thailand.[563]

P. marneffei appears to be a primary pulmonary pathogen that disseminates to other internal organs by hematogenous spread. Severity of the disease depends on the immunologic status of the host. Most patients with penicilliosis are HIV-positive. Clinical features of disseminated *P. marneffei* infection in AIDS patients are fever, anemia, weight loss, lymphadenopathy, hepatosplenomegaly, respiratory signs, and skin lesions.[560] Approximately 60% to 70% of patients have skin eruptions.[564] These usually manifest as skin-colored or pigmented papules or nodules, some of which have central umbilication or necrosis.[417] They often become generalized. *P. marneffei* can clinically resemble tuberculosis, molluscum contagiosum, cryptococcosis, or histoplasmosis.[565]

Histopathology

P. marneffei infection can lead to various tissue responses, probably reflecting the degree of cell-mediated immunity.[566] The formation of granulomas helps localize and prevent the dissemination of the infection and is seen in immunocompetent patients. The inflammatory infiltrate usually consists of multinucleated giant cells, lymphocytes, and neutrophils.[567] On the other hand, in immunocompromised patients, the granulomatous response is usually minimal or absent.[567] Instead, there is necrosis and a diffuse infiltration of macrophages engorged with proliferating yeast cells.[567] *P. marneffei* yeast-like cells can be seen both inside the cytoplasm of histiocytes and extracellularly.[560] The intracellular yeasts are oval or round cells, 2 to 3 µm in diameter, that multiply by binary fission.[560] Extracellular *P. marneffei* cells are elongated (up to 13 µm) and have one or two septa.[560]

P. marneffei can be seen in histopathologic sections stained with H&E, GMS, or PAS stain.[560] Differentiation between *P. marneffei* and *H. capsulatum* is important because of the great morphologic resemblance between the two organisms. Both are intracellular pathogens. However, *H. capsulatum* divides by budding, not by septation.[566]

Etiology and Pathogenesis

P. marneffei has been isolated from the internal organs of four species of rodents (*Rhizomys sinensis, Rhizomys pruinosus, Rhizomys sumatrensis,* and *Cannomys badius*) and from soil samples that have been collected from bamboo rat burrows.[560] However, to date no attempts to recover *P. marneffei* from environments other than those that are intimately associated with bamboo rats have been successful, and definitive proof of an environmental reservoir for *P. marneffei* within the soil or other substrates is still lacking.[560]

P. marneffei is the only known *Penicillium* species that exhibits temperature-dependent dimorphic growth.[560] At temperatures lower than 37° C, the fungus grows as mycelia with the formation of septate hyphae, bearing conidiophores and conidia typical of the genus *Penicillium*.[560] At 37° C, the fungus grows in a yeast-like form with the formation of fission arthroconidium cells.[560] The fission yeast cells represent the parasitic form of *P. marneffei*, which is seen inside macrophages. The mold-to-yeast conversion, which is thermally regulated, is a diagnostic characteristic of *P. marneffei*. In contrast to *P. marneffei*, the other *Penicillium* species are not dimorphic and are seen as hyphae in tissue, more like *Aspergillus*.[560]

Infection presumably results from inhalation of conidia from the environment.[560] On inhalation, conidia are believed to be phagocytized by alveolar macrophages, where they grow in the yeast phase. From there, the fungus can spread to other parts of the body.[560]

Hyalohyphomycoses

Hyalohyphomycosis is a term used to designate invasive fungal infections caused by hyaline septate hyphae in tissue.[568] The genus *Fusarium* and species of *Penicillium, Aspergillus, Scopulariopsis, Scedosporium, Acremonium*, and *Paecilomyces*. can be included in this group.[569]

Fusarium

Fusarium species cause a broad spectrum of disease in humans, including superficial, locally invasive, and disseminated infections, with the last occurring almost exclusively in severely immunocompromised patients.[570-572] The most common infections in immunocompetent hosts are keratitis and onychomycosis.[568,571] The infection may also occur as a result of skin breakdown (e.g., burns, wounds) or from the presence of foreign bodies, such as contact lenses (keratitis), continuous ambulatory peritoneal dialysis (peritonitis), and catheters (catheter-associated fungemia).[570,573-576] Immunocompromised patients at high risk for fusariosis are those who have prolonged neutropenia and T-cell immunodeficiency.

Disseminated fusarial infection leads to cutaneous involvement in more than 70% of patients.[577] The usual course includes fever, multiple skin lesions, myalgias, and fungemia.[577] Three forms of skin lesions can be observed: multiple subcutaneous nodules, ecthyma gangrenosum–like lesions, and target lesions consisting of ecthymiform lesions surrounded by a thin erythematous rim.[578] These lesions can involve any site, with a predilection for the extremities, and evolve rapidly, usually over a few days.[568,579] Fusariosis in immunocompromised patients usually responds poorly to antifungal therapy and is associated with a high mortality rate.[580]

In tissue, the hyphae are similar to those of *Aspergillus* species, with hyaline and septate filaments that typically dichotomize at acute and right angles (Figs. 19-79 and 19-80).[568,580] However, adventitious sporulation may be present in tissue, and the finding of hyphae and yeast-like structures together is highly suggestive of fusariosis in the high-risk population.[581] In the absence of microbial growth, the differential diagnosis between fusariosis and other hyalohyphomycoses is difficult and requires

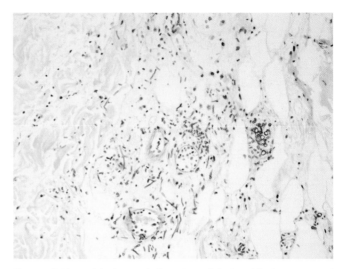

Figure 19-79. Hyalohyphomycosis (*Fusarium* sp.) (PAS stain). The presence of septate hyphae branching in acute or right angles is characteristic. Note the presence of yeast-like structures, a helpful feature for differentiating this organism from *Aspergillus* sp. (Courtesy of Mirian Sotto, MD, PhD, Department of Dermatology, Hospital das Clinicas, University of Sao Paulo.)

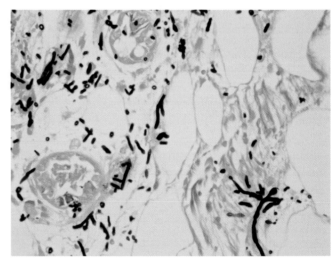

Figure 19-80. Hyalohyphomycosis (*Fusarium* sp.) (GMS stain). Hyphae and yeast-like forms infiltrate the subcutaneous fat. (Courtesy of Mirian Sotto, MD, PhD, Department of Dermatology, Hospital das Clinicas, University of Sao Paulo.)

the use of in situ hybridization in paraffin-embedded tissue specimens.[582]

Fusarium is a plant and human pathogen readily recovered from soil and water and is part of water biofilms.[568] The species most frequently causing infection in humans are *Fusarium solani, Fusarium oxysporum*, and *Fusarium moniliforme*.[581] The principal portal of entry for *Fusarium* spp. is the airways, followed by the skin at sites of tissue breakdown, and, possibly, the mucosal membranes.[568]

Cryptococcosis

Clinical Features

Cryptococcosis is caused by the yeast *C. neoformans* and has worldwide distribution.[583] *C. neoformans* is found in the excreta

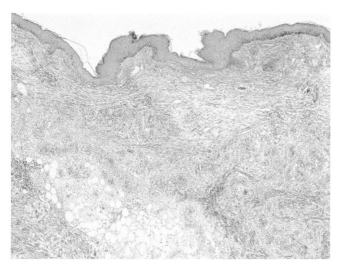

Figure 19-81. Cryptococcosis. This example illustrates the gelatinous form of the infection, which is represented by a diffuse mucoid infiltrate with a scant inflammatory infiltrate.

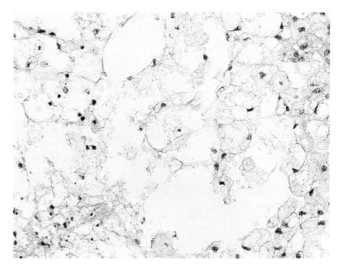

Figure 19-82. Cryptococcosis. Numerous yeast forms of *Cryptococcus neoformans* exhibit the characteristic thick capsule.

of pigeons and other birds, in soil, and in fruits.[579] Generally, the organism enters the body through the respiratory tract and may disseminate hematogenously to other sites.[584] The infection is observed mainly in immunosuppressed individuals, such as AIDS patients.[585] However, cryptococcosis can also occur in apparently immunocompetent hosts.[586]

The CNS is the most common site of extrapulmonary disease.[584,587] Meningoencephalitis has a high mortality if untreated. Other sites commonly involved in disseminated disease include the skin, bones, joints, and urinary tract.[579] Secondary skin lesions are observed in 10% to 15% of patients with disseminated cryptococcosis.[585] Cutaneous manifestations can precede and may be the only clue to disseminated disease.[363]

Skin involvement in cryptococcosis is nonspecific and produces a wide variety of lesions,[584,588] including papules, nodules, pustules, vesicles, plaques, subcutaneous abscesses, ecchymoses, and ulcers.[579] Lesions resembling those of molluscum contagiosum, Kaposi sarcoma, or acne have been described in patients with AIDS.[363,579,589] Cryptococcal cellulitis has also been reported, mostly in renal transplant recipients receiving corticosteroids.[579,587] Although lesions can be widespread, they are most commonly observed on the head and neck.[584,587]

Primary cutaneous cryptococcosis, via direct inoculation, is very rare.[583] Therefore, it is reasonable to consider any patient presenting with cutaneous lesions as potentially having disseminated cryptococcosis.[587]

Histopathology
There are two types of histologic reaction to *C. neoformans*: granulomatous and gelatinous (paucireactive).[363,584,590] Both types may be observed in the same cutaneous lesion.[363,590] In the granulomatous reaction, skin lesions display a dense infiltrate of histiocytes, giant cells, lymphoid cells, and plasma cells (Fig. 19-81).[590] Necrosis can occur and, in some cases, suppuration.[363] A small number of yeast forms are present, usually within the cytoplasm of giant cells and histiocytes (Fig. 19-82), but also free in the tissue. In the gelatinous reaction, skin lesions show

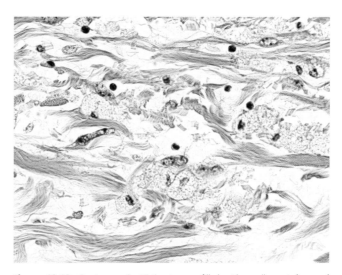

Figure 19-83. Cryptococcosis. Histiocytes are filled with small yeast forms of *Cryptococcus neoformans*.

numerous aggregated organisms with thick mucinous capsules, forming mucoid masses, and almost no inflammatory infiltrate (Fig. 19-83).[590] Palisading granulomatous response to *C. neoformans* has been described.[591,592]

C. neoformans is seen in tissues as a round to oval yeast form and may exhibit pronounced dimensional variability (range, 2-20 μm).[593] The cell wall of *C. neoformans* stains with PAS, methenamine silver, and Fontana-Masson stains (Figs. 19-84 and 19-85).[594] The capsule stains red with mucicarmine and blue with Alcian blue.[594] Fungal budding and fragmentation of the mucoid capsules can be observed.[363]

Etiology and Pathogenesis
C. neoformans is inhaled as a nonencapsulated organism measuring up to 2 μm in diameter.[584] In the human host, the size of the organism increases, and a thick gelatinous capsule develops. It reproduces by budding, which is narrow-based.[595]

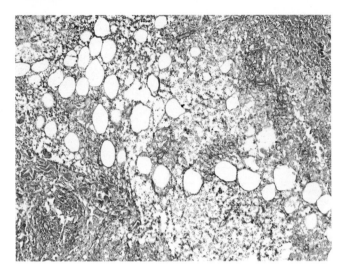

Figure 19-84. Cryptococcosis (PAS stain). Numerous fungal organisms are present in the gelatinous reaction.

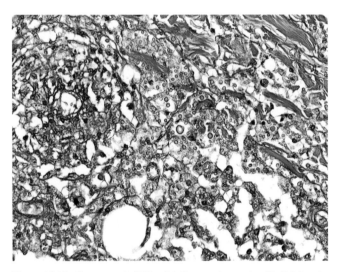

Figure 19-85. Cryptococcosis (PAS stain). The organisms stain with PAS, but the capsule, which is composed of acid mucoid polysaccharide, stains only with Alcian blue or colloidal iron.

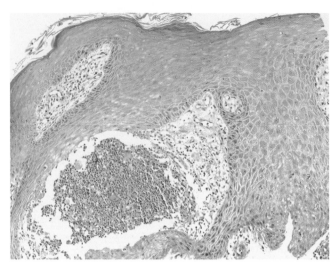

Figure 19-86. Chromoblastomycosis. There is often a pseudoepitheliomatous epidermal hyperplasia with prominent acanthosis and hyperkeratosis overlying a granulomatous infiltrate. The pigmented nature of the organisms makes them stand out even at medium power. (Courtesy of Mirian Sotto, MD, PhD, Department of Dermatology, Hospital das Clinicas, University of Sao Paulo.)

Chromoblastomycosis

Chromoblastomycosis (chromomycosis) is a chronic, suppurative, granulomatous mycosis of the skin and subcutaneous tissues.[600] It is caused by various pigmented (dematiaceous) fungi, which are observed in the tissues as sclerotic pigmented bodies. The most common fungal species associated with chromoblastomycosis are *Fonsecaea pedrosoi*, *Fonsecaea compacta*, *Phialophora verrucosa*, *Rhinocladiella aquaspera*, and *Cladosporium carrionii*.[601] *F. pedrosoi* has been isolated from approximately 95% of patients in some series.[537,602] The infection is more common in the tropics, especially in the humid areas.[601] Patients are usually healthy and without any predisposing factors.[601] The fungi are present in soil, wood, and vegetable debris and probably infect patients after trauma.[537] Those affected are mainly male rural workers.[601]

Initial lesions of chromoblastomycosis are usually erythematous papules, which slowly enlarge to display varying morphologies such as verrucous nodules, cauliflower-like tumors, and psoriasis-like plaques.[603] The cutaneous lesions are found on the feet and legs or on other exposed areas of the body.[601] Central scarring and ulceration can occur.[601] As the infection progresses, dissemination may occur by extension of the lesions as satellites along the lymphatic vessels or by autoinoculation through scratching.[604] Secondary bacterial infection is a frequent complication and can lead to lymphedema, resulting in further limb deformity.[602] Involvement of underlying tissues usually does not occur, but hematogenous spread to the CNS has been described.[605] The development of squamous cell carcinoma is a possibility in long-standing disease.[602]

Epidermal changes include hyperkeratosis with parakeratosis, acanthosis, pseudocarcinomatous hyperplasia, and papillomatosis (Fig. 19-86).[600] Intraepidermal abscesses are frequently observed, with or without fungal cells (Fig. 19-87).[600] Occasionally, the fungal bodies can be seen between keratinocytes; this has been referred to as transepithelial elimination.[606] Dematia-

C. neoformans has been traditionally classified into three varieties with five serotypes: *C. neoformans* var. *grubii* (serotype A), *C. neoformans* var. *neoformans* (serotype D), *C. neoformans* var. *gattii* (serotypes B and C), and serotype AD (a hybrid of serotypes A and D).[596] Whereas serotype A and D strains are usually isolated from pigeon droppings and cause disease mainly in immunocompromised hosts, serotype B and C strains are more commonly isolated from eucalyptus trees and more often infect hosts with normal immune status.[597]

Cell-mediated immunity plays an important role in susceptibility to infection and in dissemination of the organisms, providing an explanation for the increased incidence of infection in immunosuppressed patients.[584] The thick capsule of *C. neoformans* impairs phagocytosis[584] and is an important virulence factor.[598] The cell wall of *C. neoformans* contains melanin, which is also considered a virulence factor.[599]

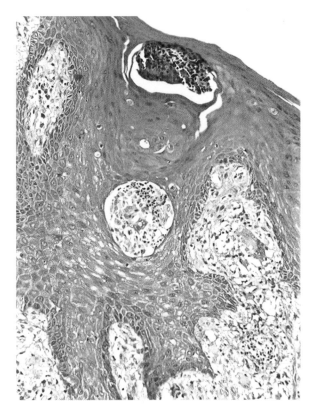

Figure 19-87. Chromoblastomycosis. In addition to the dermal granulomatous inflammatory infiltrate, there is a marked mixed inflammatory infiltrate which can affect both the dermis and the epidermis. (Courtesy of Mirian Sotto, MD, PhD, Department of Dermatology, Hospital das Clinicas, University of Sao Paulo.)

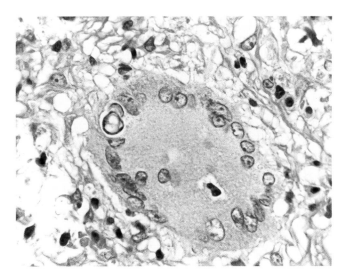

Figure 19-88. Chromoblastomycosis. High-power view of the pigmented fungal forms with the classic "copper pennies" appearance. Note the septation characteristic of this organism and evidence of cell division. This feature distinguishes this organism from those that bud. (Courtesy of Mirian Sotto, MD, PhD, Department of Dermatology, Hospital das Clinicas, University of Sao Paulo.)

ceous hyphae can rarely be seen in the stratum corneum.[600] The dermis shows a dense inflammatory infiltrate composed predominantly of neutrophils, which occasionally form dermal abscesses, and macrophages.[600] Eosinophils, lymphocytes, plasma cells, and mast cells can also be seen.[600] Both epithelioid granulomas and poorly organized granulomas formed by aggregates of macrophages and epithelioid cells with giant cells (Langhans or foreign-body type) can be observed.[600] These granulomas frequently have a suppurative center. The sclerotic bodies can be detected in the center of granulomas and within giant cells. They are dark brown and round, resembling "copper pennies," and may be seen singly or in chains or clusters (Fig. 19-88).[607] Because of their color, the fungi can be easily identified without special stains. Many cases show marked cicatricial fibrosis, which can extend from the superficial dermis to the subcutaneous fat, obliterating skin adnexa.[600] Furthermore, the sclerotic bodies are easily identified by microscopic examination of crusts and exudates from the skin lesions under potassium hydroxide.[603] However, culture is necessary for classification of the causative agent.

The sclerotic bodies are round or polyhedral, pigmented, thick-walled fungal cells that measure 5 to 12 μm in diameter.[608] They represent an intermediate vegetative form, arrested between yeast and hyphal morphology.[537] Chromoblastomycosis was previously believed to be related to blastomycosis; however, cellular division occurs by internal septation and not by budding as in blastomycosis.[601]

Mycetoma

Clinical Features

Mycetoma is a chronic granulomatous infection of the skin and subcutaneous tissues, characterized by the triad of tumefaction, draining sinuses, and the presence of grains in the exudate.[609,610] They can be caused by filamentous bacteria (actinomycetomas) or true fungi (eumycetomas).[610] These infections are most common in tropical and subtropical areas and are endemic to India and several countries in Africa and South America.[611] The organisms are present in the soil and are implanted into the host tissue through trauma.[544] The infection is most frequent in adult men, usually rural workers.[610]

The foot is the most common site of infection,[612] but any exposed area is susceptible. The lesion starts as a painless papule, which enlarges to become a discharging nodule. The disease progresses with extension to the adjacent tissues, forming multiple draining sinuses. The drainage contains grains, which can sometimes be seen with the naked eye.[544] The sinus tracts are rarely observed before 3 months but are usually present by the end of the first year.[611] The affected area becomes distorted by inflammation, edema, and fibrosis. The infection can extend to involve the underlying fascia, muscle, and bone. Eumycetomas are usually less inflammatory and less invasive and have a slower progression, compared with actinomycetomas.[544]

Histopathology

Three types of tissue reaction have been described.[610] In the type I reaction, the grains are surrounded by polymorphonuclear leukocytes, with the innermost neutrophils closely attached to the surface of the grain.[610] Outside the suppurative zone, there is granulation tissue with macrophages, lymphocytes, plasma cells, and a few neutrophils.[610] Macrophages can have large vacuolated cytoplasms.[610] Capillaries and venules are surrounded by concentrically arranged layers of fibrin, giving them an "onion skin" appearance.[610] The dermis exhibits a variable degree of fibrosis.[613]

In the type II reaction, most of the neutrophils are replaced by macrophages and multinucleated giant cells that are engulfing grain material. Other inflammatory cells and histologic changes are similar to those observed in type I reactions.[610]

The type III reaction is characterized by well-organized epithelioid granulomas that contain Langhans giant cells.[610] Occasionally, remnants of fungal material can be seen in the center of the granuloma.[610] Other inflammatory and histologic changes are similar to those seen in type I and type II reactions.[610]

The Splendore-Hoeppli phenomenon can occasionally be seen.[148] The fungal hyphae in eumycotic grains are thicker than the thin filaments seen in actinomycotic grains.[614] Special stains, such as the Gram stain, can help distinguish the subtype of mycetoma. In actinomycetoma, the grains have gram-negative centers with gram-positive, fine, radiating fringes.[614] In eumycetomas, the grains show gram-negative septate hyphae embedded in intercellular cement.[614]

Etiology and Pathogenesis

More than 20 species of fungi and bacteria have been implicated as etiologic agents of mycetoma.[615] The predominant causative organism varies by region.[614] Eumycetomas predominate in Africa and southern Asia, whereas actinomycetomas predominate in Latin America.[609]

Madurella mycetomatis is the most prevalent fungal etiologic agent worldwide,[609,612] and *Pseudallescheria boydii* is the most common cause of eumycetoma in the United States.[614,601] Other important agents include *Leptosphaeria senegalensis*, *Madurella grisea*, *Acremonium recifei*, and *Pyrenochaeta romeroi*.[612]

Worldwide, approximately 60% of all mycetomas are caused by actinomycetes, the commonest agent being *N. brasiliensis*.[544,609] Other causative organisms include *Streptomyces somaliensis*, *Actinomadura madurae*, and *Actinomadura pelletierii*.[601]

The grains are aggregates of fungal hyphae or bacterial filaments, and their size, consistency, and color provide the initial clue to the causative species (Table 19-2).[609] The black granules are seen only in eumycetomas, such as those produced by *M. mycetomatis*.[614] The consistency of most grains is soft, but those of *M. mycetomatis* and *S. somaliensis*, for example, can be hard.[544] Culture is required for accurate identification of the causal agent.

Table 19-2 Morphologic Features of Grains Associated with Microorganisms Causing Mycetomas in Humans

Agent	Color	Diameter (mm)	Consistency
Actinomadura madurae	White	1.5-2	Soft
Actinomadura pelletieri	Red	0.2-0.5	Hard
Nocardia brasiliensis	White or orange	<0.5	Soft
Nocardia asteroides	White	<0.5	Soft
Streptomyces somaliensis	Yellow	0.5-2	Hard
Madurella mycetomatis	Black	1-2	Hard

Data from Lupi O, Tyring SK, McGinnis MR: Tropical dermatology: Fungal tropical diseases. J Am Acad Dermatol 2005;53:931-951.

Phaeohyphomycosis

Phaeohyphomycosis is a term used to describe subcutaneous and systemic diseases caused by a variety of dematiaceous fungi that develop in infected tissue as darkly pigmented yeast-like cells, hyphae, pseudohyphae, or a combination of these forms.[608,616-623] Dematiaceous fungi can produce three different types of infection: phaeohyphomycosis, chromoblastomycosis, and mycetoma.[619] Unlike chromoblastomycosis or mycetoma, there are no sclerotic bodies nor grains in phaeohyphomycosis.[616,620]

More than 130 fungal species belonging to 70 diverse genera have been reported as causative agents in human and animal phaeohyphomycoses.[621] *Exophiala jeanselmei* and *Wangiella dermatitidis* are the most commonly isolated fungi in cutaneous and subcutaneous phaeohyphomycoses.[608,622] These fungi grow on soil, wood and other plant materials, and decaying organic matter.[623] The infection is usually acquired by inoculation of the organism into the skin and subcutaneous tissues through trauma.[618] However, other possible portals of entry have been suggested, including inhalation of the fungus with lung or sinus invasion, ingestion of contaminated food or water followed by penetration through the gastrointestinal tract, and contamination of vascular catheters.[618]

Phaeohyphomycosis can be divided into five groups: (1) superficial (including black piedra and tinea nigra); (2) cutaneous; (3) corneal or mycotic keratitis; (4) subcutaneous; and (5) invasive, systemic, and cerebral.[608] Disseminated infection is uncommon, but its incidence is increasing, particularly among immunocompromised patients.[624] The most important predisposing factor for cutaneous and subcutaneous infection is exposure to contaminated material present in the environment (i.e., decaying wood, plants).[618] Subcutaneous phaeohyphomycosis usually manifests as a single cyst or abscess on an extremity or another exposed area of the skin.[619] Noncutaneous phaeohyphomycosis may involve any organ or system but is most common in the sinuses, lungs, and brain.[618] In addition to invasive disease, allergic reactions to these fungi are frequent, manifested by sinusitis and pulmonary disease.[618]

Three different tissue patterns have been described in phaeohyphomycosis.[623] Keratotic plaques and nodules usually show parakeratosis and irregular epidermal hyperplasia with microabscesses.[623] The dermis is occupied by a suppurative and granulomatous inflammatory process.[623] Solid and necrotizing granulomas and microabscesses are observed.[623] Brown yeast-like cells, pseudohyphae, and true hyphae are seen among epithelioid cells and neutrophils. Some organisms are found within multinucleated giant cells. The PAS stain highlights the fungi. The yeast-like cells can be observed singly or arranged in chains of varying lengths.[623]

The second tissue pattern shows an intradermal, multiloculated cystic structure with a dense fibrous capsule.[623] Individual cystic structures are separated by broad bands of connective tissue.[623] The epidermis shows no abnormalities. The larger cysts can be empty and lined by granulomas and neutrophils.[623] The smaller cysts are usually filled with neutrophils and lined by granulomas.[623] Many dematiaceous yeast-like cells, true hyphae, and pseudohyphae are seen within the inflammatory infiltrate, as well as within giant cells.[623] Particles of wood splinter can also be seen.[623]

The third tissue pattern is that of a well-defined, dermal unilocular cyst surrounded by dense fibrous tissue.[623] The epidermis is uninvolved. The center of the cyst contains necrotic debris and neutrophils.[623] The inner lining of the cyst is composed of granulomas which contain dematiaceous organisms.[623] Fragments of vegetable material can be seen in the lumen.[623]

Chromoblastomycosis is characterized in tissues by sclerotic bodies, which are not seen in phaeohyphomycosis. The yeast-like cells in phaeohyphomycosis may resemble the sclerotic bodies of chromoblastomycosis; however, the former are lighter, have thinner walls, show septation in only one plane, and have a chain morphology.[623]

The etiologic agents of phaeohyphomycosis are characterized by yellow to brown pigmentation of their cell walls and distinctive brown to black colony morphology. In most cases, the pigment is melanin, and specifically, dihydroxynaphthalene melanin.[625]

Some species cause both phaeohyphomycosis and chromoblastomycosis. The different pathologic features produced in tissues by the same fungus are believed to be a result of undefined host factors.[623,626]

Sporotrichosis

Clinical Features

Sporotrichosis is caused by the dimorphic fungus *Sporothrix schenckii* and has worldwide distribution, especially in tropical and warm temperate climates.[611,637] Most commonly, the infection is acquired through traumatic implantation of *S. schenckii* present in organic material[627] such as wood splinters, thorns, hay, or sphagnum moss.[611,628] Pulmonary infection may result from inhalation of conidia into the lungs.[587,629,630] A cat-transmitted epidemic occurred in Rio de Janeiro, Brazil.[627]

Sporotrichosis is usually classified into four forms: lymphocutaneous, fixed cutaneous, disseminated, and extracutaneous.[627] The lymphocutaneous (or sporotrichoid) form is the most common and begins as a nontender papule on an exposed area of the skin, such as the face, hand, or arm.[601] This papule grows into a nodule and usually evolves with ulceration. Subsequently, other nodules appear along the lymphatic distribution draining the area (Fig. 19-89).[631] These lymphatic nodules may undergo suppuration and ulceration. In addition, lymphadenopathy and lymphangitis may develop.[587]

In the fixed (localized) cutaneous form of sporotrichosis, there is no lymphatic spread. A solitary plaque or a group of lesions is present on an exposed area of the skin. These lesions can be scaly, acneiform, verrucous, or ulcerative.[544]

Disseminated sporotrichosis is uncommon and results from hematogenous spread or autoinoculation.[587,632] Extracutaneous disease is also rare and can involve one or more sites such as the lungs, joints, bones, genitourinary tract, meninges, and eyes.[587] Pulmonary sporotrichosis occurs after inhalation of the organism, rather than by cutaneous inoculation.[631] Disseminated and extracutaneous sporotrichosis have been described in patients with chronic alcoholism, hematologic malignancies, chronic obstructive pulmonary disease, diabetes, use of corticosteroids, or AIDS.[587,630,633,634] Disseminated skin lesions are usually nodules or subcutaneous abscesses that later ulcerate (i.e., develop punched-out ulcerations).[633]

Histopathology

The histopathologic features include epithelial hyperplasia, with marked pseudoepitheliomatous hyperplasia and overlying hyperkeratosis and parakeratosis.[635,636] Intraepidermal neutrophilic microabscesses are common.[635] In the dermis, a characteristic arrangement of the infiltrate in three zones may occur.[637] There is a central suppurative zone composed of polymorphonuclear leukocytes, which is surrounded by an epithelioid granulomatous process.[635] A lymphoplasmacytic inflammatory infiltrate surrounds the granulomas.[635,637]

In the lymphangitic form, the inflammatory nodules are located in the deep dermis or subcutaneous tissues, and there are usually no epidermal changes.[636] Similar to the primary lesions, they consist of a central necrotic zone with neutrophils, a surrounding zone of epithelioid cells and giant cells, and an outer zone of plasma cells and lymphocytes with fibrosis.[636]

In tissues, *S. schenckii* may be identified as yeast cells that measure 3 to 5 μm in diameter, are round to cigar-shaped, and can show single or multiple buds (Fig. 19-90).[629] Although they are rare, nonseptate hyphae have also been observed.[638]

In sporotrichosis, the asteroid bodies are extracellular eosinophilic structures that measure 15 to 35 μm in diameter.[636] They are found in the center of intraepidermal or dermal abscesses.[636] Usually, one to three asteroid bodies are found in a section.[636] They consist of a central yeast-form surrounded by eosinophilic

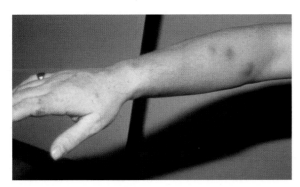

Figure 19-89. Sporotrichosis. Clinical picture illustrating the classic presentation of the lymphocutaneous form, with nodules arising along the lymphatic drainage of an ulcerated lesion.

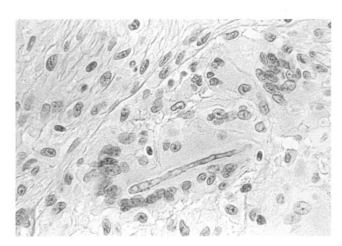

Figure 19-90. Sporotrichosis (PAS stain). Usually difficult to find in lesions from immunocompetent individuals, the fungal spores can manifest as elongated, cigar-shaped structures within giant cells and can even exhibit hyphal forms in immunosuppressed patients.

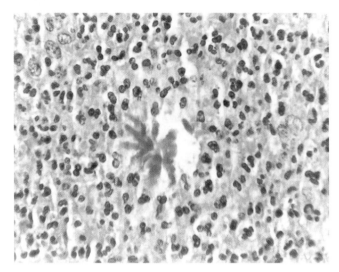

Figure 19-91. Sporotrichosis (PAS stain). Yeast forms of the organism can be found surrounded by spicules of eosinophilic material, as part of the Splendore-Hoeppli phenomenon. These structures are often found in the midst of a dermal abscess. (Courtesy of Mirian Sotto, MD, PhD, Department of Dermatology, Hospital das Clinicas, University of Sao Paulo.)

spicules (Splendore-Hoeppli phenomenon).[148] The central yeast form is positive on both PAS with diastase and GMS staining, whereas the spicules are negative for these two stains (Fig. 19-91).[636] In addition, the yeast stains with the anti-*Sporothrix* antibody, whereas the spicules do not.[248] To date, the precise nature of the eosinophilic spicules has not been entirely clarified.[636] They may represent a host defense mechanism or an antigen-antibody complex that surrounds the yeast surface.[636]

Histopathologic examination is not considered the best diagnostic method for the diagnosis of sporotrichosis, because it can be difficult to identify *S. schenckii* in histologic sections stained with routine histochemical stains such as H&E, PAS, and Gomori methenamine silver.[635] However, some studies have shown that, by careful examination of multiple serial sections, fungal elements can be found in most or even all cases.[148] Immunohistochemical staining using primary antibodies directed against *S. schenckii* may increase the percentage of cases in which the organism can be demonstrated to as much as 83%, more than double what is achieved with ordinary histochemical methods.[635]

S. schenckii can be usually grown on routine mycologic plates (e.g., Sabouraud dextrose agar, Mycosel) at 25° C, even if fungi were not observed in the tissue. Growth is commonly seen after 3 to 5 days, but cultures should be held for 4 to 5 weeks.[587,628]

Etiology and Pathogenesis
Sporotrichosis occurs after inoculation of *S. schenckii* conidia from the mold phase into the skin or subcutaneous tissues.[631] Less frequently, the conidia are inhaled, which can result in pulmonary infection.[631,634] The organism converts to the yeast form in the body.

The underlying mechanisms that explain the various clinical manifestations are not fully understood. The size of the inoculum, thermotolerance of the infecting *S. schenckii* strain, and the immune status of the host are among the possible influencing

factors.[638] Fixed cutaneous lesions seem to be caused by strains of *S. schenckii* that grow best at 35° C, whereas lymphocutaneous and extracutaneous disease are associated with strains that form colonies both at 35° C and 37° C.[639] *S. schenckii* produces melanin, which may play a role in virulence.[633,640]

The initial host response to *S. schenckii* involves neutrophils and macrophages, which are able to ingest and kill the yeast phase of *S. schenckii*.[631] T cell–mediated immunity also seems to be important in limiting the extent of infection, because sporotrichosis is more severe in athymic mice and in AIDS patients.[641]

Lobomycosis

Lobomycosis, also known as keloidal blastomycosis or Jorge Lobo disease, is caused by the fungus *Lacazia loboi*. The infection is restricted to tropical areas of Central and South America and is hyperendemic in areas of Brazil.[601] The organism is known to cause disease in humans and in dolphins.[638-640] However, the natural reservoir of *L. loboi* is unknown.[641] The infection occurs mainly in men from rural areas who work in close contact with vegetation and aquatic environments.[635] The disease is limited to the skin and subcutaneous tissues, except for the possibility of lymph node involvement.[601,638,642] Infection probably occurs by inoculation of the organism into the skin during minor trauma.[634] For this reason, lesions are mainly observed on exposed skin, such as the face, ears, and extremities.[639] These lesions have slow growth and are usually asymptomatic but can be pruritic.[636] They consist of papules, nodules, or plaques with a smooth surface that resemble keloids.[638] Verrucous lesions and ulceration can also occur.[637,638] The cutaneous lesions may be restricted to a single anatomic area, or they may be disseminated, probably reflecting the host's degree of immunity against the fungus.[637,638] Squamous cell carcinoma can occur in long-standing lesions.[638,639]

On histopathologic examination, the epidermis is commonly atrophic, with flattened rete ridges. However, hypertrophic epidermis, with hyperkeratosis or parakeratosis, is seen in some cases.[643] There is a diffuse, granulomatous dermal inflammatory infiltrate composed of numerous histiocytes and multinucleate giant cells (both foreign body and Langhans), which contain numerous fungi (Fig. 19-92).[643,644] Admixed lymphocytes, plasma cells, and, less frequently, neutrophils can be present in smaller numbers.[643] The infiltrate is separated from the epidermis by a narrow grenz zone.[645] These lesions evolve with keloidal scarring, seen as brightly eosinophilic collagen bundles. Some authors have reported destruction of skin appendages and of nerve endings as a result of invasion of the dermis by the histiocytic infiltrate.[643]

The fungi are identified in tissue as thick-walled, rounded or lemon-shaped, yeast-like cells, occurring either singly or in chains of budding cells (2-10 cells) (Figs. 19-93 through 19-95).[646-648] Individual cells, which measure 6 to 12 μm, are interconnected by thin tube-like structures to form the chain-like arrangement (see Fig. 19-94).[601,647,649-653] The fungi are PAS and methenamine silver positive and mucicarmine negative.

L. loboi has never been cultivated in vitro, but it has been successfully transmitted to mice, tortoises, and armadillos under experimental conditions.[644,654,655] The organism contains constitutive melanin in its cell wall, which seems to be associated with

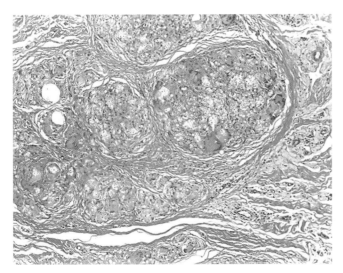

Figure 19-92. Lobomycosis. Lesions exhibit a prominent granulomatous response with the associated extensive collagenous keloidal response. (Courtesy of Mirian Sotto, MD, PhD, Department of Dermatology, Hospital das Clinicas, University of Sao Paulo.)

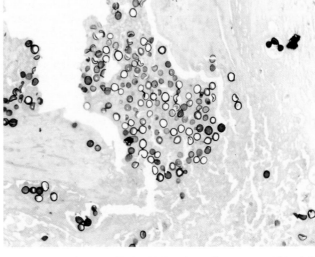

Figure 19-94. Lobomycosis (GMS stain). Fungal yeast-like structures exhibit tubular interconnections. (Courtesy of Mirian Sotto, MD, PhD, Department of Dermatology, Hospital das Clinicas, University of Sao Paulo.)

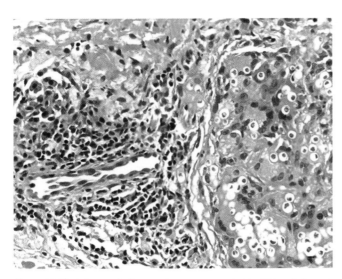

Figure 19-93. Lobomycosis. The organisms are represented by thick-walled, yeast-like cells that have a tendency to form chain-like structures. (Courtesy of Mirian Sotto, MD, PhD, Department of Dermatology, Hospital das Clinicas, University of Sao Paulo.)

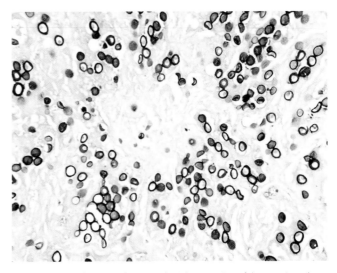

Figure 19-95. Lobomycosis (GMS stain). High-power view of the organisms shows the thick-walled, rounded or lemon-shaped, yeast-like cells that occur singly or in chains of budding cells. (Courtesy of Mirian Sotto, MD, PhD, Department of Dermatology, Hospital das Clinicas, University of Sao Paulo.)

fungal virulence, resistance to microbial attack, and greater survival under stress conditions.[643]

Zygomycosis

The term *zygomycosis* includes any infection caused by a member of the class Zygomycetes. Two orders of Zygomycetes contain organisms that cause human disease: the Mucorales and the Entomophthorales.[656] Members of these two orders produce different disease manifestations.[657] Mucorales typically cause acute, angioinvasive infections called mucormycoses, whereas Entomophthorales cause a group of infections referred to as entomophthoramycoses, which are more indolent and chronically progressive.[658]

Mucormycosis

Mucormycosis is the third most frequent invasive fungal infection, after aspergillosis and candidiasis.[659] The most commonly recovered genera are *Mucor, Rhizopus, Rhizomucor, Absidia, Apophysomyces, Cunninghamella,* and *Saksenaea.*[657] These fungi have worldwide distribution and can be found in soil and decaying organic matter.[658] The spores from these molds are transmitted by inhalation, percutaneous inoculation, or ingestion.[656] Human infection typically occurs in immunocompromised hosts as an opportunistic infection.[660] Risk factors for infection include diabetes mellitus, neutropenia, sustained immunosuppressive therapy, chronic prednisone use, iron chelation therapy, broad-spectrum antibiotic use, severe malnutrition, and primary breakdown in the integrity of the cutaneous barrier (e.g., trauma, surgical wounds, needle sticks, burns).[656] Mucormycosis is rare in immunocompetent individuals. Contamination of wounds, burns, and trauma sites is the most important modes of transmission in immunocompetent hosts.[658]

The clinical manifestations include rhino-orbito-cerebral, pulmonary, cutaneous, and gastrointestinal effects.[657] If the diagnosis is not made early, dissemination often occurs.[656] Rhino-orbital-cerebral zygomycosis originates in the paranasal sinuses and extends into the brain.[658] The overall mortality rate is approximately 62% in rhinocerebral zygomycosis and 16% in sinus infection without cerebral involvement.[661] A black necrotic eschar on the palate or nasal mucosa is a classic diagnostic clue, although this finding is not seen in all cases.[657] As the disease progresses, periorbital swelling, orbital cellulitis, blurred vision or visual loss, proptosis, eyelid gangrene, cranial neuropathies, and altered consciousness, among others symptoms and signs, can be observed.[658]

Cutaneous mucormycosis may be primary, resulting from local inoculation, or secondary, occurring after hematogenous dissemination.[662] Cutaneous mucormycoses range from superficial skin involvement, such as plaques, skin swelling, pustules, cellulitis, blisters, nodules, ulcerations, and ecthyma gangrenosum–like lesions, to deeper infections such as necrotizing fasciitis, osteomyelitis, and disseminated infection.[657] Secondary cutaneous disease usually manifests as nodular subcutaneous lesions which may ulcerate.[656]

Entomophthoramycosis

Human disease caused by Entomophthorales is seen predominantly in tropical regions, with transmission occurring by implantation of spores via minor trauma such as insect bites or by inhalation of spores into the sinuses.[656] Agents of the Entomophthorales comprise two pathogenic genera, *Conidiobolus* and *Basidiobolus,* which produce diseases called conidiobolomycosis and basidiobolomycosis, respectively.[658] The Entomophthorales are true pathogens, infecting primarily immunocompetent hosts.[656] They generally do not invade blood vessels and rarely disseminate.[656]

Basidiobolomycosis is caused by *Basidiobolus ranarum.* This organism resides in decaying plant material, soil, leaves from deciduous trees, and the intestines of fish, frogs, toads, insects, reptiles, and insectivorous bats.[657] The disease is more common in children.[663] Clinically, there is involvement of the skin and subcutaneous tissues, characterized by the formation of fluctuant, firm, and nontender swellings.[663] Usually, the overlying skin is normal and there is no bone involvement.[656] The most frequently affected parts of the body are the buttocks, thighs, and trunk.[663] Lymph node or muscle involvement can rarely occur.[656,663] Gastrointestinal infection and disseminated basidiobolomycosis in an immunocompetent host have been reported.[664-667]

Entomophthoromycosis due to *Conidiobolus coronatus* is characterized by lesions that originate in the inferior turbinate and spread through ostia and foramina to involve the facial and subcutaneous tissues and paranasal sinuses.[668] Most cases have been described from areas of tropical rainforest in West Africa, with agricultural and outdoor workers (aged 20-60 years) being the ones most commonly affected.[668] The fungus is found in soil and decaying vegetation. Patients usually present with unilateral nasal obstruction, nasal discharge, epistaxis, sinus tenderness, and swelling of the nose, upper lip, and face.[657,658] The disease usually involves subcutaneous tissue as a granulomatous infection without bone destruction or skin ulceration, and the clinical course is slowly progressive.[658] Disseminated infections, including those with fatal outcomes, have been reported with *C. coronatus* in both immunocompetent and immunocompromised hosts.[656] *Conidiobolus incongruus* is a rare agent of the disease.[668]

Histopathology

In mucormycosis, the fungi are seen as broad, ribbon-like, hyaline, pauciseptate hyphae, with a branching pattern of 45 to 90 degrees.[669] The hyphae invade blood vessels, leading to vasculitis, hemorrhage, thrombosis, infarction, and necrosis.[660] The inflammatory response is variable and can be neutrophilic (most common), pyogranulomatous, absent, or granulomatous (rare).[669] Perineural invasion may be seen.[669] The organisms are usually visualized even on H&E preparations. In addition, they can be seen with special stains for fungi.[658] The hyphae of the zygomycetes have thinner walls compared to other fungal hyphae, which possibly accounts for their weaker staining with Gomori methenamine silver and PAS techniques compared to fungi with thicker cell walls.[669] In addition, the hyphae of the zygomycetes appear more prone to twisting and folding than those of other fungi.[669]

In entomophthoromycosis, the fungi are also seen as broad, pauciseptate hyphae, with right-angled branching. However, the hyphae usually do not invade blood vessels.[656] There is granulomatous inflammation in the dermis and subcutis. The inflammatory infiltrate contains foreign-body giant cells, histiocytes, lymphocytes, epithelioid cells, and, frequently, eosinophils and plasma cells.[668] The eosinophils may be numerous, forming microabscesses.[664,668] Areas of necrosis are infrequently seen in the center of lesions.[668] The hyphae are generally visible in H&E-stained sections. They can be seen surrounded by eosinophilic material (Splendore-Hoeppli phenomenon).[148] Hyphal fragments can be found within giant cells.[663]

Protozoal Infections

Amebas

Amebas are primitive, unicellular organisms belonging to the Protista Kingdom. The species that infect humans belong to the Entamoeba and Rhizopoda classes.[670,671] A characteristic common feature of these organisms is the formation of a cyst wall when the parasite is exposed to adverse conditions, such as food deprivation, desiccation, or change in temperature or pH. The cyst form conveys resistance to biocides, chloration, and to temperature changes. However, these cysts are lysed by autoclaving or treatment with Freon or methylene oxide.[672]

Human infections are caused by the pathogenic species, which are strictly parasitic, or by the so-called free-living amebas, which are opportunistic agents and accidentally infect human beings. The majority of amebic infections in humans are caused by parasitic-pathogenic species such as *Entamoeba histolytica.* The group of free-living amebas include *Acanthamoeba* spp., *Naegleria fowleri,* and, more recently, *Balamuthia mandrillaris* and *Sappinia diploidea.*[673,674] These species affect mainly immunocompromised individuals.

Cutaneous Amebiasis

Cutaneous amebiasis is the term used for infection of the skin and soft tissue by *E. histolytica,* the only pathogenic ameba in the *Entamoeba* group. This type of amebic infection occurs mainly in the tropics and most frequently manifests with a dysenteric diarrhea and liver abscesses.[675] *E. histolytica* has a fecal-oral life cycle that involves ingestion of cysts and the subsequent development of dysenteric intestinal disease. Then, the infection can spread elsewhere, usually to the liver or the lungs. Cutaneous involvement by *E. histolytica* is a rare event[700] and can occur by direct and indirect mechanisms. Direct infection of the anus or perianal, perineal, or genital skin can occur by spread from the colon and rectum through contaminated stool. Colostomies or abdominal wounds are sometimes affected. Penile involvement results from anal intercourse. Indirect inoculation can be produced by hematogenous or contiguous spread from infectious foci in the liver or by cutaneous dissemination from scratching with contaminated hands.[676,677] Cutaneous lesions manifest clinically as painful, foul-smelling ulcers covered by gray slough. In genital and perineal areas, large exophytic ulcers can develop.[676]

Usually, the main feature of the histologic picture is the presence of extensive ulceration with necrosis and a surrounding pseudoepitheliomatous hyperplasia.[678] *E. histolytica* trophozoites can be found in the exudate singly or in clusters. They usually measure 12 to 20 μm and are strongly PAS positive. They differ from macrophages by the presence of a single, eccentrically placed nuclear chromatin with prominent karyosome.[679] Another feature, present in all cases, is the presence of phagocytosed red blood cells in the cytoplasm. This feature is useful to differentiate *E. histolytica* trophozoites from macrophages and from other species of amebas.[676] Furthermore, the *Acanthamoeba* trophozoites do not exhibit the characteristic marginally disposed nuclear chromatin. A CD59 stain can help distinguish between *E. histolytica* trophozoites (which are positive with this marker; see later discussion) and *Acanthamoeba* trophozoites. Molecular tests, such as PCR and ELISA, can be useful in difficult cases. The main differential diagnosis, both clinically and at low power, is verrucous squamous cell carcinoma, especially with lesions from the genital areas.[680] The microscopic picture can also be suggestive of a deep fungal infection, but this is promptly ruled out with visualization of the trophozoites.

The massive necrosis and invasiveness produced by this organism relates to its ability to secrete several lytic enzymes as well as the capability of phagocytizing and lysing immune cells.[676] Although the host develops humoral and cellular immune responses to the parasite, these organisms are capable of evading the immune system through several mechanisms. These include expression of *N*-acetyl-D-galactosamine (Gal/GalNCc), a specific lectin that has a similar sequence and, thus, an antigenic cross-reactivity with CD59. In humans, CD59 prevents assembly of the complement C5b-C9 membrane attack complex.[681] Also, the parasite produces serine proteases capable of cleaving IgA and IgG molecules.[671]

Acanthamebiasis

Part of the free-living ameba group, *Acanthamoeba* spp. are ubiquitous organisms. They can be isolated from soil, dust, air, natural and treated water, seawater, air-conditioning units, and

several other environments, and they have a worldwide distribution.[672] These organisms can also be found in nasal and pharyngeal mucosa of healthy individuals.[682,683] *Acanthamoeba* spp., along with *N. fowleri*, is a facultative and opportunistic human pathogen. These organisms affect mainly immunocompromised individuals, but they can cause infections in immunocompetent persons as well. The most frequent human infection with *Acanthamoeba* spp. is the amebic keratitis that is related to contact lens use. A chronic, protracted, slowly progressive CNS infection, granulomatous amebic encephalitis, has also been described.[672]

The rare event of cutaneous involvement by *Acanthamoeba* spp. is found in AIDS patients and may or may not be associated with CNS involvement.[684,685] Clinically, cutaneous lesions are described as erythematous, violaceous nodules or indurated papules that become suppurative and eventually form nonhealing ulcers. The lesions appear usually on the face, trunk, and extremities and can occur in crops.[672,686] Whether these cutaneous lesions represent a primary focus or the result of hematogenous spread from infectious foci in the respiratory tract, the maxillofacial sinuses, or the CNS, is not known.[687]

The histologic sections show mainly a granulomatous reaction with a mixed inflammatory infiltrate (Fig. 19-96). In patients with AIDS, granulomas are not always present. Abscess formation, panniculitis, and leukocytoclastic vasculitis can also be observed.[685,688,689] Both trophozoites (Fig. 19-97) and cysts (Fig. 19-98) can be observed. The cysts are PAS and GMS positive. However, *Acanthamoeba* spp. trophozoites do not stain well with PAS (Fig. 19-99). Trophozoites of *Acanthamoeba* spp. are pleomorphic and measure approximately 15 to 45 μm and have a large nucleus with a large, centrally located karyosome but no peripheral chromatin (Fig. 19-100 and 19-101). *E. histolytica* trophozoites stain well with PAS, whereas the cysts are PAS negative.[686] Also, *E. histolytica* trophozoites usually contain red blood cells within their cytoplasm.[676] *Acanthamoeba* trophozoites are negative on CD59 staining (Fig. 19-102). *N. fowleri* and

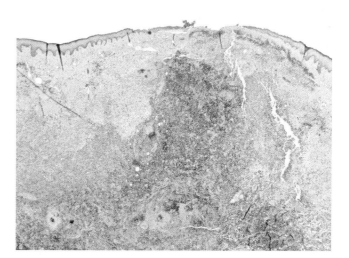

Figure 19-96. Cutaneous acanthamebiasis. Lesions tend to be irregular and very destructive. This extensive, purulent, and ulcerated, predominantly subcutaneous lesion was present in an individual undergoing post-transplantation immunosuppressive therapy.

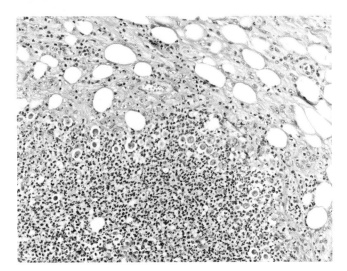

Figure 19-97. Cutaneous acanthamebiasis. At the edges of the lesion, an "advancing front" of macrophage-like organisms is identified.

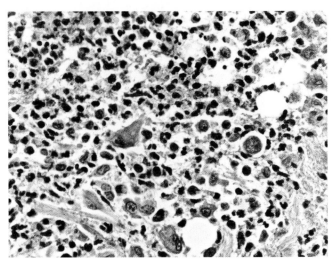

Figure 19-99. Cutaneous acanthamebiasis (PAS stain). The PAS stain weakly decorates the *Acanthamoeba* sp. trophozoites, in contrast to *Entamoeba histolytica* trophozoites, which are strongly PAS positive.

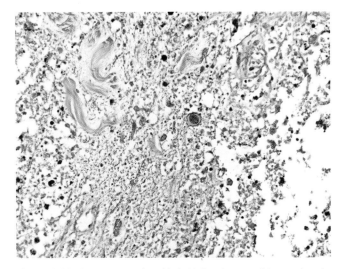

Figure 19-98. Cutaneous acanthamebiasis. Under adverse conditions, such as the predominantly necrotic area of this lesion, the organisms change to a cystic form that exhibits a prominent thick capsule, which is PAS positive.

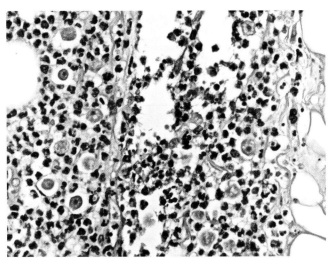

Figure 19-100. Cutaneous acanthamebiasis. Numerous trophozoites are surrounded by a dense inflammatory response.

E. histolytica express CD59 as part of their escape from the immune system.

The presence of a prominent karyosome with a surrounding halo in *Acanthamoeba* trophozoites is not found in human macrophages or any other inflammatory cell.[686] The histologic lesions can mimic fungal and viral infections or a foreign-body granulomatous response.[672] Organisms in tissue sections have been confused for yeast forms of *Blastomyces dermatitidis*, sporangia of *Rhinosporidium seeberi*, *C. neoformans*, or *Protheca wickerhamii*. Cases of acanthamebiasis have been mistaken for cat-scratch fever, Kaposi sarcoma, or even cells with CMV inclusions.[672,686]

In close similarity to *E. histolytica*, *Acanthamoeba* trophozoites are known to secrete several lytic enzymes such as proteinases, elastases, and phospholipases. Some of these proteases, the serine-proteases, are capable of degrading human IgA and IgG antibodies.[672] Inhibition of the classic pathway of complement, by blockade of C1 and by active binding of C1q, is also part of

these parasites' immune-evading repertoire.[690] Also, the active phagocytosis and destruction of leukocytes is another mechanism by which these organisms combat the immune response (Fig. 19-103).

Also noteworthy is the probable role of *Acanthamoeba* spp. as reservoirs of several bacterial species such as *Legionella pneumophila*, *M. avium*, *M. leprae*, and *Chlamydia pneumoniae*, among others.[672,691-694] Interestingly, these bacteria that can survive inside *Acanthamoeba* organisms are also mainly human intracellular pathogens that infect macrophages.

Flagellates

Trypanosomiasis

The trypanosome group is composed of several species of protozoan flagellates that belong to the Kinetoplastida order. They

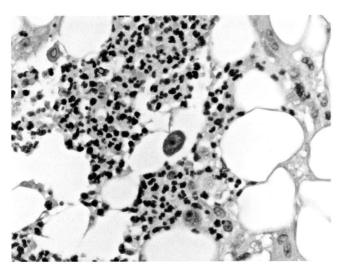

Figure 19-101. Cutaneous acanthamebiasis. High-power view of *Acanthamoeba* sp. with its prominent nucleus and nucleoli.

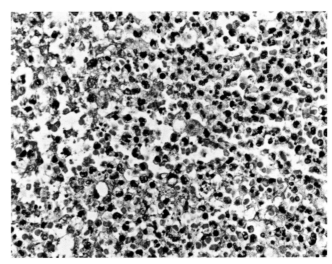

Figure 19-103. Cutaneous acanthamebiasis. A trophozoite is actively ingesting inflammatory cells.

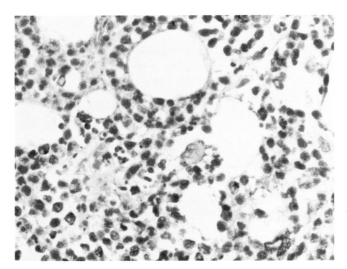

Figure 19-102. Cutaneous acanthamebiasis (CD59 immunostain). The negativity of the trophozoites with this marker (CD59, a complement inhibitor) is contrasted by the marked positivity of the inflammatory cells.

infect most species of vertebrates. The species that are known to affect humans are *Trypanosoma brucei* and subspecies in sub-Saharan Africa and *Trypanosoma cruzi* in the Americas.[695] Recently, cases of human infection with *Trypanosoma evansi* and *Trypanosoma lewisi*, which affect mainly large ungulates and rodents, respectively, have been reported in the Indian subcontinent.[696-698]

African Trypanosomiasis

Clinical Features

African trypanosomiasis is caused by the *T. brucei* and two of its subspecies, *Trypanosoma brucei gambiense*, which affects western and central Africa, and *Trypanosoma brucei rhodesiense*, which is prevalent in eastern and southern Africa. They are transmitted by flies from the Glossina group (tsetse flies), blood transfusions, contaminated needles, or congenital infection.[695,699-702] Their

known reservoirs or natural hosts comprise a large range of ungulate species, including cattle and camels. Humans also can act as reservoirs.[695]

The disease is divided into two stages, hemolymphatic and meningoencephalitic. Cutaneous involvement is present mostly in the first stage at the site of inoculation, forming an inflammatory nodule or ulcer known as the "trypanosomal chancre."[695,701] This lesion produces a 2- to 5-cm, erythematous, indurated, painful plaque, which appears within approximately 2 to 4 weeks of inoculation and heals after 3 to 4 weeks. It usually heals leaving an overlying desquamation, sometimes with altered pigmentation. The trypanosomal chancre develops in about 50% of the cases with *T. brucei rhodesiense*, but rarely in the ones with *T. brucei gambiense*.[695,702-704]

The other dermatologic manifestation that can occur later during stage 1 is a pruritic circinate maculopapular rash with pruritus, which arises usually on the trunk. This manifestation is known as trypanids and appears several weeks after inoculation.[695,703,704]

Histopathology

Microscopic examination of the trypanosomal chancre reveals a superficial and deep, perivascular lymphoplasmacellular infiltrate, somewhat resembling secondary syphilis.[703] Usually, organisms are very difficult to identify in routine stained tissue sections. Trypomastigotes can be identified in Giemsa-stained smears of the secretions found in the chancre.[673] The organisms have the classic trypanosomal morphology, measure 1.5 to 3.5 μm in width, and contain the characteristic kinetoplast with a central nucleus.[703,704]

Microscopically, the trypanid lesions exhibit mild spongiosis with exocytosis of lymphocytes, along with a superficial perivascular lymphoid infiltrate and a mild diffuse neutrophilic infiltrate with leukocytoclasis.[702] The cutaneous manifestations of African trypanosomiasis could be confused with bacterial pyoderma caused by secondary infection of a minor wound or an insect bite.[704] In the rare event that intracellular parasites are identified as amastigotes in tissue sections, they can be differentiated from other intracellular parasites such as *H. capsulatum* and *T. gondii* by the presence of the kinetoplast, which is found in both *Leishmania* and trypanosome amastigote forms.

Etiology and Pathogenesis

Trypanosomes have evolved along with humans and other vertebrate species and have developed several poorly understood mechanisms to survive despite their host's immune response. One of these unusual features is the expression of the variant surface glycoprotein (VSG). The VSG confers the ability to avoid the specific immune response via antigen variation, and it also protects them from lysis by the complement alternative pathway.[705] Because the protein coating is constantly changing, the host immune system cannot completely clear the infection before a new population of antigenically distinct parasites appears.[705-707] Furthermore, the parasites induce a massive immune dysregulation by inducing the production of autoantibodies and cytokines, which causes a polyclonal activation of B cells. The resultant secretion of large amounts of nonspecific IgM creates large amounts of circulating complexes. This phenomenon is probably partly responsible for the anemia, vascular permeability, and tissue damage observed during the infection.[695,705]

American Trypanosomiasis

T. cruzi, the agent of Chagas disease, is transmitted by infected insects of the Triatominae group (kissing bugs). The reservoirs are usually mammals such as armadillos or opossums. The disease is prevalent in 18 countries in North, Central, and South America. It is a disease strongly associated with low socioeconomic conditions.[695,708]

The trypomastigote forms of the parasite are highly concentrated in the vector's feces, which are deposited while the vector feeds and enter the host through microabrasions caused by scratching. The disease can be transmitted also through blood transfusions, by contaminated needles, and via vertical placental infection. Rare cases of transmission by contaminated food or breastfeeding have been reported.[695]

The disease has an acute and a chronic stage. The acute stage begins 6 to 10 days after the inoculation and lasts for 1 to 2 months. It is in this stage that most of the cutaneous manifestations occur. An edematous lesion, known as a chagoma, appears at the site of inoculation. If this site is the conjunctiva, a bipalpebral swelling is noticed (the Romaña sign).[695,702] The chronic phase of the disease appears usually 10 to 15 years after inoculation; it is characterized by visceral effects, such as dilated cardiomyopathy and megaviscera.[695] If an infected individual becomes immunocompromised (e.g., AIDS, transplantation), the disease can reactivate. This reactivation results in painful erythematous papules and nodules, as well as plaques, recently named reactivation chagomas, that when disseminated are known as metastatic chagomas.[709-711]

Reactivated disease, seen in immunocompromised patients, can exhibit cutaneous lesions that usually show an infiltrate of macrophages in the deep dermis and subcutaneous fat. These macrophages contain intracellular amastigote forms. Also, *T. cruzi* amastigotes can be found in surrounding blood vessel walls and arrector pili muscles.[709-711]

In tissue sections, the amastigote forms are best visualized with Giemsa stain and can be distinguished from other intracellular protozoa by the presence of the kinetoplast. They are PAS negative, which helps to differentiate them from the PAS-positive intracellular fungus, *H. capsulatum*.

Like its African counterparts, the *T. cruzi* parasite has evolved various methods to evade the host's immune system. For example, the organism expresses antioxidant enzymes such as tryparedoxin peroxidase, which enables survival of the parasites within the macrophages.[712] Also, there are *T. cruzi* products such as glycosylphosphatidylinositol and the multiple *trans*-sialidase proteins, which produce an immune dysregulatory effect in the CD8+ T cell population, macrophages, and dendritic cells.[713,714]

Leishmaniasis

Leishmaniasis is a condition with an ample geographic distribution. It is endemic in several countries of southern Europe, North Africa, the Middle East, Central and South America, and the Indian subcontinent. It is estimated that 1.5 to 2 million children and adults develop symptomatic disease annually; 1 to 1.5 million have cutaneous effects, and in 0.5 million the viscera are involved.[715] In recent years, both the reported cases and the affected geographic areas have increased,[716] probably in concert with increasing rates of deforestation and global climate change. As with most parasitic conditions, leishmaniasis is a disease of the poor, undeveloped, and neglected areas of the world, with the probable exception of southern Europe.[717]

The parasite can be transmitted by almost 70 known species of sandflies. The species most commonly involved are from the genera *Lutzomyia*, found mainly in the Americas, and *Phlebotomus*, identified in other endemic regions.[718] The disease is also spread via blood transfusion, vertical transplacental spread, and use of contaminated needles, and organ transplants.[710-721] There are a multitude of known reservoirs, including canids such as dogs and foxes, rodents, and large mammals.[722]

The disease is artificially divided into three types: cutaneous, mucocutaneous, and visceral. However, there is significant overlap among them, forming a clinical spectrum. The clinical presentation is related to the balance between factors such as host cell-mediated immunity and delayed-type hypersensitivity idiosyncrasy and the parasite burden.[718]

Cutaneous Leishmaniasis

Clinical Features Cutaneous leishmaniasis is caused by multiple *Leishmania* species and subspecies from different parts of the globe. The Old World agents include *Leishmania major*, *Leishmania tropica*, and *Leishmania* (L.) *aethiopica*, as well as *Leishmania infantum* and *Leishmania chagasi* in the Mediterranean and Caspian Sea regions. *Leishmania mexicana*, *Leishmania* (L) *amazonensis*, *Leishmania braziliensis*, *Leishmania* (V.) *panamensis*, *Leishmania* (V.) *peruviana*, and *Leishmania* (V.) *guyanensis* are prevalent in South and Central America and parts of North America.[718]

There are four recognized forms: acute, chronic, recidivous, and disseminated.[718-728] The lesion in the acute form usually begins at the site of the sandfly bite and evolves into a nodule that ulcerates after 1 to 3 months.[728,729] Affected individuals presenting with acute lesions usually exhibit several nonhealing skin lesions on nocturnally exposed skin. There are some differences according to the causative parasite. The Old World disease usually manifests as papules, nodules, or nodule-ulcers. Flat

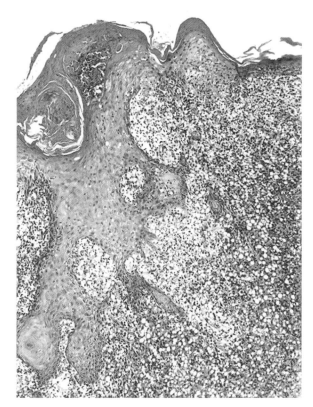

Figure 19-104. Cutaneous leishmaniasis. Pseudoepitheliomatous epidermal hyperplasia with a diffuse granulomatous inflammatory response. (Courtesy of Mirian Sotto, MD, PhD, Department of Dermatology, Hospital das Clinicas, University of Sao Paulo.)

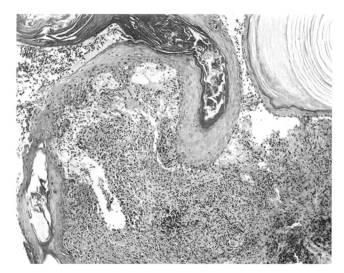

Figure 19-105. Cutaneous leishmaniasis. Ulceration and epidermal necrosis are often seen in these highly destructive lesions. (Courtesy of Mirian Sotto, MD, PhD, Department of Dermatology, Hospital das Clinicas, University of Sao Paulo.)

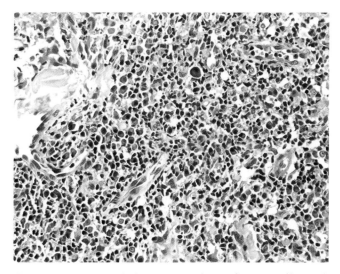

Figure 19-106. Cutaneous leishmaniasis. An exuberant inflammatory infiltrate with prominent plasma cells is found associated with the granulomatous response to the parasites. (Courtesy of Mirian Sotto, MD, PhD, Department of Dermatology, Hospital das Clinicas, University of Sao Paulo.)

plaques, hyperkeratotic, and wart-like lesions also can be found.[729] However, ulcerative lesions are more characteristic in New World disease.[730] Unusual presentations, such as paronychial, chancriform, annular, palmoplantar, zosteriform, and erysipeloid forms, have been described.[731,732] The acute lesions usually heal and leave scars.

Chronic lesions are represented by single or multiple, raised, non-ulcerated plaques that persist for 1 to 2 years. The recidivous type, part of the chronic manifestations, is also known as "lupoid" or "recidivans." It exhibits erythematous, often circinated, papules in proximity to scars of healed lesions. This type is mostly seen in Old World disease (*L. tropica*) but has also been reported in South America.[718,732-734]

The disseminated form is usually related to New World parasites. It develops in anergic individuals and consists of macules and nodules without ulceration, diffusively distributed.[735]

Histopathology Acute lesions can show either hyperkeratosis and acanthosis or atrophy. Ulceration and intraepidermal abscesses may be present.[736] As the lesions become chronic, a nonspecific pseudoepitheliomatous pattern can be found (Figs. 19-104 and 19-105). In the dermis, there is usually a prominent inflammatory infiltrate composed of CD4+ and CD8+ lymphocytes, plasma cells, parasitized macrophages, epithelioid and giant cells, and sometimes eosinophils (Fig. 19-106).[736,737] Intracellular amastigotes are identified within affected macrophages.[738,739] The amastigote forms are represented as uncapsulated 2- to 4-μm, round to oval, basophilic structures

(Fig. 19-107). These intracellular *Leishmania* forms are usually located at the periphery of the cytoplasm of the parasitized cell (marquee sign) (Fig. 19-108). The salient feature that helps in the differential diagnosis is the presence of the kinetoplast. The morphologic features are best appreciated with Giemsa stain. There are immunoperoxidase kits that use monoclonal antibodies directed to antigens present in several *Leishmania* species and are of great utility in difficult cases (Figs. 19-109 and 19-110).

Chronic lesions can show in the dermis a pattern composed of tuberculoid, noncaseating granulomas containing only rare parasitized macrophages.[739] Sometimes central necrosis can be seen.[740] The recidivous type has a histologic picture that resembles lupus vulgaris, with tubercles surrounded by histiocytes,

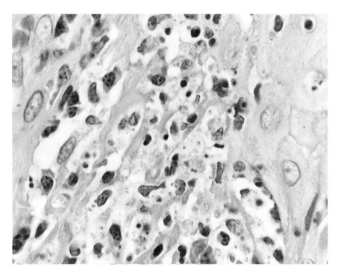

Figure 19-107. Cutaneous leishmaniasis. Amastigote forms can be identified within giant cells and macrophages and sometimes in the interstitial spaces. (Courtesy of Mirian Sotto, MD, PhD, Department of Dermatology, Hospital das Clinicas, University of Sao Paulo.)

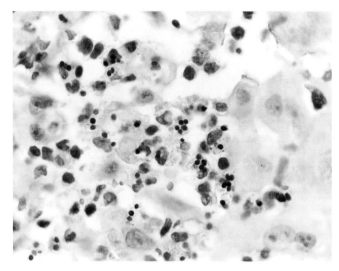

Figure 19-109. Cutaneous leishmaniasis (immunoperoxidase stain). Parasites can be highlighted by monoclonal immunoperoxidase stains. (Courtesy of Mirian Sotto, MD, PhD, Department of Dermatology, Hospital das Clinicas, University of Sao Paulo.)

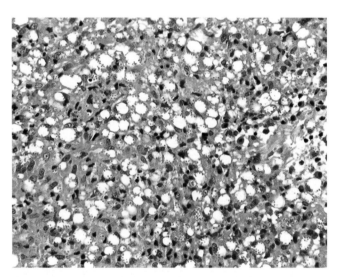

Figure 19-108. Cutaneous leishmaniasis. This is an example of the classic marquee sign, which is the placement of the parasites at the periphery of the infected cells. This feature is useful in distinguishing *Leishmania* spp. from other intracellular organisms. (Courtesy of Mirian Sotto, MD, PhD, Department of Dermatology, Hospital das Clinicas, University of Sao Paulo.)

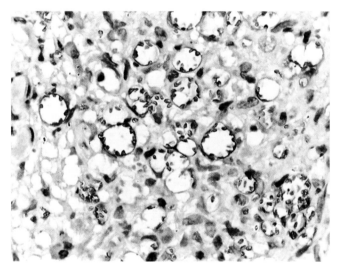

Figure 19-110. Cutaneous leishmaniasis (immunoperoxidase stain). Another example of the so-called marquee sign. (Courtesy of Mirian Sotto, MD, PhD, Department of Dermatology, Hospital das Clinicas, University of Sao Paulo.)

lymphocytes, and an occasional giant cell; parasites are hard to find.[733,738]

Disseminated cutaneous leishmaniasis, which is commonly found in anergic and immunocompromised individuals, is composed almost exclusively of parasitized macrophages with only occasional lymphocytes and sometimes eosinophils.[741,742]

Mucocutaneous Leishmaniasis

Mucocutaneous leishmaniasis is seen mainly in South and Central America (caused by *L. braziliensis, L. panamensis,* and *L. guyanensis*)[743] but has also been reported in patients with *L. infantum,*[744] *L. tropica,*[745] and *L. major*[746] infection. Mucosal dissemination

has reportedly developed in 1% to 10% of the cases of cutaneous disease caused by New World agents, most commonly *L. braziliensis.* It can occur either 1 to 5 years after the cutaneous lesions have healed or concomitantly with active skin lesions.[743,747,748]

Mucosal lesions usually begin with erythema and ulceration of the nares, which can evolve to highly destructive lesions that can perforate the nasal septum and can involve the nasopharynx and tongue, causing significant deformities.[749] This course is known as espundia and can develop up to 25 years after the primary clinical lesion.[750]

Microscopic examination of mucosal lesions usually reveals extensive ulceration flanked by pseudoepitheliomatous hyperplasia. There is a nonspecific chronic inflammation with only a few parasite-laden macrophages.[751] Tuberculoid and suppurative granulomas are often seen.[750] The presence of prominent necrosis with a reactive response is seen as a favorable prognostic feature.[752]

Visceral Leishmaniasis

The visceral variant of leishmaniasis is caused by *Leishmania donovani* in the Indian subcontinent, Asia, and Africa and affects both adults and children. *L. infantum* and *L. chagasi* affect predominantly young children in the Mediterranean region, southwest and central Asia, and South America. Occasionally, *L. tropica* and *Leishmania amazonensis* can be viscerotropic.[715,753] The course of the infection can be subclinical or oligosymptomatic or can cause a full-blown disease (kala-azar). The clinical features are fever, weakness, night sweats, anorexia, and weight loss.[718] Darkening of the skin (*kala-azar* means "black fever" in Hindi) is rather infrequent. Further progression leads to hepatosplenomegaly and serious anemia, neutropenia, and thrombocytopenia that can be lethal.[718,754] Cutaneous involvement is seen in more than 5% of cases, usually 1 to 5 years after the primary infection,[755,756] in the form of post–kala-azar dermal leishmaniasis (PKDL). PKDL is seen more frequently in the Indian subcontinent.[756,757] It consists of erythematous lesions and nodules, usually on the face, as well as hypopigmented and hyperpigmented macules on the trunk.[755,756,758] The affected skin has normal sensation, which helps to distinguish the lesions from those of leprosy. Cutaneous involvement in visceral leishmaniasis, with florid manifestations, is also seen in AIDS patients.[759,760]

Lesions in PKDL consist of an atrophic epidermis overlying a prominent inflammatory infiltrate in the upper dermis that is composed mainly of macrophages, epithelioid cells, lymphocytes, and plasma cells.[758] Tuberculoid granulomas can be seen. In some cases, the infiltrate occupies the entire dermis in a nodular fashion.[758] In patients with neuropathy, perineural inflammation can be identified.[761] Lesions of the face can show follicular plugging. Organisms are often readily found, but their quantity varies. To better appreciate the parasite morphology, Weigert iron–stained sections are superior to Giemsa-stained sections.[758]

Leishmania spp. organisms have evolved to evade humoral innate defenses and to impair macrophage and dendritic cell mechanisms.[723] The parasite achieves these effects through complex processes that manipulate intracellular molecular pathways of the host's parasitized immune cells,[719,723,724] as well as expression of virulence factors such as lipophosphoglycan and surface metalloproteinase gp 63.[725,726] Through these resources, the protozoans can orchestrate a profound dysregulation of the host's cell-mediated immunity. Even though their entire genome has been unraveled,[727] this group of parasites remain formidable adversaries because of their capacity for adaptation and the intricate nature of the immunology involved in the infection.

Trichomoniasis

Trichomonas vaginalis is a motile flagellate that usually causes genital infections that primarily affect the mucosa. Cutaneous involvement has been described as abscesses and fistulas occurring in close proximity to the genitalia, mainly the penis.[762] These lesions arise by contiguous spread from preexisting genital infections. The organisms are readily identified in wet mounts of the purulent material. An urticarial reaction has also been described and is associated with episodes of arthralgia.[763]

Giardiasis

Several skin manifestations have been described in association with intestinal *Giardia lamblia* and *Giardia intestinalis* infections. These range from lesions such as urticaria or angioedema to atopic dermatitis, vesiculopapular eruptions, and even granuloma annulare–like lesions.[764,765] The lesions usually remit on correct treatment of the intestinal infection. The protozoan has not been found in these lesions.

Other Protozoa

Cutaneous Toxoplasmosis

T. gondii can cause congenital and acquired infections. Skin lesions in toxoplasmosis are rare and usually nonspecific. Congenital toxoplasmosis can exhibit macular, hemorrhagic, and exfoliative lesions.[766] Maculopapular, hemorrhagic, lichenoid,[767] nodular, granuloma annulare–like[766,768] and dermatomyositis-like lesions[769] have been found concomitantly with acquired *T. gondii* infections.

A superficial and mid-dermal perivascular lymphohistiocytic infiltrate is often seen. Parasites are identified in the dermis as cysts of bradyzoites in the dermis or as free tachyzoite forms.[768] Occasionally, an overlying pseudoepitheliomatous hyperplasia can be found. Interestingly, in cases with dermatomyositis-like clinical presentations, the histologic picture of the lesions also resembles dermatomyositis.[768,770]

Cutaneous Pneumocystosis

The organism formerly known as *Pneumocystis carinii* was recently reclassified into the Fungi Kingdom and renamed *Pneumocystis jiroveci*. It is a well-known opportunistic agent that causes pulmonary infection in immunocompromised patients and rarely affects the skin.[771,772] Cutaneous lesions have been described in patients with advanced AIDS and concomitant cutaneous cryptococcosis. The lesions consist of polypoid lesions in the external auditory canal and necrotic papules and nodules elsewhere in the body.[772]

The amphophilic, amorphous, foamy to finely stippled material characteristically seen in pulmonary disease is found in the dermis in perivascular array. The small cysts of *P. jiroveci* are readily appreciated with silver methenamine stain. The other two forms of the parasite, the intracystic sporozoite and the encysted trophozoite, can be seen with Giemsa and Wright stains.[771,772]

Helminth Infestations

Trematodes

Schistosomiasis

Clinical Features
Schistosomiasis is caused by parasitic trematode worms that have as definitive hosts several species of vertebrates, including humans. More than 200 million people in 74 countries have the disease, and 20 million of them have severe illness.[773] The life cycle of this organism is complex and involves several species of

freshwater snails as intermediate hosts. Four major species participate in human infections: *Schistosoma mansoni, Schistosoma haematobium, Schistosoma japonicum,* and *Schistosoma mekongi.* The first two are prevalent in sub-Saharan Africa, and *S. mansoni* is also endemic in certain regions of Brazil, Venezuela, and the Caribbean. *S. japonicum* can be found in China, Indonesia, and the Philippines. *S. mekongi,* a species related to *S. japonicum,* is found in Cambodia and Laos.[774]

Several types of skin lesions have been described in schistosomiasis. The parasites penetrate the skin as cercariae forms. At the site of penetration, there is usually a pruritic erythematous and urticarial rash.[775-780] These lesions are similar to the condition known as "swimmer's itch," which is caused by larvae of other trematode species and results in less severe skin lesions and no systemic disease.[774]

Urticarial lesions can be seen in association with the dissemination of the cercariae and concomitantly with the laying of eggs by adult flukes.[774,775,780] Deposition of ova in the dermis can give rise to papular, granulomatous, or even warty genital lesions and other extragenital cutaneous manifestations.[779-782] The development of squamous cell carcinoma from genital verrucous lesions has been reported.[778] Infections with *S. japonicum* usually are associated with urticarial lesions.[783] *S. haematobium* and *S. japonicum* infections are usually complicated by extragenital cutaneous lesions,[777,783] but these rarely are seen with *S. mansoni* infection.[784]

Histopathology
The lesions related to the penetration of cercarial forms are associated with exocytosis of eosinophils and neutrophils, sometimes with microabscess formation.[784] The dermal reaction is usually mild and consists of edema, vascular dilatation, mild perivascular inflammatory infiltrate, and rare interstitial eosinophils. The larvae usually are not seen.[776]

In genital and perineal lesions, ova are easily identified in the dermis and are accompanied by a prominent granulomatous reaction or eosinophil microabscesses.[776,780] There is usually an overlying hyperkeratotic and acanthotic epidermis, sometimes with prominent pseudoepitheliomatous hyperplasia with focal ulceration and draining sinuses. Adult parasites may be identified in cutaneous vessels. Acute extragenital lesions exhibit necrobiosis and palisading granulomas around numerous ova. These features are often accompanied by an infiltrate composed of eosinophils, neutrophils, and foreign-body giant cells. Chronic lesions show degenerating and calcified ova with plasma cells and variable fibrosis.[779,785,786] In the extragenital lesions, ova are usually difficult to find.[784] The ova share an oval-shaped appearance but have specific species-related morphologic features. *S. haematobium* ova have a characteristic apical spine, whereas *S. mansoni* ova have a lateral spine, and those of *S. japonicum* have no spine.[782] *S. mansoni* and *S. japonicum* ova can be acid fast.

Cestodes

Cysticercosis

Humans are accidental hosts for *Taenia solium,* a pork tapeworm. The larvae lodge in the subcutaneous tissue, forming nodules of 1 to 3 cm.[787-793] There is certain predilection for the chest wall, arms, and thighs.[794] The nodules are composed of cystic structures containing a larva attached to one edge of a membrane. A fibrous host response surrounds the cyst.[787,789,792]

Visualization of the scolex of the cysticercus larva is helpful to make the diagnosis. The host response around the cyst is composed of fibrosis, chronic inflammatory infiltrate with eosinophils and sometimes giant cells.[789,792]

Sparganosis

Sparganosis is an infection caused by a pseudophyllidean tapeworm larva of the genus *Spirometra.*[795] The infection is more frequent in the Orient and is sporadically reported from Australia, British Guiana, Africa, Madagascar, and South America.[796,797] Rare cases have been reported in the United States and Europe, mainly among travelers.[798,799] The parasite has a complex life cycle with canids and felids as definitive hosts. Humans are usually involved as second intermediate hosts.[796] Transmission to humans usually occurs through ingestion of water contaminated with infected cyclops or consumption of contaminated meat.[795,796]

Clinically, there is a slow-growing, subcutaneous mass that is sometimes migratory.[796,797] When the parasite migrates, there is often pain and pruritus. The infection mainly affects the subcutaneous tissue, but it can spread to internal organs including brain, lungs, and bladder.[796] Examination and bisection of the nodules reveal a cyst containing a flat, thread-like worm, usually measuring 0.1 cm in thickness and several millimeters to 50 cm in length.[796,797]

Microscopically, the wall of the cyst is composed of granulation tissue and fibroadipose tissue with a variable number of inflammatory cells including eosinophils, lymphocytes, histiocytes, plasma cells, neutrophils, and foreign-body giant cells.[796] Portions of the larva are usually seen within the cavity.[798] The parasite structure is composed of a brush border of microvilli, eosinophilic tegument, two layers of smooth muscle, and a row of tegumental columnar cells. The smooth muscle bundles are often disposed in a "checkerboard" fashion. The internal structure of the parasite is also composed of a loose matrix and basophilic calcareous bodies.[796,797,800] The microscopic differential diagnosis includes trichinosis, cysticercosis, and visceral larva migrans.[796]

Echinococcosis

Echinococcosis is a zoonotic infection caused by tapeworms of the Taeniidae family. Echinococcosis still represents a public health problem in New Zealand and Australia, as well as countries of the Mediterranean, the Middle East, southern Africa, and South America.[801] The life cycle of the parasites more frequently involves sheep and canids. Four species are involved in human infection. The most important are *Echinococcus granulosus,* which causes cystic echinococcosis or hydatid disease, and *Echinococcus multilocularis,* which causes alveolar echinococcosis. Two other species, *Echinococcus vogeli* and *Echinococcus oligarthus,* rarely affect humans but are responsible for polycystic echinococcosis in Central and South America.[801-803]

Cutaneous involvement in echinococcosis is a rare event.[801,804,805] It can be a result of systemic vascular dissemina-

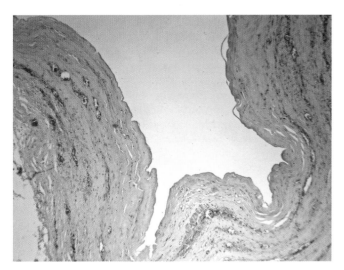

Figure 19-111. Echinococcosis. The cyst is acellular and is surrounded by fibroblasts and lymphocytic infiltrate.

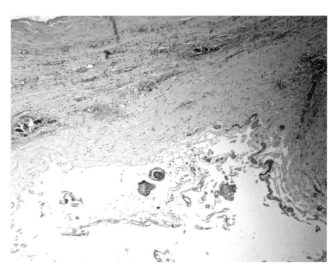

Figure 19-113. Echinococcosis. Scattered within the cyst's interior, the scolices originate from the germinal layer.

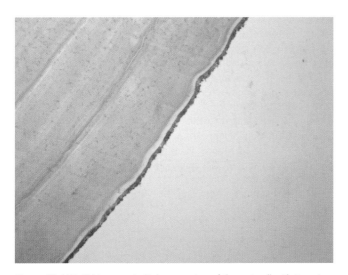

Figure 19-112. Echinococcosis. High-power view of the cyst wall with its various layers, including the inner germinal layer.

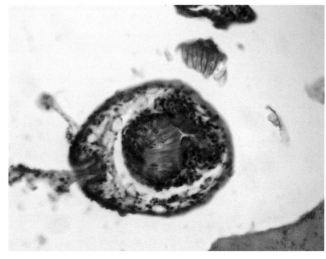

Figure 19-114. Echinococcosis. Close-up view of a scolex exhibiting its chitinous hooks.

tion,[806] diaphragmatic lymphatic drainage,[807] or contiguous spread due to rupture of viscera and cutaneous fistula formation.[807-809] Clinically, cutaneous echinococcosis manifests as painless soft tissue tumors, usually diagnosed as lipomas.[810]

The cysts of *Echinococcus* are composed of three layers. The outer host layer, or pericyst, is composed of fibroblasts, giant cells, and eosinophils. The middle, laminated membrane is an acellular, chitinous layer 2 mm thick. The inner germinal layer is thin and translucent (Figs. 19-111 and 19-112). Scolices originate from this membrane in the form of evaginations called brood capsules (Figs. 19-113 and 19-114).[811-813] In cutaneous lesions, one can find either the classic cyst with all its elements or a granulomatous palisading reaction with pseudocyst formation containing PAS-positive membrane remnants. The latter can be confused with several other palisading granulomatous reactions, such as granuloma annulare or even foreign-body reactions to keratin.[814]

Nematodes

Onchocerciasis

Human infection by *Onchocerca volvulus*, known as "river blindness," affects an estimated 17.7 million people in 34 countries in Africa, the Middle East, South America, and Central America.[815-819] The parasite has a five-stage life cycle, with the blackfly (genus *Simulium*) as an intermediate host and vector.[816,820] The habitat of these flies is the shores of rapidly flowing streams.[819]

The most common clinical presentation involves a diffuse papular dermatitis, often with intense pruritus, which is usually seen in the acute stage of the infection. Patients with chronic infection present with pruritic lesions that are heavily lichenified or with asymptomatic hypopigmented lesions in a "leopard skin" pattern.[817,820] Some chronically infected patients also have a papular eruption similar to that seen in the acute phase.[821] In cases from parts of Sudan and Yemen, there is focal involvement of one limb by the dermatitis, known as "sowda."[822] Another characteristic dermatologic manifestation is the so-called onchocercomata. These are subcutaneous nodules identified over bony prominences of the torso and hips in the African cases and on the head and shoulders in the South American cases.[823,824] The most debilitating feature of this disease is the ocular involvement by the microfilaria, which leads to blindness.[820,821]

It is noteworthy that there is an obligate endosymbiont in the female parasites, represented by bacteria of the genus *Wolbachia*, a rickettsial organism. This symbiotic relationship seems to be necessary for reproduction of the organisms.[825] This feature has also been described in dirofilariasis.[826] The release of these bacteria on lysis of the parasite has also been associated with ocular manifestations in the human hosts.[826] Therapeutic efforts have been targeted toward these bacteria.[827,828]

The onchocercal dermatitis lesions are composed microscopically of an acanthotic and hyperkeratotic epidermis overlying a mild, superficial and deep, dermal inflammatory infiltrate composed of lymphocytes and eosinophils. Microfilaria can be identified among collagen fibers in the upper dermis.[829] Degenerating parasites are usually surrounded by eosinophils showing degranulation. Chronic lesions tend to show progressive fibrosis of the dermis.[829,830] The acute lesions are Th1-type, whereas in the chronic lesions a Th2 predominance is found.[827] The subcutaneous nodules have an outer wall of dense fibrous tissue. In the center of these nodules, one can find parasites surrounded by granulation tissue and mixed inflammatory infiltrate. In chronic lesions, however, the parasites are not usually found. Calcification, chronic inflammatory infiltrate, and foreign-body giant cell response are seen instead. Eosinophils are seen in acute and in chronic lesions. Microfilaria can be identified in lymphatics adjacent to the lesions.[829-832]

Dirofilariasis

Dirofilaria is an important genus of parasites that mainly infect canids (dog heartworm) and felines. The endemic areas include the Mediterranean region and some Middle Eastern countries.[833-838] In these areas, cases of human infection by *Dirofilaria repens* and *Dirofilaria immitis* have been reported.

D. repens infection in humans usually causes solitary, erythematous, subcutaneous nodules.[839,840] These nodules are usually tender and sometimes are related to a sensation of "movement" under the skin.[841] *D. immitis* can asymptomatically involve the lungs.[840]

The nodules comprise a prominent inflammatory infiltrate composed of lymphocytes, plasma cells, histiocytes, eosinophils, and giant cells.[842] There is usually central suppuration with abundant neutrophils. In the center of the nodule, the degenerating filaria is usually identified. The parasite has a thick, laminated chitinous cuticle, longitudinal ridges, and large lateral cords, as well as a characteristic disposition of smooth muscle fibers.[835,842]

Cutaneous Larva Migrans

Cutaneous larva migrans is caused usually by hookworms and some nematode larvae that are not able to progress beyond the dermis and therefore wander in the dermis and epidermis, causing the characteristic clinical sign known as creeping eruption.[843-846] The terms *creeping eruption* and *cutaneous larva migrans* are usually used as synonyms. However, the former refers to a clinical sign and the latter to a syndrome.[847,848] Creeping eruption is a linear, serpiginous, slightly elevated, erythematous track that moves forward in an irregular pattern.[848,849] It can be caused by an animal hookworm, by other nematode larvae; by parasites such as *Gnathostoma* spp, *Loa loa*, and *Sarcoptes scabiei*; and by migratory myiasis.[848-853] The term *larva currens* is used when creeping eruption is related to *Strongyloides stercoralis* infection; the name refers to the very fast movement of the larvae.[854,855] The cutaneous larva migrans syndrome excludes creeping eruption caused by nonlarval forms of migratory parasites (i.e., dracontiasis, loiasis, or scabies). It is also not related to larvae that penetrate the dermis, such as cercarial dermatitis (schistosomiasis and swimmer's itch), onchocerciasis, or dirofilariasis.[850,856]

Hookworm-related cutaneous larva migrans, which is caused by animal hookworms such as *Ancylostoma braziliense*, *Ancylostoma caninum*, *Uncinaria stenocephala*, and *Bunostomum phlebotomum*, is quite common in tropical areas.[847,857] This infestation is endemic in poor communities and in developing countries, particularly in Brazil, India, and the West Indies.[858-862] The peak incidence usually coincides with the rainy season.[861,862] The lesions are usually located on the feet, buttocks, and thighs, but they can occur wherever unprotected skin comes in contact with contaminated soil.[857,858,863] Larvae can be transmitted through contaminated clothes or other fomites.[857] Clinically, an itchy reddish papule appears at the site of penetration of the larva.[857,849] Usually, there is a period of 1 to 5 days until the characteristic elevated tracks appear[857]; this period can last longer, especially in travelers.[863,864] Pruritus is the main symptom of the disease and can be rather intense, sometimes producing bacterial superinfection.[858,859] Vesiculobullous lesions are seen in 9% to 15% of the cases, with bullous lesions that can reach a size of several centimeters.[864] Papulopustular inflammation of the follicles and erythema annulare are rarely seen.[865-867]

The diagnosis is usually based on the clinical history and visualization of the typical creeping eruption pattern. Biopsy is usually not useful, nor is epiluminescence microscopy.[847] To the inexperienced eye, hookworm-related larva migrans may clinically mimic scabies, loiasis, myiasis, cercarial dermatitis (schistosomiasis), tinea corporis, contact dermatitis, and even VZV infection.[847] In *S. stercoralis* infestation (larva currens), the organisms migrate several centimeters per hour, much faster than in hookworm-related cutaneous larva migrans.[868] Infected immunosuppressed patients present with widespread petechiae and purpuric lesions.[855,869,870]

The parasite is rarely identified in histologic sections of the lesions. However, the tracks left by the larvae are seen as small cavities in the epidermis. There is usually a dermal mixed inflammatory infiltrate composed of neutrophils, lymphocytes, plasma cells, and numerous eosinophils.[871] In the rare event of finding a larva, there is usually no inflammation around the parasite.[871] An eosinophilic folliculitis is sometimes seen.[872,873] In larva currens, there is usually a prominent perivascular and interstitial lymphoeosinophilic infiltrate. In disseminated strongyloidiasis, which occurs in immunocompromised patients, abundant, 9- to

15-μm thick larvae are visualized amid the dermal collagen and rarely within vessels.[855,869]

Arthropod-Induced Diseases

Arachnids

Scorpions

Only a small fraction of the existing species of scorpions have a sufficiently potent venom to pose a risk to humans. Almost all of the most poisonous species are within the Buthidae family, and they are mainly found in the Middle East, Africa, and Asia.[874] Most of the scorpions have a neurotoxic venom that affects mainly the peripheral nervous system, causing intense pain at the site, altered heart activity, and paresthesia. Death is a rare event, usually resulting from respiratory failure.[874,875]

Because the majority of the effects of the venom are neurotoxic, there is virtually no dermatologic development other than edema and erythema around the sting site.[874] However, stings by *Hemiscorpion lepturus,* a species found in Iran and Iraq, cause tremendous dermatologic manifestations at the site of inoculation. The lesions begin as erythematous, purpuric plaques and then evolve to bullae, extensive cellulitis, and, later, necrotic ulcers. The venom has a prominent cytotoxic effect, producing severe vasculitis at the site of the sting. Also, prominent systemic effects may be seen.[876]

Spiders

As with the scorpions, only a small number of spider species are considered dangerous to humans. The pharmacology of spider venoms is highly variable among species, so identification of the involved spider is medically important.[874]

Spiders from the genus *Latrodectus,* popularly known as black widow spiders, are small and shiny black and have hourglass-shaped red markings in the abdomen.[874] The venom produced by these spiders contains neurotoxic peptides (mainly α-latrotoxin), which cause systemic symptoms such as contracture of the abdominal muscles (often misdiagnosed as acute abdomen), generalized muscle cramps, sweating, malaise, nausea, and hypertension.[877] At the site of inoculation, there are usually two markings, corresponding to the spider's fangs, surrounded by erythema and some petechial branching lesions.[874,878]

The other commonly medically important spiders are the ones from the genus *Loxosceles.* Also known as recluse or violin spiders, these are medium size, uniformly brown spiders with fine hairs and a violin-shaped cephalothorax. A distinctive feature is the presence of six eyes grouped in three dyads.[874] Manifestations associated with the bites from these spiders range from localized lesions to dermonecrotic, slow-healing lesions that can have life-threatening systemic manifestations, such as acute renal failure and disseminated intravascular coagulation.[879-883] The venom is overtly cytotoxic, with sphingomyelinase as its main active component, and causes disruption of the endothelial cells, massive activation of the neutrophils, and hemolysis.[880,881] Fully evolved lesions exhibit the classic bull's-eye lesion, with a central erythematous bleb separated from a peripheral cyanotic region. This lesion becomes necrotic usually 7 days after the assault, leaving a depressed ulcer.[884-886] It can be confused with various dermatologic conditions such as erythema migrans[887] and even with cutaneous manifestations of warfarin poisoning, among other conditions.[875,888]

Other medically important spiders include the so-called hobo spiders (*Tegenaria agestis*), which can cause dermonecrotic lesions similar to but somewhat less severe than those seen with *Loxosceles* spiders,[875,889] and large spiders from the genera *Phoneutria* (banana spider) and *Atrax* (Sydney funnel spider), which are found, respectively, in South America and Australia and have potent neurotoxic venoms, expressing few dermatologic manifestations.[890,891]

The term *necrotizing arachnidism* is used to designate necrotic lesions caused by spiders that produce predominantly cytotoxic venom.[892] Microscopically, the lesions usually show a prominent neutrophilic vasculitis with hemorrhage. This leads to arterial wall necrosis, eschar-covered ulceration, and even subcutaneous tissue necrosis. A prominent eosinophilic infiltrate is usually found.[893] The neurotoxic venom causes little alteration at the site of the bite.

Ticks

There are two families of ticks (Acari of the order Ixodidae) that have dermatologic importance. The Argasidae family, or soft ticks (*Ornithodoros* spp.), are usually not perceived by the host and can cause nodulohemorrhagic local lesions and even anaphylactic shock.[894,895] The Ixodidae family, or hard ticks, includes the *Ixodes* and *Dermacentor* species.[894] They are usually noticed by the host, because they remain attached to the skin while they engorge with blood. Ticks are known vectors of several agents of illnesses described elsewhere in this book.

The unique mechanism through which these arachnids feed involves the gnathosoma (capitulum), a cutting/sucking device located in the anterior portion of the tick.[894] During feeding, a substance is secreted that acts as a "cement," fixing the mouthparts to the skin.[894] This mechanical process is aided by the biologic action of several chemicals contained in the regurgitated saliva. These include vasodilators, anticoagulants, immunosuppressants, anti-inflammatory molecules, and enzymes such as hyaluronidases and metalloproteinases.[896-898]

The clinical presentation varies from local erythematous lesions to a persistent papular and nodular rash.[899] Rarely, the bites can induce panniculitis,[900] bullae, and hemorrhage. Papular urticaria is another, rather infrequent presentation of chronic nature and is usually found in children.[901]

Acute lesions show an intradermal cavity with prominent red blood cell extravasation and a rather dense inflammatory infiltrate composed predominantly of neutrophils together with lymphocytes and histiocytes. The characteristic eosinophilic infiltrate appears relatively late in the acute phase of the process.[894] The diagnosis can be difficult if the mouth parts are not identified. More evolved lesions show a tract of necrosis and perivascular fibrin deposition.[894] Sometimes, intravascular fibrin thrombi are seen. These can resemble the findings of monoclonal or mixed cryoglobulinemia.[902,903] A panniculitis may occur, with a predominant neutrophilic infiltrate.[900]

Chronic lesions are characteristically composed of a diffuse, superficial and deep, lymphoeosinophilic inflammatory infiltrate that can be wedge-shaped. This is overlain by an acanthotic and pseudoepitheliomatous epidermis. Granulomas can be found and are usually a mixed immune and foreign-body immune type. They arise in response to the strongly immunogenic, collagen-like proteins of the cement or the viable core and the sclerotized cuticle of the tick's mouthparts.[894]

The papular urticaria pattern can appear chronically as a wedge-shaped lesion involving the dermis and even subcutaneous fat.[901] The persistent nodular arthropod-bite reaction appears as a T-cell or B-cell lymphoid hyperplasia, which can be differentiated from other types of pseudolymphomatous lesions by the vascular changes and the presence of numerous eosinophils.[894] These lymphoid aggregates can express pseudoclonality in rearrangement studies.[904] Therefore, one must rely on the history and a correct clinical correlation. The histopathologic details of erythema migrans (Lyme disease), caused by a bite from the *Ixodes* group ticks, were reviewed earlier in this chapter.

A peculiar reaction to tick bites is the appearance of a patch of alopecia at the site of the bite. This unusual presentation is clinically similar to alopecia areata.[905,906] It is believed to be caused by some epilating anticoagulants injected with saliva.[905] There are several histopathologic features that one can find helpful to distinguish alopecia areata from tick bite–induced alopecia. In alopecia areata, the lymphocytic infiltrate is located mainly in the bulbs of the hair follicles. In alopecia secondary to a tick bite, the lymphoid reaction is located at the hair's isthmus.[894]

Mites

Demodicosis

Follicle mites live in the hair follicles and sebaceous glands of mammals such as cats, dogs, and horses.[907] Two species have been identified in humans: *D. folliculorum* and *Demodex brevis*.[908] These organisms colonize the pilosebaceous unit and utilize sebum as nourishment. *D. folliculorum* is the larger of the two, measuring up to 0.4 mm, and it is usually found aggregated in groups in the infundibular portion of the hair follicle (Fig. 19-115).[908,909] In contrast, *D. brevis* is usually solitary and inhabits the deeper portion of the sebaceous glands and ducts (Fig.

19-116).[910] The prevalence approximates 100% in middle-aged and older adults, although mite density is low in healthy skin.[907] The face is most often involved, and infestation is likely to occur during childhood by direct contact.[907] The mites can be found in up to 10% of skin biopsies from all sites and in 12% of all follicles of any given biopsy specimen.[911] Although they are not involved in the etiology of rosacea, with the possible exception of the granulomatous variant, the mites definitely can aggravate this disease.[907,912]

There are three basic clinical forms of *Demodex* infestation: pityriasis folliculorum, rosacea-like demodicosis, and demodicidosis gravis. Clinically, pityriasis folliculorum manifests as a diffuse but faint facial burning sensation with fine follicular plugs and scales in a "frosted" pattern. The condition is frequently seen in women who use heavy facial creams and make-up.[913] The rosacea-like demodicidosis has a sudden, rapid onset with follicular scaling, superficial small papulovesicles, and vesicopustules.[914] It can manifest with an asymmetric distribution and can affect the eyelids (demodectic blepharitis).[915] It is not related to flushing, persistent erythema, or photosensitivity, which is helpful to distinguish it from rosacea.[245] The third clinical variant of *Demodex* infestation, demodicidosis gravis, involves a clinical picture very similar to that of granulomatous rosacea.[916]

Demodex infestation has also been related to other dermatologic conditions, such as pustular folliculitis,[917] papulopustular scalp eruptions,[918] perioral dermatitis,[919] and hyperpigmented patches of the face.[913]

Microscopically, the usual picture of *Demodex* mite infestation includes follicular dilatation and the presence of dense eosin-

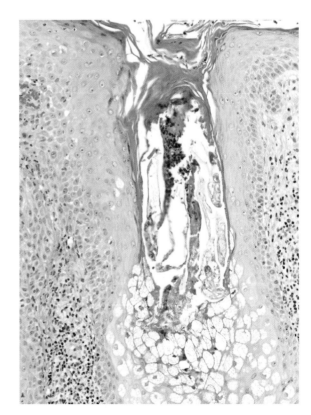

Figure 19-116. *Demodex brevis* infestation. These commonly found ectoparasites can be seen burrowed deep within the sebaceous glands.

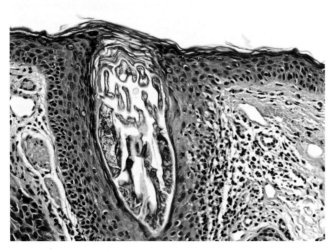

Figure 19-115. *Demodex* infestation. The chitinous exoskeleton of these organisms makes it easy to recognize them colonizing the appendages.

ophilic material around the mites (see Figs. 19-115 and 19-116). Sometimes, granulomas enveloping extrafollicular mites are seen, especially in granulomatous and pustular rosacea.[919,920]

In pityriasis folliculorum, one sees a diffuse dermal perivascular lymphocytic infiltrate with no granuloma formation.[921] The histologic picture of rosacea-like demodicosis exhibits a mononuclear, mainly perifollicular inflammatory infiltrate that can be granulomatous. Also, telangiectatic superficial vessels are seen.[907,914] Up to 10 to 15 *D. folliculorum* organisms can be seen in each follicle.[922]

Scabies

Both highly contagious and neglected, the cutaneous condition resulting from scabies infestation is an important cause of worldwide public health problems. It is usually linked to poor hygiene and overcrowded environments. The causative agent is the mite *Sarcoptes scabiei* var. *hominis,* which colonizes the upper layers of the epidermis, burrowing in the stratum corneum of the skin. Transmission can occur during direct skin contact or through contaminated fomites.[923] The primary infection induces clinical symptoms only 4 to 8 weeks after the inoculation.[924-926]

The mechanisms behind this delayed response are largely unknown. However, studies have shown that substances with immune-modulatory features are actively secreted by the mites and affect keratinocytes, fibroblasts, and endothelial cells.[927-929] Scabiosis tends to have a cyclical character, recurring at intervals of about 30 years,[930] and shows increased incidence during winter in some communities.[931,932]

There are three clinical presentations: a papulovesicular variant, a form presenting as persistent nodules, and the so-called Norwegian (crusted) scabies. The classic presentation of the papulovesicular variant includes intensely pruritic papules and papulovesicles. The pruritus is usually worse at night. The vesicles are found at the end of fine, wavy, dark lines, which represent the excreta-soiled tunnels created by the female parasite in the horny layer while depositing eggs. These burrows are specific but they may be absent.[933,934] In addition to the burrows, there is almost always a secondary rash of small papules related to autosensitization.[934,935] The most commonly involved sites are the interdigital skin folds, the palmar aspect of the hands and fingers, the wrists, the nipples, the inframammary regions, and the male genitalia.[923,933] Diagnosis of the disease relies heavily on the history and clinical features. Detection of the mites can be enhanced by epiluminesence[936] and dermoscopy without computer assistance.[937] If the diagnosis is troublesome, PCR or ELISA techniques can be used.[938]

Rarely, bullous lesions strongly resembling bullous pemphigoid are observed.[936,940] This presentation can sometimes pose a true diagnostic dilemma.[941] In some cases of bullous scabies, circulating antibodies against BP180 or BP230 or both have been detected in sera, suggesting that *S. scabiei* infection could trigger a true bullous pemphigoid.[942]

The persistent nodular form appears in about 7% of the patients, particularly in young adults and children. It manifests as reddish-brown, pruritic nodules on the lower trunk, scrotum, and thighs.[943,944] The lesions persist for a year regardless of treatment, and they usually are devoid of organisms.

At the end of the spectrum, we find the disseminated form of scabiosis, namely the crusted or Norwegian form. Heavily linked with immunocompromised states, it can occur in patients infected with HIV or human T-cell lymphotropic virus 1 (HTLV-1).[943,945] However, it has also been described in patients with previously treated leprosy, substance abuse, systemic lupus erythematosus, tuberculosis, diabetes mellitus, and hepatitis B.[946] Cases have also been reported in an otherwise healthy pregnant woman[947] and in patients with epidermolysis bullosa.[948,949] In this variant, there is extensive distribution of the mites over the body, including the neck, the scalp, and under the nails. Secondary bacterial infection, accompanied by regional lymphadenopathy, is commonly present.

There are thick hyperkeratotic scales in which one sees innumerable mites. In the dermis, there is usually a chronic inflammatory infiltrate which shows an abnormal CD8+ predominance, resulting from a Th1/Th2 imbalance. This lymphoid anomaly is probably related to psoriasis-like dysregulation of the keratinocytes and the host's inability to control the infection.[950]

On biopsy, in the classic papulovesicular scabies infestation, one usually finds a spongiotic epidermis with exocytosis of eosinophils and neutrophils. This spongiotic dermatitis overlies a superficial and deep perivascular infiltrate showing lymphocytes, histiocytes, mast cells, and eosinophils.[951,952] Some interstitial eosinophils are seen. Rarely, one can identify flame figures[953] and necrotizing vasculitis,[954] as well as subepidermal bullae.[939] If a burrow is biopsied, eggs, larvae, and even mites may be visualized.[954] The resultant secondary rash is usually nonspecific, sometimes even lacking the eosinophils.[955] Chronic lesions usually show excoriation and scale crusts.

In persistent nodular scabies, the histologic picture includes superficial and deep lymphocytes (even atypical forms), macrophages, plasma cells, eosinophils, and Langerhans cells (intermediate cells) disposed in perivascular and periappendageal array.[954,956] This infiltrate, probably directed to mite antigens,[956] can mimic reticulosis[957] and often has an overlying pseudolymphomatous pattern.[958] The infiltrate can even extend into subcutaneous fat.[959] Mites are usually not observed, but if the specimen is serially sectioned, mite parts may be found in 20% of cases.[960]

The histologic picture of Norwegian scabies is that of a massive orthokeratotic and parakeratotic scale containing innumerable mites.[949,950] Below this massive scale, there is usually a psoriasiform hyperplasia with spongiosis and exocytosis of neutrophils and eosinophils; microabscess formation may occur. The underlying dermis shows lymphocytes and eosinophils.[950]

Cheyletiella *Dermatitis*

A common cause of the so-called walking dandruff of dogs, rabbits, and cats, *Cheyletiella* spp. can also cause intensely pruritic dermatitis in humans. The disease manifests as erythematous papules and papulovesicles, which appear in areas where there is close contact with infested pets.[961-964] These mites are nonburrowing and have a "bite and run" behavior.[965] Lesions in humans probably result from delayed hypersensitivity reaction.[966] The mites are not found in humans, and the diagnosis is confirmed on examination of the pets.[963]

There is usually a superficial dermal and mid-dermal lymphoeosinophilic infiltrate with some histiocytes. In the epidermis, prominent spongiotic change is identified at the site of the bite.

Insects

Human Lice

Lice have been related to human activities since ancient times. Interestingly, the approximate date in which humans began to wear clothes has been determined by "dating" the mitochondrial DNA of the body louse.[967] These ectoparasites act as vectors of agents of conditions such as epidemic typhus (*R. prowazekii*), discussed earlier.

There are three types of human lice. The species that affects the hairs of the scalp, *Pediculus humanus capitis,* is fairly common, affecting people from all socioeconomic backgrounds. This species represents a common and recurrent problem in schools.[968] The second type, *Phthirus pubis,* has venereal transmission pattern. Infestation with *P. pubis* is strongly related to other concomitant sexually transmitted diseases.[969] This species usually infests the pubic hair, but it can be seen in the corporal hair of the trunk and limbs and even in the eyelashes.[970] The reaction to infestation of eyelashes by *P. pubis* can mimic conjunctival infections and blepharitis.[971] Erythema annulare centrifugum may develop secondary to massive infestations with *P. pubis*.[972] Both the pubic louse and the head louse cement eggs to the hairs, forming the so-called nit. The body louse, *P. humanus corporis,* lives in the host's clothes as well as in corporeal hairs. Scattered bluish spots of discoloration (maculae cerulea) can sometimes be found related to heavy body louse infestation.[973]

The saliva injected while the parasite feeds produces an allergic reaction which can become superinfected, especially after heavy scratching. One can identify lice and eggs microscopically for confirmation.

Bed Bugs

Bed bugs, part of the Cimicidae group, are hematophagous, reddish-brown insects with nocturnal feeding habits. They have a worldwide distribution, but with a greater incidence in tropical and subtropical developing countries.[974] However, there has been a dramatic increase of these parasites lately, especially in the United Kingdom and in the United States.[975]

Bed bugs are quite resistant to elimination, and adult forms can survive almost 1 year without feeding.[976] *Cimex lectularius,* the most common species, produces lesions from purpuric macules to urticarial erythematous papules. The classic presentation involves three bites in linear array, also known as "breakfast, lunch, and dinner." Lesions are commonly seen on exposed areas of the face, neck, hands, or arms.[976] In predisposed individuals, bullous lesions can be evident.[977] This is due to a late-phase response to an IgE-mediated hypersensitivity to nitrophorin, an antigen present in the *C. lenticularis* saliva.[978]

In urticarial lesions, one can see edema of the papillary dermis and a perivascular lymphoeosinophilic infiltrate with scattered mast cells. Intraepidermal and subepidermal edema is found in the vesiculobullous lesions.[976] In bullous lesions, one can find hemorrhage.[977]

Myiasis

The infestation of human tissue by fly larvae of the Diptera order is known as myiasis. Most of the cases are produced by *Derma-* *tobia hominis* or *Cordylobia anthropophaga.*[979] *D. hominis,* the so-called human botfly, is prevalent in Central and South America,[979,980] whereas the tumbu fly (*C. anthropophaga*) is found in certain parts of West and Central Africa.[981] Several other genera of flies can produce myiasis, including *Parasarcophaga,*[982] *Gasterophilus,*[983] and *Hypoderma,*[984] among others. These, however, have a more limited geographic distribution. Rarely, larvae of flies from the *Cuterebra* species infest humans.[980,985,986] The domestic fly, *Musca domestica,* can rarely infest extremely neglected and debilitated persons.[987,988]

The eggs are usually deposited directly by the flies in areas where there is damaged skin. However, ova can be transmitted and deposited by other insects, such as mosquitoes, as is the case with *D. hominis.* In the case of *C. anthropophaga,* larvae hatch on the ground or on clothing and then invade the host's skin.[981] The larvae infest the skin for a variable period, usually from about 2 weeks to 3 months, depending on the species. After that, larvae exit the host to continue their life cycle as pupae.

Myiasis infestations tend to occur during the summer and usually involve exposed surfaces, such as the feet and forearms. Other common sites are the face, scalp, neck, shoulders, and chest.[981,989] The lower body is affected in fewer than 15% of the cases.[981] Rare cases of penile infestation have been reported.[990,991] The early lesions often adopt a furuncle-like aspect or manifest as a single erythematous papule, usually with a punctum-like orifice where the larvae obtain oxygen.[985,989] The eruption can be migratory or nonmigratory. Migratory myiasis is usually related to *Gasterophilus* spp. (horse botfly) or *Hypoderma* spp. (cattle grub).[986,989] More evolved lesions manifest as ulcers or plaques with draining sinuses and fistulas. Pulsating pain can be present in large and superinfected lesions.

The developing larva is usually lodged in a cavity located in the dermis or subcutaneous fat.[985,992] Around the larva, there is a prominent host response; this is a heavy, mixed inflammatory response with lymphocytes, histiocytes, foreign-body giant cells, plasma cells, eosinophils, and neutrophils, as well as extensive fibrosis.[992,993] A sinus tract connecting the cavity to the exterior can be found. Fragmented larva parts, showing chitinous material with widely spaced spines and internal organs, can be seen inside the cavity. One can identify spinous processes emanating from the chitinous cuticle that attach the larva to the host's tissues.[981,985,989] The various species can be distinguished, especially during early development, by the location of their respiratory spiracles.[985]

Tungiasis

Tungiasis is caused by *Tunga penetrans,* a variety of free-living flea that is found in tropical environments. Originally from South and Central America, the sandfleas spread first to tropical Africa in the 19th century and then to India and Pakistan in the beginning of the 20th century.[994-996] As is the case with most of the parasitic diseases, infection is related to poor hygiene and precarious conditions, which are often found in neglected communities.[997,998] The natural habitat of these fleas are sandy and warm terrains such as beaches and arid regions, but they can also be found in stables and pigsties.[999] Infestation is commonly found in dogs, cats, and rats.[1000] In endemic regions, there is a seasonal pattern of infestations.[998] The lesions are usually located on the feet, because *T. penetrans* is a poor jumper, and they can produce

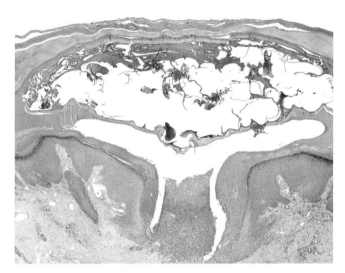

Figure 19-117. Tungiasis. The flea is usually found intraepidermally, surrounded by extensive epidermal hyperplasia with hyperkeratosis. At the site where the proboscis is inserted into the dermis, there is a prominent inflammatory response composed of lymphocytes, plasma cells, and eosinophils. (Courtesy of Mirian Sotto, MD, PhD, Department of Dermatology, Hospital das Clinicas, University of Sao Paulo.)

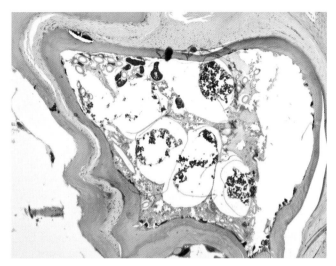

Figure 19-118. Tungiasis. Note the parasite's exoskeleton and internal organs. Eggs are found within the flea's engorged abdomen.

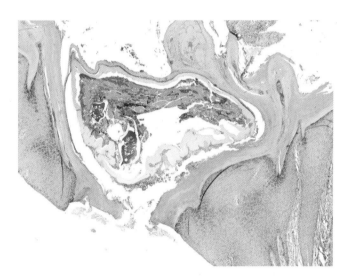

Figure 19-119. Tungiasis. Another example with exuberant epidermal hyperplasia and superinfection.

severe impairment in walking due to pain.[994,996,1001] Lesions can also be found on the hands, especially in children.[1002-1005] Other sites that may be involved are the elbows,[1004] wrists, breast, back, buttocks, thighs, knees, and legs.[1005] Periungual affectation is not uncommon.

The infestation, which usually lasts 4 to 6 weeks, begins with painless penetration of the parasite, probably with the help of keratinolyitc enzymes. This is followed by several subsequent phases: the hypertrophic phase, the "white halo" phase, the involution phase, and finally the transepidermal elimination of the residues.[1006] Overall, the lesions are usually composed of single or multiple, small, white papules that eventually develop into nodules. They can be quite pruritic, have a wart-like[1007] morphology, and can be crusted,[1008,1009] bullous,[1010] pustular,[994,1001,1003,1011] or ulcerative.[1001,1005,1008] The female flea measures about 0.1 cm at the beginning of the infection. The flea feeds and reaches a size of 0.6 cm or more, harboring up to 200 ova. At the end of the cycle, the adult flea dies, and the lesion ulcerates to release the eggs.[997] Bacterial superinfection is quite common, usually with *S. aureus* or enterobacteria; several anaerobic agents, such as *Peptostreptococcus* spp. and *Clostridium* spp., have also been isolated.[1012] The possibility of superinfection with *Clostridium tetani* is always of great concern.[1021,1037]

Although the infestation is usually suspected from the history and clinical appearance, if a biopsy is available, one can identify the parasite by its characteristic exoskeleton and internal parts, including ova (Figs. 19-117 and 19-118). The parasite is usually lodged in the upper dermis, surrounded by a pseudocystic cavity. In the surrounding and overlying skin, there is prominent hyperkeratosis, parakeratosis, and acanthosis (Fig. 19-119). The flea is surrounded with a prominent, mixed inflammatory infiltrate and fibrosis.[996,1003,1008,1013,1014] A mass of eggs can be found within the stratum corneum. In advanced lesions, there is ulceration and impetiginization.[1015]

Algal Infections

Prothecosis

Human protothecosis is a rare infection caused by members of the genus *Prototheca*. *Prototheca* species are considered to be achlorophyllic algae and are ubiquitous in nature.[1016] The disease has been reported worldwide. Trauma and inoculation with contaminated water is the most common mechanism of infection in humans.[1017] The clinical manifestations have been classified into three types: cutaneous lesions, olecranon bursitis, and disseminated or systemic disease.[1018] Infections can occur in both immunocompetent and immunosuppressed patients, although more severe and disseminated infections tend to occur in the immunocompromised.[1016] The great majority of patients with protothecosis are older than 30 years of age or elderly, although cases have also been reported in children and neonates.[1019-1021]

The cutaneous lesions are located mainly on exposed areas, such as the extremities and face.[1016] They usually have a slowly progressive course with no tendency to self-heal.[1022] The clinical presentation is variable, and the lesions can consist of erythematous plaques, pustules, papules, nodules, vesicles, verrucous lesions, ulcers, or hypopigmented or atrophic lesions.[1016,1020,1023-1028] Lesions resembling herpes, eczema, subcutaneous mycoses, and pyoderma gangrenosum have also been described.[1023,1024,1029]

The host tissue responses to *Prototheca* are variable, ranging from severe granulomatous necrosis to an absence of inflammatory changes.[1030] Usually, there is a chronic granulomatous reaction throughout the dermis, which may also involve the subcutaneous tissue, associated with a variable admixture of lymphocytes, neutrophils, plasma cells, and occasional eosinophils.[1017,1023] The granulomas can exhibit central necrosis.[1017] The epidermis can exhibit hyperkeratosis, focal parakeratosis, and pseudoepitheliomatous hyperplasia.[1016] The organisms are observed in the cytoplasm of macrophages and multinucleated giant cells, but also extracellularly. They manifest as thick-walled, spherical bodies with no budding.[1016] *Prototheca* species are not readily apparent in H&E-stained slides, but they stain with the silver methenamine and PAS stains. The sporangia of *Coccidioides* are much larger than those of *Prototheca* species, whereas the individual endospores of *Coccidioides* are smaller.[1016,1017]

Currently, the two species reported to cause infections in humans are *Prototheca wickerhamii* and *Prototheca zopfii*, with *P. wickerhamii* being more common.[1016,1020,1021,1023,1030-1032] *Prototheca* species are spherical, unicellular organisms ranging from 3 to 30 μm in diameter.[1016] Reproduction is asexual, and during cell maturation, the cytoplasm undergoes a process of cleavage to form endospores. Approximately 2 to 20 endospores are present in each mother cell. These endospores grow, causing the mother cells (sporangia) to rupture.[1016] The sporangia of *P. wickerhamii* (3-10 μm in diameter) are usually smaller than those of *P. zopfii* (7-30 μm in diameter).[1016] Another distinguishing feature of *P. wickerhamii* is the morula form of its sporangia, in which endospores are arranged symmetrically in a daisy-like appearance; other species, including *P. zopfii*, do not form these multiple septated structures.[1016,1017] Microscopic examination of the organism in culture reveals the same structures as are seen in tissue (i.e., spherical sporangia containing multiple endospores).[1020]

REFERENCES

1. Rapini RP: Bacterial infections. In Barnhill R: Textbook in Dermatopathology, 2nd ed. New York, McGraw-Hill, 2004.
2. Lucas S: Bacterial diseases. Elder DE (ed): Lever's Histopathology of the Skin. Philadelphia, Lippincott Williams & Wilkins, 2009, pp 539-578.
3. Shriner DL, Schwartz RA, Janniger CK: Impetigo. Cutis 1995;56:30-32.
4. Darmstadt GL, Lane AT: Impetigo: An overview. Pediatr Dermatol 1994;11:293-303.
5. Barnett BO, Frieden IJ: Streptococcal skin diseases in children. Semin Dermatol 1992;11:3-10.
6. Chiller K, Selkin BA, Murakawa GJ: Skin microflora and bacterial infections of the skin. J Investig Dermatol Symp Proc 2001;6:170-174.
7. Amagai M, Yamaguchi T, Hanakawa Y, et al: Staphylococcal exfoliative toxin B specifically cleaves desmoglein 1. J Invest Dermatol 2002;118:845-850.
8. Resnick SD: Staphylococcal toxin-mediated syndromes in childhood. Semin Dermatol 1992;11:11-18.
9. Cribier B, Piemont Y, Grosshans E: Staphylococcal scalded skin syndrome in adults: A clinical review illustrated with a new case. J Am Acad Dermatol 1994;30(2 Pt 2):319-324.
10. Hood AF, Kwan TH, Mihm MC Jr, et al: Primer of Dermatopathology, 3rd ed. Philadelphia, Lippincott Williams & Wilkins, 2002.
11. Lina G, Gillet Y, Vandenesch F, et al: Toxin involvement in staphylococcal scalded skin syndrome. Clin Infect Dis 1997;25:1369-1373.
12. Gemmell CG: Staphylococcal scalded skin syndrome. J Med Microbiol 1995;43:318-327.
13. Garland SM, Peel MM: Tampons and toxic shock syndrome. Med J Aust 1995;163:8-9.
14. Tierno PM Jr: Comparison of cotton and rayon/cotton tampons for efficacy of toxic shock syndrome toxin-1 production. J Infect Dis 1996;173:1289-1291.
15. Gutiérrez Rodero F, Ortiz de la Tabla V, Martínez C, del Mar Masiá M: Staphylococcal toxic shock syndrome associated with human immunodeficiency virus infection: Report of a case with bacteremia. Clin Infect Dis 1996;22:875-876.
16. Chelsom J, Halstensen A, Haga T, Høiby EA: Necrotising fasciitis due to group A streptococci in western Norway: Incidence and clinical features. Lancet 1994;344:1111-1115.
17. Forni AL, Kaplan EL, Schlievert PM, Roberts RB: Clinical and microbiological characteristics of severe group A streptococcus infections and streptococcal toxic shock syndrome. Clin Infect Dis 1995;21:333-340.
18. Travers JB, Norris DA, Leung DY: The keratinocyte as a target for staphylococcal bacterial toxins. J Investig Dermatol Symp Proc 2001;6:225-230.
19. McCormick JK, Yarwood JM, Schlievert PM: Toxic shock syndrome and bacterial superantigens: An update. Annu Rev Microbiol 2001;55:77-104.
20. Yanagisawa C, Hanaki H, Natae T, Sunakawa K: Neutralization of staphylococcal exotoxins in vitro by human-origin intravenous immunoglobulin. J Infect Chemother 2007;13:368-372.
21. Güçlüer H, Ergun T, Demirçay Z: Ecthyma gangrenosum. Int J Dermatol 1999;38:299-302.
22. Agger WA, Mardan A: *Pseudomonas aeruginosa* infections of intact skin. Clin Infect Dis 1995;20:302-308.
23. Eriksson B, Jorup-Rönström C, Karkkonen K, et al: Erysipelas: Clinical and bacteriologic spectrum and serological aspects. Clin Infect Dis 1996;23:1091-1098.
24. Chartier C, Grosshans E: Erysipelas: An update. Int J Dermatol 1996;35:779-781.
25. Green RJ, Dafoe DC, Raffin TA: Necrotizing fasciitis. Chest 1996;110:219-229.
26. Canoso JJ, Barza M: Soft tissue infections. Rheum Dis Clin North Am 1993;19:293-309.
27. Kotrappa KS, Bansal RS, Amin NM: Necrotizing fasciitis. Am Fam Physician 1996;53:1691-1697.
28. Fustes-Morales A, Gutierrez-Castrellon P, Gutierrez-Castrellon P, et al: Necrotizing fasciitis: Report of 39 pediatric cases. Arch Dermatol 2002;138:893-899.
29. Rongioletti F, Semino M, Drago F, et al: Blastomycosis-like pyoderma (pyoderma vegetans) responding to antibiotics and topical disodium chromoglycate. Int J Dermatol 1996;35:828-830.
30. Papadopoulos AJ, Schwartz RA, Kapila R, et al: Pyoderma vegetans. J Cutan Med Surg 2001;5:223-227.
31. Bianchi L, Carrozzo AM, Orlandi A, et al: Pyoderma vegetans and ulcerative colitis. Br J Dermatol 2001;144:1224-1227.
32. Hadfield TL, McEvoy P, Polotsky Y, et al: The pathology of diphtheria. J Infect Dis 2000;181(Suppl 1):S116-S120.

33. Pandit N, Yeshwanth M: Cutaneous diphtheria in a child. Int J Dermatol 1999;38:298-299.

34. Sarkany I, Taplin D, Blank H: Incidence and bacteriology of erythrasma. Arch Dermatol 1962;85:578-582.

35. Dellion S, Morel P, Vignon-Pennamen D, Felten A: Erythrasma owing to an unusual pathogen. Arch Dermatol 1996;132:716-717.

36. Montes LF, Black SH, McBride ME: Bacterial invasion of the stratum corneum in erythrasma: I. Ultrastructural evidence for a keratolytic action experted by *Corynebacterium minutissimum*. J Invest Dermatol 1967;49:474-485.

37. Wilson C, Dawber R: Trichomycosis axillaris: A different view. J Am Acad Dermatol 1989;21(2 Pt 1):325-326.

38. Wohlrab J, Rohrbach D, Marsch WC: Keratolysis sulcata (pitted keratolysis): Clinical symptoms with different histological correlates. Br J Dermatol 2000;143:1348-1349.

39. de Almeida HL Jr, de Castro LA, Rocha NE, Abrantes VL: Ultrastructure of pitted keratolysis. Int J Dermatol 2000;39:698-701.

40. Salzman MB, Rubin LG: Meningococcemia. Infect Dis Clin North Am 1996;10:709-725.

41. Neveling U, Kaschula RO: Fatal meningococcal disease in childhood: An autopsy study of 86 cases. Ann Trop Paediatr 1993;13:147-152.

42. Kirsch EA, Barton RP, Kitchen L, Giroir BP: Pathophysiology, treatment and outcome of meningococcemia: A review and recent experience. Pediatr Infect Dis J 1996;15:967-978; quiz 979.

43. Gregory B, Tron V, Ho VC: Cyclic fever and rash in a 66-year-old woman: Chronic meningococcemia. Arch Dermatol 1992;128:1645, 1648.

44. Assier H, Chosidow O, Rekacewicz I, et al: Chronic meningococcemia in acquired immunodeficiency infection. J Am Acad Dermatol 1993;29(5 Pt 1):793-794.

45. Buntin DM, Rosen T, Lesher JL Jr, et al: Sexually transmitted diseases: Bacterial infections. Committee on Sexually Transmitted Diseases of the American Academy of Dermatology. J Am Acad Dermatol 1991;25(2 Pt 1):287-299.

46. Dawe RS, Sweeney G, Munro CS: A vesico-pustular rash and arthralgia. Clin Exp Dermatol 2001;26:113-114.

47. Mofredj A, Baraka D, Madec Y, Lemaitre P: Disseminated gonococcal infection and meningitis. Am J Med 2000;109:71-72.

48. World Health Organization: Fact Sheet: Tuberculosis. 2007. Available at http://www.who.int/mediacentre/factsheets/fs104/en/ (accessed August 10, 2009).

49. Dannenberg AM Jr: Immune mechanisms in the pathogenesis of pulmonary tuberculosis. Rev Infect Dis 1989;11(Suppl 2):S369-S378.

50. Kramer F, Sasse SA, Simms JC, Leedom JM: Primary cutaneous tuberculosis after a needlestick injury from a patient with AIDS and undiagnosed tuberculosis. Ann Intern Med 1993;119(7 Pt 1):594-595.

51. Goette DK, Jacobson KW, Doty RD: Primary inoculation tuberculosis of the skin: Prosector's paronychia. Arch Dermatol 1978;114:567-569.

52. Heilman KM, Muschenheim C: Primary cutaneous tuberculosis resulting from mouth-to-mouth respiration. N Engl J Med 1965;273:1035-1036.

53. Rietbroek RC, Dahlmans RP, Smedts F, et al: Tuberculosis cutis miliaris disseminata as a manifestation of miliary tuberculosis: Literature review and report of a case of recurrent skin lesions. Rev Infect Dis 1991;13:265-269.

54. Regan W, Harley W: Orificial and pulmonary tuberculosis: Report of a case. Australas J Dermatol 1979;20:88-90.

55. Warin AP, Jones EW: Cutaneous tuberculosis of the nose with unusual clinical and histological features leading to a delay in the diagnosis. Clin Exp Dermatol 1977;2:235-242.

56. Marcoval J, Servitje O, Moreno A, et al: Lupus vulgaris: Clinical, histopathologic, and bacteriologic study of 10 cases. J Am Acad Dermatol 1992;26(3 Pt 2):404-407.

57. Haim S, Friedman-Birnbaum R: Cutaneous tuberculosis and malignancy. Cutis 1978;21:643-647.

58. Penneys NS, Leonardi CL, Cook S, et al: Identification of *Mycobacterium tuberculosis* DNA in five different types of cutaneous lesions by the polymerase chain reaction. Arch Dermatol 1993;129:1594-1598.

59. Gluckman SJ: *Mycobacterium marinum*. Clin Dermatol 1995;13:273-276.

60. Sastry V, Brennan PJ: Cutaneous infections with rapidly growing mycobacteria. Clin Dermatol 1995;13:266-271.

61. von Reyn CF, Barber TW, Arbeit RD, et al: Evidence of previous infection with *Mycobacterium avium-Mycobacterium intracellulare* complex among healthy subjects: An international study of dominant mycobacterial skin test reactions. J Infect Dis 1993;168:1553-1558.

62. Zanelli G, Webster GF: Mucocutaneous atypical mycobacterial infections in acquired immunodeficiency syndrome. Clin Dermatol 1995;13:281-288.

63. Santa Cruz DJ, Strayer DS: The histologic spectrum of the cutaneous mycobacterioses. Hum Pathol 1982;13:485-495.

64. Inwald D, Nelson M, Cramp M, et al: Cutaneous manifestations of mycobacterial infection in patients with AIDS. Br J Dermatol 1994;130:111-114.

65. Kennedy C, Lien RA, Stolz E, et al: Leprosy and human immunodeficiency virus infection: A closer look at the lesions. Int J Dermatol 1990;29:139-140.

66. Hanke CW, Temofeew RK, Slama SL: *Mycobacterium kansasii* infection with multiple cutaneous lesions. J Am Acad Dermatol 1987;16(5 Pt 2):1122-1128.

67. Owens DW, McBride ME: Sporotrichoid cutaneous infection with *Mycobacterium kansasii*. Arch Dermatol 1969;100:54-58.

68. Saxe N: Mycobacterial skin infections. J Cutan Pathol 1985;12:300-312.

69. Barbaro DJ, Orcutt VL, Coldiron BM: *Mycobacterium avium-Mycobacterium intracellulare* infection limited to the skin and lymph nodes in patients with AIDS. Rev Infect Dis 1989;11:625-628.

70. Cole GW, Gebhard J: *Mycobacterium avium* infection of the skin resembling lepromatous leprosy. Br J Dermatol 1979;101:71-74.

71. Huminer D, Pitlik SD, Block C, et al: Aquarium-borne *Mycobacterium marinum* skin infection: Report of a case and review of the literature. Arch Dermatol 1986;122:698-703.

72. Philpott JA Jr, Woodburne AR, Philpott OS, et al: Swimming pool granuloma: A study of 290 cases. Arch Dermatol 1963;88:158-162.

73. Dickey RF: Sporotrichoid mycobacteriosis caused by *M. marinum (balnei)*. Arch Dermatol 1968;98:385-391.

74. Travis WD, Travis LB, Roberts GD, et al: The histopathologic spectrum in *Mycobacterium marinum* infection. Arch Pathol Lab Med 1985;109:1109-1113.

75. van der Werf TS, Stinear T, Stienstra Y, et al: Mycolactones and *Mycobacterium ulcerans* disease. Lancet 2003;362:1062-1064.

76. Hayman J: Out of Africa: Observations on the histopathology of *Mycobacterium ulcerans* infection. J Clin Pathol 1993;46:5-9.

77. Marston BJ, Diallo MO, Horsburgh CR Jr, et al: Emergence of Buruli ulcer disease in the Daloa region of Cote d'Ivoire. Am J Trop Med Hyg 1995;52:219-224.

78. Uganda Buruli Group: Clinical features and treatment of pre-ulcerative Buruli lesions (*Mycobacterium ulcerans* infection): Report II of the Uganda Buruli Group. BMJ 1970;2:390-393.

79. Hayman J, McQueen A: The pathology of *Mycobacterium ulcerans* infection. Pathology 1985;17:594-600.

80. Torrado E, Adusumilli S, Fraga AG, et al: Mycolactone-mediated inhibition of tumor necrosis factor production by macrophages infected with *Mycobacterium ulcerans* has implications for the control of infection. Infect Immun 2007;75:3979-3988.

81. Schipper HS, Rutgers B, Huitema MG, et al: Systemic and local interferon-gamma production following *Mycobacterium ulcerans* infection. Clin Exp Immunol 2007;150:451-459.

82. Gable AD, Marsee DK, Milner DA, et al: Suppurative inflammation with microabscess and pseudocyst formation is a characteristic histologic manifestation of cutaneous infections with rapid-growing *Mycobacterium* species. Am J Clin Pathol 2008;130:514-517.

83. Britton WJ, Lockwood DN: Leprosy. Lancet 2004;363:1209-1219.

84. Abide JM, Webb RM, Jones HL, Young L: Three indigenous cases of leprosy in the Mississippi delta. South Med J 2008;101:635-638.

85. Taylor JP, Vitek I, Enriquez V, Smedley JW: A continuing focus of Hansen's disease in Texas. Am J Trop Med Hyg 1999;60:449-452.

86. Truman R: Leprosy in wild armadillos. Lepr Rev 2005;76:198-208.

87. Lane JE, Meyers WM, Walsh DS: Armadillos as a source of leprosy infection in the Southeast. South Med J 2009;102:113-114.

88. Mattila JO, Katila ML, Vornanen M: Slowly growing mycobacteria and chronic skin disorders. Clin Infect Dis 1996;23:1043-1048.

89. Nadkarni NS, Rege VL: Significance of histopathological classification in leprosy. Indian J Lepr 1999;71:325-332.

90. Cree IA, Coghill G, Subedi AM, et al: Effects of treatment on the histopathology of leprosy. J Clin Pathol 1995;48:304-307.

91. Job CK: Pathology of leprosy. In Hasting RC (ed): Leprosy. Edinburgh, Churchill Livingstone, 1994, p 193.

92. Rea TH, Ridley DS: Lucio's phenomenon: A comparative histological study. Int J Lepr Other Mycobact Dis 1979;47:161-166.

93. Pönnighaus JM: Diagnosis and management of single lesions in leprosy. Lepr Rev 1996;67:89-94.

94. Hussain R, Lucas SB, Kifayet A, et al: Clinical and histological discrepancies in diagnosis of ENL reactions classified by assessment of acute phase proteins SAA and CRP. Int J Lepr Other Mycobact Dis 1995;63:222-230.

95. Ottenhoff TH: Immunology of leprosy: Lessons from and for leprosy. Int J Lepr Other Mycobact Dis 1994;62:108-121.

96. Choudhuri K: The immunology of leprosy: Unravelling an enigma. Int J Lepr Other Mycobact Dis 1995;63:430-447.

97. Ridley MJ, Ridley DS: The immunopathology of erythema nodosum leprosum: The role of extravascular complexes. Lepr Rev 1983;54:95-107.

98. Lew D: *Bacillus anthracis*: Anthrax. In Mandell GL, Bennet JE, Dolin R (eds): Principles and Practice of Infectious Disease. New York, Churchill Livingstone, 1996, p 1885.

99. Burnett JW: Brucellosis. Cutis 1995;56:28.

100. Zuckerman E, Naschitz JE, Yeshurun D, et al: Fasciitis-panniculitis in acute brucellosis. Int J Dermatol 1994;33:57-59.

101. Walker DH, Barbour AG, Oliver JH, et al: Emerging bacterial zoonotic and vector-borne diseases: Ecological and epidemiological factors. JAMA 1996;275:463-469.

102. Ikeya T, Mizuno E, Takama H: Three cases of erythema nodosum associated with *Yersinia enterocolitica* infection. J Dermatol 1986;13:147-150.

103. Butler T: *Yersinia* infections: Centennial of the discovery of the plague bacillus. Clin Infect Dis 1994;19:655-661; quiz 662-663.

104. Straley SC, Skrzypek E, Plano GV, Bliska JB: Yops of *Yersinia* spp. pathogenic for humans. Infect Immun 1993;61:3105-3110.

105. Joseph AK, Rosen T: Laboratory techniques used in the diagnosis of chancroid, granuloma inguinale, and lymphogranuloma venereum. Dermatol Clin 1994;12:1-8.

106. Hart CA, Rao SK: Donovanosis. J Med Microbiol 1999;48:707-709.

107. Carter J, Hutton S, Sriprakash KS, et al: Culture of the causative organism of donovanosis (*Calymmatobacterium granulomatis*) in HEp-2 cells. J Clin Microbiol 1997;35:2915-2917.

108. King R, Gough J, Ronald A, et al: An immunohistochemical analysis of naturally occurring chancroid. J Infect Dis 1996;174:427-430.

109. Batsakis JG, el-Naggar AK: Rhinoscleroma and rhinosporidiosis. Ann Otol Rhinol Laryngol 1992;101:879-882.

110. Hart CA, Rao SK: Rhinoscleroma. J Med Microbiol 2000;49:395-396.

111. Kodama BF, Fitzpatrick JE, Gentry RH: Tularemia. Cutis 1994;54:279-280.

112. Senol M, Ozcan A, Karincaoglu Y, et al: Tularemia: A case transmitted from a sheep. Cutis 1999;63:49-51.

113. Jacobs RF: Tularemia. Adv Pediatr Infect Dis 1996;12:55-69.

114. Johansson A, Berglund L, Eriksson U, et al: Comparative analysis of PCR versus culture for diagnosis of ulceroglandular tularemia. J Clin Microbiol 2000;38:22-26.

115. Dennis DT, Inglesby TV, Henderson DA, et al: Tularemia as a biological weapon: Medical and public health management. JAMA 2001;285:2763-2773.

116. Scott MA, McCurley TL, Vnencak-Jones CL, et al: Cat scratch disease: Detection of *Bartonella henselae* DNA in archival biopsies from patients with clinically, serologically, and histologically defined disease. Am J Pathol 1996;149:2161-2167.

117. Avidor B, Varon M, Marmor S, et al: DNA amplification for the diagnosis of cat-scratch disease in small-quantity clinical specimens. Am J Clin Pathol 2001;115:900-909.

118. Boyce S, Peña JR, Davis DA: An ulcerated nodule associated with lymphadenopathy. Arch Dermatol 1999;135:985, 988.

119. Wong R, Tappero J, Cockerell CJ: Bacillary angiomatosis and other *Bartonella* species infections. Semin Cutan Med Surg 1997;16:188-199.

120. Fagan WA, DeCamp NC, Kraus EW, Pulitzer DR: Widespread cutaneous bacillary angiomatosis and a large fungating mass in an HIV-positive man. J Am Acad Dermatol 1996;35(2 Pt 2):285-287.

121. Webster GF, Cockerell CJ, Friedman-Kien AE: The clinical spectrum of bacillary angiomatosis. Br J Dermatol 1992;126:535-541.

122. Plettenberg A, Lorenzen T, Burtsche BT, et al: Bacillary angiomatosis in HIV-infected patients: An epidemiological and clinical study. Dermatology 2000;201:326-331.

123. Schwartz RA, Nychay SG, Janniger CK, Lambert WC: Bacillary angiomatosis: Presentation of six patients, some with unusual features. Br J Dermatol 1997;136:60-65.

124. Smith KJ, Skelton HG, Tuur S, et al: Bacillary angiomatosis in an immunocompetent child. Am J Dermatopathol 1996;18:597-600.

125. Hoffman CF, Papadopoulos D, Palmer DM, et al: A case report of bacillary angiomatosis in a patient infected with human immunodeficiency virus. Cutis 2002;69:175-178.

126. Feldmann R, Breier F, Duschet P, et al: Cutaneous malakoplakia on the forehead. Dermatology 1997;194:358-360.

127. Wittenberg PG, Douglass MC, Azam M, et al: Cutaneous malacoplakia in a patient with the acquired immunodeficiency syndrome. Arch Dermatol 1998;134:244-245.

128. Kogulan PK, Smith M, Seidman J, et al: Malakoplakia involving the abdominal wall, urinary bladder, vagina, and vulva: Case report and discussion of malakoplakia-associated bacteria. Int J Gynecol Pathol 2001;20:403-406.

129. Satterwhite TK, Wallace RJ Jr: Primary cutaneous nocardiosis. JAMA 1979;242:333-336.

130. Singh SM, Rau NV, Cohen LB, Harris H: Cutaneous nocardiosis complicating management of Crohn's disease with infliximab and prednisone. Can Med Assoc J 2004;171:1063-1064.

131. Moeller CA, Burton CS 3rd: Primary lymphocutaneous *Nocardia brasiliensis* infection. Arch Dermatol 1986;122:1180-1182.

132. Callen JP, Kingman J: Disseminated cutaneous *Nocardia brasiliensis* infection. Pediatr Dermatol 1984;2:49-51.

133. Naka W, Miyakawa S, Niizeki H, et al: Unusually located lymphocutaneous nocardiosis caused by *Nocardia brasiliensis*. Br J Dermatol 1995;132:609-613.

134. Stefano PC, Noriega AL, Kobrin AL, et al: Primary cutaneous nocardiosis in immunocompetent children. Eur J Dermatol 2006;16:406-408.

135. Chedid MB, Chedid MF, Porto NS, et al: Nocardial infections: Report of 22 cases. Rev Inst Med Trop Sao Paulo 2007;49:239-246.

136. Curry WA: Human nocardiosis: A clinical review with selected case reports. Arch Intern Med 1980;140:818-826.

137. Lee MS, Sippe JR: Primary cutaneous nocardiosis. Australas J Dermatol 1999;40:103-105.

138. Wilson JP, Turner HR, Kirchner KA, Chapman SW: Nocardial infections in renal transplant recipients. Medicine (Baltimore) 1989;68:38-57.

139. Rapaport J: Primary chancriform syndrome caused by *Nocardia brasiliensis*. Arch Dermatol 1966;93:62-64.

140. Moore M, Conrad AH: Sporotrichoid nocardiosis caused by *Nocardia brasiliensis*. Arch Dermatol 1967;95:390-393.

141. Lampe RM, Baker CJ, Septimus EJ, Wallace RJ Jr: Cervicofacial nocardiosis in children. J Pediatr 1981;99:593-595.

142. Boixeda P, España A, Suarez J, et al: Cutaneous nocardiosis and human immunodeficiency virus infection. Int J Dermatol 1991;30:804-805.

143. Merigou D, Beylot-Barry M, Ly S, et al: Primary cutaneous *Nocardia asteroides* infection after heart transplantation. Dermatology 1998;196:246-247.

144. Chung YL, Park JC, Takatori K, Lee KH: Primary cutaneous nocardiosis mimicking lupus erythematosus. Br J Dermatol 2001;144:639-641.

145. Nishimoto K, Ohno M: Subcutaneous abscesses caused by *Nocardia brasiliensis* complicated by malignant lymphoma: A survey of cutaneous nocardiosis reported in Japan. Int J Dermatol 1985;24:437-440.

146. Schreiner DT, de Castro P, Jorizzo JL, et al: Disseminated *Nocardia brasiliensis* infection following cryptococcal disease. Arch Dermatol 1986;122:1186-1190.

147. Boudoulas O, Camisa C: *Nocardia asteroides* infection with dissemination to skin and joints. Arch Dermatol 1985;121:898-900.

148. Hussein MR: Mucocutaneous Splendore-Hoeppli phenomenon. J Cutan Pathol 2008;35:979-988.

149. Patil D, Siddaramappa B, Manjunathswamy BS, et al: Primary cutaneous actinomycosis. Int J Dermatol 2008;47:1271-1273.

150. Wang YH, Tsai HC, Lee SS, et al: Clinical manifestations of actinomycosis in Southern Taiwan. J Microbiol Immunol Infect 2007;40:487-492.

151. Yeager BA, Hoxie J, Weisman RA, et al: Actinomycosis in the acquired immunodeficiency syndrome-related complex. Arch Otolaryngol Head Neck Surg 1986;112:1293-1295.

152. Brown JR: Human actinomycosis: A study of 181 subjects. Hum Pathol 1973;4:319-330.

153. Che Y, Tanioka M, Matsumura Y, et al: Primary cutaneous actinomycosis on the nose. Eur J Dermatol 2007;17:167-168.

154. Hacker P: Botryomycosis. Int J Dermatol 1983;22:455-458.

155. Mehregan DA, Su WP, Anhalt JP: Cutaneous botryomycosis. J Am Acad Dermatol 1991;24:393-396.

156. Bonifaz A, Carrasco E: Botryomycosis. Int J Dermatol 1996;35:381-388.

157. Follows GA, Mathew J, Lucas S, et al: Cutaneous botryomycosis in a patient with lupus nephritis. Nephrol Dial Transplant 1998;13:3200-3201.

158. Brunken RC, Lichon-Chao N, van der Broek H: Immunologic abnormalities in botryomycosis: A case report with review of the literature. J Am Acad Dermatol 1983;9:428-434.

159. Bishop GF, Greer KE, Horwitz DA: *Pseudomonas* botryomycosis. Arch Dermatol 1976;112:1568-1570.

160. Hoffman TE, Russell B, Jacobs PH: Mycetoma-like infection caused by previously undescribed bacterium. Arch Dermatol 1978;114:1199-1202.

161. Leibowitz MR, Asvat MS, Kalla AA, Wing G: Extensive botryomycosis in a patient with diabetes and chronic active hepatitis. Arch Dermatol 1981;117:739-742.

162. de Vries HJ, van Noesel CJ, Hoekzema R, Hulsebosch HJ: Botryomycosis in an HIV-positive subject. J Eur Acad Dermatol Venereol 2003;17:87-90.

163. Saadat P, Ram R, Sohrabian S, Vadmal MS: Botryomycosis caused by *Staphylococcus aureus* and *Pneumocystis carinii* in a patient with acquired immunodeficiency disease. Clin Exp Dermatol 2008;33:266-269.

164. Katznelsen D, Vawter GF, Foley GE, Shwachman H: Botryomycosis, a complication of cystic fibrosis: Report of 7 cases. J Pediatr 1964;65:525-539.

165. Green EG, Schwartz JN: Bacterial pseudomycosis (botryomycosis) in an otherwise normal child. South Med J 1984;77:396-399.

166. Crowson AN, Magro C, Mihm M Jr: Treponemal diseases. In Elder DE (ed): Lever's Histopathology of the Skin. Philadelphia, Lippincott Williams & Wilkins, 2009, pp 579-590.

167. Goette DK: Transepithelial elimination in botryomycosis. Int J Dermatol 1981;20:198-200.

168. Hook EW 3rd, Marra CM: Acquired syphilis in adults. N Engl J Med 1992;326:1060-1069.

169. Sparling PF: Natural history of syphilis. In Homes KK, Mardh P-A, Sparling PF, et al. (eds): Sexually Transmitted Diseases, 2nd ed. New York, McGraw-Hill, 1990, p 213.

170. Noppakun N, Dinehart SM, Solomon AR: Pustular secondary syphilis. Int J Dermatol 1987;26:112-114.

171. Stöckli HR: Neurosyphilis today. Dermatologica 1982;165:232-248.

172. Moskovitz BL, Klimek JJ, Goldman RL, et al: Meningovascular syphilis after "appropriate" treatment of primary syphilis. Arch Intern Med 1982;142:139-140.

173. Janier M, Pertuiset BF, Poisson M, et al: Early manifestations of neuromeningeal syphilis: Review of the literature apropos of 3 severe forms. Ann Dermatol Venereol 1985;112:133-140.

174. Sánchez PJ: Congenital syphilis. Adv Pediatr Infect Dis 1992;7:161-180.

175. Johnson PC, Farnie MA: Testing for syphilis. Dermatol Clin 1994;12:9-17.

176. Jeerapaet P, Ackerman AB: Histologic patterns of secondary syphilis. Arch Dermatol 1973;107:373-377.

177. Sykes JA, Miller JN, Kalan AJ: *Treponema pallidum* within cells of a primary chancre from a human female. Br J Vener Dis 1974;50:40-44.

178. Wecke J, Bartunek J, Stüttgen G: *Treponema pallidum* in early syphilitic lesions in humans during high-dosage penicillin therapy: An electron microscopical study. Arch Dermatol Res 1976;257:1-15.

179. Poulsen A, Kobayasi T, Secher L, Weismann K: *Treponema pallidum* in macular and papular secondary syphilitic skin eruptions. Acta Derm Venereol 1986;66:251-258.

180. Hartsock RJ, Halling LW, King FM: Luetic lymphadenitis: A clinical and histologic study of 20 cases. Am J Clin Pathol 1970;53:304-314.

181. Abell E, Marks R, Jones EW: Secondary syphilis: A clinico-pathological review. Br J Dermatol 1975;93:53-61.

182. Paterou M, Stavrianeas N, Civatte J, Capetanakis J: Histology of secondary syphilis. Ann Dermatol Venereol 1979;106:923-925.

183. Cochran RE, Thomson J, Fleming KA, Strong AM: Histology simulating reticulosis in secondary syphilis. Br J Dermatol 1976;95:251-254.

184. Fisher DA, Chang LW, Tuffanelli DL: Lues maligna: Presentation of a case and a review of the literature. Arch Dermatol 1969;99:70-73.

185. Degos R, Touraine R, Collart P, et al: Early malignant syphilis with a fatal course (anatomic examination). Bull Soc Fr Dermatol Syphiligr 1970;77:10-15.

186. Petrozzi JW, Lockshin NA, Berger BJ: Malignant syphilis: Severe variant of secondary syphilis. Arch Dermatol 1974;109:387-389.

187. Matsuda-John SS, McElgunn PS, Ellis CN: Nodular late syphilis. J Am Acad Dermatol 1983;9:269-272.

188. Noordhoek GT, Hermans PW, Paul AN, et al: *Treponema pallidum* subspecies *pallidum* (Nichols) and *Treponema pallidum* subspecies *pertenue* (CDC 2575) differ in at least one nucleotide: Comparison of two homologous antigens. Microb Pathog 1989;6:29-42.

189. Guderian RH, Guzman JR, Calvopiña M, Cooper P: Studies on a focus of yaws in the Santiago Basin, province of Esmeraldas, Ecuador. Trop Geogr Med 1991;43:142-147.

190. Hasselmann CM: Comparative studies on the histo-pathology of syphilis, yaws, and pinta. Br J Vener Dis 1957;33:5-12.

191. Green CA, Harman RR: Yaws truly: A survey of patients indexed under "yaws" and a review of the clinical and laboratory problems of diagnosis. Clin Exp Dermatol 1986;11:41-48.

192. Engelkens HJ, Niemel PL, van der Sluis JJ, et al: Endemic treponematoses: Part II. Pinta and endemic syphilis. Int J Dermatol 1991;30:231-238.

193. Pardo-Castello V, Ferrer I: Pinta. Arch Dermatol Syph 1942;45:843.

194. Rodriguez HA, Albores-Saavedra J, Magaña Lozano M, et al: Langerhans' cells in late pinta: Ultrastructural observations in one case. Arch Pathol 1971;91:302-306.

195. Steere AC, Grodzicki RL, Kornblatt AN, et al: The spirochetal etiology of Lyme disease. N Engl J Med 1983;308:733-740.

196. Duray PH: Histopathology of clinical phases of human Lyme disease. Rheum Dis Clin North Am 1989;15:691-710.

197. Abele DC, Anders KH: The many faces and phases of borreliosis: I. Lyme disease. J Am Acad Dermatol 1990;23(2 Pt 1):167-186.

198. Côté J: Lyme disease. Int J Dermatol 1991;30:500-501.

199. Sigal LH, Curran AS: Lyme disease: A multifocal worldwide epidemic. Annu Rev Public Health 1991;12:85-109.

200. Berger BW: Erythema chronicum migrans of Lyme disease. Arch Dermatol 1984;120:1017-1021.

201. Verweij PE, Meis JF, Eijk R, et al: Severe human psittacosis requiring artificial ventilation: Case report and review. Clin Infect Dis 1995;20:440-442.

202. Crosse BA: Psittacosis: A clinical review. J Infect 1990;21:251-259.

203. Grayston JT, Thom DH: The chlamydial pneumonias. Curr Clin Top Infect Dis 1991;11:1-18.

204. Green ST, Hamlet NW, Willocks L, et al: Psittacosis presenting with erythema-marginatum-like lesions: A case report and a historical review. Clin Exp Dermatol 1990;15:225-227.

205. Kellock DJ, Barlow R, Suvarna SK, et al: Lymphogranuloma venereum: Biopsy, serology, and molecular biology. Genitourin Med 1997;73:399-401.

206. Walker DH: Rickettsiae and rickettsial infections: The current state of knowledge. Clin Infect Dis 2007;45(Suppl 1):S39-S44.

207. Hechemy KE, Avsic-Zupanc T, Childs JE, Raoult DA: Rickettsiology: Present and future directions. Preface. Ann N Y Acad Sci 2003;990:xvii-xx.

208. Raoult D, Marrie T, Mege J: Natural history and pathophysiology of Q fever. Lancet Infect Dis 2005;5:219-226.

209. Tamura A, Ohashi N, Urakami H, Miyamura S: Classification of *Rickettsia tsutsugamushi* in a new genus, *Orientia* gen. nov., as *Orientia tsutsugamushi* comb. nov. Int J Syst Bacteriol 1995;45:589-591.

210. Walker DH, Fishbein DB: Epidemiology of rickettsial diseases. Eur J Epidemiol 1991;7:237-245.

211. Azad AF, Beard CB: Rickettsial pathogens and their arthropod vectors. Emerg Infect Dis 1998;4:179-186.

212. Dantas-Torres F: Rocky Mountain spotted fever. Lancet Infect Dis 2007;7:724-732.

213. Silber JL: Rocky Mountain spotted fever. Clin Dermatol 1996;14:245-258.

214. Lacz NL, Schwartz RA, Kapila R: Rocky Mountain spotted fever. J Eur Acad Dermatol Venereol 2006;20:411-417.

215. Helmick CG, Bernard KW, D'Angelo LJ: Rocky Mountain spotted fever: Clinical, laboratory, and epidemiological features of 262 cases. J Infect Dis 1984;150:480-488.

216. Ramos-e-Silva M, Pereira AL: Life-threatening eruptions due to infectious agents. Clin Dermatol 2005;23:148-156.

217. Kirkland KB, Marcom PK, Sexton DJ, et al: Rocky Mountain spotted fever complicated by gangrene: Report of six cases and review. Clin Infect Dis 1993;16:629-634.

218. Kaplan JE, Schonberger LB: The sensitivity of various serologic tests in the diagnosis of Rocky Mountain spotted fever. Am J Trop Med Hyg 1986;35:840-844.

219. Singh-Behl D, La Rosa SP, Tomecki KJ: Tick-borne infections. Dermatol Clin 2003;21:237-244, v.

220. Sexton DJ, Kaye KS: Rocky mountain spotted fever. Med Clin North Am 2002;86:351-360, vii-viii.

221. Parola P, Paddock CD, Raoult D: Tick-borne rickettsioses around the world: Emerging diseases challenging old concepts. Clin Microbiol Rev 2005;18:719-756.

222. Eremeeva ME, Dasch GA, Silverman DJ: Evaluation of a PCR assay for quantitation of *Rickettsia rickettsii* and closely related spotted fever group rickettsiae. J Clin Microbiol 2003;41:5466-5472.

223. Kao GF, Evancho CD, Ioffe O, et al: Cutaneous histopathology of Rocky Mountain spotted fever. J Cutan Pathol 1997;24:604-610.

224. Procop GW, Burchette JL Jr, Howell DN, Sexton DJ: Immunoperoxidase and immunofluorescent staining of *Rickettsia rickettsii* in skin biopsies: A comparative study. Arch Pathol Lab Med 1997;121:894-899.

225. Rovery C, Raoult D: Mediterranean spotted fever. Infect Dis Clin North Am 2008;22:515-530, ix.

226. Jensenius M, Fournier PE, Kelly P, et al: African tick bite fever. Lancet Infect Dis 2003;3:557-564.

227. Raoult D, Woodward T, Dumler JS: The history of epidemic typhus. Infect Dis Clin North Am 2004;18:127-140.

228. Bechah Y, Capo C, Mege JL, Raoult D: Epidemic typhus. Lancet Infect Dis 2008;8:417-426.

229. Raoult D, Ndihokubwayo JB, Tissot-Dupont H, et al: Outbreak of epidemic typhus associated with trench fever in Burundi. Lancet 1998;352:353-358.

230. Green CR, Fishbein D, Gleiberman I: Brill-Zinsser: Still with us. JAMA 1990;264:1811-1812.

231. Jeong YJ, Kim S, Wook YD, et al: Scrub typhus: Clinical, pathologic, and imaging findings. Radiographics 2007;27:161-172.

232. Kim DM, Won KJ, Park CY, et al: Distribution of eschars on the body of scrub typhus patients: A prospective study. Am J Trop Med Hyg 2007;76:806-809.

233. Kim DM, Lim SC, Won KJ, et al: Severe scrub typhus confirmed early via immunohistochemical staining. Am J Trop Med Hyg 2007;77:719-722.

234. Maurin M, Raoult D: Q fever. Clin Microbiol Rev 1999;12:518-553.

235. Madariaga MG, Rezai K, Trenholme GM, Weinstein RA: Q fever: A biological weapon in your backyard. Lancet Infect Dis 2003;3:709-721.

236. Fishbein DB, Raoult D: A cluster of *Coxiella burnetii* infections associated with exposure to vaccinated goats and their unpasteurized dairy products. Am J Trop Med Hyg 1992;47:35-40.

237. Maltezou HC, Raoult D: Q fever in children. Lancet Infect Dis 2002;2:686-691.

238. La Scola B, Raoult D: Survival of *Coxiella burnetii* within free-living amoeba *Acanthamoeba castellanii*. Clin Microbiol Infect 2001;7:75-79.

239. Raoult D, Tissot-Dupont H, Foucault C, et al: Q fever, 1985-1998: Clinical and epidemiologic features of 1,383 infections. Medicine (Baltimore) 2000;79:109-123.

240. Boele van Hensbroek M, de Vries E, Dolan G, Schneeberger P: Rash and petechiae as presenting signs of Q fever. Pediatr Infect Dis J 2000;19:358.

241. Xu X, Erickson L, Chen L, Elder DE: Diseases caused by viruses. Elder DE (ed): Lever's Histopathology of the Skin. Philadelphia, Lippincott Williams & Wilkins, 2009, pp 637-666.

242. Jenkins D: Diagnosing human papillomaviruses: Recent advances. Curr Opin Infect Dis 2001;14:53-62.

243. Mork J, Lie AK, Glattre E, et al: Human papillomavirus infection as a risk factor for squamous-cell carcinoma of the head and neck. N Engl J Med 2001;344:1125-1131.

244. Astori G, Merluzzi S, Arzese A, et al: Detection of human papillomavirus DNA and p53 gene mutations in esophageal cancer samples and adjacent normal mucosa. Digestion 2001;64:9-14.

245. Syrjänen KJ: HPV infections and lung cancer. J Clin Pathol 2002;55:885-891.

246. Jenson AB, Geyer S, Sundberg JP, Ghim S: Human papillomavirus and skin cancer. J Investig Dermatol Symp Proc 2001;6:203-206.

247. Meyer T, Arndt R, Nindl I, et al: Association of human papillomavirus infections with cutaneous tumors in immunosuppressed patients. Transpl Int 2003;16:146-153.

248. Rock B, Shah KV, Farmer ER: A morphologic, pathologic, and virologic study of anogenital warts in men. Arch Dermatol 1992;128:495-500.

249. Pereira de Oliveira WR, Carrasco S, Neto CF, et al: Nonspecific cell-mediated immunity in patients with epidermodysplasia verruciformis. J Dermatol 2003;30:203-209.

250. Berger TG, Sawchuk WS, Leonardi C, et al: Epidermodysplasia verruciformis-associated papillomavirus infection complicating human immunodeficiency virus disease. Br J Dermatol 1991;124:79-83.

251. Tieben LM, Berkhout RJ, Smits HL, et al: Detection of epidermodysplasia verruciformis-like human papillomavirus types in malignant and premalignant skin lesions of renal transplant recipients. Br J Dermatol 1994;131:226-230.

252. Morrison C, Eliezri Y, Magro C, Nuovo GJ: The histologic spectrum of epidermodysplasia verruciformis in transplant and AIDS patients. J Cutan Pathol 2002;29:480-489.

253. Muñoz N: Human papillomavirus and cancer: The epidemiological evidence. J Clin Virol 2000;19:1-5.

254. Nobbenhuis MA, Helmerhorst TJ, van den Brule AJ, et al: Cytological regression and clearance of high-risk human papillomavirus in women with an abnormal cervical smear. Lancet 2001;358:1782-1783.

255. Bai H, Cviko A, Granter S, et al: Immunophenotypic and viral (human papillomavirus) correlates of vulvar seborrheic keratosis. Hum Pathol 2003;34:559-564.

256. Della Torre G, Donghi R, Longoni A, et al: HPV DNA in intraepithelial neoplasia and carcinoma of the vulva and penis. Diagn Mol Pathol 1992;1:25-30.

257. Münger K, Howley PM: Human papillomavirus immortalization and transformation functions. Virus Res 2002;89:213-228.

258. Nahmias AJ, Lee FK, Beckman-Nahmias S: Sero-epidemiological and -sociological patterns of herpes simplex virus infection in the world. Scand J Infect Dis Suppl 1990;69:19-36.

259. Kohl S: Neonatal herpes simplex virus infection. Clin Perinatol 1997;24:129-150.

260. Whitley RJ, Roizman B: Herpes simplex virus infections. Lancet 2001;357:1513-1518.

261. Mackley CL, Adams DR, Anderson B, Miller JJ: Eczema herpeticum: A dermatologic emergency. Dermatol Nurs 2002;14:307-310, 323; quiz 313.

262. Yeung-Yue KA, Brentjens MH, Lee PC, Tyring SK: Herpes simplex viruses 1 and 2. Dermatol Clin 2002;20:249-266.

263. Jang KA, Kim SH, Choi JH, et al: Viral folliculitis on the face. Br J Dermatol 2000;142:555-559.

264. Giacobetti R: Herpetic whitlow. Int J Dermatol 1979;18:55-58.

265. Ritterband DC, Friedberg DN: Virus infections of the eye. Rev Med Virol 1998;8:187-201.

266. Prober CG, Hensleigh PA, Boucher FD, et al: Use of routine viral cultures at delivery to identify neonates exposed to herpes simplex virus. N Engl J Med 1988;318:887-891.

267. Salvini F, Carminati G, Pinzani R, et al: Chronic ulcerative herpes simplex virus infection in HIV-infected children. AIDS Patient Care STDS 1997;11:421-428.

268. Lopyan L, Young AW Jr, Menegus M: Generalized acute mucocutaneous herpes simplex type 2 with fatal outcome. Arch Dermatol 1977;113:816-818.

269. Weinberg JM, Mysliwiec A, Turiansky GW, et al: Viral folliculitis: Atypical presentations of herpes simplex, herpes zoster, and molluscum contagiosum. Arch Dermatol 1997;133:983-986.

270. Preblud SR: Varicella: Complications and costs. Pediatrics 1986;78(4 Pt 2):728-735.

271. Meythaler JM, Varma RR: Reye's syndrome in adults: Diagnostic considerations. Arch Intern Med 1987;147:61-64.

272. Pastuszak AL, Levy M, Schick B, et al: Outcome after maternal varicella infection in the first 20 weeks of pregnancy. N Engl J Med 1994;330:901-905.

273. Gnann JW Jr: Varicella-zoster virus: Atypical presentations and unusual complications. J Infect Dis 2002;186(Suppl 1):S91-S98.

274. Schmader K: Herpes zoster and postherpetic neuralgia in older adults. Clin Geriatr Med 2007;23:615-632, vii-viii.

275. Garman ME, Tyring SK: The cutaneous manifestations of HIV infection. Dermatol Clin 2002;20:193-208.

276. Al-Abdulla NA, Rismondo V, Minkowski JS, Miller NR: Herpes zoster vasculitis presenting as giant cell arteritis with bilateral internuclear ophthalmoplegia. Am J Ophthalmol 2002;134:912-914.

277. Nikkels AF, Debrus S, Sadzot-Delvaux C, et al: Comparative immunohistochemical study of herpes simplex and varicella-zoster infections. Virchows Arch A Pathol Anat Histopathol 1993;422:121-126.

278. Khoshnevis M, Tyring SK: Cytomegalovirus infections. Dermatol Clin 2002;20:291-299, vii.

279. Vancíková Z, Dvorák P: Cytomegalovirus infection in immunocompetent and immunocompromised individuals: A review. Curr Drug Targets Immune Endocr Metabol Disord 2001;1:179-187.

280. Stegmann BJ, Carey JC: TORCH infections: Toxoplasmosis, other (syphilis, varicella-zoster, parvovirus B19), rubella, cytomegalovirus (CMV), and herpes infections. Curr Womens Health Rep 2002;2:253-258.

281. Iwatsuki K, Xu Z, Ohtsuka M, Kaneko F: Cutaneous lymphoproliferative disorders associated with Epstein-Barr virus infection: A clinical overview. J Dermatol Sci 2000;22:181-195.

282. Steven NM: Epstein-Barr virus latent infection in vivo. Rev Med Virol 1997;7:97-106.

283. Cohen JL: Epstein-Barr virus infection. In Freedberg I, Eisen A, Wolff K, et al. (eds): Fitzpatrick's Dermatology in Internal Medicine, 5th ed. New York, McGraw Hill, 1999, p 2458.

284. Ikediobi NI, Tyring SK: Cutaneous manifestations of Epstein-Barr virus infection. Dermatol Clin 2002;20:283-289.

285. Su IJ, Tsai TF, Cheng AL, Chen CC: Cutaneous manifestations of Epstein-Barr virus-associated T-cell lymphoma. J Am Acad Dermatol 1993;29(5 Pt 1):685-692.

286. De Araujo T, Berman B, Weinstein A: Human herpesviruses 6 and 7. Dermatol Clin 2002;20:301-306.

287. Ranger-Rogez S, Venot C, Denis F: Human herpesviruses 6 and 7 (HHV-6 and HHV-7). Rev Prat 1999;49:2227-2231.

288. Ruzicka T, Kalka K, Diercks K, Schuppe HC: Papular-purpuric "gloves and socks" syndrome associated with human herpesvirus 6 infection. Arch Dermatol 1998;134:242-244.

289. Yasumoto S, Tsujita J, Imayama S, Hori Y: Case report: Gianotti-Crosti syndrome associated with human herpesvirus-6 infection. J Dermatol 1996;23:499-501.

290. Hengge UR, Ruzicka T, Tyring SK, et al: Update on Kaposi's sarcoma and other HHV8 associated diseases. Part 2: Pathogenesis, Castleman's disease, and pleural effusion lymphoma. Lancet Infect Dis 2002;2:344-352.

291. Slifka MK, Hanifin JM: Smallpox: The basics. Dermatol Clin 2004;22:263-274, vi.

292. Frey SE, Belshe RB: Poxvirus zoonoses: Putting pocks into context. N Engl J Med 2004;350:324-327.

293. Ryan CP: Zoonoses likely to be used in bioterrorism. Public Health Rep 2008;123:276-281.

294. Smith GL, McFadden G: Smallpox: Anything to declare? Nat Rev Immunol 2002;2:521-527.

295. Fenner F, Henderson DA, Arita I, et al: Smallpox and its eradication. In World Health Organization: The Pathogenesis, Immunology, and Pathology of Smallpox and Vaccinia. Geneva, WHO, 1988.

296. Nishiura H, Kashiwagi T: Smallpox and season: Reanalysis of historical data. Interdiscip Perspect Infect Dis 2009;2009:591935. Epub 2009 Jan 4.

297. Breman JG, Henderson DA: Diagnosis and management of smallpox. N Engl J Med 2002;346:1300-1308.

298. Greenberg RN, Kennedy JS: ACAM2000: A newly licensed cell culture-based live vaccinia smallpox vaccine. Expert Opin Investig Drugs 2008;17:555-564.

299. Martin DB: The cause of death in smallpox: An examination of the pathology record. Mil Med 2002;167:546-551.

300. Rosengard AM, Liu Y, Nie Z, Jimenez R: Variola virus immune evasion design: Expression of a highly efficient inhibitor of human complement. Proc Natl Acad Sci U S A 2002;99:8808-8813.

301. Aragón TJ, Ulrich S, Fernyak S, Rutherford GW: Risks of serious complications and death from smallpox vaccination: A systematic review of the United States experience, 1963-1968. BMC Public Health 2003;3:26.

302. Wills VL, Boorer CJ, Foster HM, et al: Vaccinia necrosum: A forgotten disease. Aust N Z J Surg. 2000;70:149-150.

303. Damaso CR, Esposito JJ, Condit RC, Moussatché N: An emergent poxvirus from humans and cattle in Rio de Janeiro State: Cantagalo virus may derive from Brazilian smallpox vaccine. Virology 2000;277:439-449.

304. Nagasse-Sugahara TK, Kisielius JJ, Ueda-Ito M, et al: Human vaccinia-like virus outbreaks in São Paulo and Goiás States, Brazil: Virus detection, isolation and identification. Rev Inst Med Trop Sao Paulo 2004;46:315-322.

305. de Souza Trindade G, Drumond BP, Guedes MI, et al: Zoonotic vaccinia virus infection in Brazil: Clinical description and implications for health professionals. J Clin Microbiol 2007;45:1370-1372.

306. Trindade GS, Guedes MI, Drumond BP, et al: Zoonotic vaccinia virus: Clinical and immunological characteristics in a naturally infected patient. Clin Infect Dis 2009;48:e37-e40.

307. Topciu V, Luca I, Moldovan E, et al: Transmission of vaccinia virus from vaccinated milkers to cattle. Virologie 1976;27:279-282.

308. MacNeil A, Reynolds MG, Damon IK: Risks associated with vaccinia virus in the laboratory. Virology 2009;385:1-4.

309. Coras B, Essbauer S, Pfeffer M, et al: Cowpox and a cat. Lancet 2005;365:446.

310. Chantrey J, Meyer H, Baxby D, et al: Cowpox: Reservoir hosts and geographic range. Epidemiol Infect 1999;122:455-460.

311. Bennett M, Baxby D: Cowpox in cats and man. Vet Q 1995;17(Suppl 1):S16.

312. Fenner F:The Florey lecture, 1983: Biological control, as exemplified by smallpox eradication and myxomatosis. Proc R Soc Lond B Biol Sci 1983;218:259-285.

313. Baxby D, Bennett M, Getty B: Human cowpox 1969-93: A review based on 54 cases. Br J Dermatol 1994;131:598-607.

314. Czerny CP, Zeller-Lue C, Eis-Hübinger AM, et al: Characterization of a cowpox-like orthopox virus which had caused a lethal infection in man. Arch Virol Suppl 1997;13:13-24.

315. Blackford S, Roberts DL, Thomas PD: Cowpox infection causing a generalized eruption in a patient with atopic dermatitis. Br J Dermatol 1993;129:628-629.

316. Vorou RM, Papavassiliou VG, Pierroutsakos IN: Cowpox virus infection: An emerging health threat. Curr Opin Infect Dis 2008;21:153-156.

317. Pahlitzsch R, Hammarin AL, Widell A: A case of facial cellulitis and necrotizing lymphadenitis due to cowpox virus infection. Clin Infect Dis 2006;43:737-742.

318. Nitsche A, Pauli G: Sporadic human cases of cowpox in Germany. Euro Surveill 2007;12:E070419.3.

319. Wolfs TF, Wagenaar JA, Niesters HG, Osterhaus AD: Rat-to-human transmission of cowpox infection. Emerg Infect Dis 2002;8:1495-1496.

320. Pelkonen PM, Tarvainen K: Cowpox with severe generalized eruption, Finland. Emerg Infect Dis 2003;9:1458-1461.

321. Byun M, Wang X, Pak M, et al: Cowpox virus exploits the endoplasmic reticulum retention pathway to inhibit MHC class I transport to the cell surface. Cell Host Microbe 2007;2:306-315.

322. Levine RS, Peterson AT, Yorita KL, et al: Ecological niche and geographic distribution of human monkeypox in Africa. PLoS ONE 2007;2:e176.

323. World Health Organization: The global eradication of smallpox: Final report of the Global Commission for the Certification of Smallpox Eradication. Geneva, World Health Organization, 1980.

324. Gispen R: Relevance of some poxvirus infections in monkeys to smallpox eradication. Trans R Soc Trop Med Hyg 1975;69:299-302.

325. Di Giulio DB, Eckburg PB: Human monkeypox: An emerging zoonosis. Lancet Infect Dis 2004;4:15-25.

326. Reynolds MG, Yorita KL, Kuehnert MJ, et al: Clinical manifestations of human monkeypox influenced by route of infection. J Infect Dis 2006;194:773-780.

327. Fleischauer AT, Kile JC, Davidson M, et al: Evaluation of human-to-human transmission of monkeypox from infected patients to health care workers. Clin Infect Dis 2005;40:689-694.

328. Hammarlund E, Dasgupta A, Pinilla C, et al: Monkeypox virus evades antiviral CD4+ and CD8+ T cell responses by suppressing cognate T cell activation. Proc Natl Acad Sci U S A. 2008; 105:14567-11472.

329. Reed KD, Melski JW, Graham MB, et al: The detection of monkeypox in humans in the Western Hemisphere. N Engl J Med 2004;350:342-350.

330. Breman JG, Kalisa-Ruti, Steniowski MV, et al: Human monkeypox, 1970-1979. Bull World Health Organ 1980;58:165-182.

331. Jezek Z, Marennikova SS, Mutumbo M, et al: Human monkeypox: A study of 2,510 contacts of 214 patients. J Infect Dis 1986;154:551-555.

332. Jezek Z, Szczeniowski M, Paluku KM, Mutombo M: Human monkeypox: Clinical features of 282 patients. J Infect Dis 1987;156:293-298.

333. Stagles MJ, Watson AA, Boyd JF, et al: The histopathology and electron microscopy of a human monkeypox lesion. Trans R Soc Trop Med Hyg 1985;79:192-202.

334. Netherton C, Moffat K, Brooks E, Wileman T: A guide to viral inclusions, membrane rearrangements, factories, and viroplasm produced during virus replication. Adv Virus Res 2007;70:101-182.

335. Lawn SD, Holwill S: Type A intracytoplasmic inclusions in human cowpox infection. J Clin Pathol 2004;57:670-671.

336. Meyer H, Damon IK, Esposito JJ: Orthopoxvirus diagnostics. Methods Mol Biol 2004;269:119-134.

337. Putkuri N, Piiparinen H, Vaheri A, Vapalahti O: Detection of human orthopoxvirus infections and differentiation of smallpox virus with real-time PCR. J Med Virol 2009;81:146-152.

338. Leavell UW Jr, Chipps HD: Milker's nodules: Presentation of three cases. J Ky Med Assoc 1962;60:362-363.

339. Leavell UW Jr, Phillips IA: Milker's nodules: Pathogenesis, tissue culture, electron microscopy, and calf inoculation. Arch Dermatol 1975;111:1307-1311.

340. Schuler G, Hönigsmann H, Wolff K: The syndrome of milker's nodules in burn injury: Evidence for indirect viral transmission. J Am Acad Dermatol 1982;6:334-339.

341. Groves RW, Wilson-Jones E, MacDonald DM: Human orf and milkers' nodule: A clinicopathologic study. J Am Acad Dermatol 1991;25:706-711.

342. Evins S, Leavell UW Jr, Phillips IA: Intranuclear inclusions in milker's nodules. Arch Dermatol 1971;103:91-93.

343. Leavell UW Jr, McNamara MJ, Meulling R, et al: Orf: Report of 19 human cases with clinical and pathological observations. JAMA 1968;204:657-664.

344. Johannessen JV, Krogh HK, Solberg I, et al: Human orf. J Cutan Pathol 1975;2:265-283.

345. Rees J, Marks JM: Two unusual cases of orf following trauma to the scalp. Br J Dermatol 1988;118:445-447.

346. Kahn D, Hutchinson EA: Generalized bullous orf. Int J Dermatol 1980;19:340-341.

347. Murphy JK, Ralfs IG: Bullous pemphigoid complicating human orf. Br J Dermatol 1996;134:929-930.

348. Macfarlane AW: Human orf complicated by bullous pemphigoid. Br J Dermatol 1997;137:656-657.

349. Sanchez RL, Hebert A, Lucia H, Swedo J: Orf: A case report with histologic, electron microscopic, and immunoperoxidase studies. Arch Pathol Lab Med 1985;109:166-170.

350. Mayet A, Sommer B, Heenan P: Rapidly growing cutaneous tumour of the right temple: Orf. Australas J Dermatol 1997;38:217-219.

351. Davis CM, Musil G, Trochet JA: Electron microscopy for the rapid diagnosis of pseudocowpox and milker's nodule. Am J Vet Res 1970;31:1497-1503.

352. Gill MJ, Arlette J, Buchan KA, Barber K: Human orf: A diagnostic consideration? Arch Dermatol 1990;126:356-358.

353. Waugh MA: Molluscum contagiosum. Dermatol Clin 1998;16:839-841, xv.

354. Connell CO, Oranje A, Van Gysel D, Silverberg NB: Congenital molluscum contagiosum: Report of four cases and review of the literature. Pediatr Dermatol 2008;25:553-556.

355. Gur I: The epidemiology of molluscum contagiosum in HIV-seropositive patients: A unique entity or insignificant finding? Int J STD AIDS 2008;19:503-506.

356. Schwartz JJ, Myskowski PL: Molluscum contagiosum in patients with human immunodeficiency virus infection: A review of twenty-seven patients. J Am Acad Dermatol 1992;27:583-588.

357. Smith KJ, Yeager J, Skelton H: Molluscum contagiosum: Its clinical, histopathologic, and immunohistochemical spectrum. Int J Dermatol 1999;38:664-672.

358. Lynch PJ, Minkin W: Molluscum contagiosum of the adult: Probable venereal transmission. Arch Dermatol 1968;98:141-143.

359. Pauly CR, Artis WM, Jones HE: Atopic dermatitis, impaired cellular immunity, and molluscum contagiosum. Arch Dermatol 1978;114:391-393.

360. Ghura HS, Camp RD: Scarring molluscum contagiosum in patients with severe atopic dermatitis: Report of two cases. Br J Dermatol 2001;144:1094-1095.

361. Toro JR, Wood LV, Patel NK, Turner ML: Topical cidofovir: A novel treatment for recalcitrant molluscum contagiosum in children infected with human immunodeficiency virus 1. Arch Dermatol 2000;136:983-985.

362. Baxter KF, Highet AS: Topical cidofovir and cryotherapy: Combination treatment for recalcitrant molluscum contagiosum in a patient with HIV infection. J Eur Acad Dermatol Venereol 2004;18:230-231.

363. Ramdial PK, Calonje E, Sing Y, et al: Molluscum-like cutaneous cryptococcosis: A histopathological and pathogenetic appraisal. J Cutan Pathol 2008;35:1007-1013.

364. Cribier B, Scrivener Y, Grosshans E: Molluscum contagiosum: Histologic patterns and associated lesions—A study of 578 cases. Am J Dermatopathol 2001;23:99-103.

365. Lee S, Park J, Kim D, Na G: Flame figures in molluscum contagiosum. Am J Dermatopathol 2004;26:441-442.

366. Moreno-Ramírez D, García-Escudero A, Ríos-Martín JJ, et al: Cutaneous pseudolymphoma in association with molluscum contagiosum in an elderly patient. J Cutan Pathol 2003;30:473-475.

367. Fields JP, Mihm MC Jr, Hellreich PD, Danoff SS: Hand, foot, and mouth disease. Arch Dermatol 1969;99:243-246.

368. Tai WC, Hsieh HJ, Wu MT: Hand, foot and mouth disease in a healthy adult caused by intrafamilial transmission of enterovirus 71. Br J Dermatol 2009;160:890-892.

369. Ho M, Chen ER, Hsu KH, et al: An epidemic of enterovirus 71 infection in Taiwan. Taiwan Enterovirus Epidemic Working Group. N Engl J Med 1999;341:929-935.

370. Chang LY, Tsao KC, Hsia SH, et al: Transmission and clinical features of enterovirus 71 infections in household contacts in Taiwan. JAMA 2004;291:222-227.

371. Zhang Y, Tan XJ, Wang HY, et al: An outbreak of hand, foot, and mouth disease associated with subgenotype C4 of human enterovirus 71 in Shandong, China. J Clin Virol 2009;44:262-267.

372. Chang LY, Lin TY, Huang YC, et al: Comparison of enterovirus 71 and coxsackie-virus A16 clinical illnesses during the Taiwan enterovirus epidemic, 1998. Pediatr Infect Dis J 1999;18:1092-1096.

373. Ishimaru Y, Nakano S, Yamaoka K, Takami S: Outbreaks of hand, foot, and mouth disease by enterovirus 71: High incidence of complication disorders of central nervous system. Arch Dis Child 1980;55:583-588.

374. Siegl G, Bates RC, Berns KI, et al: Characteristics and taxonomy of Parvoviridae. Intervirology 1985;23:61-73.

375. Cohen BJ, Buckley MM: The prevalence of antibody to human parvovirus B19 in England and Wales. J Med Microbiol 1988;25:151-153.

376. Huatuco EM, Durigon EL, Lebrun FL, et al: Seroprevalence of human parvovirus B19 in a suburban population in São Paulo, Brazil. Rev Saude Publica 2008;42:443-449.

377. Chorba T, Coccia P, Holman RC, et al: The role of parvovirus B19 in aplastic crisis and erythema infectiosum (fifth disease). J Infect Dis 1986;154:383-393.

378. Azzi A, Morfini M, Mannucci PM: The transfusion-associated transmission of parvovirus B19. Transfus Med Rev 1999;13:194-204.

379. Gay NJ, Hesketh LM, Cohen BJ, et al: Age specific antibody prevalence to parvovirus B19: How many women are infected in pregnancy? Commun Dis Rep CDR Rev 1994;4:R104-R107.

380. Brown KE, Anderson SM, Young NS: Erythrocyte P antigen: Cellular receptor for B19 parvovirus. Science 1993;262:114-117.

381. Brown KE, Hibbs JR, Gallinella G, et al: Resistance to parvovirus B19 infection due to lack of virus receptor (erythrocyte P antigen). N Engl J Med 1994;330:1192-1196.

382. Brown KE, Young NS: Parvovirus B19 in human disease. Annu Rev Med 1997;48:59-67.

383. Moore TL: Parvovirus-associated arthritis. Curr Opin Rheumatol 2000;12:289-294.

384. Brown KE, Young NS: Human parvovirus B19 infections in infants and children. Adv Pediatr Infect Dis 1997;13:101-126.

385. Levy R, Weissman A, Blomberg G, Hagay ZJ: Infection by parvovirus B 19 during pregnancy: A review. Obstet Gynecol Surv 1997;52:254-259.

386. Saulsbury FT: Petechial gloves and socks syndrome caused by parvovirus B19. Pediatr Dermatol 1998;15:35-37.

387. Young NS, Brown KE: Parvovirus B19. N Engl J Med 2004;350:586-597.

388. Magro CM, Crowson AN, Dawood M, Nuovo GJ: Parvoviral infection of endothelial cells and its possible role in vasculitis and autoimmune diseases. J Rheumatol 2002;29:1227-1235.

389. Magro CM, Nuovo G, Ferri C, et al: Parvoviral infection of endothelial cells and stromal fibroblasts: A possible pathogenetic role in scleroderma. J Cutan Pathol 2004;31:43-50.

390. Crowson AN, Magro CM, Dawood MR: A causal role for parvovirus B19 infection in adult dermatomyositis and other autoimmune syndromes. J Cutan Pathol 2000;27:505-515.

391. Magro CM, Wusirika R, Frambach GE, et al: Autoimmune-like pulmonary disease in association with parvovirus B19: A clinical, morphologic, and molecular study of 12 cases. Appl Immunohistochem Mol Morphol 2006;14:208-216.

392. Veraldi S, Mancuso R, Rizzitelli G, et al: Henoch-Schönlein syndrome associated with human Parvovirus B19 primary infection. Eur J Dermatol 1999;9:232-233.

393. Aractingi S, Bakhos D, Flageul B, et al: Immunohistochemical and virological study of skin in the papular-purpuric gloves and socks syndrome. Br J Dermatol 1996;135:599-602.

394. Dwyer JM: Manipulating the immune system with immune globulin. N Engl J Med 1992;326:107-116.

395. Dyrsen ME, Iwenofu OH, Nuovo G, Magro CM: Parvovirus B19-associated catastrophic endothelialitis with a Degos-like presentation. J Cutan Pathol 2008;35(Suppl 1):20-25.

396. Takahashi M, Ito M, Sakamoto F, et al: Human parvovirus B19 infection: Immunohistochemical and electron microscopic studies of skin lesions. J Cutan Pathol 1995;22:168-172.

397. Magro CM, Dawood MR, Crowson AN: The cutaneous manifestations of human parvovirus B19 infection. Hum Pathol 2000;31:488-497.

398. Ackerman AB, Suringa DW: Multinucleate epidermal cells in measles. Arch Dermatol 1971;103:180-181 passim.

399. McNutt NS, Kindel S, Lugo J: Cutaneous manifestations of measles in AIDS. J Cutan Pathol 1992;19:315-324.

400. Yanagihara M, Fujii T, Mochizuki T, et al: Measles virus was present in the inner cell of the acrosyringium in the skin rash. Pediatr Dermatol 1998;15:456-458.

401. Alessi E, Cusini M: The exanthem of HIV-1 seroconversion syndrome. Int J Dermatol 1995;34:238-239.

402. Kinloch-de Loës S, de Saussure P, Saurat JH, et al: Symptomatic primary infection due to human immunodeficiency virus type 1: Review of 31 cases. Clin Infect Dis 1993;17:59-65.

403. Lapins J, Lindbäck S, Lidbrink P, et al: Mucocutaneous manifestations in 22 consecutive cases of primary HIV-1 infection. Br J Dermatol 1996;134:257-261.

404. Goldman GD, Milstone LM, Shapiro PE: Histologic findings in acute HIV exanthem. J Cutan Pathol 1995;22:371-373.

405. Sapadin AN, Gelfand JM, Gumprecht J, et al: Eruption of human immunodeficiency virus seroconversion. Int J Dermatol 1998;37:436-438.

406. Barnadas MA, Alegre M, Baselga E, et al: Histopathological changes of primary HIV infection: Description of three cases and review of the literature. J Cutan Pathol 1997;24:507-510.

407. Lehloenya R, Meintjes G: Dermatologic manifestations of the immune reconstitution inflammatory syndrome. Dermatol Clin 2006;24:549-570, vii.

408. Lederman MM: Immune restoration and CD4+ T-cell function with antiretroviral therapies. AIDS 2001;15(Suppl 2):S11-S15.

409. Eisman S: Pruritic papular eruption in HIV. Dermatol Clin 2006;24:449-457, vi.

410. Rosenthal D, LeBoit PE, Klumpp L, Berger TG: Human immunodeficiency virus-associated eosinophilic folliculitis: A unique dermatosis associated with advanced human immunodeficiency virus infection. Arch Dermatol 1991;127:206-209.

411. Dlova NC, Mosam A: Inflammatory noninfectious dermatoses of HIV. Dermatol Clin 2006;24:439-448, vi.

412. Soeprono FF, Schinella RA, Cockerell CJ, Comite SL: Seborrheic-like dermatitis of acquired immunodeficiency syndrome: A clinicopathologic study. J Am Acad Dermatol 1986;14(2 Pt 1):242-248.

413. Crespo-Erchiga V, Florencio VD: Malassezia yeasts and pityriasis versicolor. Curr Opin Infect Dis 2006;19:139-147.

414. Assaf RR, Weil ML: The superficial mycoses. Dermatol Clin 1996;14:57-67.

415. Schwartz RA: Superficial fungal infections. Lancet 2004;364:1173-1182.

416. Gaitanis G, Bassukas ID, Velegraki A: The range of molecular methods for typing *Malassezia*. Curr Opin Infect Dis 2009;22:119-125.

417. Gaitanis G, Velegraki A, Alexopoulos EC, et al: Distribution of *Malassezia* species in pityriasis versicolor and seborrhoeic dermatitis in Greece: Typing of the major pityriasis versicolor isolate *M. globosa*. Br J Dermatol 2006;154:854-859.

418. Morishita N, Sei Y, Sugita T: Molecular analysis of *Malassezia* microflora from patients with pityriasis versicolor. Mycopathologia 2006;161:61-65.

419. Prohic A, Ozegovic L: *Malassezia* species isolated from lesional and non-lesional skin in patients with pityriasis versicolor. Mycoses 2007;50:58-63.

420. Morishita N, Sei Y: Microreview of pityriasis versicolor and *Malassezia* species. Mycopathologia 2006;162:373-376.

421. Thoma W, Krämer HJ, Mayser P: Pityriasis versicolor alba. J Eur Acad Dermatol Venereol 2005;19:147-152.

422. Galadari I, el Komy M, Mousa A, et al: Tinea versicolor: Histologic and ultrastructural investigation of pigmentary changes. Int J Dermatol 1992;31:253-256.

423. Nazzaro-Porro M, Passi S: Identification of tyrosinase inhibitors in cultures of *Pityrosporum*. J Invest Dermatol 1978;71:205-208.

424. Allen HB, Charles CR, Johnson BL: Hyperpigmented tinea versicolor. Arch Dermatol 1976;112:1110-1112.

425. Charles CR, Sire DJ, Johnson BL, Beidler JG: Hypopigmentation in tinea versicolor: A histochemical and electronmicroscopic study. Int J Dermatol 1973;12:48-58.

426. Karaoui R, Bou-Resli M, Al-Zaid NS, Mousa A: Tinea versicolor: Ultrastructural studies on hypopigmented and hyperpigmented skin. Dermatologica 1981;162:69-85.

427. Gupta AK, Batra R, Bluhm R, et al: Skin diseases associated with *Malassezia* species. J Am Acad Dermatol 2004;51:785-798.

428. Sina B, Kauffman CL, Samorodin CS: Intrafollicular mucin deposits in *Pityrosporum* folliculitis. J Am Acad Dermatol 1995;32:807-809.

429. Hill MK, Goodfield JD, Rodgers FG, et al: Skin surface electron microscopy in *Pityrosporum* folliculitis: The role of follicular occlu-

sion in disease and the response to oral ketoconazole. Arch Dermatol 1990;126:181-184.

430. Bufill JA, Lum LG, Caya JG, et al: *Pityrosporum* folliculitis after bone marrow transplantation: Clinical observations in five patients. Ann Intern Med 1988;108:560-563.

431. Lim KB, Giam YC, Tan T: The epidemiology of *Malassezia (Pityrosporum)* folliculitis in Singapore. Int J Dermatol 1987;26:438-441.

432. Faergemann J, Johansson S, Back O, Scheynius A: An immunologic and cultural study of *Pityrosporum* folliculitis. J Am Acad Dermatol 1986;14:429-433.

433. Parlak AH, Boran C, Topçuoglu MA: *Pityrosporum* folliculitis during pregnancy: A possible cause of pruritic folliculitis of pregnancy. J Am Acad Dermatol 2005;52:528-529.

434. Gupta AK, Chaudhry M, Elewski B: Tinea corporis, tinea cruris, tinea nigra, and piedra. Dermatol Clin 2003;21:395-400.

435. Severo LC, Bassanesi MC, Londero AT: Tinea nigra: Report of four cases observed in Rio Grande do Sul (Brazil) and a review of Brazilian literature. Mycopathologia 1994;126:157-162.

436. Pegas JR, Criado PR, Lucena SK, de Oliveira MA: Tinea nigra: Report of two cases in infants. Pediatr Dermatol 2003;20:315-317.

437. Perez C, Colella MT, Olaizola C, et al: Tinea nigra: Report of twelve cases in Venezuela. Mycopathologia 2005;160:235-238.

438. Kiken DA, Sekaren A, Antaya RJ, et al: White piedra in children. J Am Acad Dermatol 2006;55:956-961.

439. Gueho E, Smith MT, de Hoog GS, et al: Contributions to a revision of the genus *Trichosporon*. Antonie Van Leeuwenhoek 1992; 61:289-316.

440. Gueho E, Improvisi L, de Hoog GS, Dupont B: Trichosporon on humans: A practical account. Mycoses 1994;37:3-10.

441. Youker SR, Andreozzi RJ, Appelbaum PC, et al: White piedra: Further evidence of a synergistic infection. J Am Acad Dermatol 2003;49:746-749.

442. Ellner KM, McBride ME, Kalter DC, et al: White piedra: Evidence for a synergistic infection. Br J Dermatol 1990;123:355-363.

443. Lacasse A, Cleveland KO: *Trichosporon mucoides* fungemia in a liver transplant recipient: Case report and review. Transpl Infect Dis 2009;11:155-159.

444. Chowdhary A, Ahmad S, Khan ZU, et al: *Trichosporon asahii* as an emerging etiologic agent of disseminated trichosporonosis: A case report and an update. Indian J Med Microbiol 2004;22:16-22.

445. Nahass GT, Rosenberg SP, Leonardi CL, Penneys NS: Disseminated infection with *Trichosporon beigelii*: Report of a case and review of the cutaneous and histologic manifestations. Arch Dermatol 1993;129:1020-1023.

446. American Academy of Dermatology, Guidelines/Outcomes Committee: Guidelines of care for superficial mycotic infections of the skin: Piedra. J Am Acad Dermatol 1996;34:122-124.

447. Walsh TJ, Newman KR, Moody M, et al: Trichosporonosis in patients with neoplastic disease. Medicine (Baltimore) 1986;65:268-279.

448. Manzella JP, Berman IJ, Kukrika MD: *Trichosporon beigelii* fungemia and cutaneous dissemination. Arch Dermatol 1982;118:343-345.

449. Coimbra CE Jr, Santos RV: Black piedra among the Zoró Indians from Amazônia (Brazil). Mycopathologia 1989;107:57-60.

450. Figueras MJ, Guarro J, Zaror L: New findings in black piedra infection. Br J Dermatol 1996;135:157-158.

451. de Almeida HL Jr, Salebian A, Rivitti EA: Ultrastructure of black piedra. Mycoses 1991;34:447-451.

452. Weitzman I, Summerbell RC: The dermatophytes. Clin Microbiol Rev 1995;8:240-259.

453. Seebacher C, Bouchara JP, Mignon B: Updates on the epidemiology of dermatophyte infections. Mycopathologia 2008;166:335-352.

454. Svejgaard EL: Epidemiology of dermatophytes in Europe. Int J Dermatol 1995;34:525-528.

455. Aly R: Ecology and epidemiology of dermatophyte infections. J Am Acad Dermatol 1994;31(3 Pt 2):S21-S25.

456. Maraki S, Nioti E, Mantadakis E, Tselentis Y: A 7-year survey of dermatophytoses in Crete, Greece. Mycoses 2007;50:481-484.

457. Aghamirian MR, Ghiasian SA: Dermatophytoses in outpatients attending the Dermatology Center of Avicenna Hospital in Qazvin, Iran. Mycoses 2008;51:155-160.

458. Popoola TO, Ojo DA, Alabi RO: Prevalence of dermatophytosis in junior secondary schoolchildren in Ogun State, Nigeria. Mycoses 2006;49:499-503.

459. Lopes V, Velho G, Amorim ML, et al: [Three years incidence of dermatophytes in a hospital in Porto (Portugal)]. Rev Iberoam Micol 2002;19:201-203.

460. Hainer BL: Dermatophyte infections. Am Fam Physician 2003;67:101-108.

461. Degreef H: Clinical forms of dermatophytosis (ringworm infection). Mycopathologia 2008;166:257-265.

462. Davis DF, Petri WH, Hood AF: Dairy farmer with a rapidly enlarging lip lesion: Tinea barbae. Arch Dermatol 2006;142:1059-1064.

463. Xavier MH, Torturella DM, Rehfeldt FV, et al: Sycosiform tinea barbae caused by *Trichophyton rubrum*. Dermatol Online J 2008;14:10.

464. Coloe JR, Diab M, Moennich J, et al: Tinea capitis among children in the Columbus area, Ohio, USA. Mycoses 2009 Mar 17 [Epub ahead of print].

465. Fuller LC: Changing face of tinea capitis in Europe. Curr Opin Infect Dis 2009;22:115-118.

466. Cecchi R, Paoli S, Giomi A, Rossetti R: Favus due to *Trichophyton schoenleinii* in a patient with metastatic bronchial carcinoma. Br J Dermatol 2003;148:1057.

467. Havlickova B, Czaika VA, Friedrich M: Epidemiological trends in skin mycoses worldwide. Mycoses 2008;51(Suppl 4):2-15.

468. Arenas R, Toussaint S, Isa-Isa R: Kerion and dermatophytic granuloma: Mycological and histopathological findings in 19 children with inflammatory tinea capitis of the scalp. Int J Dermatol 2006;45:215-219.

469. Andrews MD, Burns M: Common tinea infections in children. Am Fam Physician 2008;77:1415-1420.

470. Bonifaz A, Archer-Dubon C, Saul A: Tinea imbricata or Tokelau. Int J Dermatol 2004;43:506-510.

471. Finch JJ, Warshaw EM: Toenail onychomycosis: Current and future treatment options. Dermatol Ther 2007;20:31-46.

472. Rongioletti F, Persi A, Tripodi S, Rebora A: Proximal white subungual onychomycosis: A sign of immunodeficiency. J Am Acad Dermatol 1994;30:129-130.

473. Mugge C, Haustein UF, Nenoff P: [Causative agents of onychomycosis: A retrospective study]. J Dtsch Dermatol Ges 2006;4:218-228.

474. Hay RJ: Chronic dermatophyte infections: I. Clinical and mycological features. Br J Dermatol 1982;106:1-7.

475. Shenoy MM, Teerthanath S, Karnker VK, et al: Comparison of potassium hydroxide mount and mycological culture with histopathologic examination using periodic acid-Schiff staining of the nail clippings in the diagnosis of onychomycosis. Indian J Dermatol Venereol Leprol 2008;74:226-229.

476. Nico MM, Rivitti EA: "Decubital candidosis": A study of 26 cases. J Eur Acad Dermatol Venereol 2005;19:296-300.

477. Segal E: Candida, still number one: What do we know and where are we going from there? Mycoses 2005;48:3-11.

478. Ali A, Natah S, Konttinen Y: Differential expression of Toll-like receptors in chronic hyperplastic candidosis. Oral Microbiol Immunol 2008;23:299-307.

479. Hay RJ: The management of superficial candidiasis. J Am Acad Dermatol 1999;40:S35-S42.

480. Mavor AL, Thewes S, Hube B: Systemic fungal infections caused by *Candida* species: Epidemiology, infection process and virulence attributes. Curr Drug Targets 2005;6:863-874.

481. Samaranayake LP, Keung Leung W, Jin L: Oral mucosal fungal infections. Periodontology 2000;49:39-59.

482. Appleton SS: Candidiasis: Pathogenesis, clinical characteristics, and treatment. J Calif Dent Assoc 2000;28:942-948.

483. Reichart PA, Samaranayake LP, Philipsen HP: Pathology and clinical correlates in oral candidiasis and its variants: A review. Oral Dis 2000;6:85-91.

484. Sitheeque MA, Samaranayake LP: Chronic hyperplastic candidosis/candidiasis (candidal leukoplakia). Crit Rev Oral Biol Med 2003;14:253-267.

485. Muzyka BC: Oral fungal infections. Dent Clin North Am 2005;49:49-65.

486. Li J, Fan SR, Liu XP, et al: Biased genotype distributions of *Candida albicans* strains associated with vulvovaginal candidosis and candidal balanoposthitis in China. Clin Infect Dis 2008;47:1119-1125.

487. Edwards S: Balanitis and balanoposthitis: A review. Genitourin Med 1996;72:155-159.

488. Tosti A, Piraccini BM, Lorenzi S, Iorizzo M: Treatment of nondermatophyte mold and Candida onychomycosis. Dermatol Clin 2003;21:491-497.

489. Darmstadt GL, Dinulos JG, Miller Z: Congenital cutaneous candidiasis: Clinical presentation, pathogenesis, and management guidelines. Pediatrics 2000;105:438-444.

490. Cosgrove BF, Reeves K, Mullins D, et al: Congenital cutaneous candidiasis associated with respiratory distress and elevation of liver function tests: A case report and review of the literature. J Am Acad Dermatol 1997;37:817-823.

491. Zaoutis T, Walsh TJ: Antifungal therapy for neonatal candidiasis. Curr Opin Infect Dis 2007;20:592-597.

492. Bluestein J, Furner BB, Phillips D: Granuloma gluteale infantum: Case report and review of the literature. Pediatr Dermatol 1990;7:196-198.

493. Tabata H, Yamakage A, Yamasaki S: Infantile gluteal granulomata mimicking mollusca contagiosa. Int J Dermatol 1997;36:157-158.

494. Kirkpatrick CH: Chronic mucocutaneous candidiasis. Pediatr Infect Dis J 2001;20:197-206.

495. Antachopoulos C, Walsh TJ, Roilides E: Fungal infections in primary immunodeficiencies. Eur J Pediatr 2007;166:1099-1117.

496. Moraes-Vasconcelos D, Costa-Carvalho BT, Torgerson TR, Ochs HD: Primary immune deficiency disorders presenting as autoimmune diseases: IPEX and APECED. J Clin Immunol 2008;28:S11-S19.

497. Lilic D: New perspectives on the immunology of chronic mucocutaneous candidiasis. Curr Opin Infect Dis 2002;15:143-147.

498. Williamson MM, Gordon RD: Severe chronic mucocutaneous candidiasis: Favorable response to oral therapy with ketoconazole. Med J Aust 1983;1:276-278.

499. Bouza E, Muñoz P: Epidemiology of candidemia in intensive care units. Int J Antimicrob Agents 2008;32:S87-S91.

500. Pedraz J, Delgado-Jiménez Y, Pérez-Gala S, et al: Cutaneous expression of systemic candidiasis. Clin Exp Dermatol 2009;34:106-110.

501. Slater DN, Wylde P, Harrington CI, Worth R: Systemic candidiasis: Diagnosis from cutaneous manifestations. J R Soc Med 1982;75:875-878.

502. Fine JD, Miller JA, Harrist TJ, Haynes HA: Cutaneous lesions in disseminated candidiasis mimicking ecthyma gangrenosum. Am J Med 1981;70:1133-1135.

503. Bougnoux ME, Dupont C, Turner L, et al: Mixed *Candida glabrata* and *Candida albicans* disseminated candidiasis in a heroin addict. Eur J Clin Microbiol Infect Dis 1997;16:598-600.

504. Bisbe J, Miro JM, Latorre X, et al: Disseminated candidiasis in addicts who use brown heroin: Report of 83 cases and review. Clin Infect Dis 1992;15:910-923.

505. Picazo JJ, González-Romo F, Candel FJ: Candidemia in the critically ill patient. Int J Antimicrob Agents 2008;32:S83-S85.

506. Naglik J, Albrecht A, Bader O, Hube B: *Candida albicans* proteinases and host/pathogen interactions. Cell Microbiol 2004;6:915-926.

507. Gugic D, Cleary T, Vincek V: *Candida glabrata* infection in gastric carcinoma patient mimicking cutaneous histoplasmosis. Dermatol Online J 2008;14:15.

508. Liu X, Hua H: Oral manifestation of chronic mucocutaneous candidiasis: Seven case reports. J Oral Pathol Med 2007;36:528-532.

509. Body BA: Cutaneous manifestations of systemic mycoses. Dermatol Clin 1996;14:125-135.

510. Woofter MJ, Cripps DJ, Warner TF: Verrucous plaques on the face: North American blastomycosis. Arch Dermatol 2000;136:547-548.

511. Assaly RA, Hammersley JR, Olson DE, et al: Disseminated blastomycosis. J Am Acad Dermatol 2003;48:123-127.

512. Mason AR, Cortes GY, Cook J, et al: Cutaneous blastomycosis: A diagnostic challenge. Int J Dermatol 2008;47:824-830.

513. Garvey K, Hinshaw M, Vanness E: Chronic disseminated cutaneous blastomycosis in an 11-year old, with a brief review of the literature. Pediatr Dermatol 2006;23:541-545.

514. Hashimoto K, Kaplan RJ, Daman LA, et al: Pustular blastomycosis. Int J Dermatol 1977;16:277-280.

515. Wilkerson A, King R, Googe PB, et al: Sweet's syndrome-like blastomycosis. Am J Dermatopathol 2003;25:152-154.

516. Taxy JB: Blastomycosis: Contributions of morphology to diagnosis—A surgical pathology, cytopathology, and autopsy pathology study. Am J Surg Pathol 2007;31:615-623.

517. Bradsher RW, Chapman SW, Pappas PG: Blastomycosis. Infect Dis Clin North Am 2003;17:21-40.

518. Walker K, Skelton H, Smith K: Cutaneous lesions showing giant yeast forms of *Blastomyces dermatitidis*. J Cutan Pathol 2002;29:616-618.

519. Moore M: Morphologic variation in tissue of the organisms of the blastomycoses and of histoplasmosis. Am J Pathol 1955;31:1049-1063.

520. Hussain Z, Martin A, Youngberg GA: *Blastomyces dermatitidis* with large yeast forms. Arch Pathol Lab Med 2001;125:663-664.

521. Atkinson JB, McCurley TL: Pulmonary blastomycosis: Filamentous forms in an immunocompromised patient with fulminating respiratory failure. Hum Pathol 1983;14:186-188.

522. Watts JC, Chandler FW, Mihalov ML, et al: Giant forms of *Blastomyces dermatitidis* in the pulmonary lesions of blastomycosis: Potential confusion with *Coccidioides immitis*. Am J Clin Pathol 1990;93:575-578.

523. Hinshaw M, Longley BJ: Fungal diseases. In Elder DE (ed): Lever's Histopathology of the Skin, 10th ed. Philadelphia, Lippincott Williams & Wilkins, 2004, pp 591-636.

524. Rutland BM, Horenstein MG: A 53-year-old man with an anterior knee fungating mass: Cutaneous blastomycosis. Arch Pathol Lab Med 2005;129:e132-e133.

525. Gray NA, Baddour LM: Cutaneous inoculation blastomycosis. Clin Infect Dis 2002;34:E44-E49.

526. Parish JM, Blair JE: Coccidioidomycosis. Mayo Clin Proc 2008;83:343-348.

527. DiCaudo DJ: Coccidioidomycosis: A review and update. J Am Acad Dermatol 2006;55:929-942.

528. Crum NF, Lederman ER, Stafford CM, et al: Coccidioidomycosis: A descriptive survey of a reemerging disease. Clinical characteristics and current controversies. Medicine (Baltimore) 2004;83:149-175.

529. Kim A, Parker SS: Coccidioidomycosis: Case report and update on diagnosis and management. J Am Acad Dermatol 2002;46:743-747.

530. Quimby SR, Connolly SM, Winkelmann RK, Smilack JD: Clinicopathologic spectrum of specific cutaneous lesions of disseminated coccidioidomycosis. J Am Acad Dermatol 1992;26:79-85.

531. Crum NF: Disseminated coccidioidomycosis with cutaneous lesions clinically mimicking mycosis fungoides. Int J Dermatol 2005;44:958-960.

532. Hobbs ER, Hempstead RW: Cutaneous coccidioidomycosis simulating lepromatous leprosy. Int J Dermatol 1984;23:334-336.

533. Chang A, Tung RC, McGillis TS, et al: Primary cutaneous coccidioidomycosis. J Am Acad Dermatol 2003;49:944-949.

534. DiCaudo DJ, Yiannias JA, Laman SD, Warschaw KE: The exanthem of acute pulmonary coccidioidomycosis: Clinical and histopathologic features of 3 cases and review of the literature. Arch Dermatol 2006;142:744-746.

535. Kaufman L, Valero G, Padhye AA: Misleading manifestations of *Coccidioides immitis* in vivo. J Clin Microbiol 1998;36:3721-3723.

536. Waldman JS, Barr RJ, Espinoza FP, Simmons GE: Subcutaneous myospherulosis. J Am Acad Dermatol 1989;21:400-403.

537. Laniado-Laborín R: Coccidioidomycosis and other endemic mycoses in Mexico. Rev Iberoam Micol 2007;24:249-258.

538. Fisher MC, Koenig GL, White TJ, Taylor JW: Molecular and phenotypic description of *Coccidioides posadasii* sp nov, previously recognized as the non-California population of *Coccidioides immitis*. Mycologia 2002;94:73-84.

539. Grayson W, Calonje E, McKee PH: Infectious diseases of the skin. In Mckee PH, Calonje E, Granter S (eds): Pathology of the Skin with Clinical Correlations. Philadelphia, Elsevier, 2005, pp 938-979.

540. Pagliari C, Sotto MN: Dendritic cells and pattern of cytokines in paracoccidioidomycosis skin lesions. Am J Dermatopathol 2003;25:107-112.

541. Ramos-E-Silva M, Saraiva Ldo E: Paracoccidioidomycosis. Dermatol Clin 2008;26:257-269.

542. Dias MF, Pereira AC, Pereira A, Alves MS: The role of HLA antigens in the development of paracoccidioidomycosis. J Eur Acad Dermatol Venereol 2000;14:166-171.

543. Nogueira MG, Andrade GM, Tonelli E: Clinical evolution of paracoccidioidomycosis in 38 children and teenagers. Mycopathologia 2006;161:73-81.

544. Lupi O, Tyring SK, McGinnis MR: Tropical dermatology: Fungal tropical diseases. J Am Acad Dermatol 2005;53:931-951.

545. García Bustínduy M, Guimerá FJ, Arévalo P, et al: Cutaneous primary paracoccidioidomycosis. J Eur Acad Dermatol Venereol 2000;14:113-117.

546. Campos MV, Penna GO, Castro CN, et al: Paracoccidioidomycosis at Brasilia's University Hospital. Rev Soc Bras Med Trop 2008;41:169-172.

547. Peres LC, Saggioro FP, Dias LB Jr, et al: Infectious diseases in paediatric pathology: Experience from a developing country. Pathology 2008;40:161-175.

548. Godoy H, Reichart PA: Oral manifestations of paracoccidioidomycosis: Report of 21 cases from Argentina. Mycoses 2003;46:412-417.

549. Golda N, Feldman M: Histoplasmosis clinically imitating cutaneous malignancy. J Cutan Pathol 2008;35(Suppl 1):26-28.

550. Kauffman CA: Histoplasmosis: A clinical and laboratory update. Clin Microbiol Rev 2007;20:115-132.

551. Daher EF, Silva GB Jr, Barros FA, et al: Clinical and laboratory features of disseminated histoplasmosis in HIV patients from Brazil. Trop Med Int Health 2007;12:1108-1115.

552. Verma SB: Chronic disseminated cutaneous histoplasmosis in an immunocompetent individual: A case report. Int J Dermatol 2006;45:573-576.

553. Saheki MN, Schubach Ade O, Salgueiro Mde M, et al: Primary cutaneous histoplasmosis: Case report on an immunocompetent patient and review of the literature. Rev Soc Bras Med Trop 2008;41:680-682.

554. Eidbo J, Sanchez RL, Tschen JA, Ellner KM: Cutaneous manifestations of histoplasmosis in the acquired immune deficiency syndrome. Am J Surg Pathol 1993;17:110-116.

555. Rodríguez G, Ordóñéz N, Motta A: *Histoplasma capsulatum* var. *capsulatum* within cutaneous nerves in patients with disseminated histoplasmosis and AIDS. Br J Dermatol 2001;144:205-207.

556. Gugnani HC, Muotoe-Okafor F: African histoplasmosis: A review. Rev Iberoam Micol 1997;14:155-159.

557. Garcia-Guiñon A, Torres-Rodríguez JM, Ndidongarte DT, et al: Disseminated histoplasmosis by *Histoplasma capsulatum* var. *duboisii* in a paediatric patient from the Chad Republic, Africa. Eur J Clin Microbiol Infect Dis 2009;28:697.

558. Loulergue P, Bastides F, Baudouin V, et al: Literature review and case histories of *Histoplasma capsulatum* var. *duboisii* infections in HIV-infected patients. Emerg Infect Dis 2007;13:1647-1652.

559. Khalil M, Ekanem IO, Gugnani HC, Attah EB: Some deep mycoses diagnosed by histopathology in South Eastern Nigeria. Rev Iberoam Micol 1999;16:221-224.

560. Vanittanakom N, Cooper CR Jr, Fisher MC, Sirisanthana T: *Penicillium marneffei* infection and recent advances in the epidemiology and molecular biology aspects. Clin Microbiol Rev 2006;19:95-110.

561. Capponi M, Segretain G, Sureau P: [Penicillosis from Rhizomys sinensis.] Bull Soc Pathol Exot Filiales 1956;49:418-421.

562. Hilmarsdottir I, Meynard JL, Rogeaux O, et al: Disseminated *Penicillium marneffei* infection associated with human immunodeficiency virus: A report of two cases and a review of 35 published cases. J Acquir Immune Defic Syndr 1993;6:466-471.

563. Supparatpinyo K, Khamwan C, Baosoung V, et al: Disseminated *Penicillium marneffei* infection in Southeast Asia. Lancet 1994;344:110-113.

564. Tsunemi Y, Takahashi T, Tamaki T: *Penicillium marneffei* infection diagnosed by polymerase chain reaction from the skin specimen. J Am Acad Dermatol 2003;49:344-346.

565. Cooper CR Jr, McGinnis MR: Pathology of *Penicillium marneffei*: An emerging acquired immunodeficiency syndrome-related pathogen. Arch Pathol Lab Med 1997;121:798-804.

566. Duong TA: Infection due to *Penicillium marneffei*, an emerging pathogen: Review of 155 reported cases. Clin Infect Dis 1996;23:125-130.

567. Yousukh A, Jutavijittum P, Pisetpongsa P, et al: Clinicopathologic study of hepatic *Penicillium marneffei* in Northern Thailand. Arch Pathol Lab Med 2004;128:191-194.

568. Nucci M, Anaissie E: Emerging fungi. Infect Dis Clin North Am 2006;20:563-579.

569. Perez-Perez L, Pereiro M Jr, Sánchez-Aguilar D, Toribio J: Ulcerous lesions disclosing cutaneous infection with *Fusarium solani*. Acta Derm Venereol 2007;87:422-424.

570. Nucci M, Anaissie E: Cutaneous infection by *Fusarium* species in healthy and immunocompromised hosts: Implications for diagnosis and management. Clin Infect Dis 2002;35:909-920.

571. Nucci M, Anaissie E: *Fusarium* infections in immunocompromised patients. Clin Microbiol Rev 2007;20:695-704.

572. Guilhermetti E, Takahachi G, Shinobu CS, Svidzinski TI: *Fusarium* spp. as agents of onychomycosis in immunocompetent hosts. Int J Dermatol 2007;46:822-826.

573. Kerr CM, Perfect JR, Craven PC, et al: Fungal peritonitis in patients on continuous ambulatory peritoneal dialysis. Ann Intern Med 1983;99:334-336.

574. Doczi I, Gyetvai T, Kredics L, Nagy E: Involvement of *Fusarium* spp. in fungal keratitis. Clin Microbiol Infect 2004;10:773-776.

575. Rippon JW, Larson RA, Rosenthal DM, Clayman J: Disseminated cutaneous and peritoneal hyalohyphomycosis caused by *Fusarium* species: three cases and review of the literature. Mycopathologia 1988;101:105-111.

576. Raad I, Hachem R: Treatment of central venous catheter-related fungemia due to *Fusarium oxysporum*. Clin Infect Dis 1995;20:709-711.

577. Gardner JM, Nelson MM, Heffernan MP: Chronic cutaneous fusariosis. Arch Dermatol 2005;141:794-795.

578. Boutati EI, Anaissie EJ: *Fusarium*, a significant emerging pathogen in patients with hematologic malignancy: Ten years' experience at a cancer center and implications for management. Blood 1997;90:999-1008.

579. Virgili A, Zampino MR, Mantovani L: Fungal skin infections in organ transplant recipients. Am J Clin Dermatol 2002;3:19-35.

580. Chi CC, Wang SH: Disseminated cutaneous *Fusarium moniliforme* infections in a leukemic child. Int J Dermatol 2007;46:487-489.

581. Nelson PE, Dignani MC, Anaissie EJ: Taxonomy, biology, and clinical aspects of *Fusarium* species. Clin Microbiol Rev 1994;7:479-504.

582. Hayden RT, Isotalo PA, Parrett T, et al: In situ hybridization for the differentiation of *Aspergillus, Fusarium,* and *Pseudallescheria* species in tissue section. Diagn Mol Pathol 2003;12:21-26.

583. Naka W, Masuda M, Konohana A, et al: Primary cutaneous cryptococcosis and *Cryptococcus neoformans* serotype D. Clin Exp Dermatol 1995;20:221-225.

584. Dimino-Emme L, Gurevitch AW: Cutaneous manifestations of disseminated cryptococcosis. J Am Acad Dermatol 1995;32:844-850.

585. Ogami N, Horino T, Arii K, et al: Primary cutaneous cryptococcosis in a patient with minimal change nephrotic syndrome. Nephrol Dial Transplant 2005;20:2578-2579.

586. Vijaya D, Kumar BH, Nagarathnamma T: Case report: Disseminated cutaneous cryptococcosis in an immunocompetent host. Mycoses 2001;44:113-114.

587. Myskowski PL, White MH, Ahkami R: Fungal disease in the immunocompromised host. Dermatol Clin 1997;15:295-305.

588. Xiujiao X, Ai'e X: Two cases of cutaneous cryptococcosis. Mycoses 2005;48:238-241.

589. Dharmshale SN, Patil SA, Gohil A, et al: Disseminated crytococcosis with extensive cutaneous involvement in AIDS. Indian J Med Microbiol 2006;24:228-230.

590. Narisawa Y, Kojima T, Iriki A, et al: Tissue changes in cryptococcosis: Histologic alteration from gelatinous to suppurative granulomatous tissue response with asteroid body. Mycopathologia 1989;106:113-119.

591. Leidel GD, Metcalf JS: Formation of palisading granulomas in a patient with chronic cutaneous cryptococcosis. Am J Dermatopathol 1989;11:560-562.

592. Su WP, Kuechle MK, Peters MS, Muller SA: Palisading granulomas caused by infectious diseases. Am J Dermatopathol 1992;14:211-215.

593. Abbott JJ, Hamacher KL, Ahmed I: In situ hybridization in cutaneous deep fungal infections: A valuable diagnostic adjunct to fungal morphology and tissue cultures. J Cutan Pathol 2006;33:426-432.

594. Lazcano O, Speights VO Jr, Strickler JG, et al: Combined histochemical stains in the differential diagnosis of *Cryptococcus neoformans*. Mod Pathol 1993;6:80-84.

595. Alfonso F, Gallo L, Winkler B, Suhrland MJ: Fine needle aspiration cytology of peripheral lymph node cryptococcosis: A report of three cases. Acta Cytol 1994;38:459-462.

596. Ito-Kuwa S, Nakamura K, Aoki S, Vidotto V: Serotype identification of *Cryptococcus neoformans* by multiplex PCR. Mycoses 2007;50:277-281.

597. Enache-Angoulvant A, Chandenier J, Symoens F, et al: Molecular identification of *Cryptococcus neoformans* serotypes. J Clin Microbiol 2007;45:1261-1265.

598. Small JM, Mitchell TG, Wheat RW: Strain variation in composition and molecular size of the capsular polysaccharide of *Cryptococcus neoformans* serotype A. Infect Immun 1986;54:735-741.

599. Eisenman HC, Nosanchuk JD, Webber JB, et al: Microstructure of cell wall-associated melanin in the human pathogenic fungus *Cryptococcus neoformans*. Biochemistry 2005;44:3683-3693.

600. Sotto MN, De Brito T, Silva AM, et al: Antigen distribution and antigen-presenting cells in skin biopsies of human chromoblastomycosis. J Cutan Pathol 2004;31:14-18.

601. Pang KR, Wu JJ, Huang DB, Tyring SK: Subcutaneous fungal infections. Dermatol Ther 2004;17:523-523.

602. Minotto R, Bernardi CD, Mallmann LF, et al: Chromoblastomycosis: A review of 100 cases in the state of Rio Grande do Sul, Brazil. J Am Acad Dermatol 2001;44:585-592.

603. Santos AL, Palmeira VF, Rozental S, et al: Biology and pathogenesis of *Fonsecaea pedrosoi*, the major etiologic agent of chromoblastomycosis. FEMS Microbiol Rev 2007;31:570-591.

604. Kondo M, Hiruma M, Nishioka Y, et al: A case of chromomycosis caused by *Fonsecaea pedrosoi* and a review of reported cases of dematiaceous fungal infection in Japan. Mycoses 2005;48:221-225.

605. Uribe F, Zuluaga AI, Leon W, Restrepo A: Histopathology of chromoblastomycosis. Mycopathologia 1989;105:1-6.

606. Batres E, Wolf JE Jr, Rudolph AH, Knox JM: Transepithelial elimination of cutaneous chromomycosis. Arch Dermatol 1978;114:1231-1232.

607. Milam CP, Fenske NA: Chromoblastomycosis. Dermatol Clin 1989;7:219-225.

608. McGinnis MR: Chromoblastomycosis and phaeohyphomycosis: New concepts, diagnosis, and mycology. J Am Acad Dermatol 1983;8:1-16.

609. Ameen M, Arenas R: Developments in the management of mycetomas. Clin Exp Dermatol 2009;34:1-7.

610. Fernandes H, D'Souza CR, Shekar JC, et al: Cytodiagnosis of actinomycetoma. Diagn Cytopathol 2009;37:506-508.

611. Queiroz-Telles F, McGinnis MR, Salkin I, Graybill JR: Subcutaneous mycoses. Infect Dis Clin North Am 2003;17:59-85.

612. McGinnis MR: Mycetoma. Dermatol Clin 1996;14:97-104.

613. Guimarães CC, Castro LG, Sotto MN: Lymphocyte subsets, macrophages and Langerhans cells in actinomycetoma and eumycetoma tissue reaction. Acta Trop 2003;87:377-384.

614. Lichon V, Khachemoune A: Mycetoma: A review. Am J Clin Dermatol 2006;7:315-321.

615. Sharma NL, Mahajan VK, Agarwal S, et al: Nocardial mycetoma: Diverse clinical presentations. Indian J Dermatol Venereol Leprol 2008;74:635-640.

616. Fader RC, McGinnis MR: Infections caused by dematiaceous fungi: Chromoblastomycosis and phaeohyphomycosis. Infect Dis Clin North Am 1988;2:925-938.

617. Matsumoto T, Matsuda T: Chromoblastomycosis and phaeohyphomycosis. Semin Dermatol 1985;4:240.

618. Silveira F, Nucci M: Emergence of black moulds in fungal disease: Epidemiology and therapy. Curr Opin Infect Dis 2001;14:679-684.

619. Silva Mdo R, Fernandes Ode F, Costa CR, et al: Subcutaneoous phaeohyphomycosis by *Exophiala jeanselmei* in a cardiac transplant recipient. Rev Inst Med Trop Sao Paulo 2005;47:55-57.

620. Rossmann SN, Cernoch P, Davis JR: Dematiaceous fungi are increasing cause of human disease. Clin Infect Dis 1996;22:73-80.

621. Kumar KK, Hallikeri K: Phaeohyphomycosis. Indian J Pathol Microbiol 2008;51:556-558.

622. Hussey SM, Gander R, Southern P, Hoang MP: Subcutaneous phaeohyphomycosis caused by *Cladophialophora bantiana*. Arch Pathol Lab Med 2005;129:794-797.

623. Ronan SG, Uzoaru I, Nadimpalli V, et al: Primary cutaneous phaeohyphomycosis: Report of seven cases. J Cutan Pathol 1993;20:223-228.

624. Brandt ME, Warnock DW: Epidemiology, clinical manifestations, and therapy of infections caused by dematiaceous fungi. J Chemother 2003;2:36-47.

625. Dixon DM, Polak-Wyss A: The medically important dematiaceous fungi and their identification. Mycoses 1991;34:1-18.

626. Wakamatsu K, Takahata Y, Tokuhisa Y, et al: Two cases of phaeohyphomycosis due to *Exophiala jeanselmei*. J Dermatol 2008;35:178-180.

627. Schubach A, Barros MB, Wanke B: Epidemic sporotrichosis. Curr Opin Infect Dis 2008;21:129-133.

628. Morris-Jones R: Sporotrichosis. Clin Exp Dermatol 2002;27:427-431.

629. Davis BA: Sporotrichosis. Dermatol Clin 1996;14:69-76.

630. Hardman S, Stephenson I, Jenkins DR, et al: Disseminated *Sporothix schenckii* in a patient with AIDS. J Infect 2005;51:e73-e77.

631. Kauffman CA: Endemic mycoses: Blastomycosis, histoplasmosis, and sporotrichosis. Infect Dis Clin North Am 2006;20:645-662.

632. Sharma NL, Mahajan VK, Verma N, Thakur S: Cutaneous sporotrichosis: An unusual clinico-pathologic and therapeutic presentation. Mycoses 2003;46:515-518.

633. Kauffman CA: Sporotrichosis. Clin Infect Dis 1999;29:231-237.

634. da Rosa AC, Scroferneker ML, Vettorato R, et al: Epidemiology of sporotrichosis: A study of 304 cases in Brazil. J Am Acad Dermatol 2005;52:451-459.

635. Marques ME, Coelho KI, Sotto MN, Bacchi CE: Comparison between histochemical and immunohistochemical methods for diagnosis of sporotrichosis. J Clin Pathol 1992;45:1089-1093.

636. Hachisuka H, Tajiri S, Hongo K, Sasai Y: Polymorphonuclear leukocyte chemotaxis in sporotrichosis. Mycopathologia 1982;79:39-41.

637. Rodríguez G, Sarmiento L: The asteroid bodies of sporotrichosis. Am J Dermatopathol 1998;20:246-249.

638. Suchitha S, Vijaya B, Sunila R, et al: Sporotrichosis in Mysore: A case report to emphasize the role of histopathology. Indian J Pathol Microbiol 2008;51:45-46.

639. Kwon-Chung KJ: Comparison of isolates of *Sporothrix schenckii* obtained from fixed cutaneous lesions with isolates from other types of lesions. J Infect Dis 1979;139:424-431.

640. Romero-Martinez R, Wheeler M, Guerrero-Plata A, et al: Biosynthesis and functions of melanin in *Sporothrix schenckii*. Infect Immun 2000;68:3696-3703.

641. De Araujo T, Marques AC, Kerdel F: Sporotrichosis. Int J Dermatol 2001;40:737-742.

642. Bullpitt P, Weedon D: Sporotrichosis: A review of 39 cases. Pathology 1978;10:249-256.

643. Vilani-Moreno FR, Belone AF, Soares CT, Opromolla DV: Immunohistochemical characterization of the cellular infiltrate in Jorge Lobo's disease. Rev Iberoam Micol 2005;22:44-49.

644. Al-Daraji WI: Cutaneous lobomycosis: A delayed diagnosis. Am J Dermatopathol 2008;30:575-577.

645. Xavier MB, Libonati RM, Unger D, et al: Macrophage and TGF-beta immunohistochemical expression in Jorge Lobo's disease. Hum Pathol 2008;39:269-274.

646. Talhari C, Oliveira CB, de Souza Santos MN, et al: Disseminated lobomycosis. Int J Dermatol 2008;47:582-583.

647. Rosa PS, Soares Ct, Belone Ade F, et al: Accidental Jorge Lobo's disease in a worker dealing with *Lacazia loboi* infected mice: A case report. J Med Case Rep 2009;3:67.

648. Burns RA, Roy JS, Woods C, et al: Report of the first human case of lobomycosis in the United States. J Clin Microbiol 2000;38:1283-1285.

649. Paniz-Mondolfi AE, Reyes Jaimes O, Davila Jones L: Lobomycosis in Venezuela. Int J Dermatol 2007;46:180-185.

650. Cowan DF: Lobo's disease in a bottlenose dolphin (*Tursiops truncatus*) from Matagorda Bay, Texas. J Wildl Dis 1993;29:488-489.

651. Lupi O, Tyring SK, McGinnis MR: Tropical dermatology: Fungal tropical diseases. J Am Acad Dermatol 2005;53:931-951, quiz 952-954.

652. Vilani-Moreno FR, Mozer E, de Sene AM, et al: In vitro and in situ activation of the complement system by the fungus *Lacazia loboi*. Rev Inst Med Trop Sao Paulo 2007;49:97-101.

653. Opromolla DV, Belone AF, Taborda PR, Rosa PS: Lymph node involvement in Jorge Lobo's disease: Report of two cases. Int J Dermatol 2003;42:938-941.

654. Vilela R, Martins JE, Pereira CN, et al: Molecular study of archival fungal strains isolated from cases of lacaziosis (Jorge Lobo's disease). Mycoses 2007;50:470-474.

655. Madeira S, Fernandes Belone Ade F, Padovani Cr, Araújo Omoprolla DV: Comparative experimental infection of *Lacazia loboi* in BALB/c and B10.A mice. Rev Iberoam Micol 2003;20:55-59.

656. Ribes JA, Vanover-Sams CL, Baker DJ: Zygomycetes in human disease. Clin Microbiol Rev 2000;13:236-301.

657. Prabhu RM, Patel R: Mucormycosis and entomophthoramycosis: A review of the clinical manifestations, diagnosis and treatment. Clin Microbiol Infect 2004;10:31-47.

658. Chayakulkeeree M, Ghannoum MA, Perfect JR: Zygomycosis: The re-emerging fungal infection. Eur J Clin Microbiol Infect Dis 2006;25:215-229.

659. Eucker J, Sezer O, Graf B, Possinger K: Mucormycoses. Mycoses 2001;44:253-260.

660. Gadadhar H, Hawkins S, Huffstutter JE, Panda M: Cutaneous mucormycosis complicating methotrexate, prednisone, and infliximab therapy. J Clin Rheumatol 2007;13:361-362.

661. Roden MM, Zaoutis TE, Buchanan WL, et al: Epidemiology and outcome of zygomycosis: A review of 929 reported cases. Clin Infect Dis 2005;41:634-653.

662. Page AV, Evans AJ, Snell L, Liles WC: Primary cutaneous mucormycosis in a lung transplant recipient: Case report and concise review of the literature. Transpl Infect Dis 2008;10:419-425.

663. Gugnani HC: A review of zygomycosis due to *Basidiobolus ranarum*. Eur J Epidemiol 1999;15:923-929.

664. Hussein MR, Musalam AO, Assiry MH, et al: Histological and ultrastructural features of gastrointestinal basidiobolomycosis. Mycol Res 2007;111:926-930.

665. Geramizadeh B, Modjalal M, Nabai S, et al: Gastrointestinal zygomycosis: A report of three cases. Mycopathologia 2007;164:35-38.

666. van den Berk GE, Noorduyn LA, van Ketel RJ, et al: A fatal pseudo-tumour: Disseminated basidiobolomycosis. BMC Infect Dis 2006;6:140.

667. Bigliazzi C, Poletti V, Dell'Amore D, et al: Disseminated basidiobolomycosis in an immunocompetent woman. J Clin Microbiol 2004;42:1367-1369.

668. Gugnani HC: Entomophthoromycosis due to *Conidiobolus*. Eur J Epidemiol 1992;8:391-396.

669. Frater JL, Hall GS, Procop GW: Histologic features of zygomycosis: Emphasis on perineural invasion and fungal morphology. Arch Pathol Lab Med 2001;125:375-378.

670. Gautom RK, Lory S, Seyedirashti S, et al: Mitochondrial DNA ?ngerprinting of *Acanthamoeba* spp. isolated from clinical and environmental sources. J Clin Microbiol 1994;32:1070-1073.

671. Haque R, Huston CD, Hughes M, et al: Amebiasis. N Engl J Med 2003;348:1565-1573.

672. Marciano-Cabral F, Cabral G: *Acanthamoeba* spp. as agents of disease in humans. Clin Microbiol Rev 2003;16:273-307.

673. Gelman BB: Amoebic encephalitis due to *Sappina diploidea*. JAMA 2001;285:2450-2451.

674. Visvesvara GS, Schuster FL, Martinez AJ: 1993. *Balamuthia mandrillaris*, n. g., n. sp., agent of amebic meningoencephalitis

in humans and other animals. J Eukaryot Microbiol 1993;40:504-514.

675. el-Zawahry M, el-Komy M: Amoebiasis cutis. Int J Dermatol 1973;12:305-307.

676. Magaña M, Magaña ML, Alcántara A, Pérez-Martín MA: Histopathology of cutaneous amebiasis. Am J Dermatopathol 2004;26:280-284.

677. Magaña ML, Fernández-Díez J, Magaña M: Cutaneous amebiasis in pediatrics. Arch Dermatol 2008;144:1369-1372.

678. Loschiavo F, Guarneri B, Ventura-Spagnolo T, et al: Cutaneous amebiasis in an Iranian immunodeficient alcoholic: Immunochemical and histological study. Dermatology 1997;194:370-371.

679. Fujita WH, Barr RJ, Gottschalk HR:. Cutaneous amebiasis. Arch Dermatol 1981;117:309-310.

680. Majmudar B, Chaiken ML, Lee KU: Amebiasis of clitoris mimicking carcinoma. JAMA 1976;236:1145-1146.

681. Braga LL, Ninomiya H, McCoy JJ, et al: Inhibition of the complement membrane attack complex by the galactose-specific adhesion of *Entamoeba histolytica*. J Clin Invest 1992;90:1131-1137.

682. Michel R, Hauroder-Philippczyk B, Muller K, Weishaar I: Acanthamoeba from human nasal mucosa infected with an obligate intracellular parasite. Eur J Protistol 1994;30:104-110.

683. Newsome AL, Curtis FT, Culbertson CG, Allen SD: Identification of *Acanthamoeba* in bronchoalveolar lavage specimens. Diagn Cytopathol 1992;8:231-234.

684. Casper T, Basset D, Leclercq C, et al: Disseminated acanthamoeba infection in a patient with AIDS: Response to 5-fluorocytosine therapy. Clin Infect Dis 1999;29:944-945.

685. Murakawa GJ, McCalmont T, Altman J, et al: Disseminated acanthamebiasis in patients with AIDS: A report of five cases and a review of the literature. Arch Dermatol 1995;131:1291-1296.

686. Wortman PD: *Acanthamoeba* infection. Int J Dermatol 1996;35:48-51.

687. Friedland LR, Raphael SA, Deutsch ES, et al: Disseminated *Acanthamoeba* infection in a child with symptomatic human immunodeficiency virus infection. Pediatr Infect Dis J 1992;11:404-407.

688. Rosenberg AS, Morgan MB: Disseminated acanthamoebiasis presenting as lobular panniculitis with necrotizingvasculitis in a patient with AIDS. J Cutan Pathol 2001;28:307-313.

689. Helton J, Loveless M, White CR Jr: Cutaneous acanthamoeba infection associated with leukocytoclastic vasculitis in an AIDS patient. Am J Dermatopathol 1993;15:146-149.

690. Kong HH, Kim TH, Chung DI: Purification and characterization of a secretory serine proteinase of *Acanthamoeba healyi* isolated from GAE. J Parasitol 2000;86:12-17.

691. Rowbotham TJ: Preliminary report on the pathogenicity of *Legionella pneumophila* for freshwater and soil amoebae. J Clin Pathol 1980;33:1179-1183.

692. Barker J, Brown MR: Trojan horses of the microbial world: Protozoa and the survival of bacterial pathogens in the environment. Microbiology 1994;140:1253-1259.

693. Krishna Prasad BN, Gupta SK: Preliminary report on the engulfment and retention of mycobacteria by trophozoites of exenically grown *Acanthamoeba castellanii* Douglas, 1930. Curr Sci 1978;47:245-247.

694. Essig A, Heinemann M, Simnacher U, Marre R: Infection of *Acanthamoeba castellanii* by *Chlamydia pneumoniae*. Appl Environ Microbiol 1997;63:1396-1399.

695. Barrett MP, Burchmore RJ, Stich A, et al: The trypanosomiases. Lancet 2003;362:1469-1480.

696. Joshi PP, Shegokar VR, Powar RM, et al: Human trypanosomiasis caused by *Trypanosoma evansi* in India: The first case report. Am J Trop Med Hyg 2005;73:491-495.

697. Powar RM, Shegokar VR, Joshi PP, et al: A rare case of human trypanosomiasis caused by *Trypanosoma evansi*. Indian J Med Microbiol 2006;24:72-74.

698. Kaur R, Gupta VK, Dhariwal AC, et al: A rare case of trypanosomiasis in a two month old infant in Mumbai, India. J Commun Dis 2007;39:71-74.

699. Robinson B, Clark RM, King JF, et al: Chronic Gambian trypanosomiasis. South Med J 1980;73:516-518.

700. Murray HW, Pépin J, Nutman TB, et al: Tropical medicine. BMJ 2000;320:490-494.

701. Spencer HC Jr, Gibson JJ Jr, Brodsky RE, Schultz MG: Imported African trypanosomiasis in the United States. Ann Intern Med 1975;82:633-638.

702. McGovern TW, Williams W, Fitzpatrick JE, et al: Cutaneous manifestations of African trypanosomiasis. Arch Dermatol 1995;131:1178-1182.

703. Cochran R, Rosen T: African trypanosomiasis in the United States. Arch Dermatol 1983;119:670-674.

704. Moore AC, Ryan ET, Waldron MA: Case records of the Massachusetts General Hospital: Weekly clinicopathological exercises. Case 20-2002: A 37-year-old man with fever, hepatosplenomegaly, and a cutaneous foot lesion after a trip to Africa. N Engl J Med 2002;346:2069-2076.

705. Vincendeau P, Bouteille B: Immunology and immunopathology of African trypanosomiasis. An Acad Bras Cienc 2006;78:645-665.

706. Gruszynski AE, DeMaster A, Hooper NM, Bangs JD: Surface coat remodeling during differentiation of *Trypanosoma brucei*. J Biol Chem 2003;278:24665-22472.

707. Donelson JE, Hill KL, El-Sayed NM: Multiple mechanisms of immune evasion by African trypanosomes. Mol Biochem Parasitol 1998;91:51-66.

708. Prata A: Clinical and epidemiological aspects of Chagas disease. Lancet Infect Dis 2001;1:92-100.

709. La Forgia MP, Pellerano G, de las Mercedes Portaluppi M, et al: Cutaneous manifestation of reactivation of Chagas disease in a renal transplant patient: Long-term follow-up. Arch Dermatol 2003;139:104-105.

710. Almeida DR, Carvalho AC, Branco JN, et al: Chagas' disease reactivation after heart transplantation: Efficacy of allopurinol treatment. J Heart Lung Transplant 1996;15:988-992.

711. Tomimori-Yamashita J, Deps PD, Almeida DR, et al: Cutaneous manifestation of Chagas' disease after heart transplantation: Successful treatment with allopurinol. Br J Dermatol. 1997;137:626-630.

712. Piacenza L, Peluffo G, Alvarez MN, et al: Peroxiredoxins play a major role in protecting *Trypanosoma cruzi* against macrophage- and endogenously-derived peroxynitrite. Biochem J 2008;410:359-368.

713. Brodskyn C, Patricio J, Oliveira R, et al: Glycoinositolphospholipids from *Trypanosoma cruzi* interfere with macrophages and dendritic cell responses. Infect Immun 2002;70:3736-3743.

714. Tarleton RL: Immune system recognition of *Trypanosoma cruzi*. Curr Opin Immunol 2007;19:430-434.

715. Desjeux P: Leishmaniasis: Current situation and new perspectives. Comp Immunol Microbiol Infect Dis 2004;27:305-318.

716. Hepburn NC: Cutaneous leishmaniasis: An overview. J Postgrad Med 2003;49:50-54.

717. Yamey G, Hotez P: Neglected tropical diseases. BMJ 2007;335:269-270.

718. Murray HW, Berman JD, Davies CR, Saravia NG: Advances in leishmaniasis. Lancet 2005;366:1561-1577.

719. Morillas-Marquez F, Martin-Sanchez J, Acedo-Sanchez C, et al: *Leishmania infantum* (Protozoa, kinetoplastida): Transmission from infected patients to experimental animal under conditions that simulate needle-sharing. Exp Parasitol 2002;100:71-74.

720. Cruz I, Morales MA, Noguer I, et al: *Leishmania* in discarded syringes from intravenous drug users. Lancet 2002;359:1124-1125.

721. Pagliano P, Carannante N, Rossi M, et al: Visceral leishmaniasis in pregnancy: A case series and a systematic review of the literature. J Antimicrob Chemother 2005;55:229-233.

722. Marsella R, Ruiz de Gopegui R: Leishmaniasis: A re-emerging zoonosis. Int J Dermatol 1998;37:801-814.

723. Sacks D, Sher A: Evasion of innate immunity by parasitic protozoa. Nat Immunol 2002;3:1041-1047.

724. Engwerda CR, Ato M, Kaye PM: Macrophages, pathology and parasite persistence in experimental visceral leishmaniasis. Trends Parasitol 2004;20:524-530.

725. Späth GF, Garraway LA, Turco SJ, Beverley SM: The role(s) of lipophosphoglycan (LPG) in the establishment of *Leishmania major* infections in mammalian hosts. Proc Natl Acad Sci U S A 2003;100:9536-9541.

726. Joshi PB, Kelly BL, Kamhawi S, et al: Targeted gene deletion in *Leishmania major* identifies leishmanolysin (GP63) as a virulence factor. Mol Biochem Parasitol 2002;120:33-40.

727. Ivens AC, Peacock CS, Worthey EA, et al: The genome of the kinetoplastid parasite, *Leishmania major*. Science 2005;309:436-442.

728. Reithinger R, Dujardin JC, Louzir H, et al: Cutaneous leishmaniasis. Lancet Infect Dis 2007;7:581-596.

729. Dowlati Y: Cutaneous leishmaniasis: Clinical aspect. Clin Dermatol 1996;14:425-431.

730. Palacios R, Osorio LE, Grajalew LF, Ochoa MT: Treatment failure in children in a randomized clinical trial with 10 and 20 days of meglumine antimonate for cutaneous leishmaniasis due to *Leishmania viannia* species. Am J Trop Med Hyg 2001;64:187-193.

731. Raja KM, Khan AA, Hameed A, Rahman SB: Unusual clinical variants of cutaneous leishmaniasis in Pakistan. Br J Dermatol 1998;139:111-113.

732. Kanj LF, Kibbi AG, Zaynoun S: Cutaneous leishmaniasis: An unusual case with atypical recurrence. J Am Acad Dermatol 1993;28:495-496.

733. Momeni AZ, Yotsumoto S, Mehregan DR, et al: Chronic lupoid leishmaniasis: Evaluation by polymerase chain reaction. Arch Dermatol 1996;132:198-202.

734. Landau M, Srebrnik A, Brenner S: Leishmaniasis recidivans mimicking lupus vulgaris. Int J Dermatol 1996;35:572-573.

735. Al-Qurashi AR, Ghandour AM, Osman M, Al-Juma M: Dissemination in cutaneous leishmaniasis due to *Leishmania major* in different ethnic groups in Saudi Arabia. Int J Dermatol 2000;39:832-836.

736. Kurban AK, Malak JA, Farah FS, Chaglassian HT: Histopathology of cutaneous leishmaniasis. Arch Dermatol 1966;93:396-401.

737. Palma GI, Saravia NG: In situ characterization of the human host response to *Leishmania panamensis*. Am J Dermatopathol 1997;19:585-590.

738. Kibbi AG, Karam PG, Kurban AK: Sporotrichoid leishmaniasis in patients from Saudi Arabia: Clinical and histologic features. J Am Acad Dermatol 1987;17(5 Pt 1):759-764.

739. Nicolis GD, Tosca AD, Stratigos JD, Capetanakis JA: A clinical and histological study of cutaneous leishmaniasis. Acta Derm Venereol. 1978;58:521-525.

740. Peltier E, Wolkenstein P, Deniau M, et al: Caseous necrosis in cutaneous leishmaniasis. J Clin Pathol 1996;49:517-519.

741. Rau RC, Dubin HV, Taylor WB: *Leishmania tropica* infections in travellers. Arch Dermatol 1976;112:197-201.

742. Bittencourt AL, Barral A, Costa JM, et al: Diffuse cutaneous leishmaniasis with atypical aspects. Int J Dermatol 1992;31:568-570.

743. Weigle K, Saravia NG: Natural history, clinical evolution, and the host-parasite interaction in New World cutaneous leishmaniasis. Clin Dermatol 1996;14:433-450.

744. Aliaga L, Cobo F, Mediavilla JD, et al: Localized mucosal leishmaniasis due to *Leishmania (Leishmania) infantum*: Clinical and microbiologic findings in 31 patients. Medicine (Baltimore) 2003;82:147-158.

745. Morsy TA, Khalil NM, Salama MM, et al: Mucosal leishmaniasis caused by *Leishmania tropica* in Saudi Arabia. J Egypt Soc Parasitol 1995;25:73-79.

746. Kharfi M, Fazaa B, Chaker E, Kamoun MR: Mucosal localization of leishmaniasis in Tunisia: 5 Cases. Ann Dermatol Venereol 2003;130(1 Pt 1):27-30.

747. Machado-Coelho GL, Caiaffa WT, Genaro O, et al: Risk factors for mucosal manifestation of American cutaneous leishmaniasis. Trans R Soc Trop Med Hyg 2005;99:55-61.

748. Blum J, Desjeux P, Schwartz E, et al: Treatment of cutaneous leishmaniasis among travellers. J Antimicrob Chemother 2004;53:158-166.

749. Farge D, Frances C, Vouldoukis I, et al: Chronic destructive ulcerative lesion of the midface and nasal cavity due to leishmaniasis contracted in Djibouti. Clin Exp Dermatol 1987;12:211-213.

750. Price SM, Silvers DN: New world leishmaniasis: Serologic aids to diagnosis. Arch Dermatol 1977;113:1415-1416.

751. Sanguenza OP, Sanguenza JM, Stiller MJ, Sanguenza P: Mucocutaneous leishmaniasis: A clinicopathologic classification. J Am Acad Dermatol 1993;28:927-932.

752. Ridley DS, Marsden PD, Cuba CC, Barreto AC: A histological classification of mucocutaneous leishmaniasis in Brazil and its clinical evaluation. Trans R Soc Trop Med Hyg 1980;74:508-514.

753. Guerin PJ, Olliaro P, Sundar S, et al: Visceral leishmaniasis: Current status of control, diagnosis, and treatment, and a proposed research and development agenda. Lancet Infect Dis 2002;2:494-501.

754. Osman OF, Kager PA, Oskam L: Leishmaniasis in the Sudan: A literature review with emphasis on clinical aspects. Trop Med Int Health 2000;5:553-562.

755. Girgla HS, Marsden RA, Singh GM, Ryan TJ: Post-kala-azar dermal leishmaniasis. Br J Dermatol 1977;97:307-311.

756. Zijlstra EE, Musa AM, Khalil EA, et al: Post-kala-azar dermal leishmaniasis. Lancet Infect Dis 2003;3:87-98.

757. Ramesh V, Mukherjee A: Post-kala-azar dermal leishmaniasis. Int J Dermatol 1995;34:85-91.

758. Mukherjee A, Ramesh V, Misra RS: Post-kala-azar dermal leishmaniasis: A light and electron microscopic study of 18 cases. J Cutan Pathol 1993;20:320-325.

759. Perrin C, Taillan B, Hofman P, et al: Atypical cutaneous histological features of visceral leishmaniasis in acquired immunodeficiency syndrome. Am J Dermatopathol 1995;17:145-150.

760. González-Beato MJ, Moyano B, Sánchez C, et al: Kaposi's sarcoma-like lesions and other nodules as cutaneous involvement in AIDS-related visceral leishmaniasis. Br J Dermatol 2000;143:1316-1318.

761. Elhassan AM, Ali MS, Zijlstra E, et al: Post-kala-azar dermal leishmaniasis in the Sudan: Peripheral neural involvement. Int J Dermatol 1992;31:400-403.

762. Pavithran K: Trichomonal abscess of the median raphe of the penis. Int J Dermatol 1993;32:820-821.

763. Purello-D'Ambrosio F, Gangemi S, Ricciardi L, et al: Urticaria from *Trichomonas* vaginalis infection. J Investig Allergol Clin Immunol 1999;9:123-125.

764. Sanchez-Carpintero I, Vazquez-Doval FJ: Cutaneous lesions in giardiasis: Report of two cases. Br J Dermatol 1998;139:152-153.

765. Pietrzak A, Chodorowska G, Urban J, et al: Cutaneous manifestation of giardiasis: Case report. Ann Agric Environ Med 2005;12:299-303.

766. Andreev VC, Angelov N, Zlatkov NB: Skin manifestations in toxoplasmosis. Arch Dermatol 1969;100:196-199.

767. Menter MA, Morrison JG: Lichen verrucosus et reticularis of Kaposi (porokeratosis striata of Nékam): A manifestation of acquired adult toxoplasmosis. Br J Dermatol 1976;94:645-654.

768. Binazzi M, Papini M: Cutaneous toxoplasmosis. Int J Dermatol 1980;19:332-335.

769. Pollock JL: Toxoplasmosis appearing to be dermatomyositis. Arch Dermatol 1979;115:736-737.

770. Leyva WH, Santa Cruz DJ: Cutaneous toxoplasmosis. J Am Acad Dermatol 1986;14:600-605.

771. Coulman CU, Greene I, Archibald RW: Cutaneous pneumocystosis. Ann Intern Med 1987;106:396-398.

772. Sandler B, Potter TS, Hashimoto K: Cutaneous *Pneumocystis carinii* and *Cryptococcus neoformans* in AIDS. Br J Dermatol 1996;134:159-163.

773. Engels D, Chitsulo L, Montresor A, Savioli L: The global epidemiological situation of schistosomiasis and new approaches to control and research. Acta Trop 2002;82:139-146.

774. Ross AG, Bartley PB, Sleigh AC, et al: Schistosomiasis. N Engl J Med 2002;346:1212-1220.

775. Obasi OE: Cutaneous schistosomiasis in Nigeria: An update. Br J Dermatol 1986;114:597-602.

776. Amer M: Cutaneous schistosomiasis. Dermatol Clin 1994;12:713-717.

777. Torres VM: Dermatologic manifestations of *Schistosomiasis mansoni*. Arch Dermatol 1976;112:1539-1542.

778. Walther RR: Chronic papular dermatitis of the scrotum due to *Schistosoma mansoni*. Arch Dermatol 1979;115:869-870.

779. Jacyk WK, Lawande RV, Tulpule SS: Unusual presentation of extragenital cutaneous *Schistosomiasis mansoni*. Br J Dermatol 1980;103:205-208.

780. McKee PH, Wright E, Hutt MS: Vulval schistosomiasis. Clin Exp Dermatol 1983;8:189-194.

781. Davis-Reed L, Theis JH: Cutaneous schistosomiasis: Report of a case and review of the literature. J Am Acad Dermatol 2000;42:678-680.

782. Wood MG, Srolovitz H, Schetman D: Schistosomiasis: Paraplegia and ectopic skin lesions as admission symptoms. Arch Dermatol 1976;112:690-695.

783. Leman JA, Small G, Wilks D, Tidman MJ: Localized papular cutaneous schistosomiasis: Two cases in travellers. Clin Exp Dermatol 2001;26:50-52.

784. Kick G, Schaller M, Korting HC: Late cutaneous schistosomiasis representing an isolated skin manifestation of *Schistosoma mansoni* infection. Dermatology 2000;200:144-146.

785. Eulderink F, Gryseels B, van Kampen WJ, de Regt J: Haematobium schistosomiasis presenting in the Netherlands as a skin disease. Am J Dermatopathol 1994;16:434-438.

786. Poderoso WL, Santana WB, Costa EF, et al: Ectopic schistosomiasis: Description of five cases involving skin, one ovarian case and one adrenal case. Rev Soc Bras Med Trop 2008;41:668-671.

787. King DT, Gilbert DJ, Gurevitch AW, et al: Subcutaneous cysticercosis. Arch Dermatol 1979;115:236.

788. Tschen EH, Tschen EA, Smith EB: Cutaneous cysticercosis treated with metrifonate. Arch Dermatol 1981;117:507-509.

789. Wortman PD: Subcutaneous cysticercosis. J Am Acad Dermatol 1991;25(2 Pt 2):409-414.

790. Schmidt DK, Jordaan HF, Schneider JW, Cilliers J: Cerebral and subcutaneous cysticercosis treated with albendazole. Int J Dermatol 1995;34:574-579.

791. O'Grady TC, Robbins BA, Barrett TL, Higginbottom PA: Subcutaneous cysticercosis simulating metastatic breast carcinoma. Int J Dermatol 1993;32:62-64.

792. Amatya BM, Kimula Y: Cysticercosis in Nepal: A histopathologic study of sixty-two cases. Am J Surg Pathol 1999;23:1276-1279.

793. Miura H, Itoh Y, Kozuka T: A case of subcutaneous cysticercosis (Cysticercus cellulosae cutis). J Am Acad Dermatol 2000;43:538-540.

794. Raimer S, Wolf JE Jr: Subcutaneous cysticercosis. Arch Dermatol 1978;114:107-108.

795. Kim SH, Park K, Lee ES: Three cases of cutaneous sparganosis. Int J Dermatol 2001;40:656-658.

796. Griffin MP, Tompkins KJ, Ryan MT: Cutaneous sparganosis. Am J Dermatopathol 1996;18:70-72.

797. Norman SH, Kreutner A Jr: Sparganosis: Clinical and pathologic observations in ten cases. South Med J. 1980;73:297-300.

798. Taylor RL: Sparganosis in the United States: Report of a case. Am J Clin Pathol 1976;66:560-564.

799. Garin YJ, Frottier J, Lavergne-Slove A, et al: Cutaneous sparganosis in France: The second case described from Europe. Case report. APMIS 1997;105:14-16.

800. Von Brand T, Nylen MU: Organic matrix of cestode calcareous corpuscles. Exp Parasitol 1970;28:566-576.

801. McManus DP, Zhang W, Li J, Bartley PB: Echinococcosis. Lancet 2003;362:1295-1304.

802. Bresson-Hadni S, Humbert P, Paintaud G, et al: Skin localization of alveolar echinococcosis of the liver. J Am Acad Dermatol 1996;34(5 Pt 2):873-877.

803. D'Alessandro A: Polycystic echinococcosis in tropical America: *Echinococcus vogeli* and *E. oligarthrus*. Acta Trop 1997;67:43-65.

804. Kismet K, Ozcan AH, Sabuncuoglu MZ, et al: A rare case: Spontaneous cutaneous fistula of infected splenic hydatid cyst. World J Gastroenterol 2006;12:2633-2635.

805. Kouskos E, Chatziantoniou J, Chrissafis I, et al: Uncommon locations of hydatid cysts. Singapore Med J 2007;48:e119-e121.

806. Isitmangil T, Toker A, Sebit S, et al: A novel terminology and dissemination theory for a subgroup of intrathoracic extrapulmonary hydatid cysts. Med Hypotheses 2003;61:68-71.

807. El Fortia M, Bendaoud M, Shaban A, et al: Subcutaneous extension of a large psoas muscle *Echinococcus* cyst. Eur Radiol 2000;10:870.

808. Parmar H, Nagarajan G, Supe A: Subcutaneous rupture of hepatic hydatid cyst. Scand J Infect Dis 2001;33:870-872.

809. Bedioui H, Ayadi S, Nouira K, et al: Subcutaneous rupture of hydatid cyst of liver: Dealing with a rare observation. Med Trop (Mars) 2006;66:488-490.

810. Marinis A, Fragulidis G, Karapanos K, et al: Subcutaneous extension of a large diaphragmatic hydatid cyst. World J Gastroenterol 2006;12:7210-7212.

811. Polat P, Kantarci M, Alper F, et al: Hydatid disease from head to toe. Radiographics 2003;23:475-494; quiz 536-537.

812. Vicidomini S, Cancrini G, Gabrielli S, et al: Muscular cystic hydatidosis: Case report. BMC Infect Dis 2007;7:23.

813. Drimousis PG, Stamou KM, Koutras A, et al: Unusual site of recurrent musculoskeletal hydatid cyst: Case report and brief review of the literature. World J Gastroenterol 2006;12:5577-5578.

814. Deonarain J, Ramdial PK, Sing Y, et al: Subcutaneous palisading granulomatous pseudocysts of *Echinococcus granulosus* origin. J Cutan Pathol 2008;36:240-245.

815. World Health Organization: Onchocerciasis (river blindness). Report from the Tenth InterAmerican Conference on Onchocerciasis, Guayaquil, Ecuador. Wkly Epidemiol Rec 2001;76:205-212.

816. Somorin AO: Onchocerciasis. Int J Dermatol 1983;22:182-188.

817. Hay RJ, Mackenzie CD, Guderian R, et al: Onchodermatitis: Correlation between skin disease and parasitic load in an endemic focus in Ecuador. Br J Dermatol 1989;121:187-198.

818. Yarzábal L: The immunology of onchocerciasis. Int J Dermatol 1985;24:349-358.

819. Murdoch ME, Hay RJ, Mackenzie CD, et al: A clinical classification and grading system of the cutaneous changes in onchocerciasis. Br J Dermatol 1993;129:260-269.

820. Richards F, Hopkins D, Cupp E: Programmatic goals and approaches to onchocerciasis. Lancet 2000;355:1663-1664.

821. Udall DN: Recent updates on onchocerciasis: Diagnosis and treatment. Clin Infect Dis 2007;44:53-60.

822. Connor DH, Gibson DW, Neafie RC, et al: Sowda—Onchocerciasis in north Yemen: A clinicopathologic study of 18 patients. Am J Trop Med Hyg 1983;32:123-137.

823. Okulicz JF, Stibich AS, Elston DM, Schwartz RA: Cutaneous onchocercoma. Int J Dermatol 2004;43:170-172.

824. Wolf R, Orion E, Matz H: Onchocerciasis (river blindness). Isr Med Assoc J 2003;5:522-523.

825. Brattig NW: Pathogenesis and host responses in human onchocerciasis: Impact of *Onchocerca filariae* and *Wolbachia endobacteria*. Microbes Infect 2004;6:113-128.

826. Grandi G, Morchon R, Kramer L, et al: *Wolbachia* in *Dirofilaria repens*, an agent causing human subcutaneous dirofilariasis. J Parasitol 2008;94:1421-1423.

827. Timmann C, Abraha RS, Hamelmann C, et al: Cutaneous pathology in onchocerciasis associated with pronounced systemic T-helper 2-type responses to *Onchocerca* volvulus. Br J Dermatol 2003;149:782-787.

828. Hoerauf A, Volkmann L, Hamelmann C, et al: Endosymbiotic bacteria in worms as targets for a novel chemotherapy in filariasis. Lancet 2000;355:1242-1243.

829. Connor DH, George GH, Gibson DW: Pathologic changes of human onchocerciasis: Implications for future research. Rev Infect Dis 1985;7:809-819.

830. Connor DH, Williams PH, Helwig EB, Winslow DJ: Dermal changes in onchocerciasis. Arch Pathol 1969;87:193-200.

831. Stingl P: Onchocerciasis: Clinical presentation and host parasite interactions in patients of southern Sudan. Int J Dermatol 1997;36:23-28.

832. Rozenman D, Kremer M, Zuckerman F: Onchocerciasis in Israel. Arch Dermatol 1984;120:505-507.

833. Payan HM: Human infection with *Dirofilaria*. Arch Dermatol 1978;114:593-594.

834. Santamaría B, Di Sacco B, Muro A, et al: Serological diagnosis of subcutaneous dirofilariosis. Clin Exp Dermatol 1995;20:19-21.

835. Gutierrez Y: Diagnostic features of zoonotic filariae in tissue sections. Hum Pathol 1984;15:514-525.

836. van den Ende J, Kumar V, van Gompel A, et al: Subcutaneous dirofilariasis caused by *Dirofilaria (Nochtiella) repens* in a Belgian patient. Int J Dermatol 1995;34:274-277.

837. Herzberg AJ, Boyd PR, Gutierrez Y: Subcutaneous dirofilariasis in Collier County, Florida, USA. Am J Surg Pathol 1995;19:934-939.

838. Jelinek T, Schulte-Hillen J, Löscher T: Human dirofilariasis. Int J Dermatol 1996;35:872-875.

839. Pampiglione S, Rivasi F, Angeli G, et al: Dirofilariasis due to *Dirofilaria repens* in Italy, an emergent zoonosis: Report of 60 new cases. Histopathology 2001;38:344-354.

840. Billups J, Schenken JR, Beaver PC: Subcutaneous dirofilariasis in Nebraska. Arch Pathol Lab Med 1980;104:11-13.

841. Shenefelt PD, Esperanza L, Lynn A: Elusive migratory subcutaneous dirofilariasis. J Am Acad Dermatol 1996;35(2 Pt 1):260-262.

842. Fisher BK, Homayouni M, Orihel TC: Subcutaneous infections with *Dirofilaria*: A report of two cases. Arch Dermatol 1964;89:837-840.

843. Williams HC, Monk B: Creeping eruption stopped in its tracks by albendazole. Clin Exp Dermatol 1989;14:355-356.

844. Davies HD, Sakuls P, Keystone JS: Creeping eruption: A review of clinical presentation and management of 60 cases presenting to a tropical disease unit. Arch Dermatol 1993;129:588-591.

845. Albanese G, Di Cintio R, Beneggi M, et al: Larva migrans in Italy. Int J Dermatol 1995;34:464-465.

846. Grassi A, Angelo C, Grosso MG, Paradisi M: Perianal cutaneous larva migrans in a child. Pediatr Dermatol 1998;15:367-369.

847. Heukelbach J, Feldmeier H: Epidemiological and clinical characteristics of hookworm-related cutaneous larva migrans. Lancet Infect Dis 2008;8:302-309.

848. Caumes E, Danis M: From creeping eruption to hookworm-related cutaneous larva migrans. Lancet Infect Dis 2004;4:659-660.

849. Hochedez P, Caumes E: Hookworm-related cutaneous larva migrans. J Travel Med 2007;14:326-333.

850. Magaña M, Messina M, Bustamante F, Cazarín J: Gnathostomiasis: Clinicopathologic study. Am J Dermatopathol 2004;26:91-95.

851. Ménard A, Dos Santos G, Dekumyoy P, et al: Imported cutaneous gnathostomiasis: Report of five cases. Trans R Soc Trop Med Hyg 2003;97:200-202.

852. Díaz Camacho SP, Willms K, de la Cruz Otero Madel C, et al: Acute outbreak of gnathostomiasis in a fishing community in Sinaloa, Mexico. Parasitol Int 2003;52:133-140.

853. Gillespie SH: Cutaneous larva migrans. Curr Infect Dis Rep 2004;6:50-53.

854. Stone OJ, Newell GB, Mullins JF: Cutaneous strongyloidiasis: Larva currens. Arch Dermatol 1972;106:734-736.

855. von Kuster LC, Genta RM: Cutaneous manifestations of strongyloidiasis. Arch Dermatol 1988;124:1826-1830.

856. Kourilová P, Hogg KG, Kolárová L, Mountford AP: Cercarial dermatitis caused by bird schistosomes comprises both immediate and late phase cutaneous hypersensitivity reactions. J Immunol 2004;172:3766-3774.

857. Beaver PC: Visceral and cutaneous larva migrans. Public Health Rep 1959;74:328-332.

858. Jackson A, Heukelbach J, Calheiros CM, et al: A study in a community in Brazil in which cutaneous larva migrans is endemic. Clin Infect Dis 2006;43:e13-e18.

859. Heukelbach J, Wilcke T, Feldmeier H: Cutaneous larva migrans (creeping eruption) in an urban slum in Brazil. Int J Dermatol 2004;43:511-515.

860. Lee CP, Bishop LJ: The incidence of cutaneous larva migrans in Montserrat, Leeward Islands, West Indies. West Indian Med J 1988;37:22-24.

861. Heukelbach J, Wilcke T, Meier A, et al: A longitudinal study on cutaneous larva migrans in an impoverished Brazilian township. Travel Med Infect Dis 2003;1:213-218.

862. Heukelbach J, Jackson A, Ariza L, Feldmeier H: Prevalence and risk factors of hookworm-related cutaneous larva migrans in a rural community in Brazil. Ann Trop Med Parasitol 2008;102:53-61.

863. Blackwell V, Vega-Lopez F: Cutaneous larva migrans: Clinical features and management of 44 cases presenting in the returning traveller. Br J Dermatol 2001;145:434-437.

864. Jelinek T, Maiwald H, Nothdurft HD, Löscher T: Cutaneous larva migrans in travelers: Synopsis of histories, symptoms, and treatment of 98 patients. Clin Infect Dis 1994;19:1062-1066.

865. Veraldi S, Bottini S, Carrera C, Gianotti R: Cutaneous larva migrans with folliculitis: A new clinical presentation of this infestation. J Eur Acad Dermatol Venereol 2005;19:628-630.

866. Caumes E, Ly F, Bricaire F: Cutaneous larva migrans with folliculitis: Report of seven cases and review of the literature. Br J Dermatol 2002;146:314-316.

867. Vaughan TK, English JC 3rd: Cutaneous larva migrans complicated by erythema multiforme. Cutis 1998;62:33-35.

868. Gill GV, Welch E, Bailey JW, et al: Chronic *Strongyloides stercoralis* infection in former British Far East prisoners of war. Q J Med 2004;97:789-795.

869. Ronan SG, Reddy RL, Manaligod JR, et al: Disseminated strongyloidiasis presenting as purpura. J Am Acad Dermatol 1989;21(5 Pt 2):1123-1125.

870. Purvis RS, Beightler EL, Diven DG, et al: *Strongyloides* hyperinfection presenting with petechiae and purpura. Int J Dermatol 1992;31:169-171.

871. Sulica VI, Berberian B, Kao GF: Histopathologic findings of cutaneous larva migrans (Abstract). J Cutan Pathol 1988;15:346.

872. Czarnetzki BM, Springorum M: Larva migrans with eosinophilic papular folliculitis. Dermatologica 1982;164:36-40.

873. Miller AC, Walker J, Jaworski R, et al: Hookworm folliculitis. Arch Dermatol 1991;127:547-549.

874. Vetter RS, Visscher PK: Bites and stings of medically important venomous arthropods. Int J Dermatol 1998;37:481-496.

875. Dehesa-Dávila M, Possani LD: Scorpionism and serotherapy in Mexico. Toxicon 1994;32:1015-1018.

876. Radmanesh M: Cutaneous manifestations of the *Hemiscorpius lepturus* sting: A clinical study. Int J Dermatol 1998;37:500-507.

877. Moss HS, Binder LS: A retrospective review of black widow spider envenomation. Ann Emerg Med 1987;16:188-192.

878. Maretić Z: Latrodectism: Variations in clinical manifestations provoked by *Latrodectus* species of spiders. Toxicon 1983;21:457-466.

879. Bernstein B, Ehrlich F: Brown recluse spider bites. J Emerg Med 1986;4:457-462.

880. Williams ST, Khare VK, Johnston GA, Blackall DP: Severe intravascular hemolysis associated with brown recluse spider envenomation: A report of two cases and review of the literature. Am J Clin Pathol 1995;104:463-467.

881. Patel KD, Modur V, Zimmerman GA, et al: The necrotic venom of the brown recluse spider induces dysregulated endothelial cell-dependent neutrophil activation: Differential induction of GM-CSF, IL-8, and E-selectin expression. J Clin Invest 1994;94:631-642.

882. Ingber A, Trattner A, Cleper R, Sandbank M: Morbidity of brown recluse spider bites: Clinical picture, treatment and prognosis. Acta Derm Venereol 1991;71:337-340.

883. Lung JM, Mallory SB: A child with spider bite and glomerulonephritis: A diagnostic challenge. Int J Dermatol 2000;39:287-289.

884. Wasserman GS, Anderson PC: Loxoscelism and necrotic arachnidism. J Toxicol Clin Toxicol 1983-1984;21(4-5):451-472.

885. Anderson PC: Necrotizing spider bites. Am Fam Physician 1982;26:198-203.

886. Sams HH, Hearth SB, Long LL, et al: Nineteen documented cases of *Loxosceles reclusa* envenomation. J Am Acad Dermatol 2001;44:603-608.

887. Rosenstein ED, Kramer N: Lyme disease misdiagnosed as a brown recluse spider bite. Ann Intern Med 1987;107:782.

888. Rees RS, Fields JP, King LE Jr: Do brown recluse spider bites induce pyoderma gangrenosum? South Med J 1985;78:283-287.

889. Fisher RG, Kelly P, Krober MS, et al: Necrotic arachnidism. West J Med 1994;160:570-572.

890. Lucas S: Spiders in Brazil. Toxicon 1988;26:759-772.

891. Sutherland S: Sydney funnel web spider bite. Aust Fam Physician 1985;14:316.

892. Sams HH, Dunnick CA, Smith ML, King LE Jr: Necrotic arachnidism. J Am Acad Dermatol 2001;44:561-573; quiz 573-576.

893. Pucevich MV, Chesney TMcC: Histopathologic analysis of human bites by the brown recluse spider (Abstract). Arch Dermatol 1983;119:851.

894. Castelli E, Caputo V, Morello V, Tomasino RM: Local reactions to tick bites. Am J Dermatopathol 2008;30:241-248.

895. Leker RR, Felsenstein I, Raveh D, et al: Ornithodoros tholozani bites: A unique clinical picture. J Am Acad Dermatol 1992;27:1025-1026.

896. Bowman AS, Sauer JR: Tick salivary glands: Function, physiology and future. Parasitology 2004;129(Suppl):S67-S81.

897. Sauer JR, McSwain JL, Bowman AS, Essenberg RC: Tick salivary gland physiology. Annu Rev Entomol 1995;40:245-267.

898. Maxwell SS, Stoklasek TA, Dash Y, et al: Tick modulation of the in-vitro expression of adhesion molecules by skin-derived endothelial cells. Ann Trop Med Parasitol 2005;99:661-672.

899. Krinsky WL: Dermatoses associated with the bites of mites and ticks (Arthropoda: Acari). Int J Dermatol 1983;22:75-91.

900. Cho BK, Kang H, Bang D, et al: Tick bites in Korea. Int J Dermatol 1994;33:552-555.

901. Jordaan HF, Schneider JW: Papular urticaria: A histopathologic study of 30 patients. Am J Dermatopathol 1997;19:119-126.

902. Stefanato CM, Phelps RG, Goldberg LJ, et al: Type-I cryoglobulinemia-like histopathologic changes in tick bites: A useful clue for tissue diagnosis in the absence of tick parts. J Cutan Pathol 2002;29:101-106.

903. Galaria NA, Chaudhary O, Magro CM: Tick mouth parts occlusive vasculopathy: A localized cryoglobulinemic vasculitic response. J Cutan Pathol 2003;30:303-306.

904. Böer A, Tirumalae R, Bresch M, Falk TM: Pseudoclonality in cutaneous pseudolymphomas: A pitfall in interpretation of rearrangement studies. Br J Dermatol 2008;159:394-402.

905. Heyl T: Tick bite alopecia. Clin Exp Dermatol 1982;7:537-542.

906. Ross MS, Friede H: Alopecia due to tick bite. AMA Arch Derm Syphilol 1955;71:524-525.

907. Baima B, Sticherling M: Demodicidosis revisited. Acta Derm Venereol 2002;82:3-6.

908. Nutting WB: Hair follicle mites (Acari: Demodicidae) of man. Int J Dermatol 1976;15:79-98.

909. Nutting WB: Pathogenesis associated with hair follicle mites (Acari: Demodicidae). Acarologia 1976;17:493-507.

910. Nutting WB, Green AC: Pathogenesis associated with hair follicle mites (*Demodex* spp.) in Australian aborigines. Br J Dermatol 1976;94:307-312.

911. Aylesworth R, Vance JC: *Demodex folliculorum* and *Demodex brevis* in cutaneous biopsies. J Am Acad Dermatol 1982;7:583-589.

912. Bonnar E, Eustace P, Powell FC: The *Demodex* mite population in rosacea. J Am Acad Dermatol 1993;28:443-448.

913. Ayres S Jr, Ayres S 3rd: Demodectic eruptions (demodicidosis) in the human: 30 Years' experience with 2 commonly unrecognized entities—pityriasis folliculorum (*Demodex*) and acne rosacea (*Demodex* type). Arch Dermatol 1961;83:816-827.

914. Ayres S: Rosacea-like demodicidosis. Calif Med 1963;98:328-330.

915. Morgan RJ, Coston TO: *Demodex* blepharitis. South Med J 1964;57:694-699.

916. De Dulanto F, Camacho-Martinez F: Demodicidosis gravis. Ann Dermatol Venereol 1979;106:699-704.

917. Purcell SM, Hayes TJ, Dixon SL: Pustular folliculitis associated with *Demodex folliculorum*. J Am Acad Dermatol 1986;15:1159-1162.

918. Miskjian HG: Demodicidosis (*Demodex* infestation of the scalp). AMA Arch Derm Syphilol 1951;63:282-283.

919. Ecker RI, Winkelmann RK: *Demodex* granuloma. Arch Dermatol 1979;115:343-344.

920. Grosshans EM, Kremer M, Maleville J: *Demodex folliculorum* and the histogenesis of granulomatous rosacea. Hautarzt 1974;25:166-177.

921. Dominey A, Tschen J, Rosen T, et al: Pityriasis folliculorum revisited. J Am Acad Dermatol 1989;21:81-84.

922. Ayres S Jr, Mihan R: *Demodex* granuloma. Arch Dermatol 1979;115:1285-1286.

923. Chosidow O: Clinical practices: Scabies. N Engl J Med 200620;354:1718-1727.

924. Orkin M: Today's scabies. Arch Dermatol 1975;111:1431-1432.

925. Orkin M: Scabies and pediculosis. Major Probl Clin Pediatr 1978;19:209-221.

926. Kemp DJ, Walton SF, Harumal P, Currie BJ: The scourge of scabies. Biologist (London) 2002;49:19-24.

927. Arlian LG, Morgan MS, Neal JS: Modulation of cytokine expression in human keratinocytes and fibroblasts by extracts of scabies mites. Am J Trop Med Hyg 2003;69:652-656.

928. Arlian LG, Morgan MS, Neal JS: Extracts of scabies mites (Sarcoptidae: *Sarcoptes scabiei*) modulate cytokine expression by human peripheral blood mononuclear cells and dendritic cells. J Med Entomol 2004;41:69-73.

929. Elder BL, Arlian LG, Morgan MS: *Sarcoptes scabiei* (Acari: Sarcoptidae) mite extract modulates expression of cytokines and adhesion molecules by human dermal microvascular endothelial cells. J Med Entomol 2006;43:910-915.

930. Mimouni D, Gdalevich M, Mimouni FB, et al: The epidemiologic trends of scabies among Israeli soldiers: A 28-year follow-up. Int J Dermatol 1998;37:586-587.

931. Mimouni D, Ankol OE, Davidovitch N, et al: Seasonality trends of scabies in a young adult population: A 20-year follow-up. Br J Dermatol 2003;149:157-159.

932. Downs AM, Harvey I, Kennedy CT: The epidemiology of head lice and scabies in the UK. Epidemiol Infect 1999;122:471-477.

933. Paller AS: Scabies in infants and small children. Semin Dermatol 1993;12:3-8.

934. Falk ES, Eide TJ: Histologic and clinical findings in human scabies. Int J Dermatol 1981;20:600-605.

935. Brenner S, Wolf R, Landau M: Scabid: An unusual id reaction to scabies. Int J Dermatol 1993;32:128-129.

936. Argenziano G, Fabbrocini G, Delfino M: Epiluminescence microscopy: A new approach to in vivo detection of *Sarcoptes scabiei*. Arch Dermatol 1997;133:751-753.

937. Prins C, Stucki L, French L, et al: Dermoscopy for the in vivo detection of *Sarcoptes scabiei*. Dermatology 2004;208:241-243.

938. Walton SF, McBroom J, Mathews JD, et al: Crusted scabies: A molecular analysis of *Sarcoptes scabiei* variety hominis populations from patients with repeated infestations. Clin Infect Dis 1999; 29:1226-1230.

939. Slawsky LD, Maroon M, Tyler WB, Miller OF 3rd: Association of scabies with a bullous pemphigoid-like eruption. J Am Acad Dermatol 1996;34:878-879.

940. Ostlere LS, Harris D, Rustin MH: Scabies associated with a bullous pemphigoid-like eruption. Br J Dermatol 1993;128:217-219.

941. Wozniacka A, Hawro T, Schwartz RA: Bullous scabies: A diagnostic challenge. Cutis 2008;82:350-352.

942. Konishi N, Suzuki K, Tokura Y, et al: Bullous eruption associated with scabies: Evidence for scabetic induction of true bullous pemphigoid. Acta Derm Venereol 2000;80:281-283.

943. Glover A, Young L, Goltz AW: Norwegian scabies in acquired immunodeficiency syndrome: Report of a case resulting in death from associated sepsis. J Am Acad Dermatol 1987;16:396-399.

944. Mollison LC, Lo ST, Marning G: HTLV-I and scabies in Australian aborigines. Lancet 1993;341:1281-1282.

945. Paterson WD, Allen BR, Beveridge GW: Norwegian scabies during immunosuppressive therapy. BMJ 1973;4:211-212.

946. Judge MR, Kobza-Black A: Crusted scabies in pregnancy. Br J Dermatol 1995;132:116-119.

947. Van Der Wal VB, Van Voorst Vader PC, Mandema JM, Jonkman MF: Crusted (Norwegian) scabies in a patient with dystrophic epidermolysis bullosa. Br J Dermatol 1999;141:918-921.

948. Torrelo A, Zambrano A: Crusted scabies in a girl with epidermolysis bullosa simplex. Br J Dermatol 2000;142:197-198.

949. Walton SF, Holt DC, Currie BJ, Kemp DJ: Scabies: New future for a neglected disease. Adv Parasitol 2004;57:309-376.

950. Walton SF, Beroukas D, Roberts-Thomson P, Currie BJ: New insights into disease pathogenesis in crusted (Norwegian) scabies: The skin immune response in crusted scabies. Br J Dermatol 2008;158:1247-1255.

951. Amer M, Mostafa FF, Nasr AN, el-Harras M: The role of mast cells in treatment of scabies. Int J Dermatol 1995;34:186-189.

952. Fernandez N, Torres A, Ackerman AB: Pathologic findings in human scabies. Arch Dermatol 1977;113:320-324.

953. Seraly MP, Shockman J, Jacoby RA: Flame figures in scabies: A case report. Arch Dermatol 1991;127:1850-1851.

954. Jarrett P, Snow J: Scabies presenting as a necrotizing vasculitis in the presence of lupus anticoagulant. Br J Dermatol 1998;139:701-703.

955. Head ES, Macdonald EM, Ewert A, Apisarnthanarax P: *Sarcoptes scabiei* in histopathologic sections of skin in human scabies. Arch Dermatol 1990;126:1475-1477.

956. Hashimoto K, Fujiwara K, Punwaney J, et al: Post-scabetic nodules: A lymphohistiocytic reaction rich in indeterminate cells. J Dermatol 2000;27:181-194.

957. Thomson J, Cochrane T, Cochran R, McQueen A: Histology simulating reticulosis in persistent nodular scabies. Br J Dermatol 1974;90:421-429.

958. Ploysangam T, Breneman DL, Mutasim DF: Cutaneous pseudolymphomas. J Am Acad Dermatol 1998;38:877-895; quiz 896-897.

959. Walton S, Bottomley WW, Wyatt EH, Bury HP: Pseudo T-cell lymphoma due to scabies in a patient with Hodgkin's disease. Br J Dermatol 1991;124:277-278.

960. Liu HN, Sheu WJ, Chu TL: Scabietic nodules: A dermatopathologic and immunofluorescent study. J Cutan Pathol 1992;19:124-127.

961. Lee BW: Cheyletiella dermatitis. Arch Dermatol 1981;117:677-678.

962. Lee BW: Cheyletiella dermatitis: A report of fourteen cases. Cutis 1991;47:111-114.

963. Powell RF, Palmer SM, Palmer CH, Smith EB: Cheyletiella dermatitis. Int J Dermatol 1977;16:679-682.

964. Wagner R, Stallmeister N: Cheyletiella dermatitis in humans, dogs and cats. Br J Dermatol 2000;143:1110-1112.

965. Shelley ED, Shelley WB, Pula JF, McDonald SG: The diagnostic challenge of nonburrowing mite bites: *Cheyletiella yasguri*. JAMA 1984;251:2690-2691.

966. Maurice PD, Schofield O, Griffiths WA: Cheyletiella dermatitis: A case report and the role of specific immunological hypersensitivity in its pathogenesis. Clin Exp Dermatol 1987;12:381-384.

967. Kittler R, Kayser M, Stoneking M: Molecular evolution of *Pediculus humanus* and the origin of clothing. Curr Biol 2003;13:1414-1417.

968. Roberts RJ: Clinical practice: Head lice. N Engl J Med 2002; 346:1645-1650.

969. Varela JA, Otero L, Espinosa E, et al: *Phthirus pubis* in a sexually transmitted diseases unit: A study of 14 years. Sex Transm Dis 2003;30:292-296.

970. Vandeweghe K, Zeyen P: Phthiriasis palpebrarum: 2 Case reports. Bull Soc Belge Ophtalmol 2006;(300):27-33.

971. Pinckney J 2nd, Cole P, Vadapalli SP, Rosen T: *Phthiriasis palpebrarum*: A common culprit with uncommon presentation. Dermatol Online J 2008;14:7.

972. Bessis D, Chraibi H, Guillot B, Guilhou JJ: Erythema annulare centrifugum induced by generalized *Phthirus pubis* infestation. Br J Dermatol 2003;149:1291.

973. Miller RA: Maculae ceruleae. Int J Dermatol 1986;25:383-384.

974. Crissey JT: Bedbugs: An old problem with a new dimension. Int J Dermatol 1981;20:411-414.

975. Ter Poorten MC, Prose NS: The return of the common bedbug. Pediatr Dermatol 2005;22:183-187.

976. Thomas I, Kihiczak GG, Schwartz RA: Bedbug bites: A review. Int J Dermatol 2004;43:430-433.

977. Tharakaram S: Bullous eruption due to *Cimex lecticularis*. Clin Exp Dermatol 1999;24:241-242.

978. Leverkus M, Jochim RC, Schäd S, et al: Bullous allergic hypersensitivity to bed bug bites mediated by IgE against salivary nitrophorin. J Invest Dermatol 2006;126:91-96.

979. Dondero TJ Jr, Schaffner W, Athanasiou R, Maguire W: Cutaneous myiasis in visitors to Central America. South Med J 1979;72:1508-1511.

980. Baird JK, Baird CR, Sabrosky CW: North American cuterebrid myiasis: Report of seventeen new infections of human beings and review of the disease. J Am Acad Dermatol 1989;21:763-772

981. Günther S: Clinical and epidemiological aspects of the dermal Tumbu-fly-myiasis in Equatorial-Africa. Br J Dermatol 1971; 85:226-231.

982. Burgess I, Spraggs PD: Myiasis due to *Parasarcophaga argyrostoma*: First recorded case in Britain. Clin Exp Dermatol 1992; 17:261-263.

983. Royce LA, Rossignol PA, Kubitz ML, Burton FR: Recovery of a second instar *Gasterophilus* larva in a human infant: A case report. Am J Trop Med Hyg 1999;60:403-404.

984. Logar J, Marini -Fišer N: Cutaneous myiasis caused by *Hypoderma lineatum*. Wien Klin Wochenschr 2008;120:619-621.

985. Delshad E, Rubin AI, Almeida L, Niedt GW: Cuterebra cutaneous myiasis: Case report and world literature review. Int J Dermatol 2008;47:363-366.

986. Cogen MS, Hays SJ, Dixon JM: Cutaneous myiasis of the eyelid due to *Cuterebra* larva. JAMA 1987;258:1795-1796.

987. Burgess I, Davies EA: Cutaneous myiasis caused by the housefly, *Musca domestica*. Br J Dermatol 1991;125:377-379.

988. Sheehan KM, Farrell BJ: A "fly in the ointment": Cutaneous infestation by *Musca domestica*. Int J Surg Pathol 2004;12:149.

989. Safdar N, Young DK, Andes D: Autochthonous furuncular myiasis in the United States: Case report and literature review. Clin Infect Dis 2003;36:e73-e80.

990. Passos MR, Barreto NA, Varella RQ, et al: Penile myiasis: A case report. Sex Transm Infect 2004;80:183-184.

991. Passos MR, Ferreira DC, Arze WN, et al: Penile myiasis as a differential diagnosis for genital ulcer: A case report. Braz J Infect Dis 2008;12:155-157.

992. Grogan TM, Payne CM, Payne TB, et al: Cutaneous myiasis: Immunohistologic and ultrastructural morphometric features of a human botfly lesion. Am J Dermatopathol 1987;9:232-239.

993. Baker DJ, Kantor GR, Stierstorfer MB, Brady G: Furuncular myiasis from *Dermatobia hominis* infestation: Diagnosis by light microscopy. Am J Dermatopathol 1995;17:389-394.

994. Reiss F: Tungiasis in New York City. Arch Dermatol 1966;93:404-407.

995. Chadee DD, Furlonge E, Naraynsingh C, Le Maitre A: Distribution and prevalence of *Tunga penetrans* in coastal south Trinidad, West Indies. Trans R Soc Trop Med Hyg 1991;85:549.

996. Veraldi S, Valsecchi M: Imported tungiasis: A report of 19 cases and review of the literature. Int J Dermatol 2007;46:1061-1066.

997. Heukelbach J, van Haeff E, Rump B, et al: Parasitic skin diseases: Health care-seeking in a slum in north-east Brazil. Trop Med Int Health 2003;8:368-373.

998. Heukelbach J, Wilcke T, Harms G, Feldmeier H: Seasonal variation of tungiasis in an endemic community. Am J Trop Med Hyg 2005;72:145-149.

999. Ugbomoiko US, Ariza L, Heukelbach J: Pigs are the most important animal reservoir for *Tunga penetrans* (jigger flea) in rural Nigeria. Trop Doct 2008;38:226-227.

1000. Heukelbach J, Costa AM, Wilcke T, et al: The animal reservoir of *Tunga penetrans* in severely affected communities of north-east Brazil. Med Vet Entomol 2004;18:329-335.

1001. Feldmeier H, Eisele M, Sabóia-Moura RC, Heukelbach J: Severe tungiasis in underprivileged communities: Case series from Brazil. Emerg Infect Dis 2003;9:949-955.

1002. Douglas-Jones AG, Llewelyn MB, Mills CM: Cutaneous infection with *Tunga penetrans*. Br J Dermatol 1995;133:125-127.

1003. Veraldi S, Camozzi S, Scarabelli G: Tungiasis presenting with sterile pustular lesions on the hand. Acta Derm Venereol 1996; 76:495.

1004. Heukelbach J, Wilcke T, Eisele M, Feldmeier H: Ectopic localization of tungiasis. Am J Trop Med Hyg 2002;67:214-216.

1005. Franck S, Feldmeier H, Heukelbach J: Tungiasis: More than an exotic nuisance. Travel Med Infect Dis 2003;1:159-166.

1006. Eisele M, Heukelbach J, Van Marck E, Mehlhorn H, et al: Investigations on the biology, epidemiology, pathology and control of *Tunga penetrans* in Brazil: I. Natural history of tungiasis in man. Parasitol Res 2003;90:87-99.

1007. Veraldi S, Schianchi R: Guess what? Tungiasis. Eur J Dermatol 1999;9:57-59.

1008. Mashek H, Licznerski B, Pincus S: Tungiasis in New York. Int J Dermatol 1997;36:276-278.

1009. Gelmetti C, Carrera C, Veraldi S: Tungiasis in a 3-year-old child. Pediatr Dermatol 2000;17:293-295.

1010. Veraldi S, Schianchi R, Cremonesi R: Bullous tungiasis. Int J Dermatol 2005;44:1067-1069.

1011. Basler EA, Stephens JH, Tschen JA: Tunga penetrans. Cutis 1988;42:47-48.

1012. Feldmeier H, Heukelbach J, Eisele M, et al: Bacterial superinfection in human tungiasis. Trop Med Int Health 2002;7:559-564.

1013. Smith MD, Procop GW: Typical histologic features of *Tunga penetrans* in skin biopsies. Arch Pathol Lab Med 2002;126:714-716.

1014. Vennos E, Burke E, Johns C, Miller S: Tungiasis. Cutis 1995;56:206-207.

1015. Zalar GL, Walther RR: Infestation by *Tunga penetrans*. Arch Dermatol 1980;116:80-81.

1016. Lass-Florl C, Mayr A: Human protothecosis. Clin Microbiol Rev 2007;20:230-242.

1017. Walsh SV, Johnson RA, Tahan SR: Protothecosis: An unusual cause of chronic subcutaneous and soft tissue infection. Am J Dermatopathol 1998;20:379-382.

1018. Thiele D, Bergmann A: Protothecosis in human medicine. Int J Hyg Environ Health 2002;204:297-302.

1019. Heney C, Greeff M, Davis V: Hickman catheter-related prothecal algaemia in an immunocompromised child. J Infect Dis 1991;163:930-931.

1020. Iacoviello VR, DeGirolami PC, Lucarini J, et al: Protothecosis complicating prolonged endotracheal intubation: Case report and literature review. Clin Infect Dis 1992;15:959-967.

1021. Torres HA, Bodey GP, Tarrand JJ, Kontoyiannis DP: Protothecosis in patients with cancer: Case series and literature review. Clin Microbiol Infect 2003;9:786-792.

1022. Dalmau J, Pimentel CL, Alegre M, et al: Treatment of protothecosis with voriconazole. J Am Acad Dermatol 2006;55(5 Suppl):S122-S123.

1023. Chao SC, Hsu MM, Lee JY: Cutaneous protothecosis: Report of five cases. Br J Dermatol 2002;146:688-693.

1024. Goldstein GD, Bhatia P, Kalivas J: Herpetiform protothecosis. Int J Dermatol 1986;25:54-55.

1025. McAnally T, Parry EL: Cutaneous protothecosis presenting as recurrent chromomycosis. Arch Dermatol 1985;121:1066-1069.

1026. Wolfe ID, Sacks HG, Samorodin CS, Robinson HM: Cutaneous protothecosis in a patient receiving immunosuppressive therapy. Arch Dermatol 1976;112:829-832.

1027. Follador I, Bittencourt A, Duran F, das Graças Araújo MG: et al: Cutaneous protothecosis: Report of the second Brazilian case. Rev Inst Med Trop Sao Paulo 2001;43:287-290.

1028. Mendez CM, Silva-Lizama E, Logemann H: Human cutaneous protothecosis. Int J Dermatol 1995;34:554-555.

1029. Zaitz C, Godoy AM, Colucci FM, et al: Cutaneous protothecosis: Report of a third Brazilian case. Int J Dermatol 2006;45:124-126.

1030. Schumann K, Hollandsworth K, Ormsby A: Nonhealing leg ulceration. Diagnosis: Protothecosis. Arch Dermatol 2000;136:1263-1268.

1031. Sudman MS: Protothecosis: A critical review. Am J Clin Pathol 1974;61:10-19.

1032. Boyd AS, Langley M, King LE Jr: Cutaneous manifestations of *Prototheca* infections. J Am Acad Dermatol 1995;32:758-764.

Index

Note: page numbers followed by f indicate figures; t, tables.

White piedra, 561
Wilder reticulin stain, 9-10, 10f
Wright stain, 24
Wuchereria bancrofti, 317. *See also* Filariasis.

X

Xanthogranulomatous pyelonephritis, 412-413, 414f

Y

Yaws
  bone infection in, 361-362
  cutaneous infection in, 541
  tertiary
    bone infection in, 362, 363f
    cutaneous infection in, 541
Yeast infections. *See* Mycoses.
Yeast lake, 161, 162f
Yeasts, capsule deficient, Fontana-Masson melanin stain of, 161, 164f
Yellow fever, liver infection in, 267-268, 268f

Yersinia enteritis, 228-229
  differential diagnosis of, 229
  histopathology of, 228-229, 229f, 243
Yersinia enterocolitica, 228, 243
Yersinia pestis, 228
Yersinia pestis pneumonia, 183-184, 184f
Yersinia pseudotuberculosis, 228, 243
Yersinia skin infections, 535-536

Z

Ziehl-Neelsen stain, 9, 10f
Zygomycetes, 579
  differentiation of mycelia of, 43-46, 47f
Zygomycosis, 579-580. *See also* Entomophthoramycosis; Mucormycosis.
  hepatic, 281
  invasive sinonasal, 107-108
  pulmonary, 172-175. *See also Fusarium; Pseudallescheria boydii* infection.
  pulmonary and renal, 48, 48f

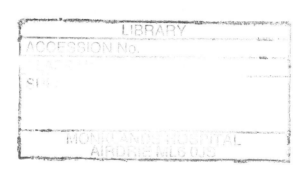

LIBRARY
ACCESSION No.

MONKLANDS HOSPITAL
AIRDRIE ML6 0JS